Pediatric Otology
and Neurotology

Pediatric Otology and Neurotology

Edited by

Anil K. Lalwani, M.D.
Assistant Professor
Director, Pediatric Otology and Neurotology and Pediatric Cochlear Implant Program
Division of Otology, Neurotology, and Skull Base Surgery
Department of Otolaryngology—Head and Neck Surgery
University of California, San Francisco
San Francisco, California

and

Kenneth M. Grundfast, M.D.
Professor of Otolaryngology and Pediatrics
Department of Otolaryngology and Pediatrics
Georgetown University Medical Center
Washington, D.C.

Illustrations by
Michael Leonard, C.M.I., F.A.M.I.
Baltimore, Maryland

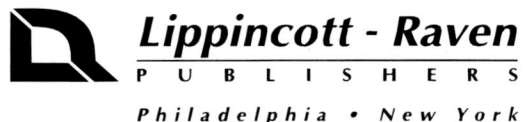

Acquisitions Editor: Danette Knopp
Developmental Editor: Juleann Dob
Manufacturing Manager: Dennis Teston
Production Manager: Kathleen Bubbeo
Production Service: Colophon, Inc.
Cover Designer: William Donnelley
Indexer: Beta Computer Indexing
Compositor: Maryland Composition
Printer: Kingsport

© 1998, by Lippincott–Raven Publishers. All rights reserved. This book is protected by copyright. No part of it may be reproduced, stored in a retrieval system, or transmitted, in any form or by any means—electronic, mechanical, photocopy, recording, or otherwise—without the prior written consent of the publisher, except for brief quotations embodied in critical articles and reviews. For information write **Lippincott–Raven Publishers, 227 East Washington Square, Philadelphia, PA 19106-3780.**

Materials appearing in this book prepared by individuals as part of their official duties as U.S. Government employees are not covered by the above-mentioned copyright.

Chapter 28, Figures 1, 2 © 1994 P.A. Wackym; Figure 3 © 1995 P.A. Wackym; Figures 4, 5, 7 © 1996 P.A. Wackym.

Library of Congress Cataloging-in-Publication Data
Pediatric otology and neurotology / editors, Anil K. Lalwani and
  Kenneth M. Grundfast ; illustrations by Michael E. Leonard.
      p.   cm.
  Includes bibliographical references and index.
  ISBN 0-397-51466-2
  1. Pediatric otology.   I. Lalwani, Anil K.   II. Grundfast,
Kenneth.
   [DNLM: 1. Ear Diseases—in infancy & childhood.   2. Ear—
pathology.   3. Ear—physiopathology.   WV 200 P371   1998]
RF122.5.C4P43   1998
618.92′0978—dc21
DNLM/DLC
for Library of Congress   97-30730
                                                           CIP

Printed in the United States of America

9 8 7 6 5 4 3 2 1

Care has been taken to confirm the accuracy of the information presented and to describe generally accepted practices. However, the authors, editors, and publisher are not responsible for errors or omissions or for any consequences from application of the information in this book and make no warranty, express or implied, with respect to the contents of the publication.

The authors, editors, and publisher have exerted every effort to ensure that drug selection and dosage set forth in this text are in accordance with current recommendations and practice at the time of publication. However, in view of ongoing research, changes in government regulations, and the constant flow of information relating to drug therapy and drug reactions, the reader is urged to check the package insert for each drug for any change in indications and dosage and for added warnings and precautions. This is particularly important when the recommended agent is a new or infrequently employed drug.

Some drugs and medical devices presented in this publication have Food and Drug Administration (FDA) clearance for limited use in restricted research settings. It is the responsibility of the health care provider to ascertain the FDA status of each drug or device planned for use in their clinical practice.

To my parents, Madan and Gulab
To my wife, Renu
To my children, Nikita and Sahil
To my teachers

                Anil K. Lalwani

I dedicate this book to my wife Ruthanne, who has supported the writing and editing of this volume as she has supported all of my time-consuming endeavors throughout my career and to my two zany and wonderful daughters, Rena and Dara, whom I love very much.

                Kenneth M. Grundfast

Contents

Contributing Authors xi
Foreword xvii
Preface xix
Acknowledgments xxi

Part I. Basic Science

1. Development of the Ear 3
   Gerald C. Goeringer

2. Anatomy, Physiology, and Pathophysiology of the Eustachian Tube 11
   Charles D. Bluestone

3. Auditory Development 29
   John H. Grose and Joseph W. Hall III

4. Development of Speech and Language 39
   Joanne E. Roberts, Ina F. Wallace, and Diane Brackett

5. Molecular Genetics: A Brief Overview 49
   Anil K. Lalwani, Eric Lynch, and Anand N. Mhatre

6. Temporal Bone Histopathology 87
   William H. Slattery III

Part II. Diagnostic Evaluation

7. Behavioral Audiologic Assessment 103
   Judith S. Gravel

8. Acoustic Immittance: Tympanometry and Acoustic Reflexes 113
   Alison M. Grimes

9. Physiologic Assessment of Hearing 127
   Yvonne S. Sininger and Carolina Abdala

10. Neonatal Hearing Screening: Early Identification 155
    Jerry L. Northern and Stephen Epstein

11. Assessment of Vestibular Function 163
    David Foyt and William H. Slattery III

12. Radiology of the Temporal Bone: Congenital Abnormalities 181
    Peter D. Phelps and Gilbert Vézina

Part III. Congenital Abnormalities

13. Congenital Anomalies of the Inner Ear 201
    P. Gerard Reilly, Anil K. Lalwani, and Robert K. Jackler

14. Skull-Base Abnormalities 211
    Todd T. Kingdom, Steven W. Cheung, and Anil K. Lalwani

Part IV. Infectious and Inflammatory Disorders

15. Otitis Media: A Spectrum of Diseases 233
    Charles D. Bluestone

16. Adenoidectomy in the Management of Otitis Media in Children 241
    George A. Gates

17. Complications of Otitis Media 251
    William H. Slattery III and John W. House

18. Acute Mastoiditis 265
    Nikolas H. Blevins and Anil K. Lalwani

Part V. Cholesteatoma

19. Congenital Cholesteatoma 279
    Jacob Friedberg

20. Acquired Cholesteatoma 295
    Simon C. Parisier, Adam J. Cohen, Bryan A. Selkin, and Jin C. Han

Part VI. Hearing Disorders

21. Nonsyndromic Hereditary Hearing Impairment 313
    Umang Khetarpal and Anil K. Lalwani

22. Syndromic Hereditary Hearing Impairment 341
    Kenneth M. Grundfast and Helga Toriello

23. Oculoauditory Syndromes 365
    Scott R. Schoem and Kenneth M. Grundfast

24. The Acquired Hearing Losses of Childhood 375
    Richard M. Irving and Robert J. Ruben

25. Central Auditory Disorders 387
    Brad A. Stach

26. Diagnosis and Management of Sensorineural Hearing Disorders 397
    Thomas J. Balkany and Michal Luntz

27. Autoimmune Inner Ear Diseases 405
    Jeffrey P. Harris

Part VII. Vestibular Dysfunction

28. Vertigo, Dizziness, and Disequilibrium 423
    Phillip A. Wackym and David G. Cyr

Part VIII. Trauma

29. Injuries of the Auricle, Middle Ear, and Temporal Bone 443
Rick A. Friedman and William M. Luxford

Part IX. Facial Paralysis

30. Disorders of the Facial Nerve 457
Barry M. Schaitkin, Andrew Shapiro, and Mark May

Part X. HIV Infection

31. Otologic Disorders in the HIV-Positive Child 479
J. Christopher Post and Garth D. Ehrlich

Part XI. Neoplasms

32. Posterior Fossa Tumors 489
Simón I. Angeli and Derald E. Brackmann

33. Tumors of the Temporal Bone 505
Karen J. Doyle

Part XII. Surgical Considerations and Reconstructive Surgery

34. Congenital Auricular Deformities: Dysmorphic and Dysplastic Ears 517
Robert O. Ruder

35. External Auditory Canal Atresia 533
Robert A. Jahrsdoerfer

36. Stapedectomy 541
Charles A. Syms, Antonio De la Cruz, and Simón I. Angeli

37. Ossicular Reconstruction 547
Robert A. Goldenberg

38. Reconstruction after Mastoidectomy 563
Juan J. Garro

Part XIII. Auditory Habilitation and Rehabilitation

39. Auditory Amplification 581
Robert W. Sweetow

40. Pediatric Cochlear Implantation 595
Richard T. Miyamoto, Karen I. Kirk, and Amy M. Robbins

Part XIV. Dilemmas, Perplexing Problems, and Controversies

41. Mixed Hearing Loss in Children 607
Ken Henry and Kenneth M. Grundfast

42. Fluctuating and Progressive Sensorineural Hearing Loss 617
Patrick E. Brookhouser

| 43. | The Cleft Palate Ear | 627 |

John P. Bent III and Richard J. H. Smith

| 44. | Perilymphatic Fistula | 635 |

Bradley F. Marple and William L. Meyerhoff

| 45. | The Atelectatic Ear | 645 |

Lisa M. Elden and Kenneth M. Grundfast

| 46. | Intact Canal Wall Versus Canal Wall Down Mastoidectomy | 663 |

Paul R. Lambert, Edward E. Dodson, and George T. Hashisaki

Part XV. The Deaf Child

| 47. | Early Intervention | 673 |

Janice C. Gatty

| 48. | Choosing the Appropriate Method for Communication | 683 |

Sue Schwartz

| 49. | Mainstreaming | 689 |

F. David Manning

| 50. | Childhood Deafness: The Complexities of Management | 697 |

Arthur Boothroyd

Appendix A: A Clinical Reference of Eye Findings in Hereditary Hearing Impairment 707
Scott R. Schoem

Appendix B: Resources 711
Sue Schwartz

Subject Index 713

Contributing Authors

Carolina Abdala, Ph.D.
Assistant Scientist
Children's Auditory Research and Evaluation Center
House Ear Institute
2100 West Third Street, Fifth Floor
Los Angeles, California 90057

Simón I. Angeli, M.D.
Clinical Fellow
House Ear Clinic
2100 West Third Street
Los Angeles, California 90057

Thomas J. Balkany, M.D., F.A.C.S., F.A.A.P.
Hotchkiss Professor and Vice Chairman
Department of Otolaryngology;
Director, University of Miami Ear Institute;
Professor of Neurological Surgery and Pediatrics
University of Miami
Box 016960 (D-48)
Miami, Florida 33136

John P. Bent III, M.D.
Assistant Professor
Surgery, Division of Otolaryngology
Medical College of Georgia
BP-4154 Laney-Walker
Augusta, Georgia 30912-4060

Nikolas H. Blevins, M.D.
Assistant Professor
Department of Otolaryngology—Head and Neck Surgery
Tufts University School of Medicine
Tufts New England Medical Center
750 Washington Street, NEMC 850
Boston, Massachusetts 02111

Charles D. Bluestone, M.D.
Eberly Professor of Pediatric Otolaryngology
Department of Otolaryngology
University of Pittsburgh School of Medicine
3705 Fifth Avenue
Pittsburgh, Pennsylvania 15213-2583;
Department of Pediatric Otolaryngology
Children's Hospital of Pittsburgh
Pittsburgh, Pennsylvania 15213

Arthur Boothroyd, Ph.D.
Distinguished Professor
Department of Speech and Hearing Sciences
Graduate School, City University of New York
33 West 42nd Street
New York, New York 10036

Diane Brackett, Ph.D.
Associate Professor
Department of Communication Sciences
University of Connecticut
850 Bolton Road, U-85
Storrs, Connecticut 06269

Derald E. Brackmann, M.D.
Associate, House Ear Clinic
2100 West Third Street
Los Angeles, California 90057

Patrick E. Brookhouser, M.D.
Director, Boystown National Research Hospital
555 North 30th Street
Omaha, Nebraska 68131;
Father Flanagan Professor and Chairman
Department of Otolaryngology and Human Communication
Creighton University School of Medicine
Omaha, Nebraska 68131

Steven W. Cheung, M.D.
Assistant Professor
Department of Otolaryngology—Head and Neck Surgery
University of California at San Francisco
350 Parnassus Avenue
A717 Box 0342
San Francisco, California 94117

Adam J. Cohen, M.D.
Resident
Internal Medicine
Staten Island University Hospital
432 East 88th Street
New York, New York 10128

David G. Cyr, Ph.D.
Director, Vestibular Laboratory
Boystown National Research Hospital
555 North 30th Street
Omaha, Nebraska 68131

Antonio De la Cruz, M.D.
Associate, House Ear Clinic
2100 West Third Street
Los Angeles, California 90057

Edward E. Dodson, M.D.
Assistant Professor
Department of Otolaryngology
The Ohio State University
4148 UMC 456 West 10th Avenue
Columbus, Ohio 43210

Karen J. Doyle, M.D., Ph.D.
Assistant Adjunct Professor
Department of Neurology
University of California, Irvine
Orange, California 92868;
Hearing and Balance Services
361 Hospital Dr., 325
Newport Beach, California 92663

Garth D. Ehrlich, Ph.D.
Professor, Department of Otolaryngology
Executive Director, Center for Genomic Sciences
Allegheny University of the Health Sciences
320 East North Avenue
Pittsburgh, Pennsylvania 15212-4772

Lisa M. Elden, B.S., M.S., M.D.
Assistant Professor
Department of Pediatric Otolaryngology
McMaster University Medical Center
1200 Main Street West
Hamilton, Ontario L8N 3Z5
Canada

Stephen Epstein, M.D., F.A.C.S.
Associate Professor of Surgery
Department of Otolaryngology—Head and Neck Surgery and Pediatrics
The George Washington University School of Medicine
11160 Viers Mill Road
Wheaton Plaza South Annex
Wheaton, Maryland 20902-2538

David Foyt, M.D.
Fellow
Department of Clinical Studies
House Ear Clinic
House Ear Institute
2100 West Third Street
Los Angeles, California 90057

Jacob Friedberg, M.D., F.R.C.S.(C)
Associate Professor
Department of Otolaryngology
University of Toronto
Hospital for Sick Children
555 University Avenue, Suite 6117
Toronto, Ontario M5G 1X8
Canada

Rick A. Friedman, M.D., Ph.D.
Assistant Professor
Department of Otology, Neurotology and Skull Base Surgery
Department of Otolaryngology
University of Cincinnati College of Medicine
231 Bethesda Avenue
Cincinnati, Ohio 45267

Juan J. Garro, M.D.
Special Consultant for Reconstructive Ear Surgery
Department of Otolaryngology
Children's National Medical Center
111 Michigan Avenue, Northwest
Washington, DC 20011

George A. Gates, M.D.
Professor
Department of Otolaryngology—Head and Neck Surgery
Virginia Bloedel Hearing Research Center
University of Washington
1959 Pacific Northeast, Box 357923
Seattle, Washington 98195

Janice C. Gatty, Ed.M., M.E.D., Ed.D.
Lecturer, Education and Child Study
Smith College
Northampton, Massachusetts 01063

Gerald C. Goeringer, M.D.
Department of Cell Biology
Georgetown University School of Medicine
3900 Reservoir Road
Washington, D.C. 20007

Robert A. Goldenberg, M.D.
Professor and Chairman
Department of Otolaryngology
Wright State University School of Medicine
Children's Medical Center
111 West First Street, Suite 600
Dayton, Ohio 45402

Judith S. Gravel, Ph.D.
Associate Professor
Department of Otolaryngology and Pediatrics
Department of Otorhinolaryngology: Division of Audiology
Albert Einstein College of Medicine
1300 Morris Park Avenue
Bronx, New York 10461

Alison M. Grimes, M.A.
Director of Audiology
Providence Speech and Hearing Center
1301 Providence Avenue
Orange, California 92868

John H. Grose, Ph.D.
Assistant Professor
Division of Otolaryngology—Head and Neck Surgery
University of North Carolina Medical School
610 Burnett-Womack Building, CB 7070
Chapel Hill, North Carolina 27599-7070

Kenneth M. Grundfast, M.D.
Professor
Department of Otolaryngology and Pediatrics
Georgetown University Medical Center
3800 Reservoir Road, Northwest
Washington, D.C. 20007

Joseph W. Hall III, M.D.
Professor, Surgery
Division of Otolaryngology—Head and Neck Surgery
University of North Carolina Medical School
610 Burnett-Womack Building, CB 7070
Chapel Hill, North Carolina 27599-7070

Jin C. Han, M.D.
Department of Otorhinolaryngology
Manhattan Eye, Ear, and Throat Hospital
210 East 64th Street
New York, New York 10021

Jeffrey P. Harris, M.D., Ph.D.
Department of Surgery
Division of Otolaryngology—Head and Neck Surgery
University of California, San Diego Medical Center
9350 Campus Point Drive
La Jolla, California 92037-1300

George T. Hashisaki, M.D.
Assistant Professor
Department of Otolaryngology—Head and Neck Surgery
University of Virginia Medical Center
P.O. Box 10008
Charlottesville, Virginia 22902-0008

Ken Henry, Ph.D.
Director, Professional Hearing Services
The Dizziness and Balance Center
6231 Leesburg Pike, 512
Falls Church, Virginia 22044

John W. House, M.D.
President, House Ear Institute
Associate, House Ear Clinic
2100 West Third Street
Los Angeles, California 90057

Richard M. Irving, M.D., F.R.C.S.
Consultant, Department of Otolaryngology
University Hospital Birmingham NHS Trust
Raddlebam Road, Selly Oak
Birmingham B29 GJD United Kingdom

Robert K. Jackler, M.D.
Professor
Departments of Otolaryngology—Head and Neck Surgery and Neurological Surgery
University of California, San Francisco
A717, 400 Parnassus Avenue, Box 0342
San Francisco, California 94143-0342

Robert A. Jahrsdoerfer, M.D.
Professor, Department of Otolaryngology—Head and Neck Surgery
University of Virginia Medical Center
P.O. Box 10008
Charlottesville, Virginia 22908-0008

Umang Khetarpal, M.D., M.S.
Clinical Instructor (Resident)
Department of Otolaryngology—Head, Neck and Craniofacial Surgery
SUNY Health Science Center
730 East Adams Street
Syracuse, New York 13210

Todd T. Kingdom, M.D.
Assistant Professor
Department of Otolaryngology—Head and Neck Surgery
Emory University School of Medicine
1365 Clifton Road, Northeast
Atlanta, Georgia 30322

Karen I. Kirk, Ph.D.
Assistant Professor
Department of Otolaryngology—Head and Neck Surgery
Indiana University School of Medicine
DeVault Otologic Research Laboratory
702 Barnhill Drive, Room 0860
Indianapolis, Indiana 46202

Anil K. Lalwani, M.D., F.A.C.S.
Assistant Professor
Director, Pediatric Otology and Neurotology and Pediatric Cochlear Implant Program
Division of Otology, Neurotology, and Skull Base Surgery
Department of Otolaryngology—Head and Neck Surgery
University of California, San Francisco
A717, 400 Parnassus Avenue, Box 0342
San Francisco, California 94143-0342

Paul R. Lambert, M.D.
Professor and Vice Chairman
Department of Otolaryngology—Head and Neck Surgery
Director Division of Otology-Neurotology
University of Virginia Medical Center
P.O. Box 10008
Charlottesville, Virginia 22908

Michal Luntz, M.D.
Senior Lecturer in Otolaryngology and Biomedical Engineering
Department of Otolaryngology
Bnai Zion Medical Center
Faculty of Medicine-Technion
P.O. Box 4940
Haifa 31048, Israel

William M. Luxford, M.D.
Associate, House Ear Clinic
2100 West Third Street
Los Angeles, California 90057

Eric Lynch, Ph.D.
Research Assistant Professor
Department of Medicine and Genetics
University of Washington
1959 Northeast Pacific Street
Seattle, Washington 98195

F. David Manning, Ed.D.
Director, The Mainstream Center
Clarke School for the Deaf
Center for Oral Education
47 Roundhill Road
Northampton, Massachusetts 01060

Bradley F. Marple, M.D.
Assistant Professor
Department of Otolaryngology
University of Texas Southwestern Medical Center at Dallas
5323 Harry Hines Boulevard
Dallas, Texas 72535-9035

Mark May, M.D.
5200 Center Avenue, Suite 211
Pittsburgh, Pennsylvania 15232

William L. Meyerhoff, M.D., Ph.D.
Arthur E. Meyerhoff Professor and Chair
Department of Otolaryngology
University of Texas Southwestern Medical Center at Dallas
5323 Harry Hines Boulevard
Dallas, Texas 72535-9035

Anand N. Mhatre, Ph.D.
Research Geneticist
Department of Otolaryngology—Head and Neck Surgery
University of California, San Francisco
533 Parnassus Avenue, U4904
San Francisco, California 94143-0526

Richard T. Miyamoto, M.D.
Arilla Spence DeVault Professor and Chairman
Department of Otolaryngology—Head and Neck Surgery
DeVault Otologic Research Laboratory
Indiana University School of Medicine
Riley Children's Hospital, Wishard
702 Barnhill Drive, Room 0860
Indianapolis, Indiana 46202

Jerry L. Northern, Ph.D., F.A.A.A.
Professor Emeritus
Department of Otolaryngology
University of Colorado School of Medicine
4200 East Ninth Avenue, B-210
Denver, Colorado 80262

Simon C. Parisier, M.D.
Clinical Professor, Chairman
Department of Otolaryngology—Head and Neck Surgery
Manhattan Eye, Ear, and Throat Hospital
Cornell University Medical Center
210 East 64th Street
New York, New York 10021

Peter D. Phelps, M.D., F.R.C.S., F.R.C.R.
Consultant Radiologist
Department of Radiology
The Royal National Throat, Nose, and Ear
 Hospital NHS Trust
Gray's Inn Road
London WC1X 8DA
United Kingdom

J. Christopher Post, M.D., F.A.C.S.
Professor, Department of Otolaryngology
Medical Director, Center for Genomic Sciences
Department of Otolaryngology
Allegheny University of the Health Sciences
320 East North Avenue
Pittsburgh, Pennsylvania 15212-4772

P. Gerard Reilly, F.R.C.S.Ed. (ORL)
Consultant Otolaryngologist
York District Hospital
Wigginton Road
York YO37HE United Kingdom

Amy M. Robbins, M.S.
Speech Language Pathologist
Department of Otolaryngology—Head and Neck
 Surgery
Indiana University School of Medicine
DeVault Otologic Research Laboratory
Riley Children's Hospital
702 Barnhill Road, Room 0860
Indianapolis, Indiana 46202

Joanne E. Roberts, Ph.D.
Research Professor
Division of Speech and Hearing Sciences
Frank Porter Graham Child Development Center
University of North Carolina at Chapel Hill
105 Smith Level Road, CB 8180
Chapel Hill, North Carolina 27599

Robert J. Ruben, M.D., F.A.C.S., F.A.A.P.
Professor and Chairman
Department of Otolaryngology
Professor, Department of Paediatrics
Albert Einstein College of Medicine
Montefiore Medical Center
111 East 210th Street
Bronx, New York 10467-2490

Robert O. Ruder, M.D.
Assistant Clinical Professor
Department of Head and Neck Surgery
University of California/Los Angeles Medical
 Center
8816 Burton Way
Beverley Hills, California 90211;
Attending Physician
Department of Head and Neck Surgery
Cedars Sinai Medical Center
8700 Beverly Boulevard
Los Angeles, California 90048

Barry M. Schaitkin, M.D.
Associate Professor
Department of Otolaryngology
University of Pittsburgh
5200 Center Avenue, Suite 211
Pittsburgh, Pennsylvania 15232

Scott R. Schoem, M.D.
Department of Otolaryngology—Head and Neck
 Surgery
National Naval Medical Center
111 Michigan Avenue
Bethesda, Maryland 20889

Sue Schwartz, Ph.D.
Family Services
Montgomery County Public Schools—Special
 Education
5121 Russett Road
Rockville, Maryland 20853

Bryan A. Selkin, M.D.
Department of Otolaryngology—Head and Neck
 Surgery
Manhattan Ear, Eye, and Throat Hospital
Cornell University Medical Center
210 East Sixth Street
New York, New York 10021

Andrew Shapiro, M.D.
Assistant Professor
Department of Surgery
Milton S. Hershey Medical Center
P.O. Box 850
Hershey, Pennsylvania 17033

Yvonne S. Sininger, M.A., Ph.D.
Director, Children's Auditory Research and
 Evaluation Center
House Ear Institute
2100 West Third Street, Fifth Floor
Los Angeles, California 90057

William H. Slattery III, M.D.
Associate, House Ear Clinic
Director, Department of Clinical Studies
House Ear Institute
Assistant Clinical Professor
Department of Otolaryngology
University of Southern California
2100 West Third Street, 5th Floor
Los Angeles, California 90057

Richard J. H. Smith, M.D.
Professor, Vice Chairman
Department of Otolaryngology
Division of Pediatric Otolaryngology
Molecular Otolaryngology Research Laboratories
The University of Iowa Hospitals and Clinics
200 Hawkins Drive
Iowa City, Iowa 52242

Brad A. Stach, Ph.D.
President and CEO
Nova Scotia Hearing and Speech Clinic
5599 Fenwick Street
Halifax, Nova Scotia B3H 1R2
Canada

Robert W. Sweetow, Ph.D.
Director of Audiology
Department of Otolaryngology
University of California, San Francisco
400 Parnassus Avenue, Room A-705
San Francisco, California 94143-0340

Charles A. Syms, III, M.D.
Assistant of Surgery
Uniformed Services University of the Health Science
59th MDW/MKCE
2200 Bergquist Drive, Suite 1
San Antonio, Texas 78236-5000

Helga Toriello, M.D.
Director, Genetic Services
Butterworth Hospital
21 Michigan Street, Suite 465
Grand Rapids, Michigan 49503

Gilbert Vézina, M.D.
Department of Diagnostic Imaging and Radiology
Children's National Medical Center
Washington, D.C. 20008

Phillip A. Wackym, M.D., F.A.C.S.
Associate Professor
Chief, Ear Service (Otology and Neuro-otology)
Department of Otolaryngology
Mount Sinai School of Medicine
Fifth Avenue and 100th Street
New York, New York 10028-6574

Ina F. Wallace, Ph.D.
Senior Research Psychologist
Center for Research in Education
Research Triangle Institute
P.O. Box 12194
Research Triangle Park, North Carolina 27709;
Visiting Associate Professor
Department of Otolaryngology
Albert Einstein College of Medicine
1300 Morris Park Avenue
Bronx, New York 10461

Foreword

The development of drugs that control bacterial infections during the fourth decade of the twentieth century profoundly altered therapy of otolaryngologic diseases, especially in children. Otitis media with effusion (middle ear catarrh) was rarely recognized in the pre-antimicrobial era. Ear disease presented as acute (painful) otitis media, requiring myringotomy, or mastoiditis necessitating surgery as a life-saving procedure.

Most bacterial infections can now be controlled, but the prevalence of otitis media with effusion and its sequelae in children has led to the emergence of physicians and allied medical personnel devoted to the care of pediatric otologic problems. Although the American Otologic Society was founded in the last century, few otolaryngologists limited their practices to otology until the development of antimicrobials. Antimicrobials made feasible otologic procedures that had previously failed because of suppuration; procedures such as fenestration, stapedectomy, closed-cavity tympanoplasty with mastoidectomy, and, more recently, neurotologic surgery.

One of us (AG) in the 1930s decided, after a residency in pediatrics, that the pediatricians were not learning enough about ears, and so completed a second residency in otolaryngology to become double boarded and an assistant professor of otolaryngology at Yale University. During World War II, experiences in England with soldiers deafened by gunfire led to a life-long interest in audiology, which in turn led to the founding and directorship of the Callier Center for Communication Disorders in Dallas, Texas in 1964.

Almost simultaneously with the emergence of otology as a subspecialty, some otolaryngologists began to limit their practices to the care of children. One of us (FL) became interested in pediatric otology during residency at Johns Hopkins and was involved in the founding of special pediatric otology and cleft palate clinics (because of the prevalence of otitis media with effusion in cleft palate [patients]) at Hopkins and upon return to Los Angeles, at the Children's Hospital.

This interest in pediatric otology came to the attention of the founders of the Otologic Medical Group (now the House Ear Clinic) who created the position of pediatric otologist for the group.

It was only natural that some other individuals practicing otology would also begin, in the fifth decade of the century, to emphasize "pediatric otology" in their practices, and several pediatric otology clinics were established in various parts of the country. Evolution of the pediatric otologist, although not a certifiable subspecialty, has been slow but steady, as evidenced by the meetings of the First International Symposium on Pediatric Otolaryngology and the First International Symposium on Otitis Media with Effusion, in 1975. Many physicians attended both symposia and have continued to do so.

In addition to the sequelae of otitis media, there are a number of conditions unique to children that are better cared for by the physician with experience and training in the care of children. The correction of microtia and congenital ossicular deformities requires astute diagnosis and a thorough knowledge of temporal bone embryology, as well as surgical expertise. Cholesteatomas tend to be more aggressive in children than in adults and must be dealt with accordingly. Vestibular disorders require special consideration because children have difficulty describing vertigo; and the usual tests of vestibular function must be carefully administered, keeping in mind the fear of the unknown that affects most children.

Skull base surgery is another recently developed subspecialty that has become a part of the armamentarium of the pediatric otologist. Some very grave types of neoplasms occurring in the temporal bone, such as rhabdomyosarcomas, fibrosarcomas, and histiocytosis, are seen in a pediatric practice and are best dealt with by individuals used to dealing with surgical problems in children.

The emergence of the pediatric otologist has occurred with the simultaneous development of ancillary services for the pediatric otologic patient, such as audiology, speech therapy, and electrophysiology, that provide diagnostic and therapeutic measures not in the area of expertise of the physician. The success of pediatric cochlear implant programs, for example, has been dependent upon such multidisciplinary coordinated services.

The development of molecular biology techniques to identify and, it is hoped, eventually treat the vast number of familial hearing losses that are being identified, makes the future of pediatric otology every more exciting. This book is a climactic amalgamation of the experience and expertise of over 50 individuals who have been involved in the evolution of pediatric otology through the years. Included are discussions of the care of the pediatric otologic patient from initial diagnosis, through therapy, and finally habilitation where indicated. Children require specialty care, for they are not just little adults. They are constantly changing, anatomically, immunologically, and psychologically, and the physician must be able to deal with these variations as they occur during the various stages of growth and maturation.

We feel very fortunate to have been a part of the evolution of modern otology and have been greatly rewarded by seeing the improvements in the treatment and habilitation of children with hearing loss.

Aram Glorig, MD
Senior Advisor, House Ear Institute
Los Angeles, California

Fred H. Linthicum Jr., MD
Head, Department of Histopathology
House Ear Institute
Clinical Professor of Otolaryngology
University of Southern California
School of Medicine
Los Angeles, California

Acknowledgments

We wish to acknowledge the time and effort spent by the contibuting authors on the writing of their chapters. We asked these authors to provide new and readily usable information focusing on otologic care for children. These scholarly experts have generously shared in this text their practical experience as well as their profound knowledge, and for this, we are extremely grateful.

We thank our editors at Lippincott-Raven Publishers, Danette Knopp and Juleann Dob, for their support and assistance throughout the development of this project.

PART I

Basic Science

CHAPTER 1

Development of the Ear

Gerald C. Goeringer

Development of the ear is at once fascinating and complex. The complexity arises from the fact that the ear anlagen arise as three separate entities. Ear development encompasses virtually all the fundamental mechanisms of development—for example, cell proliferation, migration, interaction, and death. When the spatio-temporal union of the ear anlagen is defective or if one or more of the fundamental developmental processes is compromised, any of a variety of anomalies may be anticipated. At least part of the fascination is embodied in the marvelous interaction of the seemingly disparate components involved in the differentiation of what is probably the most intricate organ of the body (insofar as both function and morphology are concerned). Indeed, when ear development is abnormal, it serves as a bellwether that may well indicate the presence of associated anomalies in other parts of the body, from the kidneys to the heart.

First, a few words about the segmental nature of embryonic development may be in order. Segmentation is obvious in the somites and in the appearance of the early brain vesicles. What is less apparent are the seven paraxial clusters of mesodermal cells in the head region, referred to as somitomeres, which never form full-blown somites. The hindbrain (rhombencephalon) likewise forms a series of nine transient vesicular structures called rhombomeres. In the developing chick, each of the first three sets of pharyngeal arches is associated with two pairs of rhombomeres. Labeling cranial nerves with fluorescent dye has revealed, for example, that motor nuclei of cranial nerve V (which services the first arch) develop in rhombomere 2. Nuclei of nerve VII (the nerve of the second arch) develop in rhombomere 4; those of nerve IX (third arch) are associated with rhombomere 6. Somitomeres seem to orient the growing cranial nerve motor fibers much as the true somites orient the outgrowing spinal nerves. It would appear then that the head region also develops in segmental fashion.

Consider the fruitfly, *Drosophila,* whose larval form is highly segmented. Each segment is associated with the activity of a particular Hox (homeotic) gene. Such genes contain a sequence of approximately 180 base pairs (bp) called a homeobox. The homeobox region produces a factor thought to interact with DNA and thereby initiate gene function. Many homeotic genes are thought to initiate a concatenation of gene expressions leading to ontogenetic changes. Interestingly, these genes are highly conserved and their activity is also associated with development in the head region of mammals. Indeed, one can map the expression of Hox genes using in situ hybridization, a technique that demonstrates the messenger RNA product of gene expression. Mapping expression of Hox and other regulatory genes reveals their activity along the rhombomeres and paraxial mesoderm. Each rhombomere differs in the combination of functioning regulatory genes with which it is associated.

In mutant experimental animals in which the Hox 1.1 gene was abnormally overactive, severe craniofacial anomalies resulted. These anomalies were quite similar to those produced in other experimental animals by injection of vitamin A analogues such as isotretinoin or retinoic acid. Is it possible that retinoids effect their teratogenic activity by causing excessive expression of Hox genes? Retinoic acid has induced Hox expression in carcinoma cells growing in vitro. This and other evidence of sequential activation of genes involved in craniofacial embryogenesis promise exciting advances in the understanding of both normal and anomalous development of that complex of structures and functions we call the ear.

Inasmuch as it is the initial component to arise, we shall first consider development of the inner ear. Then, following up a discussion of the pharyngeal (branchial) apparatus (arches, clefts, and pouches), we shall briefly describe the subsequent development of the middle and external ears.

THE INTERNAL EAR

On or about the 22nd day of development, areas of thickening surface ectoderm develop on either side of the

---

G.C. Goeringer: Department of Cell Biology, Georgetown University School of Medicine, Washington, DC 20007.

rhombencephalon. These otic placodes are the primordia of the membranous labyrinth (the sensory receptors for balance and hearing) and of at least part of the statoacoustic ganglia. The placodes sink into the underlying mesenchyme forming otic pits, which ultimately break free from the surface as the otic vesicles or otocysts. The signaling mechanism initiating this process is poorly understood, but is thought to involve an inductive interaction (probably reciprocal) between surface epithelium and underlying mesenchyme. A group of cells detaches from the medial aspect of each otocyst, and, in combination with neural crest cells, forms the statoacoustic ganglion. This ganglion subsequently resolves into vestibular and cochlear components. The fluid-filled (endolymph) otocyst undergoes as complex a series of changes as occurs in the developing body. Each otocyst grows differentially and assumes a pear shape (Fig. 1). Toward the end of week 4, endolymphatic ducts appear from their dorsal aspect. The distal ends of these outgrowths dilate as the endolymphatic sacs. During this time, differential growth results in an expanded dorsal utricle and a tapered ventral saccule. The tip of the saccule elongates and coils about itself (for 2½ turns) as the cochlear duct forms beginning in the fifth week. Again, relative growth differences leave an attenuated connection between the saccule and cochlea called the ductus reuniens. The inner ear thus subdivides into vestibular and cochlear components. The seventh week sees the differentiation of cochlear cells in the organ of Corti as well as the growth of three flangelike outgrowths from the utriculus. The central parts of these flanges undergo programmed cell death, leaving behind the semicircular canals. At one end of each semicircular canal, a dilatation (a crus ampullare) appears. Regional crests of sensory nerve endings (cristae ampullares) develop in the ampullae as well as in the utricle (maculae utriculi) and saccule (maculae sacculi). These structures function in part by recognizing accelerations and changed orientations of the head and are supplied by the vestibular ganglion of cranial nerve VIII.

Ganglion cells from the VIIIth nerve migrate along the cochlear coils forming the spiral cochlear ganglion. Processes from this ganglion terminate on the hair cells of the organ of Corti. The cochlear duct represents what many consider to be the most intricate (in terms of both morphology and function) organ in the body.

During the ninth week, the surrounding mesenchyme responds to signals from the otocyst, undergoes chondrogenesis, and forms the otic capsule. Starting in the tenth week, the cartilage adjacent to the membranous labyrinth resorbs, leaving behind a series of coalescing fluid-filled (perilymph) vacuoles. The cochlear duct thus comes to be suspended in the perilymphatic space and separates this space into a scala vestibuli and a scala tympani (Fig. 2). The duct's lateral wall attaches to surrounding cartilage by the spiral ligament while its medial aspect attaches to the modiolus. As the membranous labyrinth grows, more of the cartilaginous encasement resorbs internally, thus allowing for increase in size. Between weeks 16 and 22, the otic capsule ossifies, forming the petrous component of the temporal bone (bony labyrinth). The adult size and configuration of the inner ear is thus attained by about the 22nd week.

THE PHARYNGEAL APPARATUS

The pharyngeal apparatus consists of pharyngeal (branchial) arches, pouches, and clefts (or grooves). Congenital abnormalities of this region usually occur as the pharyngeal apparatus is converted into its adult configuration and often are due to the persistence of components that normally disappear. In the human, starting early in the fourth week, a series of five arches arises in craniocaudal sequence. For our purposes, we need emphasize only the cranial two. Neurons of the Vth (arch I), VIIth (arch II), IXth (arch III), and Xth (arches IV and VI) cranial sensory ganglia service the arches and derive from ectodermal placodes and neural crest cells.

Arches

The arches arise as a row of columns of tissue flanking the pharynx and separated from one another externally by pharyngeal clefts and internally by pharyngeal grooves. Their cores are populated by mesenchymal cells derived either from embryonic mesoderm or from the neural crest. Mesodermal cells give rise to the musculature and vascular elements; neural crest cells give rise to the connective tissue

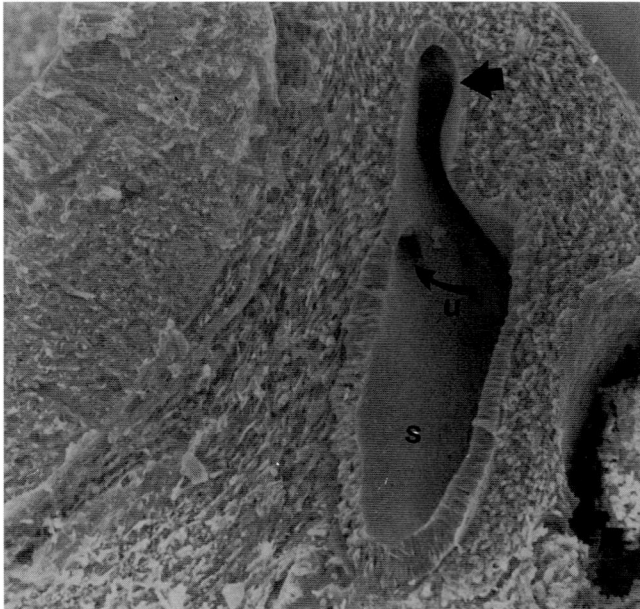

FIG. 1. Scanning electron micrograph of mouse early embryonic otocyst. *Arrowhead,* endolymphatic duct; *S,* region of forming saccule; *U,* region of forming utricle; *arrow,* opening into semicircular canal. Modified from Sadler T. *Langman's Medical Embryology,* with permission.

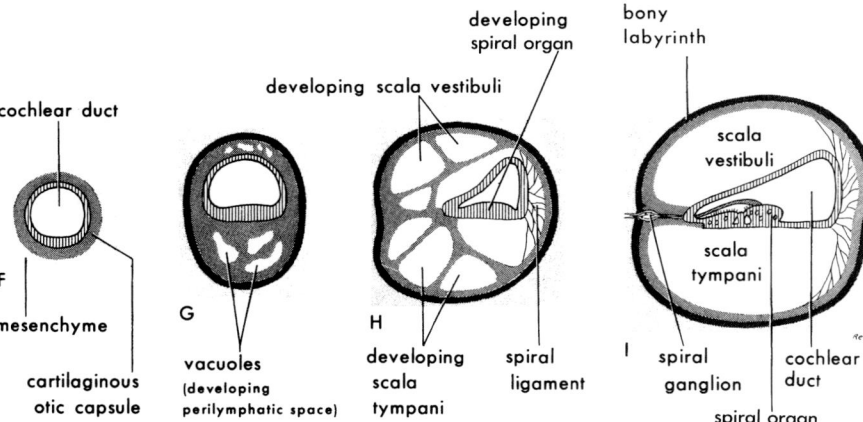

FIG. 2. Cross-sections through the cochlear duct at successive developmental stages from about 8 to 20 weeks. *F*, simple cochlear duct surrounded by a capsule of cartilage that develops from neural crest mesenchyme; *G*, cartilage adjacent to cochlear duct begins to resorb creating perilymphatic spaces while shape of duct begins to modify; *H*, scala tympani and vestibuli are forming while duct assumes a triangular profile and cells differentiate in the organ of Corti; *I*, by 20 weeks, what is essentially the adult configuration and size is achieved. The cartilaginous capsule has ossified. From Moore KL, Persaud TVN. *The developing human*, 5th ed, with permission

(including skeletal components). This mesenchymal core is covered externally by surface ectoderm and clothed internally by pharyngeal endodermal cells (Fig. 3).

The first, or mandibular, arch arises as two elevations: (a) the smaller dorsal maxillary process contributes to the maxilla, the malleus, and its anterior ligament, the zygomatic bone, and part of the temporal bone; and (b) the larger mandibular process forms the mandible and contributes to the incus. The cartilage of the first arch is named Meckel's cartilage. The mandible itself forms by intramembranous ossification around and beside Meckel's cartilage. Mesenchymal cells differentiate in the ninth week as the tensor tympani muscle.

The cartilage of the second, or hyoid, arch is called Reichert's cartilage. The skeletal elements forming here include the styloid process, parts of the hyoid bone, the stapes, and possible lesser contributions to the incus and malleus. During week 9, mesenchymal cells differentiate as the stapedius muscle, which is supplied by cranial nerve VII (the second arch nerve).

Proliferative activity in growth centers of the second (and possibly the third) arches results in caudal growth over the more posterior clefts and arches. The second arch fuses with the cardiac eminence. This results in a smoothing of the pharyngeal contours and the sequestration of the cervical sinus of His that normally completely disappears (Fig. 4).

In each pharyngeal arch a vascular element, an aortic arch, will develop. The first pair of aortic arches mainly disappears but does contribute to the formation of the maxillary arteries. Dorsal portions of the second pair of arches persist long enough to form the stapedial arteries. These vessels are, in turn, destined to disappear.

Pouches

The pharyngeal pouches are paired outpocketings of the pharynx and are numbered as the arch immediately cranial to them. Thus, on each side, the first pharyngeal pouch is situated just caudal to the first pharyngeal arch and just cranial to arch II. Each pouch corresponds to a similarly numbered pharyngeal cleft (Fig. 3).

The first pouch extends distally and unites with the first cleft at the site of the primitive tympanum. The primitive tympanic membrane then consists of layers of ectoderm and endoderm that become separated secondarily by a thin layer of fibrous mesenchyme. The elongating proximal portion of the pouch forms the auditory (eustachian) tube; its distal end expands as the cavity of the middle ear as it envelops the ossicles (Fig. 5) late in gestation. The epithelial lining of the auditory tube and cavity of the middle ear are therefore lined by cells of endodermal origin. Similarly, the ossicles are clothed with cells of endodermal origin.

Grooves or Clefts

Only the first pharyngeal clefts survive as normal adult structures (the more caudal clefts being submerged by overgrowth of the second arch). The first cleft modifies to form the external auditory meatus. Just as anomalous connections (fistulae) or cysts may persist between the cervical sinus and external surface of the neck or between the cervical sinus and pharynx, similar structures may arise in association with the first cleft.

THE MIDDLE EAR

As mentioned above, the auditory tubes and tympanic cavities form from the first pharyngeal pouches. During week 7, neural crest cells at the dorsal ends of the first arch condense and chondrify as the malleus (from mandibular process cells) and incus (maxillary process cells). The second arch cells form the stapes (with possible contributions to the first arch ossicles). The ossicles remain surrounded by mesenchyme through the eighth month. The tensor tympani and stapedius muscles differentiate from mesoderm during the ninth week.

As the ossicles are enveloped by the expanding first pouch during the ninth month, they become covered by a layer of endodermal cells. These same endodermal cells form mesen-

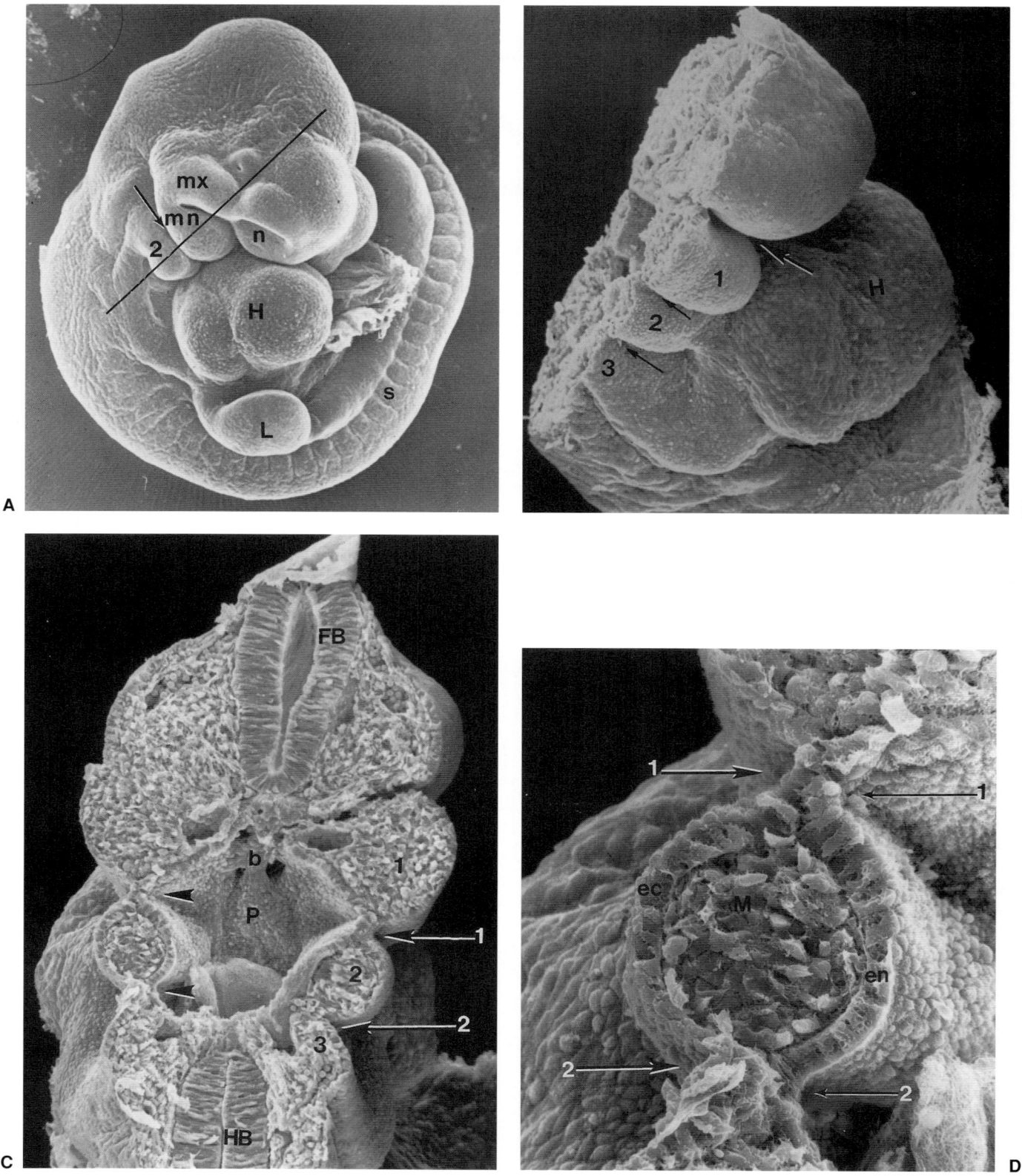

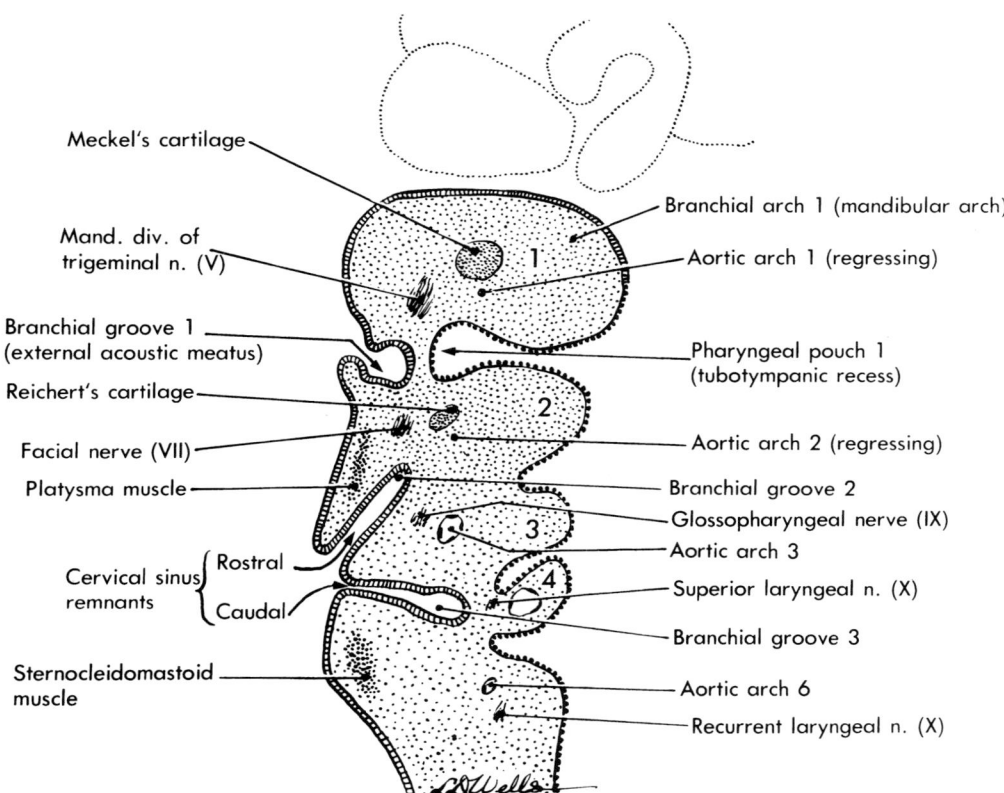

FIG. 4. A frontal section through one pharyngeal wall (near end of sixth week). Note the growth of the second branchial arch over the second pouch to fuse with the epicardial ridge (and possibly the third arch) as the cervical sinus is entrapped. This diagram makes positioning of cervical sinus fistulae relative to cranial nerves and aortic arch derivatives more apparent. From Corliss C. *Patten's human embryology,* with permission.

teries that temporarily suspend the ossicles (the mesenteries are later replaced by permanent ligaments). Late in the fetal period (ninth month), the tympanic cavity expands to form the mastoid antrum in the petromastoid portion of the temporal bone. The mastoid air cells typically form during the second year after birth.

During the ninth month, the malleus attaches to the tympanum. The footplate of the stapes associates with the oval window as the middle ear acquires its functional relationships. Failure of the annular ligament to properly attach the stapes to the oval window may result in fusion of the stapes to the bony labyrinth.

Congenital cholesteatoma, a common cause of hearing loss, forms as a rest of epithelial cells associated with the tympanic membrane. Whether the origin is from ectodermal or endodermal cells remains controversial. Whatever their origin, it would seem that programmed death of these epithelial epidermoid cells fails and thus they persist.

FIG. 3. Scanning electron micrographs of early mouse embryos (equivalent to about 4-wk human embryo) showing the pharyngeal apparatus. Fig. 3A shows an entire embryo. *mx,* maxillary process of first arch; *mn,* mandibular process of first arch; *n,* nasal pit; *H,* heart; *L,* forelimb bud; *s,* somite; *2,* second arch. *Line* indicates plane of cut seen in Fig. 3B. *1, 2, 3,* arches I through III, respectively; *small arrows* indicate pharyngeal clefts 1 and 2; *large arrow* points to site of primitive mouth. Fig. 3C shows a dorsal view of the embryo in Fig. 3B from which the dorsal portion of the head/pharyngeal region has been removed. *FB,* forebrain; *HB,* hindbrain; *b,* buccopharyngeal membrane (a transient structure separating primitive mouth cavity from primitive pharynx); *P,* floor of pharynx; *1, 2, 3,* pharyngeal arches I through III; *arrows 1 and 2,* pharyngeal clefts 1 and 2. Fig. 3D is an enlarged view showing the second arch. *ec,* surface ectoderm; *en,* pharyngeal endoderm; *M,* mesenchyme of second arch (consists of both neural crest cells and mesodermal cells); *white 1 and 2,* first and second pharyngeal clefts; *black 1 and 2,* first and second pharyngeal pouches. Pouches and clefts are separated by a region where ectoderm and endoderm fuse as a closing plate. (In developing fish, the closing plates break down to form the gill slits.)

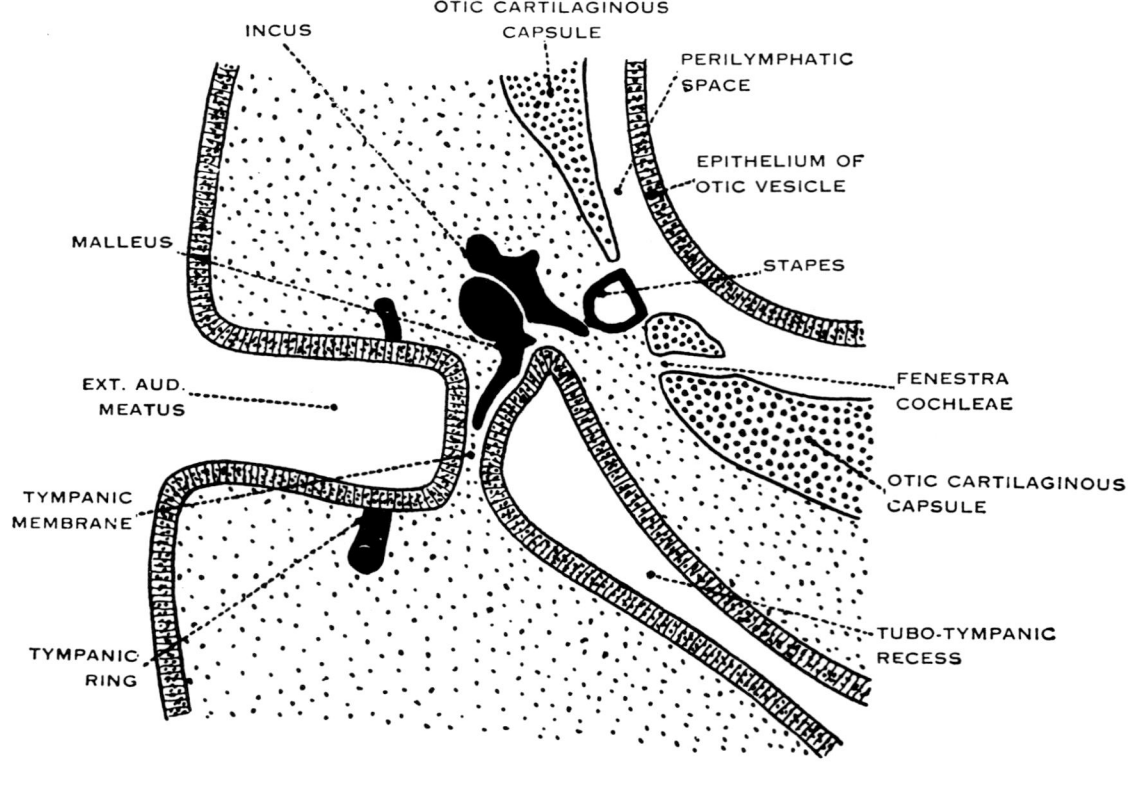
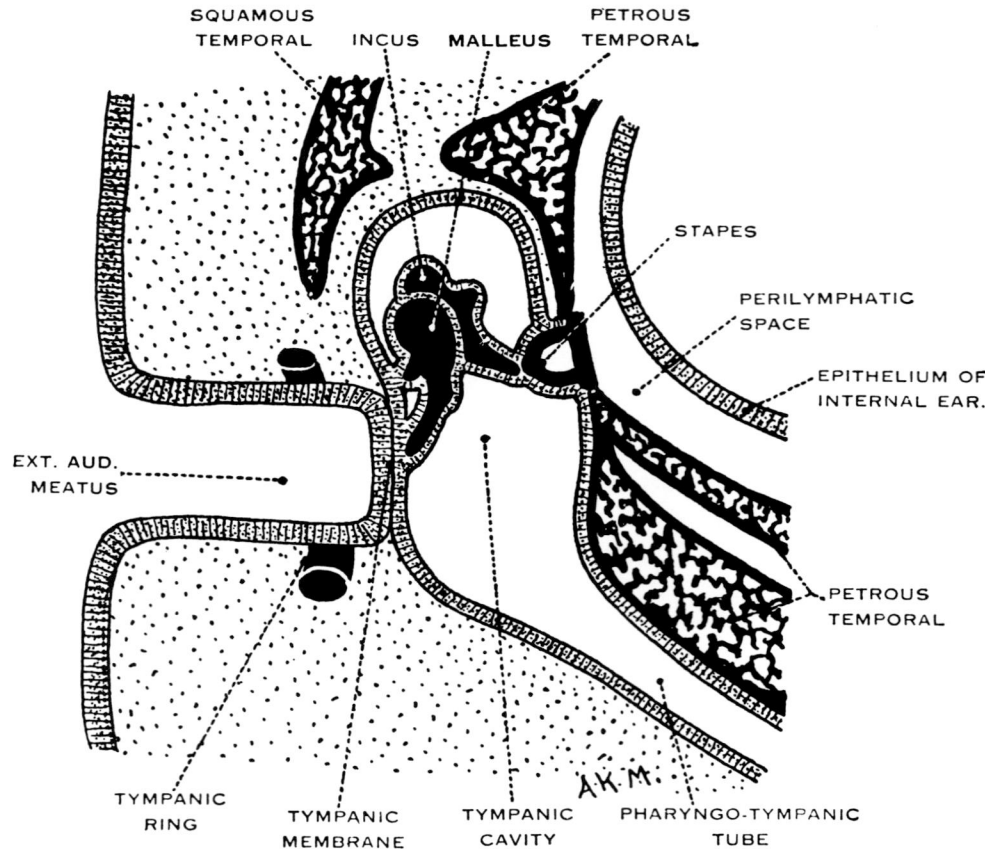

FIG. 5. The relative positions of the otocyst, forming ossicles, primitive tympanum, external auditory meatus (first cleft), and tubotympanic recess (first pouch). **A:** Positioning prior to formation of the tympanic cavity, **B:** Positioning after the tubotympanic recess has enveloped and incorporated the ossicles into the tympanic cavity. From Hamilton WJ, Boyd JD, and Mossman HW. *Human embryology,* 3rd ed, with permission.

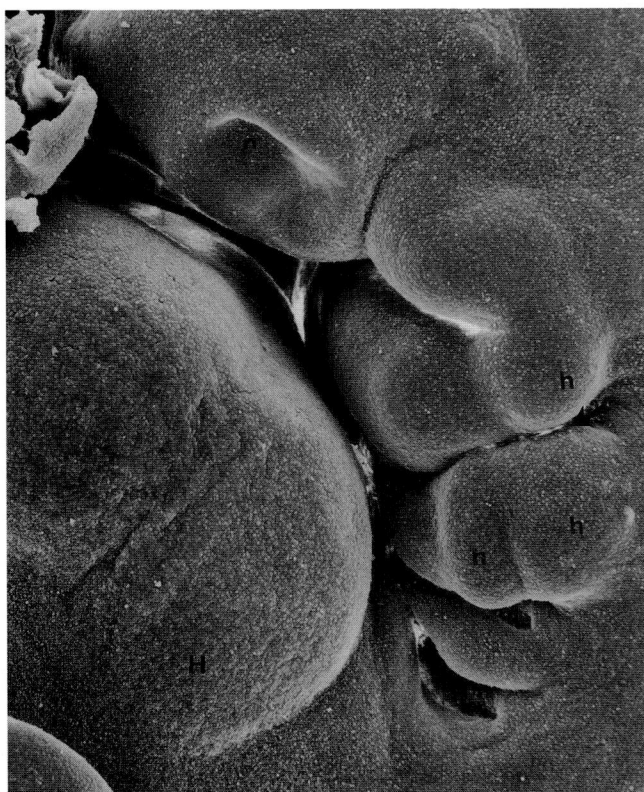 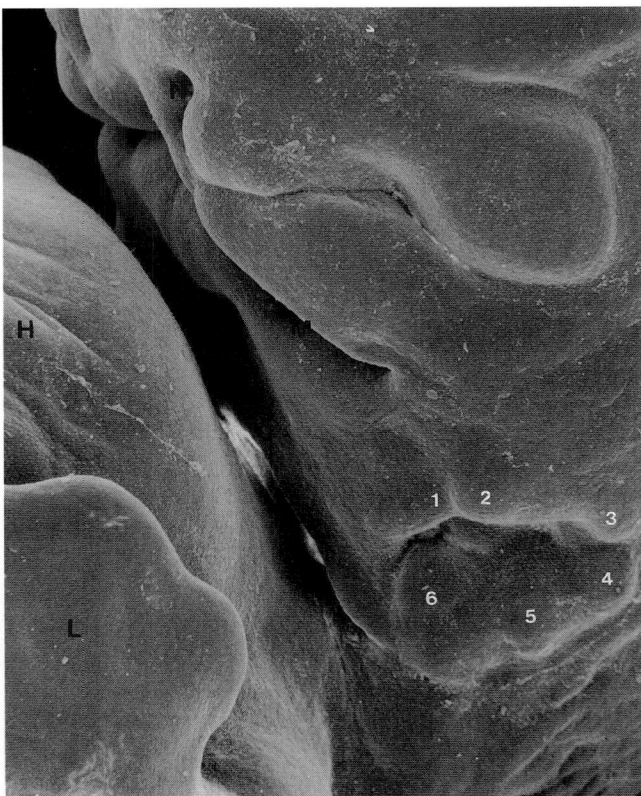

FIG. 6. Scanning electron micrographs showing early development of auricular hillocks in the human embryo. **A:** An embryo of about 5 weeks shows hillocks (*h*) forming on either side of the first cleft (*arrow*); *H*, heart; *N*, forming nasal pit. Modified from Sadler T. *Langman's medical embryology,* with permission. **B:** An embryo of about 6 weeks shows hillocks 1–6; *H*, heart; *L*, forelimb bud; *M*, primitive mouth; *N*, nasal pit. Courtesy of Dr. Kathleen Sulik.

THE EXTERNAL EAR

On the external surface of arches I and II, a set of six auricular hillocks (three per arch) arises from proliferation of mesenchymal cells on either side of the first pharyngeal cleft. These hillocks merge as the pinna forms, and the first cleft modifies as the external auditory meatus (Fig. 6). There is a relative shift in position from the pharyngeal region (at 6 wks) to the side of the head (32 wks) as the mandible develops and teeth form. As the first cleft modifies, the deep ectodermal epithelium proliferates to produce a solid plug of cells filling in the medial end of the cleft by about the 26th week (about the same time as the previously fused eyelids reopen). Apoptosis (programmed cell death) beginning at this time results in the canalization of the meatal epithelial plug, with definitive length of the meatus not being achieved until 9 or 10 years after birth. This phenomenon of epithelialization of a lumen is a common feature of embryogenesis. It characterizes development of the larynx, esophagus, duodenum, and so on. Just as apoptotic canalization of the esophagus or duodenum can fail, be incomplete, or otherwise go awry and result in, for example, esophageal atresia or double duodenum, so the first cleft may develop similar anomalies. Preauricular sinuses, which are cutaneous depressions located anterior to the auricle, tend to be familial and are often bilateral. The embryologic origin of these sinuses is uncertain but, at least in some cases, is related to anomalous union of the auricular hillocks. In some cases, development of the first pharyngeal cleft is involved. A first cleft sinus, depending on its position, may seriously compromise the facial nerve should infection occur and surgical intervention be necessary.

Apparently minor malformations of the auricle may indicate serious malformations elsewhere. Auricular appendages (tags) are common, usually unilateral, and assumed to result from supernumerary auricular hillocks. Variation in the merging of the auricular hillocks is so great as to make the morphology of the pinna an identification feature used by police in Europe.

SUMMARY

This cursory treatment of ear development emphasizes the intriguing complexity of this organ and, in many instances, our lack of understanding of the developmental mechanisms involved. Key to understanding would seem to be the spatiotemporal interaction of embryonic inductive interactions, neural crest cell migration, and programmed cell death, all of which interact on a particular genetic background. As progress in understanding the genetic mechanisms involved in embryogenesis continues, valuable clues to fathoming the molecular and morphologic genesis of the ear are to be expected. Although we are still in early days, the tools for exploring developmental mechanisms are becoming increasingly powerful. As interaction of clinicians and basic scientists becomes less uncommon, we may anticipate a satisfying sense of progress.

BIBLIOGRAPHY

Aka M. Hox and HOM: homologous gene clusters in insects and vertebrates. *Cell* 1989;57:347.

Anson B, Hanson JS, and Richany SF. Early embryology of the auditory ossicles and associated structures in relation to certain anomalies observed clinically. *Ann Otol* 1960;69:427.

Ars B. Organogenesis of the middle ear structures. *J Laryngol Otol* 1989;103:16.

Balling R, Mutter G, Gruss P, Kessel M. Craniofacial abnormalities induced by ectopic expression of the homeobox gene Hox-1.1 in transgenic mice. *Cell* 1989;58:337.

Chan VY, Tamm PPL. A morphological and experimental study of the mesencephalic neural crest cells in the mouse embryo using wheat germ agglutinin-gold conjugate as the cell marker. *Development* 1988;102:427.

Ciment G, Weston JA. Segregation of developmental abilities in neural-crest-derived cells: identification of partially restricted intermediate cell types in the branchial arches of avian embryos. *Dev Biol* 1985;111:73.

Corliss CE. *Patten's human embryology.* New York: McGraw-Hill; 1976.

Couly GF, LeDouarin N. Mapping of the early neural primordium in quailchick chimeras. II. The prosencephalic neural plate and neural folds: implications for the genesis of cephalic human congenital abnormalities. *Dev Biol* 1987;120:198.

Declau F, Jacob W, et al. Early ossification within the human fetal otic capsule: morphological and microanalytical findings. *J Laryngol Otol* 1989;103:1113.

Doutreland JJ, and Querleu D. Organogenese de l'audition. Developpement de l'oreille. *Rev Fr Gynecol Obstet* 1988;83:23.

Fraser S, Keynes R, Lumsden A. Segmentation in the chick embryo hindbrain is defined by cell lineage restrictions. *Nature* 1990;344:431.

Frenz DA, Van De Water TR, Galinovic-Schwartz V. Transforming growth factor beta: does it direct otic capsule formation. *Ann Otol Rhinol Laryngol* 1991;100:301.

Gaunt SJ, Sharpe PT, Duboule D. Spatially restricted domains of homeogene transcripts in mouse embryos: relation to a segmented body plan. *Development* 1988;103 [Suppl.]:169.

Gilbert P. The origins and development of the human extrinsic ocular muscles. *Contrib Embryol Carnegie Inst* 1957;246:61.

Goeringer GC, Vidic B. The embryogenesis and anatomy of Waldeyer's ring. *Otolaryngol Clin North Am* 1987;20:207.

Hamilton WJ, Boyd JD, Mossman HW. *Human embryology.* Baltimore: Williams & Wilkins; 1959.

Holland PW, Hogan B. Spatially restricted patterns of expression of the homeobox-containing gene Hox-2.1 during mouse embryogenesis. *Development* 1988;102:159.

Holland PW. Homeobox genes and the human head. *Development* 1988;103 [Suppl.]:117.

Irving D, Wilhite C, Burk D. Morphogenesis of isotretinoin-induced microcephaly and micrognathia studied by scanning electron microscopy. *Teratology* 1986;34:141.

Jacobson AG. Somitomeres: mesodermal segments of vertebrate embryos. *Development* 1988;104[Suppl.]:209.

Jones KL. *Smith's recognizable patterns of human malformation.* 4th ed. Philadelphia: WB Saunders; 1988.

Kirby M. Plasticity and predetermination of mesencephalic and trunk neural crest transplanted into the region of the cardiac neural crest. *Dev Biol* 1989;134:402.

LeDouarin N, Smith J. Development of the peripheral nervous system from neural crest. *Ann Rev Cell Biol* 1988;4:375.

Lewis J. Genes and segmentation. *Nature* 1989;341:382.

Lumsden A, and Keynes R. Segmental patterns of neuronal development in the chick hindbrain. *Nature* 1989;337:424.

Lumsden A, Sprawson N, Graham A. Segmental origin and migration of neural crest cells in the hindbrain region of the chick embryo. *Development* 1991;113:1281.

Marquet JE, Declau F, De Cock M, et al. Congenital middle ear malformations. *Acta Otorhinolaryngol Belg* 1988;42:117.

McPhee JR, Van De Water TR. Epithelial-mesenchymal tissue interactions guiding otic capsule formation: the role of the otocyst. *J Embryol Exp Morphol* 1986;97:1.

Meier S. Development of the chick mesoblast: formation of the embryonic axis and establishment of the metameric pattern. *Dev Biol* 1979;73:25.

Michaels L. Origin of congenital cholesteatoma from a normally occurring epidermoid rest in the developing middle ear. *Int J Pediatr Otorhinolaryngol* 1988;15:51.

Michaels L. Evolution of the epidermoid formation and its role in the development of the middle ear and tympanic membrane during the first trimester. *J Otolaryngol* 1988;17:22.

Michaels L, Soucek S. Development of the stratified squamous epithelium of the human tympanic membrane and external canal: the origin of auditory epithelial migration. *Am J Anat* 1989;184:334.

Michaels L, Soucek S. Auditory epithelial migration on the human tympanic membrane. II. The existence of two discrete migratory pathways and their embryologic correlates. *Am J Anat* 1990;189:189.

Moll M. Congenital earpits or auricular sinuses. *Acta Pathol Microbiol Scand* 1991;99:96.

Moore G, Ivens A, Chambers J, et al. The application of molecular genetics to detection of craniofacial abnormality. *Development* 1988;103[Suppl.]:233.

Moore KL, Persaud TVN. *The developing human,* 5th ed. Philadelphia: WB Saunders;1993.

Noden DM. Patterning of avian craniofacial muscles. *Dev Biol* 1986;116:347.

Noden DM. Interactions and fates of avian craniofacial mesenchyme. *Development* 1988;103[Suppl.]:121.

O'Rahilly R. The early development of the otic vesicle in staged human embryos. *J Embryol Exp Morphol* 1963;11:741.

Parrish KL, Amedee RG. Atresia of the external auditory canal. *J La State Med Soc* 1990;142:9.

Pujol R. Development of the human cochlea. *Acta Otolaryngol* (Stockh) 1991;482[Suppl.]:7.

Reid L. From gradients to axes, from morphogenesis to differentiation. *Cell* 1990;63:875.

Repressa JJ, Moro JA, Gato A, Pastor F, and Barbosa E. Patterns of epithelial cell death during early development of the human inner ear. *Ann Otol Rhinol Laryngol* 1990;99:482.

Sadler TW. *Langman's medical embryology,* 7th ed. Baltimore: Williams & Wilkins; 1995.

Slack JM. Morphogenetic gradients—past and present. *Trends Biochem Sci* 1987;12:200.

Tan S, and Morriss-Kay G. The development and distribution of the cranial neural crest in the rat embryo. *Cell Tissue Res* 1985;240:403.

Tuckett F, Lim L, Morriss-Kay G. The ontogenesis of cranial neuromeres in the rat embryo. I. A scanning electron microscope and kinetic study. *J Embryol Exp Morphol* 1985;87:215.

Van De Water TR. The morphogenesis of the middle and the external ear. *Birth Defects: Orig Artic Ser* 1980;16:147.

Van De Water TR. Tissue interactions and cell differentiation: neurone-sensory cell interactions during development. *Development* 1988;103[Suppl.]:185.

Wedden SE, Ralphs JR and Tickle C. Pattern formation in the facial primordia. *Development* 1988;103[Suppl.]:31.

CHAPTER 2

Anatomy, Physiology, and Pathophysiology of the Eustachian Tube

Charles D. Bluestone

The eustachian tube is part of a system of contiguous organs including the nose, palate, nasopharynx, middle ear, and mastoid air cells (Fig. 1). The eustachian tube, in reality, is not a tube but an *organ* consisting of a lumen with its mucosa, cartilage, surrounding soft tissue, peritubal muscles (i.e., tensor veli palatini, levator veli palatini, salpingopharyngeus, and tensor tympani), and its superior bony support, the sphenoid sulcus. An understanding of this anatomy is important so that the physiology and pathophysiology of the eustachian tube can be related to the etiology and pathogenesis of otitis media and related conditions.

ANATOMY OF THE EUSTACHIAN TUBE

The eustachian tube in the adult lies at an angle of 45 degrees in relation to the horizontal plane, whereas in infants this inclination is only 10 degrees (Fig. 2) (1). The adult tube is longer than in the infant and young child, and its length varies with race; it has been reported to be as short as 30 mm (2) and as long as 40 mm (3), but the usual range of length reported in the literature is 31 to 38 mm (1,4–8). The posterior third (11–14 mm) of the adult tube is osseous and the anterior two thirds (20–25 mm) is composed of membrane and cartilage (1,9).

The bony portion of the eustachian tube (i.e., osseous or protympanic portion) lies completely within the petrous portion of the temporal bone and is directly continuous with the anterior wall of the superior portion of the middle ear. In the adult, the juncture of the osseous tube and the epitympanum lies 4 mm above the floor of the tympanic cavity (9). This relationship, although valid, is misrepresented in the more popular descriptions and depictions of the tubal–middle-ear juncture and is of some importance in the functional clearance of middle-ear fluids. The course of the osseous tube is linear anteromedially, following the petrous apex and deviating little from the horizontal plane. The lumen in the bony portion of the tube is roughly an inverted triangular, measuring 2 to 3 mm vertically and 3 to 4 mm along the horizontal base. In the absence of the disease state, the bony portion is open at all times, in contrast to the fibrocartilaginous portion, which is closed at rest and opens during swallowing or when forced open, such as during the Valsalva maneuver. The osseous and cartilaginous portions of the eustachian tube meet at an irregular bony surface and form an angle of about 160 degrees with each other.

The fibrocartilaginous tube then courses anteromedially and inferiorly, angled in most cases 30 to 40 degrees to the transverse plane and 45 degrees to the sagittal plane (9). This portion of the tube is closely applied to the basal aspect of the skull and is fitted to a sulcus tubae between the greater wing of the sphenoid bone and the petrous portion of the temporal bone. The fibrocartilaginous portion of the tube is firmly attached at its posterior end to the osseous orifice by fibrous bands and usually extends some distance (3 mm) into the osseous portion of the tube. The inferomedial end is attached to a tubercle on the posterior edge of the medial pterygoid lamina (1,5,6,9,10–12).

The cartilaginous tube has a crook-shaped mediolateral superior wall. It is completed laterally and inferiorly by a veiled membrane, (1,4,13) which serves as the site for the attachment of the fibers of the dilator tubae, or tensor veli palatini muscle (10,14). Tubal cartilage increases in mass from birth to puberty, and this development has physiologic implications (15,16). The tubal lumen is shaped like two cones joined at their apices. The juncture of the cones is the narrowest point of the lumen and has been called the *isthmus*, and its position is usually described as at or near the juncture of the osseous and cartilaginous portions of the tube. This is not the site of the "junctional portion," as recently de-

---

C.D. Bluestone: Department of Otolaryngology, University of Pittsburgh School of Medicine, Pittsburgh, Pennsylvania 15213.

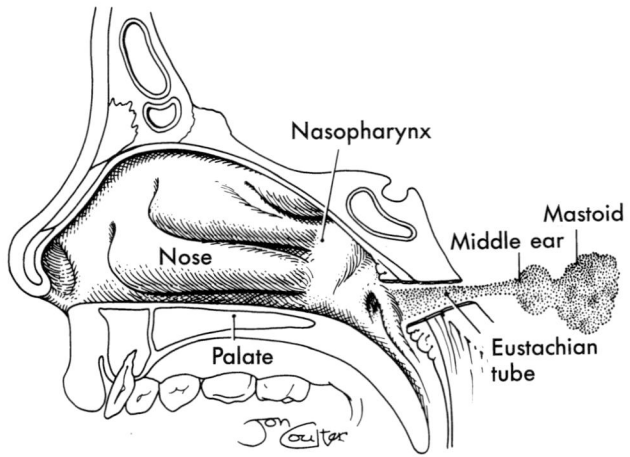

FIG. 1. Eustachian tube as part of a system of connected organs.

scribed by Sudo, Sando, and Ikui (17), which is the junction of the fibrocartilaginous portion to the more distal bony portion. The lumen at this point is approximately 2 mm high and 1 mm wide (1). From the isthmus, the lumen expands to approximately 8 to 10 mm in height and 1 to 2 mm in diameter at the pharyngeal orifice (18). The lumen has a constant height and there are only small differences between the height of the isthmus in the child and that in the adult (19,20). The isthmus portion most likely plays an important role in protecting the middle ear from nasopharyngeal secretions, as described later in this chapter.

The fibrocartilaginous portion of the eustachian tube does not follow a straight course in the adult but extends along a curve from the junction of the osseous and cartilaginous portions to the medial pterygoid plate, approximating the cranial base for the greater part of its course. The eustachian tube crosses the superior border of the superior constrictor muscle immediately posterior to its terminus within the nasopharynx. The thickened anterior fibrous investment of the medial cartilage of the tube presses against the pharyngeal wall to form a prominent fold, the torus tubarius, which measures 10 to 15 mm in thickness (1). The torus is the site of origin of the salpingopalatine muscle (21) and is the point of origin of the salpingopharyngeal muscle, which lies within the inferoposteriorly directed salpingopharyngeal fold (22). The medial lamina of the tube is attached to the lateral lamina at the hinge portion, which is rich in elastin; the lateral lamina is pulled lateral opening the lumen when the tensor veli palatini contracts (23).

The lumen of eustachian tube has mucosal lining, which is continuous with that of the nasopharynx and middle ear and is characterized as respiratory epithelium (24). Structural differentiation of this mucosal lining is evident; mucous glands predominate at the nasopharyngeal orifice, and there is graded change to a mixture of goblet, columnar, and ciliated cells near the tympanum (25). The products of these glands include active compounds (26–28). As described by Matsune, Sando, and Takahashi (29), the density of goblet cells was significantly lower in the roof of the eustachian tube than in the floor of the tube and was highest in the midcartilaginous area. The mucociliary defense system within the tube starts in fetal life and is well established soon after birth (30). Sando et al. (31) postulated that the superior portion of the tubal lumen is involved in the pressure regulation (i.e., ventilatory) function of the tube, and the inferior portion of the tubal lumen is involved in the drainage and clearance function of the tube; the inferior portion has mucosal folds, whereas the superior portion does not (Fig. 3). In addition, the hinge portion of the cartilage is in the superior part of the tube, and the tensor veli palatini muscle is attached to the lateral lamina of the cartilage in the superior portion of the tube, which is part of the active opening mechanism.

Muscles of the Eustachian Tube

There are four muscles associated with the eustachian tube: the tensor veli palatini, levator veli palatini, salpingopharyngeus, and tensor tympani. Each has at one time or another been directly or indirectly implicated in tubal function (4,7,10,32–35).

At rest, the normal eustachian tube is closed; it opens during such actions as swallowing, yawning, or sneezing and thereby permits the equalization of middle ear and atmospheric pressures. Although controversy still exists as to the mechanism of tubal dilation, most anatomic and physiologic evidence supports active dilation induced solely by the tensor veli palatini muscle (36,37). Closure of the tube has been attributed to passive reapproximation of tubal walls by extrinsic forces exerted by the surrounding deformed tissues, by the recoil of elastic fibers within the tubal wall (38), or by both mechanisms. More recent experimental and clinical data suggest that, at least for certain abnormal populations, the closely applied internal pterygoid muscle may assist tubal closure by an increase in its mass within the pterygoid fossa; this increase applies medial pressure to the tensor veli palatini muscle and consequently to the lateral membranous wall of the eustachian tube (36,39,40).

The tensor veli palatini muscle is composed of two fairly distinct bundles of muscle fibers divided by a layer of fibroelastic tissue. The bundles lie mediolateral to the tube (Fig. 4) (40a). The more lateral bundle (the tensor veli palatini proper) is of an inverted triangular design, taking its origin from the scaphoid fossa and entire lateral osseous ridge of the sulcus tubae for the course of the eustachian tube. The bundles descend anteriorly, laterally, and inferiorly to converge in a tendon that rounds the hamular process of the medial pterygoid lamina about an interposed bursa. This fiber group then inserts into the posterior border of the horizontal process of the palatine bone and into the palatine aponeurosis of the anterior portion of the velum. The more posteroinferior muscle fibers lack an osseous origin, extending instead into the semicanal of the tensor tympani muscle.

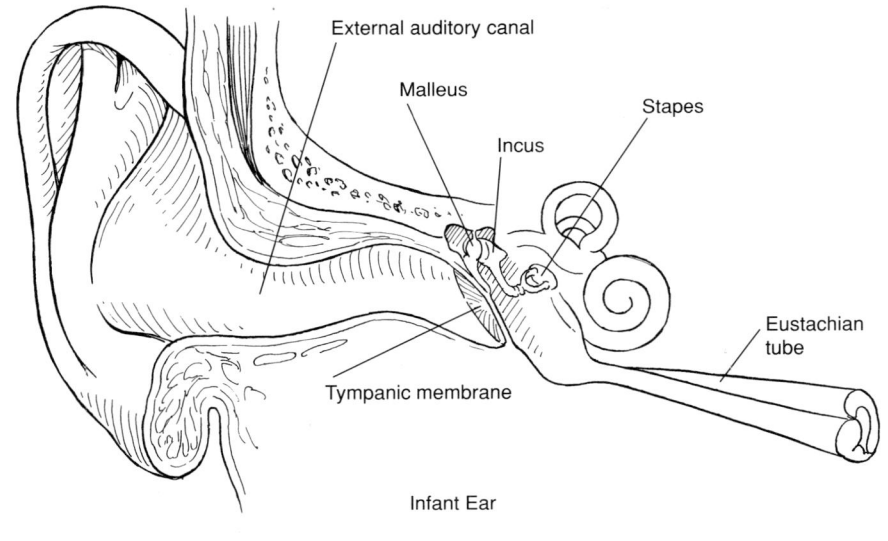

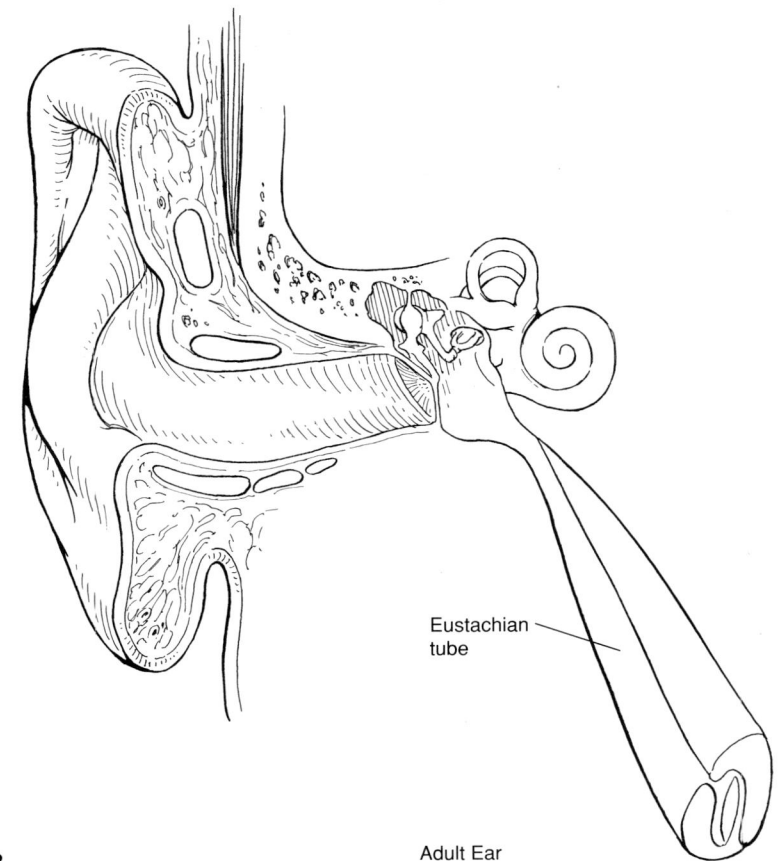

FIG. 2. Eustachian tube in the infant (A) is shorter and has less inclination than adult tube (B).

Here, the latter group of muscle fibers receive a second muscle slip, which originates from the tubal cartilages and sphenoid bone. These muscle masses converge to a tendon that rounds the cochleariform process and inserts into the manubrium of the malleus. This arrangement imposes a bipennate form to the tensor tympani muscle (14,41). The tensor tympani does not appear to be involved in the function of the eustachian tube (Fig. 5) (40a,42).

The medial bundle of the tensor veli palatini muscle lies immediately adjacent to the lateral membranous wall of the eustachian tube and is called the dilator tubae muscle (7,14). It takes its superior origin from the posterior third of the lateral membranous wall of the eustachian tube. The fibers descend sharply to enter and blend with the fibers of the lateral bundle of the tensor veli palatini muscle. It is this inner bundle that is responsible for active dilation of the

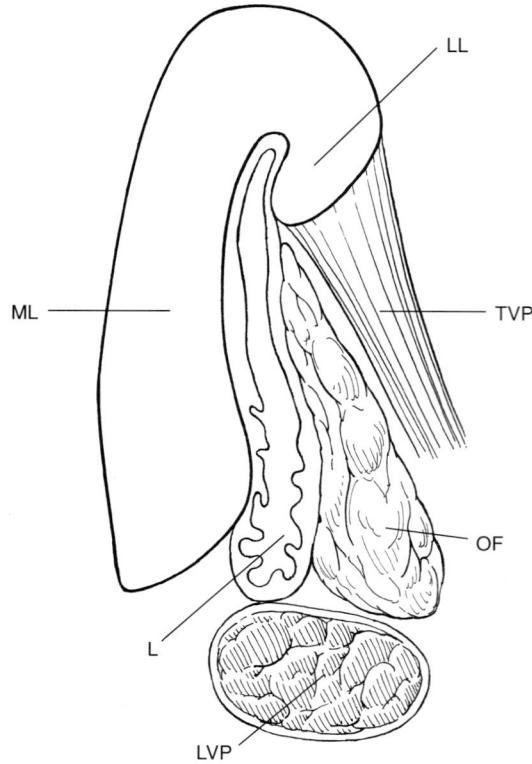

FIG. 3. Schematic representation of coronal section through left eustachian tube in the cartilaginous portion. The three physiologic functions of the eustachian tube related to the middle ear. *L*, lumen; *LL*, lateral lamina of cartilage; *ML*, medial lamina of cartilage; *TVP,* tensor veli palatine muscle; *LVP,* levator veli palatini muscle; *OF,* Ostmans's fat pad.

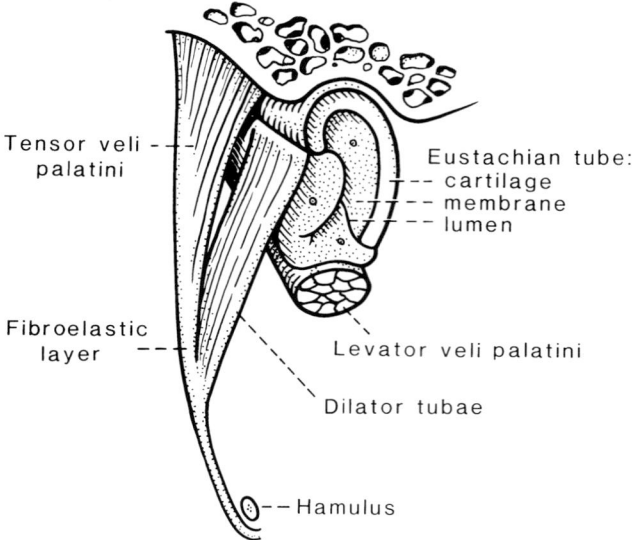

FIG. 4. Schematic representation of a coronal section through eustachian tube and the tensor veli palatini and levator veli palatini muscles. From Bluestone CD, Stool SE, Kenna MA, eds. *Pediatric Otolaryngology.* 3rd ed. Philadelphia: WB Saunders, 1996.

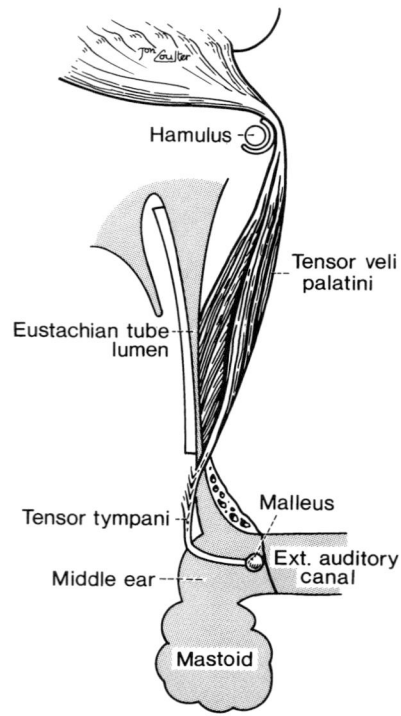

FIG. 5. Schematic representation of a transverse section through eustachian tube and the tripartite tensor veli palatini and tensor tympani muscles. From Bluestone CD, Stool SE, Kenna MA, eds. *Pediatric Otolaryngology.* 3rd ed. Philadelphia: WB Saunders, 1996.

tube by inferolateral displacement of the membranous wall (14,33,40). Swarts and Rood (20) reported that there is changing angle between the tensor veli palatini muscle and the cartilage with development, which could be related to the efficiency of tubal dilation and the increased frequency of otitis media in infants and young children.

The levator veli palatini muscle arises from the inferior aspect of the petrous apex and from the lower border of the medial lamina of the tubal cartilage. The fibers pass inferomedially, paralleling the tubal cartilage and lying within the vault of the tubal floor. They fan out and blend with the dorsal surface of the soft palate (9,10,33). Most investigators deny a tubal origin for this muscle and believe that in fact it is related to the tube only by loose connective tissue (21,43). The levator is not an active opener of the tube but probably contributes by elevating the medial arm of the cartilage at the nasopharyngeal end of the eustachian tube (12).

The salpingopharyngeal muscle arises from the medial and inferior borders of the tubal cartilage via slips of muscular and tendinous fibers. The muscle then courses inferoposteriorly to blend with the mass of the palatopharyngeal muscle (9,43). Rosen (22) examined ten hemisected human heads and identified the muscle in nine specimens. However, in all cases the muscle fibers were few in number and appeared to lack any ability to perform physiologically.

Infant Eustachian Tube

The eustachian tube in the infant is about half as long as that in the adult; it averages about 18 mm. The cartilaginous tube represents somewhat less than two thirds of this distance, whereas the osseous portion is relatively longer and wider in diameter than it is in the adult. The height of the pharyngeal orifice of the infant's eustachian tube is about half that of the adult, but the width is similar. Since the infant (and young child) has a shorter eustachian tube than does the older child or adult, nasopharyngeal secretions may reflux more readily into the middle ear through the shorter tube (44). The ostium of the tube is more exposed in the infant than it is in the adult, because it lies lower in the shallower nasopharyngeal vault. The direction of the tube varies, from horizontal to an angle of about 10 degrees to horizontal, and the tube is not angulated at the isthmus; it merely narrows (9). Holborow (45) demonstrated that in infants the medial cartilaginous lamina is relatively shorter since there is less tubal mass and stiffness in the infant tube than there is in that of the older child and adult. The tensor veli palatini muscle is less efficient in the infant. Table 1 (40a) lists the developmental differences between the anatomy of the eustachian tube in the infant with that of the adult, which most likely is related to the developmental differences in function between these two age groups, as described below.

PHYSIOLOGY OF THE EUSTACHIAN TUBE

The eustachian tube has at least three physiologic functions with respect to the middle ear: (a) *pressure regulation* of the middle ear to equilibrate gas pressure in the middle ear with atmospheric pressure; (b) *protection* from nasopharyngeal sound pressure and secretions; and (c) *clearance* (i.e., drainage) of secretions produced within the middle ear into the nasopharynx. A basic understanding of these physiologic functions will be helpful in comprehending the role of the eustachian tube in the pathogenesis of middle-ear disease.

Pressure Regulation

Regulation of pressure (ventilatory function) within the middle ear is the most important function of the eustachian tube, because hearing is optimal when the middle-ear gas pressure is relatively the same as the air pressure in the external auditory canal, that is, tympanic membrane and middle-ear compliance is physiologic. In ideal tubal function, intermittent active opening of the eustachian tube, due only to contraction of the tensor veli palatini muscle during swallowing, maintains nearly ambient pressures in the middle ear (36,37,46,47). Opening of the eustachian tube permits gas exchange and equalization of pressures between the environment and the middle ear. Under physiologic conditions, the fluctuations in ambient pressure are bidirectional (i.e., either to or from the middle ear), relatively small in magnitude, and not readily appreciated (48). These fluctuations reflect the rise and fall in barometric pressures associated with changing weather conditions and elevation, or both. However, the changes in middle-ear pressure show mass directionality, can achieve appreciable magnitudes, and can result in pathologic changes. A major reason for these conditions is that the middle ear is a relatively rigid (i.e., noncollapsible) gas pocket which is surrounded by mucous membrane in which gases are exchanged between the middle-ear space and the mucosa. Differential pressure exceeds 54 mm Hg between the middle-ear space at atmospheric pressure and the microcirculation in the mucous membrane. This represents a diffusion-driven gradient from the middle-ear cavity to the mucosa that can produce an underpressure (relative to ambient pressure) in the middle ear of more than 600 mm H_2O during equilibration.

In an important study conducted in Sweden of normal eustachian tube function using a pressure chamber, children who were considered to be otologically normal were evaluated (49). Eustachian tube function was evaluated in 53 children and compared to function in 55 adults, all of whom had intact tympanic membranes and who were apparently otologically healthy. The study revealed that 35.8% of the children could not equilibrate applied negative intratympanic pressure by swallowing, whereas only 5% of the adults were unable to perform this function. Children between 3 and 6 years of age had worse function than did children age 7 to 12 years. In this study and a subsequent one conducted by the same research group, (50) children who had tympanometric evidence of negative pressure within the middle ear

TABLE 1. *Developmental differences between anatomy of the eustachian tube in infants compared to adults*

Anatomic features	Anatomic feature in infants (compared to adults)	Reference
Length of tube	Shorter	Sadler-Kimes et al., 1989
Angle of tube to horizontal plane	10° (vs. 45°)	Proctor, 1967
Angle of TVP to cartilage	Variable vs. stable	Swarts and Rood, 1993
Cartilage cell density	Greater	Yamaguchi et al., 1990
Elastic at hinge portion of cartilage	Less	Matsune et al., 1993
Ostmann's fat pad	Relatively wider	Aoki et al., 1994

TVP, tensor veli palatini muscle.
From Bluestone CD, Klein JO. Otitis media, atelectasis, and eustachian tube dysfunction. In: Bluestone CD, Stool SE, Kenna MA, eds. *Pediatric otolaryngology*. 3rd ed. Philadelphia: WB Saunders, 1996.

had poor eustachian tube function. The conclusion from these studies is that even in apparently otologically normal children, eustachian tube function is not as good as that in adults, which is related to the higher incidence of middle-ear disease in children.

If infants have inefficient active tubal opening, how do they physiologically regulate middle-ear gas pressure? One possible explanation is that they inflate their middle ear during crying. Evidence that this occurs is the finding of positive middle-ear pressures on tympanograms when infants who have no middle-ear effusion are crying; also, a bulging tympanic membrane can be seen when pneumatic otoscopy is performed. Perhaps this is the compensatory mechanism used by infants when they are passengers in airplanes during descent. Even though pressure regulation of the middle ear is the most important of the functions of the eustachian tube, the protective and clearance functions are also important in maintaining the physiologic state.

Protective Function

The normal eustachian tube protects the middle ear due to its anatomic structure, which depends also on an intact middle ear and mastoid so that a middle-ear and mastoid gas cushion is present. The protective function has been assessed only by radiographic techniques, (51–53) which was a modification of a tubal patency test described by Wittenborg and Neuhauser (54). In these studies, radiopaque material was instilled into the nose and nasopharynx of children who had otitis media and compared to those who were otologically normal. In the physiologic state, contrast material entered the nasopharyngeal end of the eustachian tube during swallowing activity but did not enter the middle ear. By contrast, the dye did reflux into the middle ear in some patients who had middle-ear disease, especially during closed-nose swallowing. At rest, the normal eustachian tube is collapsed and the tubal lumen is closed, thus preventing liquid from entering the nasopharyngeal end of the tube. During swallowing, when the proximal end (i.e., cartilaginous portion) opens, liquid can enter this part of the tube but does not gain entrance into the middle ear due to the narrow midportion of the tube, the isthmus.

Flask Model of Protective Function

The entire eustachian tube–middle-ear system is similar in this function to a flask with a long, narrow neck, in which the mouth of the flask represents the nasopharyngeal end; the narrow neck, the isthmus; and the bulbous portion, the middle ear and mastoid–air cell system (52,55,56). Fluid flow through the neck would be dependent upon the pressure at either end, the radius and length of the neck, and the viscosity of the liquid. When a small amount of liquid is instilled into the mouth of the flask, liquid flow stops somewhere in the narrow neck owing to capillarity within the neck and the relative positive air pressure that develops in the chamber of the flask. This positive pressure in the middle ear and mastoid gas cell part of the system can be considered a gas *cushion* or *pocket,* that prevents the liquid from entering the middle ear. This basic geometric design is considered critical for the protective function of the eustachian tube–middle-ear system. The flask model is helpful in understanding how nasopharyngeal secretions can enter the middle ear when there abnormalities of the system, which is described later in the chapter (see Pathophysiology).

Clearance Function

Clearance (i.e., drainage) of secretions from the middle ear is provided by the *mucociliary* system of the eustachian tube and some areas of the middle-ear mucous membrane. Also involved in the clearance of middle-ear secretions is the *pumping action* of the eustachian tube during closing. The clearance function has been studied by instilling radiopaque material into the middle ear of children whose tympanic membranes were not intact, when the material entered the middle ear (intact tympanic membrane) from the nasopharynx (52,53), and following insertion of foreign material into the middle ear of animal models (57,58). Such material flows toward the middle-ear portion of the eustachian tube and out the tube. This movement is related to ciliary activity that occurs in the eustachian tube and parts of the middle ear; the ciliated cells in the middle ear are increasingly more active as their location becomes more distal to the opening of the eustachian tube (59). In a series of elegant experiments by Honjo (60,61), the eustachian tube was shown to pump liquid out of the middle ear in both animal models and humans.

Surface Tension Factors

Several investigators have determined certain surface tension factors that could be involved with normal eustachian tube function. Birken and Brookler (62) isolated surface tension-lowering substances from washings of eustachian tubes of dogs. They postulated that these substances could act to enhance eustachian tube functions, similar to surfactant in the lung. Rapport, Lim, and Weiss (26) described a similar substance and demonstrated the effect of washing out the eustachian tube on the opening pressure in the experimental animal; others also have demonstrated a surfactant-like phospholipid in the middle ear and eustachian tube of animals and humans (63–65). In a recent study in gerbils, Fornadley and Burns (66) produced middle-ear effusions by injecting killed *Streptococcus pneumoniae* into the middle ear through the tympanic membrane, which increased the opening pressure of the eustachian tube. When the investigators introduced exogenous surfactant, the opening pressure dropped. From these studies, it is apparent that the clearance function of the eustachian tube–middle-ear system is important in maintaining a healthy middle ear.

Because otitis media is so common in humans, efficient

removal of middle-ear effusions must depend, to a large extent, on these functions.

PATHOPHYSIOLOGY OF EUSTACHIAN TUBE

Abnormal function of the eustachian tube that can cause otitis media and related conditions can be due to (a) *impairment of pressure regulation function* of the tube; (b) *loss of protective function* of the eustachian tube–middle ear; and (c) *impairment of clearance function* of the tube and middle ear. Pathologic changes in other parts of the system, such as nasal obstruction or palatal dysfunction, may also adversely influence eustachian tube–middle-ear function.

Impairment of Pressure Regulation

Impairment of the regulation of pressure within the middle ear can be caused by either (a) *anatomic obstruction;* or (b) *failure of the opening mechanism* (i.e., functional obstruction) of the eustachian tube.

Anatomic Obstruction of Eustachian Tube

The site of anatomic (i.e., mechanical) obstruction in the tube can be either intraluminal, periluminal, or peritubal. Obstruction of the lumen or within the periluminal tissues (i.e., intrinsic obstruction) can be due to inflammation secondary to infection (67–69), or allergy (70). Obstruction within the bony portion (i.e., middle-ear end) of the tube is usually due to acute or chronic inflammation of the mucosal lining, which may also be associated with polyps or a cholesteatoma. Total obstruction may be present at the middle-ear end of the tube. Stenosis of the eustachian tube has also been diagnosed but is a rare finding. Peritubal obstruction (i.e., extrinsic obstruction) could be the result of compression caused by a tumor or possibly an adenoid mass (53,71).

Failure of Opening Mechanism of Eustachian Tube

Opening failure may be due to either persistent collapse of the eustachian tube due to increased tubal compliance (i.e., lack of stiffness, "floppy"), an inefficient active opening mechanism, or both. This has also been termed functional obstruction of the eustachian—tube the tube is not anatomically (i.e., mechanically) obstructed, but it is functionally obstructed—which was first described by Bluestone (51) in infants with unrepaired palatal clefts and who had had chronic otitis media with effusion. Failure of the opening mechanism of the eustachian tube is common in infants and younger children without cleft palate or history of middle-ear disease (50,72), but more common in those children with middle-ear disease (52,73–75).

One possible explanation for the opening failure of the tube in infants and young children may be related to the cartilage support, because the length of eustachian tube cartilage is less in the infant than in older children and adults (76), and the cell density of the cartilage decreases with advancing age (77), which could affect the stiffness of the tubal cartilage in the infant and young child (see Table 1). If the tubal cartilage lacks stiffness, the lumen may not open in response to contraction of the tensor veli palatini muscle. Also, the density of elastin in the cartilage is less in the infant, (23) and Ostmann's fat pad is less in volume in the infant than it is in the adult; the width is similar between the two age groups (78).

Another possible reason for the inefficient active opening of the eustachian tube might be related to the marked age differences in the craniofacial base. As described above, the angle of the tube in the child is different from that of the adult. In the adult, the tube is approximately 45 degrees related to the horizontal plane, but in infants the inclination is only 10 degrees (1). The difference in the angle has been thought by some to be related to possible clearance problems in children, but this hypothesis has not been confirmed. It is more likely the difference in angulation has an effect on the function of the active opening mechanism (i.e., tensor veli palatini muscle contraction). Swarts and Rood (20) found the angular relationship between the tensor veli palatini muscle and the cartilage varies in the infant but is relatively stable in the adult.

Loss of Protective Function

The eustachian tube may not protect the middle ear when (a) the tube has *abnormal patency;* (b) the tube is relatively *short;* (c) *abnormal gas pressure* develops at either end of the tube; or (d) there is a nonintact middle ear and mastoid, e.g., *perforation of the tympanic membrane,* which results in a loss of the middle-ear gas pocket or cushion.

Abnormal Patency of Eustachian Tube

In extreme cases of abnormal patency of the eustachian tube, the tube is open even at rest (i.e., patulous tube). Lesser degrees of abnormal patency result in a semipatulous eustachian tube that is closed at rest but has low resistance in comparison with the normal tube. Increased patency of the tube may be due to abnormal tube geometry or to a decrease in the peritubal pressure, such as occurs after weight loss or possibly as a result of periluminal factors. Since the eustachian tube has been found to be highly compliant in infants and young children, this increase in distensibility of the tube may result in abnormal patency, especially when there is high nasopharyngeal pressure. But, in teenagers and adults the patulous tube has been found to be too stiff compared to normal tubal compliance (79). A patulous eustachian tube usually permits gas to flow readily from the nasopharynx into the middle ear, which thus effectively regulates middle-ear pressure; however, unwanted secretions from the nasopharynx can more readily gain access (i.e., *reflux*), to the middle ear when the tube is abnormally patent. Certain special populations such as Native Americans (80), and patients who have Down syndrome and middle-ear disease have been found to have patulous or semipatulous eustachian tubes (81).

The flask model is helpful in understanding the possible consequences of an abnormally patent eustachian tube. Reflux of liquid into the body of the flask occurs if the neck is excessively wide.

The Short Eustachian Tube

Probably one of the most important differences in the structure of the eustachian tube between infants and young children and older children and adults is the length of the tube; the tube is shorter in children below the age of 7 yrs (see Table 1) (44). Young children with cleft palate have eustachian tubes that are statistically shorter than those in age-matched controls below the age of 6 yrs; also the tube is shorter in children with Down syndrome (44). The shorter the tube, the more likely secretions can reflux into the middle ear. (An analogy can be made to the length of the urethra; females of all ages have more urinary tract infections than males, because the urethra is shorter in the female.) This may be one explanation for the frequent occurrence of troublesome otorrhea in infants and young children, especially those who have a cleft palate or have Down syndrome, and the tympanic membrane is not intact.

A flask with a short neck is not as protective as a flask with a long neck. The position of the flask in relation to the liquid is another potentially important factor. In humans, the supine position enhances flow of liquid into the middle ear; thus, infants might be at particular risk for developing reflux otitis media because they are frequently supine.

Abnormal Gas Pressures

Development of high negative middle-ear pressure, secondary to obstruction of the eustachian tube, due to either anatomic obstruction, failure of active opening, or both, may result in aspiration of nasopharyngeal secretions into the middle ear. At the other end of the system, high positive nasopharyngeal pressures can result in insufflation of secretions into the middle ear, which may occur during blowing the nose, crying in the infant, or when nasal obstruction is present. Swallowing when the nose is obstructed (owing to inflammation or enlarged adenoids) results in an initial positive nasopharyngeal air pressure followed by a negative-pressure phase. When the tube is pliant, positive nasopharyngeal pressure might insufflate infected secretions into the middle ear, especially when the middle ear has a high negative pressure; with negative nasopharyngeal pressure, such a tube could be prevented from opening and could be further obstructed functionally, which has been referred to as the Toynbee Phenomenon (72,82,83). Rapid alterations in ambient pressures, which can occur during swimming, diving, airplane flying, and when patients receive hypobaric pressure treatments, may also result in aspiration or insufflation of nasopharyngeal secretions.

A flask with negative pressure applied to the bottom of the flask, results in liquid being aspirated into the vessel. In the clinical situation represented by the model, high negative middle-ear air pressure could lead to the aspiration of nasopharyngeal secretions into the middle ear. If positive pressure is applied to the mouth of the flask, the liquid is insufflated into the vessel. Nose blowing, crying, closed nose swallowing, diving, or ascent in an airplane could create high positive nasopharyngeal pressure and result in a similar condition in the human system.

One of the major differences between a flask with a rigid neck and a biological tube such as the eustachian tube is that the isthmus (neck) of the human tube is compliant. Application of positive pressure at the mouth of a flask with a compliant neck distends the neck, thereby enhancing fluid flow into the vessel. Thus, less positive pressure is required to insufflate liquid into the vessel. In humans, insufflation of nasopharyngeal secretions into the middle ear occurs more readily if the eustachian tube is abnormally distensible (has increased compliance). In this case, fluid flow occurs even if the neck is collapsed. If the negative pressure is applied suddenly, however, temporary locking of the compliant neck prevents flow of the liquid. Therefore, the speed with which the negative pressure is applied as well as the compliance in such a system appears to be a critical factor in the results obtained. Clinically, aspiration of gas into the middle ear is possible, because negative middle-ear pressure develops slowly as gas is absorbed by the middle-ear mucous membrane. On the other hand, sudden application of negative middle-ear pressure such as occurs with rapid alterations in atmospheric pressure (e.g., in the descent in an airplane, in a descent after diving, or during an attempt to test the ventilatory function of the eustachian tube), could lock the tube, and thus preventing the flow of air.

Nonintact Middle Ear and Mastoid System

Nasopharyngeal secretions are prevented from entering the middle ear when the tubal structure is normal but also occurs due to the cushion of gas that is within the intact middle-ear and mastoid–air cell system. When a perforation of the tympanic membrane is present, or in the extreme condition, when a radical mastoidectomy is present (the eardrum is absent and the middle ear, mastoid, and ear canal communicate to form a single cavity), the gas pocket is lost, which may allow secretions from the nasopharynx to reflux into the middle ear (52,73).

A flask in which reflux of a liquid into the vessel can also occur if a hole is made in the bulbous portion of the flask; this prevents the creation of the slight positive pressure in the bottom of the flask that deters reflux; that is, in this situation the middle ear and mastoid physiological cushion of air is lost. The hole is analogous to a perforation of the tympanic membrane or the presence of a tympanostomy tube that could allow reflux of nasopharyngeal secretions as a result of the loss of the middle-ear–mastoid air cushion. Similarly, following a radical mastoidectomy, a patent eustachian tube could cause troublesome otorrhea (73).

Impairment of Clearance Function

Clearance can be affected by several conditions that can occur in the eustachian tube and middle ear. Ohashi et al. (84), in studies conducted in guinea pigs, demonstrated that bacteria, their toxins, and irradiation can impair ciliary function. Also, Park et al. (85) demonstrated that influenza A virus alters the ciliary activity and dye transport function in the eustachian tube of the chinchilla. Most investigators consider impairment of the clearance function to be related to failure to resolve middle-ear effusions as opposed to being the primary cause of the disease (86). However, patients who have ciliary dysmotility in their upper respiratory tract mucous membrane have been observed to have chronic middle-ear effusions (87). Also, tubal pumping action is most likely ineffective when the opening mechanism is inadequate, and this function has been demonstrated to be impaired when negative pressure was present within the middle ear (88,89).

Certain aspects of fluid flow from the middle ear into the nasopharynx can be demonstrated by inverting a flask model. The liquid trapped in the bulbous portion of the flask does not flow out of the vessel because of the relative negative pressure that develops inside the chamber. However, if a hole is made in the vessel, the liquid drains out of the flask because the suction is broken. Clinically, these conditions occur in cases of middle-ear effusion; pressure is relieved by spontaneous rupture of the tympanic membrane or by myringotomy. Inflation of air into the flask could also relieve the pressure, which may explain the frequent success of the Politzer or Valsalva method in clearing a middle-ear effusion.

Allergy and Eustachian Tube Function

The role of allergy in the etiology and pathogenesis of otitis media has been postulated to be by one or more of the following mechanisms: (a) middle-ear mucosa functioning as a "shock" (target) organ (90,91), (b) inflammatory swelling of the mucosa of the eustachian tube (70), (c) inflammatory obstruction of the nose (Toynbee phenomenon), or (d) aspiration of bacteria-laden allergic nasopharyngeal secretions into the middle-ear cavity (92). Another possible mechanism has been proposed by Doyle (93). This hypothesis is based on the possible increase in circulating antiinflammatory mediators as the result of local allergic reactions in the mucosa of the nose or stomach, which in turn could alter the middle-ear mucosal permeability and result in altered gas exchange. Studies at the Children's Hospital of Pittsburgh involving adult volunteers have shown there is an effect on eustachian tube function when there are changes in the nose.

TABLE 2. *Evaluation of effect of nasal challenge on nasal and eustachian tube function*

Nasal provocation	Nasal function		Eustachian tube function	
	Normal	Allergic	Normal	Allergic
Allergens (pollens, mite)	No	Yes	No	Yes
Virus (rhinovirus, influenza A)	Yes	Yes	Yes	Yes
Mediators				
Histamine	Yes	Yes	No	Yes
PGD$_2$	Yes	Yes	No	Yes
Methacholine	Yes	Yes	No	No

Studies done at Children's Hospital of Pittsburgh.
Yes, adverse effect; No, little effect; PGD$_2$, prostaglandin-D synthase.
Data from Friedman et al., 1983; Ackerman et al., 1984; Doyle et al., 1984; Skoner et al., 1986; Stillwagon et al., 1987; Skoner et al., 1987; Doyle et al., 1990; Doyle et al., 1994; Buchman et al., 1994.

Table 2 shows the summary of these studies that demonstrated a relationship among intranasal challenge with allergens, virus, and mediators in volunteers who did and did not have allergic rhinitis and the effect on nasal and eustachian tube function (69,70,94–100). It seems reasonable that children with signs and symptoms of upper respiratory allergy may have otitis media as a result of the allergic condition. Most likely, however, these children also have a preexisting dysfunction of the eustachian tube. However, some investigators have concluded that allergy is not the cause of the middle-ear disease but plays a role in the persistence of effusion (86).

Eustachian Tube Function Related to Cleft Palate

Otitis media is universally present in infants with an unrepaired cleft palate (101–102). Palate repair appears to improve middle-ear status, but middle-ear disease nonetheless often continues or recurs even after palate repair (103). Studies suggest failure of the opening mechanism in the infants with an unrepaired cleft palate (39,51,104). Histopathologic temporal bone studies have confirmed that the eustachian tube of patients with cleft palate is not anatomically obstructed, which would give credence to failure of the opening mechanism (i.e., functional as opposed to anatomic obstruction), as the underlying defect. The other anatomic findings, such as the abnormal cartilage and lumen, insertion ratio of the tensor veli palatini muscle into the cartilage, deficient attachment of the tensor veli palatini muscle into the lateral lamina of the cartilage, and the deficient elastin at the hinge portion of the cartilage (105–109), most likely explain the functional obstruction identified by radiographic and manometric eustachian tube function tests. Also, animals in which the palate had been surgically split developed otitis media with effusion (110–112). From these studies in humans and animals, it appears that the high incidence of otitis media in children with cleft palate is related to failure of the opening mechanism and may also be related to the deficient length of the eustachian tube. If infants with an intact palate are able during crying, to inflate their middle ears as a physiologic compensatory mechanism for their ineffective active tubal opening, infants with an unrepaired cleft palate have an additional handicap.

Other Causes of Eustachian Tube Dysfunction

Dysfunction of the eustachian tube has also been reported to be associated with deviation of the nasal septum (113,114); trauma induced by nasogastric and nasal endotracheal tubes (115,116), trauma to the palate, pterygoid bone, or tensor veli palatini muscle; injury to the trigeminal nerve (more specifically, to the mandibular branch of this nerve) (117); and trauma associated with surgical procedures, such as palatal or maxillary resection for tumor (118). Neoplastic disease, either benign or malignant, that invades the palate, pterygoid bone, or tensor veli palatini muscle can cause otitis media (119), by causing failure of the opening mechanism of the tube (118,120,121).

CLINICAL TESTS OF EUSTACHIAN TUBE FUNCTION

Unfortunately, no completely physiologic test of eustachian tube function is yet available. But, tests that are accessible to the clinician can be helpful in distinguishing normal from abnormal function. However, no test can determine function when middle-ear effusion is present.

Tests When Tympanic Membrane Is Intact

Valsalva and Politzer Tests

Valsalva and Politzer developed methods to assess *patency,* not the function of the eustachian tube. If the tympanic membrane is intact and the middle ear inflates following one of these tests, the tube is not totally mechanically obstructed. When the tympanic membrane is not intact, passage of air into the middle ear indicates patency of the tube. The assessment is more objective with a tympanogram obtained when the tympanic membrane is intact but with a manometric observation on the impedance instrument when the tympanic membrane is not intact. Valsalva's and Politzer's maneuvers may be more beneficial as management options in selected patients than they are as methods to assess tubal function, although there is controversy about the efficacy of these procedures for treatment of middle-ear effusion (122,123).

Toynbee's Test of Function

The Toynbee test is one of the best tests of eustachian tube function. The test results are usually considered positive when an alteration in middle-ear pressure results. When negative pressure (even transitory in the absence of a patulous tube) develops in the middle ear during closed-nose swallowing, the eustachian tube function can most likely be considered normal. When the tympanic membrane is intact, the presence of negative middle-ear pressure must be determined by pneumatic otoscopy or, more accurately, by obtaining a tympanogram before and immediately following the test. When the tympanic membrane is not intact, the manometer of the immittance audiometer can be observed to determine middle-ear pressure. The test is of greater value in determining normal or abnormal eustachian tube function in adults than it is in children. However, the test is still of considerable value because, regardless of age, if negative pressure develops in the middle ear during or following the test, the eustachian tube function is most likely normal, because the eustachian tube actively opens and is sufficiently stiff to withstand nasopharyngeal negative pressure (i.e., it does not lock). If positive pressure is noted or no change in pressure occurs, the function of the eustachian tube still may be normal, and other tests of eustachian tube function should be performed.

Nine-step Tympanometric Test

At present, the most helpful method of assessing the function of the eustachian tube when the tympanic membrane is intact is the nine-step inflation-deflation tympanometric test, developed by Bluestone (124), although the applied middle-ear pressures are very limited in magnitude. The middle ear must be free of effusion. The nine-step tympanometry procedure may be summarized as follows (Fig. 6):

1. The tympanogram records resting middle-ear pressure.
2. Ear canal pressure is increased to -200 mm H_2O with medial deflection of the tympanic membrane and a corresponding increase in middle-ear pressure. The subject swallows to equilibrate middle-ear overpressure.
3. While the subject refrains from swallowing, ear canal pressure is returned to normal, thus establishing a slight negative middle-ear pressure (as the tympanic membrane moves outward). The tympanogram documents the established middle-ear underpressure.
4. The subject swallows in an attempt to equilibrate negative middle-ear pressure. If equilibration is successful, airflow is from nasopharynx to middle ear.
5. The tympanogram records the extent of equilibration.
6. Ear canal pressure is decreased to -200 mm H_2O, causing a lateral deflection of the tympanic membrane and a corresponding decrease in middle-ear pressure. The subject swallows to equilibrate negative middle-ear pressure; airflow is from the nasopharynx to the middle ear.
7. The subject refrains from swallowing while external ear canal pressure is returned to normal, thus establishing a slight positive pressure in the middle ear as the tympanic

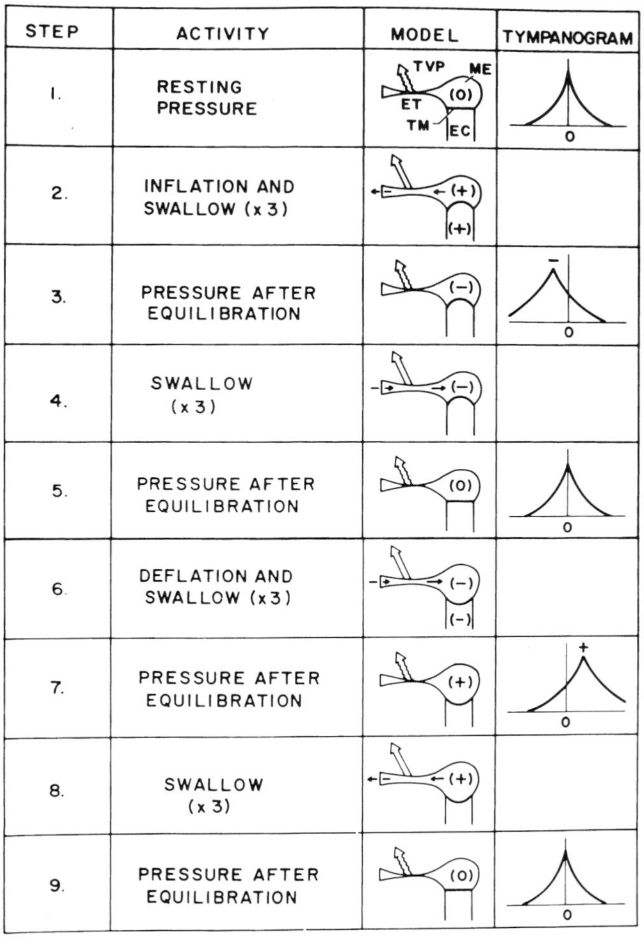

STEP	ACTIVITY	MODEL	TYMPANOGRAM
1.	RESTING PRESSURE	TVP ME ET (O) TM EC	∧ at 0
2.	INFLATION AND SWALLOW (x 3)	(+) (+)	
3.	PRESSURE AFTER EQUILIBRATION	(−)	− ∧ at 0
4.	SWALLOW (x 3)	(−)	
5.	PRESSURE AFTER EQUILIBRATION	(O)	∧ at 0
6.	DEFLATION AND SWALLOW (x 3)	(−) (−)	
7.	PRESSURE AFTER EQUILIBRATION	(+)	+ ∧ at 0
8.	SWALLOW (x 3)	(+)	
9.	PRESSURE AFTER EQUILIBRATION	(O)	∧ at 0

FIG. 6. Nine-step tympanometric test. *TVP,* tensor veli palatini muscle; *ET,* eustachian tube; *ME*-middle ear; *TM,* tympanic membrane, *EC,* ear canal.

membrane moves medially. The tympanogram records the overpressure established.
8. The subject swallows to reduce overpressure. If equilibration is successful, airflow is from the middle ear to the nasopharynx.
9. The final tympanogram documents the extent of equilibration. The test is simple to perform, can give useful information regarding eustachian tube function, and should be part of the clinical evaluation of patients with suspected eustachian tube dysfunction. In general, most normal adults can perform all or some parts of this test (68), but even normal children have difficulty in performing it. However, if a child can pass some or all the steps, eustachian tube function is considered good.

Tests When Tympanic Membrane Is Not Intact

Inflation-Deflation Test

If the tympanic membrane is not intact, the pump-manometer system of the immittance audiometer can be used to perform the modified inflation-deflation eustachian tube function test, which assesses passive as well as active functioning of the eustachian tube (125,126). The middle ear should be free of any otorrhea for an accurate assessment of eustachian tube function when this test is used. The middle ear is inflated (i.e., positive pressure is applied) until the eustachian tube spontaneously opens. At this time, the pump is manually stopped and air is discharged through the eustachian tube until the tube closes passively. The pressure at which the eustachian tube is passively forced open is called the *opening pressure,* and the pressure at which it closes passively is called the *closing pressure* (52,75). The patient is then instructed to equilibrate the middle-ear pressure actively by swallowing. The residual pressure remaining in the middle ear after swallowing is recorded. The *active function* is also recorded by applying over– and underpressure to the middle ear, which the patient then attempts to equilibrate by swallowing. The residual negative pressure that remains in the middle ear after the attempt to equilibrate applied negative pressure of -200 mm H_2O is also noted. This procedure is not performed in patients who cannot equilibrate applied overpressure. If the eustachian tube does not open following application of positive pressure using the immittance audiometer, and if no reduction in positive pressure occurs during swallowing, the eustachian tube must be assessed using a manometric system other than that available with the electroacoustic impedance audiometer. The opening pressure may be higher than 400 to 600 mm H_2O pressure or not present at all (i.e., anatomic obstruction). Failure to achieve an opening pressure is usually indicative of an anatomic obstruction somewhere in the tube, in which case a nuclear magnetic resonance image study, a computed tomogram, or both is indicated to determine the etiology of the obstruction (e.g., cholesteatoma or tumor).

Failure to equilibrate the applied negative pressure may indicate locking of the eustachian tube during the test, which may or may not be indicative of a pathologic condition. This type of tube is considered to have increased compliance or to be "floppy" in comparison to a tube with perfect function (53,79). The tensor veli palatini muscle is unable to open (dilate) the tube.

INDICATIONS FOR TESTING EUSTACHIAN TUBE FUNCTION

Assessment of eustachian tube function can be beneficial in the differential diagnosis in a patient who has an intact tympanic membrane without evidence of otitis media but who has symptoms that might be related to eustachian tube dysfunction (e.g., otalgia, snapping or popping in the ear, fluctuating hearing loss, tinnitus, vertigo). An example is a child or adolescent who has a complaint of fullness in the ear without hearing loss at the time of the examination, a symptom that could be related to abnormal functioning of the eustachian tube or could be due to an inner-ear disorder. A tympanogram that reveals high negative pressure (-50

mm H$_2$O or less) is presumptive evidence of tubal obstruction, whereas normal resting middle-ear pressure is not diagnostically significant. When the resting intratympanic pressure is within normal limits and the patient can develop negative middle-ear pressure following the Toynbee test or can perform all or some of the functions in the nine-step inflation-deflation tympanometric test, the eustachian tube is probably functioning normally. Unfortunately, failure to develop negative middle-ear pressure during the Toynbee test or inability to pass the nine-step test does not necessarily indicate poor eustachian tube function because many children who are otologically normal cannot actively open their tubes during these tests.

When there is a perforation of the tympanic membrane, especially when present bilaterally, testing the function of the eustachian tube may aid in the decision-making process to repair the defect. Normal function, as assessed using the inflation-deflation test, usually predicts a favorable outcome of tympanoplasty. However, when the child has poor active opening of the tube, the outcome still may be good, but the success rate is lower (127). The test may also be helpful when the clinician is considering removing a tympanostomy tube. Presence of normal eustachian tube function would be one factor in favor of removing the tube.

TUBAL FUNCTION RELATED TO PATHOGENESIS OF OTITIS MEDIA

The pathogenesis of otitis media is multifactorial, which includes factors such as infection (viral and bacterial); anatomic factors (e.g., eustachian tube dysfunction; host factors, such as young age, immature or impaired immunologic status, presence of upper respiratory allergy, familial predisposition, presence of older siblings in household, male sex, race (e.g., Native Americans, Australian Aborigines), and method of feeding (bottle vs. breast); and environmental factors, (e.g., day-care attendance, passive smoking). The incidence of otitis media has statistically increased during the past 2 decades in infants and young children in the United States (128). The corresponding increase in day-care attendance in this age group during the same period is the most likely cause of this dramatic rise. In the day-care environment, infants and young children develop frequent upper respiratory tract infections that commonly result in otitis media because their eustachian tubes are functionally and structurally immature, and they have immature immune systems.

Abnormal function of the eustachian tube appears to be the most important factor in the pathogenesis of middle-ear disease in all age groups. This hypothesis was first suggested more than 100 years ago by Politzer (129). However, later studies (130,131) suggested that otitis media was a disease primarily of the middle-ear mucous membrane and was caused by infection or allergic reactions in this tissue, rather than by dysfunction of the eustachian tube. But more recent studies conducted at the Children's Hospital of Pittsburgh, which involved both humans and animals, have shown that the *hydrops ex vacuo* theory as originally proposed by Adam Politzer more than a century ago is most likely the primary pathogenic mechanism in many patients; dysfunction of the eustachian tube also promotes viruses and bacteria to enter the middle ear which results in otitis media (47,52, 69,93,132).

Acute otitis media, otitis media with effusion, persistent middle-ear effusion, eustachian tube dysfunction, and chronic suppurative otitis media are the most frequent middle-ear diseases encountered by the clinician. Following the onset of either acute otitis media or otitis media with effusion, persistent middle-ear effusion may develop.

Acute Otitis Media

In most children, the pathogenesis of acute otitis media is likely to occur with the following pattern: (a) the patient has an antecedent event (usually an upper respiratory viral infection) that results in congestion of the respiratory mucosa of the upper respiratory tract, including the nasopharynx and eustachian tube; (b) congestion of the mucosa in the eustachian tube results in obstruction of the tube; (c) negative middle-ear pressure develops; (d) if negative pressure is prolonged, aspiration of potential pathogens (viruses and bacteria) from the nasopharynx into the middle ear occurs; (e) clearance of the middle-ear effusion, due to the infection, accumulates in the middle ear; (f) microbial pathogens proliferate in the secretions; (g) suppurative and symptomatic otitis media results. In a recent study conducted by Buchman et al. (133), this cascade of events was reproduced in 27 adult volunteers in whom influenzae A was inoculated into the nose. All subjects developed a nasal infection, 16 (59%) subsequently developed high negative middle-ear effusion, and in one subject an acute otitis media was present; the middle-ear aspirate revealed the virus and *S. pneumoniae*.

For children with recurrent episodes of acute otitis media or otitis media with effusion, anatomic or physiologic abnormality of the eustachian tube appears to be an important, if not the most important, factor. The child with such an underlying abnormality of the eustachian tube may be subject to recurrent episodes of acute otitis media. The pathogenesis of recurrent acute otitis media in 50 otitis-prone children (defined as more than 11 episodes of acute otitis media) was studied in Sweden by Stenstrom, Bylander-Groth, and Invarsson (74). Employing the pressure chamber to test eustachian tube function, they found the otitis-prone children to have significantly poorer active tubal function than 49 normal (controls) children who had no history of acute otitis media. This finding indicates that the pathogenesis of recurrent acute otitis media is the result of functional, as opposed to mechanical, obstruction of the eustachian tube. However, it is likely that infants and young children who have short, floppy eustachian tubes can reflux or insufflate nasopharyngeal secretions into the middle ear during a viral upper respiratory tract infection. Another possible mechanism is progressive ascending infection from the nasopharynx into the mucosa of the eustachian tube, which most likely occurs when there is an indwelling obstructing foreign object in the nasopharynx, such as a nasogastric or nasotracheal tube in place.

Otitis Media with Effusion

The acute onset of otitis media with effusion, although relatively asymptomatic in children, most likely has a similar sequence of events as described above for acute otitis media because bacteria can be isolated from middle-ear effusions of patients with otitis media with effusion (134,135), but prolonged negative pressure within the middle ear can cause a sterile middle-ear effusion. Otitis media with effusion has been produced in the monkey animal model following excision of (136), and injection of (47,132) botulinum toxin into the tensor veli palatini muscle, which resulted in an opening failure of the eustachian tube, middle-ear underpressures, and effusion. These experiments confirm the *hydrops ex vacuo* theory of the pathogenesis of middle-ear effusion. This theory postulates that in the absence of eustachian tube opening, the gas exchange from the middle ear into the microcirculation of the mucous membrane causes a middle-ear underpressure followed by transdation of effusion. Swarts et al. (137) were also able to produce middle-ear effusion in the monkey shortly after inducing middle-ear negative pressure by flushing the middle ear with carbon dioxide. Because tubal opening is possible in a middle ear with an effusion, aspiration of nasopharyngeal secretions might occur, thus creating the clinical condition in which otitis media with effusion and recurrent acute bacterial otitis media with effusion occur together. The most dramatic example of the *ex vacuo* cause of acute middle-ear effusion is following barotrauma, e.g., descent during scuba diving or airplane flying.

In two elegant studies by McBride et al. (68) and Buchman et al. (69) that involved adult volunteers, nasal challenge with rhinovirus resulted in eustachian tube obstruction, negative middle-ear pressure and, in two subjects, middle-ear effusion. The two individuals who had middle-ear effusion had negative middle-ear pressure prior to the challenge. None of the subjects who had normal middle-ear pressure before the challenge developed an effusion, which indicates that a viral infection results in middle-ear effusion if the patient has preexisting dysfunction of the eustachian tube (69). Doyle et al. (100) also demonstrated that intranasal challenge of influenza A virus in 33 healthy adult volunteers resulted in eustachian tube obstruction, negative middle-ear pressure, and in 5 of 21 infected subjects, middle-ear effusion. Most likely, influenza A virus is more virulent than rhinovirus. Periods of upper respiratory tract infection may then result in atelectasis of the tympanic membrane–middle-ear system (i.e., high negative middle-ear pressure), sterile otitis media with effusion, or acute bacterial otitis media.

In a study of eustachian tube function in 163 ears of Japa-nese children and adults who had otitis media with effusion and chronic otitis media, Iwano et al. (75) found impaired active opening function of the tube in children and adults. They concluded the tube was functionally obstructed, however, organic (i.e., mechanical or anatomic) obstruction was considered also to be involved in the pathogenesis in adults.

Persistent Middle-Ear Effusion

The pathogenesis of persistent middle-ear effusion after the initial stage of a viral or bacterial infection in the middle ear or following transudation of effusion when high negative pressure is within the middle ear is probably similar. There is stimulation of cytokines, such as interleukins 1, 2, and 6, tissue necrosis factor, and interferon-gamma from inflammatory cells of the middle-ear mucous membrane (138–143), followed by two pathways of inflammation: (a) upregulation of submucosal receptors, primarily selectins and integrins that trap lymphocytes into the mucosa, (144) which also produce cytokines and inflammatory mediators; and (b) stimulation of inflammatory mediators, such as leukotrienes, prostaglandins, thromboxane, prostacycline, and platelet activating factor (145–151), which in turn can promote fluid leakage from the mucous membrane. At this stage there is probably increase in blood flow within the mucous membrane, due to engorgement of blood vessels and angioneogenesis, which then results in further negative pressure within the middle ear due to increase in perfusion of nitrogen into the microcirculation of the mucosa (48,152). In addition, the effusion that is produced is trapped in the middle ear due to the anatomy of the system (i.e., a closed space in which there is a narrow outlet, the eustachian tube). Also, the mucociliary system and the pumping action of tubal opening and closing is most likely impaired, thus causing persistent middle-ear effusion.

Eustachian Tube Dysfunction

Dysfunction of the eustachian tube can be due to either tubal obstruction or a patulous tube and result in signs and symptoms referable to the ear, despite the lack of a middle-ear effusion. Obstruction of the tube can cause middle-ear negative pressure, retraction of the tympanic membrane, hearing loss, and, in its severe form, atelectasis of the middle ear (loss of the middle-ear space). Obstruction can be due to inflammation, failure of the opening mechanism, and can be acute or chronic, but evidently infrequent periodic tubal opening occurs to prevent the accumulation of an effusion. A patulous tube can cause patients to complain of autophony and hearing their own breathing in the ear because the eustachian tube is open at rest, that is, in the absence of swallowing activity. Both conditions have been documented during the last trimester of pregnancy (153). Eustachian tube obstruction is not uncommon in girls during puberty, which may be related to hormonal changes, but the underlying cause of this problem has not been reported.

Chronic Suppurative Otitis Media

Chronic suppurative otitis media (without cholesteatoma) is the chronic stage that follows an attack of acute otitis media in which a perforation of the tympanic membrane, or tympanostomy tube is present, followed by continuous discharge. From our studies of the pathogenesis of chronic suppurative otitis media (154,155), it appears that the sequence of events may occur in one of two ways. First, when the tympanic membrane is not intact, bacteria from the nasopharynx can gain access to the middle ear due to reflux of nasopharyngeal secretions, especially when there is inflammation (secondary to infection or possibly allergy) of the nose, nasopharynx, or paranasal sinuses, through the eustachian tube, since the middle-ear gas cushion is lost. In most instances, these bacteria (e.g., *S. pneumoniae* and *Haemophilus influenzae*), are initially the same as those isolated when acute otitis occurs behind an intact tympanic membrane, and when acute otorrhea develops when tympanostomy tubes are in place (156). Following the acute otorrhea, *Pseudomonas aeruginosa, Staphylococcus aureus,* and other organisms from the external ear canal enter the middle ear through the nonintact tympanic membrane, which results in chronic infection. The second common way in which chronic otitis media occurs is by contamination of the middle-ear cleft from organisms (e.g., *P. aeruginosa*) that are present in water that enters through the nonintact eardrum during bathing and swimming.

REFERENCES

1. Proctor B. Embryology and anatomy of the eustachian tube. *Arch Otolaryngol Head Neck Surg* 1967;86:503.
2. Speilberg W. Visualization of the eustachian tube by roentgen ray. *Arch Otolaryngol Head Neck Surg* 1927;5:334.
3. Bacher JA. The applied anatomy of the eustachian tube. *Laryngoscope* 1912;22:21.
4. Anson B, ed. *Morris' human anatomy.* New York: McGraw-Hill; 1967:1195.
5. Anson B, Donaldson J. *The surgical anatomy of the temporal bone and ear.* Philadelphia: WB Saunders; 1967:29.
6. Doyle WJ. *A functiono-anatomic description of eustachian tube vector relations in four ethnic populations—an osteologic study.* [Dissertation], Pittsburgh, PA: University of Pittsburgh, 1977.
7. Goss C, ed. *Gray's anatomy of the human body.* Philadelphia: Lea & Febiger; 1967:1087.
8. Macbeth R. Some thoughts on the eustachian tube. *Proc R Soc Med* 1960;53:151.
9. Graves GO, Edwards LF. The eustachian tube: review of its descriptive, microscopic, topographic, and clinical anatomy. *Arch Otolaryngol Head Neck Surg* 1944;39:359.
10. Bryant WS. The eustachian tube: its anatomy and its movement. With a description of the cartilages, muscles, fasciae, and the fossa of Rosenmüller. *Med Rec* 1907;71:931.
11. Rood SR, Doyle WJ. The nasopharyngeal orifice of the auditory tube: implications for tubal dynamics anatomy. *Cleft Palate J* 1982;19:119.
12. Swarts JD, Rood SR. The morphometry and three-dimensional structure of the adult eustachian tube: implications for function. *Cleft Palate J* 1990;27:374.
13. Terracol A, Corone A, Guerrier G. *La Trompe D'Eustache.* Masson; Paris, 1949.
14. Rood SR, Doyle WJ. The morphology of the tensor veli palatini, tensor tympani, and dilator tubae muscles. *Ann Otol Rhinol Laryngol* 1978;87(2):202.
15. Todhunter JS, Siegel MI, Doyle WJ. Computer-generated eustachian tube shape analysis. In: Lim DJ, Bluestone CD, Klein JO, Nelson JD, eds. *Recent advances in otitis media with effusion.* Proceedings of the third international symposium. Burlington, On: BC Decker; 1984:101.
16. Kitajiri M, Sando I, Takahara T. Postnatal development of the eustachian tube and its surrounding structures. *Ann Otol Rhinol Laryngol* 1987;96:191.
17. Sudo M, Sando I, Ikui A. *Narrowest (isthmus) portion of eustachian tube: a computer-aided 3-d reconstruction and measurement study.* Association for Research in Otolaryngology Mid-Winter Meeting, St. Petersburg, FL, February 5–9, 1995 (abst).
18. Rees-Jones GF, McGibbon JE. Radiological visualization of the eustachian tube. *Lancet* 1941;241:660.
19. Sadé J, Woldson S, Sachs Z, Levit I, Abraham S. The human eustachian tube lumen in children. *Acta Otolaryngol (Stockh)* 1985;99:305.
20. Swarts JD, Rood SR. Preliminary analysis of the morphometry of the infant eustachian tube. In: Lim DJ, Bluestone CD, Klein JO, Nelson JD, Ogra PL, eds. *Recent advances in otitis media.* Proceedings of the fifth international symposium. Hamilton, On: Decker Periodicals; 1993:111.
21. Simkins C. Functional anatomy of the eustachian tube. *Arch Otolaryngol Head Neck Surg* 1943;38:476.
22. Rosen LM. *The morphology of the salpingopharyngeus muscle.* [Thesis], Pittsburgh, PA: University of Pittsburgh, 1970.
23. Matsune S, Sando I, Takahashi H. Comparative study of elastic at the hinge portion of eustachian tube cartilage in normal and cleft palate individuals. In: Lim DJ, Bluestone CD, Klein JO, Nelson JD, Ogra PL, eds. *Recent advances in otitis media.* Proceedings of the fifth international symposium. Hamilton, On: Decker Periodicals; 1993:4.
24. Hiraide F, Inoue T. The fine surface view of the human adult eustachian tube. *J Laryngol Otol* 1983;97:149.
25. Tos M. Anatomy and histology of the middle ear. *Clin Rev Allergy* 1984;2:267.
26. Rapport PN, Lim DJ, Weiss HJ. Surface active agent in eustachian tube function. *Arch Otolaryngol Head Neck Surg* 1975;101:305.
27. Lim DJ. Functional morphology of the tubotympanum. *Acta Otolaryngol (Stockh)* 1984;98[Suppl 414].
28. Svane-Knudsen V, Larsen HF, Brask T. Secretory otitis media—a question of surface activity in the eustachian tube. *Acta Otolaryngol (Stockh)* 1988;105:114.
29. Matsune S, Sando I, Takahashi H. Distributions of eustachian tube goblet cells and glands in children with and without otitis media. *Ann Otol Rhinol Laryngol* 1992;101:750.
30. Park K, Ueno K, Lim DJ. Developmental anatomy of the eustachian tube and middle ear in mice. *Am J Otolaryngol* 1992;13:93.
31. Sando I, Takahashi H, Aoki H, Matsune S. Mucosal folds in human eustachian tube: a hypothesis regarding functional localization in the tube. *Ann Otol Rhinol Laryngol* 1993;102:47.
32. Brash J, ed. *Cunningham's textbook of anatomy.* 9th ed. London: Oxford Press; 1951.
33. Rood SR. Morphology of M. tensor veli palatini in the five-month human fetus. *Am J Anat* 1973;138:191.
34. Thomsen KA. Studies on the function of the eustachian tube in a series of normal individuals. *Acta Otolaryngol (Stockh)* 1957;48:516.
35. Van Dishoeck HAE. Resistance measuring of the eustachian tube and the ostium and isthmus valve mechanisms. *Acta Otolaryngol (Stockh)* 1947;35:317.
36. Cantekin EI, Doyle WJ, Reichert TJ, Phillips DC, Bluestone CD. Dilation of the eustachian tube by electrical stimulation of the mandibular nerve. *Ann Otol Rhinol Laryngol* 1979;88:40.
37. Rich AR. The innervation of the tensor veli palatini and levator veli palatini muscles. *Bull J Hopkins Hosp* 1920;31:305.
38. Guild SR. Elastic tissue of the eustachian tube. *Ann Otol Rhinol Laryngol* 1955;64:537.
39. Doyle WJ, Cantekin EI, Bluestone CD. Eustachian tube function in cleft palate children. *Ann Otol Rhinol Laryngol* 1980;89:34.
40. Ross M. Functional anatomy of the tensor palati. Its relevance in cleft palate surgery. *Arch Otolaryngol Head Neck Surg* 1971;93:1.
40a. Bluestone CD, Klein JO. Otitis media, alectasis, and eustachian tube dysfunction. In: Bluestone CD, Stool SE, Kenna MA, eds. *Pediatric otolaryngology.* 3rd ed. Philadelphia: WB Saunders, 1996.
41. Lupin AJ. The relationship of the tensor tympani and tensor palati muscles. *Ann Otol Rhinol Laryngol* 1969;78:792.
42. Honjo I, Ushiro K, Hajo T, Nozoe T, Matsui H. Role of tensor tympani

43. McMyn JK. The anatomy of the salpingopharyngeus muscle. *J Laryngol Otol* 1940;55:1.
44. Sadler-Kimes D, Siegel MI, Todhunter JS. Age-related morphologic differences in the components of the eustachian tube–middle-ear system. *Ann Otol Rhinol Laryngol* 1989;98:854.
45. Holborow C. Eustachian tube function: changes throughout childhood and neuro-muscular control. *J Laryngol Otol* 1975;89:47.
46. Honjo I, Okazaki N, Kumazawa T. Experimental study of the eustachian tube function with regard to its related muscles. *Acta Otolaryngol (Stockh)* 1979;87:84.
47. Casselbrant ML, Cantekin EI, Dirkmaat DC, Doyle WJ, Bluestone CD. Experimental paralysis of tensor veli palatini muscle. *Acta Otolaryngol (Stockh)* 1988;106:178.
48. Doyle WJ, Seroky JT. Middle-ear gas exchange in rhesus monkeys. *Ann Otol Rhinol Laryngol* 1994;103(8):636-45.
49. Bylander A. Comparison of eustachian tube function in children and adults with normal ears. *Ann Otol Rhinol Laryngol* 1980;89:20.
50. Bylander A, Tjernstrom O, Ivarsson A. Pressure opening and closing functions of the eustachian tube by inflation and deflation in children and adults with normal ears. *Acta Otolaryngol (Stockh)* 1983;96:255.
51. Bluestone CD. Eustachian tube obstruction in the infant with cleft palate. *Ann Otol Rhinol Laryngol* 1971;80:1.
52. Bluestone CD, Paradise JL, Beery QC. Physiology of the eustachian tube in the pathogenesis and management of middle-ear effusions. *Laryngoscope* 1972;82:1654.
53. Bluestone CD, Wittel RA, Paradise JL, Felder H. Eustachian tube function as related to adenoidectomy for otitis media. *Trans Am Acad Ophthalmol Otolaryngol* 1972;76:1325.
54. Wittenborg MH, Neuhauser EB. Simple roentgenographic demonstration of eustachian tubes and abnormalities. *Am J Roentgenol Radium Ther Nucl Med* 1963;89:1194.
55. Bluestone CD, Beery QC. Concepts on the pathogenesis of middle-ear effusions. *Ann Otol Rhinol Laryngol* 1976;85:182.
56. Bluestone CD, Klein JO. *Otitis media in infants and children.* 2nd ed. Philadelphia: WB Saunders; 1995:145.
57. Albiin N, Hellstrom S, Stenfors LE. Clearance of effusion material from the attic space—an experimental study in the rat. *Int J Pediatr Otorhinolaryngol* 1983;5:1.
58. Stenfors LE, Hellstrom S, Albiin N. Middle-ear clearance in eustachian tube function: physiology and role in otitis media. *Ann Otol Rhinol Laryngol* 1985;94:30.
59. Ohashi Y, Nakai Y, Koshimo H, Esaki Y. Ciliary activity in the in vitro tubotympanum. *Arch Otorhinolaryngol* 1986;243:317.
60. Honjo I. Experimental study of the pumping function of the eustachian tube. *Acta Otolaryngol (Stockh)* 1981;91:85.
61. Honjo I, Hayashi M, Ito S, Takahashi H. Pumping and clearance function of the eustachian tube. *Am J Otolaryngol* 1985;6:241.
62. Birken EA, Brookler KH. Surface tension lowering substance of the canine eustachian tube. *Ann Otol Rhinol Laryngol* 1972;81:268.
63. Hagan WE. Surface tension lowering substance in eustachian tube function. *Laryngoscope* 1977;87:1033.
64. White P. Effect of exogenous surfactant on eustachian tube function in the rat. *Am J Otolaryngol* 1989;10:301.
65. Karchev T, Watanabe N, Fujiyoshi T, Mogi G, Kato S. Surfactant-producing epithelium in the dorsal part of the cartilaginous eustachian tube of mice. *Acta Otolaryngol (Stockh)* 1994;114:64.
66. Fornadley JA, Burns JK. The effect of surfactant on eustachian tube function in a gerbil model of otitis media with effusion. *Otolaryngol Head Neck Surg* 1994;110:110.
67. Bluestone CD, Cantekin EI, Beery QC. Effect of inflammation on the ventilatory function of the eustachian tube. *Laryngoscope* 1977;87:493.
68. McBride TP, Doyle WJ, Hayden FG, Gwaltney JM. Alterations of the eustachian tube, middle ear, and nose in rhinovirus infection. *Arch Otolaryngol Head Neck Surg* 1989;115:1054.
69. Buchman CA, Doyle WJ, Skoner D, Fireman P, Gwaltney JM. Otologic manifestations of experimental rhinovirus infection. *Laryngoscope* 1994;104:1295.
70. Friedman RA, Doyle WJ, Casselbrant ML, Bluestone CD, Fireman P. Immunologic-mediated eustachian tube obstruction: a double-blind crossover study. *J Allergy Clin Immunol* 1983;71:442.
71. Bluestone CD, Cantekin EI, Beery QC. Certain effects of adenoidectomy on eustachian tube ventilatory function. *Laryngoscope* 1975;85:113.
72. Bluestone CD, Beery QC, Andrus WS. Mechanics of the eustachian tube as it influences susceptibility to and persistence of middle-ear effusions in children. *Ann Otol Rhinol Laryngol* 1974;83:27.
73. Bluestone CD, Cantekin EI, Beery QC, Stool SE. Function of the eustachian tube related to surgical management of acquired aural cholesteatoma in children. *Laryngoscope* 1978;88:1155.
74. Stenstrom C, Bylander-Groth A, Ingvarsson L. Eustachian tube function in otitis-prone and healthy children. *Int J Pediatr Otorhinolaryngol* 1991;21:127.
75. Iwano T, Hamada E, Kinoshita T, et al. Passive opening pressure of the eustachian tube. In: Lim DJ, Bluestone CD, Klein JO, Nelson JD, Ogra PL, eds. *Recent advances in otitis media.* Proceedings of the fifth international symposium. Hamilton, On: Decker Periodicals; 1993:76.
76. Siegel MI, Sadler-Kimes D, Todhunter JS. Eustachian tube cartilage shape as a factor in the epidemiology of otitis media. In: Lim DJ, Bluestone CD, Klein JO, Nelson JD, eds. *Recent advances in otitis media.* Proceedings of the fourth international symposium. Toronto: BC Decker; 1988:114.
77. Yamaguchi N, Sando I, Hashida Y, Takahashi H, Matsune S. Histologic study of eustachian tube cartilage with and without congenital anomalies: a preliminary study. *Ann Otol Rhinol Laryngol* 1990;99:984.
78. Aoki H, Sando I, Takahashi H. Anatomic relationships between Ostmann's fatty tissue and eustachian tube. *Ann Otol Rhinol Laryngol* 1994;103:211.
79. Sakakihara J, Honjo I, Fujita A, Kurata K, Takahashi H. Compliance of the patulous eustachian tube. *Ann Otol Rhinol Laryngol* 1993;102:110.
80. Beery QC, Doyle WJ, Cantekin EI, Bluestone CD, Wiet RJ. Eustachian tube function in an American Indian population. *Ann Otol Rhinol Laryngol* 1980;89:28.
81. White BL, Doyle WJ, Bluestone CD. Eustachian tube function in infants and children with Down's syndrome. In: Lim DJ, Bluestone CD, Klein JO, Nelson JD, eds. *Recent advances in otitis media with effusion.* Proceedings of the third international symposium. Toronto: BC Decker; 1984:62.
82. Jorgensen F, Holmquist J. Toynbee phenomenon and middle-ear disease. *Am J Otolaryngol* 1984;4:291.
83. Thompson AC, Crowther JA. Effect of nasal packing on eustachian tube function. *J Laryngol Otol* 1991;105:539.
84. Ohashi Y, Nakai Y, Furuya H, et al. Mucociliary disease of the middle ear during experimental otitis media with effusion induced by bacterial endotoxin. *Ann Otol Rhinol Laryngol* 1989;98:479.
85. Park K, Bakaletz LO, Coticchia JM, Lim DJ. Effect of influenza A virus on ciliary activity and dye transport function in the chinchilla eustachian tube. *Ann Otol Rhinol Laryngol* 1993;102:551.
86. Mogi G, Kawauchi H, Kurono Y. Tubal dysfunction or infection? Role of bacterial infection and immune response. In Mogi G, ed. *Recent advances in otitis media.* Proceedings of the second extraordinary international symposium on recent advances in otitis media. New York: Kugler 1993:73.
87. Shikowitz MJ, Ilardi CF, Gero, M. Immotile cilia syndrome associated with otitis media with effusion: a case report. In: Lim DJ, Bluestone CD, Klein JO, Nelson JD, eds. *Recent Advances in Otitis Media.* Proceedings of the fourth international symposium. Toronto: BC Decker; 1988:304.
88. Nozoe T, Okazaki N, Koda Y, Ayani N, Kumazawa T. Fluid clearance of the eustachian tube. In: Lim DJ, Bluestone CD, Klein JO, Nelson JD, eds. *Recent advances in otitis media with effusion.* Proceedings of the third international symposium. Toronto: BC Decker; 1984:66.
89. Takahashi H, Honjo I, Hayashi M, Fujita A. Clearance function of eustachian tube and negative middle-ear pressure. *Ann Otol Rhinol Laryngol* 1992;101:759.
90. Miglets A. The experimental production of allergic middle-ear effusions. *Laryngoscope* 1973;83:1355.
91. Bernstein JM, Lee J, Conboy K, Ellis E, Li P. Further observations on the role of IgE-mediated hypersensitivity in recurrent otitis media with effusion. *Otolaryngol Head Neck Surg* 1985;93:611.
92. Bluestone CD. Eustachian tube function and allergy in otitis media. *Pediatrics* 1978;61:753.
93. Doyle WJ. Panel on etiology of otitis media with effusion: role of allergy and tubal function. In: Mogi G, ed. *Recent advances in otitis*

media. Proceedings of the second extraordinary international symposium on recent advances in otitis media. Amsterdam: Kugler; 1994: 53.
94. Ackerman MN, Friedman RA, Doyle WJ, Bluestone CD, Fireman P. Antigen-induced eustachian tube obstruction: an intranasal provocative challenge test. *J Allergy Clin Immunol* 1984;73:604.
95. Doyle WJ, Friedman R, Fireman P, Bluestone CD. Eustachian tube obstruction after provocative nasal antigen challenge. *Arch Otolaryngol Head Neck Surg* 1984;110:508.
96. Skoner DP, Doyle WJ, Chamovitz AH, Fireman P. Eustachian tube obstruction after intranasal challenge with house dust mite. *Arch Otolaryngol Head Neck Surg* 1986;112:840.
97. Stillwagon PK, Doyle WJ, Fireman P. Effect of an antihistamine/decongestant on nasal and eustachian tube function following intranasal pollen challenge. *Ann Allergy* 1987;58:442.
98. Skoner DP, Doyle WJ, Fireman P. Eustachian tube obstruction (ETO) after histamine nasal provocation—a double-blind dose-response study. *J Allergy Clin Immunol* 1987;79:27.
99. Doyle WJ, Boehm S, Skoner DP. Physiologic responses to intranasal dose-response challenges with histamine, methacholine, bradykinin, and prostaglandin in adult volunteers with and without nasal allergy. *J Allergy Clin Immunol* 1990;86:924.
100. Doyle WJ, Skoner DP, Hayden F, Buchman CA, Seroky JT, Fireman P. Nasal and otologic effects of experimental influenza A virus infection. *Ann Otol Rhinol Laryngol* 1994;103:59.
101. Stool SE, Randall P. Unexpected ear disease in infants with cleft palate. *Cleft Palate J* 1967;4:99.
102. Paradise JL, Bluestone CD, Felder H. The universality of otitis media in fifty infants with cleft palate. *Pediatrics* 1969;44:35.
103. Paradise JL, Bluestone CD. Early treatment of the universal otitis media of infants with cleft palate. *Pediatrics* 1974;53:48.
104. Bluestone CD, Wittel RA, Paradise JL. Roentgenographic evaluation of eustachian tube function in infants with cleft and normal palates. *Cleft Palate J* 1972;9:93.
105. Kitajiri M, Sando I, Hashida Y, Doyle WJ. Histopathology of otitis media in infants with cleft and high arched palates. In: Lim DJ, Bluestone CD, Klein JO, Nelson JD, eds. *Recent Advances in Otitis Media with Effusion*. Proceedings of the third international symposium. Toronto: BC Decker; 1984:195.
106. Matsune S, Sando I, Takahashi H. Abnormalities of lateral cartilaginous lamina and lumen of eustachian tube in cases of cleft palate. *Ann Otol Rhinol Laryngol* 1991;100:909.
107. Matsune S, Sando I, Takahashi H. Insertion of the tensor veli palatini muscle into the eustachian tube cartilage in cleft palate cases. *Ann Otol Rhinol Laryngol* 1991;100:439.
108. Matsune S, Sando I, Takahashi H. Comparative study of elastic at the hinge portion of eustachian tube cartilage in normal and cleft palate individuals. *Ann Otol Rhinol Laryngol* 1992;101:163.
109. Shibahara Y, Sando I. Histopathologic study of eustachian tube in cleft palate patients. *Ann Otol Rhinol Laryngol* 1988;97:403.
110. Doyle WJ, Cantekin EI, Bluestone CD, Phillips DC, Kimes KK, Siegel MI. A nonhuman primate model of cleft palate and its implications for middle-ear pathology. *Ann Otol Rhinol Laryngol* 1980;89(68):41.
111. Doyle WJ, Ingraham AS, Saad M, Cantekin EI. A primate model of cleft palate and middle-ear disease: results of a one-year postcleft follow-up. In: Lim DJ, Bluestone CD, Klein JO, Nelson JD, eds. *Recent Advances in Otitis Media with Effusion*. Proceedings of the third international symposium. Toronto: BC Decker; 1984:215.
112. Odoi H, Proud GO, Toledo PS. Effects of pterygoid hamulotomy upon eustachian tube function. *Laryngoscope* 1971;81(8):1242.
113. McNicoll WD, Scanlon SG. Submucous resection: the treatment of choice in the nose-ear distress syndrome. *J Laryngol Otol* 1979;93:357.
114. McNicoll WD. Remediable eustachian tube dysfunction in diving recruits: assessment, investigation, and management. *Undersea Biomed Res* 1982;9:37.
115. Tos M, Bonding P. Middle-ear pressure during and after prolonged nasotracheal and/or nasogastric intubation. *Acta Otolaryngol (Stockh)* 1977;83:353.
116. Wake M, McCullough DE, Binnington JD. Effect of nasogastric tubes on eustachian tube function. *J Laryngol Otol* 1990;104:17.
117. Perlman HB. Observations on the eustachian tube. *Arch Otolaryngol Head Neck Surg* 1951;53:370.
118. Myers EN, Beery QC, Bluestone CD, Rood SR, Sigler BA. Effect of certain head and neck tumors and their management on the ventilatory function of the eustachian tube. *Ann Otol Rhinol Laryngol* 1984;93[Suppl 114]:3.
119. Weiss MH, Liberatore LA, Kraus DH, Budnick AS. Otitis media with effusion in head and neck cancer patients. *Laryngoscope* 1994;104:5.
120. Takahara T, Sando I, Bluestone CD, Myers EN. Lymphoma invading the anterior eustachian tube: temporal bone histopathology of functional tubal obstruction. *Ann Otol Rhinol Laryngol* 1986;95:101.
121. Yamaguchi N, Sando I, Hashida Y, Takahashi H, Myers EN. Histopathologic study of otitis media in individuals with head and neck tumors. *Ann Otol Rhinol Laryngol* 1990;99:827.
122. Chan KH, Bluestone CD. Lack of efficacy of middle-ear inflation: treatment of otitis media with effusion in children. *Otolaryngol Head Neck Surg* 1989;100:317.
123. Stangerup SE, Sederberg-Olsen J, Balle V. Autoinflation as a treatment of secretory otitis media. *Arch Otolaryngol Head Neck Surg* 1992;118:149.
124. Bluestone CD. Assessment of eustachian tube function. In: Jerger J, ed. *Handbook of Clinical Impedance Audiometry*. New York: American Electromedics Corporation; 1975:127.
125. Cantekin EI, Bluestone CD, Parkin LP. Eustachian tube ventilatory function in children. *Ann Otol Rhinol Laryngol* 1976;85:171.
126. Ingelstedt S, Ortegren U. The ear snorkel-pressure chamber technique. Volumetric determination of tubal ventilation. *Acta Otolaryngol (Stockh)* 1963;182:24.
127. Bluestone CD. Otologic surgical procedures. In: Bluestone CD, Stool SE, eds. *Atlas of pediatric otolaryngology*. Philadelphia: WB Saunders; 1995:27.
128. Schappert SM. Office visits for otitis media: United States, 1975–1990. (*Vital and Health Statistics of the Centers for Disease Control*; series 214; no 1) Hyattsville, MD: National Center for Health Statistics 1992
129. Politzer A. Ueber die willkurlichen Bewegungen des Trommelfells. *Weiner Med Halle Nr* 1862;18:103.
130. Zollner R. *Anatomie, Physiologie und klinik der Ohrtrompete*. Berlin: Springer-Verlag; 1942.
131. Sadé J. Pathology and pathogenesis of serous otitis media. *Arch Otolaryngol Head Neck Surg* 1966;84:297-305.
132. Alper CM, Tabari R, Seroky JT, Doyle WJ. Magnetic resonance imaging of the development of middle-ear effusion secondary to experimental paralysis of tensor veli palatini muscle. *Otolaryngol Head Neck Surg* 1994;111:122.
133. Buchman CA, Doyle WJ, Skoner DP, et al. Influenza A virus-induced acute otitis media. *J Infect Dis* 1995;172(5):1348–1351.
134. Bluestone CD, Stephenson JS, Martin LM. Ten-year review of otitis media pathogens. *Pediatr Infect Dis J* 1992;11:S7.
135. Post JC, Preston RA, Aul JJ, et al. Molecular analysis of bacterial pathogens in otitis media with effusion. *JAMA* 1995;273:1598.
136. Cantekin EI, Bluestone CD, Saez CA, Doyle WJ, Phillips DC. Normal and abnormal middle-ear ventilation. *Ann Otol Rhinol Laryngol* 1977;86:1.
137. Swarts JD, Alper CM, Seroky JT, Chan KH, Doyle WJ. In vivo observation with magnetic resonance imaging of middle-ear effusion in response to experimental underpressures. *Ann Otol Rhinol Laryngol* 1995;104:522.
138. Ophir D, Hahn T, Schattner A, Wallach D, Aviel A. Tumor necrosis factor in middle-ear effusions. *Arch Otolaryngol Head Neck Surg* 1988;114:1256.
139. Yellon RF, Leonard G, Marucha P, et al. Characterization of cytokines present in middle-ear effusions. *Laryngoscope* 1991;101:165.
140. Yellon RF, Leonard G, Marucha P, et al. Demonstration of interleukin 6 in middle-ear effusions. *Arch Otolaryngol Head Neck Surg* 1992;118:745.
141. Yan S, Huang C. Tumor necrosis factor alpha in middle-ear cholesteatoma and its effect on keratinocytes in vitro. *Ann Otol Rhinol Laryngol* 1991;100:1657.
142. Himi T, Suzuki T, Takezawa H, Takezawa H, Kataura A. Immunologic characteristics of cytokines in otitis media with effusion. *Ann Otol Rhinol Laryngol* 1992;101:21.
143. Juhn SK, Lees C, Amesara R, Kim Y, Le CT, Giebink GS. Role of cytokines in the pathogenesis of otitis media. In: Lim DJ, Bluestone CD, Klein JO, Nelson JD, Ogra PL, eds. *Recent advances in otitis media*. Proceedings of the fifth international symposium. Hamilton, On: Decker Periodicals; 1993:431.
144. Tedder TF, Steeber DA, Chen A, Engel P. The selectins: vascular adhesion molecules. *FASEB J* 1995;9:866.

145. Bernstein JM, Okazaki T, Reisman RE. Prostaglandins in middle-ear effusions. *Arch Otolaryngol Head Neck Surg* 1976;102:257.
146. Smith DM, Jung TTK, Juhn SK, Berlinger NT, Gerrard JM. Prostaglandins in experimental otitis media. *Arch Otorhinolaryngol* 1979;225:207–209.
147. Jung TTk, Linda L. Prostaglandins, leukotrienes, and other arachidonic acid metabolites in the pathogenesis of otitis media. *Laryngoscope* 1988;98:980.
148. Jung TTK, Park YM, Schlund D, et al. Effect of prostaglandin, leukotriene and arachidonic acid on experimental otitis media with effusion in chinchillas. *Ann Otol Rhinol Laryngol* 1990;99(Suppl 148):28.
149. Jung TTK. Arachidonic acid metabolites in otitis media pathogenesis. *Ann Otol Rhinol Laryngol* 1988;97:14.
150. Nonomura N, Giebink GS, Zelterman D, Harada T, Juhn SK. Early biochemical events in pneumococcal otitis media: arachidonic acid metabolites in middle-ear fluid. *Ann Otol Rhinol Laryngol* 1991;100:385.
151. Rhee CK, Jung TTK, Miller S, Weeks D. Experimental otitis media with effusion induced by platelet activating factor. *Ann Otol Rhinol Laryngol* 1993;102:600.
152. Doyle WJ, Seroky JT, Alper CM. Gas exchange across the middle-ear mucosa in monkeys. *Arch Otolaryngol Head Neck Surg* 1995;121:887.
153. Derkay CS. Eustachian tube and nasal function during pregnancy: a prospective study. *Otolaryngol Head Neck Surg* 1988; 99:558.
154. Kenna MA, Bluestone CD, Reilly JS, Lusk RP. Medical management of chronic suppurative otitis media with cholesteatoma in children. *Laryngoscope* 1986;96:146.
155. Kenna MA, Rosane BA, Bluestone CD. Medical management of chronic suppurative otitis media without cholesteatoma in children—update 1992. *Am J Otol* 1993;14:469.
156. Mandel EM, Casselbrant ML, Kurs-Lasky M. Acute otorrhea: bacteriology of a common complication of tympanostomy tubes. *Ann Otol Rhinol Laryngol* 1994;103:713.

CHAPTER 3

Auditory Development

John H. Grose and Joseph W. Hall III

The topic of auditory development is multifaceted and can range in content from the embryology of structures associated with hearing to the chronology with which mature listening skills are acquired. In terms of the development of "hearing," the auditory system is active in utero (1,2) and thus the early stages of audition occur prenatally. From the clinical standpoint, there is interest not only in the causes of abnormal auditory development, but also in the broader consequences of deficiencies or delays in auditory development on the acquisition of language and other higher-level cognitive processes. A particular focus of this interest is whether "critical periods" exist in auditory development. This review is confined primarily to the postnatal development of basic auditory functions in humans and to the effects of transient auditory deprivation on the development of these functions.

One of the primary challenges in creating a comprehensive description of auditory development is the appropriate integration of data that have been obtained from different age groups using a variety of age-specific measurement techniques. To differentiate real developmental changes in auditory ability from group differences due to methodologic constraints is only part of the challenge. It is also important to recognize that changes in auditory performance with age can be due to a number of factors that interrelate in a complex fashion. For example, changes in the anatomy and geometry of the external and middle ears will influence the levels of sound reaching the cochlea, while concomitant changes in nonsensory processing strategies will affect how those sounds are perceived. Both types of change are valid components of auditory development.

This chapter begins by providing a brief overview of the types of measurement techniques that have been useful in assessing auditory function in different age groups. Next, the development of some basic auditory functions are described. Finally, the effects of auditory deprivation on auditory development are considered.

MEASUREMENT TECHNIQUES

The methodologies used to measure auditory function in infants and children can loosely be divided into two categories: objective measurement techniques and behavioral measurement techniques. While objective measurement techniques are useful in assessing the functional integrity of various portions of the auditory system, they are not informative in terms of the perceptual aspects of hearing. Behavioral techniques, on the other hand, better assess the perception of sound but are subject to the myriad of factors that influence voluntary responses, such as attention, motivation, and arousal. The intent of this section is to provide a brief sampling of various techniques rather than to proffer an exhaustive review of methodology.

Objective Measurement Techniques

Each stage of the auditory system, from the periphery to the cortex, can be probed to some degree by measurement techniques that do not rely on the voluntary cooperation of the listener. The resonant characteristics of the external auditory canal can be assessed with probe microphones, a procedure integral to *real ear measures*. Because the ear canal acts like a closed end tube with resonant frequencies having wavelengths proportional to its length, an adult ear canal generates a resonance in the region of 3,500 Hz, which results in a gain of about 10 dB (3). The ear canal of an infant, however, has much smaller dimensions and therefore generates resonances at higher frequencies (4–6). This is illustrated in Fig. 1, which compares the gain characteristics of an adult ear with that of an infant ear.

The transmission of sound through the ear canal and middle ear can be gauged with a technique known generically as *immittance audiometry*. This technique measures the

---

J.H. Grose and J.W. Hall III: Division of Otolaryngology—Head and Neck Surgery, University of North Carolina Medical School, Chapel Hill, North Carolina 27599-7070.

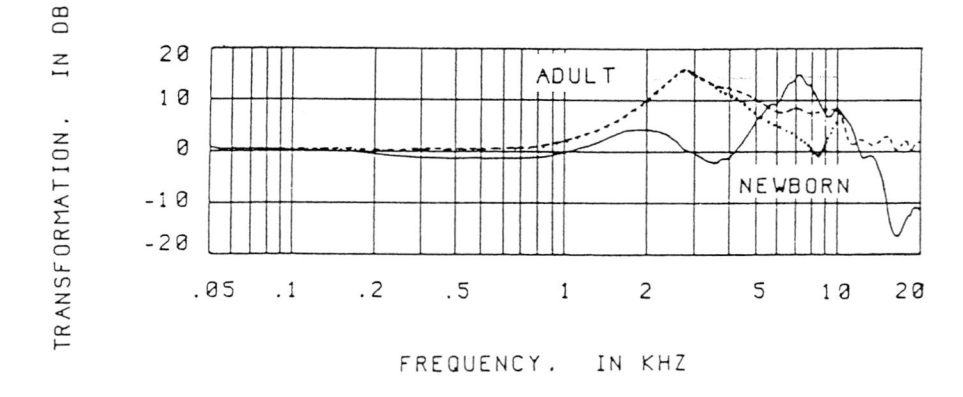

FIG. 1. Comparison of the transformation between diffuse sound field and ear canal of an adult (*dashed lines*) and a neonate (*solid line*). From Kruger B, Ruben RJ. The acoustic properties of the infant ear. *Acta Otolaryngol (Stockh)* 1987;103:578, with permission.

impedance at the plane of the tympanic membrane offered to an incoming sound. Because this impedance is due largely to the characteristics of the middle ear, reliable measures of middle ear function can be derived. Such measures in children and adults indicate that the resonance of the middle ear, where transmission of sound will be maximal, is roughly 1,500 Hz, with transmission dropping off steeply at lower frequencies (7). In terms of the acoustico-mechanical properties of the middle ear, resonance occurs in the frequency region where contributions of middle ear mass and middle ear stiffness to the total impedance are equal and opposite. A number of studies indicate that the middle-ear resonant frequencies are lower in neonates (8,9). Such an effect probably reflects differences in the elasticity and mass elements of the immature middle ear. For example, Fig. 2 depicts conductance and susceptance tympanograms for a 226-Hz probe tone measured in a neonate less than 24 hours old and in an adult. The "notching" that is present in the neonatal tympanogram but absent in the adult tympanogram indicates dissimilar middle ear characteristics. Results using a different technique involving acoustic reflectometry also point to marked differences between infant and adult middle ears in terms of the frequency dependence of sound transmission through to the cochlea (10). The net effect of these differences in middle ear characteristics is an age dependence in the transfer functions that relate adjustments in sound level en route to the cochlea as a function of frequency.

The cochlea transduces the pressure fluctuations of sound into neural impulses in a manner that maps frequency of vibration onto place of maximal stimulation. The transduction mechanism involves an active process, or amplifier, which is associated with the outer hair cells (11). An epiphenomenon of this active mechanism is the generation of pressure fluctuations within the cochlea that are transmitted out through the middle ear and are recorded in the ear canal as minute sounds termed *otoacoustic emissions* (12). Otoacoustic emissions reflect the functional integrity of the inner ear and, as such, their measurement has become an important clinical tool for the objective assessment of cochlear function. In the present context, a key point is that otoacoustic emissions are robust in infants even as young as 1 to 2 days of age, a finding that is suggestive of mature cochlear function at birth (13–19).

Following transduction into action potentials, the neural components of the auditory system can be probed with a class of techniques known as *evoked potentials*. These techniques record the EEG in the far field using surface electrodes and extract the components of the EEG that are associated with the auditory stimulus by synchronizing the averaging of the EEG to the presentation of a transient stimulus. Evoked potentials associated with structures in the brainstem are referred to as the auditory brainstem response (ABR). Middle latency and late components are evoked potentials associated with more central structures, including the auditory cortex. A wealth of developmental studies have been carried out on auditory evoked potentials (20–29). Suffice it to say that age-dependent differences exist in the various classes of auditory evoked potentials, particularly in terms of the latency with which characteristic waveform peaks occur. Such differences in latency are presumably based in part on immaturities in the myelinization of the neural elements in the auditory pathway of infants and young children (30).

In summary, this brief overview of objective measurement techniques has shown that, while external and middle ear transfer functions of neonates are likely to be different from that of adults, cochlear function appears to be largely developed at birth. Immaturities in the neural pathways are associated in part with the process of myelinization.

Behavioral Measurement Techniques

To determine whether a listener "hears," some method of measuring the response to sound must be devised. The following section provides a sampling of some age-appropriate paradigms that have generated reliable data.

Babies less than about 3 months of age who lack sufficient gross motor control can be tested using *conditioned reflexes*. The monitoring of sucking rate in response to sound is one such procedure. Sucking rate is monitored while infants habituate to a particular stimulus. The stimulus is then changed and an increase in sucking rate is interpreted as indicating

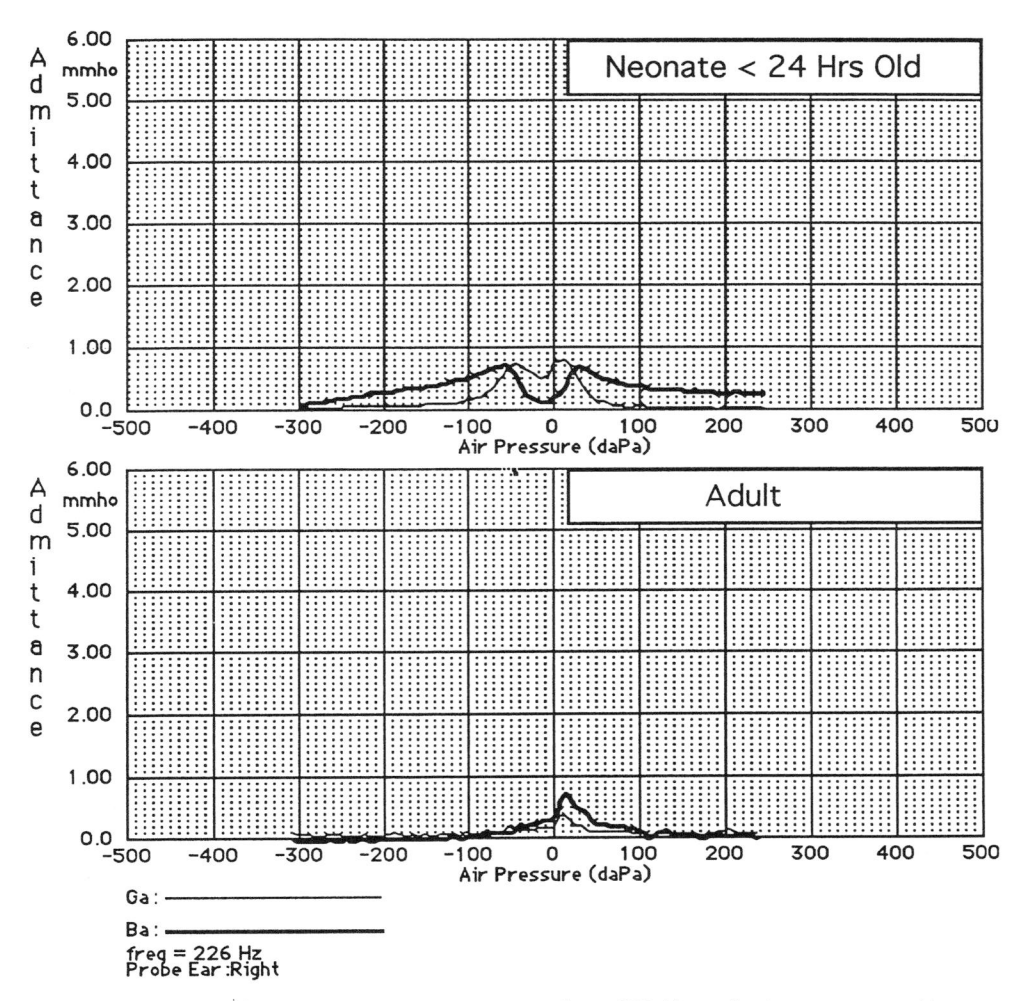

FIG. 2. Conductance and susceptance tympanograms for a 226-Hz probe tone measured in a neonate less than 24 hours old and in an adult.

that the infant has discriminated the change. This technique has been used, for example, to show different patterns of ear dominance for speech stimuli versus musical stimuli in 4-day-old infants (31).

By about 6 months of age, babies have sufficient head control to be able to turn toward a sound source. This ability has been incorporated into *visual reinforcement procedures.* In a typical procedure, the baby is situated in an upright position facing the experimenter or observer with a loudspeaker and a visually masked reinforcer (usually a mechanical toy) located on one side. Criterion head turns toward the speaker in response to signals are rewarded with illumination or activation of the visually reinforcing toy. A variant of this procedure is referred to as the Observer-based Psychoacoustic Procedure (OPP) (32). In OPP, stimuli can be delivered over headphones in an ear-specific manner, and, although head turns toward the visual reinforcer are the most usual response, a greater range of behavioral reaction can be taken into consideration when judging whether a response has occurred. This has allowed OPP to be successfully applied to babies as young as 3 months of age.

Once a child is approaching 4 or 5 years of age, basic psychophysical *forced-choice procedures* can be employed—usually in a "child-friendly" format. Studies of children in our laboratory have used a three-alternative forced-choice procedure disguised as a video game (33,34). The three observation intervals of a trial are marked by images on a video screen (e.g., three frogs). Each image in turn opens its mouth to mark the observation interval. The signal of interest occurs randomly in one of the three intervals. The child selects which image "made" the signal, and visual feedback is provided. In this example, if the child selects the correct frog, it turns into a prince; if the wrong frog is selected, the frog associated with the signal interval has a dizzy spell. The procedure is a forced-choice one in that the listener is required to enter a response whether or not the signal was actually detected. In this manner, rules for adaptively varying the signal allow the procedure to hone in on the performance level designated as threshold.

In summary, a variety of age-appropriate behavioral paradigms have been developed to study auditory function in different age groups. The following sections attempt to integrate findings generated by these various paradigms to provide a comprehensive description of changes in auditory function with age.

DEVELOPMENT OF AUDITORY FUNCTION

In describing auditory function, it is useful to classify findings according to the type of auditory information that is being processed. Five such classifications are (a) frequency processing, (b) temporal processing, (c) monaural across-frequency processing, (d) binaural processing, and (e) the perceptual organization of complex sounds. Each of these are examined in a separate section. However, the first aspect of auditory function that will be examined is absolute sensitivity.

Absolute Sensitivity

A number of studies have examined the minimum audibility of sounds as a function of frequency in different age groups in order to describe the development of absolute sensitivity (35–44). For example, Fig. 3 shows results from a study that measured thresholds across a wide frequency range in babies aged 3 to 12 months and compared them with thresholds for adults measured with the same OPP paradigm (41). A general age effect is evident wherein 3-month-old babies have higher thresholds than 6- to 12-month-old babies, who, in turn, have higher thresholds than adults. A closer look at the data reveals some additional features. While the 3-month-old infants are most different from the adults at the highest frequency, the 6- and 12-month-old babies are most different from the adults at the lowest frequency. This implies that between 3 and 6 months of age, sensitivity to high frequencies changes most rapidly. Between 1 year of age and maturity, it is the low frequencies that show the greatest change. Thus the change in absolute sensitivity with age appears to be frequency dependent and complex, a conclusion that is echoed in other studies (36,40). In terms of development after infancy, thresholds continue to improve beyond 5 years of age (43). A notable exception is the very high frequencies in the region of 20,000 Hz where 5- to 6-year-old children have better thresholds than adults (43,45,46).

Efforts to establish the basis for the developmental changes in absolute sensitivity have been only partially successful. Comparisons of behavioral thresholds and (objective) ABR thresholds in infants have shown that ABR thresholds are adultlike by 3 months of age, in contrast to behavioral thresholds (47). This suggests that factors other than cochlear function contribute to the development of auditory sensitivity. Similar work has shown that, while elevated behavioral thresholds in 3-month-old infants may be related in part to transmission through auditory brainstem structures, this is probably not the case for infants older than about 6 months of age (48).

In summary, sensitivity to sound develops in a complex, frequency-dependent manner. Development continues past 5 years of age and is, for the most part, unrelated to maturation of structures in the auditory periphery and brainstem.

Frequency Processing

Most sounds usually encountered in the real world are complex, being made up of more than one frequency. Two aspects of frequency processing that can be assessed are (a) frequency selectivity—the ability to resolve, or "hear out," one frequency component when presented against a background of other frequency components; and (b) frequency discrimination—the ability to differentiate between two different frequencies presented in succession.

Frequency selectivity appears to be mature at a very early age (49–51). Infants 6 months of age exhibit the same degree of frequency selectivity, or tuning, as do adults. This holds also for infants 3 months of age, except at high frequencies. The finding of mature frequency selectivity at an early age is supported by objective measurements of frequency selectivity using otoacoustic emissions (52) and ABR (53), at least for midfrequencies. Given these findings, it is not sur-

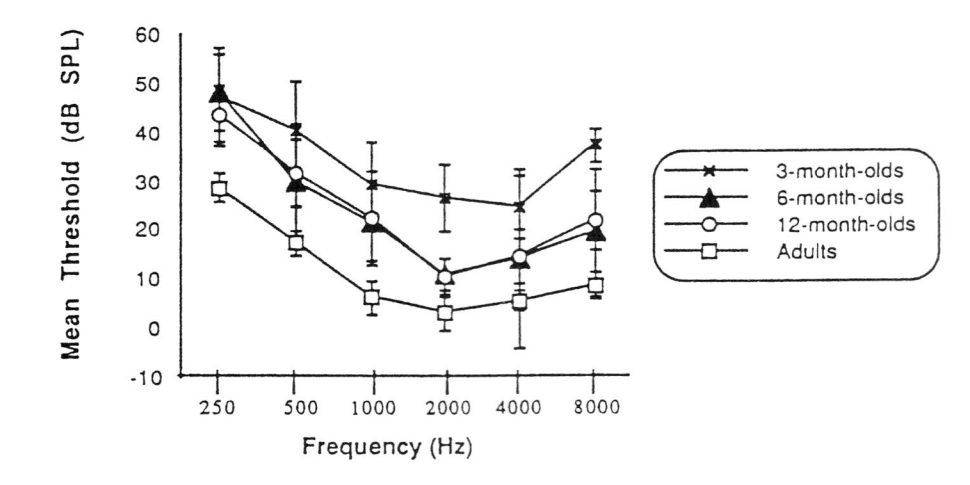

FIG. 3. Pure tone thresholds as a function of frequency for three infant age groups and adults. From Olsho LW, Koch EG, Carter EA, Halpin CF, Spetner NB. Pure-tone sensitivity of human infants. *J Acoust Soc Am* 1988; 84:1316, with permission.

prising that older children show measures of frequency selectivity on a par with adults (33,54), although this is not uniformly found (55,56). Figure 4 depicts data from a notched-noise paradigm in which the audibility of a tone is measured as a function of the amount of masking noise in the vicinity of the tone: Large changes in threshold reflect sharp auditory filtering or good frequency selectivity. Figure 4 compares data from 6-year-old children and adults, and the complete overlap of performance indicates that the auditory filters of the children are as sharp as those of the adults. This method of measuring frequency selectivity in children requires some caution because the measurement of masked thresholds in children can be influenced by factors other than the energy of the masker. For example, when the frequency selectivity of children aged 4 years is measured with the same notched-noise paradigm, the children show poorer performance than do adults, leading to the apparent paradox that infants and 6-year-olds exhibit adultlike frequency selectivity, but 4-year-olds do not. This apparent paradox is unfounded, however, because the performance of the 4-year-olds reflects reduced processing efficiency and not reduced frequency selectivity (57).

The poorer processing efficiency of infants and young children is a general feature of developmental studies (40,58–60). That is, infants and young children show a tendency to require a higher signal-to-noise ratio than do older children and adults, reflecting a reduced ability to extract target signals from noise. Because this reduction is largely unrelated to their peripheral frequency selectivity, its origin must be sought elsewhere. One candidate is the possibility that nonlinear changes in neural representation occur with age in central regions of the auditory pathway (60). Support for this comes from the observation that the time course of developmental changes in processing efficiency parallels that of changes in evoked potential measures of cortical function. A second possible contributor to reduced processing efficiency has been termed *distraction masking* (61). This refers to nonsensory effects of a masker on an infant's performance which results in an elevation of masked threshold beyond that which can be accounted for by direct energy masking of the signal.

While frequency selectivity appears to be mature by a very early age, this is not the case for frequency discrimination. The frequency difference required to differentiate between two nonsimultaneous tones in the low to middle frequencies is greater in infants aged 3 months to 1 year than it is in adults (62–64). Again, some complex frequency effects are evident, with infants aged 6 to 12 months performing like adults at a high frequency (63). Because memory plays a role in sequential comparisons, it is possible that differences in memory contribute to the adult–infant differences.

In summary, frequency selectivity appears to be well developed in human infants. Frequency discrimination, on the other hand, exhibits age-related changes.

Temporal Processing

Temporal processing refers to the ability to monitor changes in the waveform of a sound over time, including the occurrence of interruptions, energy fluctuations, and changes in duration. Infants aged 3 months to 1 year are considerably poorer than adults in detecting the occurrence of an interruption, or gap, in a stimulus (65). Gap detection in children aged 3 years to about 6 years also improves with age, with the 6-year-olds performing on a par with adults (66). Other studies put the convergence of gap detection performance to adult levels at an age later than 6 years and also show frequency effects in the developmental course (67).

Temporal processing can also be gauged by assessing sensitivity to the envelope, or fluctuation pattern, of a sound. One indirect measure of this sensitivity is to compare threshold for a tone masked by a band of noise as a function of the modulation depth of the noise. If the listener can monitor the fluctuation pattern of the noise, the tonal signal can be extracted at a better signal-to-noise ratio by "listening in the dips." Using this approach, it has been shown that by about 6 years of age, children perform at adult levels—but only for higher frequency sounds (2,000 Hz). At lower frequencies (500 Hz) even 10-year-old children exhibit poorer temporal processing than adults (68). A more direct measure of sensitivity to fluctuation pattern is to measure the depth of amplitude modulation (AM) required to just detect the presence of AM as a function of the rate of modulation. The plot of sensitivity to AM as a function of AM rate has been termed the *temporal modulation transfer function* (TMTF) (69), and examples of these obtained for different age groups are shown in Fig. 5. The key observation is that the shape of the TMTF is the same across the different age groups, although the overall sensitivity to AM generally improves with increasing age (34). The similarity in TMTF shape indi-

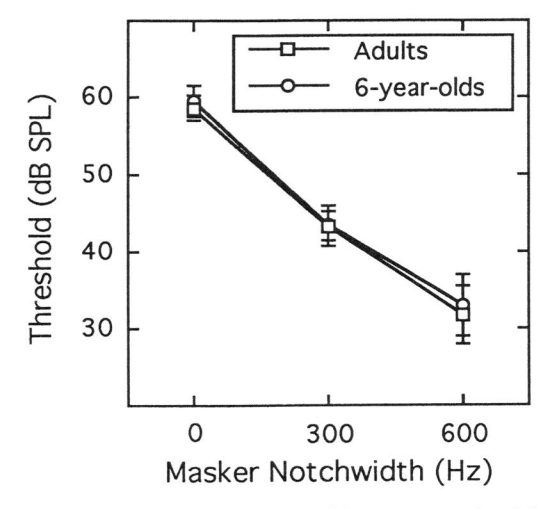

FIG. 4. Notched-noise measure of frequency selectivity from children 6 years of age (*circles*) and adults (*squares*).

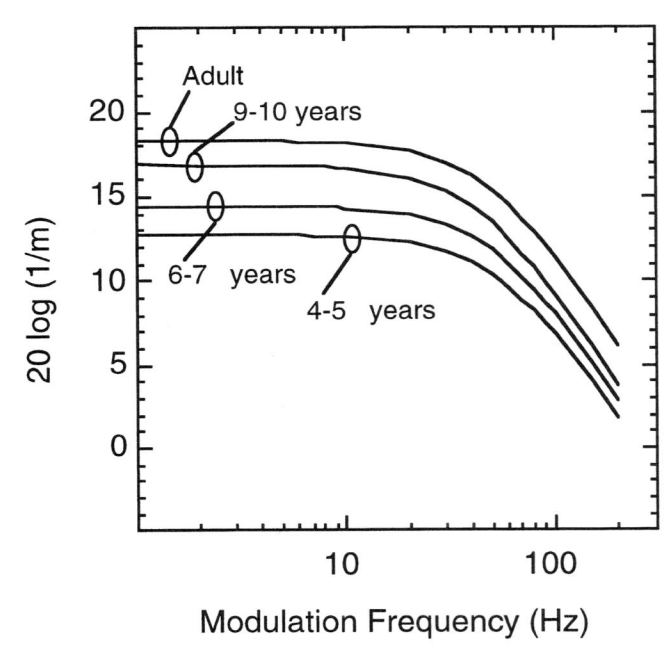

FIG. 5. Temporal modulation transfer functions from three age groups of children and adults.

cates equivalence in the time constant of temporal processing. Thus, encoding of the temporal envelope in the auditory periphery is probably mature even by 4 years of age, although the efficiency with which the modulation information is processed develops well beyond this age.

A final aspect of temporal processing is sensitivity to the duration of a sound. Infants 6 months of age require approximately double the duration changes that adults do to discriminate duration differences (70). Adult levels of duration discrimination are reached by 8 to 10 years of age (71).

In summary, the development of temporal processing depends in part on the feature of temporal processing being measured and also on the frequency region being tested. Age dependence in TMTFs reveals that the mechanism for encoding of temporal fluctuations may be intact years before the skills for processing temporal fluctuations are mature.

Monaural Across-Frequency Processing

Because the usual input to the auditory system is complex sound, it is not surprising that this system is able to combine information from across different frequency regions in processing sound. For example, a tonal signal masked by a fluctuating noise in one frequency region can be detected at a lower average signal-to-noise ratio if other frequency regions contain noise with exactly the same fluctuation pattern. This advantage of listening in correlated, or comodulated, noise has been formalized in a paradigm known as comodulation masking release (CMR). An early study of CMR in children showed that children aged 6 years were adultlike in their across-frequency processing skills (33). A later study, which included children as young as 4 years of age, also

showed no age effects in CMR at a low-frequency region (68). Further investigation revealed that this maturity of processing in listeners as young as 4 years of age held not only at a higher frequency region (2000 Hz), but also for across-frequency processing that involved dichotic presentation (72). Thus, across-frequency processing, which presumably reflects relatively central levels of analysis, appears to be mature by early childhood.

Binaural Processing

The advantages of listening with two ears (binaural hearing) over listening with one ear (monaural hearing) are evident not only in terms of localizing sources of sound, but also in terms of extracting target sounds from extraneous background noises. The ability of infants to localize sounds improves uniformly between 6 and 18 months of age but still remains poorer than that of adults (73–76). However, infants and toddlers parallel adults in that performance is better for localization near the midline than it is for the hemifields on either side of midline. This suggests that the binaural system is designed to be uniquely sensitive to processing sounds originating on the midline. Sounds originating on the midline arrive at the two ears simultaneously, and the lack of interaural differences in time and level results in a centralized image. Sensitivity to shifts of the centralized image off midline can be assessed separately for interaural differences in time and level. There is some suggestion that sensitivity to shifts due to interaural differences in time improves most rapidly between ages 4 and 6 years (77). Binaural temporal processing also features in tracking moving auditory images and, here, children aged 6 to 9 years perform significantly worse than adults, with adultlike performance being achieved by 10 to 12 years of age (78).

A laboratory test that highlights the binaural advantage for the extraction of signals from noise is the masking level difference (MLD). The MLD refers to the improvement in signal threshold when interaural differences are imposed on the signal but not on the noise. This is analogous to the noise originating on the midline but the signal originating from one side. The MLD is smaller (indicating less binaural advantage) in 7- to 8-month-old infants than in adults (79,80). Indeed, for standard conditions, the MLD does not reach adult levels until about 5 years of age (81). This is evident in Fig. 6, which shows the asymptotic improvement in MLD as a function of age, with the speckled area indicating the region of adult performance.

In summary, binaural processing appears to develop through early childhood. This development is not a simple reflection of the ability to integrate information from across the two ears because, as was mentioned in an earlier section, performance on some dichotic listening tasks can be adultlike even in 4-year-old children.

Perceptual Organization of Complex Sounds

Many of the auditory functions described so far are probed using fairly simple stimuli. The auditory system is adept at

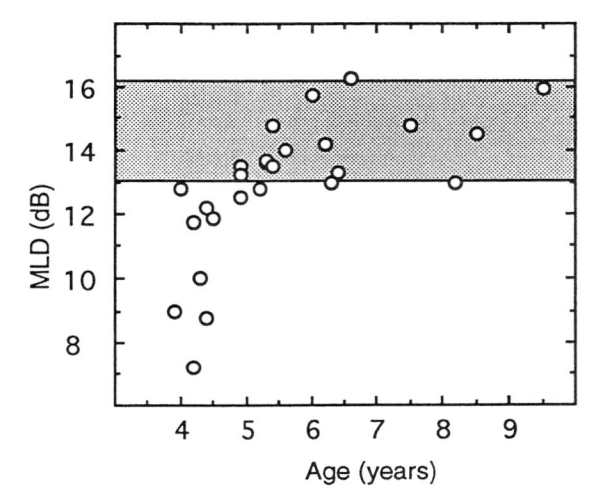

FIG. 6. Improvement of MLD with age. From Hall JW, Grose JH. The masking-level difference in children. *J Am Acad Audiol* 1990;1:81, with permission.

dealing with complex sounds made up of multiple sources, most of which are not steady state. Part of the essential task of hearing, therefore, is the correct assignment of the parts of the complex sound to their separate sources. This perceptual organization makes use of many types and levels of cues and involves learning and memory. However, an ingredient of perceptual organization is the ability to recognize and differentiate patterns in the sound. It has been shown that infants even a few months old can group sequences of sound on the basis of their pitch, make judgments about the rhythm or melodic contours of sound, and are sensitive to the number of sound elements in a sequence (82). There is also evidence that infants as young as 7 months hear the pitch of the missing fundamental, indicating that they are able to group dispersed spectral components on the basis of their harmonic structure (83). Thus, infants quickly acquire listening skills that involve pattern recognition. However, the most valuable type of sound is, of course, speech, and the acquisition of speech and language is fundamental to development as a whole. This topic is covered separately in Chapter 4.

EFFECTS OF AUDITORY DEPRIVATION ON AUDITORY DEVELOPMENT

The irreversible effects of monocular deprivation during early stages of the development of the visual system (84) have introduced the notion of "critical period" to maturational processes. Critical periods are intervals during which adequate stimulation is required in order for that modality to develop normally. There is a natural concern as to whether critical periods exist in auditory development, particularly as fluctuating, and often unilateral, conductive hearing losses are relatively common in early childhood as a frequent accompaniment to otitis media with effusion (OME) (see Chapters 15–17). Two lines of physiological work suggest that this concern is reasonable. First, monaural (conductive) deprivation studies on ferrets have shown that abnormal neural connectivity is evident at the level of the binaurally innervated inferior colliculus, but not at the level of the cochlear nucleus, which precedes binaural convergence in the auditory system (85). Second, ABR results from children with normal hearing sensitivity but positive histories of OME are abnormal (86–88). Such physiologic and electrophysiologic studies suggest that enduring effects of transient conductive hearing losses are likely even though hearing sensitivity has recovered.

To determine the perceptual consequences of fluctuating conductive hearing losses during early childhood, a number of studies have sought to assess auditory function in children with positive histories of OME. Binaural processing is an obvious choice for assessment because unilateral fluctuating hearing losses are likely to be detrimental to functions that depend critically on fine-grained interaural comparisons. A number of studies have shown that children with normal hearing but a strong history of OME have reduced MLDs (89–93). A similar result is found for children following surgical correction for congenital unilateral atresia (94). A positive history of OME is associated with both a reduced MLD and ABR abnormalities, but the relation between these two measures is complicated (90).

The general finding that transient conductive hearing losses during early childhood have enduring effects might be seen as evidence for critical periods. However, unlike the visual system, these effects of stimulatory deprivation are reversible. Longitudinal studies of children aged at least 5 years who underwent corrective surgery for chronic conductive hearing losses (tympanostomy tube placement) have shown that reductions in the MLD slowly ameliorate over time (91,93). The MLDs of most children had recovered to normal limits by about 2 years postsurgery. This is depicted in Fig. 7, which shows the recovery of MLD as a function of postsurgery time; the speckled area is the region of normal MLDs.

Although a number of studies have examined the effects of OME on binaural processing, there is some evidence that monaural auditory functions also are affected. Across-frequency processing measured with CMR is depressed before and immediately following corrective surgery for chronic hearing loss associated with OME (95). However, unlike the MLD, CMR recovers relatively rapidly and falls within normal limits about 6 to 8 months postsurgery. The suggestion that monaural sequelae of OME are evident only for relatively complex auditory functions is supported by the observation that recognition of speech signals in noise is also poorer than normal in listeners having a positive history of OME (96–98).

The recovery of normal auditory function after periods of transitory sensory deprivation during development raises the general question of plasticity within the auditory system. A number of animal studies have shown evidence for neuronal changes within the brainstem, both generative and degenerative, brought about by total sensory deprivation as a result

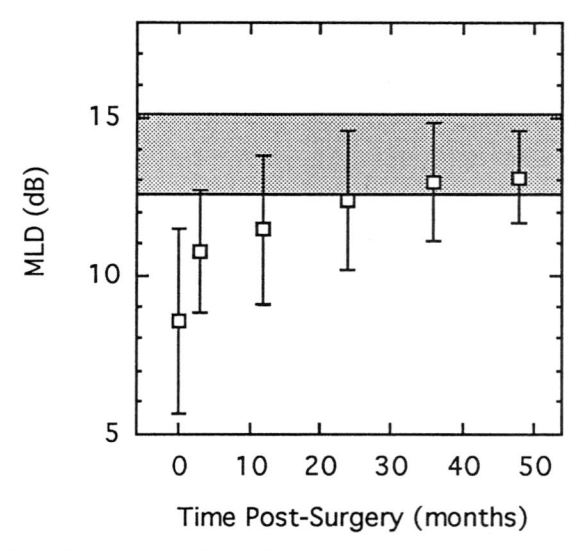

FIG. 7. Recovery of the MLD after surgical correction of hearing loss with PE tube placement.

of cochlear excision at birth (99–101). Reorganization is also evident as a result of more circumscribed sensory deprivation in neonatal animals. For example, punctate cochlear lesions resulting from the destruction of a delimited region of the organ of Corti encompassing a particular range of frequencies leads to an overrepresentation of the "edge frequencies" of the lesion in the tonotopic mapping of the auditory cortex (102–105). Physiologic and electrophysiologic findings that may be related to these edge frequencies have been noted (106–109), although the degree to which these findings may be due to alterations in the relative balance between excitation and inhibition is not clear (110). Attempts to determine functional consequences of cortical remapping have been limited (111). Although the results of neuronal plasticity are most evident in the developing auditory system, some data suggest that a form of reorganzation may exist in the mature auditory system (112–116).

In summary, fluctuating conductive hearing losses associated with childhood ear disease do appear to have enduring effects on auditory processing. The time course of hearing recovery seems to depend strongly on the specific nature of the auditory process. Because such hearing deficits appear to be reversible, a strict concept of relatively short-duration critical periods in auditory development is not supported.

SUMMARY AND CONCLUSIONS

The development of hearing begins before birth in humans and continues, for some aspects, well into late childhood. Although most measures of auditory processing show some changes with age, cochlear function appears to be relatively mature at birth. Many of the changes with age are likely to reflect a combination of factors such as anatomic or physiologic changes, changes in nonsensory and acquired processing strategies, and changes in non-auditory factors. Fluctuating conductive hearing losses in early childhood have some enduring effects, particularly on binaural hearing and speech perception in noise. However, these effects are eventually outgrown and therefore cannot be considered evidence for the existence of critical periods in auditory development. Nevertheless, there is growing interest in whether sensory deprivation at the level of the cochlea results in long-term adjustments in the neural connectivity of central stages of the auditory system, including the cortex. This has important ramifications for the provision of amplification for individuals with hearing loss of cochlear origin and for the implementation of regimens of auditory nerve stimulation in individuals with profound hearing loss who might be considered future candidates for cochlear implants.

ACKNOWLEDGMENTS

Preparation of this chapter was supported by grants R01 DC01507 and DC00397 from the National Institute on Deafness and Other Communication Disorders.

REFERENCES

1. Hepper PG, Shadidullah BS. Development of fetal hearing. *Arch Dis Child* 1994;71:F81–87.
2. Shahidullah S, Hepper PG. Frequency discrimination by the fetus. *Early Hum Dev* 1994;36:13–26.
3. Wiener FM, Ross DA. The pressure distribution in the auditory canal in a progressive sound field. *J Acoust Soc Am* 1946;18:401–408.
4. Kruger B, Ruben RJ. The acoustic properties of the infant ear. *Acta Otolaryngol (Stockh)* 1987;103:578–585.
5. Keefe DH, Bulen JC, Campbell SL, Burns EM. Pressure transfer function and absorption cross section from the diffuse field to the human infant ear canal. *J Acoust Soc Am* 1994;95:355–371.
6. Lurquin P, Magera P, Hassid S, Hennebert D. Evolution du seuil auditif durant les premiers mois de la vie liée aux modifications de la physiologie du conduit auditif externe. *Acta Otorhinolaryngol (Belg)* 1989;43:417–426.
7. Zwislocki JJ. The role of the external and middle ear in sound transmission. In: Tower DB, ed. *The Nervous System.* New York: Raven Press; 1975: 45–55. (*Human Communication and Its Disorders* vol. 3).
8. Holte L, Margolis RH, Cavenaugh RM. Developmental changes in multifrequency tympanograms. *Audiology* 1991;30:1–24.
9. McKinley AM, Grose JH, Roush J. Multi-frequency tympanometry and evoked otoacoustic emissions in neonates during the first 24 hours of life. *J Am Acad Audiol* 1997;8:218–223.
10. Keefe DH, Bulen JC, Arehart KH, Burns EM. Ear-canal impedance and reflection coefficient in human infants and adults. *J Acoust Soc Am* 1993;94:2617–2638.
11. Dallos P. Cochlear neurobiology: some key experiments and concepts of the past two decades. In: Edelman GM, Gall WE, Cowan WM, eds. *Auditory function: neurological bases of hearing.* New York: John Wiley & Sons, 1988;153–188.
12. Kemp DT. Stimulated acoustic emissions from within the human auditory system. *J Acoust Soc Am* 1978;64:1386–1391.
13. Bonfils P, Piron JP, Uziel A, Pujol R. A correlative study of evoked otoacoustic emission properties and audiometric thresholds. *Arch Otorhinolaryngol* 1988;244:53–56.
14. Chuang SW, Gerber SE, Thornton ARD. Evoked otoacoustic emissions in preterm infants. *Int J Pediatr Otorhinolaryngol* 1993;26:39–45.
15. Kennedy CR, Kimm L, Dees DC, et al. Otoacoustic emissions and auditory brainstem responses in the newborn. *Arch Dis Child* 1991;66:1124–1129.
16. Norton SJ, Widen JE. Evoked otoacoustic emissions in normal-hearing infants and children: emerging data and issues. *Ear Hear* 1990;11:121–127.

17. Stevens JC, Webb HD, Hutchinson JT, Connell J, Smith MF, Buffin JT. Click-evoked otoacoustic emissions in neonatal screening. *Ear Hear* 1990;11:128–133.
18. Uziel A, Piron JP. Evoked otoacoustic emissions from normal newborns and babies admitted to an intensive case baby unit. *Act Otolaryngol Suppl (Stockh)* 1991;482:85–91.
19. White KR, Vohr BR, Behrens TR. Universal newborn hearing screenings using transient evoked otoacoustic emissions: results of the Rhode Island Hearing Assessment Project. *Semin Hear* 1993;14:18–29.
20. Rotteveel JJ, de Graaf R, Colon EJ, Stegman DF, Visco YM. The maturation of the central auditory conduction in preterm infants until three months post term. II. The auditory brainstem reponse. *Hear Res* 1987;26:21–35.
21. Daruna JH, Rau AE. Development of the late components of auditory brain potentials from early childhood to adulthood. *Electroencephalogr Clin Neurophysiol Suppl* 1987;40:590–595.
22. Collet L, Morgon A, Soares I, Disant F, Salle B. Maturational changes in the intensity latency relation of the brainstem auditory evoked potentials in humans. *Acta Otolaryngol (Stockh)* 1988;105:473–476.
23. Gorga MP, Kaminski JR, Beauchanine KL, Jesteadt W, Neely ST. Auditory brainstem response from children three months to three years of age: normal patterns of reponse II. *J Speech Hear Res* 1989;32:281–288.
24. Eggermont JJ, Ponton CW, Coupland DG, Winklaar R. Frequency dependent maturation of the cochlea and brainstem evoked potentials. *Acta Otolaryngol (Stockh)* 1991;111:220–224.
25. Jiang DD, Zheng MS, Sun DK, Lui XY. Brainstem auditory evoked responses from birth to adulthood: normative data of latency and interval. *Hear Res* 1991;54:67–74.
26. Eggermont JJ. Development of auditory evoked potentials. *Acta Otolaryngol (Stockh)* 1992;112:197–200.
27. Lauffer H, Wenzel D. Brainstem acoustic evoked reponses: maturational aspects from cochlea to midbrain. *Neuropediatrics* 1990;21(2):59–61.
28. Enoki H, Sanada S, Yoshinaga H, Oka E, Ohtahara S. The effects of age on the N200 component of the auditory event-related potentials. *Brain Res Cogn Brain Res* 1993;1:161–167.
29. Uysal S, Renda Y, Topcu M, Erdem G, Karacan R. Evoked potentials in full-term and premature infants: a comparative study. *Childs Nerv Syst* 1993;9:88–92.
30. Reinis S, Goldman JM. *The development of the brain: biological and functional perspectives.* Springfield, IL: Charles C Thomas, 1980.
31. Bertoncini J, Morais J, Bijeljac-Babic R, McAdams S, Peretz I, Mehler J. Dichotic perception and laterality in neonates. *Brain Lang* 1989;37:591–605.
32. Olsho LW, Koch EG, Halpin CF. An observer-based psychoacoustic procedure for use with young infants. *Dev Psychol* 1987;23:627–640.
33. Veloso K, Hall JW, Grose JH. Frequency selectivity and comodulation masking release in adults and in six-year old children. *J Speech Hear Res* 1990;33:96–102.
34. Hall JW, Grose JH. Development of temporal resolution in children as measured by the temporal modulation transfer function. *J Acoust Soc Am* 1994;96:150–154.
35. Sinnott JM, Pisoni DB, Aslin RN. A comparison of pure tone auditory thresholds in human infants and adults. *Infant Behav Dev* 1983;6:3–17.
36. Berg KM. A comparison of thresholds for 1/3-octave filtered clicks and noise bursts infants and adults. *Percept Psychophysiol* 1993;54:365–369.
37. Fior R. Physiological maturation of auditory function between 3 and 13 years of age. *Audiology* 1972;11:317–321.
38. Leninhan JMA, Christie JF, Russell TS, Orr NM, Hamilton MD, Konz EC. The threshold of hearing in school children. *J Laryngol Otol* 1971;85:375–385.
39. Maxon AB, Hochberg I. Development of psychoacoustic behavior: sensitivity and discrimination. *Ear Hear* 1982;3:301–308.
40. Nozza RJ, Wilson WR. Masked and unmasked pure-tone thresholds of infants and adults: Development of auditory frequency selectivity and sensitivity. *J Speech Hear Res* 1984;27:613–622.
41. Olsho LW, Koch EG, Carter EA, Halpin CF, Spetner NB. Pure-tone sensitivity of human infants. *J Acoust Soc Am* 1988;84:1316–1324.
42. Roche AF, Siervogel RM, Hines JH, Johnson DL. Longitudinal study of hearing in children: baseline data concerning auditory thresholds, noise exposure, and biological factors. *J Acoust Soc Am* 1978;64:1593–1601.
43. Schneider BA, Trehub SE, Morrongiello BA, Thorpe LA. Auditory sensitivity in preschool children. *J Acoust Soc Am* 1986;79:447–452.
44. Trehub SE, Schneider BA, Endman M. Developmental changes in infants' sensitivity to octave-band noises. *J Exp Child Psychol* 1980;29:283–293.
45. Schecter MA, Fausti SA, Rappaport BZ, Frey RH. Age categorization of high-frequency auditory threshold data. *J Acoust Soc Am* 1986;79:767–771.
46. Trehub SE, Schneider BA, Morrongiello BA, Thorpe LA. Developmental changes in high-frequency sensitivity. *Audiology* 1989;28:241–249.
47. Werner LA, Folsom RC, Mancl LR. The relationship between auditory brainstem response and behavioral thresholds in normal hearing infants and adults. *Hear Res* 1993;68:131–141.
48. Werner LA, Folsom RC, Mancl LR. The relationship between auditory brainstem response latencies and behavioral thresholds in normal hearing infants and adults. *Hear Res* 1994;77:88–98.
49. Olsho LW. Infant auditory perception: Tonal masking. *Infant Behav Dev* 1985;8:371–384.
50. Schneider BA, Morrongiello BA, Trehub SE. Size of critical bands in infants, children, and adults. *J Exp Psychol* 1990;16:642–652.
51. Spetner NB, Olso LW. Auditory frequency resolution in human infancy. *Child Dev* 1990;61:632–652.
52. Bargones JY, Burns EM. Suppression tuning curves for spontaneous otoacoustic emissions in infants and adults. *J Acoust Soc Am* 1988;83:1809–1816.
53. Folsom RC, Wynne MK. Auditory brain stem response from human adults and infants: wave V tuning curves. *J Acoust Soc Am* 1987;81:412–417.
54. Soderquist DR. Auditory filter widths in children and adults. *J Exp Child Psychol* 1993;56:371–384.
55. Allen P, Wightman F, Kistler D, Dolan T. Frequency resolution in children. *J Speech Hear Res* 1989;32:317–322.
56. Irwin RJ, Stillman JA, Schade A. The width of the auditory filter in children. *J Exp Child Psychol* 1986;41:429–442.
57. Hall JW, Grose JH. Notched-noise measures of frequency selectivity in adults and children using fixed-masker-level and fixed-signal-level presentation. *J Speech Hear Res* 1991;34:651–660.
58. Quaranta A, Salonna I, Bellomo F. Pyschoacoustical performance in children. *Scand Audiol* 1992;21:265–267.
59. Bull D, Schneider BA, Trehub SE. The masking of octave-band noise by broad-spectrum noise: a comparison of infant and adult thresholds. *Percept Psychophysiol* 1981;30:101–106.
60. Schneider BA, Trehub SE, Morrongiello BA, Thorpe LA. Developmental changes in masked thresholds. *J Acoust Soc Am* 1989;86:1733–1742.
61. Werner L, Bargones J. Sources of auditory masking in infants: distraction effects. *Percept Psychophysiol* 1991;50:405–412.
62. Sinnott JM, Aslin RN. Frequency and intensity discrimination in human infants and adults. *J Acoust Soc Am* 1985;78:1986–1992.
63. Olsho LW, Koch EG, Halpin CF. Level and age effects in infant frequency discrimination. *J Acoust Soc Am* 1987;82:454–464.
64. Aslin RN. Discrimination of frequency transitions by human infants. *J Acoust Soc Am* 1989;86:582–590.
65. Werner LA, Marean GC, Halpin CF, Spetner NB, Gillenwater JM. Infant auditory temporal acuity: gap detection. *Child Dev* 1992;63:260–272.
66. Wightman F, Allen P, Dolan T, Kistler D, Jamieson D. Temporal resolution in children. *Child Dev* 1989;60:611–624.
67. Irwin RJ, Ball AK, Kay N, Stillman JA, Bosser J. The development of auditory temporal acuity in children. *Child Dev* 1985;56:614–620.
68. Grose JH, Hall JW, Gibbs C. Temporal analysis in children. *J Speech Hear Res* 1993;36:351–356.
69. Viemeister NF. Temporal modulation transfer functions based upon modulation thresholds. *J Acoust Soc Am* 1979;66:1364–1380.
70. Morrongiello B, Trehub S. Age-related changes in auditory temporal perception. *J Exp Child Psychol* 1987;44:413–426.
71. Elfenbein JL, Small AM, Davis JM. Developmental patterns of duration discrimination. *J Speech Hear Res* 1993;36:842–849.
72. Grose JH, Hall JW, Mendoza L. Developmental effects in complex sound processing. In: Manly GA, Klump GM, Köppl C, Fastl H, Oeckinghaus H, eds. *Advances in Hearing Research.* Singapore: World Scientific Publishers, 1995:97–104.

73. Ashmead DH, Clifton RK, Perris EE. Precision of auditory localization in human infants. *Dev Psychol* 1987;23:641–647.
74. Morrongiello BA. Infants' localization of sound along the horizonal axis: estimates of minimum audible angle. *Dev Psychol* 1988;24: 8–13.
75. Morrongiello BA, Rocca PT. Infants' localization of sounds in the horizontal plane: effects of auditory and visual cues. *Child Dev* 1987; 58:918–927.
76. Morrongiello BA, Rocca PT. Infants' localization of sounds within hemifields: estimates of minumum audible angle. *Child Dev* 1990; 61:1258–1270.
77. Kaga M. Development of sound localization. *Acta Paediatr Jpn* 1992; 34:134–138.
78. Cranford J, Morgan M, Scudder R, Moore C. Tracking of "moving" fused auditory images by children. *J Speech Hear Res* 1993;36: 424–430.
79. Nozza RJ. The binaural masking level difference in infants and adults: developmental change in binaural hearing. *Infant Behav Dev* 1987; 10:105–110.
80. Nozza RJ, Wagner EF, Crandell MA. Binaural release from masking for a speech sound in infants, preschoolers, and adults. *J Speech Hear Res* 1988;31:212–218.
81. Hall JW, Grose JH. The masking-level difference in children. *J Am Acad Audiol* 1990;1:81–88.
82. Trehub SE. Temporal auditory processing in infancy. *Ann N Y Acad Sci* 1993;682:137–149.
83. Clarkson MG, Clifton RK. Infant pitch perception: evidence for responding to pitch categories and the missing fundamental. *J Acoust Soc Am* 1985;77:1521–1528.
84. Weisel TN, Hubel DG. Comparison of the effects of unilateral and bilateral eye closure on cortical unit responses in kittens. *J Neurophysiol* 1965;28:1029–1040.
85. Moore DR, Hutchings ME, King AJ, Kowalchuk NE. Auditory brainstem of the ferret: some effects of rearing with unilateral ear plug on the cochlea, cochlear nucleus, and projections to the inferior colliculus. *J Neurosci* 1989;9:1213–1222.
86. Anteby I, Hafner H, Pratt H, Uri N. Auditory brainstem evoked potentials in evaluating the central effects of middle ear effusion. *Int J Pediatr Otorhinolaryngol* 1986;12:1–11.
87. Chambers R. Auditory brain-stem responses in children with previous otitis media. *Arch Otolaryngol Head Neck Surg* 1989;115:452–457.
88. Folsom RC, Weber BA, Thompson G. Auditory brainstem responses in children with early recurrent middle ear disease. *Ann Otol Rhinol Laryngol* 1983;92:249–253.
89. Besing JM, Koehnke J, Goulet C. Binaural performance associated with a history of otitis media in children. 15th Midwinter Research Meeting of the Association for Research in Otolaryngology, St Petersburg Beach, FL 1993:15.
90. Hall JW, Grose JH. The effect of otitis media with effusion on the masking level difference and the auditory brainstem response. *J Speech Hear Res* 1993;36:210–217.
91. Hall JW, Grose JH, Pillsbury HC. Long-term effects of chronic otitis media on binaural hearing in children. *Arch Otolaryngol* 1995;121: 847–852.
92. Moore DR, Hutchings ME, Meyer SE. Binaural masking level differences in children with a history of otitis media. *Audiology* 1991;30: 91–101.
93. Pillsbury HC, Grose JH, Hall JW. Otitis media with effusion in children: Binaural hearing before and after corrective surgery. *Arch Otolaryngol* 1991;117:718–723.
94. Wilmington D, Jahrsdoerfer R, Gray L. Binaural processing after corrected congenital unilateral conductive hearing loss. *Hear Res* 1994; 74:99–114.
95. Hall JW, Grose JH. The effect of otitis media with effusion on co-modulation masking release in children. *J Speech Hear Res* 1994;37: 1441–1449.
96. Gravel JS, Wallace IF. Listening and language at 4 years of age: effect of early otitis media. *J Speech Hear Res* 1992;35:588–595.
97. Jerger S, Jerger J, Alford BR, Abrams S. Development of speech intelligibility in children with recurrent otitis media. *Ear Hear* 1983; 4:138–145.
98. Schilder AGM, Snik ADM, Straatman H, van den Broek P. The effect of otitis media with effusion at preschool age on some aspects of auditory perception at school age. *Ear Hear* 1994;15:224–231.
99. Russell FA, Moore DR. Afferent reorganization within the superior olivary complex of the gerbil: development and induction by neonatal, unilateral cochlear removal. *Comp Neurol* 1995;352:607–625.
100. Moore DR. Auditory brainstem of the ferret: long survival following cochlear removal progressively changes projections from the cochlear nucleus to the inferior colliculus. *Comp Neurol* 1994;339:301–310.
101. Moore DR, King AJ, McAlpine D, Martin RL, Hutchings ME. Functional consequences of neonatal unilateral cochlear removal. *Prog Brain Res* 1993;97:127–133.
102. Harrison RV, Nagasawa A, Smith DW, Stanton S, Mount RJ. Reorganization of auditory cortex after neonatal high frequency cochlear hearing loss. *Hear Res* 1991;54:11–19.
103. Rajan R, Irvine DRF, Wise LZ, Heil P. Effect of unilateral partial cochlear representation of lesioned and unlesioned cochleas in primary auditory cortex. *J Comp Neurol* 1993;338:17–49.
104. Robertson D, Irvine DRF. Plasticity of frequency organization in auditory cortex of guinea pigs with partial unilateral deafness. *J Comp Neurol* 1989;282:456–471.
105. Willott JF, Aitkin LM, McFadden SL. Plasticity of auditory cortex associated with sensorineural hearing loss in adult C57BL/6J mice. *J Comp Neurol* 1993;329:402–411.
106. Gerken GM, Solecki JM, Boettcher FA. Temporal integration of electrical stimulation of auditory nuclei in normal-hearing and hearing-impaired cat. *Hear Res* 1991;53:101–112.
107. Willott JF, Lu S. Noise-induced hearing loss can alter neural coding and increase excitability in the central nervous system. *Science* 1982; 216:1331–1332.
108. Harrison RV, Stanton SG, Ibrahim D, Nagasawa A, Mount RJ. Neonatal cochlear hearing loss results in developmental abnormalities of the central auditory pathway. *Acta Otolaryngol* 1993;113:296–302.
109. Salvi RJ, Saunders SS, Gratton MA, Arehole S, Powers N. Enhanced evoked response amplitudes in the inferior colliculus of the chinchilla following acoustic trauma. *Hear Res* 1990;50:245–258.
110. Boettcher FA, Salvi RJ. Effect of short duration acoustic trauma on activity of single neurons in the ventral cochlear nucleus. In: Cazals Y, Horner K, Demany L, eds. *Auditory physiology and perception.* Oxford: Pergamon Press; 1992:599–606.
111. Harrison RV, Smith DW, Nagasawa A, Stanton S, Mount RJ. Developmental plasticity of auditory cortex in cochlear hearing loss: physiological and psychophysical findings. In: Cazals Y, Horner K, Demany L, eds. *Auditory physiology and perception.* Oxford: Pergamon Press; 1992:625–634.
112. Silverman CA, Silman S. Apparent auditory deprivation from monaural amplification and recovery with binaural amplification: two case studies. *J Am Acad Audiol* 1990;1:175–180.
113. Silman S, Silverman CA, Emmer MB, Gelfand SA. Adult-onset auditory deprivation. *J Am Acad Audiol* 1992;3:390–396.
114. Silman S, Gelfand SA, Silverman CA. Late-onset auditory deprivation: Effects of monaural versus binaural hearing aids. *J Acoust Soc Am* 1984;76:1357–1362.
115. Robinson K, Gatehouse S. Changes in intensity discrimination following monaural long-term use of a hearing aid. *J Acoust Soc Am* 1995; 97:1183–1190.
116. Gatehouse S. The time course and magnitude of perceptual acclimatization to frequency response; evidence from monaural fitting of hearing aids. *J Acoust Soc Am* 1992;92:1258–1268.

CHAPTER 4

Development of Speech and Language

Joanne E. Roberts, Ina F. Wallace, and Diane Brackett

It is through communication that people make requests, share their ideas, and express their feelings. Successful interactions in life are greatly affected by one's ability to communicate. The first few years of life provide an important foundation for the development of communication skills. Children learn to listen to caregivers and others in their environment with whom they have daily interactions and thereby learn to use speech and language to communicate. When hearing is impaired, either from sensorineural or conductive causes, there may be a disruption in the communicative process. Although it is well documented that children with moderate to severe permanent hearing loss display communication difficulties, the effects of the mild conductive fluctuating hearing loss associated with chronic otitis media are less clear (1,2).

This chapter defines terminology related to children's communication development; describes the speech and language development of young children, including important developmental milestones; and then examines the role of hearing in normal language and learning. The effects of both conductive and sensorineural hearing loss on speech and language development of children are also described.

SPEECH AND LANGUAGE DEVELOPMENT

Communication, Speech, and Language

Although sometimes used interchangeably, communication, speech, and language are terms important to distinguish. *Communication* is the process of exchanging information, ideas, and feelings between individuals. It can be intentional, (e.g., when a person asks someone for directions) or unintentional (e.g., someone inadvertently frowns to indicate displeasure). Language is a socially shared code used to communicate and is composed of arbitrary symbols (e.g., *p, b*) and rules for combining those symbols (*p* and *z* never occur next to each other in the same word). To communicate and express *language* a mutually understood mode or system of motor acts is needed. *Speech,* the production of vocal sound patterns, is the most common mode of human communication. However, communication can occur nonverbally through other modes of communication such as signing (e.g., American Sign Language), facial expressions (e.g., smiling) vocalizations (e.g., "baba"), nonspeech sounds (e.g., laughter), gestures (e.g., pointing), and writing (e.g., "Dear Matthew"). Another important distinction is between expressive communication/language and receptive communication/language. *Expressive communication* is the ability to produce speech, vocalizations, and gestures; *receptive communication* is the ability to receive and comprehend the speech, vocalizations, and gestures of others.

Components of Language

When acquiring language, children learn rules about its sounds, grammar, meanings, and uses. These rules are reflected in four components of language: (a) *phonology*—rules for the formation of speech sounds (e.g., *p, s*) and how sounds are combined into words (e.g., *rd* can occur in words but not *qa*; (b) *syntax*—the rule system for combining morphemes (i.e., units of meaning) into phrases and sentences (e.g., "I like to go dancing" not "dancing to go like I"); (c) *semantics*—the rules for meanings of individual words and word classes (e.g., "I want to eat an apple" not "I want to eat dancing"); and (d) *pragmatics*—rules for the use of language in social contexts (e.g., when you want something, you request it).

Development of Speech and Language

The major achievements of language acquisition occur during the first 5 years. To identify atypical speech and

---

J.E. Roberts: Frank Porter Graham Child Development Center, Division of Speech and Hearing Sciences, University of North Carolina at Chapel Hill, Chapel Hill, North Carolina 27599.
I.F. Wallace: Center for Research in Education, Research Triangle Institute, Research Triangle Park, North Carolina 27709; Department of Otolaryngology, Albert Einstein College of Medicine, Bronx, New York 10461.
D. Brackett: Department of Communication Sciences, University of Connecticut, Storrs, Connecticut 06268.

language development it is critical to first know the milestones of speech and language. Figure 1 highlights some of the major milestones in language comprehension as compared to language production.

Birth to 1 Year

During the first year of life, infants do not produce meaningful words. However, their early interactions with people and objects provide the foundations for the development of language. In the first few months, infants orient to sounds, learn to recognize familiar voices, "coo" and "gurgle," and produce some single syllables such as "*ba*." Caregivers then respond to infants' unintentional signals (e.g., eye gaze, facial expressions, body movements) as if the communication is purposeful. For example, crying is often interpreted as a purposeful indication of a desire to be picked up; repetitive sucking is interpreted as hunger. When a baby smiles in response to a tickle from her mother, the mother smiles and says "tickle, tickle, tickle" and tickles the child again. These early nonverbal interchanges between a child and a caretaker during the first few months of life form the basis for later conversational interactions. Throughout infancy, the baby increasingly participates in interactions with caregivers, uses more varied and readable signals, and has a greater ability to participate in reciprocal turn taking sequences. By 4 mo, infants can localize to sounds. At 6 mo, infants typically begin to babble using consonant-vowel combinations (e.g., "mamma" "dada") and produce non-speechlike vocalizations ("raspberries" and squeals). Initially, the sounds that infants can discriminate and produce include sounds from their native language as well as other languages.

At about 9 to 10 mo, a change in communication typically occurs. The infant begins to intentionally communicate, resulting in the infant's purposeful communication having a planned effect on the behavior of others. For example, if a child wants a cookie from the cookie jar, the child will pick up an adult's hand and move it toward the cookie jar. The child also begins to use word-like sounds consistently (e.g., "a" for something he wants) and gestures consistently (e.g., extending arms to be picked up) so that others can understand what the infant is communicating. Yet unlike a few months before, infants now discriminate and produce sounds only in their own language, not sounds in other languages. By the end of their first year, infants consistently vocalize and use gestures to request objects and actions (e.g., child points to a desired truck), seek attention (e.g., child runs to Mom and pats her arm), protest something (e.g., child pushes adult's hand away), and comment on objects and actions (e.g., child holds up toy car and smiles).

1 to 2 Years

During the second year, children's communication becomes more frequent, consistent and clear, resulting in greater success in getting needs met. Children also are able to respond more consistently to the language around them. Around 12 to 13 mo, children's first words emerge. Early words are words that have the most meaning for the child, such as the names of important people and objects ("Mommy" and "milk") in the child's environment. The words are used to express the same intentions that were previously conveyed through gestures and vocalizations. For example, when a child wants to be picked up, in addition to raising his arms, the child now will say "up." A close relationship has been found between a child's previous babbling and early words. Often, children who displayed limited babbling repertoires have restricted vocabularies in comparison to children with more extensive babbles. At this point, gestures and vocalizations still comprise a large proportion of the child's communication. Children respond consistently to simple familiar action words (e.g., "no"). Between 12 and 18 mo, acquisition of new words is slow and unstable, with some words dropping out of the vocabulary.

At 18 mo, two major shifts in development occurs. First, vocabulary begins to expand dramatically, particularly word comprehension. Children may use about 50 words, but they may understand as many as 300 words. Children now talk about things that exist (e.g., "car") and no longer exist (e.g., pointing to missing wheel on car). Toddlers also begin to combine two or more words into multiword utterances (e.g., "Doggie bark" and "Mommy eat cookie"). Children are generally able to request information (e.g., "What that?") and answer (e.g., child says "juice" in response to "What do you want?"). They also show increasing ability to participate in a conversation. However, they are able to maintain the topic of a conversation only about 50% of the time, and their conversational interactions are generally short and focus on observable events. Other linguistic achievements include following directions, finding familiar objects, and identifying body parts (e.g., "show me your nose").

2 to 3 Years

Between 2 and 3 yr, children acquire basic sentence grammar and syntax, expand their vocabulary, articulate sounds correctly more of the time, and use language in a more precise and descriptive fashion. In the first half of their third year, children tend to speak in utterances of two and three words (e.g., "I like cake" or "block on chair"), but also still use single word utterances and occasionally produce ones that are six words long. As children begin to use three-word utterances, they typically add morphological markers to their utterances. These include *s* for plurals (hats), *s* for possessive (Sue's), *ed* for past (walked), and *ing* for present progressive (running). There is considerable variation in the rate of acquisition of morphemes; however, the order of acquisition remains generally constant across children. Although children's early sentences are not grammatically correct (e.g., "no go eat" or "dog not big"), a few months later, their language becomes more similar to adult language ("That is not a big dog").

| QQ | SINGLE Fr | IP |

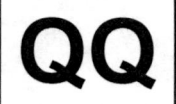

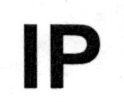

Customer:
Z. H. Christian Bartesch
R201a

L MON PM

Pediatric Otology and Neurotology

Lalwani MD, Anil K., Grundfast MD, Kenneth M.

E1-N014-K5

W2-DDM-915

No CD
Used - Very Good
9780397514663

Picker Notes:
M _____ 2 _____
WT _____ 2 _____
CC _____

65279873

[AmazonDE] betterworldbooks__: 302-8303815-5592317

1 Item   1064922510

Friday Expedited Singles

Ship. Created: 4/25/2019 6:17:00 AM
Date Ordered: 4/25/2019 7:58:00 AM

check one YES NO	Hearing and Understanding	Child's Age	Talking	check one YES NO
	Does your child hear and understand most of what is said at home and in school? Does everyone who knows your child think he/she hears well (teacher, baby sitter, grandparent, etc.)? Does your child pay attention to a story and answer simple questions about it?	4½–5 YEARS	Does your child communicate easily with other children and adults? Does your child say all sounds correctly except maybe one or two? Does your child use the same grammar as the rest of the family?	
		4–4½ YEARS	Does your child's voice sound clear like other children's? Does your child use sentences that give lots of details (e.g., "I have two red balls at home")? Can your child tell you a story and stick pretty much to the topic?	
	Does your child hear you when you call from another room? Does your child hear television or radio at the same loudness level as other members of the family? Does your child answer simple "who," "what," "where," "why" questions?	3–4 YEARS	Does your child talk about what he/she does at school or at friends' homes? Does your child say most sounds correctly except a few, like r, l, th and s? Does your child usually talk easily without repeating syllables or words? Do people outside your family usually understand your child's speech? Does your child use a lot of sentences that have 4 or more words?	
	Does your child understand differences in meaning ("go-stop"; "in–on"; "big-little"; "up–down")? Does your child continue to notice sounds (telephone ringing, television sound, knocking at the door)? Can your child follow two requests ("get the ball and put it on the table")?	2–3 YEARS	Does your child have a word for almost everything? Does your child use 2–3 word "sentences" to talk about and ask for things? Do you understand your child's speech most of the time? Does your child often ask for or direct your attention to objects by naming them?	
	Can your child point to pictures in a book when they are named? Does your child point to a few body parts when asked? Can your child follow simple commands and understand simple questions ("Roll the ball," "Kiss the baby," "Where's your shoe?")? Does your child listen to simple stories, songs, and rhymes?	1–2 YEARS	Is your child saying more and more words every month? Does your child use some 1–2 word questions ("where kitty?" "go bye-bye?" "what's that"?)? Does your child put 2 words together ("more cookie," "no juice," "mommy block")? Does your child use many different consonant sounds at the beginning of words?	
	Does your child recognize words for common items like "cup," "shoe," "juice"? Has your child begun to respond to requests ("Come here," "Want more?")?	7 MONTHS–1 YEAR	Does your child have 1 or 2 words (bye-bye, dada, mama, no) although they may not be clear?	
	Does your child enjoy games like peek-a-boo and pat-a-cake? Does your child turn or look up when you call his or her name? Does your child listen when spoken to?		Does your child's babbling have both long and short groups of sounds such as "tata upup bibibibi"? Does your child imitate different speech sounds? Does your child use speech or non-crying sounds to get and keep your attention?	
	Does your child respond to "no"? Changes in your tone of voice? Does your child look around for the source of new sounds, e.g., the doorbell, vacuum, dog barking? Does your child notice toys that make sound?	4–6 MONTHS	Does your child's babbling sound more speech-like with lots of different sounds, including p, b, and m? Does your child tell you (by sound or gesture) when he/she wants you to do something again? Does your child make gurgling sounds when left alone? When playing with you?	
	Does your child turn to you when you speak? Does your child smile when spoken to? Does your child seem to recognize your voice and quiet down if crying?	0–3 MONTHS	Does your child repeat the same sounds a lot (cooing, gooing)? Does your child cry differently for different needs? Does your child smile when he/she sees you?	
	Does your child listen to speech? Does your child startle or cry at noises? Does your child awaken at loud sounds?	BIRTH	Does your child make pleasure sounds? When you play with your child, does he/she look at you, look away, & then look again?	
	Total		Total	

Instructions:
Read each question through your chlid's age group and check *yes* or *no*. Add the total and see below.

ALL YES: Good-Your child is developing hearing, speech, and language normally.

1-2 NO: CAUTION! Your child may have delayed hearing, speech, and language development.

3 or more NO: ACTION! Take your child for professional help.

FIG. 1. Major milestones in language comprehension. Adapted with permission from the brochure *How Does Your Child Hear and Talk?* © American Speech-Language Hearing Association.

By age 2, children generally produce vowels and many types of sounds (*p, b, t, d, k, g*). However, the words children produce often fail to match the sound of the words produced by adults. For example, the 2 year old may say "do" for dog and "nana" for "banana." At the same time, children's word knowledge expands greatly. Children in the second half of their third year frequently have a vocabulary of 500 words and can comprehend as many as 1,000 words. During this same time period, children's understanding of abstract relations also increases dramatically. Children usually can understand and talk about spatial ("under the chair"), temporal ("after dinner"), quantity ("two cats"), and color concepts ("blue hat"). They begin to use words referring to objects or people not in their immediate environment, including past and future events ("Joe at school").

3 to 5 Years

Between 3 and 5 years, more fine-tuning and growth in all aspects of speech and language occurs. At about age 3, children begin to use complex sentences in which clauses are conjoined and embedded into one another. At this point, sentences sound like those used by adults: "My mommy says that the stove is hot," "I know what we can sing," and "Why don't you like jelly on it?" Errors in children's speech sounds decrease dramatically after 3½ years, and by 4 years of age, children can produce accurately most of the sounds of their native language, although some errors persist (e.g., "bwead" for "bread," "pwane" for "plane"). Continued refinements of sounds in words with consonant clusters (e.g., street, bread) and multisyllables (e.g., spaghetti, elephant) takes place during the next few years. The 3½-year-old is also a more skilled conversationalist, frequently maintaining a topic of conversation 75% of the time, including providing new information on the topic.

By 4 years, children's language use shifts from a focus on the present to talk about events and people more distant in time. The 4-year-old is able to report on present and past events, imagine situations, identify his own and others feelings, plan events, and anticipate what will happen. Children of age 4 generally can recognize and respond appropriately to requests for repetitions or clarifications in conversations. At about 4 years, children also develop metalinguistic knowledge (i.e., the competence to focus on the form and content of language). *Metalinguistic skills* include the ability to identify grammatical versus ungrammatical utterances, segment words into phonemes and sentences into words, recognize word beginnings and endings, distinguish correctly produced from incorrectly produced sounds, judge whether two sounds or words are the same, define words, and use the multiple meaning of words for humor. The 4-year-old child also becomes sensitive to the language skills of the listener and can modify speech and language accordingly. At this age, children can tell jokes, tease, and provide warnings. They show increasing ability to use language for abstract purposes that are removed from the present context.

Role of Hearing in Language Learning

Although language acquisition often appears to be effortless, there are many underlying prerequisites for it to develop smoothly. For instance, cognitive achievements such as object permanence and symbolic thought are tied to the emergence of language. Information acquired through sight, hearing, touch, and taste each contribute to the cognitive structures from which language develops. Yet, of all of the sensory systems involved in acquiring the knowledge base, hearing plays the pivotal role in language development. A young child acquires speech and language through listening and interacting with people in the environment. From the continuous flow of surrounding speech, the child learns to detect and organize speech into units, categorize these units, attach meaning to them, and then abstract the rules for the syntax, semantics, phonology and pragmatics of language.

However, conversational speech is not always a consistent and clear source of information. Conversational speech typically occurs so very rapidly that words are often glossed over. The precision of producing sounds varies greatly among speakers, and even within the same speaker. For example, adjacent speech sounds, stress patterns, a speaker's style, and the environmental context all affect a speaker's articulation. These, in turn, affect the ability of a listener to understand a message. The comprehension of speech is also greatly influenced by the distance between the talker and the listener. For example, at 3 feet, average conversational speech is 45 dB hearing level (HL) (65 dB sound pressure level [SPL]) and can vary by approximately 30 dB. As the distance between the talker and listener increases, there is a corresponding decrease in the intensity of the speech signal (at 6 ft, 39 dB HL; at 12 ft, 33 dB HL). The comprehension of speech is also influenced by background noise, which ideally should be 10 to 15 dB less than the intensity level of speech, but is often equal to or greater than the level of speech making speech hard to understand.

The typical challenges experienced by a listener with intact peripheral, conductive, and central auditory systems are magnified for individuals who have an impairment at any level in auditory system. Moreover, hearing loss may place an additional burden on children in the early stages of language learning. Young children do not have the same ability as older children and adults to use contextual cues or previous experience to decipher a message, even when the message is clear. Thus, segmenting communication, categorizing it into meaning of units, and acquiring rules may be particularly difficult for a young child with a hearing loss.

HEARING LOSS AND COMMUNICATIION

Having full access to all auditory aspects of the speech signal is the first prerequisite for acquiring spoken language. The second requires supplying the child with abundant and rich caregiver input on which to base the rule system of the native language.

Variables Affecting Communication

Many factors affect the development of a child's communication skills including factors related to the child's hearing status and input from the child's environment. Child-related variables that most affect the development of communication skills include type of loss (e.g., conductive, sensorineural, mixed), degree of hearing loss (e.g., mild, moderate, severe), and laterality (unilateral or bilateral). The configuration of the hearing loss (whether the loss is in the low or high frequencies or across all frequencies) also affects children's communication. Other important variables affecting children's communication include the age of onset of the hearing loss (children who lose their hearing later in the formative years of language learning tend to have better communication skills) and the age of identification of hearing loss (earlier identification of hearing loss often results in earlier intervention and improved communication). In addition, the child's cognitive and emotional abilities also greatly affect a child's communication.

The caregiver-child interaction style is another important factor shown to affect children's communication development. Although it is generally acknowledged that maternal input is important for both typically developing children and children with hearing impairments, there is some controversy concerning how parental language style affects children's communication skills. Several studies have shown that the mothers of children with hearing impairment are more controlling, demanding, use more questions, and use more commands than do caregivers of children with normal hearing (3,4). Yet, other studies indicate that when children with hearing impairments and typically developing children were matched on language level rather than age (most previous studies used age matches) mothers in both groups were similar in their interactional style (5). Further, Marfo (6) suggests that a directive style of interaction may be facilitative for children with disabilities because it helps children focus on the language learning task.

Finally, the type, quality, and onset of auditory habilitation and rehabilitation also greatly affects children's communication skills. Discussion of amplification, cochlear implants, and their effects on language outcomes are discussed in detail in chapters by Sweetow (Chapter 39), Miyamoto (Chapter 40), and Irving and Ruben (Chapter 24) in this book.

Permanent Sensorineural/Conductive Hearing Loss

The extent to which spoken language skills are affected by permanent sensorineural/conductive hearing loss depends on the many factors described in previous sections. If these factors are held constant, it is possible to isolate the potential effects of mild, moderate, moderately severe, severe, and profound hearing loss and unilateral loss. The description offered below of hearing loss categorized by severity reflects the scheme described by Flexor (7). It is important to note that the type and degree of hearing loss do not necessarily predict the level of a child's communication skills. The multiple factors described in the previous section greatly affect development. Further, provision of amplification or a cochlear implant can make a child function like a child with a lessor degree of hearing loss, thereby altering a child's communication skills. Each section below describes a different level of hearing loss, includes a case description of a child, information about the child's communication characteristics, and some implications for classroom functioning. The focus of this discussion is on spoken language; signs are discussed in other chapters (Chapter 48).

Minimal or Slight Hearing Loss

Case History

Sarah is 5 years old and is functioning at a level commensurate with her kindergarten classmates. She has a 25 dB flat sensorineural hearing loss that was diagnosed in a kindergarten hearing screening program. Her parents report that Sarah is less fatigued at the end of school and has better grades since seating accommodations that allow easier access to the teacher's voice were made.

A minimal hearing loss (16–25 dB HL) tends to have a mild impact on a child's communication skills. According to Northern and Downs (8), the child with a minimal hearing loss may have difficult accessing distant speech, following fast-paced conversational exchanges, and hearing morphological markers such past tense and plurals. Although the effects of minimal hearing loss are unclear, Dobie and Berlin (9) stated that a child's hearing sensitivity must be 15 dB or better at all frequencies in both ears for the child to detect the complete signal even at soft conversational levels.

Thus, children with minimal hearing loss usually learn language from conversational input that is typically 20 dB above their threshold (conversational speech is about 45 dB HL). Given this minimal intensity, increased effort is required to maintain attention for learning. With modifications in teaching style resulting in decreased classroom instructional distances and use of classroom sound field amplification or personal listening systems, an efficient learning environment for children with minimal hearing loss can be maintained.

Mild Hearing Loss

Case History

Timothy, is a 3-year-old whose bilateral thresholds slope from 25 dB HL in the low frequencies to 40 dB HL in the high frequencies in both ears. His hearing has been monitored regularly since birth following anoxia. Despite the confirmation at 18 months of a mild hearing loss, he achieved most speech and language milestones within normal limits. Mild gain amplification was recommended and full time use achieved by 2 years of age. His development continues to be monitored every 6 months.

The child with a mild hearing loss (26–40 dB HL) has difficulty hearing faint or distant speech. Vowels sounds are heard clearly, but voiceless consonants are hard to hear. Typically, these students display slight delays in phonological, semantic, and syntactic skills.

School-age students with mild hearing loss have difficulty when functioning in the poor acoustic environment of the regular classroom. Blair, Petersons, and Viehweg (10) demonstrated poorer academic achievement of children with hearing losses less than 40 dB, when compared to their classmates. Their inability to access the complete speech signal compromised academic achievement to the extent that they performed at levels less than expected for their potential. Matkin (11) and Northern and Downs (8) reported that a mild hearing loss left unmanaged may result in academic performance or grade placement at least one grade below same-aged peers.

Moderate Hearing Loss

Case History

> Leah is 6 years old with a bilateral sensorineural hearing loss sloping from 30 dB HL in the low frequencies to 60 dB HL in the high frequencies. Due to her ability to hear the low frequency aspects of speech, this hearing loss was not identified until 4 years at a preschool screening. At that time, it was determined that she had a language delay of approximately 1 year and only fair speech intelligibility. Her parents were initially reluctant to follow through on the recommendation for hearing aids because Leah has been able to "get by" without them.

Children with moderate hearing loss (41–55 dB HL) miss much of the speech signal. Those with loss of 40 to 50 dB miss an average of 62% of the speech signal and those with a 50 dB hearing loss miss 80% to 100% of the signal (12). Communication deficits for children with moderate hearing loss include limited vocabulary, delays in syntax and many speech errors. Poor social adjustment and academic performance.

Since these children can hear loud speech without amplification, the hearing loss may not be noticed until the child enters an organized educational program. As soon as amplification is fitted, many children make dramatic progress, some are able to close the existing gaps in a short time given appropriate input. Children with mild to moderate hearing loss often challenge their caregivers about the need for amplification when they can already hear some of what is being said. Also, parents of this group may find it difficult to insist on full time hearing aid use when they notice that the child can "hear" without them. Thus, this group of children, who could benefit dramatically from wearing amplification, are often the poorest hearing aid users; some of them never achieve full time use.

Moderately Severe Hearing Loss

Case History

> Brandon was 26 months old before seeing an audiologist. Although his mother had reported inconsistent responses to speech as well as delays in learning vocabulary for a full year prior to this time, Brandon was not referred until 2 years of age because "boys often talk late." He readily accepted his binaural ear-level hearing aids and is making excellent progress in achieving age appropriate language skills.

Without amplification, children with moderately severe hearing loss (56–70 dB HL) can hear only very loud speech presented close to the ear. When wearing amplification, they have the capability of detecting and discriminating all aspects of speech at normal conversational levels in quiet. Vocabulary (e.g., use of synonyms, multiple mearnings) syntax, pragmatics, and speech are affected by a moderate hearing loss resulting typically in academic achievement delays of 1 year or more in language-based subjects. The language delays are related to age of identification, full time use of amplification, and early intervention.

Severe Hearing Loss

Case History

> Kevin is 3 years old and has been wearing binaural ear-level hearing aids since his severe hearing loss was identified at 1 year of age. His mother was aware of his lack of auditory responsiveness because she had the comparison of two older children. Kevin was immediately enrolled in an early intervention program that stressed spoken language acquisition through parent guidance. While he still displays considerable communication delays relative to normally hearing peers, Kevin is able to express himself intelligibly to siblings, peers, and adults.

Children with severe hearing loss (71–90 dB HL) have difficulty understanding even loud and amplified speech. Their syntax is delayed and inflexible, their vocabulary restricted, and pragmatic difficulties occur (e.g., frequent interruptions, topic shifts, poor topic maintenance, and failure to adapt to the listener). Speech deficits may include sound omissions, substitutions, and distortions and errors on vowels. Voice quality can be hypernasal, high pitched, have flat intonation, and inaccurate stress (13). In language-based subjects, children show academic delays of 2 or more years.

Children with severe hearing loss are typically identified earlier (i.e., at 12–18 months) than are children with lesser degrees of hearing loss, due to the dramatic effect of hearing loss on their ability to respond to language. The advantage of early identification is counteracted by the lack of auditory input during infancy. For example, the child who is not identified until 1 year of age, must, when amplified, progress through auditory learning that is easily accomplished from birth to 1 year but is much more difficult when the child is 12 to 18 months of age. For children with a severe hearing loss (and for those with profound loss), caregiver input becomes critical to their achievement. This requires that caregivers capitalize as much as possible on all language-learning aspects of daily activities.

Profound Hearing Loss

Case History

> Ryan, age 3, has a congenital profound bilateral hearing loss which was diagnosed at 1 year of age. Once it was determined that Ryan was able to access some of the speech signal through his superpower post-auricular hearing aids, his parents decided to concentrate on the acquisition of spoken language on a 6-month trial. If, at the end of that time, Ryan had not made progress toward understanding and using words, they would reevaluate their choice and consider other communication modalities (total communication or cued speech) and amplification options (cochlear implant). At age 3 Ryan has a large repertoire of single words and is generating word combinations. His parents are investigating a cochlear implant for the purpose of increasing the amount of speech input Ryan could potentially receive.

Fewer children with profound hearing loss (110+ dB HL), compared to the other categories of hearing loss, achieve intelligible speech. When spoken language is chosen as the primary communication modality, it is frequently characterized by poor speech intelligibility and severe delays in syntax, semantics, and pragmatics. This then results in poor achievement in language-based subjects.

There is a subgroup of profoundly hearing impaired individuals who do develop intelligible speech, age-appropriate spoken language skills, and are high achievers in regular class environments. There are several factors which characterize these children. First, they have families, teachers, and other caregivers who are committed to maximizing the child's residual hearing through amplification. Second, hearing aids are used consistently and function optimally and frequency modulation (FM) listening devices are used regularly to improve the quality of the speakers voice. When maximum audibility can not be obtained through traditional amplification, cochlear implants are considered. Third, children are placed in rehabilitation/educational programs that have high expectations and children are in communicative environments in which speech is expected and used. When these approaches are coupled with early identification, children with profound hearing loss often become effective spoken language communicators.

Unilateral Hearing Loss

A child with unilateral hearing loss has one ear with normal hearing sensitivity and the other with at least a mild permanent hearing loss (any degree).

Case History

> Megan is a 4½-year-old with a recently identified 60 dB hearing loss in her right ear. Her left ear tested within normal limits. Megan was referred for audiologic testing by her preschool teacher who noted Megan's lack of responsiveness in large group instructional settings, on the playground, and in the gym. Seating accommodations and attention to the acoustics of the learning environment have resulted in Megan's increased level of attention in these difficult listening situations.

For the student with unilateral hearing loss, audibility is compromised by the masking effects of noise rather than loudness of the speech signal. In quiet, it is possible to attend to the speaker by orienting the unimpaired ear toward the source of sound. When noise is present, noise competes with speech for prominence in the normally hearing ear. If listening takes place in continually noisy environment, one may see an effect on social (withdrawal) and academic (not achieving to potential) areas (14). Early identification is critical so that extra vigilance can be applied to maintain normal hearing in the unimpaired ear.

Otitis Media, Fluctuating Hearing Loss, and Communication Development

The hearing loss associated with chronic otitis media with effusion (OME) is a special case of conductive hearing loss. Because OME is so prevalent in young children, the auditory consequences of OME have become an important consideration for otolaryngologists and other heath-care professionals. Yet, the research basis for understanding the consequences of OME is often contradictory. By way of illustration, we present a fairly common situation with a discussion of why there is no straight-forward rationale for the options.

Case History

> David is 2 years old and has had chronic otitis media for 4 months. A hearing test indicated a mild hearing loss. He has begun to use some words communicatively, but his rate of language development appears to be behind that of the other children in his childcare center. His doctor has recommended that he have pressure-equalizing tympanostomy tubes placed in his ears. His parents cannot decide whether David should have tubes. They want to know whether the fluid in his ear is affecting his speech and language and will continue to affect later developing skills.

Unlike sensorineural hearing loss, conductive hearing loss secondary to OME, is often fluctuating. Thus, it is not surprising there is no one-to-one correspondence between OME, hearing loss, and communication development. Studies that have examined the relationship between persistent OME in early childhood and later speech and language skills have shown mixed findings. Several have found a relationship (15–19), but others have not found a relationship between an early history of OME and later communication outcomes (1,20,21,22). It is important to note that in each of these studies the middle-ear status of the children was prospectively documented using accepted techniques of pneumatic otoscopy, tympanometry, or both. However, except for two studies (15,21) the hearing status of children was not always considered. That is, it was not uniformly known whether children had experienced a hearing loss. The importance of this is illustrated by considering the models linking OME and speech–language impairments.

Several hypothesized causal mechanisms have been offered to explain the relationship between persistent or recurrent OME during early childhood and the development of speech and language. Such hypotheses are not mutually exclusive and none has been unequivocally endorsed by research.

A child with OME may experience a mild to moderate fluctuating hearing loss and thus receive a partial or inconsistent auditory signal (see Chapter 7 by Gravel for a discussion of hearing loss occurring with OME). Persistent (prolonged) or frequent (and varied) disruptions in auditory input may impede discrimination and processing of speech. Certain sounds (e.g., *t, k, s, sh*), unstressed syllables (e.g., *ba* in banana), final consonants (e.g., *t* in hat) are brief, have low intensity and are difficult to hear. Further, morphological markers (e.g., *s* to mark plurality or possessive) and short words (*is, the*), which are spoken rapidly and are of brief duration, don't carry much meaning. Stress and patterns of intonations that carry subtle nuances of language (e.g., questions) may also be difficult to perceive. As a result of the partial or distorted auditory input, the child may encode information incompletely and inaccurately into the database from which speech and language develop. In many ways, the hearing loss typical of children with a conductive loss is similar to that of children with mild to moderate sensorineural losses, except that the loss fluctuates.

In a computer simulation of the hearing losses common to those experienced during OME, Dobie and Berlin (9) found such patterns evident in adults listeners. Thus, given that the ability to discriminate speech is a precursor to the development of later speech and language development, even mild hearing losses associated with OME may place infants at a distinct disadvantage for recognizing, comprehending, and then producing speech and language during the developmental years. In fact, Nozza (23) suggested that because infants have a developmental requirement for a greater stimulus intensity before being able to discriminate speech, even a mild hearing loss has a profound effect on their speech processing abilities.

Another model also hypothesizes auditory effects of recurrent and persistent OME but suggests that mechanisms other than hearing may be effected. This model suggests that prolonged or frequent OME could lead to problems in attending to auditory-based communication. Children may experience frequent changes in the intensity of signals, learn to tune out, and therefore develop attention difficulties specifically to auditory-based information. A few studies have found results compatible with this model. Feagans, Kipp, and Blood (24) found that the percentage of time toddlers had otitis media was associated with nonattentional behaviors during a language-based task (i.e., book reading). Gravel and Wallace (25) found that preschoolers with positive histories of early otitis media performed more poorly than did preschoolers without histories of early otitis media when listening to sentence material in the presence of background competition. Roberts et al. (26) and Roberts, Burchinal, and Campbell (27) found that children with a history of OME during early childhood were described by their teachers in elementary school as being less attentive, receiving less talk and being more dependent compared to children who did not have history of otitis media. In all of these studies, no differences were found in global measures of language development as a function of otitis media.

There is another model in which the effects of OME do not involve the auditory system. Rather, the illness associated with OME (i.e., the stuffy congested feeling and general malaise) may affect the child's interactions in the environment such that the child has fewer opportunities to establish the knowledge base from which speech and language develop. Although there has been some research that has found that interactions between children and their caregivers are affected as a function of OME (21), others have shown that the language of parents with otitis-prone children did not differ from the language of parents with otitis-free children (28). Moreover, the illness hypothesis itself has not been tested, and because OME is often "silent" (few observable manifestations such as a runny nose or fever), this explanation is probably not sufficient.

Because findings relating OME and communicative outcomes have not reached a consensus, the nature of the relationship continues to be controversial (2,29,30). However, it is clear that to adequately examine this issue, more attention needs to be directed toward the mediating role of hearing.

CONCLUSIONS

For all children, hearing plays a critical role in the development of speech and language. The effects of permanent sensorineural hearing loss on speech and language development can be considerable, depending on the degree of hearing loss and other child and environmental factors. Although the effects of otitis media on children's speech and language are controversial, for some children frequent episodes of chronic otitis media and associated hearing loss may affect later development.

Identifying the type and degree of hearing loss as early as possible is essential. Regardless of the type of hearing loss, it is important to inform parents and caregivers about how hearing loss can potentially affect the development of communication skills. Parents and caregivers should be informed about modification in the environment and in their own interaction skills to minimize the impact of hearing loss on speech and language development.

For children with permanent sensorineural hearing loss, the importance of early intervention and use of amplification or other assistive listening devices is without question. Whether a child is taught oral or manual instruction using signs, total communication, simultaneous speech and signs, or speech only depend on the most appropriate modality for the child and the wishes of the family (see Chapter 24 by Irving and Ruben for further discussion of these issues). Amplification devices such as hearing aids and FM units should also be adapted to needs of each child and family. Cochlear implants are an option for children with profound sensorineural hearing loss after traditional amplification has been deemed ineffective. For more information about management of sensorineural hearing loss, see Flexor (7) and Northern and Downs (8).

For a child with a conductive hearing loss due to chronic otitis media, hearing should be monitored. Modifications made to improve the listening environment can also be helpful. Recent guidelines published on management of middle ear fluid recommend that children's hearing be tested after 3 months of middle-ear fluid (2). For more details about management of otitis media in young children, see Stool et al. (2), Roberts and Medley (31), and Roberts and Wallace (32).

Many health-care professionals deal with management of young children with hearing impairment. Pediatricians, family physicians, and nurses may screen hearing and speech and language. Children should be referred to an audiologist when there are concerns about hearing, so they may undergo audiological testing, and when decisions need to be made about habilitation and rehabilitation. It must be emphasized that hearing can be reliably assessed even in newborns. A child should be referred to a speech-language pathologist when there are concerns about a child's speech and language development (see Figure 1 for milestones that children should achieve at early ages).

In summary, it is essential that all children with hearing loss receive a solid foundation for communication development. Knowledge by health-care professionals and caregivers of speech and language milestones as well as options for treatment are essential. Regardless of the type and degree of hearing loss, every child should be individually assessed and, when appropriate, have an intervention program implemented.

ACKNOWLEDGMENTS

Supported by Maternal and Child Health Program (MCJ-370599 and MCJ-370649, Title V, Social Security Act), Health Resources and Services Administration, U.S. Department of Health and Human Services.

REFERENCES

1. Roberts JE, Burchinal MR, Davis BP, Collier AM, Henderson FW. Otitis media in early childhood and later language. *J Speech Hear Res* 1991;34: 1158–1168.
2. Stool SE, Berg AO, Berman S, Carney CJ, Cooley JR, Culpepper L, et al. Otitis media with effusion in young children. Rockville, MD: U.S. Department of Health and Human Services; 1994. Clinical Practice Guideline, no 12. AHCPR publication no. 94-0622.
3. Heggeler SW, Watson SM, Cooper PF. Verbal and nonverbal maternal controls in hearing mother-deaf child interaction. *J App Dev Psychol* 1984; 5:319–329.
4. Meadow KP. *Deafness and child development.* Berkeley: University of California Press; 1980.
5. White SJ, White REC. The deaf imperative: Characteristics of maternal input to hearing-impaired children. *Top Lang Disord* 1984;4:38–49.
6. Marfo K. Correlates of maternal directiveness with children who are developmentally delayed. *Am J Orthopsychiatry* 1992;62:219–233.
7. Flexor, C. *Facilitating hearing and listening in young children.* San Diego: Singular Publishing Group; 1994.
8. Northern JL, Downs MP. *Hearing in children* 4th ed. JP Butler, ed. Baltimore: Williams & Wilkins; 1991.
9. Dobie R, Berlin C. Influence of otitis media on hearing and development. *Ann Otol Rhino Laryngol* 1978;88:46–53.
10. Blair JC, Peterson MD, Viehweg SH. The effect of mild hearing loss on academic performance of young school-age children. *Volta Rev* 1985;87:87–93.
11. Matkin N. Amplification for children: current status and future priorities. In: Bess F, Freeman B, Sinclair J, eds. *Amplification in Education.* Washington, DC: Alexander Graham Bell Association for the Deaf; 1981.
12. Mueller JG, Killion MC. An easy method for calculating the articulation index. *Hear J* 1990;43:14–22.
13. Monson RB. General effects of deafness on phonation and articulation. In Hochberg I, Levitt H, Osberger MJ, eds. *Speech of the hearing impaired.* Baltimore: University Park Press; 1983:23–34.
14. Bess F, Klee T, Culbertson J. Identification, assessment and management of children with unilateral sensori-neural hearing loss. *Ear Hear* 1986;7:43–51.
15. Friel-Patti S, Finitzo-Hieber T. Language learning in a prospective study of otitis media with effusion in the first two years of life. *J Speech Hear Res* 1990;33:188–194.
16. Teele DW, Klein JO, Rosner BA, The Greater Boston Otitis Media Study Group. Otitis media with effusion during the first three years of life and development of speech and language. *Pediatr* 1984;74: 282–287.
17. Teele DW, Klein JO, Chase C, et al., and the Greater Boston Otitis Media Study Group. Otitis media in infancy and intellectual ability school achievement, speech and language at age 7 years. *J Infect Dis* 1990;162:685–694.
18. Wallace IF, Gravel JS, McCarton CM, Stapells DR, Bernstein RA, Ruben RJ. Otitis media, auditory sensitivity and language outcomes at 1 year. *Laryngoscope* 1988;98:64–70.
19. Roberts JE, Burchinal MR, Koch MA, Footo MM, Henderson FW. Otitis media in early childhood and its relationship to later phonological development. *J Speech Hear Disord* 1988;53:424–432.
20. Lous J, Fiellau-Nikolajsen, Jeppesen AL. Secretory otitis media and language development: a six-year follow-up study with case-control. *Int J Pediatr Otorhinolaryngol* 1988;15:185–203.
21. Roberts JE, Burchinal MR, Medley LP, Zeisel SA, Mundy M, Roush J, et al. Otitis media, hearing sensitivity, and maternal responsiveness in relation to language during infancy. *J Pediatr* 1995;126:481–489.
22. Wright PF, Sell SH, McConnell KB. Impact of recurrent otitis media on middle ear function, hearing, and language. *J Pediatr* 1988;113: 581–587.
23. Nozza RJ. Auditory deficit in infants with otitis media with effusion: More than a mild hearing loss. In: Lim DJ, Bluestone CD, Klein JO, Nelson JD, eds. *Recent Advances in Otitis Media* Proceedings of the fourth international symposium. Toronto: BC Decker; 1988:376–379.
24. Feagans LV, Kipp E, Blood I. The effects of otitis media on the attention skills of day-care-attending toddlers. *Dev Psychol* 1994;30:701–708.
25. Gravel JS, Wallace IF. Listening and language at 4 years of age: effect of early otitis media. *J Speech Hear Res* 1992;35:588–595.
26. Roberts JE, Burchinal MR, Collier AM, Ramey CT, Koch MA, Henderson FW. Otitis media in early childhood and cognitive, academic, and classroom performance in the school-aged child. *Pediatrics* 1989;83: 477–485.
27. Roberts JE, Burchinal MR, Campbell F. Otitis media in early childhood and patterns of intellectual development and later academic performance. *J Pediatr Psychol* 1994;19:347–366.
28. Wallace IF, Gravel JS, Schwartz RG, Ruben RJ. Otitis media, caregiver communication style of primary caregivers, and language skills of 2-year olds: A preliminary report. *J Dev Behav Pediatr* 1996;17:22–35.
29. Paradise JL, Rogers KD. On otitis media, child development, and tympanostomy tubes: new answers or old questions? *Pediatrics* 1986;77: 88–92.
30. Ruben RJ, Dagger-Sjoback D, Chase C, Feagans LV, Friel-Patti S, Gravel JS, et al. Complications and sequelae. *Ann of Otol Rhino Laryngol* 1994;103 (164, P2).
31. Roberts JE, Medley L. Otitis media and speech-language sequelae in young children: current issues in management. *Am J Speech Language Pathol* 1995;4:15–24.
32. Roberts JE, Wallace IF. Language and otitis media. In: Roberts JE, Wallace IF, Henderson FW, eds. *Otitis media, language and learning in young children.* Baltimore: Brookes 1997;133–161.
33. Davis J. Performance of young hearing impaired children on a test of basic concepts. *Speech Hear Res* 1974;17:342–351.
34. Davis J. *Our forgotten children: hard of hearing pupils in school* (2nd ed.). Washington, DC: Self Help for the Hard of Hearing; 1990.

CHAPTER 5

Molecular Genetics

A Brief Overview

Anil K. Lalwani, Eric Lynch, and Anand N. Mhatre

Rapid progress in the fields of molecular biology and molecular genetics has added a new dimension to analysis of human disease. Previously, understanding the genetic etiology of disease required knowledge of its biochemical basis. This requirement precluded deciphering the genetic basis of a variety of disorders, hearing disorders in particular, to biochemical analysis of their pathology. Development of powerful analytical techniques, such as the polymerase chain reaction (PCR), and the concomitant development of a number of critical resources, including the "linkage map" of the human genome, have led to a more direct, rapid, and powerful means of studying the genetic etiology of a variety of human diseases, independent of any prior knowledge of their biochemical basis. Identification of disease-causing genes through molecular–genetic approaches and their subsequent characterization are essential for understanding pathophysiology of the disease and for development of appropriate therapeutic intervention(s).

This brief review has a twofold purpose:

1. To outline the principles of inheritance of a disease phenotype through review of mendelian genetics and its extensions
2. To describe principles and methodologies used for localizing and identifying disease genes via genetic linkage analysis and physical mapping studies, respectively.

The descriptions of these principles and their applications will be illustrated using examples from genetic analysis of syndromic and nonsyndromic hearing disorders.

A.K. Lalwani and A.N. Mhatre: Department of Otolaryngology—Head and Neck Surgery, University of California, San Francisco, California 94143.
E. Lynch: Department of Medicine and Genetics, University of Washington, Seattle, Washington 98195.

CONSTITUTION OF THE HUMAN GENOME

The Nuclear Genome

The eukaryotic genome exists in association with proteins or histones in a highly ordered structure. This DNA–protein complex is also known as chromatin. The chromosomes represent a highly condensed form of chromatin that is present following DNA replication and preceding cell division. The highly condensed organization of the DNA within the chromosomes is necessitated by size constraint—the need to pack a relatively long DNA strand within a relatively small nucleus. The human genome, 3×10^9 bp in size, represents a physical distance of approximately 2 m in length, while the nucleus is approximately 0.06 μm in diameter. Hence, the DNA is condensed extensively to meet its size constraint. A schematic of the hierarchical structural organization of DNA is illustrated in Fig. 1. The beadlike units of the chromatin are called nucleosomes. The nucleosome is composed of several different types of histones with DNA wrapped around them. This structural unit is refolded on itself to yield the highly condensed chromosomes.

The nucleated human cell contains 23 pairs of chromosomes. Each chromosome pair in its condensed form (observed during the metaphase stage of the cell cycle) can be distinguished from all other pairs by size, location of the centromere, and its banding pattern when subjected to a particular stain (e.g., the Giemsa stain). Figure 2, panel A, illustrates a photograph or digitized image of Giemsa-stained metaphase chromosomes that yield distinct yet reproducible banding patterns in each of the chromosome pairs. These chromosome-specific banding patterns can be used to determine the presence of gross structural abnormalities or chromosomal aneuploidies within the individual's karyotype (chromosome pairs arranged in a standardized format). Fig-

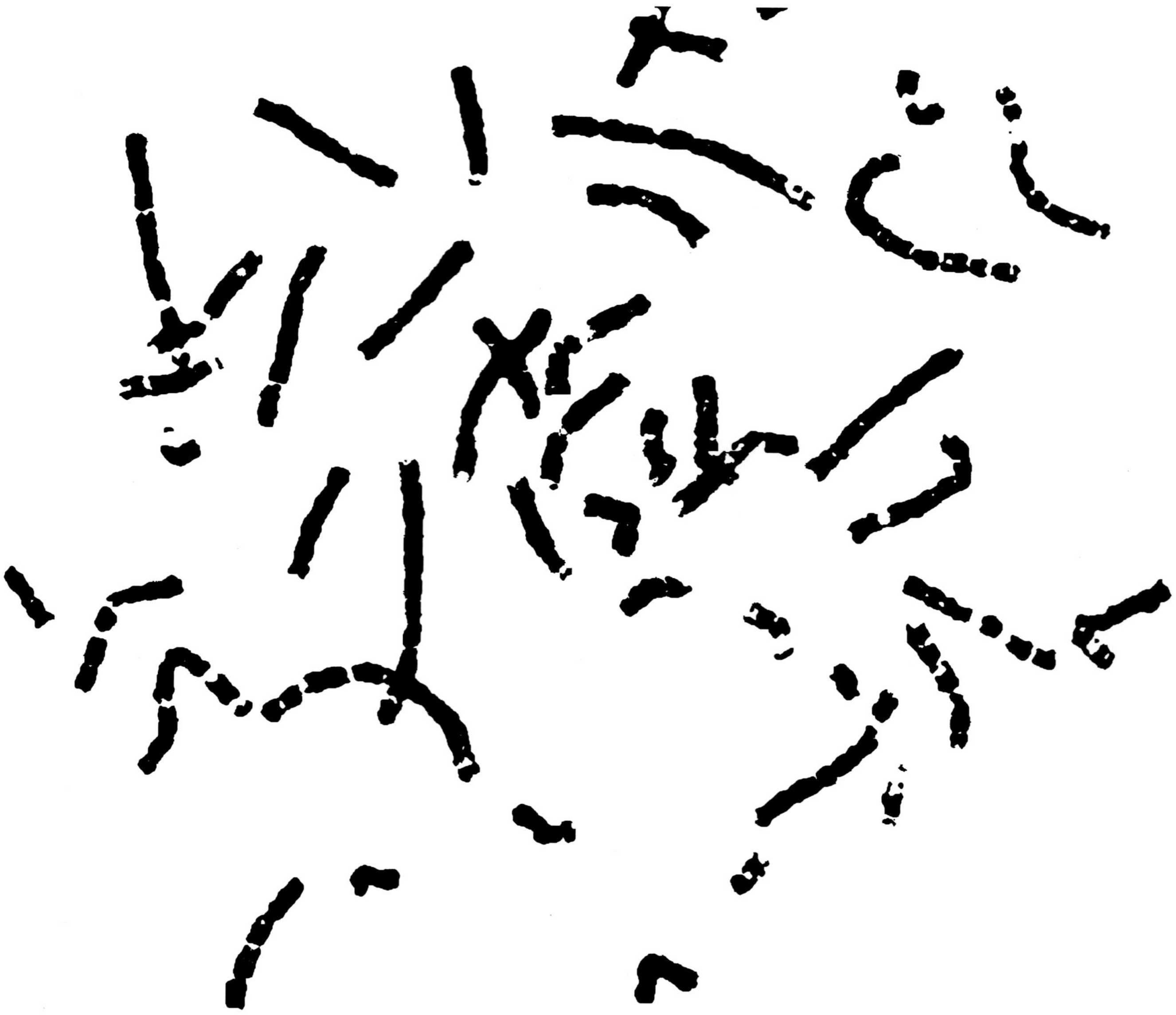

FIG. 1. Constitution of the Human Genome. **A:** Photomicrograph of Giesma stained human chromosomes in metaphase. Peripheral blood lymphocytes arrested in metaphase and stained with Giesma. A photomicrograph of these chromosomes can then be subsequently used for the preparation of the karyotype where the individual chromosomes are paired and arranged. The karyotype serves to assess the constitutional and structural integrity of the chromosomes from their numbers and banding patterns.

ure 2, panel B, illustrates the ideogram of a complete set of 24 human chromosomes. Their band designations are delineated to the left of each chromosome.

In a karyotype, images of the autosomal chromosome pairs are arranged in decreasing size and numbered from 1 to 20. The nomenclature for chromosomes 21 and 22 strays from this trend, with chromosome 21 being slightly smaller than chromosome 22, a subtle size difference that was not readily recognized during the early days of cytogenetics. The remaining pair of chromosomes are referred to as the sex chromosomes and are designated X and Y. The nucleated somatic cells in our bodies have two sets of the autosomes and the sex chromosomes, each set inherited or acquired from the parents of the individual. Females (46, XX) have a pair of X chromosomes, so they are diploid for the X chromosome, while males (46, XY) have only one X chromosome and are haploid for the X chromosome as they are for their single Y chromosome Each chromosome contains two arms, the "p" (or petite) arm and the longer "q" arm, which are separated by the centromere. The banding patterns for each chromosome have been characterized and are numbered in accordance with the standards set by the International Society for Cytogenetics Nomenclature.

The banding pattern of the chromosomes reflects the gross

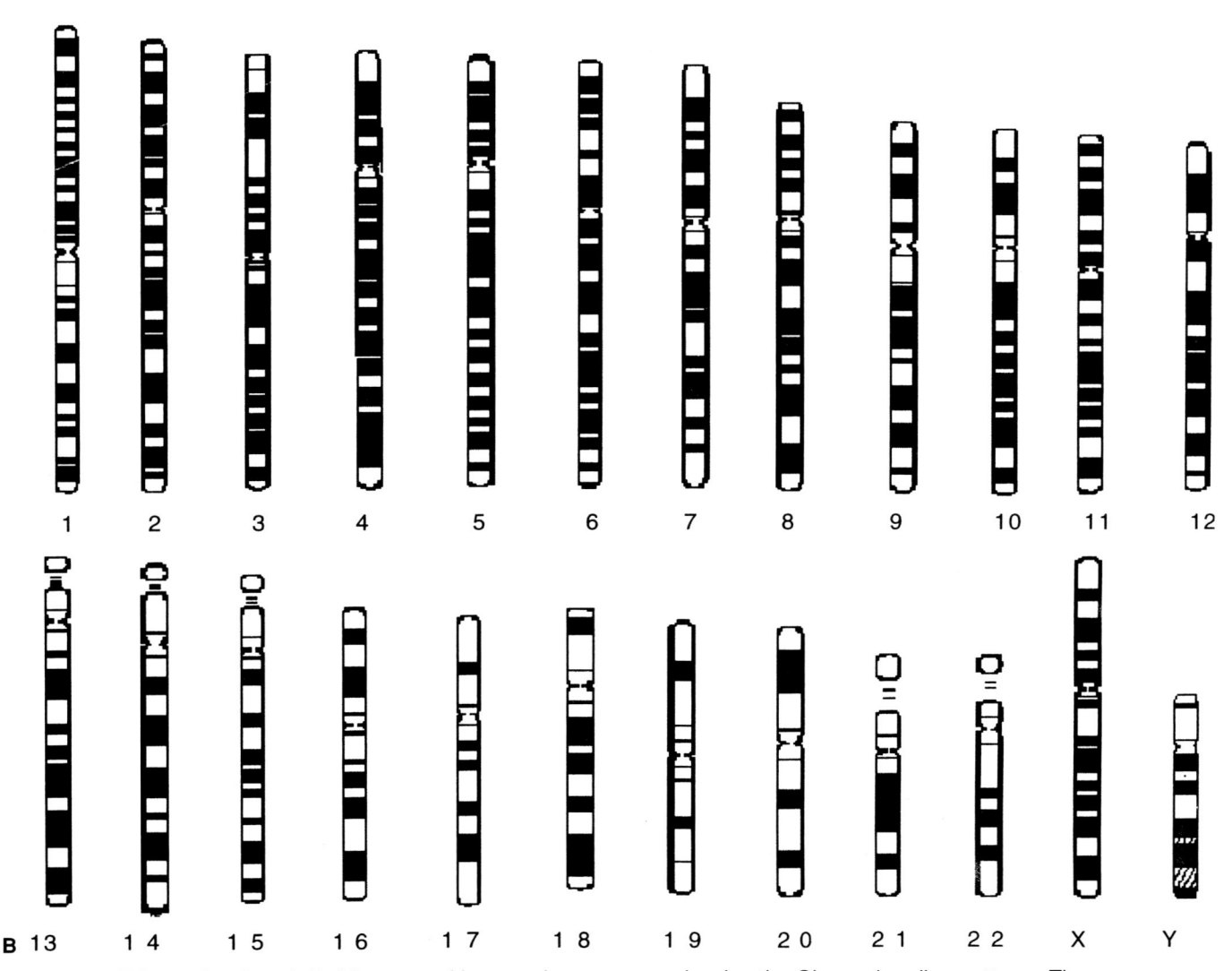

FIG. 1. *Continued.* **B:** Ideogram of human chromosomes showing the Giesma banding patterns. The chromosomes are arranged and numbered according to the Paris classification of 1971.

structural organization and characteristics of the chromatin (1). The chromatin may be divided into two distinct states: euchromatin and heterochromatin. These two states reflect the degree of compression or condensation of the chromatin. The heterochromatin region remains compressed or highly condensed throughout the cell cycle, replicates late, and is considered to contain repetitive noncoding sequences. The major heterochromatic region is adjacent to the centromere, while smaller blocks are located near the ends of the chromosome arms, called the telomeres, and also interspersed within the euchromatin. It is estimated that greater than 95% of the genome represents a noncoding sequence. In comparison, the euchromatin regions are relatively decondensed in the interstate (the state that precedes DNA synthesis), replicate early in the cell cycle, and are considered to contain expressed sequences or genes. The coding sequence, less than 5% of the total genome, is estimated to encode 100,000 genes (2), whose integrity is vital to health and well being.

The study of mutations causing human disease began with the study of chromosomes and chromosomal aneuploidies (aberration from the normal diploid constitution) in the late 1950s with the identification of abnormal chromosome numbers and relatively few structural aberrations. Syndromes such as Down (trisomy 21, 47XX-21 or 47XY-21) and Klinefelter's (47XXY) were recognized long before the chromosomal abnormalities associated with them were identified. It was almost fifteen years after the publication of a paper characterizing Down syndrome, which now bears his name, that data was presented in 1959 supporting the correlation of Down syndrome with the inheritance of an extra chromosome 21.

Chromosome banding techniques began in the 1970s and allowed researchers a much more refined level of analysis of the chromosomes. Shortly after the introduction of chromosome banding to cytogenetics, a large number of chromosomal rearrangements were discovered, including deletions,

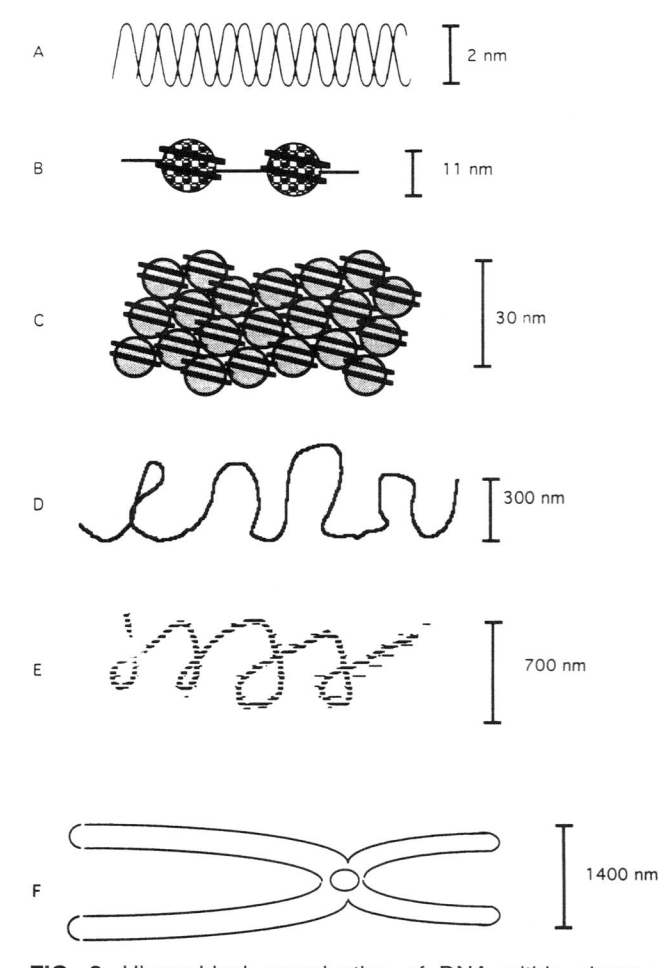

FIG. 2. Hierarchical organization of DNA within chromosomes. A schematic of the structural organization of DNA **A:** within various stages of condensation or packaging, from nucleosomes to chromosomes. These organizational structures contribute both functionally as well as structurally by regulating gene expression and facilitating division and transmission of the enormous length of genomic DNA. The nucleosome structure **B:** consisting of histones, positively charged proteins, around which DNA is wrapped, represents the first level of packaging. This is followed by further coiling of the DNA-protein complex **C–E:** that ultimately yields the highly condensed DNA that is present within the metaphase chromosome **F**. The approximate width of each of the structural units is also indicated in the figure.

translocations, and inversions. Prior to chromosome banding, researchers had to identify these rearrangements on the basis of an increased or decreased length of the chromosome arm(s) involved. With the aid of banding techniques, subtle changes in the structure and/or content of the chromosomes in a karyotype could be identified.

More recently, in the late 1980s and early 1990s, techniques for more refined analysis of chromosomes have been developed that utilize the staining patterns of the less condensed prometaphase chromosomes. These refinements in the banding techniques have helped to identify relatively subtle chromosomal alterations and thus localize the disease locus. Employing such techniques, an inversion spanning a relatively small region was identified at the telomeric end of chromosome 2 in an individual with Waardenburg type I syndrome. This rare de novo inversion, 2q35-q37, is illustrated in Fig. 3, panel A (3). Identification of this inversion contributed toward localizing the disease locus and subsequently the responsible gene, PAX-3. In Norrie's disease a reciprocal translocation at t(X;10)(p11;p14) was noted in a female infant exhibiting typical clinical and histopathologic features of vitreoretinal dysplasia, while her siblings and parents had normal karyotypes (4). This karyotype analysis, illustrated in Fig. 3 (panel B) suggested that the Norrie's disease locus may be on Xp and band Xp11. This rare de novo translocation assisted in the eventual cloning of the responsible gene by acting as a reference point to refine the map position of the suspect gene. Norrie's Disease Protein (NDP) was subsequently cloned using positional cloning techniques by Berger et al. (5); its function is under investigation.

Chromosomal analysis at high resolution is generally performed on patients with multiple phenotypic abnormalities, because these may be caused by a number of genes being disrupted or lost at once. This is often the case in chromosomal deletions and translocations. Patients with marked developmental or psychological deficiencies are also excellent candidates for chromosomal analysis because their phenotype is consistant with the presance of a gross genetic imbalance resulting from chromosomal abnormalities. Identification of chromosomal breakpoints through karyotypic analysis can greatly accelerate the mapping and cloning of the gene or genes causing the observed phenotype.

The Mitochondrial (Extranuclear) Genome

An additional source of genetic material resides within each mitochondria of nucleated somatic cells. There are several hundred mitochondria in each somatic cell, and all are strictly inherited through the maternal lineage. Each mitochondria contains a small circular chromosome that encodes for approximately 5% of the total gene products required for proper mitochondrial function. The remainder of the proteins used by mitochondria are encoded by genes on nuclear chromosomes. A human mitochondrial chromosome contains 16,569 bp of DNA (6) and is not observable by standard cytogenetic techniques. Mutations of mitochondrial DNA have been identified in various human diseases (7). Deficiencies or DNA mutations in the mitochondrial genome have been shown to play a role in several forms of inherited and acquired hearing loss. The mitochondrial-associated mutations are described in the following sections.

COMPOSITION AND STRUCTURE OF DNA

The DNA in each chromosome in human cells generally exists as a long double-stranded right-handed helix formed by a series of repeating deoxyribonucleotides. Each deoxyribonucleotide is comprised of a five-carbon sugar ring with a hydroxyl group covalently bound to the 3′ carbon atom, a phosphate group covalently bound to the 5′ carbon atom, and one of four bases—guanine, adenine, thymine, or cytosine—covalently bound to the 2′ carbon atom of the deoxyribose sugar ring. The deoxyribonuclotides of a single strand of DNA are bound together in a long unbranched polymer by a series of phosphodiester bonds between the sugar and phosphate groups to form the backbone of the long DNA molecule. Information encoded by DNA is contained in a specific order of four DNA nucleotide bases in a single strand.

The two DNA strands of the double helix are held together by hydrogen bonds with an adenine base on one strand always hydrogen bonding to a thymine base on the opposite strand or a guanine base on one strand always hydrogen bonding to a cytosine base on the other strand. The specificity of base pairing allows for a single DNA strand to act as the template for synthesis of another strand with a complementary sequence. Bonds holding two DNA strands together are relatively weak hydrogen bonds that can be easily broken and reformed without disrupting the covalent bonds holding each strand together. This feature in conjunction with the

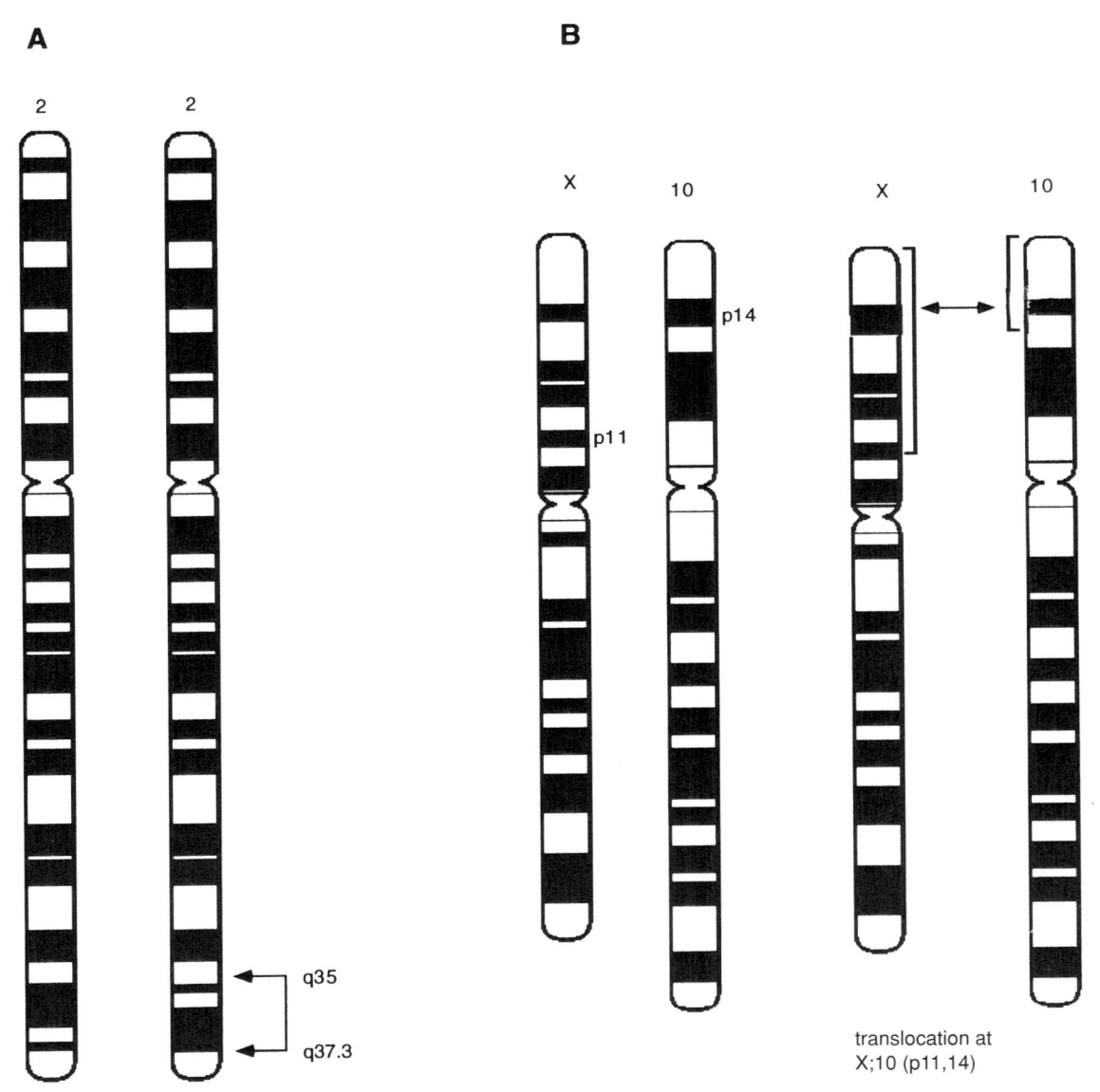

FIG. 3. Chromosomal abnormalities identified via the karyotype. **A:** Ideogram of the human chromosome two from an individual with the Waardenberg's syndrome. Analysis of the banding patterns illustrates an inversion at the telomeric end of the q arm in one of the two homologues of chromosome 2 in an individual with Waardenberg's syndrome. Detection of this chromosomal abnormality contributed towards the determination of the Waardenberg locus. **B:** Ideogram of chromosomes X and 10 from an affected female with Norrie disease. A reciprocal translocation (exchange of fragments) between telomeric regions of the short arms of chromosomes X and 10 was identified in this individual. This reciprocal translocation is designated as t(X;10)(p11;p14).

base pairing rules allows for the opening up of DNA double helix and enzymatic replication of each DNA strand by proteins encoded within the genome. Each strand acts as the template for the synthesis of a new strand with a complementary sequence—a process referred to as semiconservative replication.

Each strand of DNA has an orientation that is defined by position of the deoxyribose ring of each nucleotide and the 5′–3′ phosphodiester bond that is formed between two adjacent nucleotides. A two-dimensional representation of the double-stranded DNA is illustrated in Fig. 4, panel A. The two strands of DNA in a double helix are arranged in an antiparallel direction with the 5′ end on one strand being opposite the 3′ end of the other strand. In general, there are approximately 10 bp per turn of the DNA helix. A three-dimensional helical structure of DNA is illustrated in panel B of Fig. 4. As a double-helical molecule, the two strands of DNA are arranged such that the sugar phosphate backbone forms the rails of a right-handed turning ladder, while the bases are facing each other, allowing the hydrogen bonds to form between the complementary bases (guanine to cytosine and adenine to thymine).

BIOLOGY OF GENE EXPRESSION

Replication

During DNA replication in a living cell, the hydrogen bonds between the two DNA strands are enzymatically broken in a localized manner, creating what is known as a replication bubble. Free nucleotides are then paired with the complementary nucleotide on each of the DNA strands by replicating enzymes present in the cell, known as DNA polymerases. A schematic of the replication process is illustrated in Fig. 5. In synthesizing new polymers of DNA, bases are added to the unbound 3′ hydroxyl group at the 3′ end of a growing DNA strand. Thus a growing strand of DNA is extended in the 5′ to 3′ direction. There are many origins of replication present on each of the very long DNA strands and when one section of replicating DNA comes into contact with an adjacent section, the two are covalently bound together by enzymes known as DNA ligases in order to form a single long chain of DNA. The multiple replication origins ensure a rapid synthesis of the entire genome. When the entire chromosome has been replicated, each of the two original DNA strands has a newly synthesized complementary strand. DNA replication occurs prior to cell division or mitosis but does not occur in cells that are not dividing. The combination of highly specialized enzymes and the ability to proofread during the synthesis of a new strand of DNA make this a remarkably reliable process. The integrity of the genome in nondividing cells is also maintained using a host of scanning, editing, and repair enzymes. The double-stranded nature of DNA helps to ensure that a mutation in one strand will be rapidly detected and repaired by the cell.

Transcription

The information encoded by the DNA double helix in the form of a string of the bases guanine, adenine, cytosine and thymine, is transcribed into RNA in a manner similar to that of the DNA replication. Although DNA and RNA appear chemically similar (both composed of a long unbranched polymer consisting of a series of four nucleic acids), there are two distinct differences between them. In RNA, the sugar portion of the molecule has a hydroxyl group (OH) on the 2′ carbon. In DNA, the 2′ hydroxyl group is missing from the sugar group. In addition, the base thymine used in DNA synthesis is substituted by the base uracil. For RNA transcription to occur, a DNA-binding enzyme recognizes a specific sequence of DNA bases on the chromosome and causes the two strands of DNA to unwind. This allows RNA polymerase to bind to a specific DNA sequence, called a promoter, and subsequently synthesize an RNA copy of one strand of the DNA region. A schematic of the transcription process is illustrated in Fig. 6.

The mechanisms controlling recognition and attachment of RNA polymerase to the starting point of a gene are critical determinants of the pattern of gene expression in a cell. For example, specific DNA-binding proteins, known as transcription factors, can attach to a promoter region upstream from the starting point of the gene. Depending on the type of transcription factor, this may either promote or inhibit binding of the RNA polymerase and subsequent transcription. Similarly, other upstream regions, known as enhancer or repressor sites, can also influence transcriptional activity. Thus, cellular identity and its function is an expression of the repertoire of its transcribed genes.

There are three RNA polymerases active in nucleated cells. All transcribe DNA to RNA using only a single strand of the DNA as a template. This strand is known as the sense strand. The direction of growth is 5′ to 3′, with newly attached nucleotides found at the 3′ end. RNA polymerase type I is responsible for the transcription of precursor ribosomal RNA (rRNA) only. The pre-rRNA molecules are then processed by the cell into rRNA molecules, which are then integrated into the construction of new ribosomal complexes. RNA polymerases II and III are responsible for the transcription of many different genes with a variety of gene products. The distinguishing feature between these two RNA polymerases is that RNA polymerase III is responsible for the transcription of all transfer RNAs (tRNAs). The tRNAs are subsequently linked with an amino acid via an enzyme, aminoacyl synthetase, thus preparing them for their role as the "translators" of genetic information.

RNA polymerase II does not transcribe the tRNA genes or the rRNA genes, but it does act as the major transcriptional polymerase for the class of RNAs known as messenger RNAs (mRNAs). The mRNA transcribed for the majority of protein-encoding genes in mammals and other higher organisms is generally precursor mRNA, or pre-mRNA. Pre-mRNA contains both exons (the expressed regions of

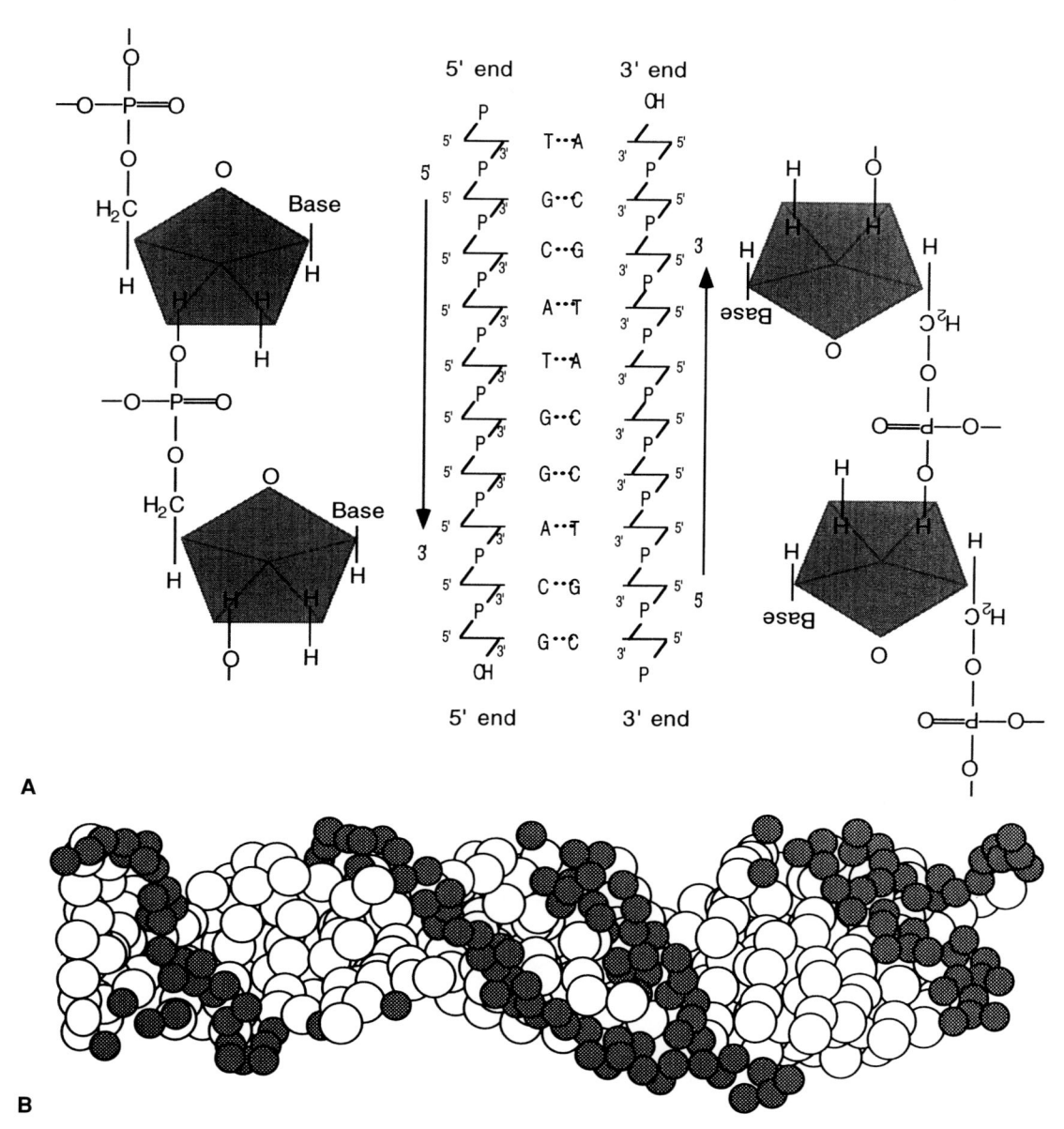

FIG. 4. The double stranded deoxyribonucleic acid (DNA). **A:** A two dimensional representation of a segment of double stranded DNA. DNA is comprised of a linear series of nucleotides (deoxyadenosine—A, deoxythymidine—T, deoxycytidine—C, deoxyguanosine—G) which all have the same basic structure comprised of a heterocyclic ring of carbon and nitrogen atoms, a five carbon pentose sugar, and a phosphate group. The nucleotides in DNA are joined by phosphodiester linkages, which are covalent bonds between the phosphate group (P) on one nucleotide and a hydroxyl group on the deoxyribose portion of the adjacent nucleotide. DNA normally exists as a double-stranded molecule, with one strand being complementary to the other by virtue of the precise pairing of complementary basepairs (i.e. A with T and C with G). Each nucleotide has a 5′ site and a 3′ site, referring to the numbering of carbon molecules in the pentose deoxyribose sugar. Nucleotides are strung together by their deoxyribose chains at the 5′ and 3′ sites. Therefore one end of a DNA strand is referred to as the 5′ end, while the other is the 3′ end. Complementary strands of DNA have opposite 5′ to 3′ orientations. The two strands of a DNA molecule can be easily separated (for example, with heat) since they are held together by relatively weak hydrogen bonds. **B:** A three dimensional space filling model of the double stranded DNA. The sugar phosphate backbones (filled balls) of the antiparallel strands wind around the outside while the bases (open balls), attached to the backbone at 1′ position of the sugar ring, are stacked upon top of each other within the helix.

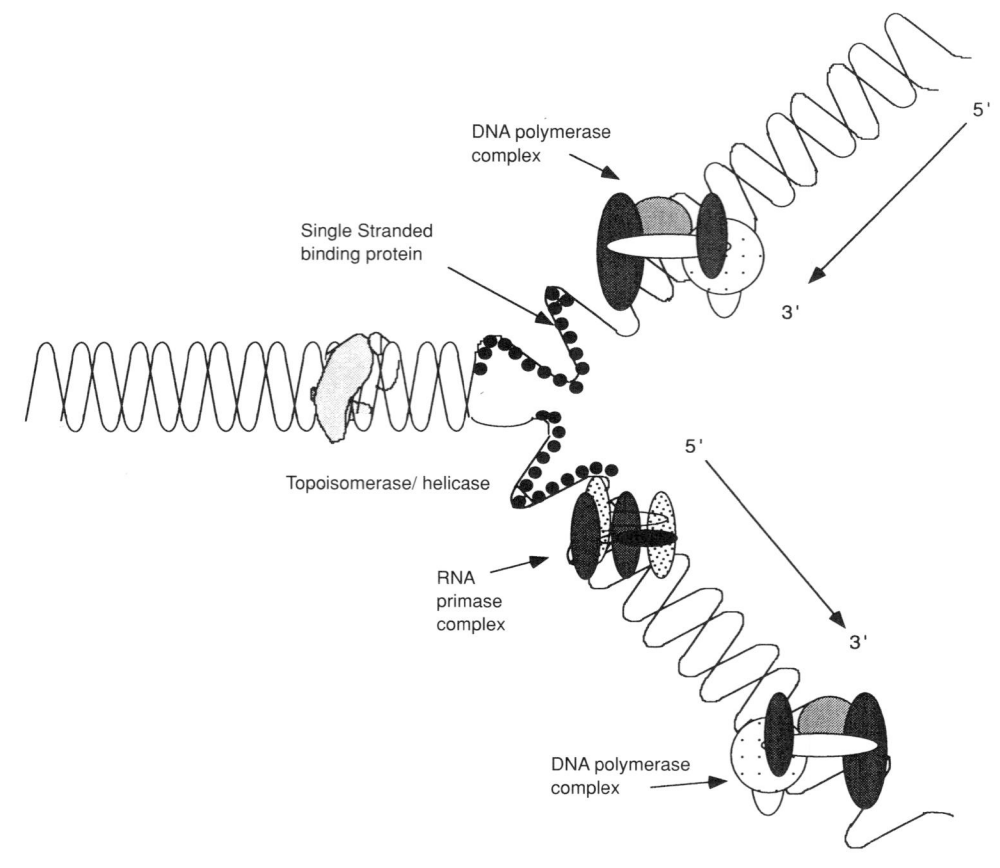

FIG. 5. Mechanism of DNA replication. Replication (or duplication) of DNA involves a complex sequence of events and enzymes that includes unraveling and strand separation of the DNA (topoisomerase/ helicase), attachment of DNA binding proteins, annealing of small primer fragments, and the creation of new complementary strands via DNA polymerase enzymes. Because each strand is replicated once, the process is termed 'semiconservative', The combination of highly specialized enzymes and the ability to "proofread" during the synthesis of a new strand of DNA makes this a highly reliable process.

the gene) and introns. which do not code for amino acids used in the resulting protein. The introns or intervening sequences must be removed from the pre-mRNA and the exons spliced together in the proper order and with exact precision for the mRNA to yield a stable template for its translation into a functional protein. Specific nucleotide sequences at the boundaries of introns and exons, usually a GU at the 5′ beginning of an intron and AG at the 3′ end of an RNA intron, guide the nuclear enzyme complex responsible for mRNA splicing. The mRNAs act as templates for translation of the sequence information into proteins, the effector molecules that mediate cellular functions.

Why have the genes divided into exons and introns, a phenomenon not observed in the prokaryotes? An explanation that has been postulated is derived from structure-function analysis of genes that have been cloned, sequenced, and characterized. These studies have revealed that the exons often correspond to a discrete structural or functional protein domain. Thus, the exons that can potentially encode an independent functional domain in a protein may then be mixed and matched during the course of evolution to create new genes, with different combinations of functional domains encoding a product displaying a novel function. This strategy for developing proteins with distinct functions is much more efficient than having to evolve a new gene from scratch. Meiotic recombination represents a mechanism for generating novel combinations of exons. This mechanism is aided by the relatively greater length of intron sequence than exon sequence; thus recombination of two separate genes is more likely to occur between introns creating at least one hybrid intron. The hybrid intron would not affect the splicing machinery, however, because the internal sequences of introns are not highly crucial to their function, while their terminal splice junction sequences are conserved and generally interchangeable. For genes without introns, the recombination would have to occur precisely in frame to yield a functional hybrid gene. This nearly impossible alternative may provide the sufficient evolutionary force to develop and maintain the intron–exon structure present in vast numbers of protein-encoding genes in higher organisms.

Translation

Transcribed mRNA is subsequently converted, or translated, into protein, the molecular mediator of the information encoded within the DNA. This interpretive process involves two different types of RNA as well as variety of proteins that facilitate the process, such as initiation factors and elongation factors. Protein synthesis begins with the attachment of the mRNA to a ribosome (rRNA plus proteins) near the "start codon." A codon is a triplet of RNA bases that codes for either a specific amino acid or a start or stop to the translation procedure. A tRNA, which carries a particular amino acid, then joins the complex based on the complementary nucleotide sequence of the mRNA (codon) and tRNA (anticodon). The polypeptide chain is created by sequentially bringing pairs of tRNAs together on the ribosome using the mRNA as a template. A peptidyl transferase reaction forms a new peptide bond between the two amino acids on the tRNAs. This process continues until the end of the mRNA encoding sequence is reached, and the newly formed polypeptide is released in the cell with the aid of specific release factors. A schematic of the translation process is illustrated in Fig. 7.

There are 4 different ribonucleotide (G, A, U, C) possibilities at any base position in an mRNA, and three bases in series form a functional unit called a codon. This creates the possibility of **64 (4 × 4 × 4)** different codons while there exist 20 amino acids that are available for construction of human proteins. Methonine, the initial amino acid in a polypeptide chain, is encoded by a single codon AUG. With the additional exception of tryptophan, encoded by UGG, all other amino acids are encoded by a minimum of two alternative codons. This degeneracy in the genetic code allows for some level of mutation in the DNA sequence of a gene to occur without affecting the final amino acid sequence of the resulting protein. Three of the possible 64 triplet codons do not code for any amino acids; they code instead for the termination of the growing polypeptide chain.

MUTATIONS: AGENTS OF EVOLUTION AND DISEASE

The survival of an organism depends on its ability to faithfully transmit its genetic information from one generation to the next. The organism's survival also depends on its ability to adapt to the changing environment, a condition that may not be satisfied by a static genome. These apparent contradictory requirements are addressed primarily through nondirected, random, and low-frequency sequence alterations in the organism's genome during the replication process. These sequence alterations, or mutations, represent a primary source of genetic variation without which evolution would not take place. A mutation may vary in size, ranging from a chromosomal aneuploidy to a single base-pair change. The alterations at the chromosomal level (involving a large number of base pairs) in the form of inversions, translocations, and deletions (discussed previously) may be detected through karyotype analysis. These mutations occur largely at the post-DNA synthesis stage (e.g., during meiosis). On the other hand, sequence alterations that are relatively subtle, so as to require refined, high-resolution analysis (e.g., sequencing), are the result of errors by the DNA polymerase during replication of the genome. These replication errors are relatively infrequent due to the 3' to 5' proofreading activity of the enzyme. The error rate for human

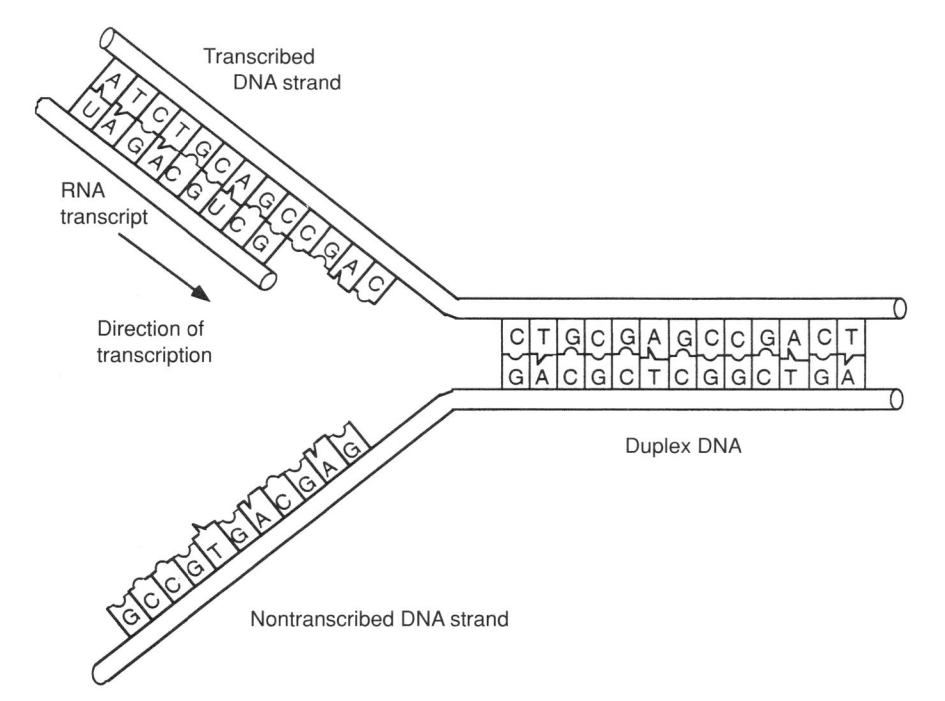

FIG. 6. Transcription of DNA. RNA is transcribed off a single strand of a double stranded DNA termed the sense strand, i.e. the strand in which the nucleotide sequences "make sense" when read in a 5' to 3' direction (the opposing DNA strand is termed "antisense". RNA polymerase synthesizes a single-stranded RNA molecule (messenger RNA or mRNA) that is complementary to the DNA template, with the exception that ribonucleic acids are substituted for deoxy ribonucleic acids, and the Uracil (U) replaces Thymidine in the coding process. This process is mediated by the enzyme RNA polymerase that recognizes and attaches to a specific region at the starting point of a gene. Transcription proceeds without the need for a primer.

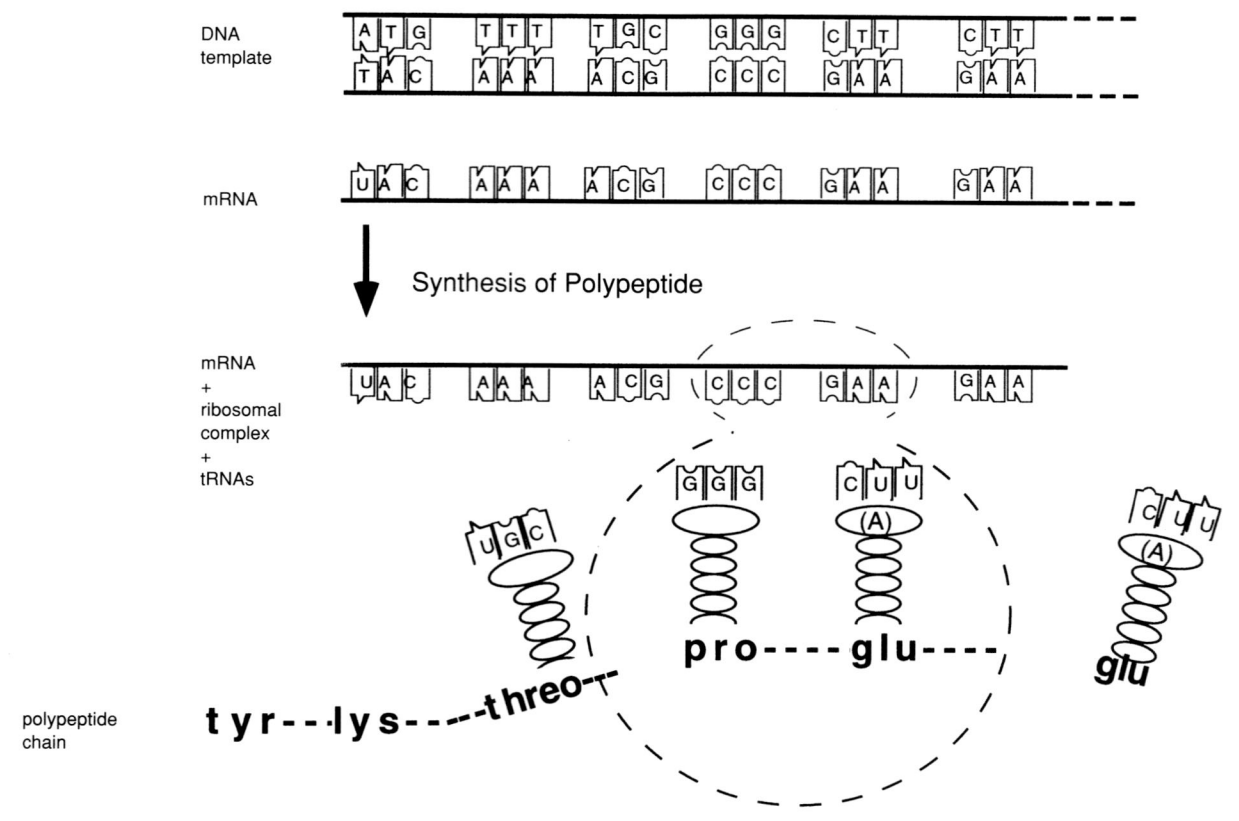

FIG. 7. Information flow from DNA to RNA to proteins. mRNA, transcribed from DNA, is translated into protein by an interpretive process involving ribosomes (dashed lines), transfer RNA (tRNA), and a variety of other proteins that facilitate the process. Protein synthesis begins with the attachment of the mRNA to a ribosome near the 'start codon'. A tRNA, which carries a particular amino acid, then joins the complex based on the complementary nucleotide sequence of the mRNA (codon) and tRNA (anticodon). The polypeptide chain is created by sequentially bringing pairs of tRNAs together on the ribosome using the mRNA as a template. A peptidyl transferase reaction forms a new peptide bond between the two amino acids on the tRNAs. This process continues until the end of the mRNA encoding sequence is reached, and the newly formed polypeptide is released in the cell with the aid of specific release factors.

DNA polymerase is estimated to be as low as 10^8. Replication error rates of the DNA polymerase vary between species as well as genes.

Several different types of mutations that reflect subtle errors in fidelity of DNA replication have been categorized. A large number of these have been identified within the coding sequence of genes. These include single base-pair alterations within a coding sequence that either result in a substitution of one amino acid with another in the translated protein, known as missense mutation, or introduce a stop signal, resulting in premature truncation of the translated protein, known as nonsense mutation. The missense mutation can have varying effects on the translated product of the gene that can range from complete dysfunction to a null effect, depending on the location of alteration and the nature of amino acid substitution. A missense mutation within an "active site" of an enzyme or a highly conserved transmembrane region of a channel protein that causes a "nonconservative" amino acid substitution (e.g., exchanging an amino acid with a polar side chain with an amino acid containing a nonpolar side chain) can potentially cause a major dysfunction in the protein. A sudden truncation of the translated protein can also occur as a consequence of "frameshift" mutation within the gene. These frameshift mutations occur when one or more bases (nonmultiples of 3) are added or deleted from the coding sequence, thus altering the reading frame and generating a stop signal nearby.

Mutations within specific nucleotide sequences at the boundaries of introns and exons have also been documented. These "splice site" mutations can cause aberrant splicing of the pre-mRNA, generally resulting in a loss of function for the encoded protein. Several splice mutations in the PAX3 gene, causing Waardenburg type I, have been identified. Tassabehji et al. (8) identified a mutation in the donor splice site of intron 3 that replaces the invariant GT dinucleotide sequence with a TT dinucleotide. This mutation prevents efficient splicing out of intron 3. When the ribosomal complex translates this aberrantly spliced transcript, translation is terminated prematurely due to the presence of a stop codon in intron 3. The resulting truncated protein is missing half of the critical paired box domain of the native protein and is presumed to be nonfunctional. Another splice site mutation within the PAX3 gene also involves intron 3 of PAX3. However, the change occurs at the 3' end splice acceptor wherein the AG dinucleotide is replaced by a GG dinucleotide. This mutation is predicted to cause the splicing out of intron 3, exon 4, and intron 4. The next functional splice acceptor site occurs at the 3' end of intron 4. The resulting protein is missing the amino acids normally encoded by exon 4, which includes half of the paired box domain known to be integral to the ability of PAX3 protein to bind DNA and act as a transcriptional regulator early in embryogenesis.

Prior to the identification of PAX3 as the disease gene in Waardenburg type I, Epstein et al. (9) identified a splice mutation in the mouse homologue, PAX3. This mutation was identified in a spontaneously arising Splotch mouse, which models the patchy skin coloring but not the hearing loss or heterochromia seen in many cases of Waardenburg Syndrome type I. The mutation in the Sp allele of the mouse PAX3 gene is a transversion of an A to T at the invariant 3' AG splice acceptor of intron 3, which disrupts normal splicing of intron 3. The mutation bearing pax3 transcript is alternatively spliced in four different ways, each of which results in the generation of aberrantly spliced mRNA transcripts that are not predicted to result in functional PAX3 proteins. It is interesting to note that nearly identical mutations in the same gene in both mouse and human can lead to such disparity in the overall phenotype exhibited by each species.

Mutations outside of the coding region or the intron–exon boundary region can also affect protein function. These mutations are considered to occur within regions that regulate expression of these proteins, such as promoters, enhancers, or repressors. These mutations are generally defined by an absence of RNA transcribed from the affected gene. Not all sequence alterations affect function of the gene product. These variant sequences, within or outside of the coding region, referred to as polymorphisms, have proven to be extremely helpful for identifying transmission of alleles from parents to offspring.

If the DNA sequence alterations occur within the reproductive or germ cells (eggs or sperm), these mutations are potentially transmissible to the next generation. Analysis of the patterns of transmission of a variety of disorders caused by these mutations and their subsequent identification is described in the following sections.

INHERITED DISORDERS AND THEIR INHERITANCE PATTERNS

Roughly half of the observed severe hearing loss seen in childhood has been attributed to genetic factors. Approximately one in every 1,000 children is born with a severe hearing impairment, with the estimated prevalence of genetic hearing loss around 1 in 2,000. Of these cases, approximately 75% exhibit an inheritance pattern that is consistent with an autosomal recessive trait, 23% exhibit autosomal dominant inheritance, 2% appear to be X-linked, and less than 1% is caused by deleterious mutations in the mitochondrial genome. A combination of environmental and genetic factors can complicate pedigree analysis and, to date, most genes and chromosomal regions identified as being involved in syndromic and nonsyndromic hearing loss have been monogenic in origin for the majority of the phenotype and with little environmentally induced effect.

The observed familial inheritance of disorders that cause hearing loss has been validated at the molecular level with the cloning of several genes expressing pathogenic mutations for the disease phenotype under investigation. Several of the genes recently cloned include MITF in Waardenburg syndrome type II, PAX3 in Waardenburg syndrome type I, POU3F4 in X-linked mixed deafness (DFN3), FGFR2 in Crouzan's syndrome, FGFR1 and FGFR2 in Pfeiffer's syndrome, and the mitochondrial 12S rRNA gene in aminoglycoside hypersensitivity–induced deafness. A large body of statistical evidence implying the inheritance of a mutant copy of a gene or genes in a particular chromosomal region being coinherited with a hearing loss phenotype has also grown dramatically over the past few years.

To map and clone a gene responsible for an inherited trait such as hearing loss, pedigrees exhibiting that trait need be identified for study. Individuals with cytogenetically detectable chromosomal aberrations expressing the same disease phenotype greatly aid the localization of the disease locus. Thus, a single patient with a cytogenetically detectable rearrangement involving a gene for hearing loss is potentially sufficient for the identification and characterization of the responsible gene and may provide valuable insights for familial studies of pedigrees without aberrant karyotypes but with a similar phenotype.

Autosomal Recessive Inheritance

An autosomal recessive trait is characterized by two unaffected parents who are heterozygous carriers for mutant forms of the gene in question but in whom the phenotypic expression of the mutant allele is masked by the normal allele. These heterozygous parents (A/a) can each generate two types of gametes, one carrying the mutant copy of the gene (a) and the other having a normal copy of the gene (A). Of the four possible combinations of these two gamete types from each of the parents, only the offspring that inherits both mutant copies (a/a), will exhibit the trait. Of the three remaining possibilities, all will have a normal hearing phenotype, but two of the three will be heterozygous carriers for the mutant form of the gene, similar to the carrier parents.

Although relatively uncommon, it is permissible for more distant relatives, such as first or second cousins, to marry and have children. This practice, known as consanguineous mating, greatly increases the potential to produce a child

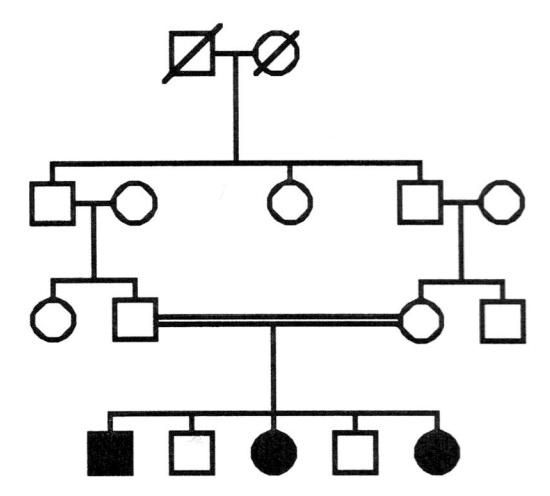

FIG. 8. A pedigree pattern illustrating transmission of an autosomal recessive trait. The affected individuals (shaded) have parents who are first cousins as well as carriers of the recessive trait. The double horizontal line between the parents of the affected children indicates that this is a consanguious mating between first cousins. When the recessive allele is rare it is more likely to become homozygous through inheritance from a common ancestor than from parents who are completely unrelated.

affected by a recessive disorder. Figure 8 illustrates the inheritance pattern of an autosomal recessive trait in offspring of consanguineous mating in a pedigree spanning several generations. A consanguineous mating of first cousins can generate a risk of 1 in 64 for having a child affected with an autosomal recessive disorder from unaffected parents with a common grandparent. With approximately 1 in 2,000 children born with a genetic form of hearing loss and 75% of these due to autosomal recessive inheritance, a generalized risk of having such an affected child is on the order of 1 in 2,700 for any two unaffected parents. Thus, the increased risk for a consanguineous mating producing a child with autosomal recessive hearing loss is 1:64 divided by the frequency of autosomal recessive hearing loss within the general population (random mating) 1:2,700. This represents a 42-fold increase in the odds of two unrelated individuals giving rise to a child with autosomal recessive hearing loss.

Autosomal recessive deafness is extremely heterogeneous, as inferred from frequent examples of normal-hearing children in families in which both parents are deaf. Thus, the generalized risk of having such an affected child as stated earlier is a simplification based on an assumption of a single causative locus and consequently an overestimate. In certain cases, individuals considered to be affected by autosomal recessive deafness may in fact be noncomplementary double heterozygotes. Such "digenic" individuals have been identified within several families affected with retinitis pigmentosa. Mutations within unlinked photoreceptor-specific genes ROM1 and peripherin/RDS were identified in members of the affected family (10). Only the double heterozygotes were observed to develop retinitis pigmentosa. These cases represent the first example of digenic inheritance in human disease.

Autosomal Dominant Inheritance

For autosomal dominant disorders, the transmission of a rare allele of a gene by a single heterozygous parent is sufficient to generate an affected child. A heterozygous parent can produce two types of gametes. One gamete will carry the mutant form of the gene of interest, and the other, the normal form. Each of these gametes then has an equal chance of being utilized in the formation of a zygote. Thus, the chance that an offspring of an autosomal dominant affected parent will itself be affected is 50%. Equal numbers of affected males and females are expected for an autosomal dominant trait and roughly half of the offspring of an affected individual will be affected. If male-to-male transmission of the trait is observed, the possibility that the trait is X-linked can be eliminated. Figure 9, panel A, illustrates the inheritance pattern of an autosomal dominant trait with complete penetrance. Thus, all carriers of the disease allele express the disease trait.

The ability of an autosomal dominant gene to be transmitted is influenced by the genetic fitness of those carrying the mutation. If the mutation greatly reduces the chance of mating and or reduces the viability of the gametes produced by the affected individual, it may be difficult to identify pedigrees transmitting the disorder. One example of this is Apert's syndrome, which is now known to be caused by mutations in the fibroblast growth factor receptor type 2 (FGFR2) gene. Apert's syndrome is a severe autosomal dominant malformation syndrome with a birth prevalence of 1 in 65,000. It is characterized by craniosynostosis and severe syndactyly, with a variety of abnormalities of the brain, skin, skeleton, and other internal organs at lower frequency. Very few instances of Apert's syndrome adults known to have children have been recorded, and the syndrome is most commonly identified as a new mutation.

Due to a low number of pedigrees useful for genetic linkage analysis to map the Apert's syndrome locus, a candidate gene approach was employed. The FGFR2 gene had previously been shown to be involved in Crouzon's syndrome (11), Pfeiffer's syndrome (12), and Jackson-Weiss syndrome (13), all of which are autosomal dominant disorders that share craniosynostosis as a feature in common with Apert's syndrome. When tested in 40 unrelated Apert's syndrome patients, mutations were identified in the FGFR2 gene in all 40 patients (14). Although linkage analysis of Apert's syndrome was not attempted, careful attention to the phenotype and correlation with other disease led to the identification of the responsible gene. Thus, mutations in the FGFR2 gene may result in any one of several disease phenotypes (15). Furthermore, the same mutation may result in any one of several disease phenotypes. The occurrence of different phenotypes with the same mutations reflects the role of genetic background (i.e., other genes and gene products) in phenotype expression. The FGFR2 belongs to a family of receptors. The other fibroblast growth factors that have been identified include FGFR1, FGFR3, and FGFR4. Mutations within FGFR3 have been causally linked to achondroplasia (16).

Autosomal dominant traits often exhibit incomplete penetrance and variable expressivity. *Variable expressivity* refers to the differences in the observed effects of a given allele in related and unrelated individuals. Incomplete penetrance is an extreme form of variable expressivity and is characterized by the total absence of expression in persons known to carry the mutant allele. Variation in the age of onset for symptoms associated with a genetic disorder is common for traits that are not expressed at birth or prenatally. Variation in age of onset is often treated as incomplete penetrance in linkage analysis. An example of this variation is seen in a single, large pedigree from Costa Rica that is affected by nonsyndromic autosomal dominant hearing loss. In that nine-generation pedigree all affected individuals have one affected parent, a hallmark of autosomal dominant disorders with high penetrance. Also, the ratio of affected males to affected females approaches unity and male-to-male transmission of the hearing loss phenotype is observed, thus ruling out X-linked inheritance. All affected offspring developed bilateral sensory neural hearing loss greater than 80 dB by their mid-30s to early 40s and had normal intelligence and fertility. Thus, the penetrance of the mutant allele was shown to be complete in older individuals. However, the age of onset of the hearing loss was variable. All affected individuals were born with normal hearing followed by its degeneration beginning between the ages of 6 and 16 years and continuing into their third decade of life, when the rate of hearing loss plateaus. The gene for this type of hearing loss, DFNA1, has been mapped to chromsome 5q31 by genetic linkage analysis of this family (17). In the initial mapping of the DFNA1 gene, children under the age of 16 years were not included in the linkage analysis to avoid problems of misdiagnosing carriers of the mutant allele who had not yet expressed the phenotype.

If the mutant phenotype is always expressed in individuals carrying the disease allele, its penetrance is said to be complete; otherwise it is incomplete. Where penetrance of the affected gene is complete or 100%, the pattern of its inheritance may be discerned in a relatively straightforward manner. Complete penetrance of the dominant allele will result in expression of the disease phenotype in all carriers of that allele without skipping generations. However, with incomplete penetrance of the affected gene, the inheritance pattern of the affected trait becomes relatively harder to discern; that is, one cannot easily distinguish between dominant inheritance with reduced penetrance and more complicated modes of inheritance. If the penetrance of an allele is very low, the parents of the affected child may not initially recognize the existence of similarly affected relatives who are distantly related. Figure 9, panel B, illustrates a pedigree expressing transmission of an autosomal dominant trait with incomplete penetrance. Note that not all carriers of the disease allele are affected. The presence of low-penetrance dominant alleles causing the phenotype to be transmitted through unaffected carriers cannot be ruled out without a thorough pedigree analysis that includes the ancestors and relatives of the affected individual. The failure of the gene to express itself may be due to variety of reasons. The most common rationale put forth to explain reduced penetrance is the effect of genetic background. Factors such as genetic redundancy, presence of more than one gene for the performance of a given function, and modifiers affect a variety of genes. Incomplete penetrance also can be seen in traits that

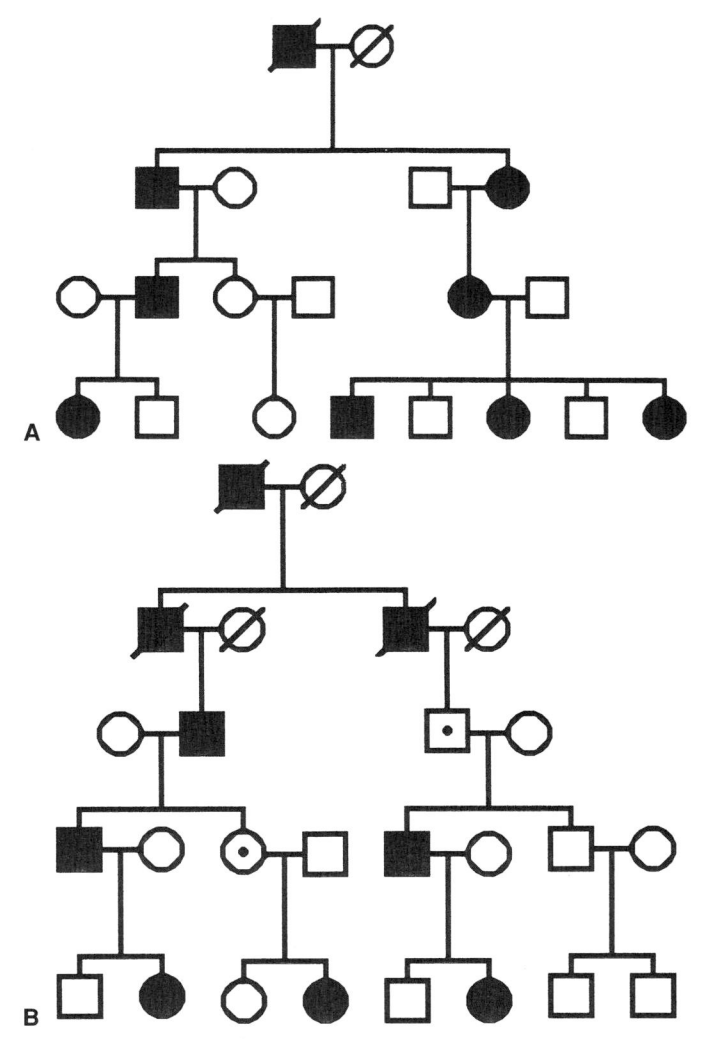

FIG. 9. A: A pedigree pattern illustrating transmission of autosomal dominant trait. The autosomal dominant trait is transmitted from the affected parent to their offsprings, who have 50% probability of inheriting the disease allele. All carriers of the mutant gene express the disease trait, indicating complete penetrance of the mutant allele. **B:** A pedigree pattern illustrating transmission of autosomal dominant trait with incomplete penetrance. Not all carriers of the mutant gene () are affected indicating incomplete penetrance of the mutant allele.

are inherited in an autosomal recessive, X-linked recessive, and X-linked dominant manner.

Variable expression of different aspects of syndromes including hearing loss is common. Some aspects may be expressed in a range from mild to severe, and/or different combinations of associated symptoms may be expressed in different individuals carrying the same mutation within a single pedigree. An example of variable expressivity is seen in families transmitting autosomal dominant branchio-otorenal (BOR) syndrome. For BOR syndrome, aplasia or stenosis of the lacrimal duct is reported in approximately 10% of cases, diagnosed structural anomalies of the renal system occur in 12% to 20% of cases; branchial cysts or fistulae are present in approximately 60% of cases, anomalies of the inner ear occur in 30% to 60% of reported cases, and hearing loss is found in approximately 75% of reported cases. Of the hearing loss seen in BOR syndrome, 50% is mixed loss, 30% is conductive, and 20% is sensorineural. All three forms of hearing loss have been seen in affected members of the same family. In several individuals, the type of hearing loss appears to differ between the two ears. The genetic locus for BOR syndrome has been mapped (18), but the disease gene(s) remains to be identified.

The range of variation observed in dominant disorders is generally wider than in recessive disorders. A major contributing factor to the variation observed in the dominant disorders is the presence of a functional product from the wild-type allele. Variable regional concentration of the functional product may lead to the variable phenotype in the affected individuals. The wide range of phenotypic expression of the syndrome may also reflect the epistatic effects of different genetic backgrounds in the affected individuals (i.e., different alleles for other genes) interacting with the major causative gene or genes. Additionally, variable expression may be influenced by environmental exposures and/or random stochiastic events, which occur during development.

The ability of a single mutant allele to express its aberrant phenotype, despite the presence of a normal allele, as observed in transmission of dominant disease traits, can occur via several mechanisms. These in turn depend on the nature of the protein encoded by the gene and the nature of the pathogenic mutation. If the mutant protein is involved in transcriptional regulation or functions that are sensitive to its quantity, its dysfunction would reduce the available product by a half. This pathologic reduction in total amount of the active product is referred to as haploinsufficiency. For example, PAX3 is considered to encode a transcription factor, and its haploinsufficiency resulting from a mutant allele is postulated to cause the expression of the disease phenotype, the dominantly transmitted Waardenburg syndrome type I. Another group of genes that can cause expression of the disease phenotype are those encoding structural proteins. Mutations within genes encoding collagens represent an example of such dominantly inherited disorders (19). Disruption of normal structural interaction between proteins by the mutant product is considered to be the mechanism of dominance expressed by genes encoding structural proteins. However, not all mutations in structural genes are dominant. For example, both dominant and recessive forms of a disease result from different mutations in the same gene. This has been demonstrated for autosomal dominant and recessive forms of Stickler's syndrome, a syndromic sensorineural deafness, which results from different mutations within the COL11A2 gene.

X-Linked Inheritance

In humans, females have 22 pairs of autosomes and a pair of X chromosomes (46XX), males have 22 autosomes, one X chromosome, and one Y chromosome (46XY). Accordingly, males always receive their Y chromosome from their father and their X chromosome from their mother, while females receive one of their X chromosomes from each of their two parents. Because males have one copy of the X chromosome, they are hemizygous for genes on the X chromosome and the X chromosome is active in all their nucleated cells. In general, only one of the two X chromosomes carried by a female is active in any one cell, while the other is rendered inactive by a natural process known as lyonization. This random inactivation process makes all females, who are heterozygous for X-linked traits, mosaic at the tissue level, resulting in variable expression of the mutant gene. Diseases that are rarely expressed clinically in heterozygous females are called X-linked recessive. In female tissues, various proportions of cells may exist in which one or the other of two alleles for an X-linked locus is expressed. Occasionally, a carrier female may manifest some symptoms of an X-linked recessive disorder due to this mosaicism if she, by chance, has an abundance of cells with the mutant allele being expressed. Transmission of an X-linked recessive trait in a pedigree is illustrated in Fig. 10.

The X-linked disease was one of the first well-docu-

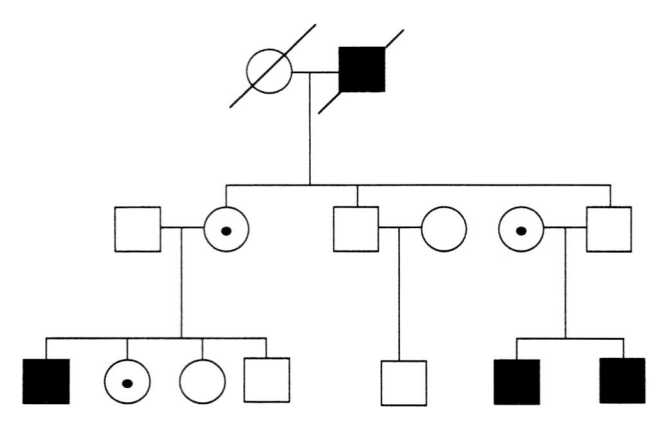

FIG. 10. A pedigree pattern illustrating transmission of X-linked recessive trait. The affected males inherit the X-linked recessive disease allele from their unaffected carrier mother. The X-linked trait is characterized by absence of male to male transmission while all daughters of the affected male are heterozygous or carriers for the disease allele.

mented genetic disorders in humans due to its unique inheritance patterns. Hemophilia A is one the most well-known X-linked human diseases resulting from deficiency in a blood clotting factor—factor VIII encoded by its gene located on the X chromosome. While comprising only approximately 2% of cases, X-linked transmission of alleles involved in inherited hearing loss is significant. Examples of such disorders include Norrie's syndrome, X-linked congenital sensorineural hearing loss, and X-linked high-frequency sensorineural hearing loss. In pedigrees exhibiting X-linked recessive traits, many more males than females are affected because males have only one X chromosome. Thus, a recessive allele for hearing loss is not masked in males. Females have two X chromosomes allowing the masking of a recessive allele on one X chromosome by a normal allele of the gene on their other X chromosome. Females who express a true X-linked recessive trait have either inherited a mutant form of the gene from both parents, in which case the father should be affected, or the process of lyonization allowed a sufficient number of cells to express the mutant allele, resulting in the complete or partial expression of the phenotype. Approximately half of the sons are affected and half are unaffected when a female carrier of an X-linked recessive gene has children with a normal man. No affected offspring will result from the mating of a man affected by an X-linked recessive disorder with a homozygous normal woman; however, all of his daughters will be carriers.

In certain rare conditions, females may express a disease phenotype that is considered to be X-linked recessive. Translocation of regions of X chromosome to an autosome represents one possible mechanism for expression of X-linked recessive disorders in females. This phenomenon of X chromosomal translocation has been shown to occur in females that expressed X-linked Duchenne's muscular dystrophy (20). Also, an apparent X-linked recessive trait in females may be due to a mutation of an autosomal gene that can cause a similar phenotype.

For an X-linked dominant trait with complete penetrance, all of the daughters of an affected man will be affected, while all of his sons will be unaffected, assuming that the mother is homozygous for the normal allele of the gene in question. X-linked dominant inheritance with reduced penetrance in heterozygous carriers may make clinical identification of symptoms in carrier females difficult to establish in some cases due to the mosaic nature of female tissues with respect to cellular X chromosome activity. For X-linked dominant inheritance of a fully penetrant allele, half of the daughters and half of the sons of an affected mother should themselves be affected. An affected father should produce no affected sons and only daughters who are affected. The absence of father-to-son transmission is a unique characteristic of all X-linked traits, because males always receive their X-chromosome from their mothers. An example of X-linked dominant inheritance is seen in families transmitting Alport's syndrome, which is characterized by hematuria, progressive renal failure, and sensorineural hearing loss. The gene for X-linked Alport's syndrome has been identified as the basement membrane–specific type IV collagen alpha-5 chain (COL4A5) (21). It should be noted, however, that an autosomal recessive form of Alport's syndrome has been mapped to chromosome 2q35-2q37, and the genes COL4A3 and COL4A4 have been shown to play a causative role. Examples of similar or identical clinical phenotypes caused by mutations in different genes are known as genetic heterogeneity.

DFN3 represents one of the most frequent forms of X-linked deafness. Affected males have conductive hearing loss (as a result of stapes fixation) and progressive sensorineural deafness. The DFN3 gene has been cloned and is referred to as POU3F4, a member of a multigene family encoding nuclear transcription factors (22). POU3F4 represents the first cloned gene that has been found to be mutated in individuals with nonsyndromic deafness.

VARIATIONS ON MENDELIAN PRINCIPLES

Mendel established the two fundamental principles of genetics: segregation of genes and their independent assortment. These principles refer to processes that occur in the formation of germ cells, known as meiosis. *Segregation* refers to separation of homologous genes, representing the paternal and the maternal contributions to the individual's genotype, into two separate daughter cells. Thus, the diploid genome is reduced to haploid state in the germ cells. The principle of independent assortment states that segregation of one gene occurs independently of other genes. These principles have served well for analysis and understanding of inheritance of traits through a single locus. However, a number of variations on these principles exist, some of which have already been stated implicitly. These variations and their underlying principles have contributed to increasing our understanding of genetic etiology of disease.

Linkage and Recombination

Not all genes assort independently of each other. This variation on the mendelian principle was identified initially by Thomas Morgan through analysis of transmission of selected traits in fruit flies. Experiments showed inheritance of a specific pair of alleles in a combination not present in the parental phenotype. This new combination of alleles was considered to result from crossing over and exchange of genetic material between two homologous chromosomes, known as homologous recombination, yielding the new combination of alleles not present in the original parental chromosomes. Analysis of recombination frequencies between two traits considered to be controlled by genes residing on the same linkage group (i.e., the same chromosome) provided two essential concepts that led to the development of the genetic map: Genes are arranged in a linear order, and the frequency with which two alleles are inherited together is a function of the relative physical distance to each other.

Thus, the closer the two genes, the greater the chance that they will remain linked postmeiosis. The relative chromosomal positions of genes may be readily mapped through the application of these principles of linkage and recombination to generate genetic maps. The genetic distance between two linked genes, as measured through frequency of recombinants between the two alleles, is measured in centimorgans (cM). These two loci are 1 cM apart on the genetic map if there is a 1% chance of a recombination between them in meiosis. Thus, genes that are far apart on a chromosome will assort in an apparent independent manner, while genes that are close together will tend to remain linked postmeiosis. These concepts are illustrated in Fig. 11. Applying the principles of genetic linkage, Morgan and his colleagues were able to order over several hundred genes in *Drosophilia melanogaster* via recombination analysis by 1922.

Mitochondrial Inheritance

Not all genes are inherited equally from both parents. The extranuclear genome is inherited solely through the mother. Male mitochondria are not contributed to newly formed zy-

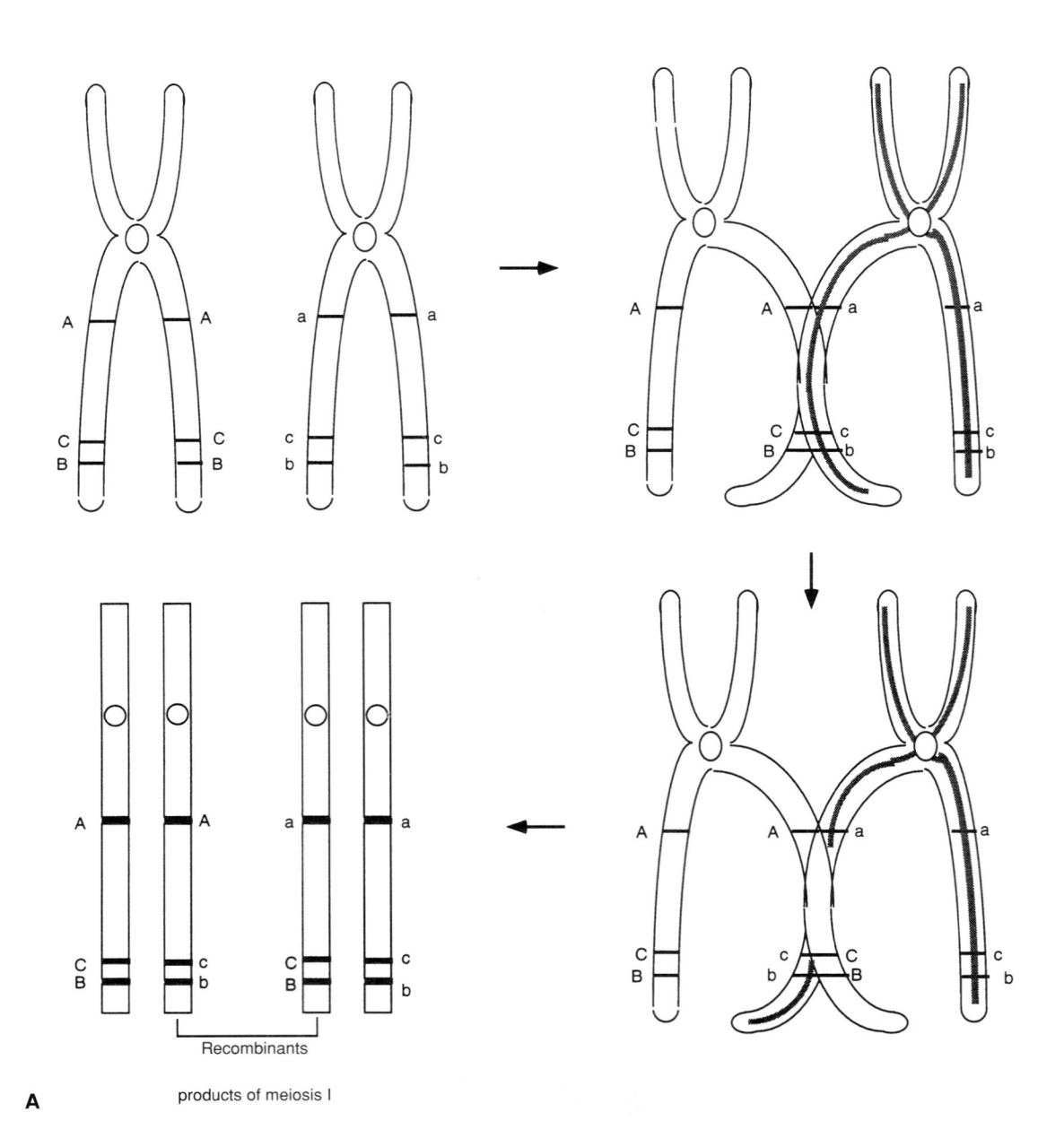

FIG. 11. A: Recombination between homologous chromosomes in meiosis. A schematic of a recombination event between three loci (A/a, B/b and C/c) on homologous chromosomes. While the distant loci are recombined in the meiotic products, the loci that are near to each other remain linked. Note that 50% of the meiotic products are recombinants-accounting for the 2 of the 4 chromatids that are involved at any one meiotic crossover event.

gotes. This inheritance pattern, illustrated in Fig. 12, gives rise to pedigrees in which all the children of an affected mother may be affected and none of the children of an affected father will be affected. In practice, the expression of mitochondrially inherited disorders is often variable and may be incompletely penetrant. This observation is possibly due in part to the fact that a population of mitochondria which can itself be genetically heterogeneous is actually transmitted by the mother. If all of the mitochondria transmitted by the mother are of the same genotype, it is called homoplasmia; if there are genetic differences between them, it is call heteroplasmia.

To date there are 326 syndromes, disorders, or peculiar phenotypes associated with mutations in the mitochondrial genome. Twenty-one of these disorders have some involvement with sensory neural hearing loss (23), indicating that the requirement for a healthy population of mitochondria is very important to the cells involved in normal hearing. One of the most striking examples of a mitochondrially inherited trait whose expression is environmentally affected is that for hearing loss caused by hypersensitivity to aminoglycosides. The aminoglycoside hypersensitivity phenotype is the result of a single base transition of A to G at position 1555 in the mitochondrial 12S rRNA. This mutation causes a portion of the 12S rRNA transcript structure to closely resemble the binding site of aminoglycosides to bacterial rRNA. When an aminoglycoside such as streptomycin is administered to patients carrying this mutation, it binds to the mutant 12S rRNA and prevents it from functioning in the translation of mitochondrially transcribed genes. This results in the loss of mitochondria in cells, which may lead to cell death or impairment of their normal function.

X Chromosome Inactivation

The inactivated X chromosome can be identified in nondividing cells of females (within the interphase nuclei) as a darkly staining mass called a Barr body attached to a nuclear membrane. The Barr body represents the X chromosome that has been inactivated and thus appears as a condensed mass (heterochromatization). This X chromosome inactivation in females is also known as lyonization, named after Mary Lyon, who first offered an explanation for its presence in females. Thus, lyonization represents a dosage

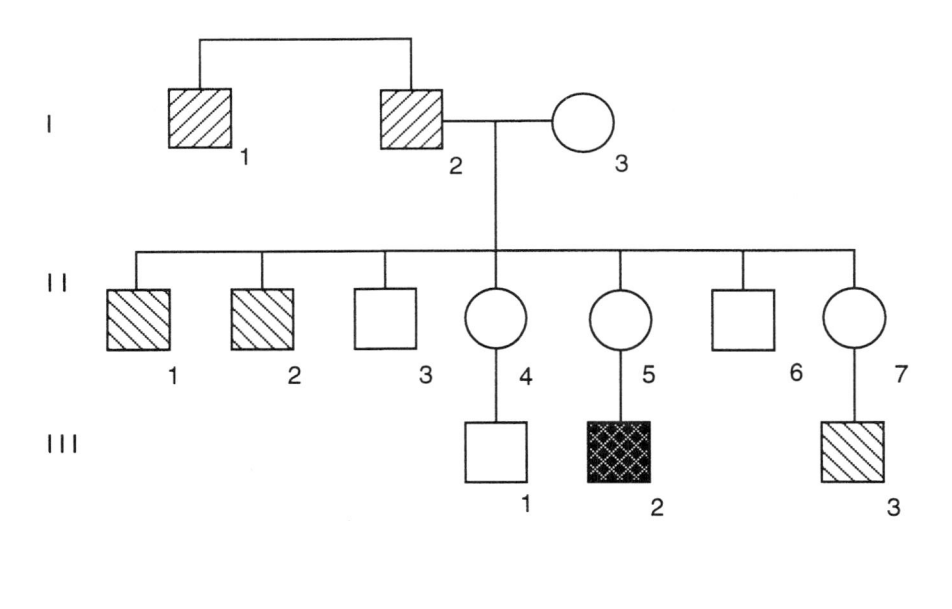

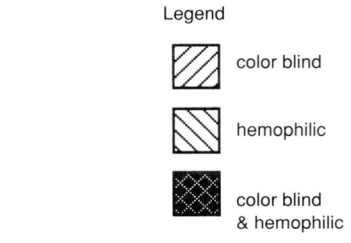

FIG. 11. *Continued.* **B:** A pedigree illustrating a recombination event between two X-linked recessive traits. Both hemophilia and color blindness are X-linked recessive. The individual II.5 is heterozygous for the two traits carried on two separate X chromosomes. A meiotic crossover between these two loci yields an X chromosome carrying both recessive alleles. This recombinant X chromosome is inherited by her offspring III.2 who is both a hemophiliac and color blind.

compensation mechanism to correct for differences in sex chromosome constitution between sexes and targeted toward the X chromosome. This mechanism ensures that genes located on the X chromosome are not expressed in proportion to the number of X chromosomes but are equivalent to a single X chromosome that is present in both male and female cells. Thus, both male and female cells are balanced with respect to the expression of their X-linked genes. (The consequence of X-inactivation in females and hemizygous expression of X-linked genes in males as it relates to inheritance patterns of familial mendelian disorders was discussed under the heading, X-Linked Inheritance.)

Genomic Imprinting

Frequency of some genetic diseases depend upon the sex of the transmitting parent. This occurrence is considered to result from genomic imprinting (24). This phenomenon runs counter to the teachings of mendelian genetics, which emphasize equal contribution from paternal and maternal genes, with the obvious exception of genes on the sex chromosomes. Thus, in certain instances, despite the presence of both the paternal and maternal alleles, only one of the parental alleles is expressed. This differential expression of the parental alleles is detected in certain disease states when inheritance of that disorder is dependent on sex of the parent that transmits the mutant gene.

The gene-specific imprinting, as with X inactivation (described previously) is presumed to be the consequence of reversible "epigenetic" modification of the parental allele during gametogenesis, leading to its differential expression. The precise mechanism of imprinting and its evolutionary significance remain unknown. Imprinting is considered to be established prior to or during gametogenesis and is known to persist stably throughout somatic cell divisions. Hypermethylation of the imprinted gene represents one possible mechanism. This process involves the covalent addition of a methyl group to the C5 position of the cytosine ring. The role of methylation for mediating the imprinting process is supported by the observations that all of the imprinted sequences that have been analyzed are methylated. It is possible that methylation of the imprinted gene is secondary to a prior imprinting step, and its role may be as a stabilizer of the imprinted signal.

The gene encoding insulin-like growth factor (IGF-II), a potent growth factor and a mitogen, was the first identified example of an autosomal imprinted gene (25,26). The expression of IGF-II was shown to be restricted to its paternal allele; the maternally derived allele was transcriptionally silent. Several other imprinted loci or genes have been identified in humans based on inheritance patterns of familial disorders that are consistent with imprinting phenomenon. These include Prader-Willi syndrome, in which the affected gene is maternally imprinted, and Angelman's syndrome, in which the affected gene is paternally imprinted. A pedigree

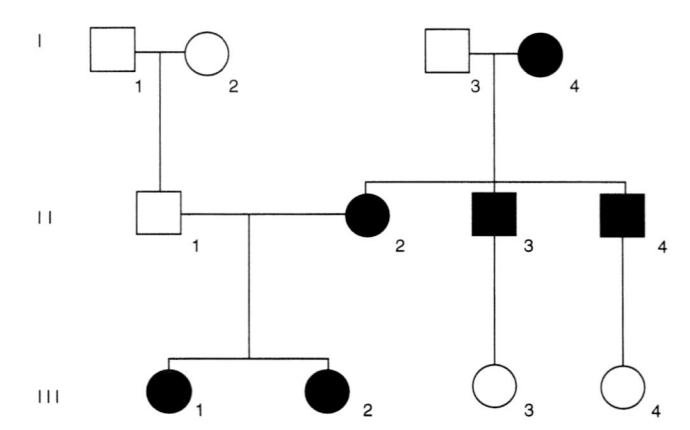

FIG. 12. A pedigree pattern illustrating mitochondrial inheritance of the disease trait. The disease trait is transmitted maternally, through its mitochondrial genome, to both male and female offsprings.

transmitting a maternally imprinted disease gene is illustrated in Fig. 13.

An example of genomic imprinting at the level of a specific gene has also been identified in familial cases of non-chromaffin paragangliomas, benign tumors of the paraganglionic cells. Although benign, their enlargement can cause deafness and or facial palsy. Familial cases of paragangliomas (glomus tumors) have shown an autosomal dominant inheritance with genomic imprinting of the maternal allele. Thus, the transmission of the disease occurs via the affected paternal allele and not the maternal allele. Two distinct, imprinted genes for glomus tumur have been mapped on 11q, 11q13.1, and 11q22.3-q23.3, by linkage analysis in two unrelated families (27,28).

Trinucleotide Repeat Expansion

Another type of deviation from mendelian genetics has been identified through analysis in six different neurologic disorders that are characterized by increased severity and or an earlier onset of the disease in successive generations. This phenomenon, unique to these disorders, is termed *anticipation*. These include the fragile X syndrome (FRAXA), spinal and bulbar muscular atrophy, Huntington's disease, and muscular dystrophy. Mutation analysis within the affected individuals has revealed a pathologic expansion of an region of DNA (trinucleotide repeats) beyond the normal range observed in the unaffected, within genes linked to disorders characterized by anticipation. A progressive increase in the size of these trinucleotide repeats is correlated with the increased severity and or age of onset of the disease. The mechanism of pathophysiology caused by this dominantly inherited pathologic mutation remains relatively unknown.

In patients affected by fragile X-linked syndrome, the syndrome can be transmitted not only by heterozygous female carriers, but also by unaffected (hemizygous) males. The carrier males possess expanded trinucleotide repeats ranging from 60 to 230, relative to normal controls, who possess an average trinucleotide repeat number of 29. The unaffected paternal carriers of X-linked disorders or the phenomenon of anticipation associated with trinucleotide repeat expansion could not have been predicted from principles of mendelian genetics.

MULTIFACTORIAL INHERITANCE

An expression of a phenotype whose outcome is determined by a single gene is termed a *mendelian trait*. Its pattern of transmission within a pedigree can be readily discerned in most cases, as described in previous sections. On the other hand, most common human disease and traits show irregular inheritance patterns. These traits are considered to be determined from the action of multiple genes and or nongenetic factors. A phenotype that is an outcome of both genetic and environmental factors is called a multifactorial or complex trait. The low proportion of mendelian traits relative to the number of multifactorial traits in humans is better illustrated by considering the proportion of the total number of mendelian traits known, approximately 6,000 according to McKusiak's *Mendelian Inheritance in Man,* to the total number of genes that are estimated to exist, approximately 50 to 100,000. It should be emphasized that classification of mendelian traits as being "determined" by single genes is an oversimplification. As more mendelian disorders are identified and their phenotype investigated, their phenotypic variability and complexity are becoming increasingly clear and concomitantly their distinction from complex or multifactorial traits is becoming increasingly blurred. Phenotype variability or variable expression seen in a single gene disorder such as Waardenburg's syndrome may reflect interaction of that major gene, such as PAX3, with "modifier" genes. Identification of these modifier genes has important implications in the understanding and treatment of mendelian disorders with variable expressivity.

One of the clearest examples of interaction of other genes and their products (termed *epistatic effects*) or nongenetic factors during development of a particular mendelian phenotype is provided by the large variation of the clinical phenotype observed in individuals with an identical mutation in a given gene. A classic example of a single mutant allele yielding a varying phenotype is the hemoglobin beta-S mutation that results in substitution of valine or glutatmine at position 6 of the beta-globin chain. In the homozygous state, this mutation usually causes sickle cell anemia of varying clinical severity. The identity of the modifying genetic factors that interact to yield the variable clinical severity in sickle cell anemia remain undetermined. Such phenotypic heterogeneity despite the identity of the mutation has been described in a number of disorders, including Waardenburg's syndrome, cystic fibrosis, phenylketonuria, Duschenne's muscular dystrophy, retinitis pigmentosa, Marfan syndrome, and XY gonadal dysgenesis. Thus, mutation analysis alone is insufficient in predicting the clinical phenotype of the affected individual. Conversely, the phenotypic outcomes do not depend on the nature of mutations only. As seen in the examples cited, the primary structural change in the DNA sequence can result in a spectrum of consequences, depending on the genotype or the genetic background of the individual. This can range from complete blocking of the pathway to complete compensation of the defect, depending on interactions with other genes and their products and their relative influence for the specific process or the role that is mediated by the mutant gene.

The relatively irregular mode of inheritance that characterizes a multifactorial trait is presumed to result from interaction of multiple genes (polygenic) (29). This interaction is apparently distinct from that presumed for mendelian traits. This distinction, however, may be at a quantitative rather than a qualitative level. For example, instead of a predominant influence or effect of one gene on expression of the phenotype, the multifactorial trait is characterized by a num-

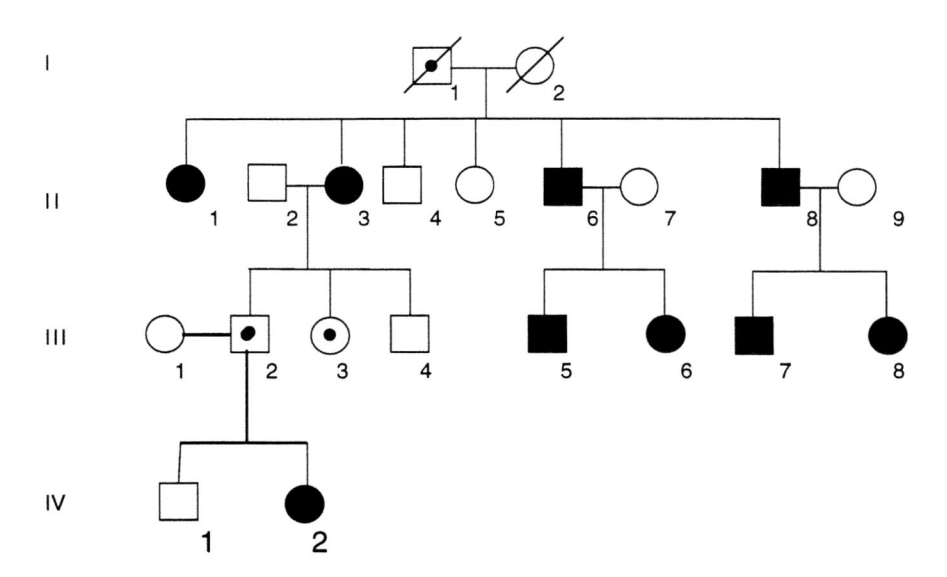

FIG. 13. A pedigree pattern illustrating transmission of autosomal dominant trait that is genomically imprinted. A pedigree demonstrating a maternally imprinted autosomal dominant transmission of a disease allele. Individuals are affected only if they receive the mutant allele through paternal and not maternal transmission. Furthermore, the affected individuals can receive the mutant. Both, the affected and the unaffected carrier male who has received the mutant allele through maternal inheritance can then transmit the allele.

ber of genes with equivalent influence or effect. The genetic component of multifactorial traits is referred to by terms such as *increased risk, predisposition, or susceptibility*. Because of their complexity, the factors that contribute to the multifactorial traits are poorly defined. Two well-studied diseases that are classified as multifactorial include cardiovascular conditions and diabetes, as well as distinct behavioral disorders. The influence of nongenetic factors, such as environmental agents or stochastic processes during developmental outcome of a variety of traits, is also clearly illustrated in the studies of identical twins.

MAPPING AND IDENTIFICATION OF DISEASE GENES

Prior to the development of the human linkage map, the genetic etiology of human disease was identified by focusing on the biochemical and physiologic differences between normal and affected individuals. A large number of genes whose mutation results in human disease have been identified subsequent to the understanding of their biochemical basis (30). Specifically, knowledge of structural or functional information of the aberrant protein associated with the disease was applied toward cloning the gene that encoded the protein. To clone a gene is to isolate it in a form that allows its replication into multiple copies for subsequent study and manipulation. Identification and cloning of specific genes utilizing knowledge of the protein involved in the pathophysiology of the disorder is termed *functional cloning*. However, functional cloning cannot be applied to a large number of disorders, including those affecting hearing, because their underlying biochemical defects remain uncharacterized. The relative absence of knowledge concerning the biochemical basis of these disorders stems from a number of reasons. For example, the relative inaccessibility of the inner ear combined with its small size has deterred biochemical analysis of hearing and its dysfunction. Under these circumstances, where the information on pathophysiology of the disorder cannot be obtained or detected using current diagnostics techniques, the use of the genetic approach has been fruitful for identifying the disease gene in a variety of human disorders. This approach of gene identification is termed *positional cloning* (31). In this method, the disease gene is initially localized to a small region on the chromosome. Information on the chromosomal position of the gene is then subsequently used to identify the disease gene, using methods of molecular biology (described within the following sections).

Classically, localization of the chromosomal position of the human disease gene was tentatively determined through the identification of associated but relatively rare chromosomal abnormalities, such as deletions or translocations. These assignments were relatively low in the power of their resolution, spanning from a width of a chromosomal band to the length of an entire chromosomal arm. Currently, localization of the disease gene is accomplished through the principles used in the development of the genetic linkage map (described under Linkage and Recombination). This process, referred to as linkage analysis, determines which of the known genetic markers is most closely "linked" to the disease phenotype, thus the disease gene. Identification of the "linked" marker, whose map position is well established, reveals the approximate location of the disease locus. The disease gene may then be identified, and its role in the etiology of the disease can then be studied. The ability to identify the gene responsible for the disease in absence of all but genetic information, through the analysis of coinheritance of an observed trait with a previously characterized genetic marker, underlines the power of the genetic approach.

The key development that has made this strategy widely applicable and fruitful is the construction of the human genetic map, also known as linkage map, with closely spaced landmarks. The current high-resolution linkage map consists of genetic markers spaced less than 1 cM apart on average and distributed across the human genome (32–36). The development of this high-resolution linkage map has in turn been due to identification and characterization of highly polymorphic genetic markers. A description of these genetic markers and their use in mapping or identifying the chromosomal position of the disease gene (linkage analysis) are described in the following section.

Genetic Markers and Genetic Maps

Any inherited characteristic that differs among individuals and is easily detectable is a potential genetic marker. Some forms of these variations are observed in relatively simple traits such as eye or hair color or more complex traits such as disease susceptibility. The underlying basis of these phenotype variations in a given trait resides within the inherited DNA sequence. The human genome is characterized by such variations distributed throughout its length, within both coding and noncoding sequences. The sequence variations within a given chromosomal location or locus are termed *polymorphisms,* while a specific sequence variant is referred to as an *allele*. Formally, a locus is considered to be polymorphic if it contains more than one allele in the population, with a frequency greater than 1%. It is estimated that one third of the loci are polymorphic in the human genome. It is this extensive polymorphism at the geomic level that forms the basis of human diversity and uniqueness.

Classically, polymorphisms at the molecular level were identified within proteins. Variation between similar proteins among different individuals was identified through analysis of their physical properties. These include the differing antigenicity of cell surface proteins, as exemplified in the ABO blood types, as well as the histocompatibility antigens or their differing electrophoretic properties, as observed in the varying migration rates of subunits of the enzyme aldehyde dehydrogenase.

Polymorphism within coding seqences or within noncoding sequences arises from mutations within the genomic

DNA. It is estimated that a greater degree of polymorphism exists within a noncoding sequence relative to coding sequence as a consequence of its presumed null effect on the phenotype of the individual. The variation in the noncoding sequence, more prevalent and extensive than within the coding sequence, is representative of a genetic marker and has been cleverly utilized by the geneticist to construct a linkage map to dissect the genetic etiology of specific phenotypic traits. These genetic markers are mapped on the genome relative to each other based on how frequently they are coinherited. If these markers are "close together," then they are much less likely to be separated by recombination than are markers that are located far apart. If two markers or loci are physically near each other on the same chromosome, the probability that they will be coinherited will be greater than 50%. If two loci are seen to recombine in only 1 out of 100 meioses, they are said to be at 1% recombination or 1 cM apart, the genetic distance between two loci. If two loci are seen to recombine in 25 of 100 meioses, they are said to be 25 cM apart on that chromosome. Alternatively, if two markers are on different chromosomes, the probability that they will be coinherited is 50% due to a random assortment of chromosomes in meiosis in accordance with Mendel's second law. In the case of two loci separated by a 50% probability of a crossover event between them, it cannot be determined whether they are on the same chromosome or on two different chromosomes. In such a case, the loci are said to be unlinked.

The relative order and genetic distance between markers is determined in well-characterized, extended human pedigrees in a process known as segregation analysis—determining if a given genetic marker is coinherited with another marker and how frequently to assess its genetic distance. The detection of a meiotic crossover between two loci requires that the parent generating the recombinant chromosome, inherited by the offspring, be heterozygous at each locus. If the parent is homozygous at the loci being tested, a crossover event between the two loci will be undetected. The closer the markers are to each other, the more tightly linked they are and the less likely they will have a recombination crossover occur between them. A genetic distance of 1 cM between two markers (i.e., separated by recombination 1% of the time) is roughly equal to a physical distance of 1 million bp (1 Mb). It should be noted that recombination frequencies vary considerably, depending on the chromosomal region involved and the sex of the individual in which the meiosis is generated. Telomeric regions in general have higher recombination frequencies than centromeric regions, and recombination frequencies are generally higher in females than in males, yielding a longer genetic linkage map in females.

The principles of linkage analysis used in the construction of the genetic map can then be readily used to identify an unknown locus controlling an observable trait, such as a disease phenotype (i.e., hearing loss). Using a panel of genetic markers that are closely spaced and distributed throughout the genome, one can carry out a genome-wide search, at any particular location, for a specific marker that cosegregates with or is linked to the disease phenotype in the affected individuals. Identification of such a linked marker localizes the disease locus. Thus, the utility and application of linkage analysis to determine an unknown disease gene locus is a function of distribution and character of the genetic markers and the linkage map that is constructed from them. The physical location of these genetic markers is determined through hybridization analysis, described within the section, Physical Mapping.

Sequence analysis of DNA has identified several types of sequence variations or genetic markers within the population. An example of such sequence variation includes single base pair alterations that affect cleavage or noncleavage by restriction endonucleases. The consequence of the presence or absence of a restriction site is known as restriction fragment length polymorphisms (RFLPs). Another sequence alteration that has become the dominant choice for the construction of a linkage map is known as simple sequence repeat polymorphism (SSRP). The polymorphism of the SSRPs results from variation in the number of repeat units, either two, three, or four nucleotides long. Thus, SSRPs are also known as length polymorphism.

Restriction Fragment Length Polymorphism

Restriction enzymes provide a tool for cutting or cleaving DNA at sequence-specific sites. These enzymes, isolated from bacteria where they serve to protect against exogenous DNA, are characterized by the specificity of the sequence they recognize and cleave. If a mutation changes a base in the recognition site, the enzyme will no longer recognize and cut this site. When coupled with gel electrophoresis, a technique that permits separation of DNA fragments according to their length, restriction enzymes can be used to detect heritable variations in the DNA sequence of individuals, reflecting the presence or absence of a specific restriction site within a given region. A schematic of an RFLP and its detection are illustrated in Fig. 14. Such germline variations in RFLPs can be correlated with a given phenotype to make statistical statements regarding the probability that a particular size of fragment, or allele, is coinherited with a particular phenotype.

The extensive sequence variation in the human genome and the identification of a large number of restriction enzymes have led to the detection of numerous RFLPs. Specific RFLPs have been identified to be linked to certain disease loci. For example an RFLP closely associated with sickle cell anemia has been used for predictive diagnosis of potential carriers of the disease gene. Limitations of RFLP as a genetic tool are twofold. An absence or presence of a given restriction site represents a maximum of two alternate forms of that allele in the population. This limited polymorphism or dimorphism represents a major drawback of an RFLP as an informative genetic marker for following its

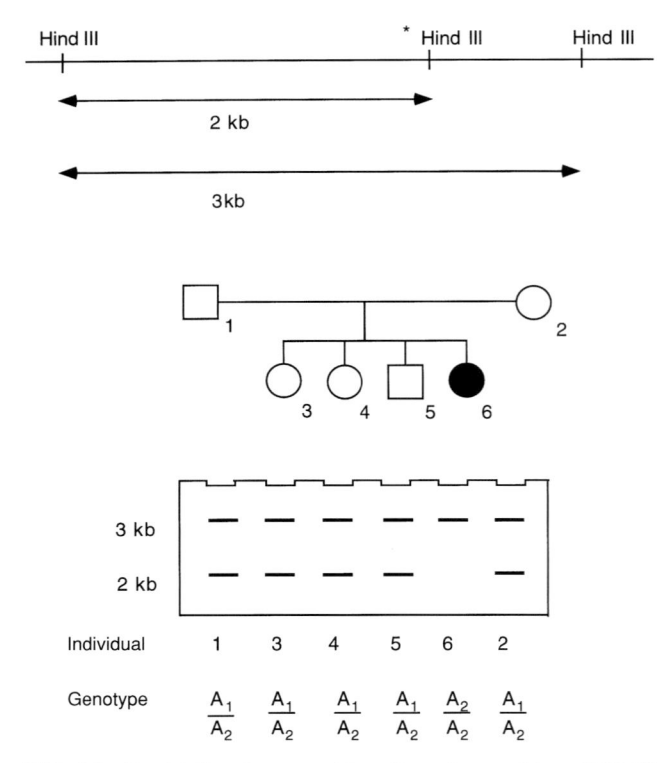

FIG. 14. Restriction fragment length polymorphism (RFLP) and its analysis. The top panel depicts a schematic of two alleles that are detected by presence or absence of a restriction site surrounding a gene locus and the distance between them in Kb. Genotype analysis of this polymorphism in a pedigree is carried out through the following steps: 1) digestion of genomic DNA from family members with the given restriction enzyme, 2) resolution of the products via gel electrophoresis followed by its transfer to a matrix such as a nitrocellulose membrane, referred to as the Southern Blot, 3) hybridization of the blot with a radioactive DNA probe, prepared from DNA that is encompassed within the restriction sites, and then 4) analysis of hybridization by exposing the blot to a radioactive film. The results of this analysis are illustrated in the bottom panel. Homozygous genotype (A1/A1 or A2/A2) yields a single fragment, while the heterozygous genotype (A1/A2) yields two fragments.

transmission from parent to offspring. An "informativeness" of a genetic marker is predicated by its degree of polymorphism, also known as its heterozygosity index. The heterozgosity index predicts the likelihood of any individual in a population being heterozygous for a given locus. The higher the index for a given locus, the more likely that the tested individual will be hetereozygous for that locus. A second shortcoming of RFLP is that its analysis relies on hybridization-based approaches that are labor intensive, expensive, and require large amounts of DNA.

Simple Sequence Repeat Polymorphism

The recognition of length variation or polymorphism resulting from variation in an SSRP unit and the ability to readily detect them via PCR (described later within the section) represent the two fundamental advances toward construction of a high-resolution genetic linkage map. The development of the linkage map utilizing the SSRPs has greatly accelerated identification of disease genes in a variety of human disorders

The length polymorphism was initially identified within relatively large repeat units termed *variable number of tandem repeats* (VNTRs), detected as RFLPs. The repeat units within the VNTRs were shown to range in length from several base pairs to several kilobases. A particular type of length polymorphism identified through the VNTRs was composed of either 2, 3, or 4 base pair repeats. These were referred to as simple sequence repeats (SSRs) or microsatellites and were found to be both abundant and highly polymorphic. In addition, the utility of these SSRs derives from their relatively simple assay via PCR (discussed in the following section) without the added time-consuming, labor-intensive hybridization step that is necessary to detect the RFLPs or the VNTRs. The combination of three key attributes of the SSRs has led to their predominant use in the construction of the high-resolution linkage map of the human genome and in identification of the disease genes. These attributes include relatively wide and uniform distribution throughout the genome, a high degree of polymorphism (necessary for following transmission of an allele so as to establish its parental origin and/or its linkage to the disease trait), and the relative simplicity of detection.

The best characterized class of SSRs is the $[CA]_n$ family and is often referred to as a CA repeat. These dinucleotide repeats generally reside within a noncoding sequence. However, a class of trinucleotide repeats, [CAG], has been found within gene sequences. Pathogenic expansion of these repeat units has been associated with several human diseases. Although less frequent than di-, and trinucleotide repeats, tetranucleotide repeats have also been identified and represent a widely used set of genetic markers. Collectively, the di-, tri-, and tetranucleotide repeats markers, in view of their relative high density in the mammalian genome, can conceivably provide a tag for every gene within the human genome. For example, the density of CA repeats alone is considered to be approximately every 20 Kb. Thus, the CA repeats alone can potentially tag every gene in the human genome.

Identification and mapping of SSRPs have enabled the development of high-resolution, genome-wide genetic maps. For the human genome, three major centers have provided maps and reagents in the form of highly polymorphic SSRPs to map disease genes. Up to 200 markers, spaced an average of 20 cM apart (spanning the entire genome that is 3.0×10^9), may have to be tested to find a marker linked to the disease locus. The availability of these markers and maps has increased linkage mapping efficiency and now made it possible for numerous laboratories to perform linkage studies.

Assay of Simple Sequence Repeat Polymorphisms via the Polymerase Chain Reaction

The SSRPs are assayed by first amplifying them from genomic DNA to increase their copy number followed by resolution of the product on a polyacrylamide gel to assess for its length variation. The methodology used for amplification of the alleles is known as polymerase chain reaction (PCR) is a powerful technique for making many copies of DNA from a piece of target DNA. Rather than relying on cloning vectors such as plasmids or phage λ, PCR uses an enzyme called Taq DNA polymerase to repeatedly copy the original DNA fragment present in the reaction. A schematic of PCR is illustrated in Fig. 15. The PCR reaction mixture includes four basic components: (a) the target DNA, which can be as little as a single copy of DNA and derived from almost any source (e.g., cells, tissue, plasmids); (b) oligonucleotide "primers," which are each designed to hybridize at the 5' end of the sequence of DNA to be amplified; (c) an excess of individual nucleotides (dATP, dCTP, dTTP, dGTP); and (d) Taq polymerase, a DNA polymerase derived from the bacterium *Thermus aquaticus* that is extremely stable at a wide range of temperatures. Using an automated heating block, this mixture is cycled through a series of temperature changes that are designed to allow the polymerase to repeatedly duplicate the target DNA. Each cycle begins at a denaturing temperature (e.g., 94°C) to separate the strands of target DNA (strand separation phase). The temperature is then decreased (i.e., 42–60°C, depending on reaction conditions) to allow the oligonucleotides to anneal (primer annealing phase). Following annealing, the temperature is increased to 72°C, the optimal temperature for Taq polymerase activity, to enable amplification or replication of the target DNA using the oligonucleotides as the primers (primer extension phase). Figure 16 illustrates the application of PCR to characterize or type the identity of a particular SSRP for a given genomic DNA.

Linkage Analysis

Linkage analysis represents the genetic approach of identifying the chromosomal location of gene(s) responsible for an inherited trait, relative to a known marker locus. Linkage is determined by assessing whether a marker and the disease locus do or do not segregate (separate) independently after a meiotic crossover. Analysis of coinheritance of the marker and disease trait allows one to determine the probability of their physical proximity or linkage to each other. The statistical probability of linkage is expressed in terms of LOD score, the *l*ogarithm to the base 10 of the *od*s that the markers are linked at a recombination distance of N centimorgans. The more frequently two markers are seen to cosegregate, the higher the LOD score. Two markers are considered to be linked at a confidence level of 95% when the LOD score reaches 3.0 or, equivalently, when the odds in favor of linkage are 1,000 to 1. Conversely, if the odds of two markers that appear linked reaches 100:1 against linkage, a lod score of −2, then those two markers are said to be unlinked. For a disease locus with a clear, fully penetrant phenotype and no genetic heterogeneity, these levels of statistical significance are acceptable for confirming or ruling out linkage at the particular locus under analysis. Linkage analysis of complex phenotypes may need to take into account some modifications of these conventions.

The utility and power of linkage analysis is dependent on polymorphism of the genetic maker that is being identified, or "typed" in an individual. The greater the polymorphism, the more likely that an individual will be heterozygous for the marker whose transmission and inheritance is followed relative to the disease trait. The capacity to "trace" the pa-

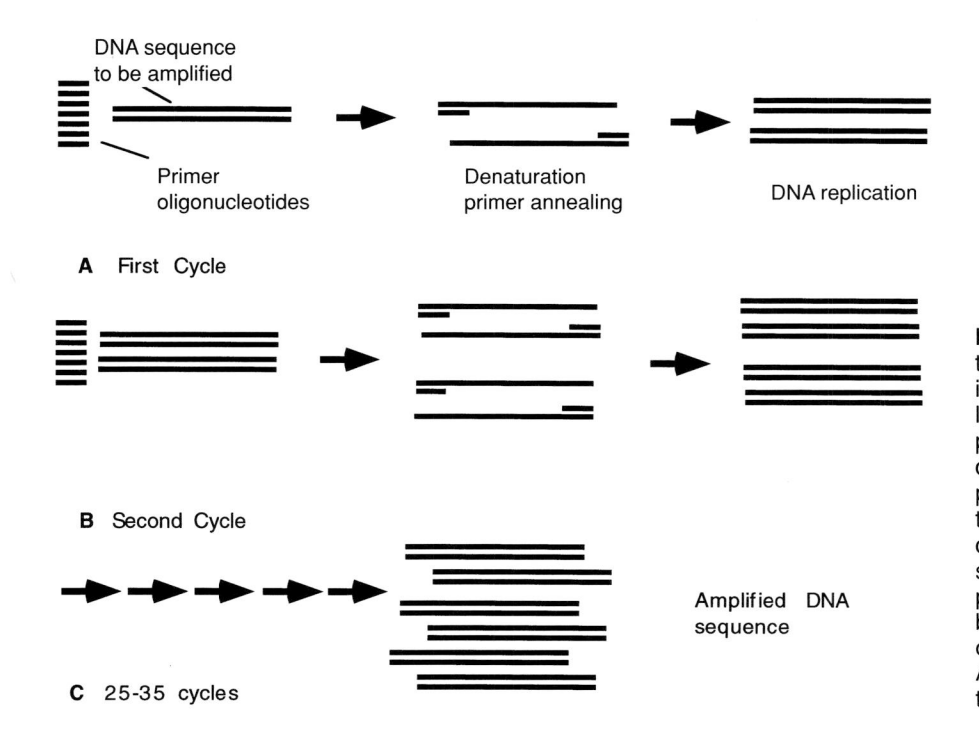

FIG. 15. The polymerase chain reaction (PCR). Double stranded target DNA is mixed with short, single stranded polynucleotides or primers that are complementary to the target. The mixture is denatured and then cooled to an appropriate temperature allowing the primers to anneal to their complementary sequence. The annealed primers then serve to initiate synthesis of new complementary DNA strands by thermostable DNA polymerase. Repeated cycles of DNA synthesis (25 to 35 cycles) using A and B primers exponentially amplifies the DNA flanked by these primers.

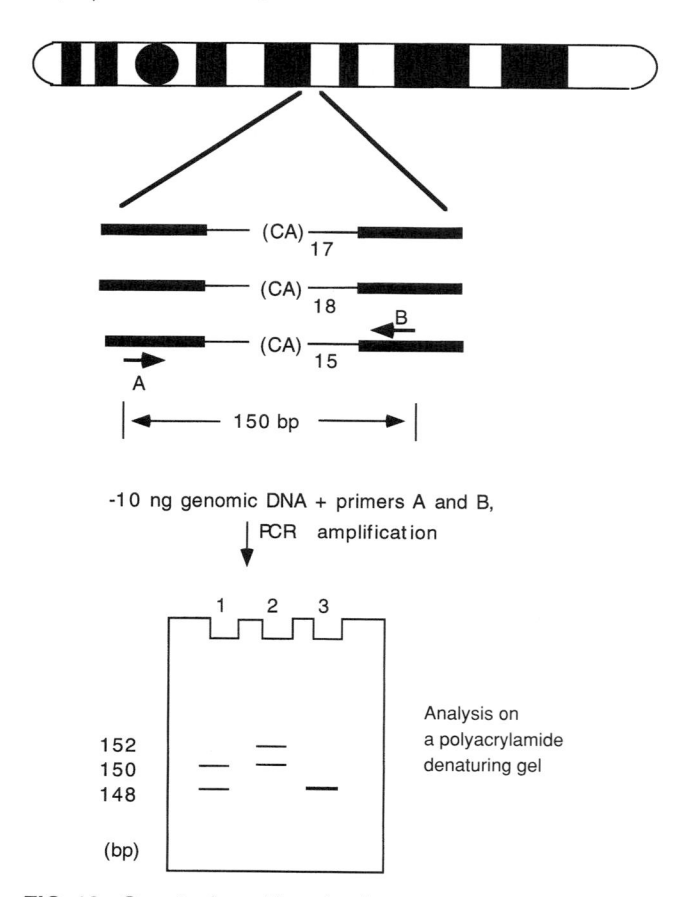

FIG. 16. Genotyping with a simple sequence repeat polymorphism (SSRP). Mapped SSRP are used to genetically identify or genotype an individual in a pedigree for the purpose of linkage analysis. The upper panel in the figure illustrates the chromosomal location of a mapped SSRP containing the dinucleotide 'CA' as the repeat unit. Also shown below the chromosome are several alleles of this SSRP that vary in the length of their repeat unit, from 15 to 18. The lower panel illustrates how the identity of these polymorphic alleles in an individual is determined. The polymorphic locus is amplified from genomic DNA by PCR using oligonucleotides (arrows) that recognize the surrounding nonpolymorphic, single copy sequence. The amplification products are then analysed on a high resolution polyacrylamide gel. Since the polymorphism is based on variation in the number of dinucleotide repeat unit, the observed alleles differ from each other by a multiple of two base pairs. Note that individuals 1 and 2 are heterozygotes at this locus while individual 3 is a homozygous.

rental origin of a marker in the offspring is essential for orientation of the marker and the disease locus on the same or opposite chromosomes. If the relationship between the marker, its parental origin and the disease phenotype can be established (known as linkage phase) the meiosis or the mating is said to be fully informative for that marker. For an autosomal dominant disorders, fully informative meiosis requires the affected parent to be heterozygous for the linked locus. On the other hand, determination of linkage phase in recessively inherited disorders requires both parents of the affected individual(s) to be heterozygous for the linked

locus. Confounding technical factors in linkage analysis include the misdiagnosis of individuals within the family under study and nonpaternity. The presence of genetic heterogeneity or phenocopies within the pedigree can also skew linkage analysis. *Genetic heterogeneity* refers to similar phenotypes produced by mutations in different genes. It is imperative that sporadically affected cases be distinguished from those that occur through the inheritance of the putative disease gene. Phenocopies represent identical or indistinguishable phenotypes caused by or simulated by an environmental agent.

The first key step in linkage analysis, prior to genotyping using genetic markers that span the genome, is the identification and clinical characterization of the study sample. This process involves initial identification of individuals and family with the disorder, accurate construction of pedigrees, accurate clinical evaluation, and proper handling of the DNA samples extracted from each individual. Once this step has been established, one may proceed with genotyping and linkage analysis. Linkage analysis of genetic traits has allowed the positional cloning of genes causing diseases such as retinoblastoma and cystic fibrosis (37,38).

Statistical Methods of Linkage Analysis and Their Application

The statistical methods of linkage analysis may be classified as parametric and nonparametric. The parametric method is based on segregation analysis of marker alleles. It is the method of choice for family pedigrees that span several generations when the mode of inheritance is straightforward, as in mendelian traits. This method involves the assumption of a genetic model as well as specification of certain parameters. The major requirement for a successful application of linkage analysis for mapping a disease trait of a family pedigree requires a large, well-defined family. A LOD score of 3 is considered evidence of linkage (i.e., there is cosegregation of the locus with deafness), and a LOD score of -2 is considered evidence against linkage (i.e., the deafness is unlikely to be located at the tested locus). For X-linked families, a LOD score of 2 is considered significant evidence of linkage. For a disease that is transmitted in an autosomal dominant fashion, each affected and unaffected informative individual contributes a LOD score of approximately 0.3; therefore, a family needs to have at least ten informative individuals to provide evidence for linkage (LOD score of 3). For recessive disorders, each affected individual contributes approximately 0.6 to the LOD score; therefore, one needs only five affected members to identify the disease gene locus.

The nonparmetric method does not require prior knowledge of the parameters that are associated with or define the inheritance of the disease within a family or among a "select" population. The nonparametric method is particularly applicable in situations in which the family is not large enough to yield sufficient recombinants for high-resolution mapping. It is also applicable when the probable mode of inheritance (autosomal dominant, recessive, or X-linked) cannot be assumed, as in nonmendelian or complex traits. Several different nonparametric methods have been described including sib-pair analysis and affected-pedigree-member analysis (39). The sib-pair method is based on the principle that siblings who share a specific phenotype would also share the same marker alleles more frequently than randomly expected, if the loci encoding the trait and the marker allele are linked. Conversely, if the two loci are linked, siblings that do not share the linked marker would not share the same trait. Thus, the putative disease locus may be mapped without segregation analysis or tracing transmission of a marker in multiple generations. This method is useful in situations in which individuals within the family under study are in a single generation or are scattered in an extended kindred. Because this method does not involve segregation analysis and hence detection of recombinants, the genetic distance between the marker and the disease loci cannot be determined; nor can one estimate the relative order of multiple loci. Extensions to the method of sib-pair analysis include use of sibling pairs in unrelated families having an identical trait, with the underlying assumption that these families also share the same disease gene (i.e., genetic homogeneity). This approach allows the use of smaller families with fewer affected members as well as not having to assume a genetic model of inheritance. A major disadvantage of this methodology is its relative lack of power to detect linkage; that is, a substantially greater number of affected individuals are required for analysis.

An application of the parametric approach of linkage analysis is illustrated in Fig. 17. Each individual in the three-generation pedigree expressing autosomal dominant inheritance of the disease trait is typed for a genetic marker with two distinct alleles. Analysis of the pedigree indicates that allele 1 carried by the individual I-1 is linked with the disease trait in this family. This marker allele is identified in all affected individuals with the exception of III-7, who has inherited allele 2 from his affected father. Mathematic analysis of this segregation pattern to assess linkage and the genetic distance between the marker and the disease loci is then presented in the form of LOD scores. These values are presented in a table format below the pedigree in Fig. 17. At a recombination fraction of 0, the LOD score is less than infinity. This value indicates that the probability that the marker and the disease locus are identical is zero, consistent with the presence of a recombination event identified in the individual III-7. As θ increase, the LOD score becomes positive, expressing a maxim value of 3.4 with equal to 0.07. As θ increases above 0.07, the LOD score decreases, indicating that increasing the genetic distance between the marker and the disease locus makes the mathematic estimate less likely with the observed results. This is known as two-point analysis, and the maximum LOD score obtained at $\theta = 0.07$ (7% recombination) indicates that the most likely distance between the marker and the location of the disease gene is 7 cM. This value, based on percent recombination between the two loci, may also be simply calculated by dividing the number of recombinant meiotic crossovers (individual III-7) by the total number of meiotic crossovers assessed. This ratio is 1:15 or 0.07. The LOD score of 3.4 thus provides strong evidence of linkage of the marker and disease locus in this particular pedigree.

Following linkage of the disease trait to a marker locus, one may then proceed to define the position of the disease locus within a narrow interval. This may be realized through linkage analysis of multiple markers relative to each other and to the disease locus. This analysis, known as multipoint mapping, allows one to develop a genetic map across the disease locus, thereby establishing identity, order, and the relative distance of markers that flank the disease locus on its proximal and terminal sides.

Applications of the Linkage Principles for Mapping Genes Responsible for Nonsyndromic Hearing Loss

As indicated earlier, a constraint in mapping disease genes is the requirement for relatively large pedigrees with a relatively clear pattern of the disease transmission. An additional factor that makes this requirement even more difficult to meet for mapping genes that cause nonsyndromic hearing loss (NSHL) is the relatively frequent occurrence of marriages between deaf individuals. The affected families resulting from these marriages are likely to have more than one gene for deafness (genetic heterogeneity). The possibility of phenocopies, hearing loss due to nongenetic factors, within these families also cannot be excluded. As a consequence, large pedigrees with a clear pattern of segregation of only one factor responsible for the hearing loss are relatively uncommon. One way to overcome this problem is to study families from relatively isolated populations. There is a relatively greater degree of genetic homogeneity within these isolated populations as a consequence of its origins from limited number of individuals and relative absence of immigration from outside, thus precluding a change in the constitution of its gene pool.

Such large isolated populations with incidence of NSHL have been extremely valuable for mapping several different deafness genes. The autosomal dominant form of NSHL has been linked with a number of different loci. This includes linkage to 5q31 in a large Costa Rican family (17), to 1p32 in an extended Indonesian family (40) and to 13q12 in a French family (41). Mapping autosomal recessive disorders has also relied upon the use of large isolated populations with an altered selection criteria. These studies have selected pedigrees with occurrence of autosomal recessive NSHL in which marriages between cousins (consanguinity) is relatively common. The relative isolation of the population as well as consanguinity ensures the presence of a single mutant locus and relatively high frequency of its homozygosity. Thus, within the offspring of consanguineous marriages, a fraction of the genome would be expected to be homozygous

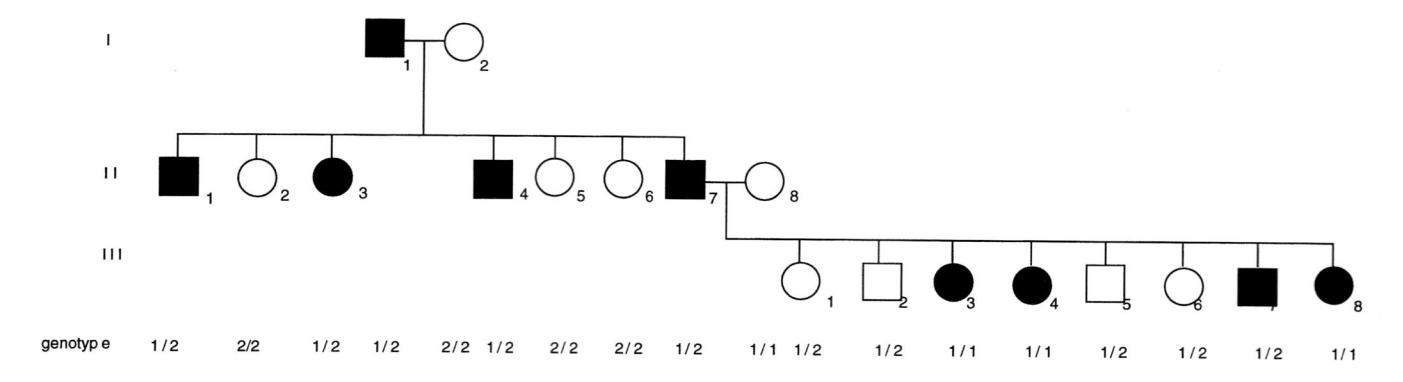

	LOD (Z) Scores for various θ				
θ =	0.00	0.05	0.10	0.20	$\bar{\theta}$ (0.07)
Distance vs marker	−∞	3.0	3.1	2.2	$\bar{Z}$ (3.4)

FIG. 17. Analysis of a linked marker in a pedigree transmitting an autosomal dominant trait and determination of its LOD score. The genotype of the dimorphic marker (alleles 1 and 2) is shown below each member of the pedigree with autosomal dominant transmission of disease. The disease trait can be seen to be consegregating with the marker allele 1 except for individual III-7 who does not carry that allele descended from I-1. Individual III-7 is thus a recombinant for the disease gene and the marker loci. Note that heterozygosity of the 'linked' marker locus in the affected grandfather (I-1) and father (II-7) enables one to determine its 'phase' or chromosomal orientation of the marker alleles with respect to the disease locus. Determining the linkage phase of marker alleles 1 and 2 aids in distinguishing their parental origin in generations II and III. The mathematical analysis of the probability of linkage between the marker and the disease loci (Z) at various values of recombination fraction (θ), computed using LINKAGE program, is given in the table below the pedigree.

because of common descent. The regions of identity would be expected to be random between different offspring of these matings, except at the common disease locus shared by the affected offspring. This strategy has been used to map an autosomal recessive form of NSHL to several different loci, including 13q12 in a Northern Tunisian family (42), 17p11.2-q12 in an Indonesian family (43) and 21q22 in a large consanguineous group of kindred from Pakistan (44). This strategy of determining a shared region of the genome among offspring of consanguineous marriages is also referred to as homozygosity mapping (45). It is widely applied in the mapping of various other autosomal recessive disorders, specifically within isolated inbred populations in which the problem of genetic heterogeneity is partially overcome. It should be noted that among the numerous isolated populations that are available, the relatively recently founded populations are likely to require a relatively low density screen of its genome for linkage analysis than a population that has been established for many generations. The greater the number of generations, the greater the amount of meiosis that would yield a relatively small shared segment containing the disease gene, thus requiring a relatively high-density screen with the genetic markers.

A consequence of the identity of descent of a disease gene is that there exist associated markers and alleles that descend with the disease gene. Thus, affected individuals that share a region of their genome also display a unique combination of linked alleles that span that region. This combination of alleles across a region is known as haplotype. The preferential association of a particular allele in individuals with the disease trait, more frequently than that predicted by chance, is referred to as linkage disequilibrium. Analysis of linkage disequilibrium mapping may also be used to narrow the interval once the general location of the gene has been identified. The use of linkage disequilibrium is limited to disease genes that have descended from a single individual. Haplotype analysis of region spanning the disease can determine which combination is more frequent in the affected individuals than predicted from haplotype combinations in the nonaffected individuals. This information on linkage disequilibrium may then be used to further narrow the disease locus. The gene causing diastrophic dysplasia was fine mapped and subsequently identified using linkage disequilibrium data (46).

Advancing from the Linked Locus to the Disease Gene

Linkage of a given disease trait to a genetic marker and its subsequent localization within a defined region of the chromosome represents the first stage in identifying the disease gene. Mapping of the locus within flanking genetic markers narrows the search to a limited region relative to the entire genome. However, the length of DNA sequence to be analyzed, contained within flanking markers, is still extremely large. For example, the closest marker may be a megabase apart from the disease gene from either the centromeric (proximal) or the telomeric (terminal) side. Thus, the region that can potentially contain the disease gene is several megabases in length.

At this stage, one may assess the genetic linkage map for the presence of previously cloned genes that map to the linked locus. If any genes are mapped within the linked region, they represent candidate disease genes for mutation analysis. This strategy of characterizing a previously cloned gene based on its location within the linked region is known as the positional candidate gene approach.

If no positional candidate genes are present in the linked region (a situation that is relatively common) and if the pedigree under study is relatively large with numerous informative meioses, then it is possible to map the disease locus to within 0.1 to 0.2 cM. This genetic distance corresponds to approximately 100 to 200,000 bases (physical distance). At this level of resolution of the linked locus, positional cloning of the disease gene may be considered (i.e., cloning of the disease gene entirely from information on its position). This method, unlike the positional candidate gene approach, identifies unknown genes that map within the linked locus. The following section describes the molecular methodology involved in analyzing large regions of DNA, up to 1 million bp (or 1 Mb) for presence of the disease gene. The alternative approach of candidate gene analysis, that sidesteps the highly time-consuming and labor-intensive positional cloning strategy, will also be discussed.

Positional Cloning

Once the disease region has been sublocalized to 1 Mb, it can be isolated in overlapping large and small capacity cloning inserts for further characterization. Currently, the yeast artificial chromosome (YAC) is utilized as the large-capacity cloning vector. The YACs permit cloning of large genomic DNA fragments that can vary in size from 200 kb up to 1 Mb, hence providing a bridge between linkage or cytogenetic analysis (a chromosome band contains approximately 5 to 15 Mb of DNA) and subsequent cloning of the target locus (47). A physical map of the linked region is then developed through characterization of the YAC clones that encompass the flanking markers. Physical mapping includes determining the size of the YAC insert and localization of various polymorphic markers, such as SSRPs or restriction enzyme sites, and nonpolymorphic markers, such as sequence tag sites, anonymous sequences that serve as landmarks and expressed sequence tags, short sequences that are identified from cDNA libraries. Development of the physical map facilitates subdivision of the YAC clone and thus aids in the identification of candidate genes spanning the cloned region. Various methods exist for identifying expressed sequences in the linked region. These procedures include hybridization-based as well as function-based assays. Identification of expressed sequences is then followed by mutation analysis to determine identity of the disease gene. Figure 18 illustrates the steps that are utilized in the positional cloning approach, advancing from a linked locus to physical maps to candidate genes to the pathogenic mutation. Note the increasing level of resolution that is achieved at each successive stage of the cloning procedure. The following sections describe the steps that are utilized in this approach.

Physical Mapping

Physical maps differ from genetic maps in the types of information they yield. Genetic maps yield relative positions of a number of polymorphic hereditary characters and their relative distance from each other based on segregation analysis of these traits. Physical maps provide a more direct description of all landmarks, both polymorphic and nonpolymorphic traits, in terms of their precise sequence and distance in base pairs from each other. Figure 19 illustrates the relationship between genetic and physical maps. Note that the linear order of markers or genes on both maps is the same but the relative distance between the markers is not necessarily proportional between the two maps. Physical mapping facilitates further subdivision of that region so that the genes contained within the linked region may be identified and then characterized for the pathogenic mutation. Development of the physical map spanning the linked region requires the generation and localization of markers as reference points. This facilitates localization of genes within or expressed sequences within the region. The ultimate aim in the development of this physical map is to obtain the nucleotide sequence of a candidate gene contained within the region, the sequence representing the highest resolution of the physical map.

The first step in physical mapping of a linked locus is its isolation within a cloning vector. The YAC vector, as with other cloning vectors, contains the elements necessary for its replication and maintenance in the host cell. These include the segment that encodes the origin of replication function, a segment that encodes the centromere function (CEN), and two segments encoding the chromosome ends that permit the replication and maintenance of the linear DNA molecule, the YAC. Genomic or chromosome specific YAC libraries have been constructed. These libraries can be readily screened for the presence of DNA markers via PCR, enabling one to isolate a cloned genomic segment containing the region of interest. The YACs that span the linked region may be readily identified from an arrayed YAC library that is available through the human genome project. If the linked region cannot be isolated within a single YAC clone, several overlapping, contiguous YACs will need to be isolated and ordered (also known as contig building). This contig or the

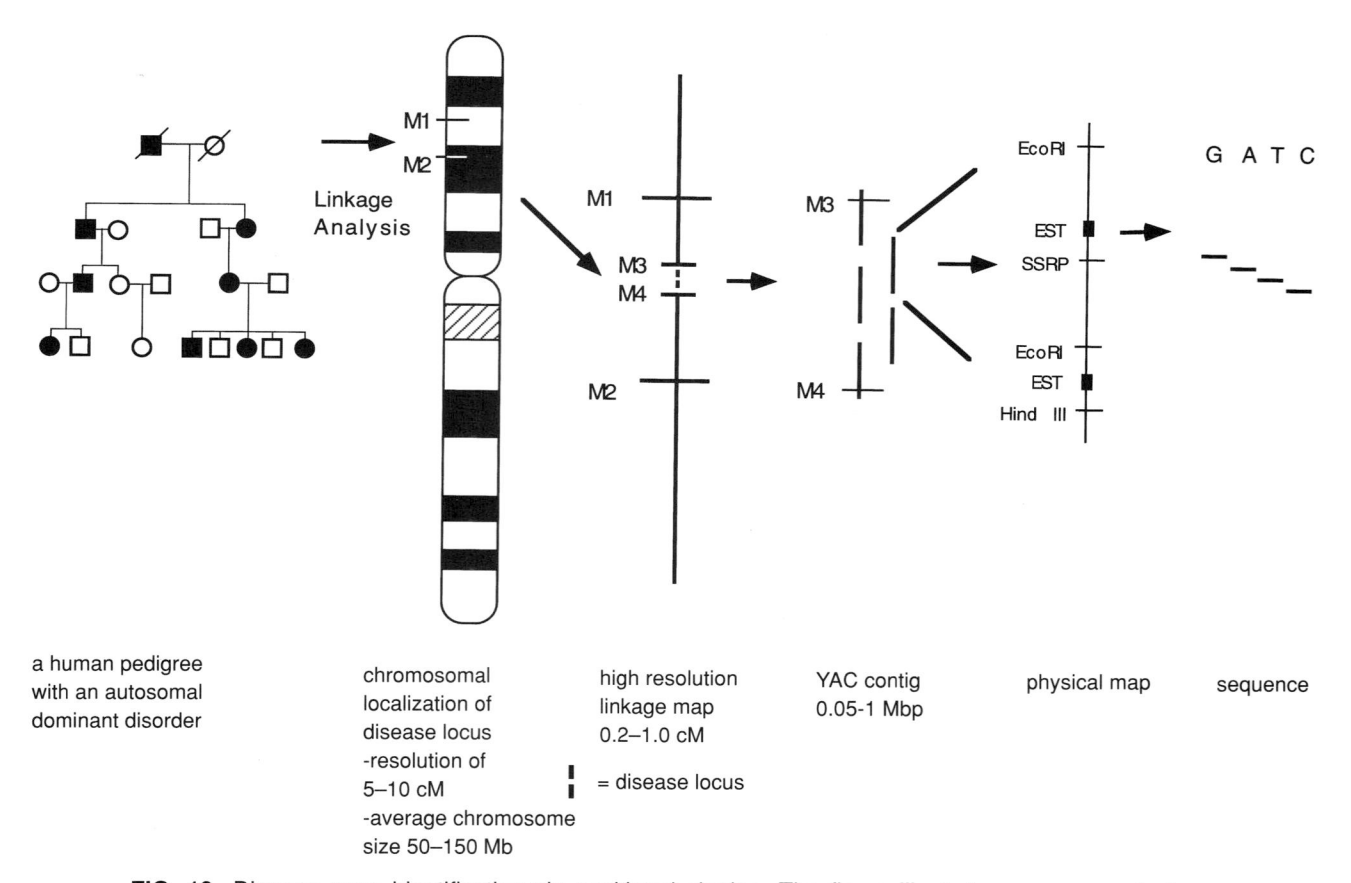

FIG. 18. Disease gene identification via positional cloning. The figure illustrates sequence of steps involved in disease gene identification via the positional cloning approach—from localization of the disease locus within the banding patterns of the chromosomes to its isolation within clones of overlapping segments of DNA and ultimately to the nucleotide sequence of the disease gene. The process is initiated with the identification of a 'linked' marker in an affected family via linkage analysis. Linkage serves to map the chromosomal location of the disease locus. The mapped region is narrowed to within genetic distance of 0.2 cM (approximately, 2 Mb in physical distance) on a linkage map. A panel of overlapping YAC clones or a contig that spans the mapped disease locus may then be identified. A physical map for the cloned genomic region is then developed by localizing various types of markers, including restriction enzyme sites, expressed sequence tags (EST) and sequence tagged sites (STS) and determining the relative physical distance between these markers. The physical map serves to identify genes that lie within the disease locus. Identity of the disease gene is established through the demonstration of pathogenic sequences alteration. These candidate genes are then sequenced. Also illustrated is levels of detail present at each stage of gene mapping and identification process.

YAC spanning the linked region may then be further characterized through a restriction map, thus adding another level of detail to the physical map. The sizes of the restriction fragments as well as the total size of the insert may be determined through pulse field gel electrophoresis, which is capable of resolving large DNA fragments. The next stage of the process is to generate subclones of the primary YAC clone(s) and identify or generate DNA markers that can be mapped onto the cloned region. The subclones that span the primary YAC clone are usually cosmids, whose insert is generally 40 kb.

There are several limitations to the use of YACs, and recognition of these limitations is critical to their efficient use. One of the frequent problems with the use of YACs is their chimerism. These chimeras are thought to arise by recombination in vivo between repeated sequences present within the human genomic DNA. Over 40% of YACs in most libraries are chimeric according to variety of criteria. These include analysis of its termini via PCR to assess that the two ends are contiguous (not derived from two different chromosomes) as well as hybridization of YACs to the genome, via the high-resolution direct mapping technique of fluorescence in situ hybridization, to assess for a single hybridization site to ensure its fidelity. Thus, YACs that have been isolated need to be initially characterized for presence of chimerism. In addition to their chimerism, the YACs are difficult to use; it is not easy to separate YAC DNA from yeast background and colony hybridization, to detect a specific sequence, is much more difficult due to the low copy number of YACs and the small number of cells in the colony.

E. coli-based vector systems have been developed in recent years that provide a more easily accessible source of DNA than YACs. These include the bacteriophage P1 cloning system, the bacterial artificial chromosome, and the P1-derived artificial chromosome. These vectors allow propagation of genomic DNA that is intermediate in size between the inset capacity of YACs and cosmids. Nevertheless, YACs remain the preferred vector for large-scale cloning or for contig building (generation of overlapping clones spanning a contiguous region of genomic DNA) despite the difficulties of fidelity (chimeras) and technical drawbacks (low copy number, etc.) (48).

A good strategy for generating markers that span the contig is to identify SSR within the YACs or the subclones (49). If such markers can be identified, they are mapped onto the contig and the pedigree retested for cosegregation of the marker and the disease phenotype. If a recombination is detected between the disease phenotype and the marker, the disease locus is localized further. If no recombination is detected, then the chances are that the disease locus is near the polymorphic marker. More polymorphic markers may be generated for mapping and genotyping that would generate a high-resolution map and aid in the sublocalization of the disease locus.

Mapping of the DNA markers on to the contig may be accomplished in several different ways. Classic mapping techniques utilized well-characterized somatic cell hybrids between humans and mice for mapping human genes and unique DNA probes. Such hybrids, also referred to as mapping panels, have been constructed for each individual chromosome and consist of a collection of hybrids that retain different subfragments of that chromosome. A greater degree of resolution in mapping may be obtained through the use of radiation hybrids. These constructs are hybrids formed between subfragments of human chromosome generated using radiation and the mouse genome, unlike the somatic cell hybrids that are formed using unmodified whole genome. A panel of radiation hybrids that span a given chromosomal interval may be used for a higher-resolution mapping. The use of these panels can be relatively cumbersome.

A relatively rapid and high-resolution mapping technique that is currently in favor is fluorescence in situ hybridization. This technique, in which the DNA probe is labeled with a fluorescence label and hybridized with metaphase chromosome, allows direct, rapid, and high-resolution visualization of the chromosomal location of a DNA marker (50). Commercially available whole chromosome paint probes are useful to identify or exclude unknown chromosomes or chromosome fragments in an aberrant karyotpye. DNA probes for a specific chromosomal region are also available for some of the more commonly identified submicroscopic DNA deletion/duplication syndromes.

To help identify genes through the positional cloning method, physical maps are being constructed across the human genome. This is being achieved by developing YAC contigs that span the genome and the mapping of various DNA markers on these contigs (51). The generation of such a physical map is an essential step prior to sequencing analysis. Premature large-scale sequencing would be of little use without knowing its precise location on the genome. Such a physical map would also allow for selective sequencing. A major factor that should simplify gene identification is the development and map assignment of expressed sequence tags (ESTs), short cDNA sequences developed to identify expressed genes (52,53).

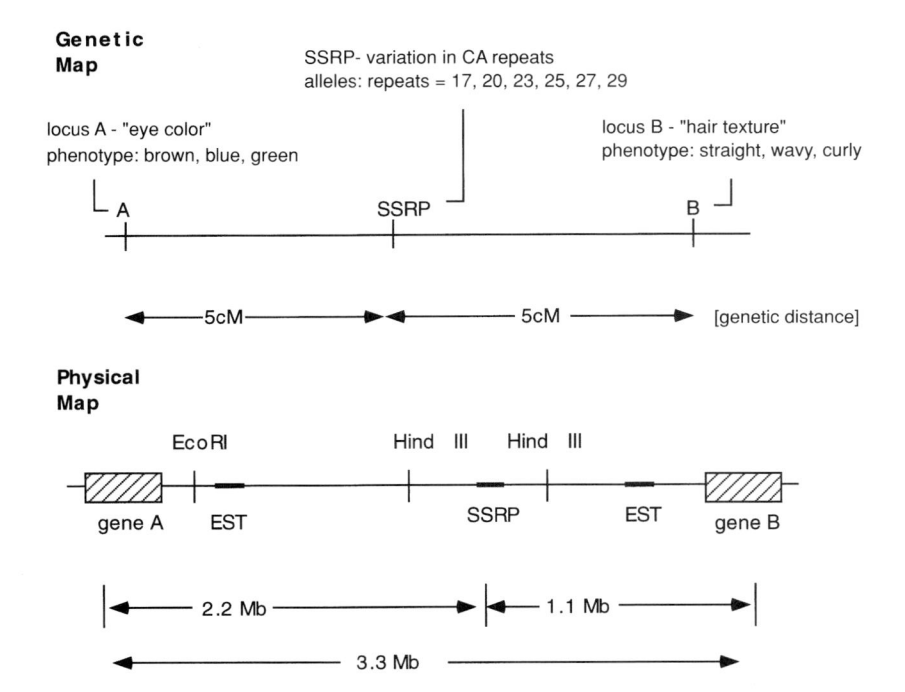

FIG. 19. Relationship between linkage map and physical map. The genetic linkage map shows the relative locations of polymorphic markers. These include both the phenotypic and DNA sequence based markers. A physical map on the other hand incorporates both the nonpolymorphic (expressed sequence tag (EST)) and polymorphic markers. While the linear order of loci on both maps is the same the distances between them are not necessarily proportional, i.e., centiMorgans on a genetic map cannot be directly translated into base pairs on the physical map.

Identifying Genes Within the Linked Region

The detection of coding sequence within genomic DNA represents one of the major tasks of positional cloning approach. The difficulty of this task stems from the noncontiguous nature of the genes, the fact that the coding sequence occupies a small fraction (3–5%) of the total sequence under study, that relatively large number of genes that can potentially exist within the linked locus and that no single assay exists that can simply and reliably identify all of these genes. It is estimated that there may be as many as 30 genes per megabase of DNA, the size of the genome that is generally faced within positional cloning studies. A number of strategies exist for identifying an expressed sequence. These methods, (listed and described in the following sections) fall into two general groups. Methods that utilize a structural or functional feature associated with the transcribed sequence (e.g., promoters, exons and polyadenylation sites) for its detection. The other group of techniques is directed toward identifying mRNAs transcribed from the disease locus. Direct selection of cDNA from an appropriate cDNA library probed with the genomic DNA under analysis represents an example of this class of techniques. In principle, both of these groups of methods should identify all of the expressed sequences. However, each technique within each group is subject to constraints inherent in its applications. Thus, no single method has been shown to be 100% efficient; hence a combination of several methods can help to complement each other's limitations. These constraints are emphasized in description of the methods. Description of these methods also illustrates their technically difficult and time-consuming nature.

CpG Islands. Regions rich in CpG residue islands are frequently associated with 5′ flanking sequences of some genes. The presence of these regions may be an indication of a potential downstream gene sequence. These sites are unmethylated and therefore accessible to cleavage by methylation-sensitive enzymes. Digestion of genomic DNA clones with such enzymes can lead to identification of a cluster of these cleavage sites, indicating the presence of CpG islands. Through this method, previously unknown genes can be recognized within the physical map under analysis. Markers associated with these islands can then be used to screen for genes.

Exon Trapping. This method makes use of the functional cis-acting elements required for RNA splicing. Yeast artificial chromosome or cosmid clones are digested and then shotgun-cloned into a vector containing an exon-trapping cassette. Such a vector can consist of a splice donor site, and the genomic insert is tested for the presence of a splice acceptor site. A drawback of this method is the relatively high frequency of cryptic splice acceptor sites, thus yielding numerous false-positives.

Tissue-Specific cDNA Library Screening. An apparently straightforward method for identifying the disease gene is to screen the cDNA library of the affected tissue with the linked region cloned into YAC or cosmid contigs. This approach is based on the rationale that affected tissue would be selectively expressing the disease gene. However, this method is plagued with a selection of highly repetitive sequences that hybridize to the immobilized YAC or cosmid clones. If an expressed sequence is selected, it is characterized initially by first confirming its presence within the linked region before becoming a candidate for mutation detection.

Zoo Blots and Northern Blots. These hybridization methods are used to detect highly conserved sequences that are likely to be protein coding. Genomic subclones are labeled and then hybridized with Zoo blots of genomic DNA from various species. Hybridizing clones are selected and screened for conserved exons via sequence analysis. Similarly, clones also can be hybridized with Northern blots of normal RNA isolated from multiple tissue types, including the affected tissue to identify fragments containing coding sequences.

At present, it is not possible to predict with high confidence the presence of coding regions in large-scale sequencing projects. A confirmation by one of the aforementioned methods is still required.

Identifying the Pathogenic Mutation

Once a gene has been identified within the disease locus, the next and final task is its analysis for the pathogenic mutation. The search for the sequence alteration is mostly localized to the coding sequence of the gene, although under certain circumstances the search may need to be extended to its noncoding sequence. Prior to the mutation search, several properties of the potential disease gene need to be determined to assess if they are compatible with the disease phenotype and its pattern of inheritance. Analysis of the expression pattern, within a tissue and cell type, represents one of the initial characterizations of the potential disease gene. Identification of its expression within the affected tissue represents a starting point for subsequent analysis of the gene. One need not necessarily look for selective expression in the candidate gene for diseases with high tissue specificity. Several examples exist of genes that are ubiquitously expressed but whose mutation can result in a tissue-specific disorder; these include the widely expressed STA gene that is responsible for Emery-Dreifuss muscular dystrophy as well as the RB1 gene responsible for retinoblastoma.

If the complete coding sequence of the potential disease gene has been determined, one may search for functional domains that correspond to the biochemical defect predicted or identified in the affected tissue. Developmental defects as well as inheritance patterns of the disease under study may also be considered for analysis of candidate disease genes. The genes responsible for developmental defects would be expected to exhibit the expression only at a certain developmental stage within the affected tissue or its embryonic predecessor. Diseases that show imprinted inheritance patterns would predicate genes with imprinted expression pattern. Disorders that are characterized by progressive increases in the severity of the phenotype (anticipation) would predicate genes that contain trinucleotide repeats within its coding or noncoding sequence. Thus, the probability that a gene within the region of interest represents the disease gene depends on how well its properties match up with the disease pathology and its inheritance pattern. Such criteria may be utilized when faced with characterization of multiple potential disease genes, located within the linked locus, for the pathogenic sequence alteration.

Identification of pathogenic sequence alteration within expressed sequences or candidate genes that map within the linked locus represents a challenging finishing touch in the disease diagnosis process. The degree of difficulty in identifying the mutation depends on the length of the coding sequence to be screened and the nature of its pathogenic DNA alteration. When the disease results from a large DNA rearrangement, such as a deletion, this altered form may be readily detected in the physical map of the region. However, when the disease results from a single base alteration that leads to missense or nonsense mutation, the task of identifying the disease gene can be extremely difficult. Not every sequence alteration in a candidate gene for a mendelian disorder represents the pathogenic mutation. It is very likely that the pathogenic mutation represents a normal polymorphism within the given population. An example of this situation is illustrated by a report of a 300-bp deletion within the gene encoding an alpha chain subunit of type II collagen among individuals affected with type II osteogenesis imperfecta. This deletion was considered to be pathogenic because it was not detected in the "control" population. It has subsequently been shown that this apparent deletion probably represents normal polymorphism common in persons of Asian Indian origin. Thus, when a sequence alteration is identified, its pathogenicity needs to be confirmed with absolute confidence. This includes demonstration of coinheritance or cosegregation of the sequence alteration with the disease phenotype. In vitro studies demonstrating dysfunction of the mutant protein, containing the altered sequence variation, also supplement our understanding of how the sequence alteration affects protein function. This concept may be further extended by correcting the suspected DNA alteration in the mutant cell with corresponding reversion to the normal phenotype. Such a demonstration may constitute the ultimate proof of identity of the pathogenic mutation.

The simplest strategy for identifying the pathogenic mutation is to sequence the candidate gene from both the affected and the nonaffected individuals. Figure 20 illustrates the dideoxy chain termination method of DNA sequencing. Dideoxy sequencing (also called chain termination or the Sanger method) uses an enzymatic procedure to synthesize DNA chains of varying lengths, stopping DNA replication at one of the four bases, and then determining the resulting fragment lengths. Figure 20 demonstrates a sequence variation between two individuals at a single base pair that results in a missense/nonsense mutation. Direct sequencing is highly time consuming and expensive and has low throughput. Several methods with relatively higher throughput exist that scan for the presence of an aberrant sequence. Most such procedures rely on altered conformation of the DNA containing the mutation. These include hybridization-based as well as function-based assays. In addition, methods that localize the site of the altered sequence also have been developed.

Conformation-based methods of mutation detection utilize migratory properties of DNA fragments that are dependent on its length and nucleotide sequence under certain conditions of gel electrophoresis. Thus, an altered mobility of DNA fragments between affected and nonaffected individuals within a family implies the presence of a sequence alteration between the two. But, this analysis does not indicate the precise position of the mutation. The location and precise nature of the sequence alteration may then be determined through sequence analysis. These methods have moderate sensitivity for detecting rare mutations that can vary from 70% to more than 95%.

One of the methods that is most widely used for rapid mutation detection is the technique referred to as single-stranded conformational polymorphism (SSCP). This method is developed on the principle that secondary structure contributes to the mobility of single-stranded DNA in electrophoresis gels under nondenaturing conditions. This technique can detect up to 70% mutations under single gel condition, and 95% of mutations using multiple gel conditions. Another conformation-based method of mutation analysis with a greater detection rate is denaturing gradient gel electrophoresis (DGGE). This method is based on the principle that regions of single-stranded DNA within double-stranded fragments greatly retard its migration through polyacrylamide gels. Thus, bands representing the heteroduplexes (mismatched mutant and normal strands) always appear above the bands representing the normal strands, or the homoduplexes.

In addition to the conformation-based techniques, methods based on base mismatch recognition also are being used. A representative example of this method is the ribonuclease protection assay. The mismatched base is recognized by the ribonuclease enzyme that cleaves single-stranded RNA. The presence of a mismatch, and hence cleavage of the RNA probe, is detected by analysis of the products on an acrylamide gel.

All of these methods have been used successfully to identify alleles that cause disease. Yet, SSCP, because of its simplicity, and DGGE, because of its high sensitivity, are the favored techniques.

Candidate Gene Analysis

As emphasized in the preceding section, relatively large pedigrees are required for use of positional cloning to be feasible. A minimum of 100 informative meioses are required to map the disease locus to within a minimum of 0.2 cM (or 200 kb). Most linkage studies do not have such large pedigrees to analyze. These studies usually manage to map the disease locus within 5 to 10 cM or roughly 5 to 10 Mb,

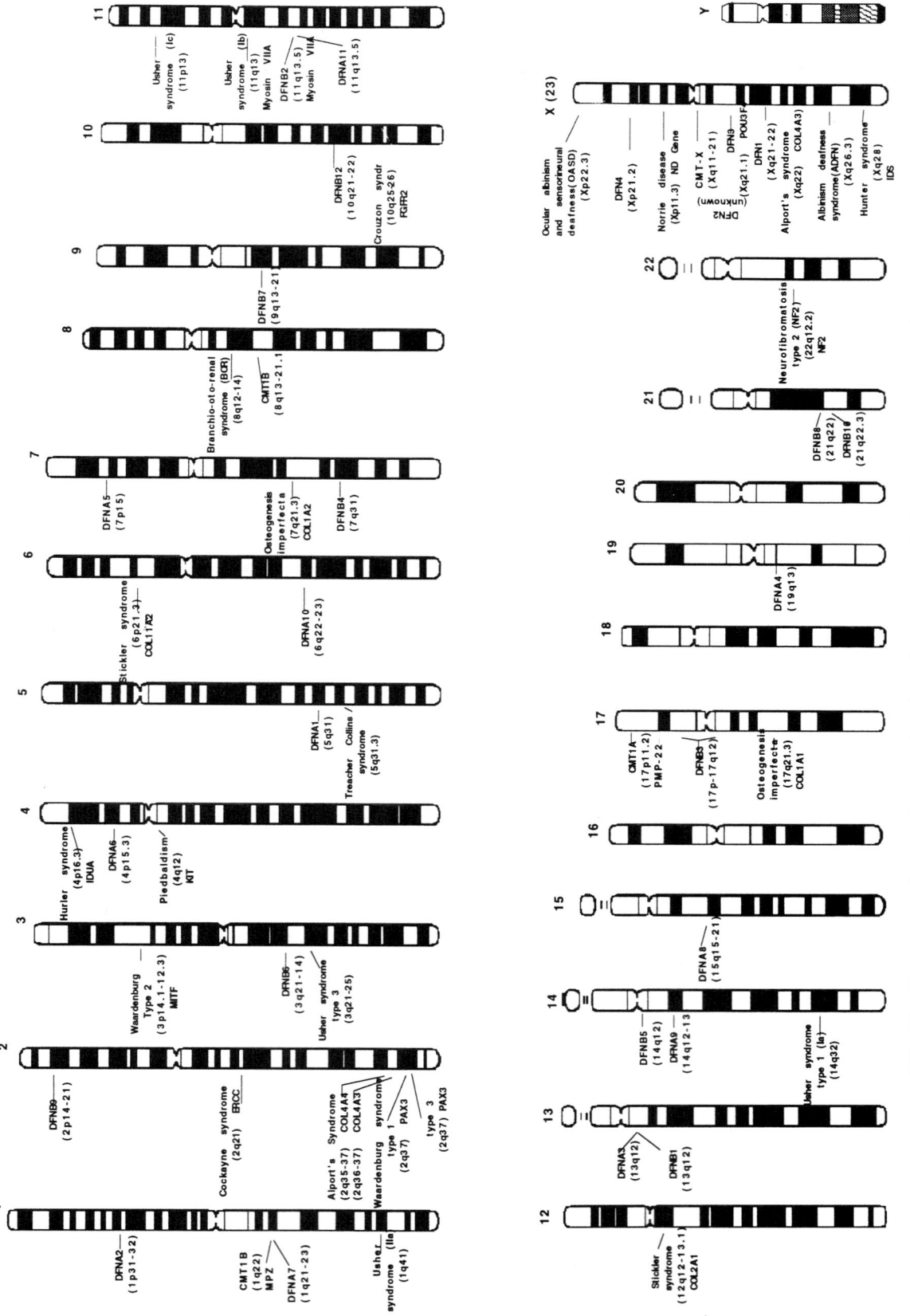

FIG. 20. Chromosomal map of nonsyndromic and syndromic deafness loci and genes. Map of the chromosomal location of loci or genes that have been identified in Nonsyndromic and Syndromic Deafness. While many nonsyndromic deafness loci have been identified through linkage analysis, only one nonsyndromic deafness gene has been cloned. In comparison many syndromic deafness genes have been cloned.

due to the limited number of available meioses. This is an extremely large area, roughly the size of a chromosomal band, to be feasibly characterized for a disease gene via the large-scale cloning approach described previously. In this situation, the best recourse is to search the human genome database for previously cloned genes or ESTs that have been mapped within the linked locus. Any genes that are mapped within the linked locus are referred to as positional candidates. They represent potential disease genes and should be characterized first for linkage to the disease locus and then for the pathogenic mutation. This approach has been successfully applied toward identifying a number of disease genes without the exhaustive search and cloning of the region circumscribed by the linked markers. For example, the candidate gene approach was used for identifying the disease gene in Alport's syndrome, a neuropathy with progressive sensorineural hearing loss and eye anomalies. The gene encoding collagen type IV was mapped to the same locus as the disease locus for Alport's syndrome, thereby becoming a logical candidate gene. In addition, this gene was found to be expressed in basement membranes of the eye, kidney, and inner ear. Sequence analysis of the Col4A5 gene in Alport's patients confirmed the presence of pathogenic mutations linked to the disease.

As more genes are cloned and mapped, the probability of finding a gene in a linked region will improve significantly. In most cases, the linked locus is relatively free of previously cloned genes. Nevertheless, for families too small for positional cloning, the candidate gene approach may be the only viable strategy for the identification of the disease gene. The key difference between the purely positional cloning method and the candidate gene method is that no new genes need to be isolated or cloned in the latter, because it relies on information available from previously cloned and mapped genes.

A major effort that is being carried out by the human genome project is the sequencing and mapping of ESTs from the brain cDNA library (52). Nearly 4,000 genes been mapped. Of these, almost a fourth represent ESTs, while the other three fourths represent full-length cDNA sequences. (Most of the short human cDNA sequences that have been isolated and sequenced have not been mapped.) Assuming the presence of 100,000 genes in the human genome, 4% of the genes have been mapped, thus underlining the relative sparsity of the human gene map. Not surprisingly, most of the loci that have been linked for various disorders are without candidate genes. For example, linkage analysis of inherited nonsyndromic hearing loss (NSHL) in selected and well-defined human pedigrees has led to identification of a number of loci. However, with the exception of POU3F4, the DFN3 gene, no previously cloned gene has been identified within loci that have been linked with NSHL. The limited sample sizes of the affected families with familial NSHL has precluded positional cloning of the linked loci. Thus, the mutant genes causing deafness and their role in mediating hearing remain unknown.

To facilitate the identification of the disease genes within the linked loci several strategies have been developed. These strategies may be subdivided into two overlapping classes. The first group of approaches utilizes animal models with a variety of inherited disorders that parallel human diseases. Because of the difficulties and limitations of genetic analysis in humans, various animal models are used for genetic analysis of variety of disorders diagnosed in humans. For example, in hearing disorders, the mouse represents an excellent model system. Mouse strains with auditory and vestibular disorders are readily detected and may be easily studied. Given the similarity of their auditory apparatus and the observed homology and conservation at the genetic level, mice represent a popular model system for the study of abnormal development and or function of the inner ear. Cloning genes for deafness is a more feasible goal in mice because a large number of recombinants that span the disease locus may be generated through selective matings. The disease locus can then readily be resolved to within 100 kb that would enable cloning of the mutant gene. Mapping and identification of the underlying genetic factors can then be used to predict the corresponding human genes and their chromosomal locations. The underlying principle for predicting the chromosomal location of the corresponding human gene from the map location of a mouse gene is the relative conservation of gene order within small linkage groups in the course of mammalian evolution. Thus, analysis of chromosomal gene maps in different species has revealed regions of cross-species conservation or synteny. The best comparative map is between mice and humans, as a consequence of an intense effort to map the genome of both species. These comparative maps are an excellent resource for identifying candidate disease genes and their chromosomal locations in humans.

Identification of the DFN3 gene represents an example of the use of comparative chromosomal maps between mice and humans. The mouse gene pou3f4, encoding a transcription factor, was found in the region that is evolutionarily conserved in both mice and humans. This region in humans corresponds to the interval Xq13-q22 to which the X-linked mixed deafness with perilymphatic gusher was mapped. Further, the rat homologue of pou3f4, rhs2, was found to be expressed during embryonic development of the brain, the neural tube, and the otic vesicle. Thus, the map position and its temporal/spatial expression pattern rendered the human homologue of the mouse gene, pou3f4, a likely candidate for DFN3. The identity of POU3F4 as the DFN3 gene was confirmed through the demonstration of gene deletions, point mutations within the coding sequence, as well as gene rearrangements within the regulatory region that is upstream of the coding sequence in DFN3 patients (22).

Techniques of molecular biology may also be used to identify potential disease genes. Direct analysis of genes expressed within the auditory neuroepithelia, using techniques of molecular biology, represents an alternative approach being used for understanding the mechanism of hearing. A major strategy that is used in this approach is to identify and characterize "differentially" expressed genes within the cochlea and specifically within the neurosensory epithelia. Genes expressed specifically or selectively within the cochlea represent excellent candidates for subserving a critical function in the auditory apparatus and thus also represent potential candidates genes responsible for NSHL.

Animal Models

Several naturally occurring genetic diseases of animals have been identified that parallel human disease. These include hemophilia in dogs due to a defect in Factor IX, hypercholesterolemia in rabbits due to a defect in low density lipoprotein (LDL) receptor and atherosclerosis in pigs due to variation in their apolipoproteins. Analysis of these diseases in the model organisms has been critical to our understanding of their molecular pathology and the development of therapeutic interventions. As mentioned, the mouse has been the model organism of choice in the analysis of hearing disorders. Mice with hearing disorders are readily detected through their circling behavior. Physiologic studies of these circlers through auditory brainstem response confirms their auditory dysfunction, and histopathologic study of their inner ear localizes its cause to the degeneracy of the cochlear architecture, at the level of development of the bony labyrinth or the integrity of the membranous labyrinth.

Molecular and genetic analysis of Waardenberg syndrome, a dominantly inherited craniofacial disorder with hearing dysfunction and pigmentory abnormalities, represents one of the first examples of a candidate disease gene for a human disorder derived through its corresponding animal model. Mice, heterozygous for the splotch mutation, display white spotting on their coats. However, when homozygous, the mutation causes severe neural tube defects and inner ear malformations. Epstein et al. (9) identified and cloned the gene responsible for the splotch mutation. This gene, designated pax3 mapped to mouse chromosome 1, is in a region that is homologous to the locus for Waardenberg's syndrome. Thus PAX3, the human homologue of pax3, became a candidate disease gene for WS. Sequence analysis of PAX3 in the affected individuals within the family under study for linkage analysis revealed several different mutations (8,54,55). The similarities between the mouse and the human disorders resulting from a mutation in the same gene include pigmentory abnormalities and vestibular/hearing dysfunction. Several major differences also exist, however, including the lack of dominance effect of the pax3 mutation in mice. The splotch mutant represented the first application of genetic knowledge of a hearing defect in a model animal organism toward understanding the genetic basis of hearing dysfunction in humans.

Shaker 1 represents another mouse deafness model, the genetic analysis of which aided identification of the disease gene in recessively inherited Usher's syndrome type Ib, characterized by profound congenital deafness and prepubertal retinitis pigmentosa. The shaker 1 mutant is recessive and causes deafness as well as hyperactivity and circling behavior in the affected animal. Histopathologic analysis of the inner ear demonstrated neuroepithelial degeneration. Weil et al. (56) used positional cloning to identify the disease gene, isolated from a mouse inner ear cDNA library using an exon-trapped product derived from the linked region. Sequence analysis of this clone established its identity as myosin VIIA, and its analysis within shaker 1 identified the presence of pathogenic mutation in the region of the myosin head (57). This gene encodes an "unconventional" myosin, a motor molecule that mediates movement via its adenosine triphosphatase-activated sliding action along actin filaments. Its classification as an unconventional myosin stems from its highly divergent tail. The combination of cytoskeletal abnormalities in Usher's syndrome patients within the microtubules of their photoreceptor cells and the degeneration of the organ of Corti and mapping of the human homologue of myosin VIIA within the disease locus for Usher type Ib prompted its analysis in the human disorder. Different mutations were identified within the myosin VIIA gene in several families affected with Usher type Ib that likely result in the absence of a functional protein (56). In situ hybridization studies have shown expression of this gene within human embryonic cochlear and vestibular neuroepithelia, suggesting that the auditory and vestibular dysfunction observed in the patients stems from morphogenetic defect of the neurosensory tissue. Interestingly, the shaker 1 phenotype differs from Usher's syndrome by the absence of retinal degeneration. The underlying basis of this phenotype variation remains unknown and further emphasizes the effects of differing genetic backgrounds on phenotype expression.

Positional cloning approach also has been used by Avraham et al. (58) to identify another unconventional myosin gene, myosin VI, as the mutant gene in another mouse deafness model, Snell's Waltzer. Histopathologic analysis of the inner ear from Snell's Waltzer demonstrated degeneration of the auditory sensory epithelium. This histopathologic observation has provided a molecular explanation, with studies demonstrating expression of myosin VI specifically within the sensory hair cells. The inferred role of myosin VI is in maintaining the structural integrity of the hair cell. The human Myo6 gene maps to the centromeric region of chromosome 6. As yet, neither a syndromic or nonsyndromic deafness locus has been mapped to this region. Nevertheless, the degeneration of the auditory sensory epithelium in Snell's Waltzer linked to the mutation of the gene encoding myosin VI underscores its importance to the mammalian hearing process and makes it an excellent target for a mutation leading to deafness in humans. The identification of two unconventional myosins with critical roles in hearing may be predicative of involvement of additional unconventional myosins in our auditory function. Figure 21 illustrates the map positions of all nonsyndromic hearing disorders, the disease loci of which have been mapped and/or the disease genes of which have been cloned through the two major approaches described previously.

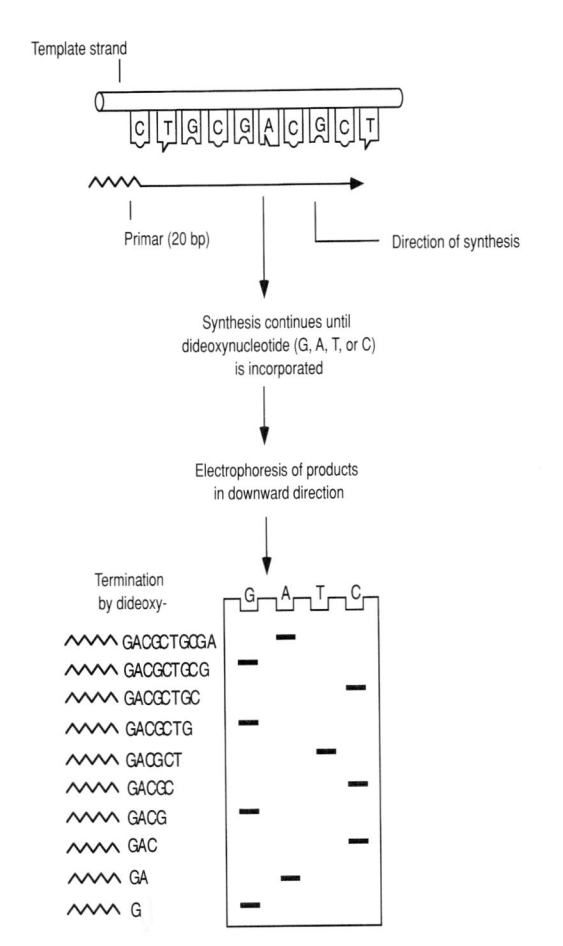

FIG. 21. Chain termination method of DNA sequencing. Using a primer that is homologous to one end of the target DNA to be sequence, the complementary DNA strand is synthesized using DNA polymerase. The template extension takes place in presence of dNTPs and ddNTPs. Incorporation of ddNTP in place of dNTP, terminates chain extension. Incorporation of ddNTP occurs randomly.

Two other mouse deafness mutants have been mapped, shaker 2 and whirler (59). The map location of shaker 2, recessive mouse mutation, is homologous to 17p12-q12 the region of the human genome to which DFNB3 is mapped (60). Thus, the shaker 2 gene may be the mouse homologue of DFNB3.

In addition to hearing disorders, a variety of other diseases are modeled in humans. These include the developmental disorders that affect the neural tube craniofacial and skeletal formations and defects as well as obesity. Identification of their underlying genetic basis will contribute significantly to understanding the cause of corresponding human disorders.

Molecular Approaches

Molecular analysis of tissue-specific functions represents another potential source of candidate genes. Dysfunction of specific tissue or cell types may be traced to genes that are specifically or selectively traced in that tissue or cell. For example, genetic analysis of cardiac myopathies as well as disorders of RBCs has been greatly aided by knowledge of the predominant proteins expressed within the tissue or cell types. However, biochemical analysis of such predominant and selectively expressed proteins is feasible with a relatively large tissue size. These biochemical methods cannot be applied to study the repertoire of proteins within a tissue of limited size, such as the organ of Corti, the auditory sensory neuroepithelia. Instead, the repertoire of proteins expressed by a given tissue type may be readily studied by analysis of their gene expression.

The first task in analysis of gene expression in a tissue for the purpose of cloning and characterizing specific genes is to construct cDNA from the tissue under study. This requires the enzymatic conversion of the single-stranded mRNA isolated from the tissue into its complementary single-stranded DNA copy, or cDNA. The conversion of RNA into cDNA produces a relatively stable substrate that is resistant to degradation and open to numerous enzymatic analyses. Direct analysis of this cDNA may then proceed by its amplification via PCR and/or insertion into an independently replicating vector, such as bacterial plasmid, transfected into bacteria for amplification. Thus, a tissue-specific cDNA library is a collection of independently replicating "clones" of all genes that are expressed within that tissue. Such a library represents a valuable resource for selection, identification, and characterization of genes expressed by the tissue.

Molecular studies to identify the genes critical for hearing have been initiated through the construction of cDNA libraries derived from fetal cochlea in humans (61), adult cochlea in rats (62) and microdissected cochlear neuroepithelia and vestibular epithelia in guinea pigs (63,64). The differential expression approach has been used to isolate and identify several cDNA clones with cochlear-specific or -selective expression. Robertson et al. (61) have identified several such genes with cochlear-specific expression using the fetal cDNA library they constructed. These include several previously cloned genes as well as several 'novel' cDNAs, including Coch-5b2, the sequence of which suggests a protein involved in cell–cell interaction. A caveat associated with work involving a fetal human cDNA library is the need to assess its expression in adult cochleae. Resolution of this issue will need to be addressed using cochleae from animal models, either rat or guinea pig, and the corresponding species-specific homologues of this gene.

The cDNA subtraction or differential expression analysis is optimal for isolating messages that are present in moderate-to-high abundance. Candidate clones that are selected through this approach then need to be characterized for tissue distribution and cellular localization of the RNA and subcellular localization of the translated product. Those confirmed to be organ of Corti–specific or –selective may then be further characterized for their sequence, chromosomal location, and function. Genes identified through this direct molecular analysis provide tissue-specific or -selective candidate genes

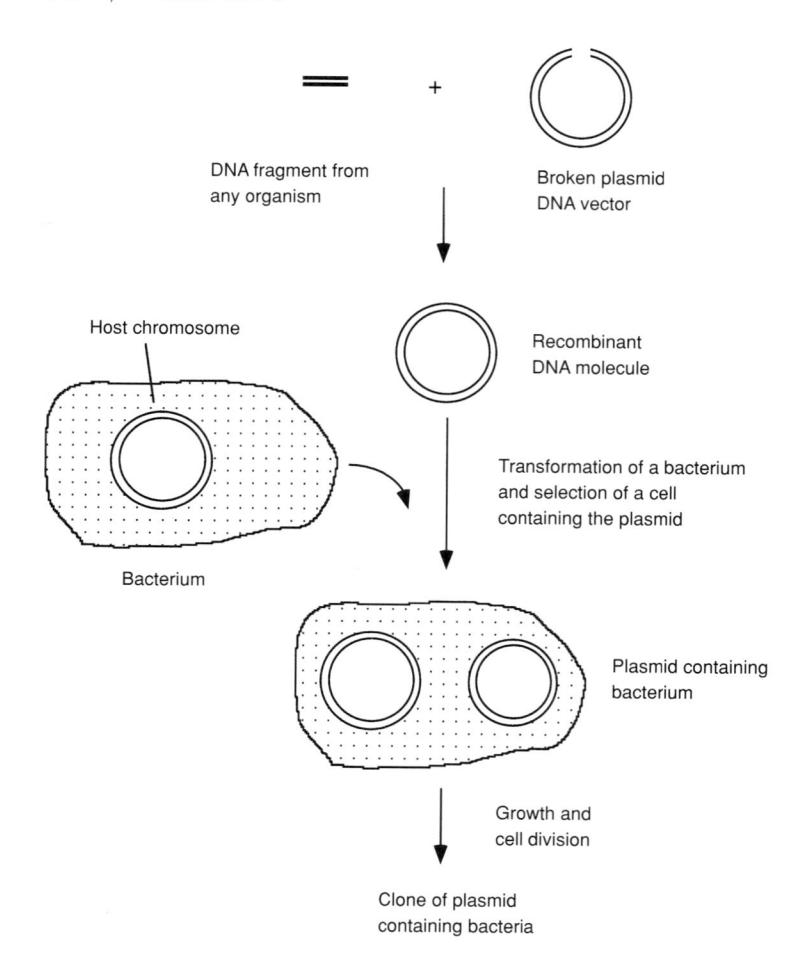

FIG. 22. Cloning. A DNA fragment is joined or 'ligated' to an autonomously replicating vector such as plasmid or a viral genome and the recombinant vector introduced into an appropriate host cell for amplification of the 'cloned' fragment.

that may represent targets of mutation resulting in tissue-specific disorders. Several basic techniques critical for gene identification and its characterization are described next.

DNA Cloning. In studying a particular piece of DNA, it is often important to clone or copy the DNA in order to have an abundant supply. This is done relatively easily by inserting the fragment into cloning vehicles or "vectors" that are able to self-replicate in bacteria. The two vectors most commonly used for cloning are plasmids (circular pieces of DNA that are taken up by bacteria) and bacteriophages (viruses that infect bacteria). The choice of vector rests primarily on the sizes of DNA fragments to be cloned weighed against the degree of difficulty in working with the vector. Plasmids are extremely easy to work with but can handle only pieces up to 5,000 to 10,000 bps; larger fragments tend to become unstable and are unreliable during cloning procedures. Standard bacteriophages require slightly more effort but accomodate fragments up to 20,000 bp; certain variants of bacteriophages, known as cosmids can accept up to 45,000 bp fragments.

The cloning process is usually straightforward and illustrated in Fig. 22. The DNA fragment of interest (foreign DNA) is first modified at the 5' and 3' ends to contain a predetermined sequence of bases (termed *adapters* or *linkers*). Next, the modified DNA is introduced into a vector (e.g., plasmid). This is done by cutting the circular plasmid with restriction endonucleases, which cleave the plasmid at predetermined locations to create a linear plasmid with ends that match the ends of the modified foreign DNA. Finally, the foreign DNA is inserted into the plasmid with a ligation reaction, which also serves to recircularize the vector. The plasmid, along with its foreign insert, is then placed into bacteria designed to allow plasmids to replicate at very high efficiency. The plasmids usually encode an antibiotic resistance gene, so that only bacteria that have been "transformed" with the plasmid are able to replicate in the presence of the antibiotic. The bacteria are plated out on agar plates containing the antibiotic, and individual colonies of bacteria (which contain thousands of bacteria, which each contains thousands of copies of the plasmid) are picked and allowed to replicate even more. A large quantity of the cloned plasmid is then obtained by doing a "plasmid prep" to separate the plasmid DNA from the rest of the bacterial components. Finally, copies of the original foreign DNA are isolated by cutting the plasmid DNA with restriction enzymes that will cut out the insert, running the fragments on an electrophoretic agarose gel, and purifying the insert (identified by its predicted size) from the gel.

Nucleic Acid Probes. DNA probes are pieces of DNA used to detect the presence of a specific complementary sequence of DNA or RNA (the target). (RNA probes can also be used for this same purpose.) The underlying principle is based on the likelihood of a complementary match between a piece of single-stranded DNA and its target. For example, a very short DNA probe with the sequence 5'-AGCT-3' would find its complementary sequence 3'-TCGA-5' in the target DNA once every 256 bp (i.e., 4^4) if the target sequence were random. However, using a typical minimal probe length of 16 bp, the likelihood of a match is only one in 4^{16}, or 4.3×10^9 bp, and this is sufficient for most situations. The identification of the target is typically accomplished by allowing a radioactively labeled probe to mix with the target DNA and then identifying the probe–target hybrid by autoradiography. Nonradioactive means for labeling probes have been developed and will probably become the preferred method once the sensitivity of detection is improved.

Northern, Southern, and Western Analysis. Northern analysis is a method for detecting the presence of a particular mRNA transcript in a population sample. Either total RNA or purified mRNA is isolated from tissue or cells using a standard extraction process, and the RNA is separated by size via electrophoresis through a formaldehyde/agarose gel. The size-separated RNA is transferred to a membrane, and the membrane is then exposed to a radiolabeled probe. If the mRNA of interest is in the sample, the probe will specifically hybridize to the mRNA and produce a signal at the predicted size on the autoradiogram.

If DNA is used in place of RNA, a Southern blot is produced. The only significant distinction between these two types of analyses is the type of ribonucleic acid on the nylon membrane being probed. Similarly, if proteins are used in the place of RNA or DNA, the blot is termed a *Western blot*. In the case of Western blots, radioactive or luminescent antibodies to a protein antigen are used to identify the protein of interest on the blot. Using a combination of Southern, Northern, and Western blots, changes in gene expression, mRNA transcription, and protein translation can be quantified across a variety of experimental states.

In situ Hybridization. In situ hybridization provides a means of determining the pattern of mRNA expression at the cellular level. Whereas Northern analysis uses mRNA derived from homogenized tissue, in situ hybridization uses fixed tissue sections so that the cellular anatomy is preserved. Otherwise, the technique uses the same concepts described for Northern analysis. The tissue sections are mounted on slides and prepared in a way that allows the probe to have access to the cellular compartments and hybridize with the mRNA. The sections are washed to remove the nonhybridized probe, dried, and placed directly on autoradiograph film to detect the overall pattern of hybridization in the tissue. To obtain cellular detail, the slides are coated with a very thin layer of photograph emulsion, such that the radiolabeled probe will expose the emulsion directly overlying the cells. The slides are then developed in the same manner as film. When the slides are viewed under a microscope, the exposed silver grains in the emulsion are seen as black specks, and the presence of this signal signifies the presence of the specific mRNA transcript.

ACKNOWLEDGMENT

We would like to thank Jeremy S. Faust for his contribution to the preparation of the chapter illustrations.

REFERENCES

1. Bickmore WA, Sumner AT. Mammalian chromosome banding—an expression of genome organization. *Trends Genet* 1989;5:144–8.
2. Fields C, Adams MD, White O, Venter JC. How many genes in the human genome? [news] [see comments]. *Nat Genet* 1994;7:345–6.
3. Ishikiriyama S, Tonoki H, Shibuya Y, et al. Waardenburg syndrome type I in a child with de novo inversion (2)(q35q37.3). *Am J Med Genet* 1989;33:505–7.
4. Ohba N, Yamashita T. Primary vitreoretinal dysplasia resembling Norrie's disease in a female: association with X autosome chromosomal translocation. *Br J Ophthalmol* 1986;70:64–71.
5. Berger W, Meindl A, van de Pol TJ, Cremers FP, Ropers HH, et al. Isolation of a candidate gene for Norrie disease by positional cloning. *Nat Genet* 1992;2:84.
6. Anderson L. Identification of mitochondrial proteins and some of their precursors in two-dimensional electrophoretic maps of human cells. *Proc Natl Acad Sci U S A* 1981;78(4):2407–11.
7. Lestienne P, Bataill N. Mitochondrial DNA alterations and genetic diseases: a review. *Biomed Pharmacother* 1994;48:199–214.
8. Tassabehji M, Read AP, Newton VE, et al. Waardenburg's syndrome patients have mutations in the human homologue of the Pax-3 paired box gene [see comments]. *Nature* 1992;355:635–6.
9. Epstein DJ, Vogan KJ, Trasler DG, Gros P. A mutation within intron 3 of the Pax-3 gene produces aberrantly spliced mRNA transcripts in the splotch (Sp) mouse mutant. *Proc Natl Acad Sci U S A* 1993;90:532–6.
10. Kajiwara K, Berson EL, Dryja TP. Digenic retinitis pigmentosa due to mutations at the unlinked peripherin/RDS and ROM1 loci. *Science* 1994;264:1604–8.
11. Reardon W, Winter RM, Rutland P, Pulleyn LJ, Jones BM, Malcolm S. Mutations in the fibroblast growth factor receptor 2 gene cause Crouzon syndrome. *Nat Genet* 1994;8:98–103.
12. Rutland P, Pulleyn LJ, Reardon W, et al. Identical mutations in the FGFR2 gene cause both Pfeiffer and Crouzon syndrome phenotypes [see comments]. *Nat Genet* 1995;9:173–6.
13. Jabs EW, Li X, Scott AF, et al. Jackson-Weiss and Crouzon syndromes are allelic with mutations in fibroblast growth factor receptor 2 [published erratum appears in *Nat Genet* 1995 Apr;9(4):451]. *Nat Genet* 1995;8:275–9.
14. Wilkie AO, Slaney SF, Oldridge M, et al. Apert syndrome results from localized mutations of FGFR2 and is allelic with Crouzon syndrome [see comments]. *Nat Genet* 1995;9:165–72.
15. Mulvihill JJ. Craniofacial syndromes: no such thing as a single gene disease [news; comment] [published erratum appears in *Nat Genet* 1995 Apr;9(4):451]. *Nat Genet* 1995;9:101–3.
16. Shiang R, Thompson LM, Zhu YZ, et al. Mutations in the transmembrane domain of FGFR3 cause the most common genetic form of dwarfism, achondroplasia. *Cell* 1994;78:335–42.
17. Leon PE, Raventos H, Lynch E, Morrow J, King MC. The gene for an inherited form of deafness maps to chromosome 5q31. *Proc Natl Acad Sci U S A* 1992;89:5181–4.
18. Kumar S, Kimberling WJ, Kenyon JB, Smith RJ, Marres HA, Cremers CW. Autosomal dominant branchio-oto-renal syndrome—localization of a disease gene to chromosome 8q by linkage in a Dutch family. *Hum Mol Genet* 1992;1:491–5.
19. Prockop DJ, Kivirikko KI. Collagens: molecular biology, diseases, and potentials for therapy. *Annu Rev Biochem* 1995;64:403–34.
20. Miller G, Wessel HB. Diagnosis of dystrophinopathies: review for the clinician. *Pediatr Neurol* 1993;9:3–9.

21. Antignac C, Zhou J, Sanak M, et al. Alport syndrome and diffuse leiomyomatosis: deletions in the 5′ end of the COL4A5 collagen gene. *Kidney Int* 1992;42:1178–83.
22. de Kok YJ, van der Maarel, SM, Bitner-Glindzicz M, et al. Association between X-linked mixed deafness and mutations in the POU domain gene POU3F4. *Science* 1995;267:685–8.
23. Gold M, Rapin I. Non-Mendelian mitochondrial inheritance as a cause of progressive genetic sensorineural hearing loss. *International J of Ped Otorhinolaryngol* 1994;30(2):91–104.
24. Tycko B. Genomic imprinting: mechanism and role in human pathology. *Am J Pathol* 1994;144:431–43.
25. Lee JE, Tantravahi U, Boyle AL, Efstratiadis A. Parental imprinting of an Igf-2 transgene. *Mol Reprod Dev* 1993;35:382–90.
26. Giannoukakis N, Deal C, Paquette J, Goodyer CG, Polychronakos C. Parental genomic imprinting of the human IGF2 gene. *Nat Genet* 1993;4:98–101.
27. Heutink P, van der Mey AG, Sandkuijl LA, et al. A gene subject to genomic imprinting and responsible for hereditary paragangliomas maps to chromosome 11q23-qter. *Hum Mol Genet* 1992;1:7–10.
28. Mariman EC, van Beersum SE, Cremers CW, Struycken PM, Ropers HH. Fine mapping of a putatively imprinted gene for familial non-chromaffin paragangliomas to chromosome 11q13.1: evidence for genetic heterogeneity. *Hum Genet* 1995;95:56–62.
29. Lander E, Kruglyak L. Genetic dissection of complex traits: guidelines for interpreting and reporting linkage results [see comments]. *Nat Genet* 1995;11:241–7.
30. McKusick VA, Amberger JS. The morbid anatomy of the human genome: chromosomal location of mutations causing disease. *J Med Genet* 1993;30:1–26.
31. Collins FS. Positional cloning: let's not call it reverse anymore [news]. *Nat Genet* 1992;1:3–6.
32. Murray JC, Buetow KH, Weber JL, et al. A comprehensive human linkage map with centimorgan density. Cooperative Human Linkage Center (CHLC). *Science* 1994;265:2049–54.
33. Dib C, Faur S, Fizames C, et al. A comprehensive genetic map of the human genome based on 5,264 microsatellites [see comments]. *Nature* 1995;380:152–4.
34. Weissenbach J. Microsatellite polymorphisms and the genetic linkage map of the human genome. *Curr Opin Genet Dev* 1993;3:414–7.
35. Weissenbach J. A second generation linkage map of the human genome based on highly informative microsatellite loci. *Gene* 1995;135:275–8.
36. Gyapay G, Morissette J, Vignal A, et al. The 1993-94 Généthon human genetic linkage map [see comments]. *Nat Genet* 1994;7:246–339.
37. Friend SH, Horowitz JM, Gerber MR, Wang XF, Bogenmann E, Li FP, Weinberg RA. Deletions of a DNA sequence in retinoblastomas and mesenchymal tumors: organization of the sequence and its encoded protein [published erratum appears in *Proc Natl Acad Sci U S A* 1988;85(7)2234]. *Proc Natl Acad Sci U S A* 1987;84(24):9059–63.
38. Rommens JM, Zengerling-Lentes S, Kerem B, Melmer G, Buchwald M, Tsui LC. Physical localization of two DNA markers closely linked to the cystic fibrosis locus by pulsed-field gel electrophoresis. *Am J Hum Genet* 1989;45(6):932–41.
39. Weeks DE, Lange K. The affected pedigree member method of linkage analysis. *Am J Hum Genet* 1988;42:315–26.
40. Coucke P, Van Camp G, Djoyodiharjo B, et al. Linkage of autosomal dominant hearing loss to the short arm of chromosome 1 in two families [see comments]. *N Engl J Med* 1994;331:425–31.
41. Chaib H, Lina-Granade G, Guilford P, et al. A gene responsible for a dominant form of neurosensory non-syndromic deafness maps to the NSRD1 recessive deafness gene interval. *Hum Mol Genet* 1994;3:2219–22.
42. Guilford P, Ben Arab S, Blanchard S, et al. A non-syndrome form of neurosensory, recessive deafness maps to the pericentromeric region of chromosome 13q. *Nat Genet* 1994;6:24–8.
43. Guilford P, Ayadi H, Blanchard S, et al. A human gene responsible for neurosensory, non-syndromic recessive deafness is a candidate homologue of the mouse sh-1 gene. *Hum Mol Genet* 1994;3:989–93.
44. Veske A, Oehlmann R, Younus F, et al. Autosomal recessive non-syndromic deafness locus (DFNB8) maps on chromosome 21q22 in large consanguineous kindred from Pakistan. *Hum Mol Genet* 1996;5:165–8.
45. Lander ES, Botstein D. Homozygosity mapping: a way to map human recessive traits with the DNA of inbred children. *Science* 1987;236:1567–70.
46. Hästbacka J, de la Chapelle A, Mahtani MM, et al. The diastrophic dysplasia gene encodes a novel sulfate transporter: positional cloning by fine-structure linkage disequilibrium mapping. *Cell* 1994;78:1073–87.
47. Burke DT, Carle GF, Olson MV. Cloning of large segments of exogenous DNA into yeast by means of artificial chromosome vectors. 1987 [classical article]. *Biotechnology* 1992;24:172–8.
48. Monaco AP, Larin Z. YACs, BACs, PACs and MACs: artificial chromosomes as research tools. *Trends Biotechnol* 1994;12:280–6.
49. Rotman G, Vanagaite L, Collins FS, Shiloh Y. Rapid identification of polymorphic CA-repeats in YAC clones. *Mol Biotechnol* 1995;3:85–92.
50. Flejter WL, Barcroft CL, Guo SW, et al. Multicolor FISH mapping with Alu-PCR-amplified YAC clone DNA determines the order of markers in the BRCA1 region on chromosome 17q12-q21. *Genomics* 1993;17:624–31.
51. Cohen D, Chumakov I, Weissenbach J. A first-generation physical map of the human genome. *Nature* 1993;366:698–701.
52. Adams MD, Kerlavage AR, Fields C, Venter JC. 3,400 new expressed sequence tags identify diversity of transcripts in human brain [see comments]. *Nat Genet* 1993;4:256–67.
53. Adams MD, Soares MB, Kerlavage AR, Fields C, Venter, JC. Rapid cDNA sequencing (expressed sequence tags) from a directionally cloned human infant brain cDNA library. *Nat Genet* 1993;4:373–80.
54. Baldwin CT, Hoth CF, Amos JA, da-Silva EO, Milunsky A. An exonic mutation in the HuP2 paired domain gene causes Waardenburg's syndrome [see comments]. *Nature* 1992;355:637–8.
55. Baldwin CT, Hoth CF, Macina RA, Milunsky A. Mutations in PAX3 that cause Waardenburg syndrome type I: ten new mutations and review of the literature. *Am J Med Genet* 1995;58:115–22.
56. Weil D, Blanchard S, Kaplan J, et al. Defective myosin VIIA gene responsible for Usher syndrome type 1B. *Nature* 1995;374:60–1.
57. Gibson F, Walsh J, Mburu P. A type VII myosin encoded by the mouse deafness gene shaker-1. *Nature* 1995;374:62–4.
58. Avraham KB, Hasson T, Steel KP, et al. The mouse Snell's Waltzer deafness gene encodes an unconventional myosin required for structural integrity of inner ear hair cells. *Nat Genet* 1995;11:369–75.
59. Fleming J, Rogers MJ, Brown SD, Steel KP. Linkage analysis of the whirler deafness gene on mouse chromosome 4. *Genomics* 1994;21:42–8.
60. Friedman TB, Liang Y, Weber JL, et al. A gene for congenital, recessive deafness DFNB3 maps to the pericentromeric region of chromosome 17. *Nat Genet* 1995;9:86–91.
61. Robertson NG, Khetarpal U, Gutiérrez-Espeleta GA, Bieber FR, Morton CC. Isolation of novel and known genes from a human fetal cochlear cDNA library using subtractive hybridization and differential screening. *Genomics* 1994;23:42–50.
62. Ryan AF, Batcher S, Brumm D, O'Driscoll K, Harris JP. Cloning genes from an inner ear cDNA library. *Arch Otolaryngol Head Neck Surg* 1993;119:1217–20.
63. Wilcox ER, Fex J. Construction of a cDNA library from microdissected guinea pig organ of Corti. *Hear Res* 1992;62:124–6.
64. Wilcox ER, Fex J. Construction of a cDNA library from microdissected guinea pig crista ampullaris. *Hear Res* 1994;73:65–6.

CHAPTER 6

Temporal Bone Histopathology

William H. Slattery III

The surgical and microscopic anatomy of the ear must be understood to appreciate the physiology of hearing and to understand the diseases which affect the structures of the temporal bone. This chapter reviews the normal microscopic anatomy of the ear and the histopathologic processes that may affect hearing.

NORMAL ANATOMY

External Auditory Canal

The S-shaped external auditory canal is composed of a lateral cartilaginous portion and a medial bony portion. The lateral end of the cartilaginous canal has numerous hair follicles with associated sebaceous and modified apocrine glands. Ear wax, which contains lysozymes, immunoglobulins, and lipids, is believed to be secreted by the sebaceous and modified apocrine glands. The variety of ear wax (sticky brown vs. dry crust) is believed to be determined by the relative concentration of the sebaceous glands to modified apocrine glands. The acini of the sebaceous glands are connected to form a single duct, which empties into the hair follicles (Fig. 1). The modified apocrine glands are located in the deep dermis below the hair follicles and sebaceous gland. The modified apocrine gland is composed of secretory myoepithelial and ductal cells that empty into the hair follicles via the follicular ducts (1).

The skin of the cartilaginous ear canal is composed of an epidermis with stratified squamous epithelium with papillae. There is a well-developed dermis and subcutaneous layer. Active migration of the skin occurs in the stratified epithelium. The anterior and inferior wall of the cartilaginous canal is formed by cartilage. There are two or three vertical fissures between the cartilaginous sheaths. These form the fissures of Santorini through which the neurovascular structures emerge. The superior and posterior wall is formed by firm connective tissue.

W.H. Slattery III: House Ear Clinic and Department of Clinical Studies, House Ear Institute, Los Angeles, California 90057; Department of Otolaryngology, University of Southern California, Los Angeles, California 90057.

The medial one third of the external auditory canal is composed of squamous epithelium with no subcutaneous layer. The bony external auditory canal rarely has accumulation of cerumen due to the lack of sebaceous and apocrine glands in this area. The temporal mandibular joint is located anterior to the bony canal, as is the parotid gland. Neurovascular structures enter through the foramen of Luschka located in the anterior inferior medial aspect of the bony canal.

Tympanic Membrane

The conical tympanic membrane is thicker in the center and periphery with a thinner intermediate area. The tympanic membrane can be divided into the larger pars tensa and smaller superior pars flaccida. Both areas have three layers consisting of the epidermis, lamina propria, and mucosal layers. Lim (1) described the characteristics of the pars tensa. The epidermal layer contains the four layers characteristic of normal skin: the corneum, granulosum, spinosum, and basal layers. The lamina propria contains collagen fiber arranged in four distinct layers. A subepidermoid connective tissue layer, which contains nerve fibers, capillaries, and loose connective tissue, is lateral to an outer radial collagenous layer and inner circular collagenous layer. Medial to the collagenous layer is a submucosal connective tissue layer that is thinner than the subepidermoid connective tissue layer but also contains loose connective tissue with nerves and capillaries. The mucosal layer, found on the middle-ear surface, consists of a single layer of squamous epithelial cells. At the margin, it is composed of cuboidal cells.

The pars flaccida is much thicker than the pars tensa and has an epidermal layer that is 5 to 10 cells thick. The lamina propria has irregular collagenous fibers, not the highly organized radial and circular collagenous fibers found in the pars tensa. There is also a more extensive extracellular amorphous ground substance found within the lamina propria. The substance may be responsible for its translucent characteristics. The mucosal layer is similar to the pars tensa.

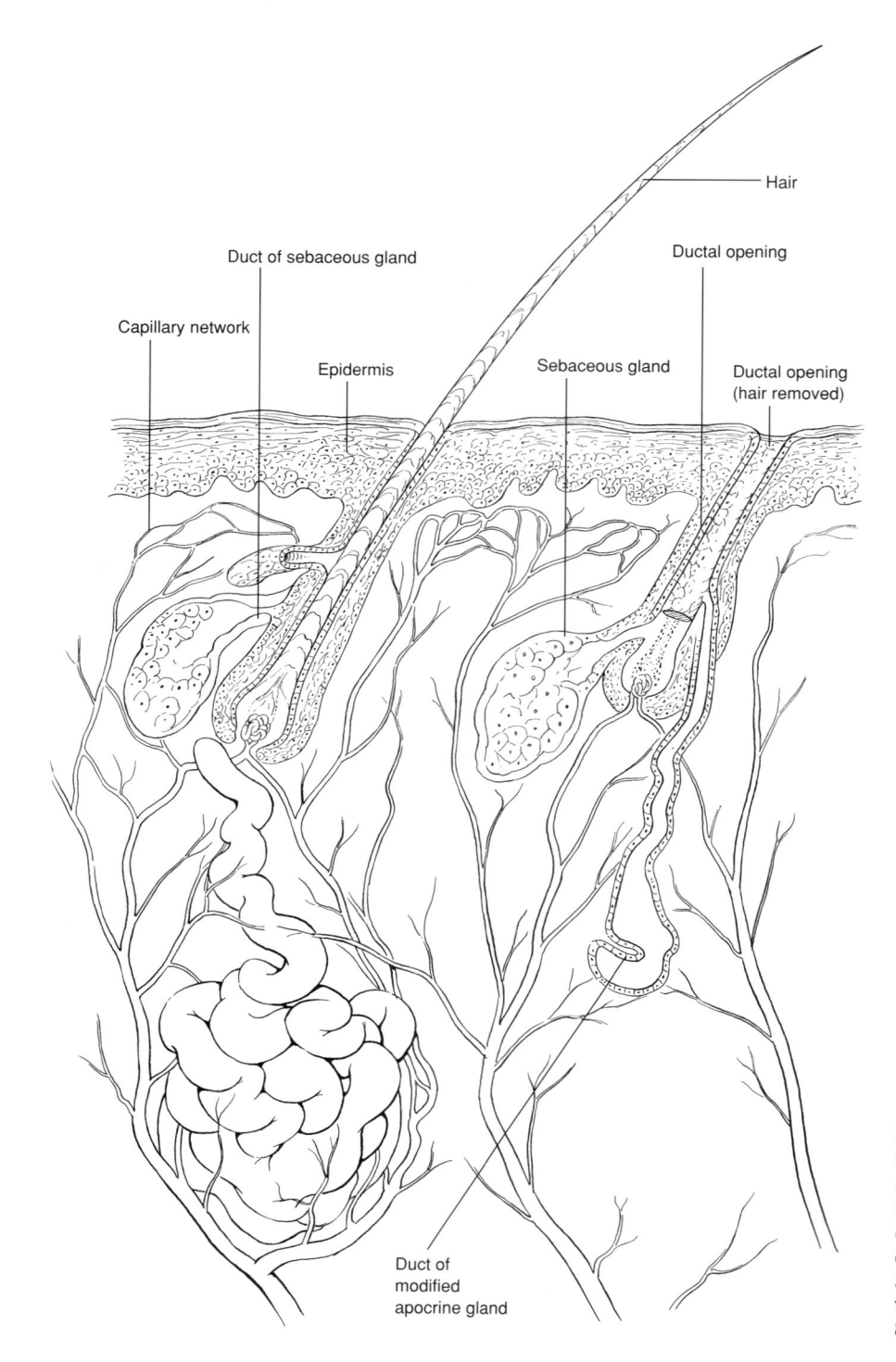

FIG. 1. Cross section through the external auditory canal demonstrating secretory systems. The sebaceous gland is more superficial to the modified apocrine gland but both secrete into the hair duct. From Main T, Lim D. The human auditory canal secretory system—an ultrastructoral study. *Laryngoscope* 1976; 86:1164–1176.

Middle Ear

Sound travels through the middle ear via the ossicular amplification system, which connects the tympanic membrane to the inner ear. This aerated area communicates with the nasopharynx via the eustachian tube. Posteriorly, it communicates with the sinus tympani and facial recess (Fig. 2). These cavities are important during surgery for cholesteatoma. Superiorly, the epitympanic recess communicates with the pneumatized air-cell tract. The middle-ear mucosa is a modified respiratory epithelium containing five types of cells: nonciliated cells without secretory granules, nonciliated cells with secretory granules, ciliated cells, intermediate cells, and basal cells (2). Ciliated cells and secretory cells are found in the mucosa more commonly in the eustachian tube area. Contrasted with most bones of the body which are surrounded by muscu-

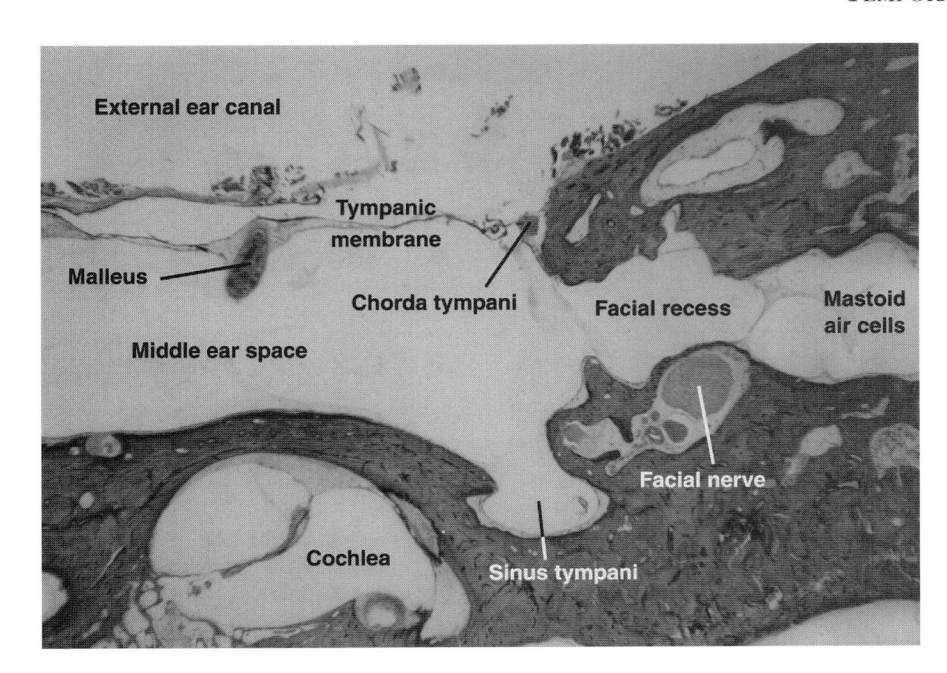

FIG. 2. Normal histology of middle ear at the level of the sinus tympani, just inferior to the oval window area. Jacobsen's nerve can be seen on the promontory. Keratin debris is in external auditory canal. Reprinted with permission of House Ear Institute.

lature, the middle-ear ossicles are suspended in an aerated cavity. The ossicles have a thin endosteal layer of bone on the outer surface that surrounds a central interosseous segment. The blood supply to the ossicle lies within the mucosa surrounding the endosteal bone and enters through numerous channels into the central marrow space. The anterior tympanic artery, a branch of the mandibular portion of the internal maxillary artery, provides the main blood supply to the malleus and incus. The blood supply to the stapes originates from the arterial plexus within the fallopian canal, which is supplied by the stylomastoid artery.

The malleus and incus are connected by a diarthrodial joint, which is an incomplete cartilaginous surface in adults. The incudostapedial joint is another diarthrodial joint. In children, this joint has cartilage, but it ossifies in adults. The stapes oval window is a syndesmotic joint, and within the annular ligament is a small bursa commonly found in the posterior aspect of the joint.

The middle ear contains two muscles: the stapedius and tensor tympani. The stapedius muscle lies medial to, and is innervated by, the facial nerve. The muscular fibers arise from the bony sulcus and attach to a central tendon core. This tendon emerges at the pyramidal process to attach to the head of the stapes and superior margin of the posterior crus (Fig. 3). The tensor tympani also has peripheral muscle fibers that are attached to a central tendon core which

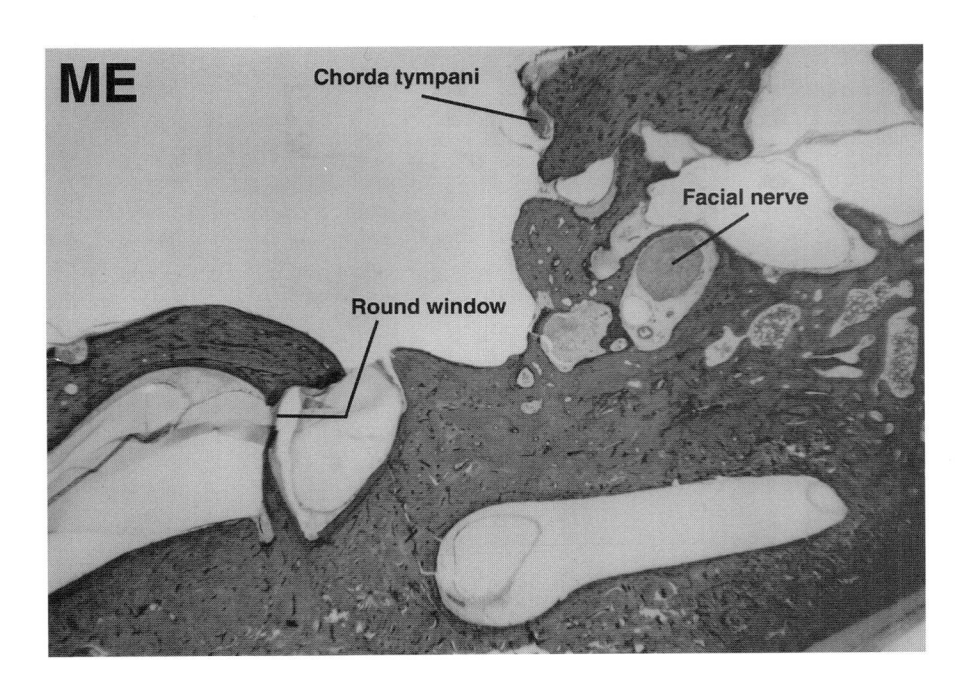

FIG. 3. Normal round window niche (2×) with bony overhang and round window membrane. Stapedius muscle is found medial and anterior to the facial nerve. Middle ear *(ME)*. Reprinted with permission of House Ear Institute.

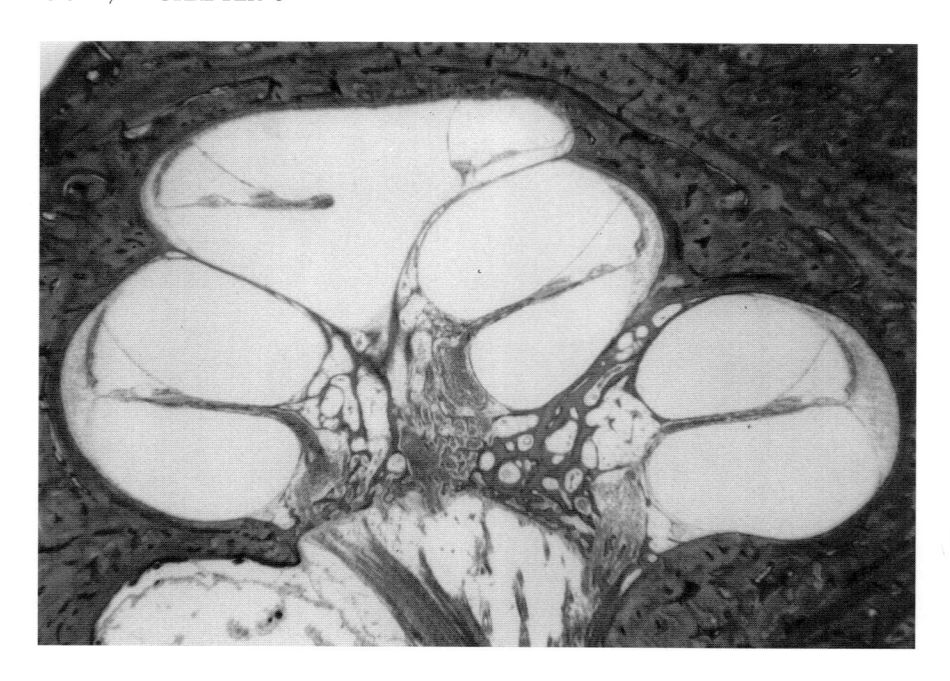

FIG. 4. Normal cochlea demonstrating 2½ turns. Numerous ganglion cells are found throughout the lower 1½ turns of the modiolus. Peripheral processes of the ganglion cells travel through the osseous spiral lamina to reach the hair cells and the organ of Corti. Reprinted with permission of House Ear Institute.

emerges at the cochleariform process to attach to the medial surface of the neck of the malleus.

Inner Ear

The membranous labyrinth is suspended within the bony labyrinth. The space between the two contains perilymph. The otic capsule or labyrinthine bone is a hard nonpneumatized bone. A thin endosteum layer is found along the bony labyrinth. Cartilaginous rest from development may be found along the endosteal edge, especially in the apex of the cochlea and along the walls of the semicircular canals.

The cochlea twists 2¾ the way around a central modiolus and is approximately 33 mm in length (Fig. 4). It is divided into three chambers: the scala vestibuli, scala media and scala tympani. The scala vestibuli begins at the vestibule and extends around the modiolus to communicate with the scala tympani at the apex of the cochlea. This area of communication is called the helicotrema. The scala vestibuli and scala media are separated by a thin bony plate, the osseous spiral lamina. The scala vestibuli is separated from the scala media by Reissner's membrane, and the scala tympani and scala media are separated by the basilar membrane and the organ of Corti.

The central bony modiolus contains cochlear nerve ganglion cells. In contrast to animal species in which the ganglion cells are distributed in the modiolus throughout all the turns of the cochlea, human ganglion cells are only located within the basal 1½ turns of the modiolus. Fibers from the ganglion cells pass through Rosenthal's canal to extend into the organ of Corti (Fig. 5). Fibers enter into the internal auditory canal and maintain a spatial orientation as they travel through the cochlear nerve to the cochlear nucleus. There are two types of cochlear neurons. Type I are large bipolar cells that connect exclusively to the inner hair cells. These constitute approximately 95% of the total population. Ten to 15 type I cochlear neurons innervate one inner hair cell. Type II cochlear neurons are pseudomonopolar and have small fibers that extend to approximately 10 outer hair cells (3).

The basilar membrane extends from the osseous spiral lamina to the spiral ligament and supports the organ of Corti (Fig. 6). The spiral ligament arises from the bony labyrinth and extends from the scala vestibuli to the scala media. The basilar membrane and Reissner's membrane are suspended from this structure. The stria vascularis separates the spiral ligament from the scala media. The spiral ligament is composed of a loose connective tissue that contains the vascular supply to the organ of Corti.

The stria vascularis is composed of three layers and lies on the external surface of the scala media. It is thought to be responsible for endolymph metabolism. Marginal cells are found in the endolymphatic surface. The next layer is composed of intermediate cells, but there are numerous blood vessels also found in this area. The basilar cells lie on the spiral ligament, and tight junctions separate this layer from the spiral ligament.

The spiral limbus is located on the internal area of the scala media, resting on the osseous spiral lamina and the basilar membrane. This area may also be responsible for active fluid transport. The organ of Corti rests on the basilar membrane in the central portion of the scala media. It is composed of both inner and outer hair cells and their supporting cells (Fig. 7). The human cochlea has approximately 12,000 outer hair cells and 3,500 inner hair cells (4). The single layer of inner hair cells is pear-shaped and surrounded by a border of cells, inner phalangeal cells and inner pillar cells. The stereocilia project toward the tectorial membrane.

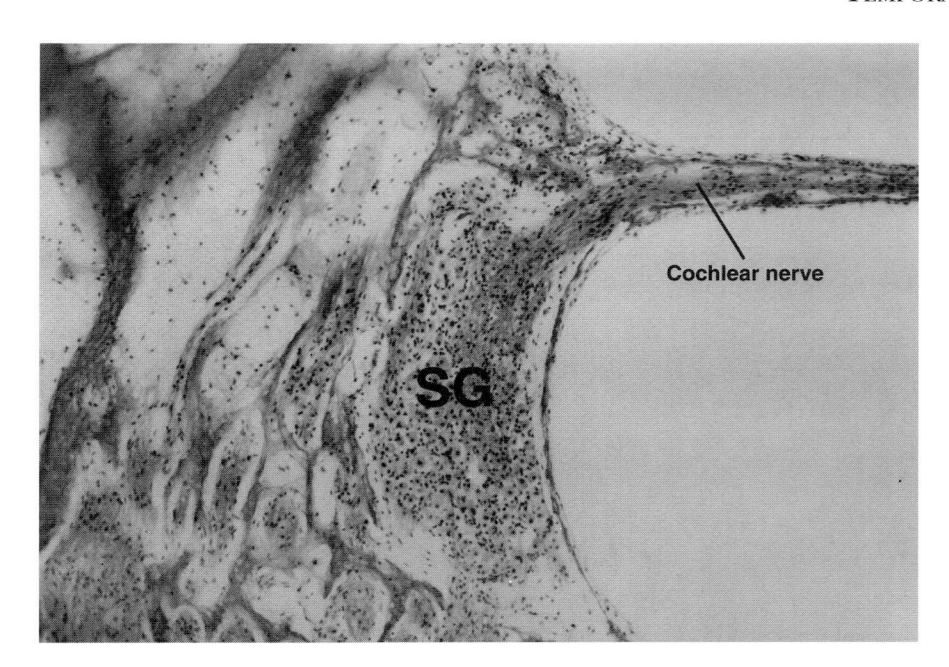

FIG. 5. Spiral ganglion (SG) with peripheral processes traveling through the osseous spiral lamina to innervate the organ of Corti cochlear hair cells (10×). Reprinted with permission of House Ear Institute.

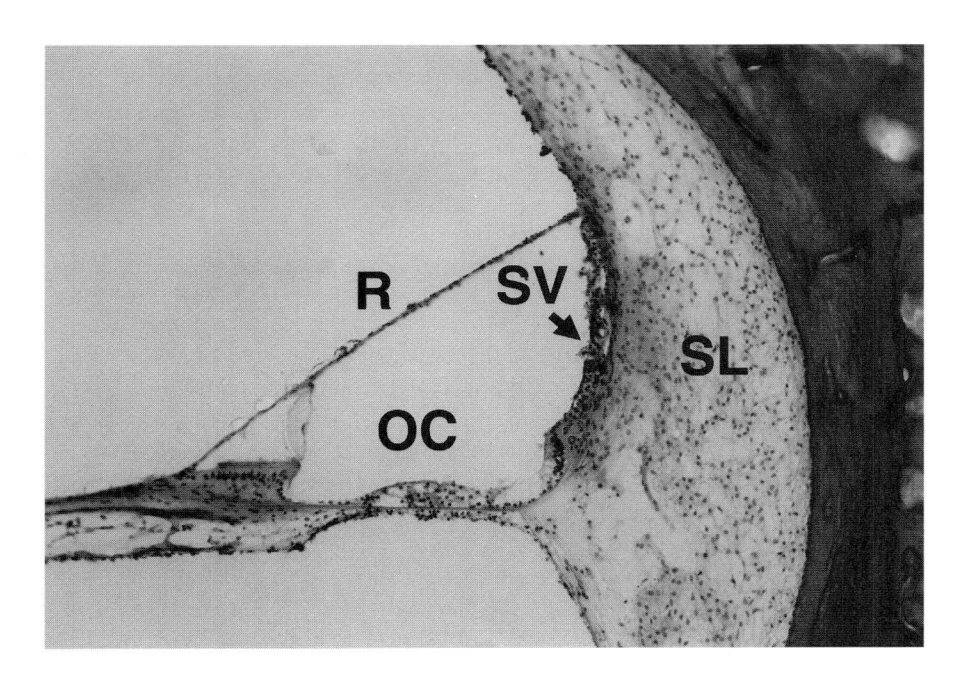

FIG. 6. Organ of Corti *(OC)* and stria vascularis *(SV)* found in scala media. Reissner's membrane *(R)* separates the scala media from the scala vestibuli. The spiral ligament *(SL)* arises from the bony labyrinth and extends from the scala media to scala vestibuli (6×). Reprinted with permission of House Ear Institute.

The three-layer outer hair cells are supported by Deiter's cells. The stereocilia arise from within the cuticular plate. The long stereocilia are imbedded in the tectorial membrane.

The vestibule contains the saccule and utricle. The walls of these structures contain three layers: a loose connective layer, the basilar membrane, and the internal epithelium. At the macule, the epithelium is thickened to form the sensory organ. The structure of the macule is similar to that of the cristae of the semicircular canals.

There are two types of sensory receptor cells found within the vestibular epithelium. The lateral semicircular canal cristae have the kinocilium directed toward the utricle, as opposed to the superior and posterior canals in which the cilia are directed away from the utricle.

The vestibular aqueduct is a bony channel that exits the vestibule directed medial to the posterior semicircular canal and toward the posterior fossa. The membranous endolymphatic duct and sac are contained within this area, which is divided into three segments. The proximal segment is composed of epithelial cells and provides a conduit toward the intermediate segment. The intermediate segment lies within the bony canal and has irregular-shaped channels with a highly differentiated villi structure. Proteinaceous material found in these areas, are believed to be a part of active fluid

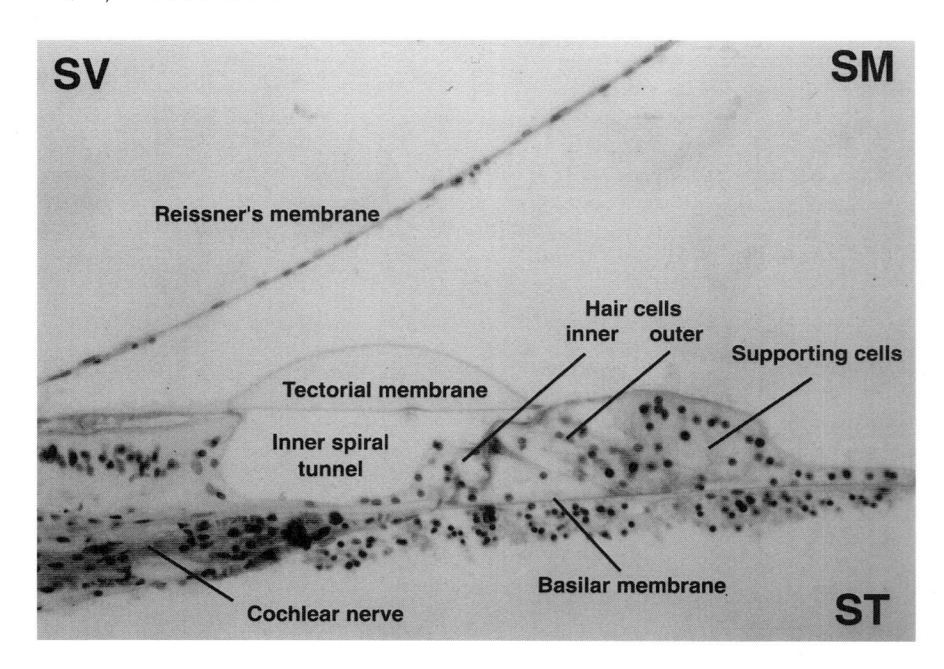

FIG. 7. Organ of Corti with the corresponding hair cells. Scala vestibuli *(SV)*, scala media *(SM)*, and scala tympani *(ST)* are identified (40×). Reprinted with permission of House Ear Institute.

transport (5). The distal segment contains the sac, which is found within the layers of the dura. Epithelium in this area is more cuboidal in form. A potential space exists in this area but the space is normally collapsed.

NORMAL DEVELOPMENT

A detailed summary of normal temporal bone development is presented in Table 1. The ectoderm from the branchial groove forms the external auditory canal. The otic placode arises from surface ectoderm and invaginates mesenchymal tissue to form the otic pit. The mesenchymal tissue later becomes the cartilage that forms the otic capsule. The otic placode forms three parts, which become the membranous labyrinth. The cranial section becomes the endolymphatic duct and sac. The intermediate becomes the utricle, saccule, and semicircular canals, and the caudal swelling becomes the cochlear duct. The intermediate segment has three outpouchings that form the semicircular canals. As the swelling enlarges, the center area is obliterated, forming a circular canal. The first two arches form the auricle. Endoderm of the pharynx from the first pharyngeal pouch forms the eustachian tube and tympanic cavity. The mesenchymal tissue or mesoderm forms muscles for the ossicles and the fibrous layer of the middle ear. The cochlear duct differentiates in a basal to apical fashion.

The otic capsule undergoes three stages of development. First, condensation of mesenchymal tissue occurs to form the cartilage structure. Next, formation of the perilymphatic spaces occurs, surrounding the membranous labyrinth. Finally, ossification of the otic capsule occurs.

The mesodermal elements of the first and second branchial arches form the ossicles. Meckel's cartilage from arch 1 forms the malleus and incus, which are generally shaped by 9 weeks. Reichert's cartilage from arch 2 forms the stapes superstructure. This is usually adult size by 15 weeks of gestation. The medial surface of the footplate develops from the mesenchyme of the otic capsule. The lateral surface is formed from Reichert's cartilage. The stapes is slightly slower to develop and ossify than are the malleus and incus.

At 9 weeks of development, the primitive membranous labyrinth has formed in an identifiable adult shape. However, the cochlear duct is only 1½ turns long. The middle ear is a slit-like opening communicating with the first pharyngeal pouch. The membranous labyrinth, although formed, is still contained within mesenchymal tissue because the otic capsule has not formed perilymphatic spaces. At 21 weeks of gestation, the cochlea is fully formed with endolymphatic and perilymphatic spaces complete. The ossicles are adult size, as are the semicircular canals. Ossification of the cartilaginous precursors occurs during the remaining fetal development. The cochlea is adult size by 25 weeks of gestation. Mastoid development begins late in fetal life and continues until approximately 2 years of age. The external auditory canal is fully ossified by age 2 but continues to grow to adult size by age 9. The auricle is nearly adult size by age 4 and reaches full adult size at age 9.

ABNORMAL MORPHOLOGY

Defects in the developmental process may yield a wide range of inner ear abnormalities. Although widely discussed, these abnormalities are responsible only for a small percentage of congenital deafness. These abnormalities are typically bilateral. Computed tomography has been very helpful in delineating inner-ear abnormalities.

Michel first described complete aplasia of the inner ear.

TABLE 1. *Human ear development*

Fetal week/age	Inner ear	Middle ear	External ear
3	Otic placode forms	Ectoderm of pharyngeal pouch appears	
4			Tissue thickening
5	Utricle, saccule, semicircular canals form		Six hillocks form; EAC sulcus begins
6	Superior semicircular canal complete		
7		Formation of eustachian tube; Meckel's & Reichert's cartilage differentiate to form ossicles	
8	Cochlear duct differentiation begins; cochlear duct one turn; ductus reuniens forms; otic capsule—cartilage	Stapes ring forms	Outer one-third EAC formed
9		Incus and malleus generally shaped	Ectoderm of first groove contacts epithelium of first pharyngeal pouch
10	Cochlear duct two turns	Tympanic ring fully fused	
11	Macule and cristae development complete		
15		Incus and malleus adult size	
16	Otic capsule ossification begins	Incus and malleus ossification begins; stapes adult size and ossification begins	
19	Superior semicircular canal adult size		
20		Stapes adult size	Auricle adult shape
21			Epithelial cells reforming canal
22	Lateral superior semicircular canal adult size and shape	Epitympanum begins to form	
23	Cristae adult size and shape		
24		Pneumatization of apex air cells begins	
25	Cochlear duct 2½ turns and adult shape; Organ of Corti completely formed; otic capsule ossification complete	Incus and malleus ossification complete	
27		Stapes ossification complete	
28			EAC fully formed
32		Pneumatization of middle ear almost complete	
Late fetal life		Antrum and mastoid development begin in later fetal life and continue until approximately 2 yr	
2 yr			EAC fully ossified
4–5 yr			Auricle near adult size
9 yr			Full adult size

EAC, external auditory canal.

This is usually associated with an absence of the cochlear and vestibular nerve. The facial nerve is usually normal (6).

Mondini abnormalities refer to an incomplete development of the bony and membranous labyrinth (Fig. 8). There are a variety of morphologic abnormalities that may be seen. They have been classified by radiographic studies by Jackler and Luxford (Table 2) (7). Abnormalities such as aplasia of the cochlea, common cavity, hypoplasia and incomplete partition are recognized as radiographically distinct entities. The incomplete partition refers to fusion of the middle and upper turns of the cochlea (Fig. 9). Hypoplasia occurs when only the basal turn has developed. A common cavity exists when the otic capsule is severely hypoplastic. The vestibular system is classified as aplastic with small buds and dysplasia of the canals. Histologically, the modiolus may be hypoplastic if the intrascalar septae between the middle and apical turns are absent. The hearing loss associated with this dysplasia may also vary, depending on the extent of the abnormalities. The organ of Corti may be normal or underdeveloped. Varying degrees of the sensorineural hearing loss

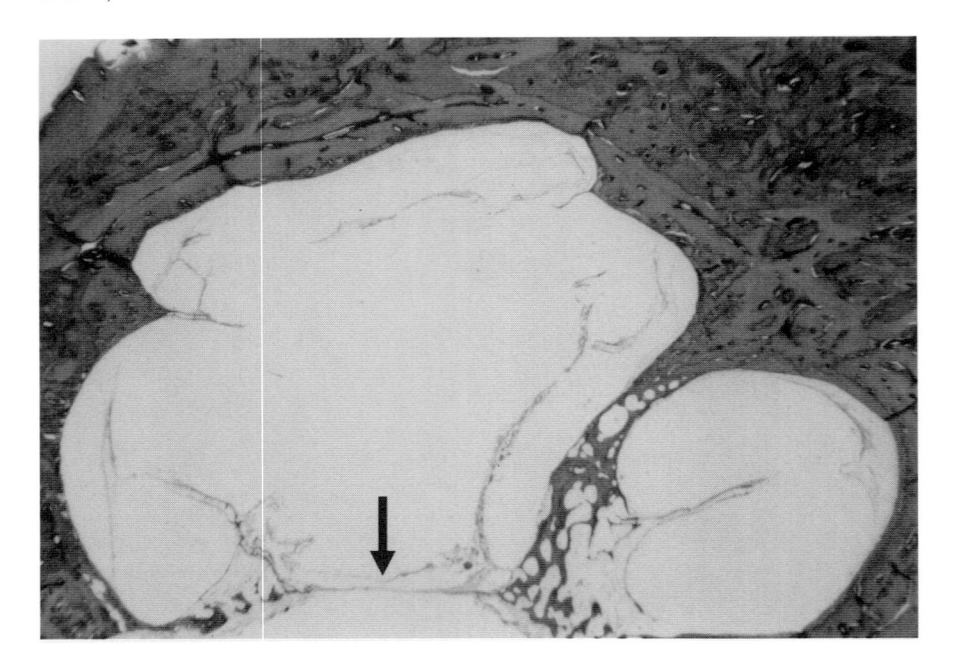

FIG. 8. Mondini deformity of the cochlea demonstrating fusion of middle and apical turns. Basilar turn has normal osseous form but abnormal membranous structures. Thin bony septum separates the cochlea from the internal auditory canal. Absence of osseous modiolus is evident in this diagram (2×) Reprinted with permission of House Ear Institute.

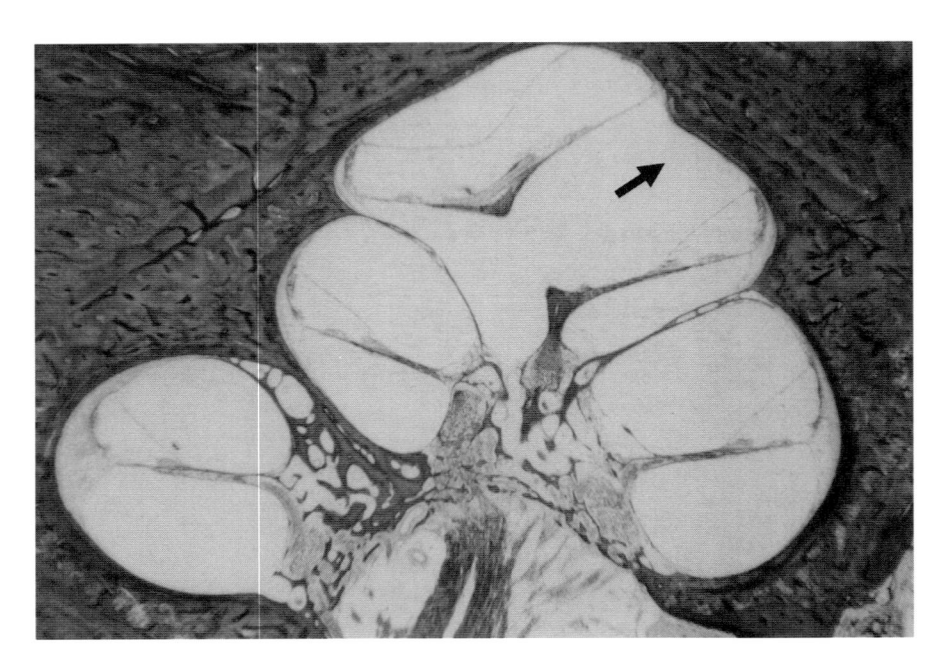

FIG. 9. Arrow indicates intrascalar septal defect. This cochlea has three turns with a fusion of the scala tympani and scala media due to the absence of the intrascalar septum. Reprinted with permission of House Ear Institute.

TABLE 2. *Mondini deformity*

Cochlea
    Complete aplasia
    Common cavity
    Hypoplasia
    Incomplete partition
Vestibular
    Aplasia
    Small buds
    Dysplasia

usually correlates with the degree of gross overall abnormal morphology.

Scheibe deformity is also known as cochleosaccular dysplasia (Fig. 10). The bony otic capsule is normal in these cases. This is thought to be the most common pathologic process associated with sensorineural deafness. It may occur as a congenital abnormality or as a result of degeneration in a normal-hearing cochlea. Phylogenically, the cochlea and saccule are the newer part of the membranous labyrinth. Presumably, then, the Scheibe deformity represents a defect in later fetal development. Characteristic findings include stria vascularis dysplasia (Fig. 11). Alternating areas of hy-

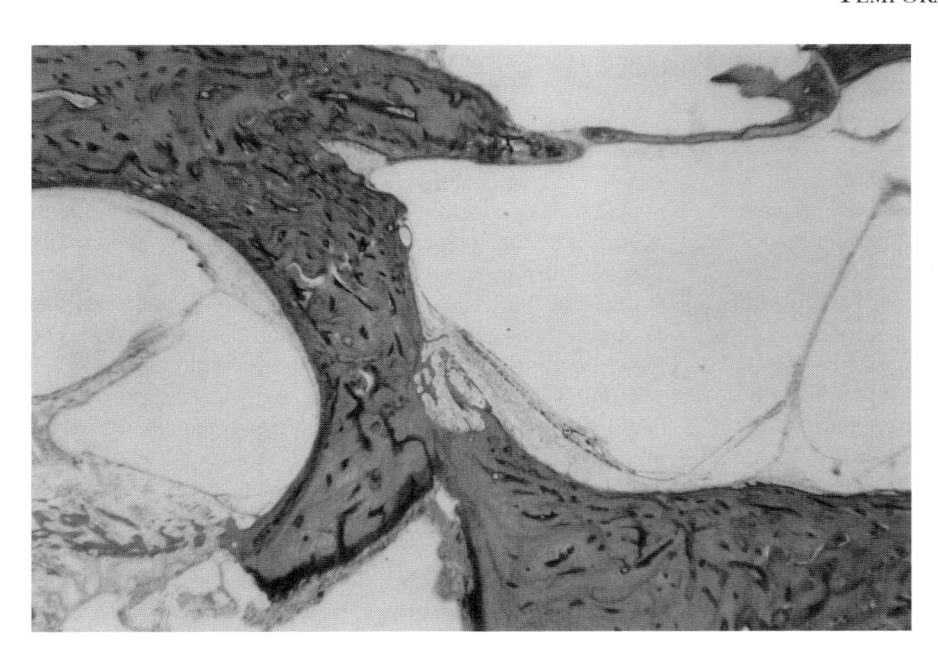

FIG. 10. Scheibe deformity evidence of cochlear and saccular degeneration is present. Flattening of the saccule is seen in this photomicrograph. The membranous utricle is normally shaped in the far right side of the diagram. Reprinted with permission of House Ear Institute.

perplasia and aplasia with absence of cells is seen. There is severe degeneration of the organ of Corti, with an absence of hair cells and supporting cells. The saccule is collapsed with absence of the neurosensory elements. The utricle and three semicircular canals are normally shaped and have normal function. The ganglion cell population of the cochlea is usually normal.

Developmental anomalies of the middle ear and external auditory canal may also occur. The most common deformity is congenital aural atresia. This may also be associated with other anomalies of the middle-ear space. Congenital aural atresia is thought to result from failure of the ectodermal pit to degenerate, which may result in a soft tissue or bony stenosis of the external auditory canal.

Isolated anomalies of the ossicles are unusual. The most common anomalies are associated with stapes malformation. The most frequent anomaly is a bulky stapes (8).

CAUSES OF HEARING LOSS

Alport syndrome is associated with a slow, progressive, bilateral, sensorineural hearing loss and progressive renal failure. It is an X-linked, dominant, inherited disorder that has been linked to the middle of the Xq22 chromosome.

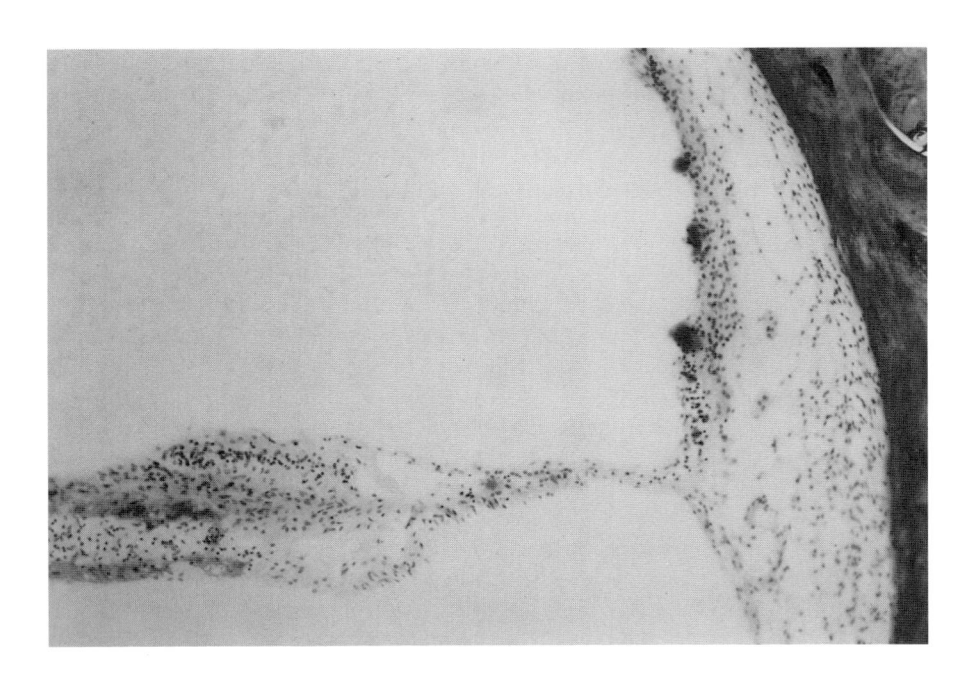

FIG. 11. Scheibe deformity of the cochlea with strial vascular dysplasia. There is severe degeneration of the organ of Corti with absence of normal hair cells and supporting cells. Reprinted with permission of House Ear Institute.

Type IV collagen has been found to be abnormal in the glomerular basement membrane, and it is possible that abnormal type IV collagen is responsible for the sensorineural loss. Temporal bone studies have found no consistent histopathology that can be directly attributed to the disease.

Branchio-otorenal syndrome consists of abnormalities of the lateral branchial sinuses, hearing loss, and renal malformations. Since the hearing loss may be conductive, mixed, or sensorineural, Mondini s deformity and abnormalities of the ossicles have been described with this syndrome.

Crouzon's disease is inherited in a dominant heterozygous genetic pattern. The hearing loss associated with Crouzon's disease is usually conductive, with middle-ear abnormalities and occasionally congenital atresia.

Jervell and Lange-Neilsen syndrome is an autosomal recessive disease with severe sensorineural hearing loss associated with cardiac abnormalities. Deaf children will usually present with syncopal episodes in early life. Sudden death may be seen if this syndrome is not identified early and treatment instituted. Abnormalities seen on electrocardiograms include large T waves and a prolonged QT interval. The histopathology reveals severe degeneration of the entire auditory and vestibular neurosensory epithelium. There is atrophy of the entire organ of Corti and a decreased number of spiral ganglion cells. The bony labyrinth is normal. Periodic acid-Schiff deposits are found in the atrophic stria vascularis. This suggests the material is a mucopolysaccharide. The vestibular system has degeneration of the utricle, saccule and three cristae (9).

The *mucopolysaccharidoses* are a group of inherited disorders that result in abnormal deposition of mucous polysaccharides. Deposition within the middle ear may be associated with conductive hearing loss.

Hurler syndrome is an autosomal recessive inherited disease with a deficiency of 2-L-iduronidase enzyme. Partial retention of mesenchyme in the middle-ear space and basophilic deposits in the stria vascularis may be seen (10).

Hunter's syndrome is an X-linked inherited recessive disease. The main defect is a deficiency of iduronate-2-sulfatase. Incomplete mesenchyme resorption within the middle ear is responsible for the conductive hearing loss associated with this syndrome.

Pendred's syndrome is an autosomal recessive disorder that presents with profound sensorineural hearing loss and is associated with the development of a thyroid goiter in childhood. Children with this syndrome are usually euthyroid. The thyroid goiter may develop in later childhood or be present at birth. The hearing loss is usually a severe to profound sensorineural hearing loss that affects the high frequencies more than the low frequencies. A Mondini deformity is typically associated with this disorder. There is usually a fusion of the middle and apical turns with loss of intrascalar septae. There is severe atrophy of the neuroepithelial element and a lack of ganglion cells. The entire cochlea is usually shortened.

Pierre Robin syndrome is inherited as an autosomal dominant disorder with variable penetrance. This typically involves the first arch, and classic findings include a receded mandible with shortened chin. The hearing loss is usually conductive, with abnormalities of the middle-ear ossicle.

Treacher Collins syndrome is usually inherited as an autosomal dominant disorder. The classic clinical facial symptoms include an underdeveloped mallear bone and a receded mandible. The external auditory canal is usually stenotic or atretic. The tympanic membrane is usually abnormally shaped. The tympanic cavity is usually abnormal with abnormalities of the ossicles present. This may include absence of the malleus and incus, and a rudimentary stapes. The facial nerve can frequently have an aberrant course (11).

Usher's syndrome consists of congenital sensorineural hearing loss with progressive retinitis pigmentosa. It may be inherited as an autosomal recessive, autosomal dominant or X-linked recessive disorder. It has been divided into three groups on the basis of its clinical characteristics. Histologically, degeneration of the organ of Corti and spiral ganglion cells are seen. This is typically severe in the basal turn. Despite the clinical loss of vestibular function, no histopathologic changes have been reported with this disorder (12).

Waardenburg syndrome is an autosomal dominant disorder with classic clinical facial characteristics and sensorineural hearing loss. Patients with this syndrome typically have several of the following characteristics: dystrophic canthi, broad nasal root, hypertrichosis of the eyebrows, white forelock, heterochromia of the irides, and associated sensorineural hearing loss. The histologic abnormalities were described by Fisch in 1959 (13). The bony labyrinth is usually normal. There is atrophy of the organ of Corti and a decreased number of spiral ganglion cells. The stria vascularis also atrophies, and there is a normal vestibular system.

Infectious Causes

Infectious cytomegalovirus is a ubiquitous viral infection of pregnant women. It is believed to be present in 1% to 2% of all live births. It may be completely asymptomatic or act as a teratogen for the infant. The hearing loss associated with cytomegaloviral infection is variable. The loss may be profound or may be progressive. The histopathologic characteristics are that of an endolymph viral infection. Cytomegaloviral inclusions are found in the epithelial cell lining of the cochlear duct. The organ of Corti and perilymphatic spaces appear normal. The exact pathogenesis of the hearing loss is as of yet unknown. Other organ systems may also be affected by cytomegaloviral infections (14).

Measles infection may be associated with sensorineural hearing loss. The clinical hearing loss is usually bilateral and may range from moderate to profound. Endolymphatic labyrinthitis may occur from measles infection by a hematogenous route, whereas perilymphatic labyrinthitis may occur from the meninges associated with meningeal encephalitis. The histopathologic characteristics include an organ of Corti that is shrunken with absence of the hair cells. This may be more severe in the basal turn. There is severe atrophy of the stria vascularis with displacement of Reissner s membrane towards the basilar membrane.

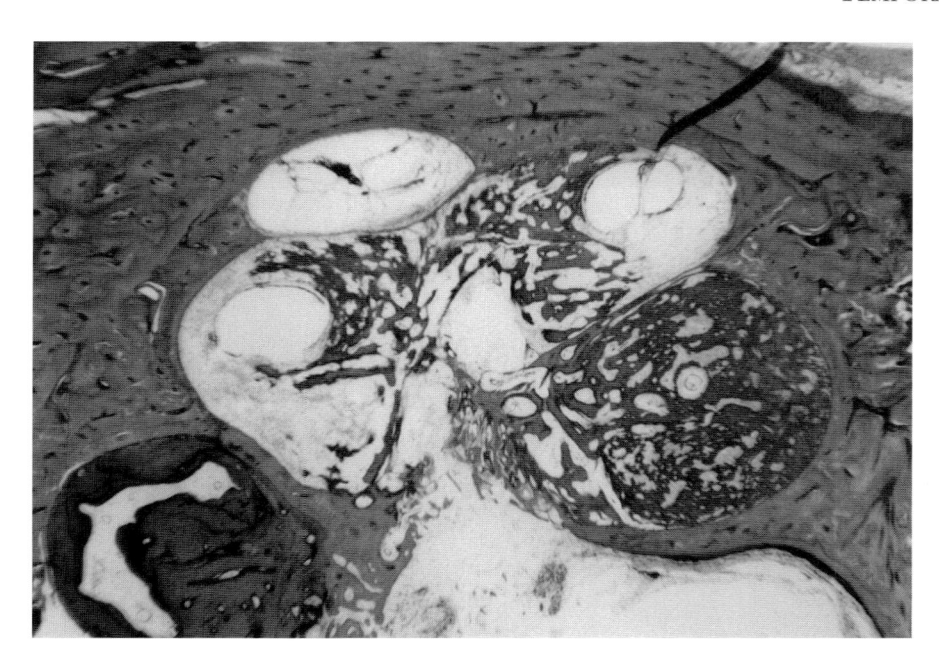

FIG. 12. Severe ossification of the cochlea in the basal and middle turns. Soft tissue fibrosis is also seen in both scala tympani and the middle turns. Reprinted with permission of House Ear Institute.

Meningitis can cause sensorineural hearing loss. Otitis media may lead to meningitis by hematogenous spread. The meningitis usually resolves after the otitis episode has been treated. Suppurative labyrinthitis may develop as meningitis spreads to the labyrinth via the internal auditory canal or by the cochlear aqueduct. Most histopathologic specimens of meningitis have been acquired when an individual has died of the disease process. An acute inflammatory infiltration of the labyrinth is usually found. The most significant sequelae in individuals who survive meningitis with associated hearing loss are those of fibrosis and new bone formation, which may occur as a result of the labyrinthitis. New bone formation usually occurs within the perilymphatic spaces but may involve the entire cochlea with obliteration of neurosensory elements. This is especially important in considering cochlear implants in individuals with profound deafness following meningitis. The ossification process occurs within the first year following the onset of hearing loss (Fig. 12).

Mumps is probably the most common viral infection responsible for sensorineural hearing loss. Characteristically, it is unilateral in nature and may occur at any time throughout childhood. Lindsey (15) described the pathology found in a child with bilateral sensorineural loss presumably due to mumps. There was severe degeneration of the cochlear duct and organ of Corti. A loss of the spiral ganglion cells was also noted especially in the basal turn. There was severe atrophy of the stria vascularis.

Maternal *rubella* infection may have severe teratogenic effects, especially during the first and second trimesters. The United States epidemic of 1963–1965 is in some ways responsible for our understanding of this disease due to the number of individuals involved. Possible damage includes sensorineural hearing loss, cataracts, heart defects, mental retardation, thrombocytopenia, and mild brain damage. The histopathologic abnormalities are characteristic of cochleo-saccular dysplasia. There is atrophy of the organ of Corti and loss of hair cells. Hemorrhage into the cochlea is a common finding. There is typically inflammation and thrombosis within the stria vascularis.

Syphilis may be responsible for hearing loss and may be acquired through sexual contact or contracted through exposure from the placenta. The latter is commonly referred to as congenital otosyphilis. The pathologic changes may occur in two ways. Goodhill (16) described the meningeoneurolabyrinthitis and osteitis of the temporal bone that may occur followed by a secondary membranous labyrinthitis. Periosteitis may be caused by microgumma that cause destruction of the bony labyrinth and ossification. Multinucleated giant cells with lymphocytic infiltration produce endarteritis. Progressive degeneration of the membranous labyrinth may also occur with an inflammatory fibrosis and atrophy of the organ of Corti. Endolymphatic hydrops may occur due to endolymphatic duct obliteration (Fig. 13) (17). This is responsible for clinical symptoms similar to those of Ménière's disease.

Sudden idiopathic sensorineural hearing loss remains an etiological mystery. The pathologic changes resemble that of other viral disorders in that the principal abnormalities are related to the organ of Corti. Loss of hair cells and supporting cells is found in the majority of cases (Fig. 14). Other abnormalities include atrophy of the stria vascularis and loss of cochlear neurons. There is an absence of fibroproliferative response. This absence of fibrosis points to viral etiology as the cause of sudden hearing loss.

Cholesteatoma

Cholesteatoma is the most common acquired condition of the ear, secondary only to otitis media with effusion that

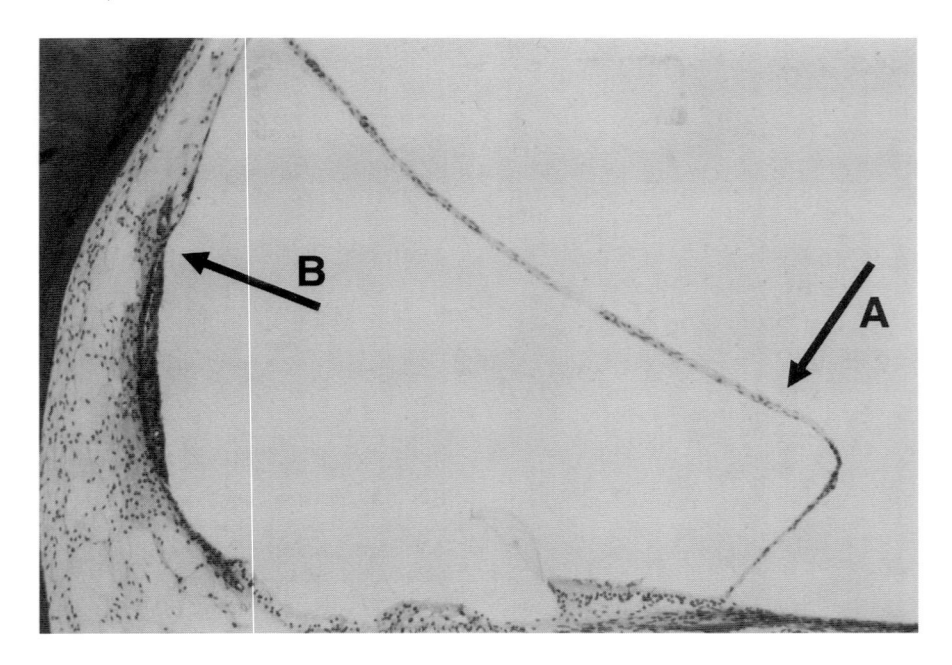

FIG. 13. Endolymphatic hydrops with ballooning of Reissner's membrane (A). Arrow B demonstrates the upper limit of the stria vascularis where Reissner's membrane normally originates. Reissner's membrane is adherent to the spiral ligament. Reprinted with permission of House Ear Institute.

requires surgical intervention. Cholesteatomas may develop from retraction pockets of the pars flaccida or at perforations of the tympanic membrane. The ingrowth of surface epithelium into the middle ear and epitympanic space continues along paths of least resistance. Keratin debris collects in the center, which increases the size of the cholesteatoma. Bone resorption may occur due to enzyme production by the expanding epithelial lining. This may lead to bony erosion of the ossicle, otic capsule, and mastoid air cells. The epithelium of the keratinized layer is similar to the skin of the external auditory canal. Acute and chronic inflammatory cells are associated with fibroblasts and capillaries in the subepithelial region.

Ototoxic Agents

Aminoglycosides are perhaps the most common drug responsible for ototoxicity. Their indications for certain life-threatening disorders require their persistent use today. The main histologic pathology associated with aminoglycoside ototoxicity is loss of cochlear hair cells. The outer hair cells are thought to be more susceptible than inner hair cells. The damage appears to be dose dependent. Hair cells for the higher frequencies appear more sensitive.

Loop diuretics (ethacrynic acid and furesomide) may cause sensorineural hearing loss. The major effects appear to be on the stria vascularis of the cochlea and dark cells of

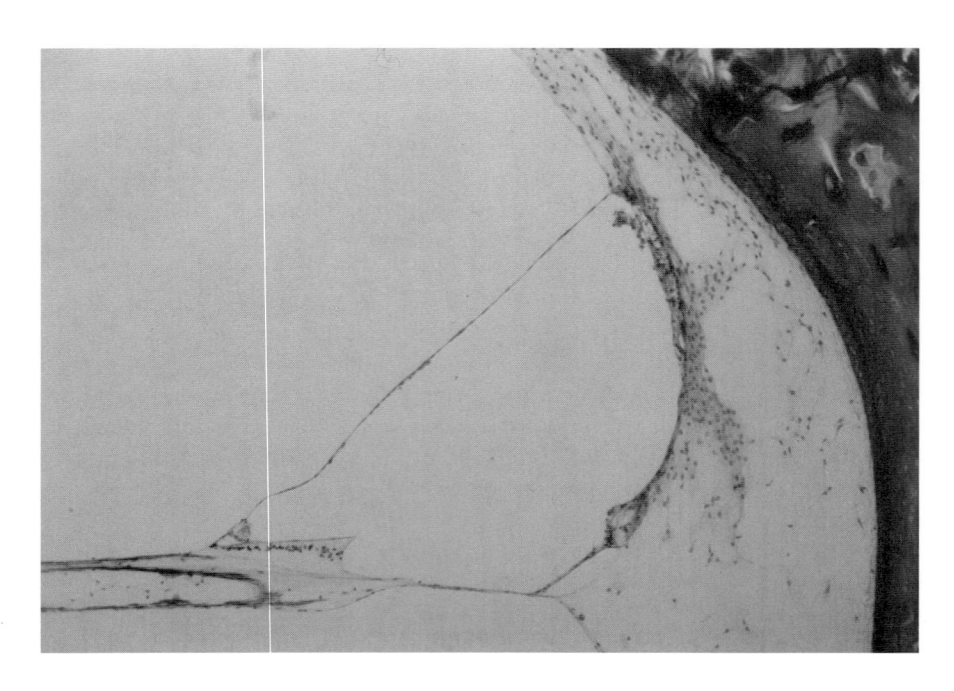

FIG. 14. Complete absence of the organ of Corti. This case illustrates the pathology of a sudden hearing loss. Reprinted with permission of House Ear Institute.

the vestibular system. Furosemide may increase the nephrotoxicity of aminoglycoside antibiotics (18).

COCHLEAR IMPLANTATION

Cochlear implantation has become the standard treatment for congenitally profoundly deaf children who receive no benefit from hearing aids. Current devices available for implantation have long electrodes inserted through the round window into the scala tympani. The site of stimulation appears to be the ganglion cells of the modiolus. Patients with absence of hair cells and peripheral processes still receive benefit from cochlear implantation. The magnitude of the neuronal cell loss may correlate with the patient's ability to receive information from the cochlear implant, but this has not been documented in temporal bone studies. Ossification of the labyrinth may occur with multiple etiologies of hearing loss. The most common, mentioned earlier, is meningitis. This may cause obliteration of the scala tympani and inhibit implantation. New bone growth is most severe in the basal turn. The electrodes enter the scala tympani, and it is common for them to pierce the basilar membrane and travel through the cochlear duct, entering into the scala vestibuli. Injury to the cochlea in this manner does not appear to affect performance (19).

SUMMARY

Knowledge of the normal temporal bone histology is required for understanding of the histopathology. Histopathology of the temporal bone has allowed the pathophysiology of many etiologies of hearing loss to be understood. Future development and refinement of biochemical techniques will unlock our further understanding at the molecular level to the causes of many of presently unknown etiologies of hearing loss.

REFERENCES

1. Lim DJ. Tympanic membrane. Electron microscopic observation. Part I: pars tensa. *Acta Otolaryngol (Stockh)* 1968;66:181.
2. Hentzer E. Ultrastructure of the normal mucosa in the human middle ear, mastoid cavities, and eustachian tube. *Ann Otol Rhinol Laryngol* 1970;79:1143.
3. Schuknecht HF. Anatomy. eds. *Pathology of the ear.* 2nd ed. Philadelphia: Lea & Febiger, 1993:66.
4. Schuknecht HF. Anatomy. eds. *Pathology of the ear.* 2nd ed. Philadelphia: Lea & Febiger, 1993:47.
5. Tian Q, Rask-Andersen H, Linthicum FH Jr. Identification of substances in the endolymphatic sac. *Acta Otolaryngol (Stockh)* 1994;114:632.
6. Michel EM. Mémoire sur les anomalies congénitales de l'oreille interne avec la premiére observation authentique d'absence compléte d'oreilles internes eustachian tube de nerfs auditifs, eustachian tube de l'absence partielle de le'oreille moyenne chez un sourd et muet de naissance, mort à l'âge de onze acoustic neuromas. *Gaz Méd Strasb* 1863;23:55.
7. Jackler RK, Luxford WM, eds. Congenital malformations of the inner ear. *Laryngoscope* (Suppl 40) 1987;97:1.
8. Sando I, Wood RP II. Congenital middle ear anomalies. *Otolaryngol Clin North Am* 1971;4:291.
9. Friedmann I, Fraser GR, Froggatt P. Pathology of the ear in the cardioauditory syndrome of Jervell and Lange-Nielsen (recessive deafness with electrocardiographic abnormalities). *J Laryngol Otol* 1966;80:451.
10. Schachern PA, Shea DA, Paparella MM. Mucopolysaccharidosis I-H (Hurler's syndrome) and human temporal bone histopathology. *Ann Otol Rhinol Laryngol* 1984;93:65.
11. Sando I, Hemenway WG, Miller DR, Black FO. Vestibular pathology in otosclerosis temporal bone histopathological report. *Laryngoscope* 1974;84:593.
12. Belal A Jr. Usher's syndrome. (Retinitis pigmentosa and deafness.) A temporal bone report. *J Laryngol Otol* 1975;89:175.
13. Fisch L. Deafness as part of an hereditary syndrome. *J Laryngol Otol* 1959;73:355.
14. Strauss M. Human cytomegalovirus labyrinthitis. *Am J Otolaryngol* 1990;11:292.
15. Lindsay JR, Davey PR, Ward PH. Inner ear pathology in deafness due to mumps. *Ann Otol Rhinol Laryngol* 1960;69:918.
16. Goodhill V. Syphilis of the ear: a histopathologic study. *Ann Otol Rhinol Laryngol* 1939;48:676.
17. Linthicum FH Jr, El-Rahman AGA. Hydrops due to syphilitic endolymphatic duct obliteration. *Laryngoscope* 1987;97:568.
18. Arnold W, Nadol JB Jr, Weidauer H. Ultrastructural histopathology in a case of human ototoxicity due to loop diuretics. *Acta Otolaryngol (Stockh)* 1981;91:399.
19. Linthicum FH Jr, Fayad J, Otto SR, Galey FR, House WF. Cochlear implant histopathology. *Am J Otol* 1991;12:245.

PART II
Diagnostic Evaluation

CHAPTER 7

Behavioral Audiologic Assessment

Judith S. Gravel

Appropriate and timely otologic and audiologic management strategies can be initiated once a child's hearing has received comprehensive assessment. The evaluation techniques selected for use with the pediatric population must be accurate, specific, and efficient so that medical and audiologic monitoring, intervention and follow-up may be focused and comprehensive. This chapter examines the behavioral audiologic test techniques that are currently available—procedures that can provide the requisite audiometric information to achieve the aforementioned goals. Behavioral audiometry is one critical component of the pediatric audiologic test battery. However, an armamentarium of test procedures is the best means of ensuring the validity of the assessment outcome. Concordance of the findings from a battery of test procedures (behavioral, electrophysiologic, acoustic immittance, and otoacoustic emissions [OAEs]) is sought to determine the accuracy of audiologic assessment. This "cross-check principle" has long been the tenant of pediatric audiology practice (1).

The effects of hearing loss on the speech and language development of children are addressed in this volume by Roberts, Wallace, and Brackett (Chapter 4). Consequently, the purpose of the audiologic evaluation is to provide a timely and individualized assessment that accurately delineates the type, degree, configuration, and symmetry of any hearing impairment in the child (2,3). The audiologic assessment should include measures of sensitivity, and function (speech audiometry), whenever possible.

The critical role of auditory evoked response procedures, such as the auditory brainstem response (ABR) in the assessment of audition in children, cannot be overemphasized. Indeed, one chapter that follows thoroughly overviews these important auditory assessment strategies (Chapter 9). However, in day-to-day practice, the routine use of the ABR each time a child requires hearing threshold assessment is not practical, nor is it time- or cost-efficient. Moreover, traditional electrophysiologic test procedures may not provide frequency-specific threshold information for follow-up and amplification fitting. Acoustic immittance (tympanometry and acoustic reflex threshold measures) provides invaluable information regarding middle ear function and suprathreshold auditory responsivity. However, information regarding sensitivity and hearing loss type is unavailable from the results of such studies. Finally, while evoked OAEs provide valuable insight into cochlear function, their usefulness in predicting hearing sensitivity, regardless of the degree of hearing loss, is limited. Thus, behavioral audiometry is the procedure of choice for the routine clinical assessment of hearing in children.

BEHAVIORAL AUDIOLOGIC ASSESSMENT TECHNIQUES

The primary concern raised by professionals regarding behavioral hearing assessment of children is whether audiologic data acquired through behavioral audiometry are reliable and valid. This concern has frequently turned practitioners away from "subjective" behavioral approaches and toward more "objective" physiologic and electrophysiologic test methods. Indeed, some clinicians still believe that children must have developed speech and language before behavioral audiometry can be completed successfully. Hence, reports that hearing assessment has been postponed "until the child can talk" are still not uncommon. In reality, currently available clinical behavioral test procedures meet the requirements of efficiency, accuracy, and, in some circumstances, objectivity. For routine clinical use, behavioral test techniques are simple, reliable, pleasant, cost- and time-efficient for the vast majority of children from infancy through school age.

Infants and young children who are otherwise developing normally have the cognitive and motor capacity to provide reliable audiometric data, beginning at about 6 mo of age (4). However, test procedures must be made developmentally

---

J.S. Gravel: Department of Otorhinolaryngology: Division of Audiology, Albert Einstein College of Medicine, Bronx, New York 10461.

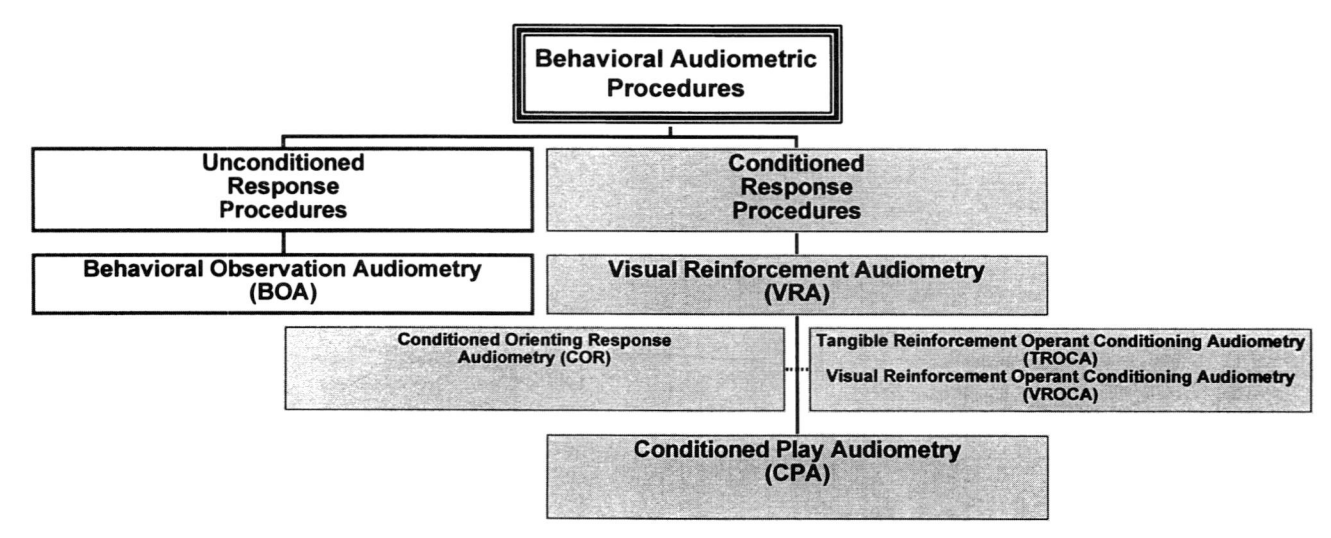

FIG. 1. A classification scheme for considering various pediatric behavioral audiometric test methods as unconditioned or conditioned response procedures.

appropriate and optimized, through the use of reinforcement, to maximize the probability of obtaining repeatable responses. One cannot expect to comprehensively assess the hearing of children using test equipment or a test environment designed for adults— some changes to the typical audiologic test setting are necessary. Included in the discussion that follows are specific suggestions regarding the modifications that can optimize the audiologic assessment of infants and young children.

Behavioral assessment procedures fall into two general categories: those that rely on overt, unconditioned responses to auditory signals, and those that use conditioned response procedures to examine hearing function. Considering these alternatives, this chapter addresses three age ranges of children for whom behavioral audiometry can be used effectively for audiometric assessment: infants and toddlers, preschool children, and school-aged children. Figure 1 depicts a classification scheme for conceptualizing behavioral audiometric procedures.

Behavioral Assessment of Infants and Toddlers

Behavioral Observation Audiometry

For many years, behavioral observation audiometry (BOA) was the procedure typically used to screen and evaluate hearing in neonates and infants (5,6). Behavioral observation audiometry relies on the fact that a novel or interesting sound presented to an infant generally elicits some overt, observable behavioral response. Behaviors accepted as evidence that the infant has heard the signal range from those that are easily defined and clearly observable; such as a head turn or eye shift toward the signal source. However, both gross and subtle responses, such as a startle, limb movements, eye-blink, or cessation or initiation of sucking activity, have also been used as response indicators. Traditionally, an audiologist presenting test stimuli and observing from the adjacent test suite, as well as one situated inside the test booth with the infant and parent, had to agree on the presence or absence of a response. Rarely were examiners or parents "deafened" to the presence of the test signals; thus, the opportunity for observer bias was high.

Behavioral responses elicited during BOA are *unconditioned* responses in that no reward or reinforcement is provided. Therefore, rapid habituation (cessation) of responding to the presence of the test stimulus usually occurs; dishabituation requires the introduction of a new (novel) test stimulus. Unfortunately, these auditory signals (speech, environmental noises, or music) tend to be broadband, lacking frequency specificity. Thus, clear definition of the configuration of any hearing loss is usually precluded. Moreover, presentation intensities required to startle the infant or attract the baby's attention are often well above the young child's threshold of hearing. When the intent is to delineate hearing thresholds across the audiometric speech frequency range, the significant drawbacks of BOA are obvious.

As conventionally practiced, BOA provides a means for grossly estimating an infant's auditory responsivity. Indeed, behavioral observations of very young babies' (0–4 mo) responses to sound should always be incorporated into hearing evaluations, even when ABR or OAE results are available. The concordance among electrophysiologic, physiologic, and behavioral measures provides assurance that the clinical impression of auditory function is valid. In circumstances in which the measures do not agree, further exploration of hearing should be undertaken (7). However, because of unacceptable response variability (even in infants with normal hearing), BOA cannot distinguish among various degrees and configurations of hearing loss with sufficient accuracy for it to be used as the primary measure of hearing sensitivity in very young babies.

Visual Reinforcement Audiometry

Another test method, visual reinforcement audiometry (VRA, or the conditioned head-turn procedure), has allowed audiologists to reliably determine hearing thresholds in infants beginning at about 5 to 6 months of age. Indeed, empiric studies of the applicability of the VRA procedure have found that 85% to 90% of infants who are developmentally 5 to 6 months of age and older can be successfully tested using the technique (4,8). Visual reinforcement audiometry has been described extensively in several publications (3,4,7–13). The principles of VRA are fundamentally the same, regardless of procedural modifications including those using logic systems (8), computer mediation (4,9,12,14–16), and manual (3,7,11) approaches.

Visual reinforcement audiometry is a conditioned (operant) test technique that uses one or more visual reinforcers to maintain responding; the behavioral response is a 45- to 90-degree head turn. Visual reinforcement is made contingent on a "correct" response during or immediately after the presentation of a signal trial (an interval containing a stimulus)—in signal detection theory, a "hit." If the head turn is made during a catch trial (an interval containing no signal), reinforcement is not provided (a false alarm). Neither is reinforcement provided when the infant fails to turn to a signal trial (a "miss"), nor when the infant does not respond to a catch trial (a correct rejection).

Because responding is supported by a visual reinforcer, any intrinsic interest value the test signal might have is irrelevant. Thus, conventional audiometric test stimuli that are frequency-specific (pure tones, FM tones, narrow bands of noise) can be used for the assessment. Moreover, once the response contingency (stimulus-response-reward) has been established, commonly used psychometric procedures, such as the conventional up–down adaptive staircase, can be used to estimate the infant's threshold.

Thresholds obtained from infants using VRA are approximately 10 to 15 dB poorer than those of adult listeners (8,9). Further, average threshold values for normally hearing children remain relatively stable throughout infancy (6–18 mo) (8). Thus, it is not necessary to apply correction factors according to the child's age. Minimal response variability in infants who are hearing normally allows even mild degrees of hearing loss to be detected (8,10). Figure 2 shows audiograms from four babies, all 9 months of age, that were obtained using VRA. Threshold estimates obtained in infancy using VRA have been found to be reliable in the longer term, demonstrating good agreement with audiograms obtained at older ages (10). Finally, behavioral thresholds obtained with VRA show excellent agreement with auditory sensitivity es-

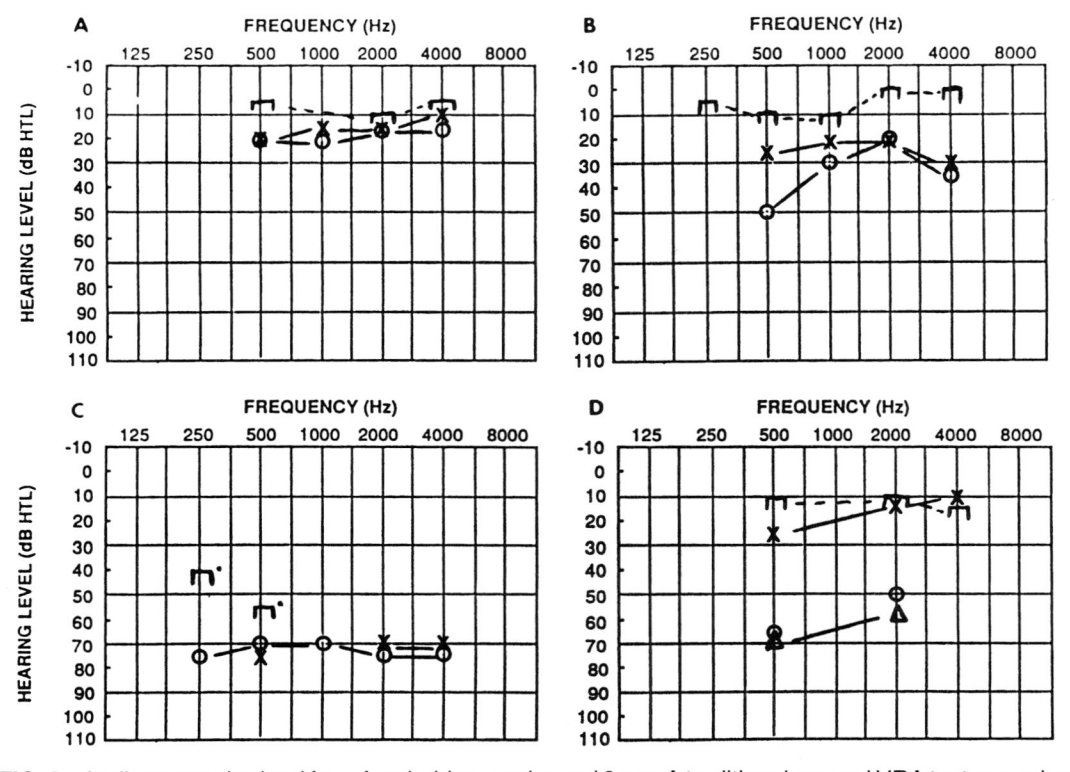

FIG. 2. Audiograms obtained from four babies, each aged 9 mo. A traditional manual VRA test procedure was used to obtain the thresholds. O, right ear; X, left ear; Π, unmasked bone-conduction threshold (best bone); △, masked threshold, right ear; * indicates a vibrotactile (nonauditory) response. From Gravel JS. Behavioral assessment of auditory function. *Semin Hearing* 1989; 10:216–28. Reprinted with permission.

timates obtained using a frequency-specific ABR procedure (17).

VRA Test Protocol

"Efficiency" is the motto of VRA testing; no trial should be considered extraneous (18). Infants can sometimes tire quickly and cease responding. Thus, the initial phases of VRA take advantage of behaviors that occur naturally (e.g., head orienting in the direction of a novel signal) to teach the baby the required response. Simultaneously, these intial responses provide valuable audiometric information.

To initiate VRA testing, the infant's attention is brought to the midline position. This is accomplished through the manipulation of a simple but interesting distraction toy (handled by an examiner or the parent). When the infant is looking forward and is quiet and attentive, a suprathreshold test signal is presented through a loudspeaker that is positioned to one side of the baby. Ninety percent of infants with normal hearing will orient toward a 500-Hz, 30-dB HL test signal by looking in the direction of its source (19). When the head turn occurs, a toy reinforcer located near the loudspeaker is activated and illuminated. Following the response, the infant's attention is brought back to the midline position. Another test signal at the same intensity is presented. Infants who oriented to the initial presentation of the test signal and saw the reinforcer will generally turn once more to the presentation of the second stimulus. Once again, reinforcement for the response is provided. After two reinforced head turns at 30 dB HL, threshold acquisition begins (18).

Because the baby has responded twice correctly to the 30-dB HL signal, the intensity of the next stimulus is lowered by 20 dB. If the infant responds, reinforcement is delivered and the intensity of the next stimulus is lowered again by 20 dB. If the baby does not respond to the stimulus, the intensity of the subsequent presentation is increased by 10 dB. The threshold search is instituted using an up–down (a decrease in intensity following a hit, an increase in intensity following a miss) adaptive test procedure (20). Instead of the traditional 5-dB interval commonly used with adults, a 10-dB step size is often used for threshold assessment of infants. This larger step size provides a means of approximating threshold quickly. In addition, only three response reversals (hit-miss-hit) following the first miss on the initial descent are sufficient for estimating threshold at a particular frequency (15). Following successful acquisition of threshold at 500 Hz, testing continues at higher frequencies (2,000 or 4,000 Hz). Minimally, a soundfield audiogram that characterizes hearing at low-, mid-, and high-frequency regions is completed. The soundfield audiogram provides an overall impression of the degree and configuration of any existing hearing loss, at least for one (the better) ear.

After soundfield assessment has been completed, bone conduction thresholds are obtained in a similar manner for low-, mid-, and high-frequency regions. Next, individual-ear air-conduction thresholds are obtained. Determining the symmetry of hearing sensitivity is important for medical and surgical or audiologic intervention that must be initiated. A pediatric headset assembly coupled to standard earphone receivers may be used. While many clinicians do not attempt audiometry using earphones with infants, the majority of infants between the ages of 6 and 24 months can be assessed with these conventional transducers (21). Currently, a better means of obtaining ear-specific thresholds from infants is through the use of insert receivers. These transducers are lightweight and comfortable and do not interfere with the head-turn response. Moreover, for the purposes of masking, insert earphones provide greater inter-aural attentuation than conventional earphones, and leakage of the acoustic signal is greatly reduced.

Masking can be used with infants if their audiogram suggests the need for it. Initially, babies may be confused by, or even respond to, the masking noise. However, after a shaping period during which the masking is gradually introduced and suprathreshold test signals are presented and reinforced, it is possible to establish contingent responding only to the test signal.

Returning to our initial VRA protocol, if an infant does not respond to the 30 dB HL, 500 Hz test signal after two presentations (as described previously), the level of the test signal is raised by 20 dB. If no head orientation toward the loudspeaker occurs following two presentations of the signal at 50 dB HL, the level of the stimulus is raised to 70 dB HL. If the infant does not respond to either of two presentations at this intensity, soundfield testing is discontinued. Of course, if the infant does respond at either the 50-dB or 70-dB HL levels, the up–down staircase procedure (as described earlier) is initiated.

When an infant demonstrates no response to the soundfield signals at 70 dB HL, the bone oscillator is placed on either the baby's left or right mastoid: The side is chosen to correspond with the side closest to the visual reinforcer display. At this point, classic response shaping is begun. The presentation of a 40- to 50-dB HL bone-conducted 500-Hz narrowband noise will produce a vibrotactile sensation, if not an auditory one. Consequently, even if the infant were to have a profound loss of hearing, the signal would be *felt,* even if it were not heard. With the knowledge that the signal is salient (detectable through vibration), the audiologist can provide reinforcement immediately after the presentation of the bone-conducted test signal. The parent is requested to turn the infant's head in the direction of the reinforcer after the presentation of the stimulus if the infant does not turn automatically when the toy reinforcers are illuminated and activated. The infant's attention is then brought back to the midline position. Again, the bone-conducted stimulus is presented, and the visual reinforcer illuminated. After several such classical shaping presentations, the infant generally learns the response contingency (stimulus-response-reward), and bone-conduction thresholds are obtained using the up–down staircase procedure.

Some audiologists prefer to begin VRA using a speech stimulus instead of a tonal signal. This may be useful for rapidly teaching the baby the VRA task. Indeed, as discussed previously, babies find speech more interesting than tonal signals and thus spontaneously turn when they hear a human voice. However, a threshold for speech provides a gross estimate of hearing sensitivity, and it is only with the use of frequency-specific stimuli that a comprehensive audiogram can be developed.

Infants who cannot be conditioned (even when the bone-conduction procedure is used) may not have achieved a developmental age appropriate for VRA. Neuromotor deficits or severe visual impairments may also preclude VRA assessment. If the audiologist is unable to obtain reliable responses from an infant after two visits (on closely spaced test days), and if other measures, observations, or case history suggest the infant is at risk for hearing loss, auditory threshold estimates should be pursued using the ABR. Postponing behavioral testing for weeks or months ''until the child is older'' can often delay the identification of significant hearing loss.

VRA Test Suite Arrangement and Equipment

Various VRA test suite arrangements are depicted in Fig. 3. The specific arrangement selected will depend on the

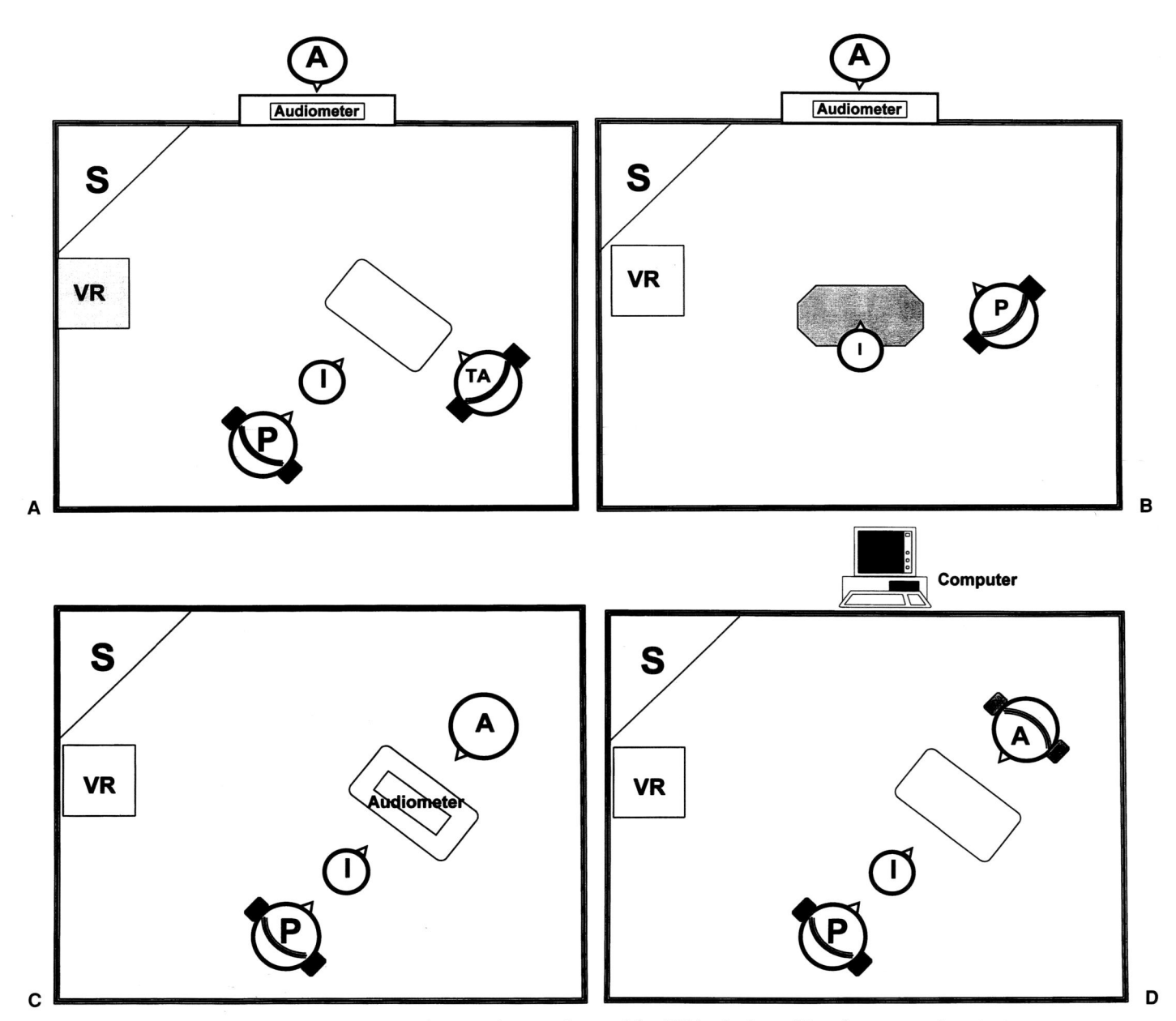

FIG. 3. Test suite arrangements that are frequently used for VRA. **A:** A traditional two-examiner test arrangement. **B, C:** Arrangements that require only one audiologist for VRA. **D:** The test suite arrangement when a computer-assisted VRA test procedure is employed. *S*, loudspeaker; *VR*, visual reinforcer; *A*, audiologist; *TA*, test assistant; *P*, parent; *I*, infant.

needs and resources of a given facility. Centers that routinely evaluate infants and children often have instrumentation dedicated to pediatric assessment. However, even in settings that only occasionally evaluate infants, the optimization of the test suite and equipment to accommodate VRA is equally important.

In traditional VRA, the test suite is arranged as depicted in Fig. 3A. The parent or caretaker is seated with the infant placed on the parent's lap. A visual reinforcer display is located to one side and a loudspeaker is located immediately adjacent to the visual reinforcer. An assistant is seated toward the baby's opposite side. A small table located in front of the infant is used by the assistant for the manipulation of distraction toys. An audiologist located outside the test suite is responsible for the presentation of test signals. To reduce observer bias, both the parent and the examiner within the test booth wear earphones. The parent listens to masking noise (usually music), while the examiner in the test suite hears a noise each time a trial (regardless of the type) is presented.

If one audiologist is used for VRA, Fig. 3B, and C depicts arrangements that are most optimal. In Fig. 3B, the audiometer is outside the test booth and the baby in the examination room is seated in a highchair facing the observation window. The mother is seated slightly to one side of the baby and performs the function of the assistant, maintaining the infant's gaze in the midline position between test trials. In Fig. 3C, the audiologist and the audiometer are located within the test suite. The audiologist controls all signal presentations and also is responsible for the between-trial midline distraction. If the test is being mediated by a computer (usually located outside the test booth; Fig. 3D), the arrangement is the same. In this circumstance, a handheld control allows interaction with the computer (see following discussion).

In all of the arrangements (Fig. 3A–D), note the location of the loudspeaker and visual reinforcer display. Primus (22) demonstrated that the placement of the loudspeaker and visual reinforcer display is critical to the success of VRA. The loudspeaker should be located immediately adjacent to the visual reinforcer display rather than on the side opposite to the reinforcer, or above the infant's head.

Appealing visual reinforcers are crucial. The complexity and novelty of the reinforcers helps to maintain the motivation and attention of the infant across repeated test trials (8). Brightly illuminated mechanical toys are the most useful. The toy reinforcers are housed in individual dark, smoked plexiglas boxes, so that when not illuminated, the toy is completely out of the infant's view. While VRA can be completed with only one reinforcer, having more than one toy heightens the novelty of the reinforcement because a different reinforcer is activated after each correct response (24). Improving the visual reinforcers used with VRA is a simple and economical means of enhancing the effectiveness of the procedure in the clinical setting.

A computer-mediated test procedure is one means of implementing VRA in the clinical setting. Several investigators have described procedures that use the computer as a test assistant (9,14,15). The advantages of computer-mediated VRA are multiple. Observer bias is greatly reduced, because the computer determines (based on a specified probability) whether a signal trial or catch trial is presented. The audiologist in the test booth with the baby interacts with the computer via a hand or foot switch, signaling the computer when the infant is ready for a trial and when a head-turn response has been made. The computer delivers reinforcement only when appropriate (for a head turn to a signal trial). The computer initiates the up–down adaptive procedure, maintaining a trial-by-trial record of performance, and the rate of false-positive responding. The false alarm rate allows the audiologist to estimate the reliability of the threshold. Randomly interspersed probe trials (higher-intensity test signals introduced to assess the baby's attention and motivation during testing) can also be included in the protocol. The computer provides the opportunity to optimize test algorithms, such as the interleaving of test frequencies during a single test run (20). In this manner, more than one frequency can be tested during one run, rather than determining threshold for one frequency before beginning another (14,16).

Currently, a PC-based VRA system (Intelligent Visual Reinforcement Audiometry [IVRA]) is available commercially (Intelligent Hearing Systems, Inc., Miami). It provides three protocols useful for both screening and assessment purposes (15,16,23). The CAST (Classification of Audiograms by Sequential Testing) screening and OHTA (Optional Hearing Test Algorithm) assessment procedures available on IVRA utilize Bayesian mathematic theory to efficiently screen hearing and determine threshold sensitivity. The only disadvantage of computer-controlled procedures may be lack of clinical flexibility that can restrict the audiologist's ability to diverge from the test protocol when deemed necessary.

Manual VRA assessment can also be optimized using a simple paper and pencil technique with one or two examiners (3) or through the use of simple logic circuitry (8). The use of a second examiner, naive as to the occurrence of a test trial, is the only means of ensuring a bias-free threshold estimate when using manual VRA. This may be the only reason to justify the use of two clinicians in the audiologic assessment of infants.

COR Audiometry

Visual reinforcement audiometry is often confused with the conditioned orienting response (COR) procedure. Both methods use visual reinforcement of correct responding but differ in methodology and information obtained. In VRA, a unidirectional head turn serves as the response indicator. This response remains invariant regardless of the type of signal transduction (loudspeaker, earphones, insert receivers, or bone oscillator). In COR, a head orientation toward the source of the sound emanating from loudspeakers located to the right and the left side of the infant is the desired response. The visual reinforcers are located next to (or on

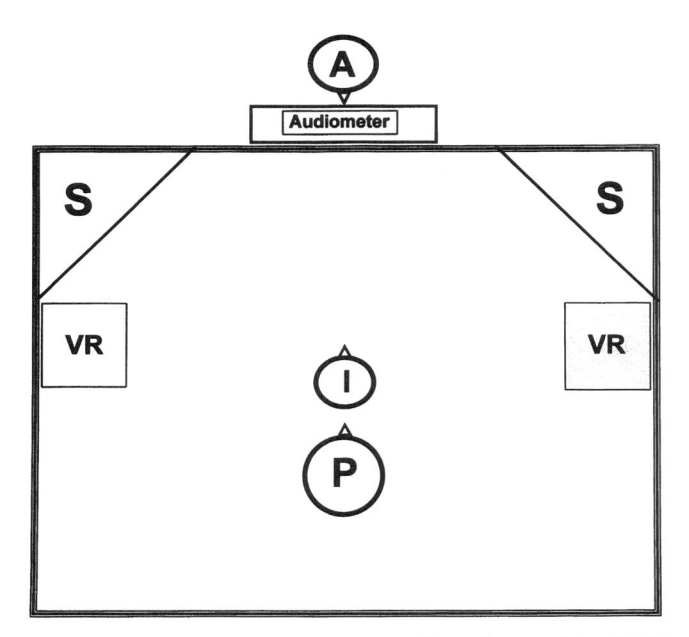

FIG. 4. Test suite arrangement traditionally used for COR audiometry. *S*, loudspeaker; *VR*, visual reinforcer; *A*, audiologist; *P*, parent; *I*, infant.

top of) the soundfield speakers. Figure 4 depicts the COR arrangement. In COR, the infant must first detect the presence of the test signal, and second, turn his or her head in the correct direction in order to be reinforced for the response. While COR provides qualitative information about the baby's ability to localize sound, ear-specific data are usually not available. Thus, while including COR in the test battery may be useful for the assessment of localization ability, it is not the procedure of choice for threshold assessment.

In summary, VRA is the most useful clinical procedure for the behavioral audiometric evaluation of infants and young children aged 5 to approximately 24 mo. When a specified test protocol is followed, babies and toddlers (even those with severe or profound hearing loss) are readily assessed. Moreover, the procedure can distinguish between normal hearing and mild degrees of hearing loss, such as impairments often associated with otitis media with effusion. Through the assessment of air- and bone-conducted thresholds, the type (conductive, sensorineural, or mixed) and degree of hearing loss present may be determined.

Behavioral Assessment of Preschool Children

The audiologic assessment of young preschool-aged children involves test methods that continue to use reinforcement of the behavioral response. While, the motor task (response) is changed to take advantage of maturing motor and cognitive abilities, the use of reinforcement to maintain attention and motivation during audiometry is still important. Young children, beginning at about the age of 24 months, often lose interest in VRA (24). Consequently, a more engaging test procedure is useful for obtaining their thresholds.

The TROCA and VROCA Procedures

Tangible reinforcement operant conditioning audiometry (TROCA), or its variant visual reinforcement operant conditioning audiometry (VROCA), is a useful procedure for the audiometric assessment of young children from about 24 to 36 months of age. TROCA and VROCA require the young child to push a button, or a response bar, each time a stimulus is detected. Reinforcement for a correct response is either tangible (e.g., a piece of cereal or a raisin, dispensed through a specially constructed TROCA test unit), or visual (the illumination of a mechanical toy reinforcer on top of the unit) (8). Clinics often develop a response button arrangement mounted on a plywood board for VROCA. The button can be interfaced with the same computer or visual reinforcers as are used for VRA.

In the classical TROCA arrangement, the manipulandum on the front of the TROCA box is made of clear plexiglas. A light bulb coupled to a dimmer switch allows the audiologist to present an auditory signal and a visual signal simultaneously. The child is taught to push the manipulandum each time the signals are presented. After learning this response, the light cue is faded. If the child hears the auditory stimulus, responding continues and the standard threshold search procedure is initiated. If when the visual cue is eliminated, the child stops responding, the auditory and visual cues are presented again, with the auditory presented at a significantly higher intensity level. Unfortunately, because TROCA and VROCA are useful for a relatively narrow age range of children, the procedures are not in widespread clinical use. However, experience suggests that in the "transition" period between when VRA is no longer useful but play audiometry (discussion follows) is not yet appropriate, the TROCA/VROCA procedures may be very useful.

Conditioned Play Audiometry

Play audiometry is a frequently used procedure for the audiologic assessment of preschool children. The age at which play audiometry is useful begins at about 24 to 30 months of age. However, the variation is quite marked, and some younger children can be tested with the method, while, at times, children who would be considered appropriate candidates for play audiometry cannot be taught the response. In traditional play audiometry, the child learns to respond to a test stimulus by performing a "play" motor task, such as dropping a block in a bucket or stacking a ring. Although the understanding of verbal instructions is not mandatory for successful play audiometry, a certain level of maturity is required.

In most test situations, verbal praise is provided as reinforcement. Changing the play response frequently also serves to maintain the child's attention to the task. However, providing visual reinforcement for correct responding is also very useful in maintaining a child's motivation and attention (3). Thus, the same visual reinforcers that are used in the VRA procedure can easily be used for play audiometry as well. Again, once responses have become contingent (thus, the term *conditioned play audiometry*) on the presentation of the test stimulus, standard threshold search procedures can be instituted.

The test booth arrangement is similar to that described for VRA. A parent or assistant can be used to move the child's arm during a training period of successive approximations of the play response. Gradually, after several trials, the manual or verbal prompts are diminished, until the child is responding to the signal independently.

Behavioral Assessment of School-Aged Children

By the time a child is of kindergarten to elementary school age, he or she is usually ready for conventional audiometry procedures. The same motor responses (a hand raise or button push) as used with adults are appropriate. Verbal praise, a delighted facial expression, or hand clapping can serve as reinforcement of correct responses for younger children. Older children may require only intermittent positive verbal reinforcement. The child is encouraged to listen for low-level signals either verbally or through gestures or manual (sign) communication. The test booth arrangement is similar to that used for adults. Sometimes the child is turned to face one side (away from the observation window of the test booth) so that he or she is less likely to use any visual cues that may be inadvertently provided.

A comprehensive audiologic assessment should be possible to complete in one test session. Assessing air- (250–8,000 Hz) and bone-conducted thresholds (250–4,000 Hz) across the range of frequencies depicted on the conventional audiogram is encouraged. As with audiometry with adults, the child's hearing is assessed for the presence of any hearing loss. When present, the type, degree, and symmetry of the impairment are delineated. Because a 5-dB step size is usually used in audiometry with preschool and school-aged children, variations in thresholds of ±10 dB are considered indicators of a change in hearing status.

Speech Measures

Speech perception measures should assess auditory detection, discrimination, recognition, and comprehension whenever possible (2,25). Speech test procedures are selected to examine these aspects of the auditory continuum in order to monitor the developing functional use of audition for aural/oral communication. With children, monitored live-voice presentations of the test materials are most frequently used. However, some measures require the use of recorded speech materials.

Speech awareness or speech detection thresholds can be obtained for words or individual phonemes ("ah," "ee," "oo," "sh," "s"). A speech detection threshold, however, does not provide details about audiometric configuration, nor does it provide information on how the child is developing functional audition. Thus, as soon as possible, it is important, to assess the speech recognition (identification) abilities of young children. While these measures are commonly referred to as speech discrimination procedures, most traditional materials require more than a same-different determination. Rather, a more complex identification or recognition of the speech material is sought. Standardized clinical tools useful for examining the speech recognition abilities of young children are scarce. Indeed, some procedures that are commonly used with children are developmentally inappropriate because they depend on the size of the child's vocabulary and/or their speech production proficiency (as in a "repeat the word" response task). The simplest speech recognition procedures are limited (closed) sets of words or sentences. For children, the test items are often pictorialized or actual objects are used.

The speech reception threshold requires the child to identify (either by repeating the word or, by pointing to the appropriate picture or object) spondee (two-syllable) words (e.g., baseball, hot dog, ice cream). The threshold level (in dB HL) at which half of the spondee words are identified correctly is determined. Other pediatric speech test procedures that are presented at a fixed suprathreshold intensity examine the young child's ability to recognize speech at comfortable listening levels. Some speech recognition materials are closed-set tests that require a picture-point response. Materials such as the Pediatric Speech Intelligibility (PSI) test (26) and the Northwestern University Children's Perception of Speech (NU-Chips) test (27) are useful for children as young as 36 mo of age. The Word Intelligibility by Picture Identification (WIPI) test (28) can also be used with children of this age range; however, receptive vocabulary level must always be considered in the selection and interpretation of any of these test materials. Other materials commonly used with children, such as the PBK-50 monosyllabic word lists (29) are used with older children because they require the child to repeat the test item heard.

Despite the limitations inherent in many speech materials currently available for use with children, measures of speech recognition should be included in the audiometric evaluation of young children (2). These measures provide an important means of monitoring the development of audition and determining the influence of any loss of hearing or speech understanding. Speech measures, however, should not be used in place of behavioral threshold assessment for determining the degree of hearing loss.

A FINAL COMMENT

This chapter has reviewed the behavioral audiometric assessment procedures that are available for use with infants and children. While the test procedures have been studied and refined, the successful assessment of hearing in young children requires the skills and knowledge of an experienced clinician. Requisite to the practice of audiology with infants and children is academic preparation in normal auditory development and disorders of hearing in childhood, as well as clinical experience in the assessment and management of infants and young children with impaired auditory function. As in the practice of pediatric otology, the unique requirements of the audiologic assessment of infants and children have resulted in the specialization of a group of professionals who consider themselves pediatric audiologists. In addition to the audiologic assessment of the pediatric population, counseling of parents regarding communication and educational options is an important function of these professionals. Parents must be kept apprised of the outcome of each audiologic assessment and understand the implications of the findings for determining the immediate and longer-term communication and educational needs of their child. The selection, evaluation, and long-term monitoring of appropriate amplification for home and classroom use are additional roles that pediatric audiologists fulfill (30). The importance of a strong relationship between pediatric otologists and audiologists cannot be overemphasized.

REFERENCES

1. Jerger J, Hayes D. The cross-check principle in pediatric audiometry. *Arch Otolaryngol* 1976;102:614–20.
2. American Speech-Language-Hearing Association. Guidelines for the audiologic assessment of children from birth through 36 months of age. *ASHA* 1991;33(Suppl 5):37–43.
3. Gravel JS. Audiologic assessment of infants and toddlers. *ASHA* 1992; 21:55–62.
4. Widen JE. Behavioral screening of high-risk infants using visual reinforcement audiometry. *Semin Hear* 1990;11:342–56.
5. Northern JL, Downs MP. *Hearing in children.* 3rd ed. Baltimore: Williams & Wilkins; 1984.
6. Northern JL, Downs MP. *Hearing in children.* 4th ed. Baltimore: Williams & Wilkins; 1991.
7. Gravel JS. Behavioral assessment of auditory function. *Semin Hear* 1989;10:216–28.
8. Wilson WR, Thompson G. Behavioral audiometry. In: Jerger J, ed. *Pediatric audiology* San Diego, CA: College-Hill; 1984:1–44.
9. Nozza RJ, Wilson WR. Masked and unmasked puretone thresholds of infants and adults: development of auditory frequency selectivity and sensitivity. *J Speech Hear Res* 1984;27:613–22.
10. Diefendorf AO. Behavioral evaluation of hearing-impaired children. In: Bess F, ed. *Hearing impairment in children.* Parkton, MD: York; 1988:133–51.
11. Gravel JS. Auditory assessment of infants. *Semin Hear* 1994;15:100–13.
12. Widen JE. Adding objectivity to infant behavioral audiometry. *Ear Hear* 1993;14:49–57.
13. Primus M. Repeated infant thresholds in operant and nonoperant audiometric procedures. *Ear Hear* 1991;12:119–22.
14. Bernstein RS, Gravel JS. A method for determining hearing sensitivity in infants: The interweaving staircase procedure (ISP). *J Am Acad Audiol* 1990;1:138–45.
15. Eilers RE, Widen JE, Urbano R, Hudson T, Gonzalez L. Optimization of automated hearing test algorithms: a comparison of data from simulations and young children. *Ear Hear* 1991;12:199–204.
16. Eilers RE, Ozdamar O, Steffins ML. Classification of audiograms by sequential testing: reliability and validity of an automated behavioral hearing screening algorithm. *J Am Acad Audiol* 1993;4:172–81.
17. Stapells DR, Gravel JS, Martin B. Thresholds for auditory brain stem responses to tones in notched noise from infants and young children with normal hearing or sensorineural hearing loss. *Ear Hear* 1995;16:361–71.
18. Tharpe AM, Ashmeade DH. Computer simulation technique for assessing pediatric auditory test protocols. *J Am Acad Audiol* 1993;4:80–90.
19. Thompson G, Folsom RC. A comparison of two conditioning procedures in the use of visual reinforcement audiometry (VRA). *J Speech Hear Disord* 1984;49:241–45.
20. Levitt H. Adaptive testing in audiology. In: Ludvigsen C, and Barford J, eds. Sensorineural hearing impairment and hearing aids. *Scand Audiol* 1978(Suppl 6):241–91.
21. Gravel JS, Trequina D. Experience with audiologic assessment of infants and toddlers. *Int J Pediatr Otorhinolaryngol* 1992;23:59–71.
22. Primus M. The role of localization in visual reinforcement audiometry. *J Speech Hear Res* 1992;35:1137–41.
23. Ozdamar O, Eilers R, Miskiel E, Widen J. Classification of audiograms by sequential testing using a dynamic Bayesian procedure. *J Acoust Soc Am* 1990;88:2171–2179.
24. Thompson M, Thompson G, McCall A. Strategies for increasing response behavior of 1- and 2-year-old children during visual reinforcement audiometry (VRA), *Ear Hear* 1992;13:236–40.
25. Erber NP. *Auditory training.* Washington, DC: AG Bell; 1982:29–71.
26. Jerger S, Jerger J. *Pediatric speech intelligibility test.* St. Louis: Auditec; 1984.
27. Elliot L, Katz D. *Development of a new children's test of speech discrimination.* St. Louis: Auditec; 1980.
28. Ross M, Lerman J. A picture identification test for hearing-impaired children. *J Speech Hear Res* 1970;13:44–53.
29. Haskins H. *A phonetically balanced test of speech discrimination for children* [Master's thesis]. Northwestern University, Evanston, 949.
30. Chase P, Gravel J. Hearing aids for children. In: Goldenberg R, ed. *Hearing aids: a manual for clinicians.* Philadelphia: Lippincott-Raven. 1996;215–23.

CHAPTER 8

Acoustic Immittance

Tympanometry and Acoustic Reflexes

Alison M. Grimes

The measurement of acoustic immittance, an objective assessment of the tympanic membrane, middle ear, cochlea, cranial nerves VII and VIII, and the auditory centers in the lower brainstem, is an integral part of the evaluation of auditory function in children. Because this test battery, comprising tympanometry and the measurement of the acoustic reflex, is neither a behavioral nor a strictly electrophysiologic assessment, it merits separate consideration. Although no voluntary behavioral response is required of the child to complete tympanometry and acoustic reflex measurements (simply that the child sit relatively quietly for a short period of time), there is also nothing electrophysiologic in the test battery in the sense that there is no direct measure of electrical auditory potentials as in the measurement of electrocochleography, the auditory brainstem response (ABR), or cortical evoked potentials. Acoustic immittance is best described as an objective measure of the anatomy and physiology of many of the peripheral auditory structures.

Considered a standard part of the diagnostic audiologic evaluation since at least the mid-1970s, acoustic immittance measures are quick to obtain, reliable, valid, and yield enormous information for a small investment in time and effort. The test battery provides an objective assessment of the status and physiology of the peripheral and the retrocochlear auditory system. It is important to keep in mind, however, that acoustic immittance measures do not test hearing per se. Perception and understanding of acoustic stimuli are not necessary and cannot be inferred from normal acoustic immittance test results. A deaf child can have a completely normal tympanogram; a child with a small perforation of the eardrum may have little loss in hearing sensitivity, yet a distinctly abnormal tympanogram. A patient with significant stapedial fixation and conductive hearing loss can have a normal tympanogram. Acoustic reflexes will be absent in all three of these patients, however, for completely different reasons.

The terminology used to describe the immittance test battery has evolved over time as equipment and test protocol have changed. Acoustic *immittance* is the term preferred to *impedance,* the term that was initially used in describing this test procedure. Immittance encompasses both impedance (resistance and reactance) and admittance (conductance and susceptance), which are reciprocal values. Although early equipment measured only impedance, today many devices measure admittance. Its components, conductance and susceptance, are also frequently assessed in advanced diagnostics and in research. With the adoption of the American National Standard Institute (ANSI) standard for aural-impedance/admittance instruments (1), the terminology used to refer to immittance measures was standardized, along with the procedures for calibration, instrument specifications, and the format of the tympanogram.

The acoustic immittance test results are most valuable and yield the greatest diagnostic strength when interpreted side by side with a complete behavioral audiogram. In this fashion, many ambiguities that may arise when immittance measures are examined in isolation are clarified. A conductive hearing loss can be confirmed, and its nature determined, through examination of the tympanogram, and the acoustic reflex pattern. Conversely, the reason for elevated or absent acoustic reflexes is often made clear when the behavioral audiogram is available for comparison and confirmation. Although a tympanogram may be abnormal, it is not possible to infer the degree of hearing loss accompanying the abnormal tympanogram. One may choose to treat an ear with an abnormal tympanogram and a 45-dB hearing loss very differently

---

A.M. Grimes: Director of Audiology, Providence Speech and Hearing Center, Orange, California 92868.

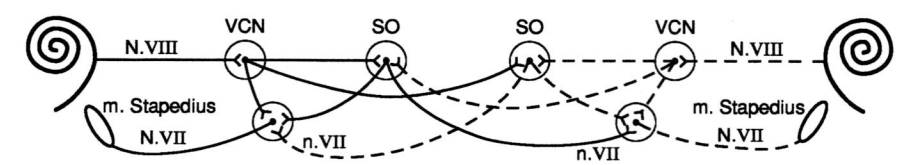

FIG. 1. Acoustic reflex arc. Ipsilateral (____): first order neuron, eighth nerve from the hair cells the ventral cochlear nuclei; second order neuron, to the ipsilateral facial-nerve nuclei (or first to the ipsilateral superior olivary complex then to the ipsilateral facial-nerve nuclei); third order neuron, to the ipsilateral stapedius muscle. Contralateral (_____): first order neuron, eighth cranial nerve from the hair cells to the ventral cochlear nuclei; second order neuron, to the ipsilateral and to the contralateral superior olivary complex; third order neuron, to the contralateral facial nerve nuclei; fourth order neuron, to the contralateral stapedius muscle (27).

from an ear with an abnormal tympanogram and a 15-B hearing loss.

Acoustic immittance measures are sensitive to abnormalities in the structure and function of the tympanic membrane (TM), the middle-ear space, the ossicles, the eustachian tube, and the function of the middle-ear muscles (tensor tympani and, primarily, the stapedius muscles) in response to either auditory or tactile stimulation. In addition, these measures yield information about the function of the cranial nerves VII and VIII, and the auditory pathway in the lower brainstem (Fig. 1). Finally, indirect and somewhat imprecise information about the cochlear perception of loudness can be inferred from the acoustic reflex thresholds.

Interpretation of the acoustic immittance battery aids in the differential diagnosis of conductive or cochlear hearing loss and distinguishes among conductive pathologies (e.g., middle-ear effusion [MEE] vs. ossicular fixation vs. ossicular discontinuity). In addition, immittance tests can assesses the patency of transtympanic tubes, and can identify the presence of TM perforations. Immittance helps differentiate cochlear from neural pathology and can indicate the presence of pseudohyperacusis. Facial nerve function can be assessed through the use of either auditory or tactile stimulation. The function of the eustachian tube can be inferred from middle-ear pressure, and the ability of the eustachian tube to open in response to pressure change or swallow can be rapidly ascertained. Finally, the acoustic reflex can be used to predict the degree of hearing loss in children. Before ABR and otoacoustic emissions (OAE) assessments came into widespread use as objective measures of hearing sensitivity, the acoustic reflex was one of the only objective measures of peripheral hearing sensitivity clinically available.

In children, one of the primary values of tympanometry and acoustic reflex measurements is the assessment of middle-ear function. Middle-ear effusion is one of the most common health impairments in children. Its diagnosis can be made more reliably and efficiently through the assessment of acoustic immittance. This objective test battery, which may take less than 30 seconds per ear to administer to a cooperative child, is highly reliable and is both sensitive and specific in the diagnosis of MEE when the test protocol and interpretation are carefully controlled.

Each measure, tympanometry and acoustic reflex assessment, has a specific underlying physical basis, test procedure, and interpretation. By using appropriate protocols for testing and applicable normative data and by examining specific aspects of both the tympanogram and the reflex, confirmation of conductive hearing loss, otoscopic impressions, and behavioral signs and symptoms can be realized. The combination of tympanometry and acoustic reflex data strengthens the findings of either alone; an absent acoustic reflex is highly significant in the presence of a normal tympanogram, yet is the predicted finding when the tympanogram is abnormal. On the other hand, a finding of present acoustic reflex when the tympanogram is clearly abnormal is most indicative of artifact or equipment malfunction.

TYMPANOMETRY

A tympanogram is a physical measurement of the movement of the eardrum and middle-ear system. Simply stated, the tympanogram is a pressure-compliance function, a description of the movement of the eardrum as varying degrees of air pressure are applied against it. The tympanogram is shown as a graph with air (middle ear) pressure, expressed in dekaPascals (daPa) on the abscissa and admittance, expressed in millimhos (mmho) on the ordinate (Fig. 2). The

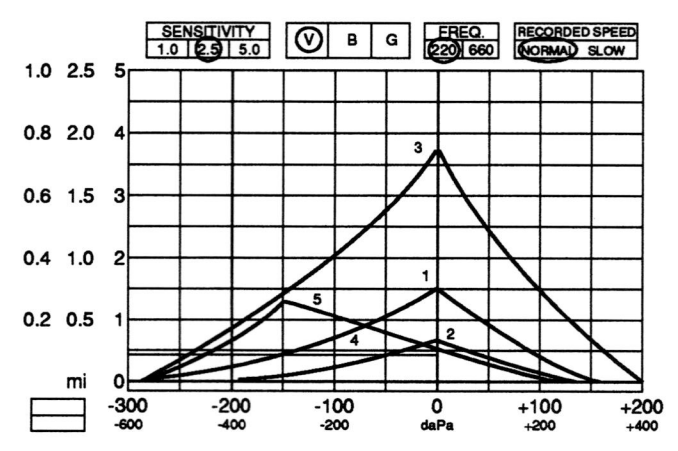

FIG. 2. Normal tympanogram showing ordinate and abscissa.

height (ordinate), the point of peak pressure (abscissa), and the overall shape of the tympanogram are examined for interpretation. Early immittance meters measured acoustic impedance, but it is more common today that acoustic admittance (or its components, susceptance and conductance) is the metric. Normative data are typically expressed in terms of static acoustic admittance (SAA) (the amount of sound energy admitted through the tympanic membrane into the middle-ear system), equivalent volume (expressed in mmho or cm^3), and tympanometric width (TW) or gradient, expressed in daPa.

The procedure for obtaining a tympanogram is relatively simple. An ear-canal probe equipped with an appropriately sized rubber tip is secured into the outer portion of the ear canal. This typically involves pulling the pinna up and back to straighten the canal and using a gentle screwing motion to insert the probe tip fully. For a tympanogram to be obtained the probe tip must be completely sealed in the canal so that air pressure can be successfully built up between the end of the probe tip and the TM (hermetically sealed).

The probe assembly typically has three or four components:

1. Pneumatic system (air pump) to vary the air pressure in the ear canal, monitored by a manometer. Air pressure can typically be varied from $+400$ to -600 daPa.
2. Probe-tone system, which is a driver or small loudspeaker located in the probe box used to send the probe tone into the probe tip. The probe tone is a sinusoid, typically of low frequency (220–226 Hz), although higher frequencies are often used.
3. Monitoring microphone, which is located in the probe box and monitors the intensity of the probe tone as it changes with changes in immittance (as air pressure is varied) at the TM.
4. Stimulus generator or acoustic reflex activator system for assessment of ipsilateral acoustic reflexes. A second stimulus generator is located in an earphone placed on or in the contralateral ear for contralateral acoustic reflex recordings. Some simple tympanometers do not allow measurement of the acoustic reflex.

After securing the probe tip in the child's ear canal, air pressure (either positive or negative, typically $+200$ daPa) is introduced into the canal to exert pressure on the tympanic membrane. The positive pressure is reduced, passing through zero (ambient pressure) and extending down to a negative pressure, typically -400 daPa. The intensity change with air pressure change is continuously recorded. The change in intensity is a result of the stiffening of the TM, with a stiffer TM reflecting a greater percentage of acoustic energy from the probe tone back to the probe microphone. The resultant curve, the pressure-compliance function, depicts the point (daPa) and degree (mmho) of maximum compliance of the tympanic membrane.

Tympanograms are generally described by shape (TW or gradient), height, equivalent ear-canal volume Vec, and positive, normal or negative tympanometric peak pressure (TPP).

When the conventional low-frequency probe tone is used, typical tympanogram configurations include:

normal: TPP at approximately 0 daPa, although it may be as low as -100 daPa or may be slightly positive; SAA not less than 0.5 cm^3 in children

normal/shallow: TPP as above, with reduced SAA (this pattern is seen as a normal variant, but may also indicative of ossicular fixation when conductive hearing loss is present)

normal/deep: TPP as above, with higher than normal SAA (this pattern is seen as a normal variant, but also may be seen in ears with healed TM perforations or, when conductive hearing loss is present, in ears with ossicular discontinuity). It has been noted (2) that when the TM is extremely thin or scarred, tympanometry as a diagnostic tool is seriously impaired.

flat: minimal or no compliance peak, very low SAA, TW greater than 150 daPa in children (this is consistent with MEE and is also seen in ears with nonpatent transtympanic tubes)

negative pressure: normal SAA with negative TPP (-100 to -200 daPa or greater) (considered indicative of retracted TM or eustachian tube dysfunction)

non-intact tympanic membrane: (no peak compliance, abnormally wide gradient, high Vec (this is seen in ears with patent transtympanic tubes or with TM perforations)

notched or double-peaked: more typically seen when higher-frequency probe tones are used

In older nomenclature (3), normal tympanograms were called Type A (shallow indicated by As and deep by Ad), flat tympanograms Type B, and negative Type C. Subsequent to the adoption of a standard for immittance meters (1), these terms have been replaced by more objective descriptions that use actual values of pressure (daPa), admittance (mmho), Vec (cm^3) and gradient (daPa). This allows for a more careful determinations of normalcy, and facilitates comparisons among different immittance meters. It also aids in documenting the progression or resolution of MEE over a period of time.

In general, test–retest reliability of tympanometry is high. Certain characteristics of the tympanogram are known to be more reliable and therefore more indicative of the status of the TM and middle ear than others. The SAA was found to have the highest reliability and TPP the lowest in a group of young adults studied by Wiley and Barrett (4).

Tympanometry is increasingly being used as a technique to screen hearing and middle-ear function in preschool and school-age children. A primary reason for the use of screening tympanometry is that screening low-frequency hearing sensitivity (e.g., 500 Hz) to identify MEE is often not possible due to the high ambient noise environment present in screening sites. Due to high noise, the 500-Hz stimulus may have to be presented at 25 to 30 dB hearing level (HL) or higher, which can easily result in failing to identify significant low-frequency conductive hearing loss. Indeed, it is well known that pure-tone screening alone is largely ineffective in identifying children with MEE (5). When tympanometry is used as a screening technique (e.g., in mass hearing screenings in school settings), a chronic problem has been overreferral. A single tympanogram, particularly if slight deviations from normal are used as referral criteria, may not be a reliable indicator of the chronic status of the ear. Silman, Silverman, and Arick (6) investigated the efficacy of pure-tone assessment in detecting MEE and found that current screening guidelines of the American Speech-Language-Hearing Association (ASHA) (7) (which do not call for 500-Hz screening), fail to identify a significant number of these children. In this study, acoustic immittance screening was not performed, however, MEE was confirmed through the use of pneumotoscopy or microscopy. The inclusion of 500 Hz as a screening frequency was advised.

Current guidelines (7) for the use of tympanometry as a screening tool call for the examination of three characteristics of the tympanogram to determine normalcy:

1. Static acoustic admittance ("peak height" of the tympanogram): a measure of the height of the tympanogram relative to the tail value (Fig. 3) expressed in mmho or cm^3 and formerly referred to as static compliance (8). Only low SAA relative to the normative data is cause for referral, because high SAA without conductive hearing loss may be seen in minor eardrum abnormalities not associated with active ear disease. Interim normative data (Table 1) for children presented in the ASHA guidelines are a mean of 0.5 mmho or cm^3; with a 90% range of 0.2 to 0.9 mmho or cm^3.

The measurement of SAA is obtained by subtracting the SAA value obtained with the TM "clamped" by positive ($+200$) or negative (-400) pressure from the TPP value (9). This subtraction is performed automatically in contemporary immittance meters, although formerly it was necessary to generate each of the two values separately by introducing the appropriate pressure and then subtracting one value from another.

2. Equivalent ear canal volume (in cm^3): an estimate of the enclosed volume of air between the probe tip and the tympanic membrane. It is measured by introducing significant positive ($+200$ daPa) or negative (-400 daPa) air pressure into the ear canal and measuring the admittance. In the presence of a TM perforation or a patent transtympanic tube, Vec represents the volume of air both in front of and behind the TM, and the measurement is therefore substantially larger than normal. A flat tympanogram in the presence of Vec exceeding the 90% normal range (mean, 0.7 cm^3; 90% range, 0.4–1.0 cm^3) is indicative of TM perforation. The Vec value was shown to increase with increasing age in a

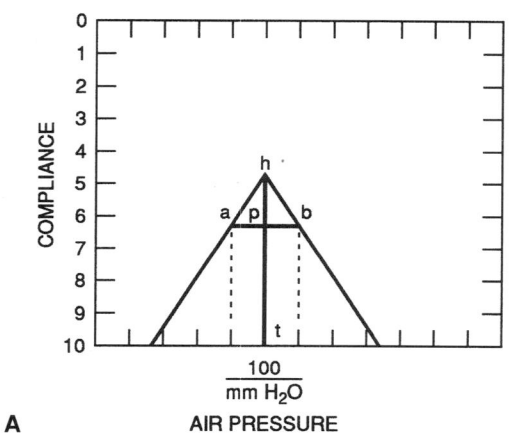

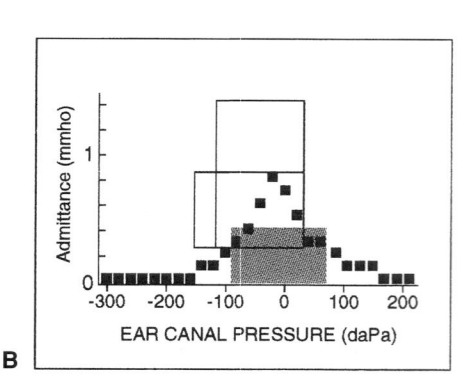

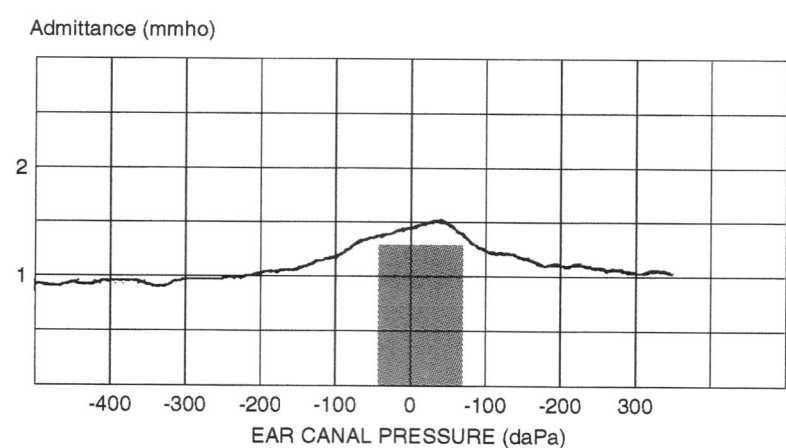

FIG. 3. Two methods for calculating gradient.

TABLE 1. ASHA preliminary normative data

	Peak Y (mmho or cm^3)		V$_{ec}$ (cm^3)		TW (daPA)	
	Mean	90% range	Mean	90% range	Mean	90% range
Children	0.5	0.2–0.9	0.7	0.4–1.0	100	60–150
Adults	0.8	0.3–1.4	1.1	0.6–1.5	80	50–110

Suggested interim norms (means and 90% ranges) for static admittance (Peak Y), equivalent ear-canal volume (V$_{ec}$), and tympanometric width (TW). The values were extracted from Margolis and Heller (1987) who employed an acoustic immittance screening instrument (226-Hz probe tone; pump speed −200 daPa/s) that automatically compensated for ear-canal volume by subtracting the admittance at 200 daPa from all values. Normative values for children were obtained from preschool-aged children (3–5 years).
American Speech-Language-Hearing Association Guidelines for Screening for Hearing Impairments and Middle Ear Disorders. ASHA 32(Suppl 2):17–24.

large group of school-age children ages 7 to 13. The younger group showed a median Vec of 0.65 cc, older children a median Vec of 1.0 (10).

3. Tympanometric width (gradient): a description of the shape of the tympanogram in the vicinity of the peak. Gradient is a quantitative expression of the "flatness" or "peakness" of the tympanogram. It is measured either by the pressure interval corresponding to a 50% reduction in peak SAA or by the ratio of the peak to the points of intersection on the tails of the tympanogram corresponding to a width of 100 daPa or TW expressed in daPa to the total height of the tympanogram (see Fig. 3). Tympanometric gradient is expressed in daPa in either method. An abnormally small gradient (flat tympanogram) or an abnormally wide TW appears to be a good indicator of MEE. Only wider than normal values constitute a referral, because a narrow gradient is not indicative of active ear disease. In the ASHA document, preliminary normative data for TW for children are mean of 100 daPa and a 90% range of 60 to 150 daPa.

On the basis of these three criteria, decisions are made about whether the child passes screening, should be rescreened at a 4 to 6 week interval, or should be referred for medical evaluation immediately (Fig. 4). Abnormalities in SAA, gradient, or both are rescreened after a 4 to 6 week period. Only after two successive abnormal findings during this interval should medical referral be made. On the other hand, an abnormally large Vec is cause for immediate referral, because this finding is indicative of TM perforation.

Use of TW was found to have the highest sensitivity and specificity values of any single acoustic admittance measure in a group of 171 children, ages 1 to 12 years (11). The authors note, however, that although the screening criteria presented in the ASHA document are appropriate in the general population, there is a high false-positive rate in a sample of children with chronic or recurrent MEE. In ears with a history of chronic MEE, therefore, normative data based on ears without chronic MEE may not be applicable and may lead to high rates of false positives and thus have poor positive predictive value. It is important that the normative data be based on a subject group that is similar, including history of MEE, to the sample being assessed.

One other aspect of the tympanogram, which is descriptively useful but was not specified in the ASHA screening document, is TPP, an indicator of retraction (or bulging) of the TM. Long believed to be an indicator of eustachian tube dysfunction, TPP is an indirect measure of the air pressure in the middle ear because it gives the point at which the air pressure on either side of the TM is equal. The pressure behind the TM must be inferred from TPP. In a normal tympanogram, the point of maximal compliance (middle-ear pressure) is observed at approximately the same pressure as the ambient air pressure. The reliability of the measure and the correlation of negative TPP with MEE, however, is not strong (12). Further, Silman and Silverman (9) caution that, particularly in children, the presence of negative TPP cannot be assumed to signify negative middle-ear pressure; its presence should therefore be evaluated with caution in children. The use of TPP was not recommended by the ASHA committee as a screening procedure. In clinical test administration and interpretation, TPP is often viewed as one of several diagnostically significant features of the tympanogram. When TPP is greater (more negative) than −100 to −150 daPa, particularly when it is accompanied by low SAA, absent acoustic reflexes, conductive hearing losses, or both, the finding is viewed by many as cause for referral. Agreement regarding the exact degree of negative middle-ear pressure that is considered abnormal is not unanimous. While normal middle ear pressure in adults is considered to be +50 to −50 daPa, if, for instance, −100 daPa is considered abnormal and grounds for referral, the false-positive rate may be unacceptably high. One important variable in examining TPP is the direction of air-pressure change (positive–negative or negative–positive) used in obtaining the tympanogram. Hall and Chandler (13) studied 182 patients and compared the effects of air-pressure-direction change on tympanogram interpretation. In 13% of ears, altering the direction of air-pressure change altered the classification of tympanograms based on the Jerger system(3).

The ASHA screening guidelines present preliminary normative data for tympanometric gradient, SAA and Vec (see Table 1). Nozza, Bluestone, and Karadatzke (14) found that these criteria appeared to be appropriate when examining an

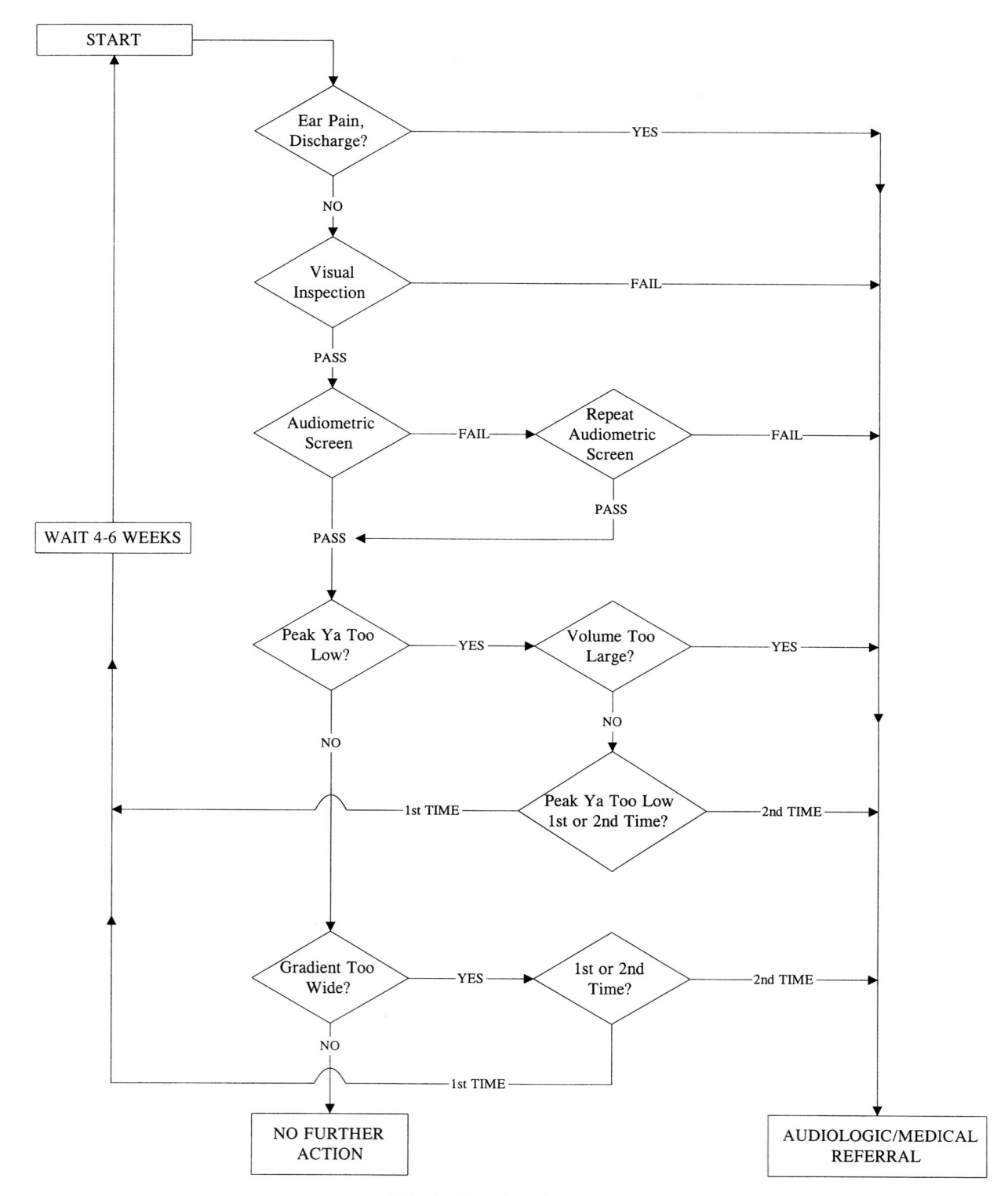

FIG. 4. Flowchart for referral.

unselected group of children (i.e., without regard to their history of MEE). A slightly different mean and 90% range for both SAA and Vec was reported by Hanks and Rose (15). In measuring tympanometric SAA values in 158 children ages 6 to 15, these authors found a mean value of 1.0 cm^3 and 90% range of 0.6 to 1.5 cm^3. The mean SAA value in this group of children was 0.7 mmho, with a 90% range of 0.3 to 1.5 mmho, as compared with the upper admittance value of 0.9 mmho reported as preliminary normative data in the ASHA screening guidelines.

In a study of 171 children ages 1 to 12 (mean age, 4 yr), 249 ears were examined via otoscopy, acoustic immittance measures and surgically (14). The SAA, gradient, and TW were found to be superior to measures of TPP and acoustic reflexes for distinguishing between ears with and without MEE in the subgroup of children with chronic or recurrent MEE.

Some screening test protocols call for the use of the acoustic reflex in addition to tympanometry, presumably to increase detection of middle ear abnormality. Because the reflex can be elevated or absent for a number of reasons other than abnormal middle-ear function, acoustic reflex assessment, is not included in ASHA's screening protocol. Acoustic reflexes can be elevated or absent due to conductive pathology (in either the stimulated or recorded ear), cochlear hearing loss of greater than a mild to moderate degree, neural pathology of cranial nerve VII (recorded ear) or VIII (stimulated ear), or brainstem lesions. Thus, accurate interpretation of the acoustic reflex can take place only in the presence of a complete, bilateral audiogram (including appropriately masked bone-conduction thresholds) and bilateral tympanograms.

Silman, Silverman, and Arick (16) stated that mass acoustic immittance screening with any single acoustic immittance measure to detect MEE may be associated with an unacceptably high false-positive rate. These authors stated that use of the ASHA guidelines results in unacceptably high false-positive rates and low true-positive (''hit'') rates. It was proposed that the best acoustic immittance screening protocol would be based on a combined assessment of TW, SAA, and TPP, assessment of the ipsilateral acoustic reflex at 110 dB HL, and pure-tone screening.

Eustachian Tube Function

Another tympanometric measure which is often useful in pediatric as well as adult diagnosis is the assessment of eustachian tube function. This can be accomplished either in the presence of a TM perforation or when the TM is intact. Although eustachian tube function can be inferred from the TPP, the dynamic ability of the eustachian tube to open as a result of air pressure changes or swallow can be an important diagnostic and prognostic indicator. To assess eustachian tube function when the TM is perforated, positive air pressure is introduced into the ear canal (middle ear) to determine whether the eustachian tube can be forced open. A sudden change (decrease) in air pressure occurs when the tube spontaneously opens. The patient can also be requested to swallow or perform a Toynbee or Valsalva maneuver to see whether air pressure at the probe changes in response to such manipulations. A series of tympanograms can be recorded behind an intact eardrum as the patient swallows or performs the Toynbee or Valsalva maneuver, and changes in peak pressure can be recorded as serial attempts are made to alter middle-ear pressure. A significant change in middle-ear pressure indicates that the eustachian tube has been successfully opened.

Transtympanic Tube Patency

Another useful application of tympanometry is the assessment of the patency of transtympanic tubes. When a transtympanic tube is open, large Vec, relative either to the contralateral ear or to established normative data, is observed because the Vec value reflects both the volume of the ear canal and the middle-ear space. To assess tube patency, positive air pressure of +200 daPa is introduced into the canal. In the case of an intact TM, this value reflects Vec only; however, when the TM is perforated or in the presence of a patent transtympanic tube, the Vec measurement also takes into account the entire middle-ear space. Shanks et al. (17) suggested that a criterion value equal to or greater than 1.0 cm^3 as an indicator of a TM perforation is appropriate for children ages 0 to 7. When preoperative and postoperative comparisons can be made, a difference equal or greater than 0.4 cm^3 suggests a patent transtympanic tube.

Multifrequency Tympanometry

Generating tympanograms with a variety of probe-tone frequencies is increasingly being utilized to describe the dynamic characteristics of the middle-ear system more completely. Traditionally, tympanometry has been accomplished by using a single probe-tone frequency of 220 or 226 Hz. Tympanograms measured in this fashion are invariably single-peaked, leading to simple classification and interpretation. When a higher-frequency probe tone is utilized, multiple peaks (''notching'') are observed in both normal and pathologic ears. It is well known that tympanograms recorded with higher-frequency probe tones (e.g., 660–678 Hz) allow determination of the resonance frequency of the middle ear (that point at which the contributions of mass and stiffness elements of the middle ear are equal). The primary advantage of multifrequency tympanometry is to assess middle-ear resonance, and by so doing, distinguish among different types of middle-ear pathologies.

Increasingly, contemporary acoustic immittance measurement devices allow sweep frequency tympanometry up to 2,000 Hz to determine middle-ear resonance. For example, if stiffness is increased (e.g., otosclerosis), the resonant frequency is shifted to a higher than normal frequency. Conversely, if a mass pathology (e.g., ossicular discontinuity) is present, the resonant frequency is decreased (18). Tympanograms obtained with higher-frequency probe tones often have notching or double peaks, and as equipment and software allowing multiple probe tones have become more commonly used, it has been observed that many normal ears display such notching. A disadvantage to using a high-frequency probe tone for standard tympanometric assessment, however, is that normal ears typically display notching, or an undulating tympanometric pattern, thus rendering interpretation of gradient, admittance, or pressure more difficult.

To examine the possibility that deaf children have different middle-ear resonance than that of normal-hearing children (e.g., that deaf children might have a higher incidence of ossicular pathology that could not be measured with traditional audiometric tests), multifrequency tympanometry was compared between 90 children with normal hearing and 68 deaf children (15). No significant difference between groups was observed, leading these authors to conclude that tympanometric measures can be successfully used with deaf children to examine middle-ear abnormalities.

Special Considerations for Infants

Developmental changes in both tympanometric characteristics and acoustic reflex thresholds are well known. Younger children have tympanometric forms that vary markedly from those in older children, probably as a result of differences in Vec, ear-canal composition, middle-ear resonance, and vibration. It has been observed that neonates with MEE often show normal tympanometric patterns. In infants, use of a probe tone at a frequency above 220 Hz (e.g., 660–668 Hz or 800 Hz), may prove more sensitive to the detection of MEE than use of lower-frequency probe tones. Even at 220 Hz, tympanograms in infant ears may be double peaked, unlike tympanograms of older children and adults. This factor makes it difficult to interpret infant tympanograms by use of conventional measures. For this reason, the routine use of tympanometry in young infants is not common clinical practice, although when children are 2 to 4 months old, tympanograms assume a single-peaked shape (19).

In infants, tympanometry using the conventional 220-Hz pure tone may appear abnormal. Conversely, what appears to be a normal tympanogram may be recorded from an abnormal ear when one uses a 220-Hz probe tone in young children. The use of a 660-Hz probe tone, separating susceptance and conductance elements of the tympanogram, has been shown in some studies to yield more usable information in children under the age of 6 months. There is not uniform agreement on this point, however. For example, Holte, Margolis, and Cavanaugh (20) evaluated the maturational course of tympanometric shape and admittance in young infants over a 4-month period. These authors found that tympanograms recorded with the 220 Hz probe tone was preferable to a higher-frequency probe tone for two reasons: (a) there was less individual maturational difference present, and (b) the tympanograms were easier to interpret.

Tympanometry using a 226-Hz probe tone is least affected by normal developmental changes in normal infants. However, it has been noted that this is not the case with pathologic ears (L. Holte, personal communication). For this reason, it is not believed that use of the higher-frequency probe tone is preferable in infants. Marchant et al. (21) examined infants age 5 months and younger with susceptance tympanograms with a 660-Hz probe tone. These authors found that this measure, coupled with ipsilateral acoustic reflexes, was very efficient in separating ears with MEE from normal ears in this young population.

Using video otoscopy and multifrequency tympanometry, Holte, Margolis, and Cavanaugh (20) examined 23 young infants. Among other findings, it was noted that use of negative-to-positive pressure change frequently resulted in ear-canal collapse and consequently uninterpretable tympanograms. It was therefore recommended that positive-to-negative pressure change be used with this population. It was further concluded that with increasing age in infancy, the contribution of acoustic admittance increased, indicating a growing contribution of compliant elements in the first 4 months of life, although considerable variability was found to exist among the infants tested.

Roush et al. (22) noted significant age effects in SAA and TW in a population of 88 children ages 6 to 30 months. The SAA was found to be significantly lower, and the TW significantly greater in younger children. It is clear from these studies and others that the use of normative data that differentiate very young children from other groups leads to better sensitivity and specificity.

Several factors other than pathology can influence the shape and amplitude of the tympanogram. The SAA was shown to be significantly increased on test–retest in a group of 116 children (mean age, 7.2 yr). No significant changes in TW, TPP, or estimates of Vec were noted (23). Direction of pressure change (positive to negative vs negative to positive) affects the measured SAA, with greater admittance seen in tympanograms recorded in the negative-to-positive direction (24). Rate of ear-canal pressure change can result in changes in measured immittance either as a result of measurement artifact or as a result of the nonlinear behavior of the middle ear (25). As the rate of ear-canal pressure change increases, the difference in peak pressure for the two directions of pressure change increases. The use of a higher-frequency probe tone results in notched (double-peaked) tympanograms in both normal and pathological ears, whereas notched tympanograms are rare when one uses a low-frequency probe tone.

In summary, assessment of tympanometry in children as young as 2 to 4 months can yield important objective information about the status of the TM and middle-ear space. When appropriate test protocol (choice of probe-tone frequency, pump direction, and pump speed) and normative data are employed, diagnosis of a number of pathologic conditions can reliably be made.

ACOUSTIC REFLEX

The acoustic reflex is an involuntary contraction in response to intense sound or to tactile stimulation of the muscles of the middle ear, the tensor tympani, and, primarily, the stapedius muscle. In humans, the contraction in response to auditory stimulation is believed to be of the stapedius muscle only (26). The contraction is bilateral and simultaneous; the reflex can be elicited by stimulating one ear and measuring the change in immittance in the contralateral ear. It is most typically elicited by pure tone stimuli of 500, 1,000, or 2,000 Hz, although in some applications, narrowband and broadband noise may also be used. The stapedius muscle, which is innervated by cranial nerve VII, attaches to the posterior side of the stapes. The contraction of the acoustic reflex, resulting in a stiffening of the ossicular chain, causes an increase in impedance at the TM (inferred by an increased in sound pressure reflected off the TM back to the probe assembly) which is time locked to the presentation of the acoustic stimulus.

The auditory centers responsible for the acoustic reflex are the ventral cochlear nucleus, the trapezoid body and the medial superior olive. There is both an ipsilateral and a contralateral reflex arc (see Fig. 1) (27).

Persons with normal hearing sensitivity and cochlear hearing loss to approximately 50 dB HL show acoustic reflex thresholds in the 70 to 100 dB HL range. With this degree of hearing loss, acoustic reflex thresholds occur at the same intensity level. As hearing loss increases, the acoustic reflex threshold increases up to 100 to 115 dB HL (Fig. 5), and with more severe loss, the reflex is absent (28). The proportion of acoustic reflex absence is dependent on the degree of hearing loss, activator frequency, and equipment limitations. Silman and Gelfand (1981) concluded that acoustic reflexes are rarely absent for cochlear impairments less than 80 dB HL.

As the contraction of the stapedius muscle in the acoustic reflex causes a only small decrease in mobility of the TM, measurement of the reflex is obtained when the TM is in its most mobile position, that is, at the point of maximal compliance (TPP). Maximal compliance of the TM occurs when the air pressure on the lateral aspect of the TM (in the ear canal) is approximately equal to the air pressure on the medial aspect of the TM (in the middle ear). For example, if the tympanogram showed TPP of −150 daPa, acoustic reflex measurements would be conducted with air pressure introduced into the ear canal equal to −150 daPa. An exception to this procedure is in the case of a very flaccid TM in which the resting immittance shows erratic or fluctuating values. This can be observed in hypermobile TMs. In such a case, it is often helpful to introduce very mild positive or negative pressure relative to the TPP (+/− 50 daPa) to slightly "tighten" the TM, thus making the time-locked change in immittance easier to observe.

Measurement of the acoustic reflex is accomplished by introducing a stimulus, either through the probe assembly (ipsilateral, the reflex is measured in the same ear to which the stimulus is presented) or through an earphone on the opposite ear (contralateral, in which the reflex is elicited by stimulation of the ear opposite the probe). The term contralateral acoustic reflex is used somewhat ambiguously in some centers; that is, the ear stimulated is the ear referenced (e.g., "right contralateral reflexes" refers to the situation in which the earphone was in the right ear, the probe in the left ear, and the activator was presented to the right ear). Either visual observation of needle deflection or, preferably, generating a graphic display of the change in immittance following the stimulus, is used to determine the presence of the reflex. The reflex appears as a significant, time-locked response (increase in impedance) that grows in amplitude and shortens in onset time as intensity is increased.

A number of aspects of the acoustic reflex have been stud-

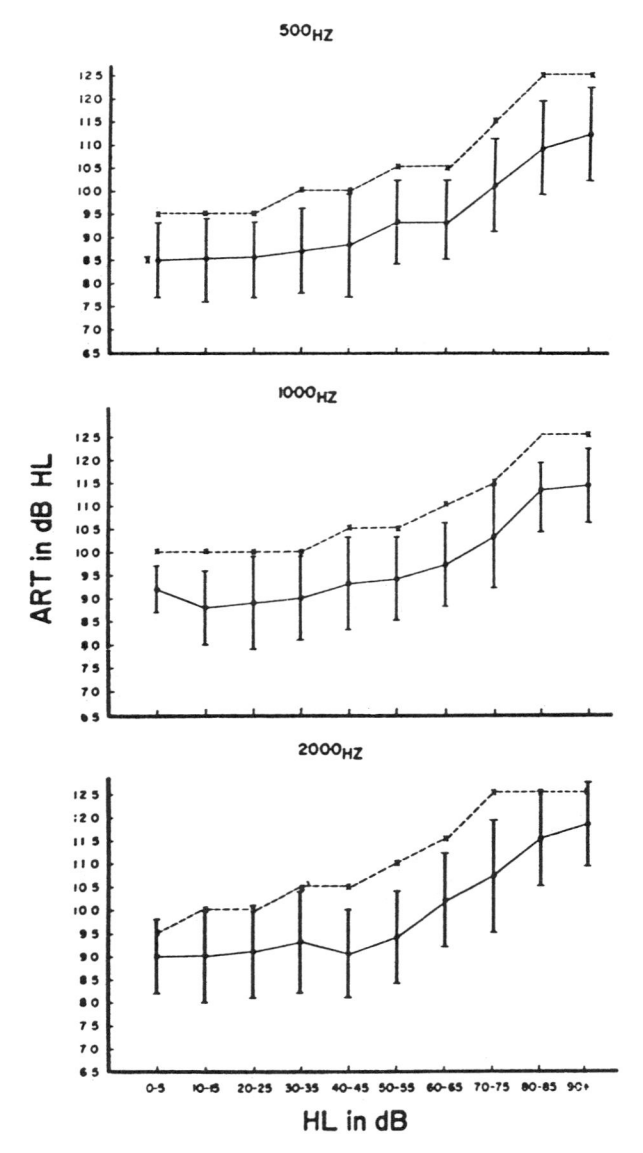

FIG. 5. Silman chart of acoustic reflex threshold by hearing loss.

ied: effect of activating stimulus (frequency, bandwidth), latency of the onset, amplitude of the reflex, time course (brief activators, decay of reflex during prolonged stimulation) of the reflex, relationship between ipsilaterally and contralaterally elicited reflexes, and others.

Presence of the acoustic reflex when results of behavioral hearing evaluation show no measurable hearing, or show profound hearing loss suggests nonorganicity. In general, acoustic reflex thresholds are not observed at less than 15 to 20 dB sensation level (i.e., dB above the voluntary threshold) and certainly are not seen at or below admitted threshold. In patients in whom unequivocal acoustic reflex responses are seen near or below the voluntary threshold, nonorganic hearing loss should certainly be suspected.

Gelfand (29) investigated the use of the acoustic reflex threshold in identifying functional hearing impairment. He noted that tonal acoustic reflex thresholds are an effective nonbehavioral tool for identifying functional hearing loss when hearing thresholds are equal to or greater than 60 dB HL, but that one cannot reliably identify a functional component when thresholds are equal to or less than 55 dB HL.

Acoustic Reflex Assessment by High-Frequency Probe Tones

As is seen with tympanometry, acoustic reflex determinations are more reliably and validly made when one uses a higher-frequency probe tone in neonates and young infants. With use of using a 220-Hz probe tone, the acoustic reflex is often not observed in infants; however, with a higher-frequency probe tone, the presence of the reflex increases. At 800 Hz, the infant reflex is present in the same proportion as that seen in the adult population (30). The acoustic reflex to a broadband noise was found to be present in 100% of cases (45 full-term neonates) older than the age of 12 hours in a study conducted by Geddes (31) with a 660-Hz probe tone. Bennett (32) suggested that a probe-tone frequency of 1,400 Hz is optimal in the detection of infant acoustic reflexes, because at lower frequencies the reduced impedance of the eardrum precludes measurement of the small impedance changes that occur with the contraction of the acoustic reflex.

In a study comparing ipsilateral and contralateral acoustic reflexes in neonates, use of a 660-Hz probe tone tripled the observance of the reflex as compared with use of a 220-Hz probe tone (33). Ipsilateral acoustic reflexes were detected in 76% of the ears tested with the 660-Hz probe tone. It was theorized that the reason for the improved detectability with use of the higher-frequency probe tone is that raising the probe-tone frequency has the effect of moving away from the resonant peak of the middle ear into a region in which the neonatal eardrum has an impedance similar to that of the adult. In so doing, the reflex can be reliaby detected.

Prediction of Hearing Loss from the Acoustic Reflex

Due to the relationship between loudness perception and the threshold of the acoustic reflex, several methods for prediction of hearing loss from the acoustic reflex have been developed. Use of the acoustic reflex to predict hearing loss, particularly in young or difficult-to-test children, has the appeal of a quick, reliable, objective approach to quantification of the presence and degree of hearing impairment. General statements about the probable degree of loss (mild, moderate, severe, profound) and probable shape (slope) of the hearing loss can be made with some degree of accuracy. The various methods for prediction of hearing loss rest on the discrepancy between acoustic reflexes to pure-tone stimuli and acoustic reflexes to broadband noise. Acoustic reflexes in normal and cochlear-impaired ears are lower in threshold for broadband activators than they are for pure-tone activators. It is known that in cochlear hearing loss, the normal difference between thresholds to pure tones and broadband noise is diminished in direct proportion to the degree of hearing loss. Approaches to predicting hearing loss from acoustic reflex thresholds are based on the work of Niemeyer and Sesterhenn (34) who noted that an estimate of audibility can be calculated from pure-tone, broadband, and low-pass and high-pass filtered noise activators. Several methods for prediction of hearing loss from the acoustic reflex thresholds have been proposed. The modified sensitivity prediction with the acoustic reflex (SPAR) developed by Jerger et al., (35) compared acoustic reflexes at 500, 1,000, and 2,000 Hz with broadband noise to predict normal hearing compared with mild or moderate sensorineural loss and severe sensorineural loss. Use of this method gained some degree of acceptance in the late 1970s and early 1980s, but at least three problems were noted (37):

1. High false-positive rates, ranging from 25% to 40%
2. High false-negative rates
3. In accuracy of prediction of the hearing-loss categories when actual hearing loss is low

A second method, the bivariate plot, was designed to separate normal from nonnormal ears. The bivariate plotting procedure (37) allows separation between normal and impaired ears on the basis of the pure-tone/broadband noise acoustic reflex difference. The separation between normal and abnormal ears is assessed by two factors: (a) the ratio of the average acoustic reflex threshold for pure-tone activators to the threshold for a broadband activator, and (b) the average acoustic reflex thresholds for pure-tone activators (500, 1,000, and 2,000 Hz). By use of this comparison, a dichotomous categorization of normal and nonnormal can be made. The modified bivariate plot (36) was shown to have good sensitivity and specificity, and was a better choice for prediction of hearing loss than was SPAR.

Although ABR and OAE have largely supplanted use of the acoustic reflex as an objective predictor of hearing sensitivity in children, Northern and Gabbard (26) note that, in difficult-to-test patients, use of the acoustic reflex to predict hearing sensitivity remains a simple, economic, and efficient method. Conductive hearing loss, so common in children, obscures the acoustic reflex, but this is also true for OAE and, depending on the degree of conductive loss for air-conducted ABR. Recently, Margolis (38) reviewed methods for detecting hearing impairment by using the acoustic reflex. He concluded that the acoustic reflex is effective in detecting hearing impairment in excess of 30 dB HL when procedural variables are carefully controlled. Further, he stated that, if a high-frequency probe tone is employed, the use of the acoustic reflex to detect hearing impairment in infants is theoretically feasible.

The acoustic reflex can be also used as a gross indicator of level of loudness discomfort. There is an imperfect relationship between the acoustic reflex threshold and the perception of loudness discomfort. This application can be useful as a gross measure of aided response for selecting maximal output levels for hearing aids and in fitting hearing aids on young children (39). Evaluation of hearing aids with use of acoustic reflexes as an objective measure was discussed by McCandless and Keith (40). They offered guidelines for five aspects of hearing-aid fitting by using acoustic reflex thresholds: setting the saturation sound pressure level, setting gain, measuring real-ear gain, estimating Vec to estimate modification of 2-cm^3 coupler gain, and determining appropriate frequency response. Due to the imperfect correlation between loudness and the acoustic reflex, however, reliance on the reflex for hearing-aid parameters is not a generally accepted technique.

Contralaterally Elicited and Ipsilaterally Elicited Acoustic Reflexes

Comparison of ipsilaterally and contralaterally elicited acoustic reflexes constitutes an important of the diagnostic immittance test battery. An acoustic reflex may be absent for one of several reasons.

In the probe ear, there may be MEE or other conductive pathology or dysfunction of cranial nerve VII. In the stimulated ear, there may be conductive hearing loss, severe to profound hearing loss, dysfunction of cranial nerve VIII, or collapsed ear canal.

By comparing contralaterally and ipsilaterally elicited reflexes, particularly in conjunction with examination of the patient's audiogram, a more complete understanding of the probable disorder can be reached. For example, in the case of a conductive 30-dB, left-sided hearing loss, the left ipsilateral, left contralateral, and right contralateral reflexes would be absent; if the loss is cochlear, however, all reflexes would be present. Jerger and Jerger (41) noted that comparison of the two modes of reflex assessment can also differentiate between cranial nerve VIII and brainstem pathology.

Other measures of the acoustic reflex, which are not commonly performed in routine pediatric testing, include:

acoustic reflex decay: a measure of the decay, or relaxation of the acoustic reflex, to stimulation of prolonged duration (typically 10 sec). In adults, acoustic reflex decay greater than 50% in 10 seconds is indicative of retrocochlear disease.

acoustic reflex latency: a measure of the latency of the onset of the contraction of the stapedial muscle. Similar to decay, increased latency has been shown to correlate with auditory neural pathology.

ADDITIONAL CONSIDERATIONS IN IMMITTANCE MEASUREMENT

Sensitivity and Specificity

An ongoing problem in the use of tympanometry and acoustic reflex measures for screening middle-ear function in children is the balance between sensitivity and specificity. Sensitivity of a measure refers to the percentage of patients who test positive and who truly have the disease. Specificity is the percentage of patients who test negative and who do not have the disease. Sensitivity refers to the ability of a measure to identify disease, specificity to the ability of a test to identify normalcy. Increasing sensitivity (e.g., by using a more inclusive criterion for what is deemed pathologic) carries with it the increased probability of overidentification (false positive), in which normal ears are mistakenly identified as pathologic.

In a comparison of two screening procedures (ASHA's and a traditional procedure based on measurements of TPP and acoustic reflexes), Roush et al. (42) examined 204 children, ages 3 to 4 years. It was found that the two procedures differed significantly in sensitivity and specificity. Among other findings, it was shown that the ASHA procedure generally had much higher specificity. In addition, these authors noted that the addition of acoustic reflex thresholds to the screening protocol appeared to significantly lower the specificity and contributed little to sensitivity.

The inclusion in the ASHA guidelines of a waiting period between the first identification of an abnormal tympanogram and the referral for medical care was an attempt to reduce the well-known incidence of false-positive findings with tympanometric screening. To decrease the false-positive rate, that is, to improve the specificity by using a more stringent criterion for pathology, an increased number of abnormal ears will be identified as normal. This trade-off is inevitable in any screening protocol, and the costs of both overreferral, and failing to identify true pathology must be weighed in considering whether to conduct screening and in specifying the criteria for pass and fail.

Calibration

Immittance meters must be calibrated at least annually to ensure that their performance falls within the ANSI S3.39—1987 standard. Calibration includes a check of the frequency and intensity of the probe tone(s) with acceptable levels of distortion and noise. Acoustic reflex activator stimuli are calibrated for frequency, intensity, linearity of the attenuator, and distortion. The accuracy of the pneumatic air-pressure system to ensure that the rate of air-pressure change and the accuracy of the manometer are within specifications must be checked. The immittance meter itself is calibrated with fixed cavity volumes, taking into account the ambient air pressure and altitude.

Personnel

In using tympanometry as a screening technique for preschool and school-age children, previous (pre-1996) ASHA screening guidelines called for supervision of the screening protocol by an audiologist. This requirement was primarily to ensure that techniques of otoscopy (necessary to avoid performing immittance screening on ears with pressure-equalization tubes, obvious ear-canal blockage, or other gross pathology) and tympanometric interpretation were performed correctly. It is common, however, to have either speech-language pathologists or trained volunteers conduct hearing screening programs in schools. It continues to be important that the protocol, normative data, equipment calibration, training of screeners, and interpretation of test outcome be monitored by an audiologist.

Condition of the Child for Evaluation

It is not uncommon for young children to resist the audiologist's attempts to insert the probe tip for immittance measurements. Although the ideal circumstance for measuring the tympanogram and acoustic reflex thresholds is to have the child sitting quietly, it is not impossible to obtain good information from a squirming or crying child. The parent can be asked to hold the child firmly, including the child's hands. The child can be distracted by use of a quiet toy or puppet; some tympanometric screeners use an interesting display that the child can watch while the tympanogram is being generated (e.g., one manufacturer has a tympanogram display that shows a car driving into a garage as the tympanogram is run). Good information can be obtained from a nursing child or one that is sucking a bottle or pacifier.

CONCLUSION

Tympanometry and acoustic reflex assessment comprise a rapid, reliable, and valid measure of many aspects of the ear and of auditory function. In infants, acoustic reflex measures can help in identifying the presence of cochlear hearing loss. Tympanometry provides a quick diagnosis of MEE in children older than the age of 2 to 4 months. Acoustic reflex measurements can help to substantiate functional hearing loss. Conditions of TM, such as perforation and patency of transtympanic tubes, can be rapidly assessed by using tympanometric values. Immittance measures should be considered an integral part of the audiologic evaluation. Including these measures, in conjunction with auditory sensitivity measures (pure-tone and speech-threshold measures), will improve the diagnostic capability of either measure alone.

REFERENCES

1. American National Standards Institute. *Specifications for instruments to measure aural acoustic impedance and admittance (aural acoustic immittance),* ANSI S3.39—1987. New York: American National Standards Institute; 1988.
2. Van Camp K, Shanks J, Margolis R. Simulation of pathological high impedance tympanograms. *J Speech Hear Res* 1986;29:505–514.
3. Jerger JF. Clinical experience with impedance audiometry. *Arch. Otolaryngology* 1970;92:311–324.
4. Wiley T, Barrett K. Test-retest reliability in tympanometry. *J Speech Hear Res* 1991;34:1197–1206.
5. Roush J, Tait C. Pure-tone and acoustic immittance screening of preschool-aged children: an examination of referral criteria. *Ear Hear* 1985;6:245–250.
6. Silman S, Silverman C, Arick D. Pure tone assessment and screening of children with middle-ear effusion. *J Amer Acad Audiol* 1994;5:173–182.
7. American Speech-Language-Hearing Association. Guidelines for screening for hearing impairment and middle-ear disorders. *ASHA* 1990;32(Suppl 2):17–24.
8. Northern J, Grimes A. Impedance audiometry. In: Katz J, ed. *Handbook of clinical audiology.* 2nd ed. Baltimore: Williams & Wilkins; 1977.
9. Silman S, Silverman C. *Auditory diagnosis: principles and applications.* San Diego: Academic Press; 1991.
10. Haapaniemi J. Immittance findings in school-aged children. *Ear Hear* 1996;17:19–27.
11. Nozza R, Bluestone C, Kardatzke D, Bachman R. Identification of middle ear effusion by aural acoustic admittance and otoscopy. *Ear Hear* 1994;15:310–323.
12. Margolis R, Hunter L. Audiologic evaluation of the otitis media patient. Otitis Media: the pathogenesis approach. *Otolaryngol Clin North Am* 1991;24:877–899.
13. Hall J, Chandler D. Tympanometry in clinical audiology. In J. Katz, ed. *Handbook of clinical audiology,* 4th ed. Baltimore: Williams and Wilkins; 1994
14. Nozza R, Bluestone C, Karadatzke D. Sensitivity, specificity and predictive value of immittance measures in the identification of middle ear effusion. In: Bess F, Hall J, eds. *Screening children for auditory function.* Nashville: Bill Wilkerson Center Press; 1992.
15. Hanks W, Rose K. Middle ear resonance and acoustic immittance measures in children. *J Speech Hear Res* 1993;36:218–222.
16. Silman S, Silverman C, Arick D. Acoustic-immittance screening for detection of middle-ear effusion in children. *J Amer Acad Audiol* 1992;3: 262–268.
17. Shanks J, Stelmachowicz P, Beauchaine K, Schulte L. Equivalent ear canal volumes in children pre- and post-tympanostomy tube insertion. *J Speech Hear Res* 1992;35:936–941.
18. Shanks J, Wilson R, Cambron N. Multiple frequency tympanometry: effects of ear canal volume compensation on static acoustic admittance and estimates of middle ear resonance. *J Speech Hear Res* 1993;36:178–185.
19. Margolis R, Popelka G. Static and dynamic acoustic impedance measurements in infant ears. *J Speech Hear Res* 1975;18:435–453.
20. Holte L, Margolis R, Cavanaugh R. Developmental changes in multifrequency tympanograms. *Audiology* 1991;30:1–24.
21. Marchant C, McMillan P, Shurin P, et al. Objective diagnosis of otitis media in early infancy by tympanometry and ipsilateral acoustic reflex thresholds. *J Pediatr* 1986;109:590–595.
22. Roush J, Bryant K, Mundy M, Zeisel S, Roberts J. Developmental changes in static admittance and tympanometric width in infants and toddlers. *J Am Acad Audiol* 1995;6:334–338.
23. Karzon RG, Validity and reliability of tympanometric measures for pediatric patients *J Speech Hear Res* 1991;34:386–390.
24. Shanks J, Wilson R. Effects of direction and rate of ear-canal pressure changes on tympanometric measures. *J Speech Hear Res* 1986;29:11–19.
25. Shanks J, Lilly D, Margolis R, Wiley T, Wilson R. Tympanometry. *J Speech Hear Disord* 1988;53:354–377.
26. Northern J, Gabbard S. The acoustic reflex. In: Katz J, ed. *Handbook of clinical audiology.* 4th ed. 1994.
27. Borg E. On the neuronal organization of the acoustic middle ear reflex. *Arch Otolaryngol* 1974;99:172–176.
28. Silman S, Gelfand S. The relationship between magnitude of hearing

loss and acoustic reflex threshold levels. *J Speech Hear Disord* 1981;46:312–316.
29. Gelfand S. Acoustic reflex threshold tenth percentile and functional hearing impairment. *J Am Acad Audiol* 1994;5:10–16.
30. Weatherby M, Bennett M. The neonatal acoustic reflex. *Scand Audiol* 1980;9:103–110.
31. Geddes N. Tympanometry and the stapedial reflex in the first five days of life. *Int J Pediatr Otorhinolaryngol* 1987;13:293–297.
32. Bennett M. Impedance concepts relating to the acoustic reflex. In: Silman S, ed. *The acoustic reflex.* Orlando: Academic Press; 1984.
33. McMillan P, Bennett M, Marchant C, Shurin P. Ipsilateral and contralateral acoustic reflexes in neonates. *Ear Hear* 1985;6:320–324.
34. Niemeyer W, Sesterhenn G. Calculating the hearing threshold from the stapedius reflex threshold for different sound stimuli. *Audiology* 1974;13:421–427.
35. Jerger J, Burney P, Mauldin L, Crump B. Predicting hearing loss from the acoustic reflex. *J Speech and Hearing Disorders.* 1974;39:11–22.
36. Silman S, Gelfand S, Piper N, Silverman C, Van Frank L. Prediction of hearing loss from the acoustic-reflex threshold. In: Silman S, ed. *The acoustic reflex.* Orlando: Academic Press; 1984.
37. Popelka G. *Hearing assessment with the acoustic reflex.* New York: Gruen and Stratton; 1981.
38. Margolis R. Detection of hearing impairment with the acoustic stapedius reflex. *Ear Hear* 1993;14:3–10.
39. Mueller H, Grimes A. Amplification systems for the hearing impaired. In: Alpiner J, McCarthy P, eds. *Rehabilitative audiology: children and adults.* Baltimore: Williams & Wilkins; 1987.
40. McCandless G, Keith R. The use of impedance measures in hearing aid fitting. In: Jerger J, and Northern J, eds. *Clinical impedance audiometry.* 2nd ed. Acton, MA: American Electromedics Press; 1980.
41. Jerger S, Jerger J. Diagnostic value of crosses vs uncrossed acoustic reflexes. *Arch Otolaryngol* 1977;103:445–453.
42. Roush J, Drake A, Sexton J. Identification of middle ear dysfunction in young children: a comparison of tympanometric screening procedures. *Ear Hear* 1992;13:63–69.

CHAPTER 9

Physiologic Assessment of Hearing

Yvonne S. Sininger and Carolina Abdala

Accurate assessment of hearing and auditory function is critical for management and treatment of otologic and audiologic disorders. Assessment of auditory function can be particularly challenging in a pediatric population. As we are faced with the need to define hearing thresholds and other aspects of auditory function in very young children and newborn infants or in children with developmental delays or other handicapping conditions, it becomes increasingly important to include objective, physiologic-based assessment tools in the diagnostic battery. This chapter discusses the use of otoacoustic emissions and auditory evoked potentials, with particular emphasis on the auditory brainstem response in otologic-audiologic assessment of infants and children.

AUDITORY EVOKED POTENTIALS

Measurement of auditory evoked potentials (AEPs) involves presenting an appropriate acoustic stimulus to the ear and sampling and averaging the resulting neural activity by means of externally placed electrodes. Auditory evoked potentials are categorized by the poststimulus time of neural activity measured and/or the generators of the response. Each type of AEP has characteristic spectral content and requires specific stimuli for optimal generation. In general, the earliest evoked potentials are smaller in amplitude and require more averaging and amplification for measurement, have more high-frequency energy, and require more rapid onset stimuli.

Figure 1 shows a schematic of AEPs using a log time scale to show detail. Not shown in this diagram are cochlear potentials, which occur immediately after stimulation and are measured by means of electrocochleography. Each segment of AEP involves progressively ascending neurons in the central auditory system. Consequently, an AEP battery can help to delineate the site of a lesion or neoplasm involving the central auditory pathway (1–3).

Important distinctions exist in the function of the various types of AEPs. Responses generated before about 60 to 100 ms are considered exogenous potentials. These potentials are determined and controlled primarily by external stimuli, have a characteristic response that depends on the auditory signal, and, consequently, are excellent for assessing sensory function such as auditory sensitivity. Later AEPs (past 60–100 ms) are considered endogenous potentials; that is, they are influenced primarily by internal cognitive processes rather than by external stimuli. A good example is the P300, or "expectancy wave." This potential is produced only when an unexpected or surprising stimulus is encountered, and the P300 is observed equally well with visual or auditory stimuli. Endogenous potentials are used to assess cognitive function and processing of stimuli but are *less helpful* in evaluation of specific sensory systems. Some of the late AEPs continue to develop and change throughout adolescence, making it necessary to correct for age-specific factors. For these reasons, this chapter focuses on the early evoked potentials, known as the auditory brainstem response (ABR).

Electrocochleography

The earliest evoked potentials are generated in the cochlea and the auditory nerve. Measurement of this activity by electrodes is termed *electrocochleography* (ECochG). Receptor potentials include the *cochlear microphonic,* an immediate, amplified representation of the stimulus and the *summating potential,* a dc shift in the resting cochlear potential in response to sound. The *whole nerve action potential* (AP), representing the composite firing of first-order neurons, can also be recorded during ECochG.

Whenever the recording electrode is moved closer to the cochlea than the typical mastoid placement, the resultant recording is considered ECochG. At one time ECochG involved measurement from a transtympanic needle that contacted the promontory. While this recording set-up results

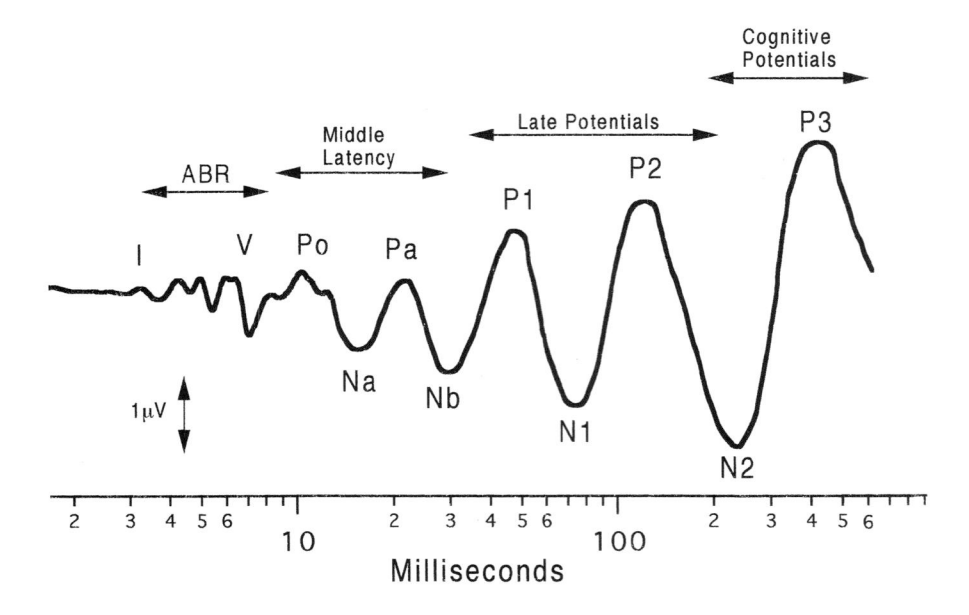

FIG. 1. Human AEP in log time scale.

in excellent recordings because of the proximity of the electrode to the generators, this measure requires sterile procedure and is rarely used in the U.S. due to cost and discomfort to the patient. Several ear canal electrodes have been employed with varying degrees of success. In general, the foam-plug ear canal electrodes are only slightly better than a surface electrode on the mastoid or ear lobe in terms of signal-to-noise ratio.

An electrode that is placed on the tympanic membrane has been described by Stypulkowski and Staller (4). This electrode is a foam plug embedded with silver wire. The foam is impregnated with conductive gel and placed directly on the tympanic membrane. The gel makes contact with the wire, which creates the electrode lead. Although little has been published on the use of this electrode in children, Ferraro and Ferguson (5) have found it to be an excellent alternative to transtympanic recording that may be comfortable enough for use in cooperative and/or sedated children. An example of an ABR recorded with this electrode is shown in Fig. 2. Because this electrode is closer to the cochlea, wave I, which is the same as the whole nerve AP, is considerably larger with this configuration than is generally found with mastoid, earlobe, or ear canal electrodes.

Auditory Brainstem Response

The ABR occurs during the first 10 to 20 ms after the stimulus, and, as the name implies, it is generated in the auditory nerve and brainstem auditory pathway (6,7). This AEP is present as early as 25 weeks gestational age (8) and can be reliably recorded regardless of sleep state. Consequently, the ABR is the most commonly used measure of hearing sensitivity in newborns and young children. Auditory brainstem response has two major functions in assessment of auditory function in children: (a) It can be used as a measure of functional integrity of the auditory nerve and brainstem auditory pathway, and (b) it can be applied to predict hearing level.

An example of ABR recorded for neurologic analysis can be found in Fig. 3. The vertex-positive peaks of the ABR are labeled with roman numerals I through VI or VII. The work of Möller, using direct recordings from the human auditory nerve and brainstem structures during surgical procedures, has been invaluable in characterizing the structures associated with the peaks of the scalp-recorded ABR. By comparing simultaneous intra- and extracranial recordings, Möller and Jannetta have determined that the first two positive peaks of the human ABR are associated with auditory nerve activity (6) and the negativity following wave II and

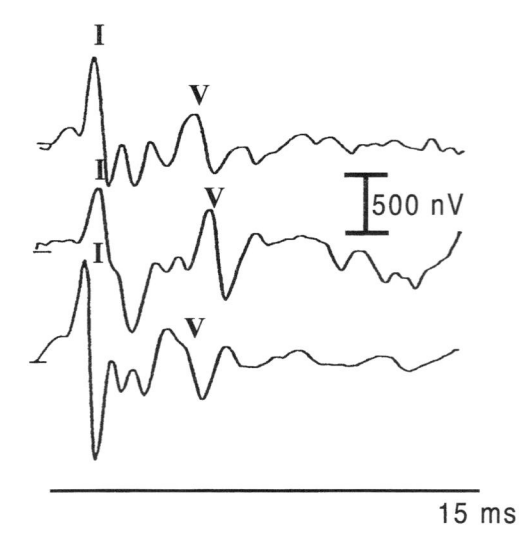

FIG. 2. Combined CochG and ABR recorded from vertex to tympanic membrane electrode in three adult subjects. The stimulus was 80 dB nHL clicks. Wave I is larger than wave V in all cases.

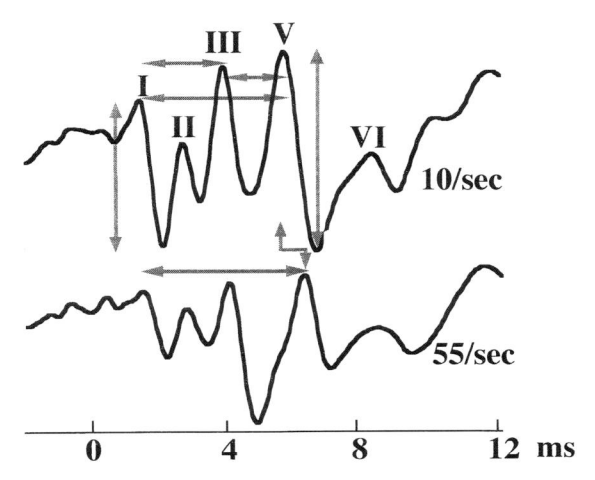

FIG. 3. Auditory brainstem response recorded in response to 60-dB nHL click stimulus and 100- to 3,000-Hz bandpass filter for assessment of brainstem integrity. The top trace was recorded with slow stimulus rate and the bottom at a high rate to stress the auditory system. Peak latency (I, III, V) and amplitude (I, V) as well as interpeak latencies (I–III, I–V, III–V) are measured and compared with normative data. A wave V latency shift with increased rate is also evaluated.

ear of an individual patient (2). In the absence of hearing loss, extended peak latency, especially extended interpeak latency (I–V or III–V), can be indicative of brainstem pathology or VIII nerve tumor. In the case of VIII nerve tumor, the extent of abnormality can be slight, such as a delayed wave V latency or as severe as a complete loss of waveform morphology. Demyelinating disease, such as multiple sclerosis or peripheral nerve neuropathy, can desynchronize activity in the VIII nerve and brainstem and cause deletion of waves or prolongation of latencies as well (13,14).

Interpretation of ABR waveform morphology must be done carefully when cochlear hearing loss is present. Because the ABR is dominated by activity in the highly-synchronous, high-frequency fibers of the auditory nerve, high frequency sensory loss can be particularly deleterious to ABR morphology. Wave I is most sensitive to high-frequency hearing loss (15) and interpeak latency measures may be impossible if wave I is obliterated by sensory loss (16). However, because the effect of high-frequency hearing loss on wave V latency is predictable, one can correct the expected latency of wave V, based on the amount of high-frequency hearing loss seen on the audiogram. For example, Selters and Brackmann (2) suggest that the expected wave V latency be adjusted by 0.1 ms for every 10 dB that the 4,000-Hz threshold exceeds 50 dB HL. When comparing interaural wave V latency, a maximum difference of 0.3 ms is usually allowed before suspicion of neoplasm is aroused (2,17). Interaural latency differences can also be corrected for asymmetrical hearing loss if necessary.

the peak of wave III are associated with activity from the cochlear nucleus, although there may be other contributions to wave III (9,10). The complexity of fiber decusations and staggered cochlear output make association of ABR peaks with individual brainstem structures unlikely past wave II. In humans, the negativity following wave V, sometimes referred to as the SN10 (11), is generated during the same poststimulus time frame as activity in the inferior colliculus (10,12). This is the most robust segment of the ABR and can be recorded with the very low stimulus levels necessary in establishing ABR threshold for hearing-level prediction.

Analysis of ABR for assessment of brainstem system integrity involves measurement of peak latency, amplitudes, and relative peak latency and amplitude as shown in Fig. 3. An additional measure that is important in the determination of low brainstem and VIII nerve disorders is the comparison of absolute and interpeak latencies in ABRs elicited from each

The second use of ABR in children is in the prediction of hearing level. In this application, the threshold for detection of wave V (as a function of stimulus level) is determined for wide-band and/or narrow-band stimuli. In the absence of neurologic disorder, ABR thresholds are directly related to psychophysical thresholds for like stimuli (18,19). An example of an ABR from a normally hearing child is shown in Fig. 4. This topic is covered in detail later in the chapter.

Middle Latency Response

Middle latency response (MLR) occurs during the first 100 ms after stimulation. Middle latency response is a larger,

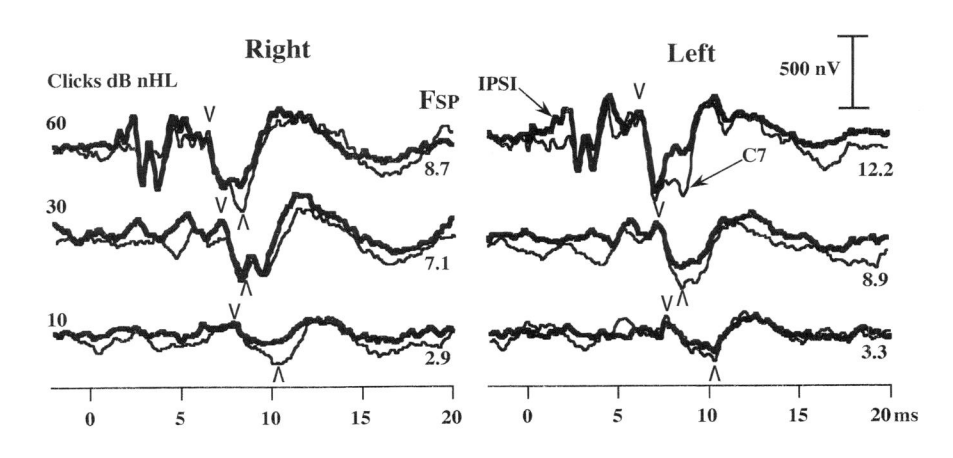

FIG. 4. Auditory brainstem response input-output series for click stimuli of 60, 30, and 10 dB nHL in the left and right ear. Light lines are recordings from vertex to seventh cervical vertebra (C7) and heavy lines from vertex to ipsilateral mastoid (IPSI). The patient was a 2-year-old child with poor speech and language development and poor response to behavioral audiometry. The audiogram was later determined to be normal.

slower AEP than the ABR and can also be used in evaluation of both neural integrity and hearing level. There are advantages and disadvantages to MLR relative to the ABR in either of these applications. The auditory MLR is generated primarily in the thalamus and primary auditory cortex (20). Unlike the ABR, MLR is affected by the sleep state of the patient and is not consistently recorded until after about 12 years of age (21) unless careful monitoring of sleep state is conducted (22). At the same time, the MLR is less dependent on rapid stimulus onset than the ABR and, consequently, may be helpful in detecting auditory response to low-frequency stimuli. A combined approach using lower filter settings and a longer recording window than traditionally used for ABR recording may allow for an optimal recording of AEPs to tonal stimuli in children. This approach is discussed later.

AUDITORY EVOKED POTENTIAL MEASUREMENT PRINCIPLES

Signal-to-Noise Ratio

Scalp-recorded neural potentials from humans can be an order of magnitude smaller than the other activity (noise) picked up by electrodes. The most important principle to consider when measuring AEPs is the relationship between the magnitude of the neural potential and the background noise. This relative quantity is termed the signal-to-noise ratio (SNR). It is not possible to make an exact measurement of the SNR in any recording, but there are ways of estimating the individual quantities and enhancing signal and/or reducing noise. A general overview of these techniques is given and specific ways of enhancing recordings for infant and pediatric populations are discussed in the appropriate sections.

The level of "signal" in an averaged response is estimated by the overall amplitude of the AEP, with the understanding that some residual noise is always present in the recording. Specific recording parameters can influence the SNR of any given response. Response amplitude is influenced by stimulus level, type and location of electrodes, and response filtering. Noise level in the averaged response will be influenced by subject state, filtering, number of sweeps averaged, electrode placement and electrode-to-scalp impedance.

Fsp and Auditory Brainstem Response Detection Routines

Several routines that help to estimate the SNR of an AEP recording have been described. The technique known as Fsp, developed by Elberling and Don (23,24) has been in use in our center for 10 years and has proven to be quite valuable in determining the quality of our recordings and threshold of ABR. The technique provides a value that approximates the SNR 11 by calculating the variance of the averaged response (estimate of the averaged signal + noise) divided by the variance of the amplitude of a single point at a given time in each sweep that makes up the average (estimate of the background noise in the response). An example of the procedure used to calculate the Fsp is shown in Fig. 5.

The variance across the averaged window relates to the overall amplitude in the average, which contains either evoked potential and residual noise or noise alone. Because the AEP that is buried in any given single sweep of data is time-locked to the stimulus, it will not contribute to the variance of the single point from sweep to sweep. That value will estimate the amount of noise that contributed to the average. Fsp is calculated by dividing the signal plus noise by the estimate of the noise, which gives a value that is approximately the SNR + 1. This value has an F-distribution, and when the degrees of freedom are known, the confidence that a true response exists can be determined by looking up the Fsp value on an F table. For example, an Fsp value of 3.1 is associated with 99% confidence of true response for a toddler (assuming 5 and 250 degrees of freedom), and a 95% confidence is found for a response with an Fsp of 2.25. These values change as the degrees of freedom change. This happens with different populations, such as infants or when filtering or window length change.

Fsp, which is updated every 256 sweeps, will grow as the noise is reduced by the averaging process. For a small amplitude response, such as those generated with low-level stimuli, many sweeps may be needed to reach the predefined confidence that a true response exists. However, the reverse is also true. When a large response is present and noise is low, a given confidence may be reached very quickly. For this reason, when using Fsp, we do not fix the number of sweeps averaged. Rather, we allow the averaging to continue until a criterion Fsp is reached, and if not reached, we stop after the noise is sufficiently low or we have reached 6,000 sweeps.

Besides optimizing the number of sweeps averaged and providing an objective measure of response confidence, an-

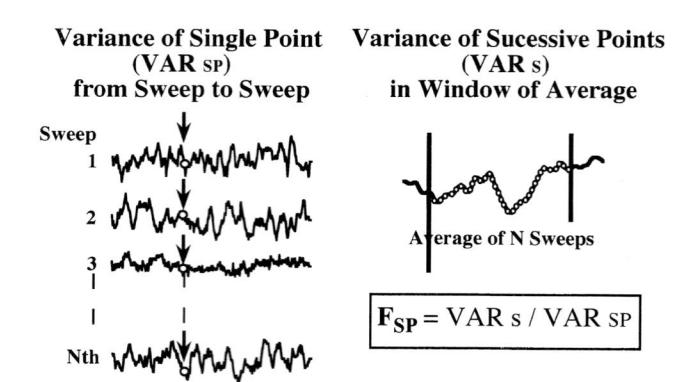

$$F_{SP} = VAR_s / VAR_{SP}$$

FIG. 5. The calculation of Fsp values involves calculation of the variance of a single point in N (usually 256) successive raw sweeps of ABR, as shown at left. At the completion of each block of 256 sweeps, the average response is computed and the variance across an appropriate window of the average is computed (*right side*).

other advantage of using Fsp for ABR measures in children is that response repetition is no longer necessary. Without this type of measure, a response and a replication are compared by visual cross-correlation to determine if a true response exists. Because the confidence can be derived off-line with Fsp, this time-consuming replication is avoided.

Electrode Placement

Auditory evoked potential recording systems generally utilize a differential recording amplifier to enhance SNR. Activity is sampled from two electrode locations on the scalp. The differential amplifier subtracts the two signals before averaging to eliminate any large common signals, such as muscle activity from movement, or large extraneous electrical noise, such as 60-Hz line noise from the recording. At the same time, by placing the two electrodes at sites that will "see" different aspects of the tiny, internally generated AEP, those signals will be enhanced by the subtraction technique. Orienting the electrode array in the plane of the dipole source of the neural component of interest can enhance the recorded amplitude, especially for far-field recordings such as the ABR (25,26). For example, wave I generated by the auditory nerve will be optimally recorded from a horizontally arranged electrode pair (ear to ear) while wave V of the ABR will be optimally recorded in line with the neural axis (vertex to neck) (25,26). In the same way, it is possible to eliminate certain AEP components from a recording by orienting differential electrodes at 90 degrees from the axis of the dipole source.

Auditory Brainstem Response Electrode Placement for Pediatric Evaluation

We have been using a two-channel recording montage for ABR evaluation with infants and children. One channel is recorded from the vertex to the seventh cervical vertebra (C7) or from the hairline over the spine for newborns. The second channel (referred to as IPSI) is recorded from the vertex to the ipsilateral mastoid or ear lobe. For most recordings, the ABR results in these channels are reasonably predictable. As shown in Fig. 4, recordings from the IPSI channel have a larger wave I and a smaller wave V than the C7 channel in most subjects. When evaluating ABRs from both full-term and premature infants in these two channels, the C7 channel generally shows larger wave V amplitude. However, the Fsp in these channels was not significantly larger across subjects than found in the IPSI channel (27). This is the result of much higher noise in the C7 channel from the pick-up of cardiac activity because of the proximity of the C7 electrode to the chest cavity in newborns. Consequently, larger amplitude is sometimes overshadowed by the higher noise in the C7 channel. Myogenic pick-up is alleviated somewhat by moving the C7 electrode up the neck to the hairline. We have chosen to record from both channels in all pediatric evaluations. However, it is not clear which channel will produce the lowest threshold on any given infant or child.

Recording from two channels simultaneously allows for a type of response replication (see Fig. 4). When using Fsp, we gain confidence in response detection from the statistic. However, it is helpful to see a replication of expected waveform morphology across the two channels, for correct interpretation. No extra time is required for this type of replication because the two channels are recorded simultaneously.

Filtering

When AEP and noise components of an averaged recording have different spectral properties, filtering of electrode activity can be used to reduce noise components and enhance the SNR. Unfortunately, the spectra of the neural signal often overlap with the spectra of the noise, and, in these instances, filtering must be used cautiously and bandpass parameters must be selected carefully. In addition, analog filters can distort signals and will affect waveform morphology and peak latencies. Care must be taken in the proper selection of both filter slopes and bandpass frequencies.

Filtering for Pediatric Auditory Brainstem Response Assessment

The waveform morphology and the spectral content of the ABR undergoes dramatic changes between infancy and adulthood. The most dramatic developmental changes in the ABR occur up to the age of 18 to 24 months. Figure 6 illustrates those changes. Spectral analysis of these waveforms demonstrates that the infant ABR has considerable energy below 100 Hz and may require different bandpass filtering to avoid removing this slow, low-frequency activity in these ABRs. Sininger (28) has shown that using a 30-Hz high-pass filter for recording ABR in full-term newborns can dra-

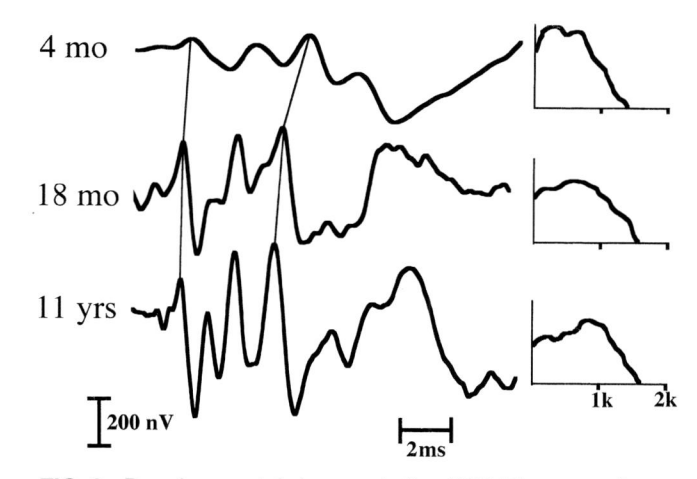

FIG. 6. Developmental changes in the ABR. Time waveforms are shown at left and spectral analysis of each is shown at right, showing the shift in major spectral energy with age.

present (61), and suggests that the presence of SOAEs may be a positive indicator for normal or near-normal hearing. However, difficulty in interpretation occurs when the SOAE is not present, because this is not necessarily an indicator of

as a microphone to measure it. Stimuli are presented the transducer in the probe assembly, and the microphone-measured response to many stimuli is averaged in the time domain to improve the SNR. The averaged response is amplified, and low-frequency noise is reduced with a high-pass filter.

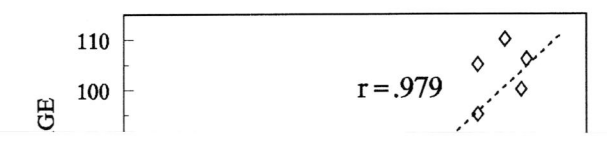

Stimulus artifact is a serious problem when measuring TEOAEs, because the stimulus ringing may overlap with early components of the echo. At present, the only commercial system available for measuring TEOAEs is the otodynamics ILO system, which provides, as an option, the use of a nonlinear click stimulus train. This technique utilizes the non-linearity of the response to cancel stimulus artifact. Like the cochlear microphonic, an OAE will reflect the polarity of the stimulus input. The ILO unit presents a click train that contains three equal-level clicks of a given polarity, followed by a fourth click that is three times the amplitude of the first three but inverted in polarity. Because the stimulus level is near to the level that shows saturation of the TEOAE, response amplitude does not grow significantly for the fourth click, and only about one third of the original OAE response is canceled by the polarity inversion. The stimulus artifact, in contrast, grows linearly, and the fourth inverted stimulus cancels the majority of stimulus artifact. The remaining artifact is eliminated by setting the first 2.5 ms of response to zero. Sweep rejection strategies also help improve the signal clarity by eliminating sweeps that contain high levels of noise.

A TEOAE is typically evaluated by observing two aspects of the response: (a) replicability of two simultaneously collected TEOAE time waveforms and (b) comparison of noise and response of spectral amplitude across a broad frequency range. These spectra can be sectioned into octave-wide bands for frequency-specific evaluation. Figure 10 displays these two forms of response analysis.

Figure 10A shows 12 ms of two TEOAE time waveforms superimposed. The first part of the waveform represents high-frequency energy from the basal cochlea and the later portion, mid- to low-frequency energy. During data collection, the response is alternatively sent to one of two buffers (buffer A or B) for averaging. Therefore, two separate waveforms are collected simultaneously under almost identical conditions. After acquisition, these waveforms undergo a cross-correlation to evaluate their similarity. If a robust emission is present, buffers A and B will contain similar waveforms, and the correlation, expressed as a percentage reproducibility score, will be high. The time waveforms in Fig. 10A are highly similar (99% reproducibility), confirming the presence of a robust response. Kemp et al. (60) recommended at least a 50% reproducibility score to consider a response present. If no response is present, buffers A and B will contain only uncorrelated noise, and a low correlation score will be obtained. If a response is present in limited spectral regions, the overall correlation may be low but will be high in those octave bands that contain emission. When responses in A and B are subtracted from one another, a residual waveform is provided (A-B). Any common response in A and B should cancel, and the residual should indicate the approximate amount of noise left in the recording. The residual waveform undergoes spectral analysis in the same way as the response and gives an estimate of noise level. The noise level combined with the measured response level provides an estimate of the SNR.

Figure 10B displays the TEOAE amplitude spectrum from 0 to 5,000 Hz. The black portion at the base of the graph represents noise energy, and the white outline rising above the noise represents energy in the TEOAE. In this figure, it is clear that there is greater energy in the response than the

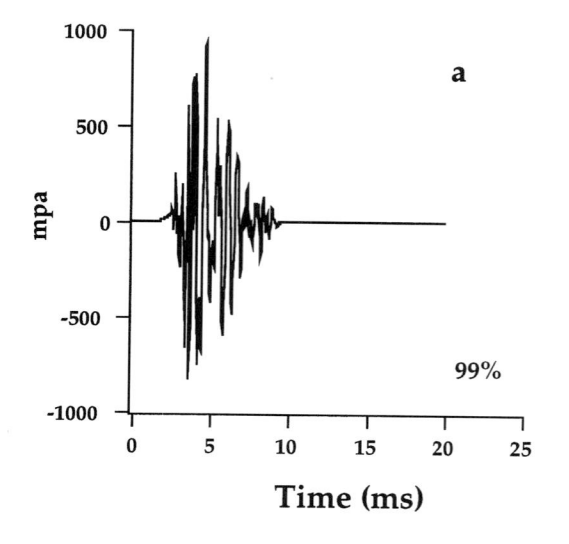

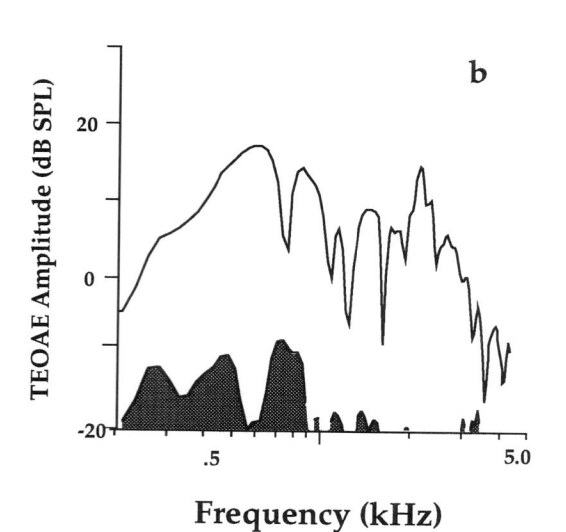

FIG. 10. A: Two superimposed traces of TEOAE time waveforms recorded simultaneously from the ear canal of an adult. The two traces are indistinguishable from one another because response replication was excellent. The correlation between these two traces is shown in the lower right corner as a reproducibility score. **B:** A TEOAE amplitude spectrum for the same individual. The noise floor is shown in solid black and the response is the white outline rising above the noise. Both A and B demonstrate that a TEOAE is present and robust in this individual.

noise floor and a TEOAE is judged to be present. The response is broadband with energy present from 1,000 to 5,000 Hz (60), and robust with an overall level of 18 dB SPL. Note: The judgment of response presence or absence depends heavily on the level of the noise floor and not solely on the absolute amplitude of the TEOAE. For example, if a child is breathing heavily due to congestion, or an infant is sucking on a pacifier, biologic noise will be high. If the acoustic environment around the patient is also noisy, this will likewise contribute to the noise floor. Under these poor conditions, if a small OAE is present, it may be difficult to extract it from the noise. However, if the same low-level TEOAE is present under ideal biologic and acoustic conditions, it may be detected as a response.

The TEOAE can be analyzed in octave-wide bands to allow for an evaluation of response reproducibility within specific frequency regions. This analysis provides a gross comparison of response components originating in low-, mid-, or high-frequency regions of the cochlea.

Distortion-Product Otoacoustic Emissions

Distortion-product otoacoustic emissions are produced when two pure tones of different frequency are presented simultaneously to the ear. These primary tones are referred to by their frequency (f1 and f2) or level (L1 and L2). The nonlinear nature of the cochlea modifies the signal and creates additional frequencies that are not present in the initial stimulus. The most common and robust DPOAE in the human auditory system is found at $2f1 - f2$. For example, if pure tones of 2,000 Hz (f1) and 2,400 Hz (f2) were presented to the ear, a third tone would be produced by the cochlea at 1,600 Hz.

Distortion-product otoacoustic emissions are present in virtually all normally hearing ears. Lonsbury-Martin and Martin (67) reported DPOAEs present in 44 ears from 22 normally hearing adult subjects. Similar figures have been reported by others (65).

Figure 11A displays the spectrum of f1, f2, and the DPOAE at $2f1 - f2$. The response is generated near the region of f2 where the two tones interact on the basilar membrane (55,69,70), and measurement of the DPOAE evaluates cochlear integrity primarily in this region. The response is measured, however at $2f1 - f2$ frequency region. This allows for simultaneous presentation of stimuli and measurement of response without contamination from the primary tones. Figure 11B displays the hypothesized pattern of traveling wave displacement occurring within the cochlea when a distortion product is generated. The spectral level at the frequency of the DPOAE is compared with the level measured in adjacent spectral regions. Average measures at off-frequencies allow for an estimate of the recording "noise floor," which is then compared with the level of the DPOAE to estimate the SNR of the response. If no response is present, or if the noise is excessive, the noise floor and DPOAE will have similar levels.

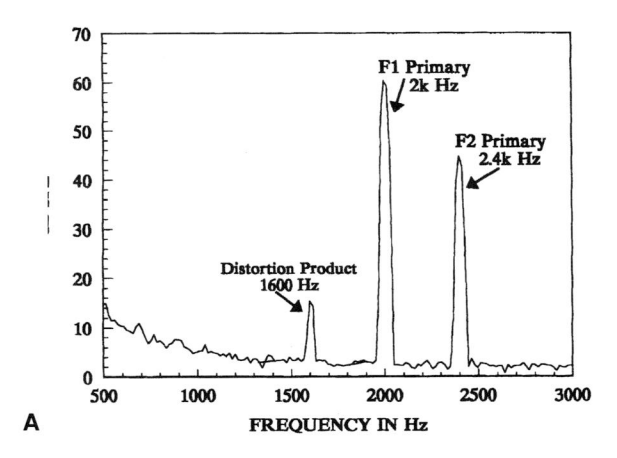

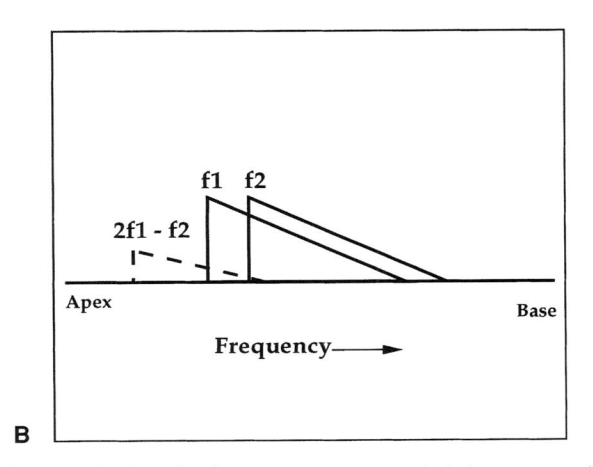

FIG. 11. A: Amplitude spectrum recorded from an adult showing two simultaneously presented primary tones at 2,000 and 2,400 Hz and the resulting DPOAE at $2f1 - f2$, 1,600 Hz. **B:** The hypothesized pattern of basilar membrane displacement during the generation of the $2f1 - f2$ DPOAE.

Distortion-Product Otoacoustic Emission Measurement and Evaluation

The probe assembly required to record DPOAEs includes a low-noise microphone and two receivers to present the primary tones. The receivers must have a fairly flat frequency response from about 200 to 10,000 Hz (67). The response recorded in the ear canal can be averaged in the time domain, spectral domain, or both, to improve the SNR. Spectral analysis is performed at $2f1 - f2$ and at the frequency of the two primaries to monitor the levels of the eliciting tones and measure the level of the DPOAE.

The amplitude of the DPOAE depends on two stimulus-related factors: (a) frequency separation between f1 and f2 and (b) stimulus level—both the absolute levels and level difference between the two stimulating tones. In general, the closer the frequency of the two primary tones, the more they interact on the basilar membrane. Conversely, as f1 and f2 are moved apart, their interaction becomes limited and the amplitude of the DPOAE is smaller. An optimal average frequency ratio of 1.22 has been found in human adults although this ratio varies slightly with primary tone frequency (70,71). A recent study verified that this frequency separation generally produces optimal amplitude DPOAE in newborn term infants as well (73).

Optimal level separation of the primary tones in both infants and adults (L1, L2) has been determined to be approximately 10 to 15 dB with L1 greater than L2 (70,72,73).

The absolute level of the primary tones is critical as well. If the clinical objective is to detect the presence of DPOAEs at any given frequency, the primary tones will be presented at suprathreshold levels. Default stimulus levels of up to 75 dB SPL are used by some clinical units. The clinician is typically attempting to use the optimal stimulus parameters (F2/F1 ratio and L1-L2 absolute level and level separation) to generate the most robust DPOAE. In other cases, it may be desirable to generate a DPOAE using a low-level stimulus to evaluate the growth rate and threshold of DPOAE amplitude.

Two clinical procedures for evaluation of DPOAEs have been described: (a) DP audiogram, and (b) DPOAE input/output function or growth test. The most common application is known as the DP audiogram. To generate a DP audiogram, primary tone levels are fixed and DPOAE amplitude is measured at various audiometric frequencies using parameters designed to evoke a robust response. However, because the level of the stimulus is not changed for measures at each frequency, as is done with standard audiometry, the term *audiogram* is somewhat misleading.

A DP audiogram for the left or right ear of a normally hearing subject is shown in Fig. 12A. The solid black area represents the noise floor plus 2 SDs. Any signal that rises above this noise floor is considered a response. Clinics must apply their own criteria, but a DPOAE at least 3 dB above the noise floor is typically considered a response (67). Lonsbury-Martin and Martin have designated an acceptable template for DPOAE response levels based on a large normative base of data, and they use these guidelines to evaluate the normalcy of DPOAE responses in their laboratory. The dark solid lines shown on Fig. 12A represent a template of normal DPOAE levels for adult subjects. Because the noise floor can change dramatically with equipment and recording environment, each testing site should generate its own normative standards.

The second measure used to evaluate DPOAE is the input/output (I/O) function or growth rate. To generate a DPOAE I/O function, one F2/F1 combination is presented while the level of the eliciting primary tones is varied between 25 and 85 dB SPL, typically in 5-dB steps. A DPOAE I/O function for F2 = 2000 Hz is shown in Fig. 12B. These functions provide information about DPOAE amplitude at both suprathreshold and threshold levels. The *DPOAE threshold* is defined as the lowest stimulus level at which the DPOAE is

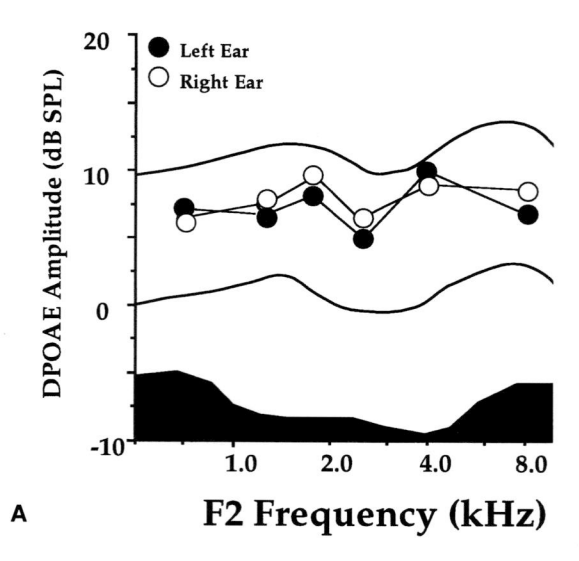

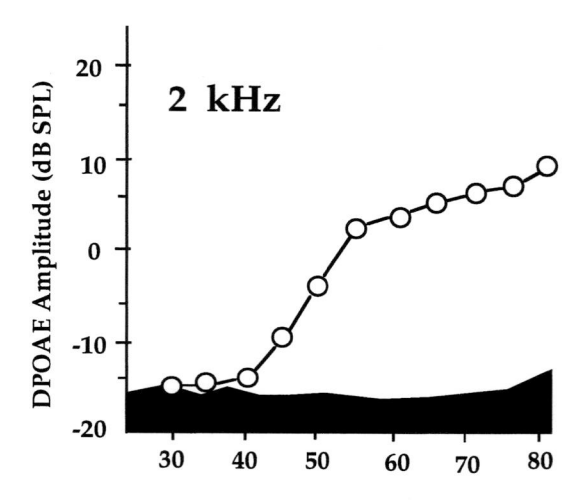

FIG. 12. A: Distortion-product audiogram for the right and left ear of an adult. The thick black lines represent the range of expected DPOAE amplitude for each F2 frequency and are based on data collected from a group of normal-hearing individuals. The black area on the bottom of the graph represents the noise floor + 2 SDs. The response is between 10 and 15 dB higher than the noise floor across all frequencies. **B:** A DPOAE input/output function or growth test for F2 = 2 kHz. The level of the primary tones is decreased in 5-dB steps until the amplitude of the DPOAE can no longer be distinguished from the noise floor.

clearly differentiated from the noise floor. This threshold value is influenced heavily by the level of the noise floor and the sensitivity of the instrumentation used (73) and considerable DPOAE threshold variability exists among normal hearing subjects. Lonsbury-Martin and Martin (67) found DPOAE detection thresholds at approximately 35 to 40 dB SPL for a group of normally hearing adults. Others have devised techniques to reduce the noise floor substantially and, consequently, lower the DPOAE threshold (74). At present, the relationship between pure-tone audiometric threshold and DPOAE threshold is not clearly understood.

The slope of the I/O function reflects the growth rate of DPOAE amplitude with stimulus level. This is another aspect of this graph that can be evaluated. Popelka et al. (74) reported that at low levels, DPOAE level grows approximately 1 dB for each 1-dB increase in the stimulus level in normal-hearing adults. At higher levels, response saturation occurs, and growth in DPOAE amplitude slows considerably or plateaus. It is not known, at present, how this slope value should be interpreted or applied in the identification of hearing impairment. This area warrants further investigation to evaluate clinical applicability.

OTOACOUSTIC EMISSIONS AND MIDDLE EAR FUNCTION

The objective of OAE testing is to assess cochlear/OHC function. To do this, however, it is necessary to rule out influence of the middle ear on the measurement, so that confounding factors do not interfere with cochlear evaluation. The status of the middle ear is critical to the measurement of OAEs (60,75,76). With middle ear pathology, OAEs may not be measurable because transmission of the evoking signal into the cochlea, as well as transmission of the OAE from the cochlea back to the ear canal, is attenuated as it travels through the dysfunctional middle ear system (60,75).

Few reports have carefully documented the effect of middle ear disease on OAEs in pediatric patients (75,77). The alteration in middle ear loading that occurs when middle ear fluid is present can prevent the detection of the OAE in most cases (60). Generally, if an air-bone gap is greater than 30 to 35 dB, an OAE will not be detected (78). The viscosity of the fluid in the middle ear may relate to the detection of OAEs. For example, low-level OAEs have been recorded when thin, watery liquid is present in the middle ear (75). In contrast, a recent investigation found that TEOAEs were absent in 100% of ten ears with mucoid effusion (77). In this same investigation, TEOAEs were present in nearly 90% of ears with serous otitis. These findings suggest that TEOAE absence may be related to the type of middle ear effusion rather than the simple presence of effusion (77).

The presence of negative or positive pressure, in the absence of middle ear effusion, can reduce emission energy and alter the spectral content of the response. Kemp, Ryan, and Bray (60) reported that emission energy below 2,000 Hz is reduced significantly, and, in some cases, energy above 3,000 Hz is also attenuated with abnormal pressure in the middle ear. Even small amounts of negative middle ear pressure (-100 daPa) can eliminate OAE detection (75). Otoacoustic emission results vary widely in patients that have had pressure equalization (PE) tubes inserted into the tympanic membrane. The presence of PE tubes appears to enhance low-frequency noise, making OAE detection impossible in this frequency range. At mid and high frequencies, the OAEs are often detectable in these patients, but they show reduced amplitude (75). The reason for this amplitude reduction is unclear, but it may relate to an increase in ear canal volume due to a patent PE tube and a subsequent reduction in stimulus level arriving at the cochlea.

Figure 13 displays the audiogram and OAE results of a 4-year-old child with serous otitis media in the right ear and relatively normal function in the left. A low-amplitude TEOAE is clearly present in the left ear, while no response is observed in the ear with middle ear disease. Likewise, the DP audiogram is below the normal range for the right ear, while the left ear DP audiogram falls within the normal template.

The effect of middle ear dysfunction on OAEs warrants thorough investigation because the pediatric population is particularly susceptible to this type of pathology (79), yet this is the very patient population that will benefit most from OAE evaluation. The existing data thus far suggest that the presence of middle ear effusion, specifically mucoid effusion, makes OAEs undetectable, and pressure abnormalities as well as the presence of PE tubes alter OAE amplitude and spectral content.

OTOACOUSTIC EMISSIONS IN INFANTS AND CHILDREN

Infants and children have the same prevalence of SOAEs as adults. Prevalence figures range from 38% to 62% (80–82), depending on how age categories are defined and other methodologic variables. Regardless of age, SOAEs are more prevalent in females and in right ears. Females also show bilateral SOAEs and multiple SOAE in the same ear more often than males for adults (83) or infants (81).

Although prevalence is comparable, differences have been observed between infant and/or child and adult SOAEs. Infant SOAEs occur at higher frequencies than adult. Adult SOAEs usually occur in the frequency range from 1,000 to 2,000 Hz, whereas infant responses are typically in the 3,000 to 4,500-Hz range (80–82,84–86). In addition, SOAEs from infants are generally greater in amplitude than SOAEs from adults (81,87). Most investigations of SOAE age effects have not distinguished between infants and young children; consequently, this age difference has not been adequately defined. The limited results available suggest that SOAE frequency and level appears to be adultlike by the time children reach the age of 5 to 7 years old (82).

Both TEOAEs (57,64,88–93) and DPOAEs (92,94–97) have been recorded with great success in infants. Elberling et al. and Don (64) reported present TEOAEs in 199 of 200 newborn ears. Others have reported similar prevalence figures. Response differences have been observed, however, between adult and infant OAEs. The overall level of both OAEs and DPOAEs from infants and young children is higher than levels measured in older children and adults (60,88,91,94,96). Healthy newborns tested in our laboratory have consistently shown DPOAEs that are 4 to 5 dB larger than adult responses for high-frequency stimuli

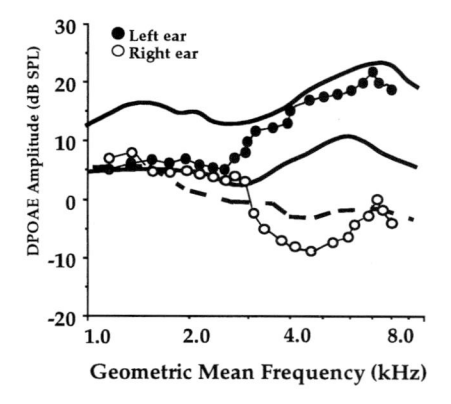

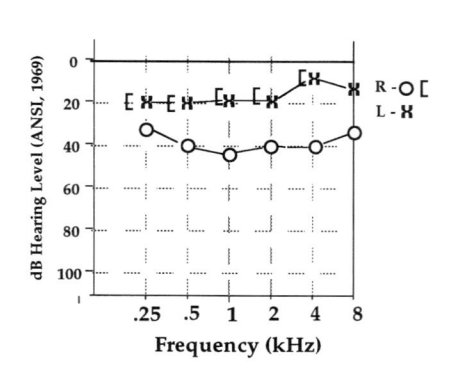

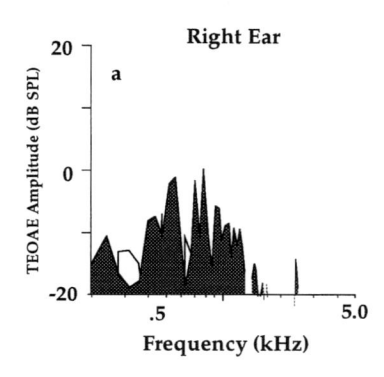

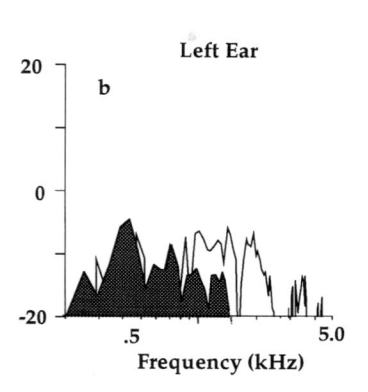

FIG. 13. The DP audiogram and TEOAE amplitude spectra for a 4-year-old child with serous otitis media in the right ear and a relatively normal-functioning left ear. The solid lines on the DP audiogram represent the range of normal DPOAE amplitude, and the dashed line represents the noise floor. Consistent with the pure-tone audiogram, the DP audiogram demonstrates abnormal DPOAEs in the right, while DPOAEs are within normal range for the left ear. The TEOAE amplitude spectra show an absent TEOAE on the right and present TEOAE in the normally functioning left ear. Adapted from JJ Owens, MJ McCoy, BL Lonsbury-Martin, GK Martin (1992): Influence of Otitis Media on Evoked Otoacoustic Emissions in Children. Seminars in Hearing 13(1): 53–66.

(3,000–6,000 Hz). Low- to mid-frequency DPOAEs appear to be more comparable between adults and infants, showing an average difference of 1.5 dB (95). Similarly, Prieve (98) reported mean TEOAE levels of 32.8 for 0 to 4-year-old subjects, compared to 14.6 to 16.5 dB SPL for 4- to 12-year-olds and 8.4 to 11.6 dB for young adults. Figure 14 displays TEOAE time waveforms from our laboratory showing comparable age trends.

Other studies have shown that as the age of the subject increases, the high-frequency spectral content in the response decreases (60,91). As a consequence of this decrease in high-frequency energy, the bandwidth of the response is also reduced with age. Infant TEOAEs tend to be present from 1,000 to 5,000 Hz with almost equal energy at each frequency band. Adult responses are less flat and full and have notches of decreased or absent energy at discrete frequency regions (60). Figure 15 displays TEOAE spectra from a healthy neonate and a normal-hearing adult for comparison.

The DP audiogram recorded from healthy neonates is also generally flatter than the adult DP audiogram (95). The adult DP audiogram consistently shows a dip in DPOAE amplitude between 1,000 and 3,000 Hz, while infants show fewer dips; if dips occur, they are present at higher frequencies than the adult response. Smurzynski et al. (97), for example, reported a trough or dip between 3,400 and 4,000 Hz in the

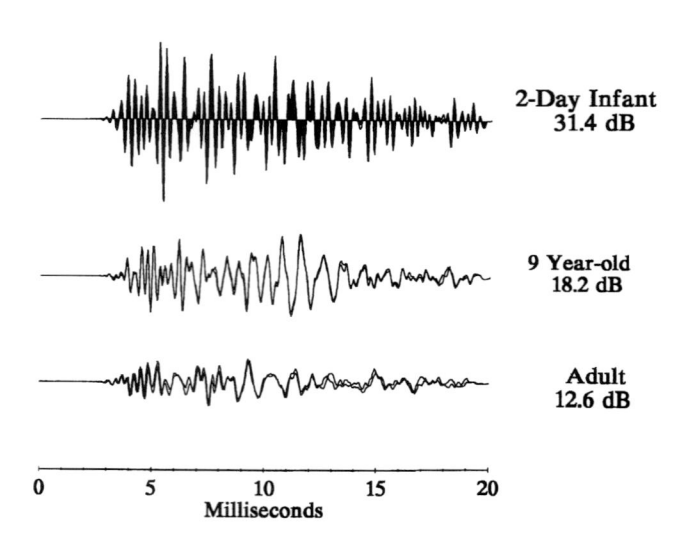

FIG. 14. A TEOAE time waveform for a healthy neonate, a 9-year-old child, and an adult. Amplitude of the response progressively decreases with age. From YS Sininger (1993): Clinical Applications of Otoacoustic Emissions. Advances in Otolaryngology-Head and Neck Surgery 7:247–269.

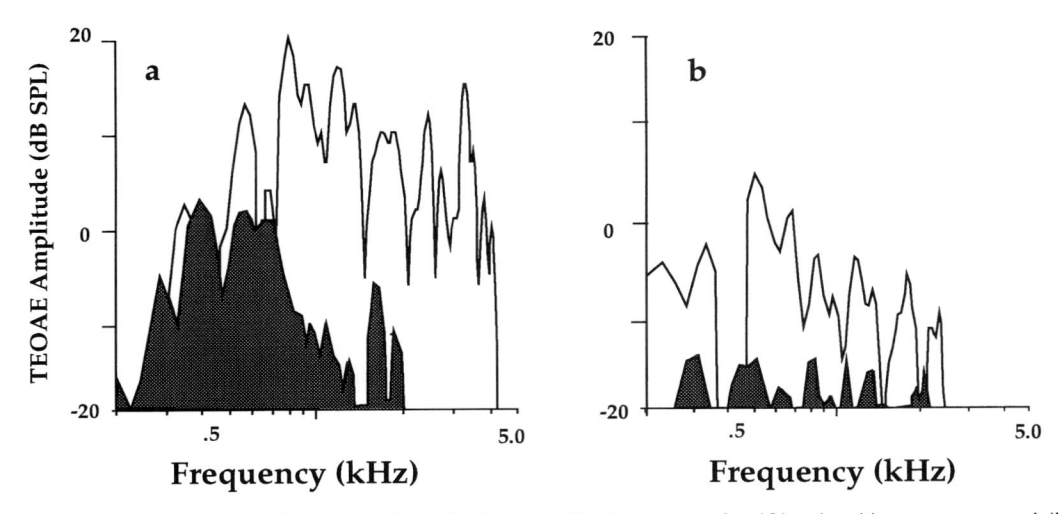

FIG. 15. Transient-evoked otoacoustic emission amplitude spectra for (**A**) a healthy neonate and (**B**) a normal-hearing adult. The infant response is present and robust from 500 to 5,000 Hz. The adult response is also present but is lower-level and narrower in bandwidth, showing a response through approximately 2,800 Hz. The adult TEOAE also has more notches or frequency regions of absent or diminished response.

DP audiogram of neonates. Figure 16 displays DP audiograms from a healthy neonate, a 6-year-old child and a 34-year-old adult. In contrast to the DP audiogram, DPOAE I/O functions from premature neonates appear to be comparable to adult functions in slope and shape (99).

The reason for the large OAE amplitudes and increased high-frequency contribution in infants and young children is not clear. Differences in infant and adult outer and middle ear resonance may contribute (100–103). The smaller volume of the ear canal in the infant and the resonance characteristics may provide additional gain in the high-frequency region (104). Also, the infant middle ear demonstrates lower compliance, and resistance is higher, contributing to relatively poor power transfer into the infant middle ear (100,101). These differences in the conductive mechanism of infants and adults may contribute to the OAE age differences reported. Cochlear immaturity may also account for some differences between OAEs recorded from infants and adults; however, several investigations of cochlear morphology and physiology suggest that the human cochlea is basically mature at birth (72,80,94,105–108).

HEARING LOSS PREDICTION FROM OTOACOUSTIC EMISSIONS

Hearing Loss and Cochlear Pathology

Otoacoustic emissions reflect processes in a normally functioning cochlea in response only to low- or moderate-level stimuli. When cochlear damage causes hearing impair-

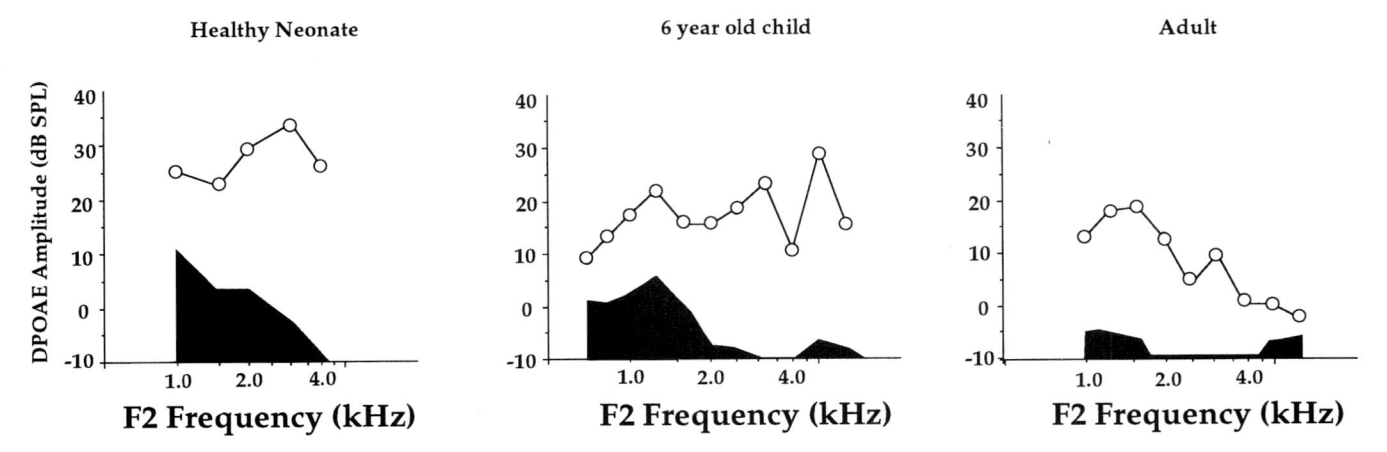

FIG. 16. Distortion-product audiograms for a healthy neonate, a normally hearing 6-year-old child, and a 34-year-old adult. Amplitude of the response progressively decreases with age, and the high-frequency components become less prominent.

ment in the moderate-to-profound range, emissions will be absent and are of little or no use in predicting actual hearing level, other than to confirm that a significant loss may be present. It is not clear exactly how much cochlear damage or hearing loss will obliterate an OAE. Estimates range from 20 to 50 dB as an upper limit of hearing loss before OAEs are obliterated (48,65,78,88,109,110). Differences appear to exist between DPOAEs and TEOAEs with respect to the amount of hearing loss tolerated. An example of this difference is shown for patient DC, in the case study section at the end of this chapter. This patient has present DPOAEs and absent TEOAEs with a mild, relatively flat sensorineural hearing loss (SNHL).

In the current state of the art, OAEs are often used in a categorical fashion to identify hearing impairment. That is, if they are present, cochlear function is considered normal, or, at most, a mild hearing loss may exist. If they are not present, hearing loss may range from moderate to profound. As mentioned earlier, when OAEs are absent, it is not possible to describe the hearing loss with precision based only on these results. For this reason, the absence of an OAE must be combined with additional information, such as patient history, behavioral testing, and click and tone burst ABR testing, in order to estimate auditory thresholds.

Transient-Evoked Otoacoustic Emissions and Hearing Loss

Few studies have systematically examined the effects of hearing loss on TEOAE in children. Kemp (48) initially reported that TEOAEs are absent in adults with hearing losses of greater than 30 dB HL. Bray and Kemp (88) found that all of their 79 subjects, ranging in age from 6 weeks to 13 years, had detectable TEOAEs if their hearing loss was less than 20 dB HL. In neonates, the upper limit of cochlear hearing loss that can coexist with a TEOAE appears to be approximately 40 dB (111,112). Several investigators have found 40 dB to be the upper limit of hearing loss for recording TEOAEs at 1,000 Hz, and 35 dB the upper limit if using a mean audiometric threshold at 500, 1,000, 2,000, and 4,000

Hz (65,109,110). These findings are dependent on stimulus level. If higher level stimuli are used to elicit the emission (≥85 dB SPL), TEOAEs may be measurable in patients with up to 40 to 50 dB of hearing loss (78).

TEOAEs can be present in frequency regions where cochlear sensitivity is normal and absent where it is not (60,110,113). Also, in some cases, depending on the nature of the pathology, TEOAEs may be able to track the progress of a fluctuating hearing loss. Hinz and Von Wedel (114) evaluated five patients with sudden SNHL of unknown etiology. Transient-evoked otoacoustic emissions were absent following the onset of hearing loss, but after recovery of hearing, they were detected in all five patients.

Noise-induced high-frequency hearing loss is associated with a reduced incidence of TEOAEs (110). When individuals with noise-induced hearing loss (NIHL) were compared to individuals with comparable hearing loss of other etiologies, the spectral peaks of the TEOAEs were more sparse in the group with NIHL. It has been suggested that TEOAE testing may be able to identify subclinical OHC loss before audiometric thresholds reflect this damage (73).

Distortion-Product Otoacoustic Emissions and Hearing Loss

Distortion-product otoacoustic emissions are absent when hearing loss due to cochlear etiology is 45 to 50 dB or greater (67,115,116). The DP audiogram has proven useful in estimating audiometric configuration (67,117). Researchers at the Miami Ear Institute report that the frequency pattern of DPOAE amplitude reduction or absence often follows the configuration of hearing loss in the audiogram, as shown in Fig. 17.

Predicting audiometric configuration in infants and children from DP audiograms has not been systematically studied or described, but Lonsbury-Martin and Martin (67) have presented various case studies showing promising results and possible application to pediatric diagnosis. For example, they report a 6-year-old patient with progressive high-frequency SNHL. The DP audiogram was grossly able to

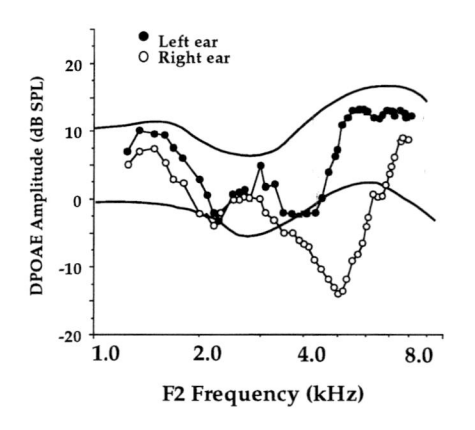

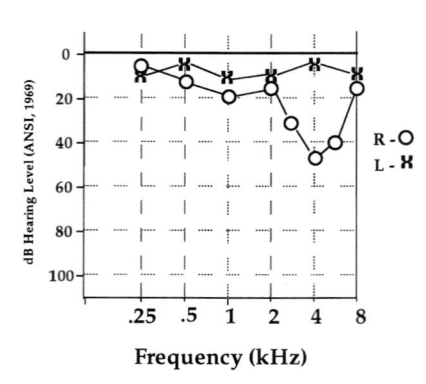

FIG. 17. A DP audiogram for an individual with mild-to-moderate high-frequency SNHL in the right ear and normal hearing in the left. The DP audiogram for the left ear is within the range of normal. The contour of the DP audiogram on the right follows the pure-tone audiogram for that ear and is clearly below normal levels, between 3,000 and 6,000 Hz. Adapted from BL Lonsbury-Martin and GK Martin (1990): The Clinical Utility of Distortion Product Otoacoustic Emissions. Ear and Hearing 11(2):144–154.

predict the shape and threshold of this child's behavioral audiogram. The DPOAE I/O function recorded from the child's normal-hearing sibling also showed an abnormal pattern of response amplitude, suggesting that DPOAEs may provide prognostic information in cases of subclinical cochlear dysfunction (67). However, this potential application of DPOAE data has not been systematically studied.

The DP audiogram can also be useful for tracking changes in fluctuating hearing loss and has successfully reflected glycerol-induced changes in hearing in Meniere's patients (67). Lonsbury-Martin and Martin, for example, described a case in which audiometric thresholds actually worsened postglycerol in one subject. The corresponding DPOAE amplitude also decreased to reflect this threshold change.

Low- to moderate-level DPOAEs have been shown to be vulnerable to ototoxic drugs in animals (73,78,118) and may also prove effective for monitoring auditory status during administration of ototoxic drugs in humans (67). Recent reports are promising. Hotz, Harris, and Probst (119) monitored cochlear status in nine patients receiving aminoglycoside treatment. They observed a reversible reduction in TEOAE level after 16 days of treatment in most of their patients. Others have reported that OAEs are clearly affected by aspirin intake (120,121). One report found that, in guinea pigs, DPOAE changes occurred before actual changes in hair cell morphology (122). This suggests that OAE evaluation may be an effective method for the early identification of ototoxic effects and the possible prevention of permanent hearing loss. Continued research is needed in this promising area. The use of OAEs to monitor auditory status in pediatric patients taking ototoxic medication may prove to be a powerful application.

Otoacoustic emission testing has also been recommended as an initial neonatal screen, followed by a second-stage screening with ABR (78). Several large-scale projects are currently ongoing in the United States and Europe investigating the utility of OAEs as screening tools for hearing loss prior to discharge from the hospital nursery (93,123,124). Neonatal hearing screening is discussed in greater depth in another chapter.

OTOACOUSTIC EMISSIONS AND SITE OF LESION TESTING

Both TEOAEs and DPOAEs are typically present in ears with hearing loss due to retrocochlear disorders (58,67). In patients with acoustic neuromas, the factor determining the absence or presence of OAEs appears to be whether the vascular supply to the cochlea is interrupted (67,73,125).

The use of OAEs in children, combined with the ABR, can aid in site of lesion testing. Otoacoustic emissions are useful in assessing cochlear function, specifically OHC integrity, while the ABR is useful in evaluating VIIIth nerve, as well as brainstem auditory pathway function. If OAEs and ABRs are present with normal click and tone burst thresholds, a clinician may conclude that the child has a normally functioning cochlea, auditory nerve, and brainstem auditory pathway. In the absence of a specific cortical deficit, this combination of findings would indicate normal signal transduction and conduction through the auditory system.

If OAEs are normal and no ABR is present in a pediatric patient, this set of findings may indicate a lesion central to the OHC. It is not possible to distinguish between IHC, spiral ganglion, VIIIth nerve, or brainstem pathology with this result, but an VIIIth nerve tumor is not likely in pediatric patients. This type of auditory neuropathy has been described in a growing population of children and is currently being studied by various audiologic centers (126–128). These children also demonstrate absent acoustic reflexes and, occasionally, fluctuating audiometric thresholds. It is likely that this type of pathology has existed with similar prevalence during the last 20 to 30 years, but the tools to observe cochlear function independent of neural function in the human auditory system were not widely used. The ability to diagnose this auditory neuropathy poses new problems related to the development of appropriate rehabilitation for neurally deaf children (127).

If middle ear conduction is normal, OAEs are absent and the ABR shows an elevated click-evoked threshold at 50 to 60 dB HL bilaterally, a moderate to moderate-to-severe SNHL is likely. As discussed previously, the absence of OAEs, without ABR data, indicates that hearing loss is at least moderate level (if middle ear function is normal). Using the OAE alone, it is not possible to estimate auditory thresholds, but in combination with the click- and tone burst–evoked ABR, audiometry thresholds can be estimated. These two tools, together, can offer a comprehensive picture of hearing loss and auditory pathology. Clinics will often screen a patient with OAEs. If they are normal and robust, it may be unnecessary to perform an ABR. However, if they are not present or if they are of low amplitude, an ABR will be performed to estimate auditory thresholds. Finally, if OAEs are absent and the tympanogram is flat or shows negative pressure, there is a confounding factor that needs to be eliminated before relying on these results to define cochlear status.

CASE STUDIES OF AUDITORY BRAINSTEM RESPONSE AND OTOACOUSTIC EMISSIONS APPLIED TO A PEDIATRIC POPULATION

JF is a 2-year, 10-month-old developmentally delayed boy. He was hospitalized at 5 months of age with sepsis and respiratory arrest. He currently has chronic otitis media and is functioning at an 18-month-old level with a limited, single-word vocabulary. Because of the developmental delay, he was unable to condition for either visual reinforcement or play audiometry. Consequently, an ABR/OAE evaluation was conducted to rule out hearing loss as a contributing factor to his speech and language delay.

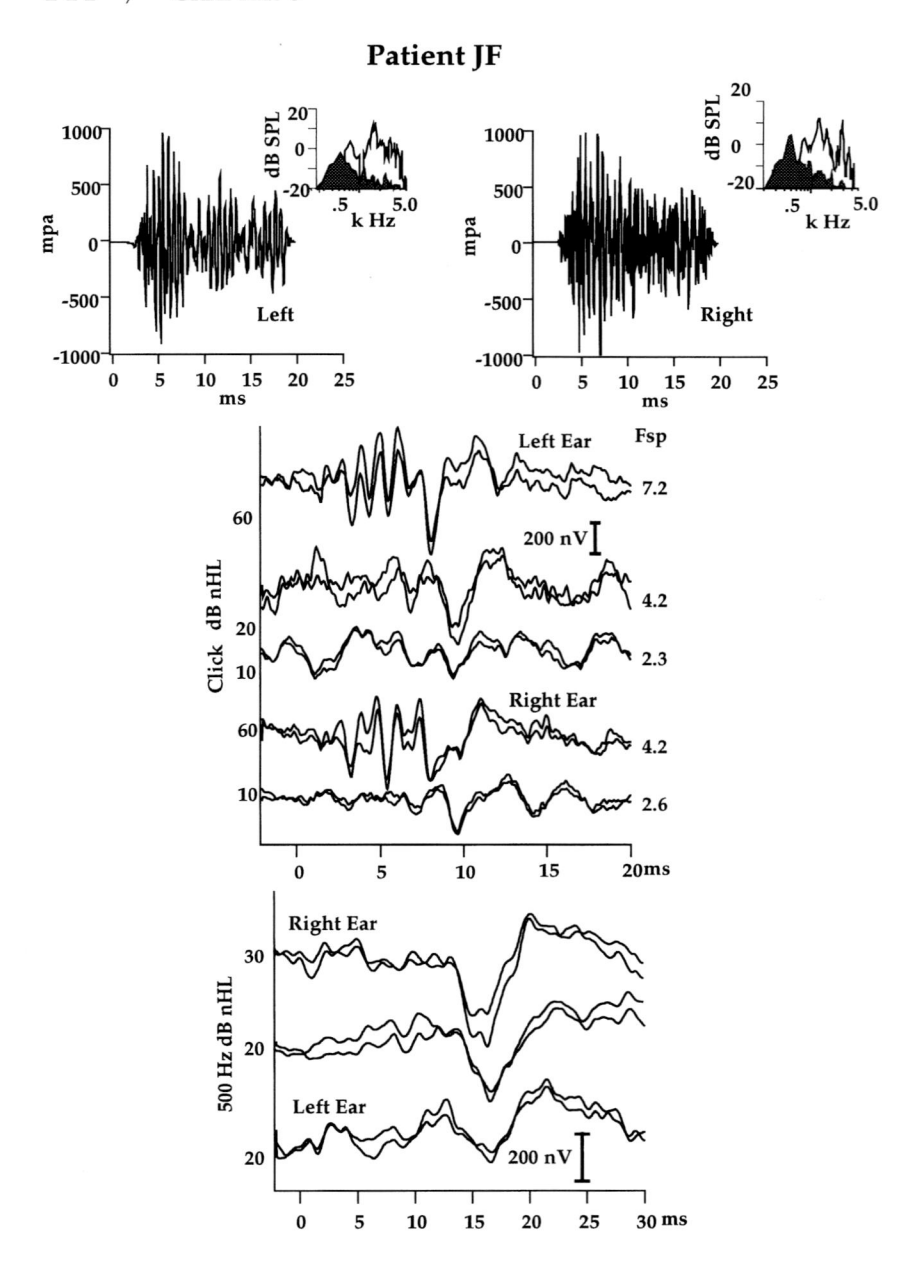

FIG. 18. JF results.

ABR Results: Test results are shown in Fig. 18. morphology. Click-evoked ABRs were seen at 10 dB HL bilaterally, with excellent morphology and robust amplitude; 500-Hz ABRs were observed at 20 dB HL bilaterally, with excellent morphology.

TEOAE Results: Transient-evoked OAEs were present and robust bilaterally with click stimulation of 84 dB SPL.

Impression: The ABR is consistent with normal hearing in low- and high-frequency ranges; 500-Hz tone burst thresholds are expected to be 15 to 20 dB above the actual behavioral threshold for that frequency. Present TEOAEs combined with normal ABR thresholds suggest normal hearing sensitivity bilaterally. These results illustrate a completely normal evaluation, with excellent ABR and OAE responses.

Audiogram: An audiogram on JF had not been obtained yet. The patient is scheduled to return to the CARE Center for behavioral audiometric testing to confirm physiologic tests.

BM is a 4-year-old boy with speech and language delay. His medical history is positive for three to four cases of otitis media and upper respiratory problems, such as asthma and bronchitis. He was referred to the clinic by an otolaryngologist for ABR/OAE testing to rule out hearing loss as a contributing factor to his speech and language delay. (Note: At this age, it would have been more appropriate to refer for

Patient BM

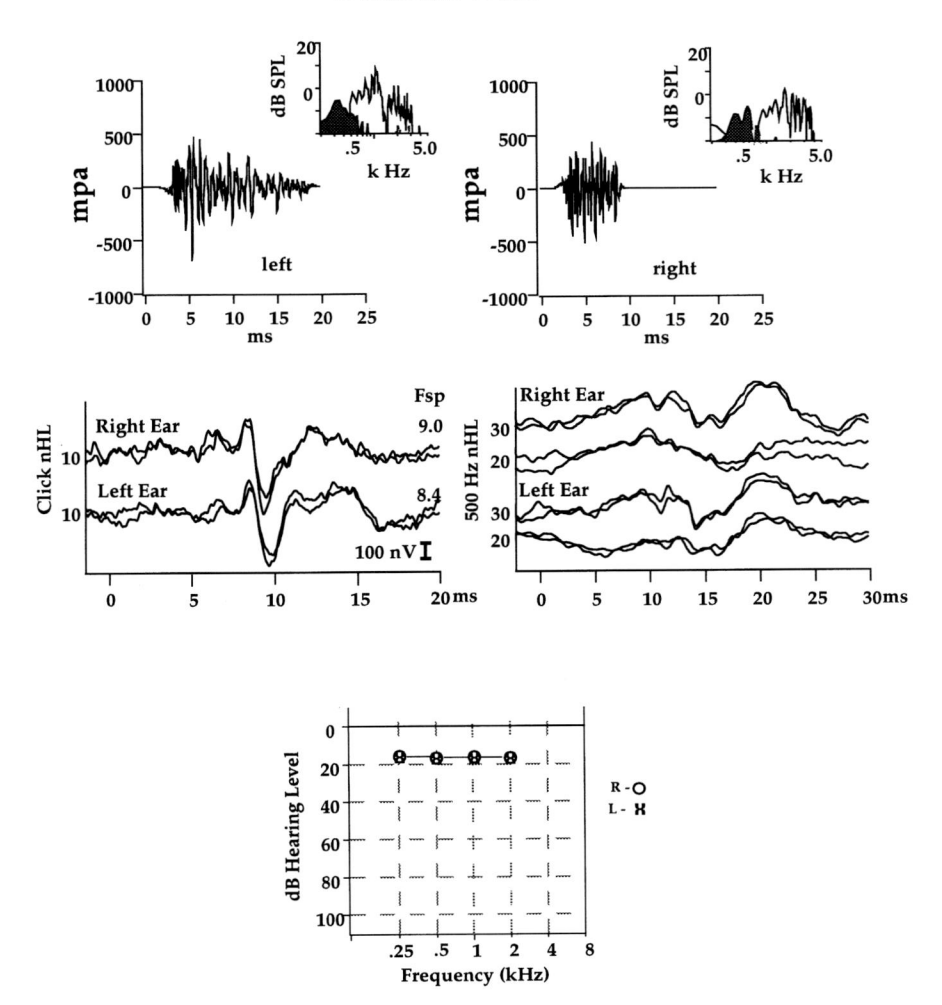

FIG. 19. BM results.

behavioral audiometry, but results are used here to illustrate a normal finding).

ABR Results: Test results are presented in Fig. 19. Click-evoked ABRs were seen at 10 dB HL in both the right and left ears. Response morphology was excellent, with robust amplitude; 500 Hz tone burst–evoked ABRs were clearly present at 20 dB HL bilaterally.

TEOAE Results: Transient-evoked OAEs were present and robust, with click stimulation between 83 and 86 dB SPL bilaterally.

Impressions: The ABR is consistent with normal hearing in the low- and high-frequency ranges. 500-Hz tone burst thresholds are typically obtained 15 to 20 dB above the actual behavioral threshold for this frequency. Present TEOAEs, combined with normal ABR thresholds, suggest normal hearing sensitivity bilaterally.

Subsequent Audiogram: An air-conduction audiometric screen was conducted 2 weeks after the initial ABR/OAE evaluation to verify normal hearing. BM responded at 15 dB HL from 500 to 8,000 Hz.

KM is a 2½-year-old girl with chronic otitis media. Pressure equalization tubes were inserted 1 year ago. Visual reinforcement and conditioned-play audiometry have been attempted repeatedly with little success. This child's speech is highly unintelligible, and the mother reports poor receptive skills as well. Because various attempts at behavioral audiometry had not been successful, she was referred for an ABR/OAE evaluation to estimate hearing sensitivity.

ABR Results: Results are shown in Fig. 20. Click-evoked ABRs were present at 10 dB HL bilaterally, with excellent morphology and robust amplitude. Responses were obtained only in the C_2–C_7 channel.

TEOAE Results: Transient-evoked OAEs were present bilaterally, with click stimulation of 80 to 82 dB SPL. Reduced high-frequency spectral content was observed.

DPOAE Results: Distortion-product OAEs were present from 1,000 to 6,000 Hz bilaterally, with pure tone stimuli of 70/55 dB SPL.

Impressions: The ABR is consistent with normal auditory thresholds in the 2- to 4-kHz range. Present transient and

Patient KM

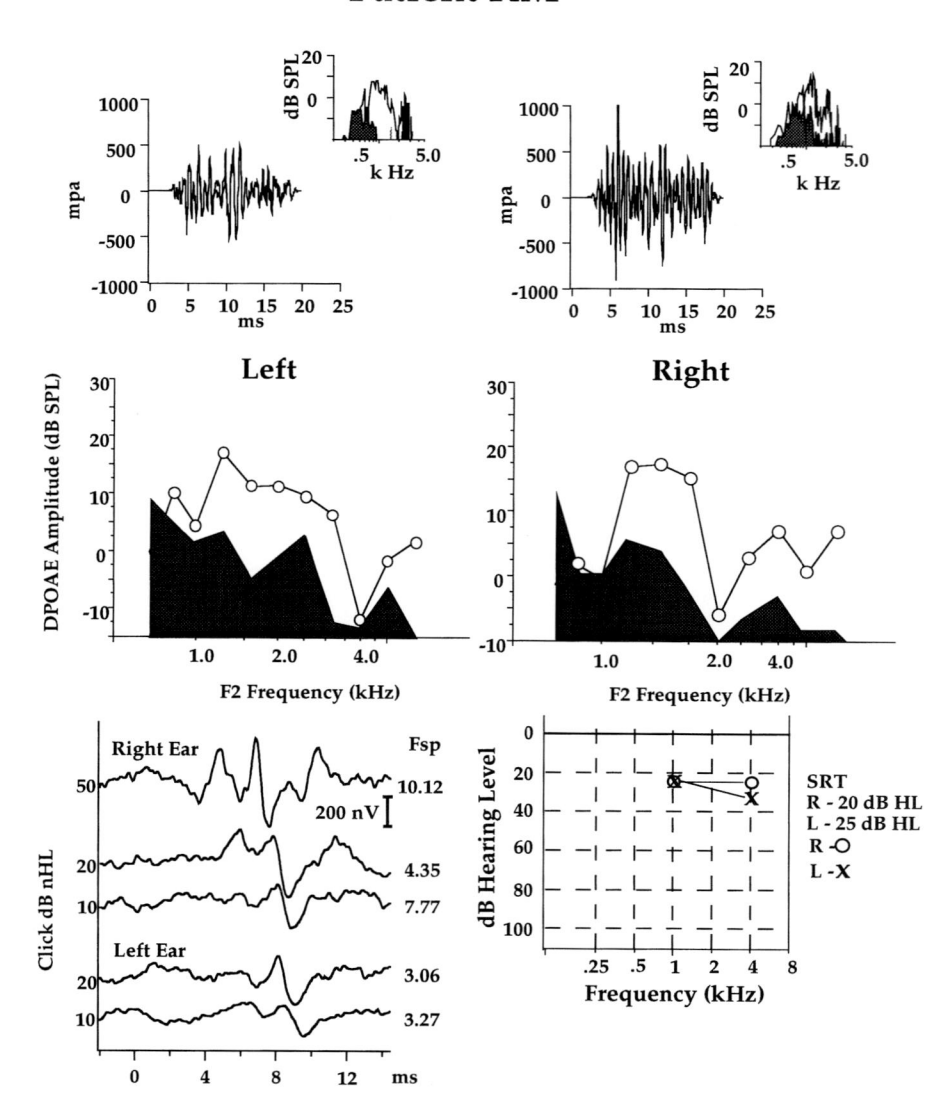

FIG. 20. KM results.

distortion-product OAEs from 1,000 to 6,000 Hz, combined with the ABR thresholds, are consistent with normal cochlear function and hearing sensitivity bilaterally. The fairly low-level TEOAEs and reduced high-frequency spectral content may be due to the presence of PE tubes.

Behavioral responses continue be very difficult to condition in this child; therefore, physiologic tests have been important for establishing normal hearing sensitivity.

Subsequent Audiogram: A limited audiogram was obtained 2 months following ABR/OAE evaluation using visual reinforcement audiometry under earphones. The patient had speech reception thresholds of 20 and 25 dB HL for the right and left ears respectively. Thresholds for 1,000 and 4,000 Hz were between 25 and 30 dB HL.

DC is a 6-year-old boy with previously confirmed hearing loss. He was referred to the CARE Center for a complete hearing aid evaluation and fitting. A repeat audiogram and OAE testing were conducted prior to hearing aid evaluation. Results are shown in Fig. 21.

TEOAE Results: Transient-evoked OAEs were absent bilaterally, with click stimulation of 87 dB SPL.

DPOAE Results: A DP audiogram revealed low- to moderate-level responses in the mid- (1,500–2,400 Hz) and high- (4,000–6,000 Hz) frequency regions bilaterally. DPOAE I/O function at 6,000 Hz revealed DPOAE thresholds of 55 for the right ear and 65 for the left ear.

Audiogram: Mild- to borderline-moderate SNHL, left slightly worse than right in the mid- to high-frequency range.

Impressions: Transient-evoked otoacoustic emissions were not measurable in the presence of mild SNHL. Distortion-product otoacoustic emissions were present bilaterally but at reduced levels. The DPOAE threshold obtained from the 6,000-Hz I/O function was 10 dB better in the right

Patient DC

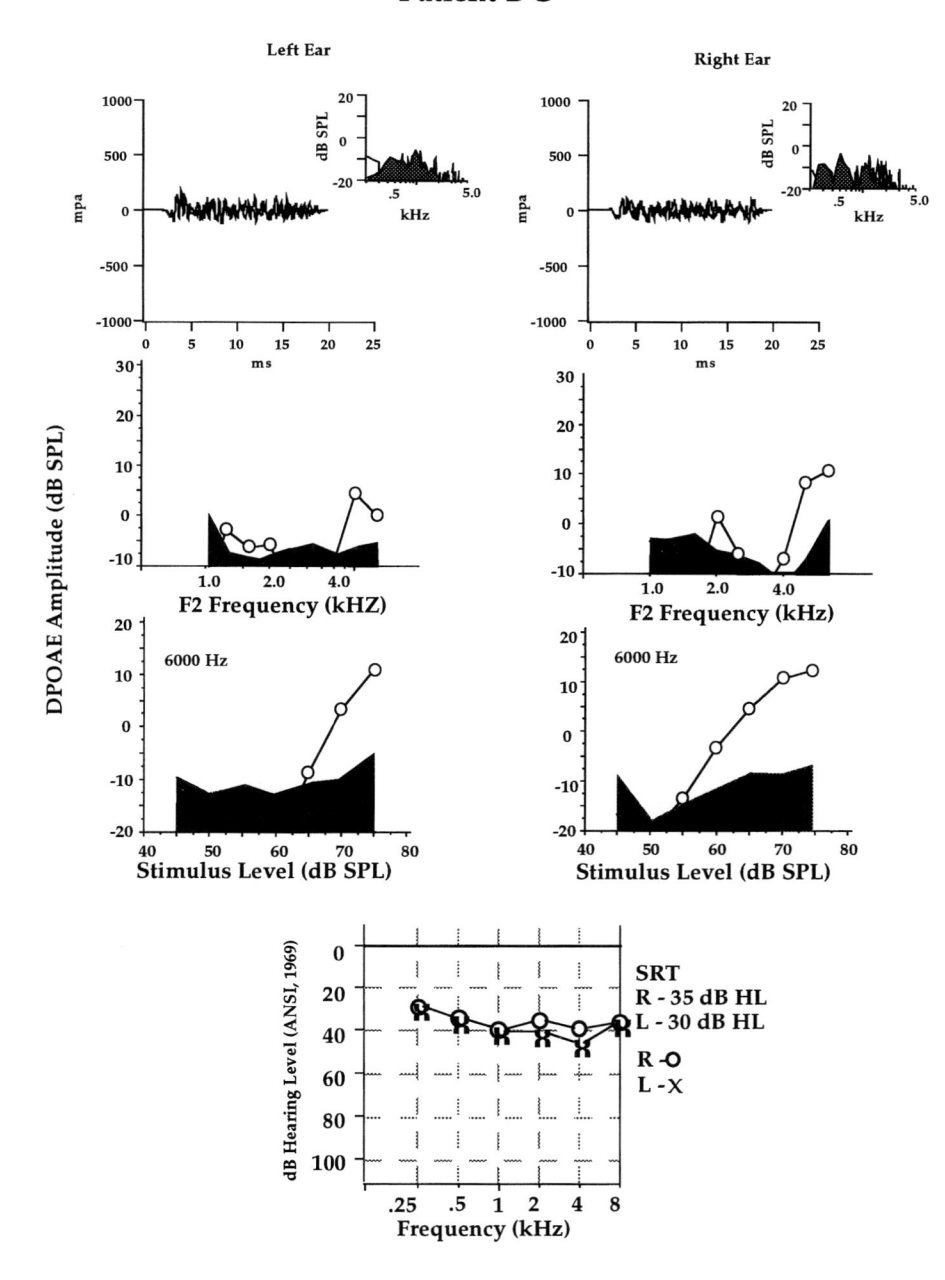

FIG. 21. DC results.

ear. This is consistent with slightly better audiometric thresholds at 6,000 Hz for the right ear.

EA is a 1-month-old boy with two older congenitally hearing-impaired siblings. He was evaluated with ABR/OAE testing because of this high-risk factor for hearing loss. He was tested without sedation and slept only 20 minutes, thus limiting the auditory evaluation.

ABR Results: Results are shown in Fig. 22. Click-evoked ABR thresholds were 40 dB HL bilaterally.
TEOAE Results: Transient-evoked OAEs were absent bilaterally, with click stimulation of 86 to 87 dB SPL.
Impressions: The ABR is consistent with a mild-to-moderate hearing loss bilaterally. Auditory brainstorm response morphology is abnormal and response latency is extended. Long latency may reflect the apical generation of the response from 500- or 1,000-Hz regions. We are always cautious about labeling peaks when using ABR for audiometric purposes. Cochlear loss will often create abnormal waveform morphology in the ABR. Therefore, we use consistent response detection as our threshold predictor, rather than simply wave V detection or latency. The absence of TEOAEs bilaterally is consistent with hearing loss greater than 35 to 40 dB HL.
Subsequent Audiogram: An audiogram was obtained using visual reinforcement audiometry with insert phones at 6

Patient EA

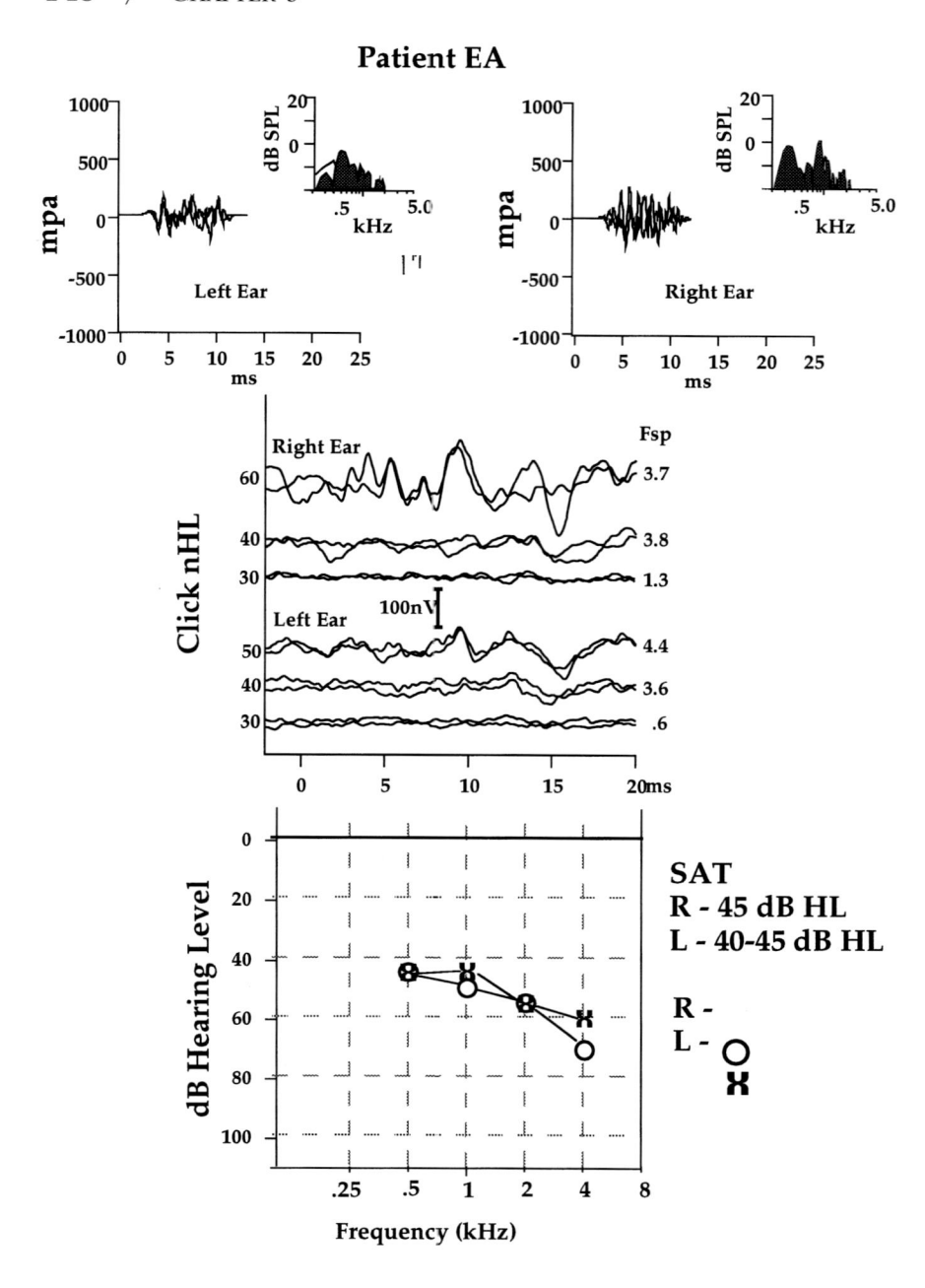

FIG. 22. EA results.

months of age. This audiogram showed a moderate sloping to moderate-to-severe SNHL bilaterally. Binaural AGC BTE hearing aids with compression were fit. The patient will return for a repeat hearing test and hearing aid check in 6 weeks.

HF is a 2 year, 9-month-old girl. Previous sound field visual reinforcement audiometry had indicated mild-to-moderate hearing loss in the better ear. Ear-specific thresholds could not be obtained. Her parents reported that she has hearing difficulty and responds only to loud sounds. Speech is delayed slightly. Because behavioral results suggested hearing loss but were limited, ABR/OAE evaluation was conducted to assess hearing sensitivity in each ear.

ABR Results: Results are shown in Fig. 23. Click-evoked ABR thresholds were 45 in the right ear and 50 in the left ear. Auditory brainstorm response thresholds for 500-Hz toneburst stimuli were 60 dB in the right ear and 50 dB in the left.

TEOAE Results: Transient-evoked OAEs were absent bilaterally, with click stimulation of 86 dB SPL.

Impressions: Auditory brainstorm response is consistent with relatively flat, moderate SNHL bilaterally; TEOAE

Patient HF

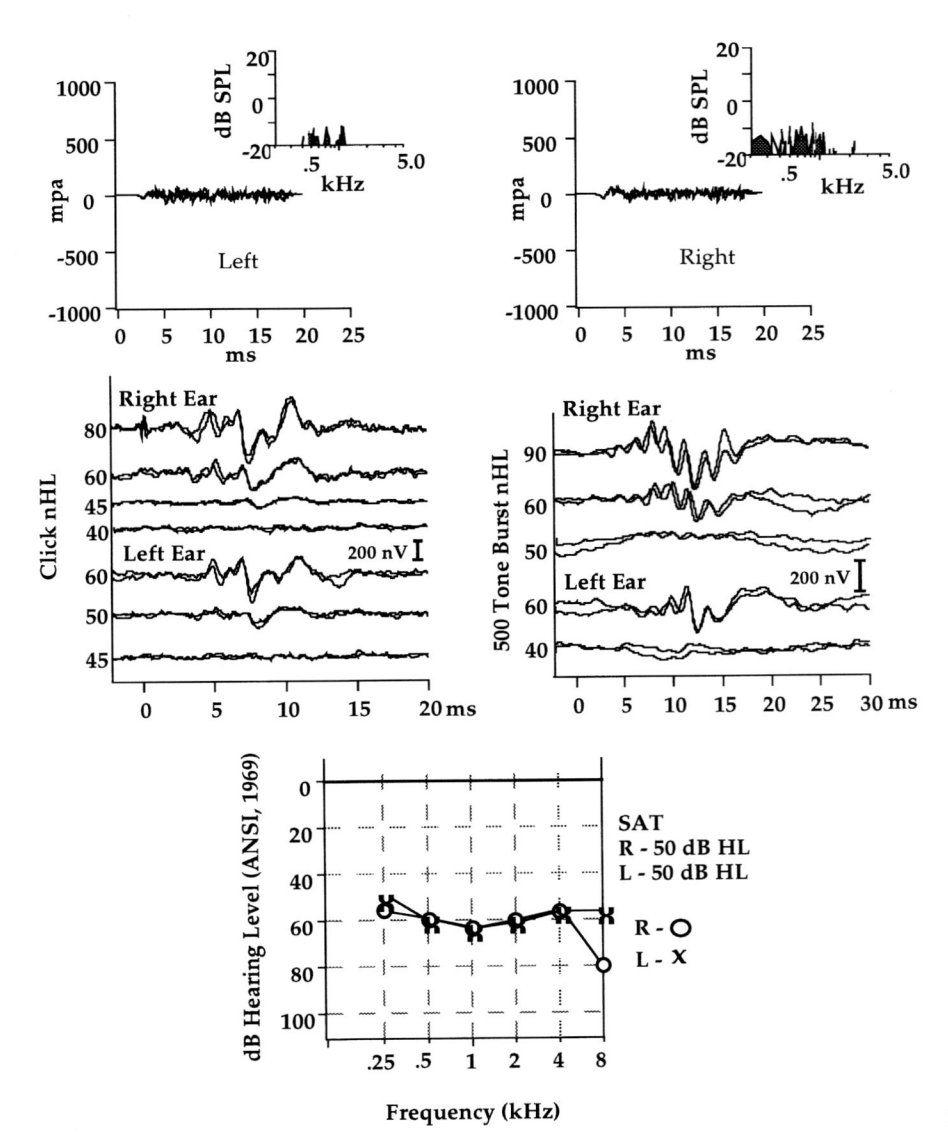

FIG. 23. HF results.

results are consistent with hearing loss greater than 35 to 40 dB HL.

Subsequent Audiogram: A full audiogram was obtained 1 month following ABR/OAE evaluation and revealed a moderate-to-severe 50- to 60-dB HL SNHL from 250 to 4,000 Hz bilaterally.

KF is a 2-year, 4-month-old girl born with a heart defect and unilateral repaired cleft lip and palate. She has a history of otitis media with PE insertion at 2 months of age. She is delayed in speech and language, with only a one- to two-word vocabulary at present. Because behavioral responses to auditory stimuli were not reliable, an ABR/OAE evaluation was conducted to assess hearing sensitivity.

ABR Results: Test results are shown in Fig. 24. Click-evoked ABR thresholds were 70 dB HL in both right and left ears. Given the history of middle ear disease, an unmasked bone-conduction ABR was also performed to confirm the sensorineural nature of the loss. The ABR bone-conduction threshold was 60 dB HL.
TEOAE Results: Transient-evoked OAEs were absent bilaterally, with click stimulation of 83 dB SPL
DPOAE Results: Distortion-product OAEs were absent bilaterally, with pure-tone stimuli at 70/55 dB SPL.
Impressions: The click-evoked ABR is consistent with a moderately severe SNHL bilaterally. The OAEs are consistent with this finding because they are expected to be absent in the presence of hearing loss greater than 35 to 45 dB.

Patient KF

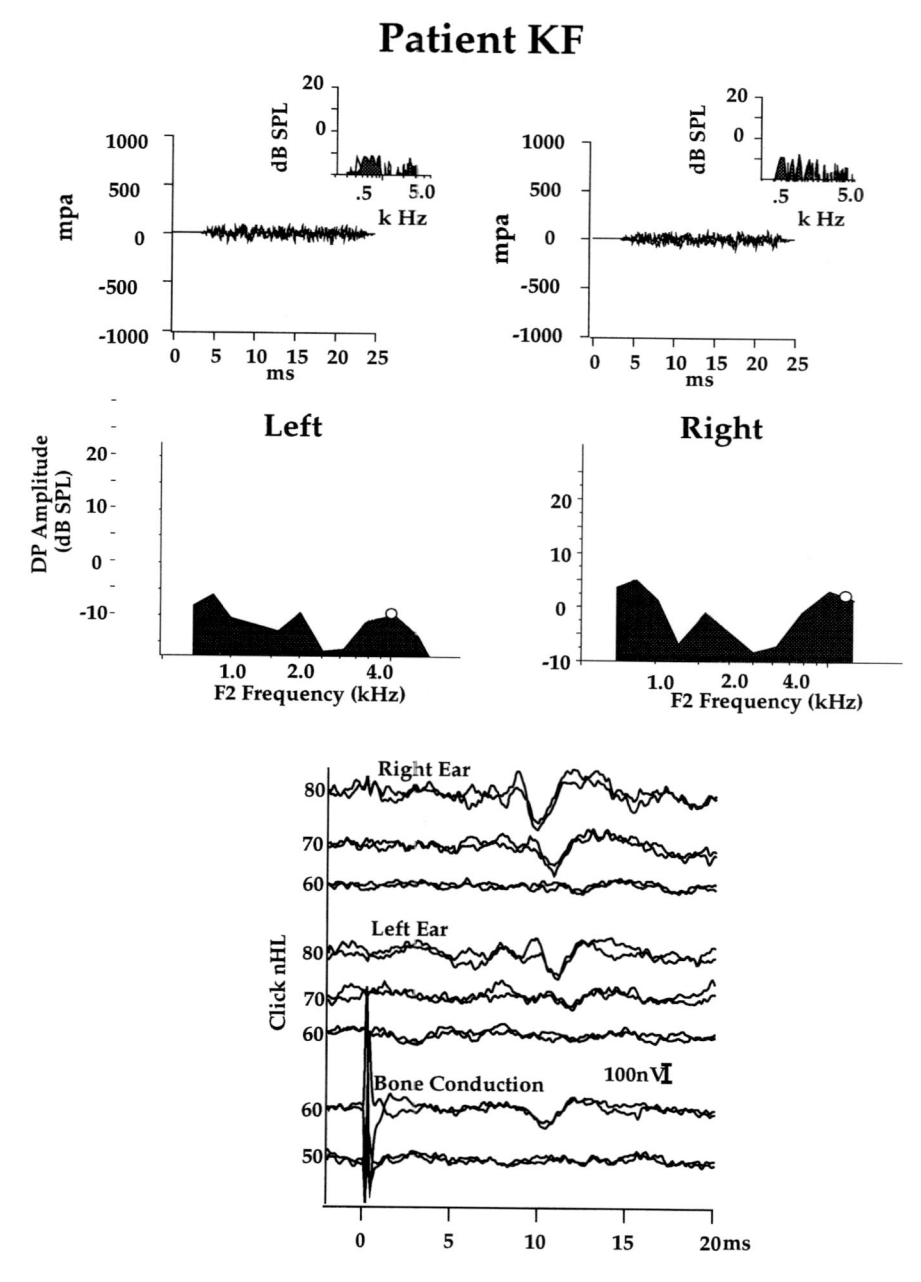

FIG. 24. KF results.

 This case shows the usefulness of bone-conducted ABR to distinguish conductive from SNHL. Conductive loss was suspected due to the presence of cleft palate. An air-bone gap of no more than 10 to 15 dB may exist in this patient.

Audiogram: No audiogram was obtained at the CARE Center because this patient was followed at another clinic closer to her home.

 JG is a 12-year-old boy with normal speech and language development and IQ but very poor school performance. He is suspected of having attention deficit disorder. There is evidence of multiple CNS disorders, including optic atrophy with progressively decreased vision, absent deep tendon reflexes, and lateral gaze nystagmus. He was referred to the CARE Center for a complete evaluation of auditory function.

ABR Results: Results are shown in Fig. 25. Click-evoked ABRs were absent bilaterally at 90 dB HL.

TEOAE Results: Transient-evoked otoacoustic emissions were present bilaterally, with click stimulation of 84 dB SPL.

Audiogram: The audiogram shows a moderate to moderate-to-severe low-frequency SNHL rising to borderline normal hearing in the mid and high frequencies bilaterally.

Impressions: This child appears to have normal cochlear function, at least through the OHC system. Absent ABRs suggest pathology central to the cochlea.

Patient JG

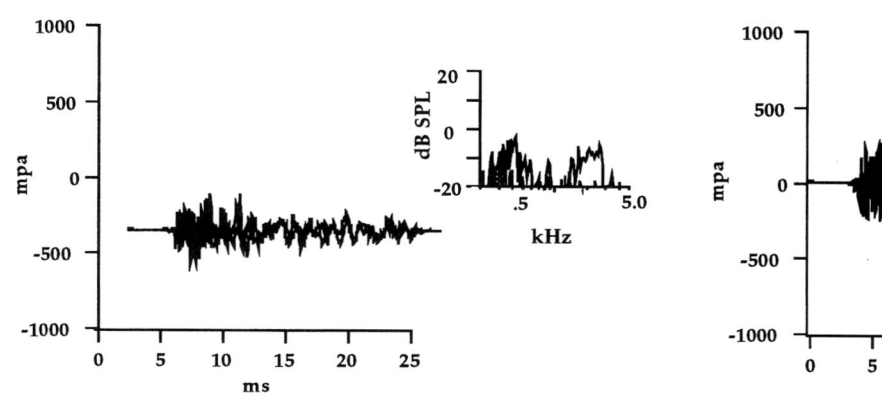

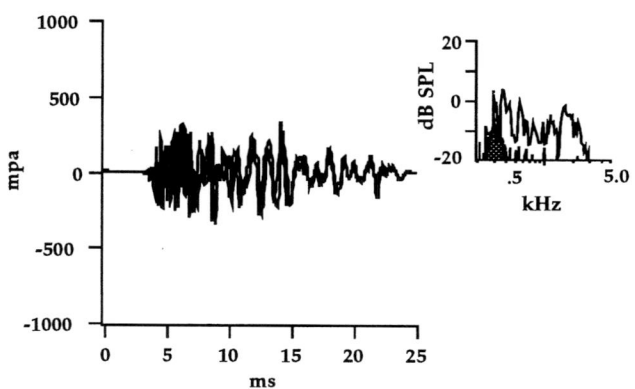

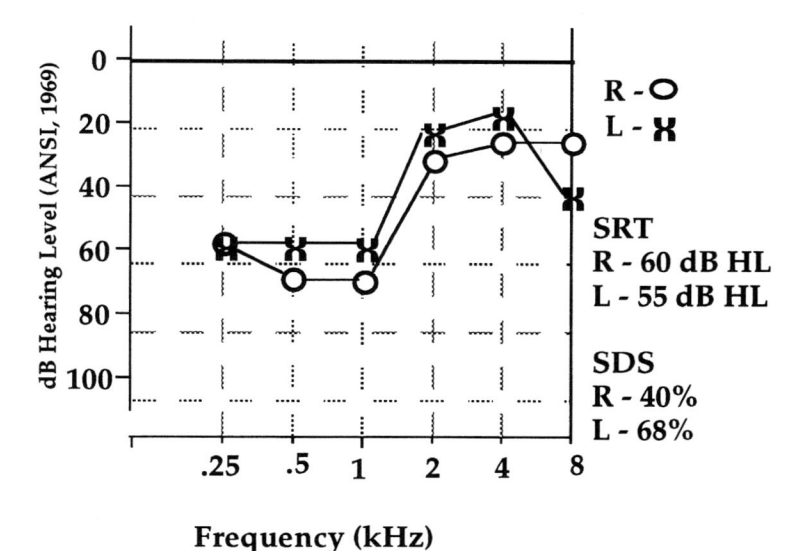

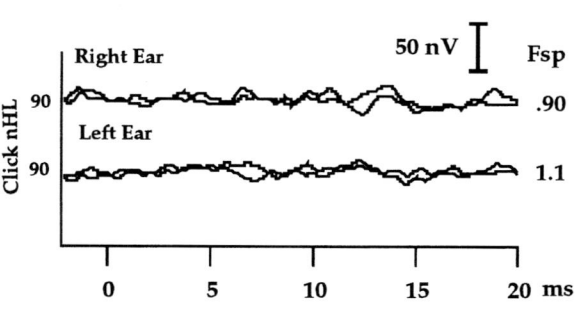

FIG. 25. JG results.

This collection of symptoms is rare and comprises what is being termed, *auditory neuropathy*. The etiology and course of this disorder is not known or clearly understood. The patient typically shows normal OAEs, absent ABR, and low-frequency flat or often fluctuating hearing loss. Speech discrimination scores are disproportionately poor relative to auditory thresholds, and acoustic reflexes are absent. Hearing aids are typically not helpful to these individuals, although FM systems, which enhance the SNR have proven useful.

REFERENCES

1. Eggermont JJ, Don M, Brackmann DE. Electrocochleography and auditory brainstem electric responses in patients with pontine angle tumors. *Ann Otol Rhinol Laryngol* 1980;(Suppl 75),89:1–19.
2. Selters WA, Brackmann DE. Acoustic tumor detection with brain stem electric response audiometry. *Arch Otolaryngol* 1977;103:181.
3. Tallal P, Piercy M. Developmental aphasia: rate of auditory processing and selective impairment of consonant perception. *Neuropsychologica* 1974;12:83–93.
4. Stypulkowski PH, Staller SJ. Clinical evaluation of a new ECoG recording electrode. *Ear Hear* 1987;8:304.
5. Ferraro J, Ferguson R. Tympanic ECochG and conventional ABR: A combined approach for the identification of wave I and the I-V interwave interval. *Ear Hear* 1989;10:161–6.
6. Moller AR, Jannetta PJ. Compound action potentials recorded intracranially from the auditory nerve in man. *Exp Neurol* 1981;74:862–74.
7. Moller AR, Jannetta PJ, Moller MB. Neural generators of brainstem evoked potentials results from human intracranial recordings. *Ann Otol Rhinol Laryngol* 1981;90:591–6.
8. Starr A, Amlie RN, Martin WH, Sanders S. Development of auditory function in newborn infants revealed by auditory brainstem response. *Pediatrics* 1977;60:831–9.

9. Moller AR, Jannetta PJ. Auditory evoked potentials recorded intracranially from the brainstem in man. *Exp Neurol* 1982;78:144–57.
10. Moller AR, Jannetta PJ. Interpretation of brainstem auditory evoked potentials: Results from intracranial recordings in humans. *Scand Audiol* 1983;12:125–33.
11. Davis H, Hirsh S. The audiometric utility of brain stem responses to low-frequency sounds. *Audiology* 1976;15:181–95.
12. Moller AR, Jannetta PJ. Evoked potentials from the inferior colliculus in man. *Electroencephalogr Clin Neurophysiol* 1982;53:612–20.
13. Robinson K, Rudge P. Auditory evoked responses in multiple sclerosis. *Lancet* 1975;1:1164–66.
14. Starr A, Picton TW, Sininger YS, Hood LJ, Berlin CI. Auditory neuropathy. *Brain* 1996;119:741–53.
15. Coats AC, Martin JL. Human auditory nerve action potentials and brain stem evoked responses: Effects of audiogram shape and lesion location. *Arch Otolaryngology* 1977;103:605–22.
16. Jerger J, Mauldin L. Prediction of sensorineural hearing level from the brain stem evoked response. *Arch Otolaryngol* 1978;104:456–61.
17. Clemis JD, McGee T. Brain stem electric response audiometry in the differential diagnosis of acoustic tumors. *Laryngoscope* 1979;89:31–42.
18. Sininger YS. Auditory brainstem response for objective measures of hearing. *Ear Hear* 1993;14:23–30.
19. Stapells DR, Gravel JS, Martin BA. Thresholds for auditory brainstem responses to tones in notched noise from infants and young children with normal hearing or sensorineural hearing loss. *Ear Hear* 1995;16:361–371
20. Kraus N, Kileny P, McGee T. Middle latency auditory evoked potentials. In: Jacobson JT, ed. *Principles & applications in auditory evoked potentials.* Boston: Allyn and Bacon; 1994:387–405.
21. Kraus N, Smith DI, Reed NL, Stein LK, Cartee C. Auditory middle latency responses in children: effects of age and diagnostic category. *Electroencephalogr Clin Neurophysiol* 1985;62:343–51.
22. McGee T, Kraus N, Killion M, Rosenberg R, King C. Improving the reliability of the auditory middle latency response by monitoring EEG delta activity. *Ear Hear* 1993;14:76–84
23. Don M, Elberling C, Waring M. Objective detection of averaged auditory brainstem responses. *Scand Audiol* 1984;13:219–28.
24. Elberling C, Don M. Quality estimation of averaged auditory brainstem responses. *Scand Audiol* 1984;13:187–97.
25. Sininger YS, Gardi JN, Morris JHI, Martin WH, Jewett DL. The 3-channel Lissajous' trajectory of the auditory brainstem response. VII. Planar segments in humans. *Electroencephalogr Clin Neurophysiol* 1987;68:368–79.
26. Starr A, Squires K. Distribution of auditory brainstem potentials over the scalp and nasopharynx in humans. *Ann N Y Acad Sci* 1982;388:427–42.
27. Sininger YS, King AJ. Effect of electrode configuration on amplitude of the auditory brainstem response to low intensity stimuli. Abstracts of the Twelfth Midwinter Research Meeting of the Association for Research in Otolaryngology 1989 (abst.)
28. Sininger YS. Filtering and spectral characteristics of averaged auditory brainstem response and background noise in infants. *J Acoust Soc Am* 1995;98(4)2048–2055.
29. Hall JWI. *Handbook of auditory evoked Responses.* Boston: Allyn and Bacon; 1992.
30. Hyde ML. Frequency-specific BERA in infants. *J Otolaryngol* 1985;(Suppl 14):19–27.
31. Stapells DR. Auditory brainstem response assessment of infants and children. *Semin Hear* 1989;10:229–51.
32. Gorga MP, Kaminski JR, Beauchaine KA, Jesteadt W. Auditory brainstem responses to tone bursts in normally hearing subjects. *J Speech Hear Res* 1988;31:87–97.
33. Hayes D, Jerger J. Auditory brainstem response (ABR) to tone-pips: results in normal and hearing-impaired subjects. *Scand Audiol* 1982;11:133–42.
34. Don M, Eggermont JJ. Analysis of the click-evoked brainstem potentials in man using high-pass noise masking. *J Acoust Soc Am* 1978;63:1084–92.
35. Picton TW, Ouellette J, Hamel G, Smith AD. Brainstem evoked potentials to tone pips in notched noise. *J Otolaryngol* 1979;8:289–314.
36. Don M, Eggermont JJ, Brackmann DE. Reconstruction of the audiogram using brain stem responses and high-pass noise masking. *Ann Otol Rhinol Laryngol* 1979;88(Suppl 57):1–20.
37. Hooks RG, Weber BA. Auditory brain stem responses in premature infants to bone-conducted stimuli: a feasibility study. *Ear Hear* 1984;5:42–6.
38. Stapells DR, Ruben RJ. Auditory brain stem responses to bone-conducted tones in infants. *Ann Otol Rhinol Laryngol* 1989;98:941–9.
39. Yang EY, Rupert AL, Moushegian G. A developmental study of bone conduction auditory brainstem response in infants. *Ear Hear* 1987;8:244–51.
40. von Bekesy G. *Experiments in hearing.* New York: McGraw-Hill; 1960.
41. Rhode WS. Observations of the vibration of the basilar membrane in squirrel monkeys using the Mossbauer technique. *J Acoust Soc Am* 1971;49:1218–31.
42. Sellick PM, Patuzzi R, Johnstone BM. Measurement of basilar membrane motion in the guinea pig using the Mossbauer technique. *J Acoust Soc Am* 1982;72:131–41.
43. Kiang NY-S, Moxon EC, Levine RA. Auditory nerve activity in cats with normal and abnormal cochleas. In: Wolstenholme GEW, Knight J, eds. *Sensorineural Hearing Loss.* London: Churchill; 1970:241–73
44. Ashmore JF. A fast motile response in guinea-pig outer hair cells: the cellular basis of the cochlear amplifier. *J Physiol* 1987;388:323–47
45. Brownell WE, Bader CR, Bertrand D, De Ribaupierre Y. Evoked mechanical responses of isolated cochlear outer hair cells. *Science* 1985;227:194–6.
46. Zenner HP. Motile responses in outer hair cells. *Hear Res* 1986;22:83–90.
47. Brownell WE. Outer hair cell electromotility and otoacoustic emissions. *Ear Hear* 1990;11:82–92.
48. Kemp DT. Stimulated acoustic emissions from within the human auditory system. *J Acoust Soc Am* 1978;64:1386–91.
49. Plinkert PK, Gitter AH, Zenner HP. Tinnitus associated spontaneous otoacoustic emissions. Active outer hair cell movements as a common origin? *Acta Otolaryngol* 1990;110:342–7.
50. Neely ST, Kim DO. A model for active elements in cochlear biomechanics. *J Acoust Soc Am* 1986;1472:1480.
51. Wilson JP. Evidence for cochlear origin for acoustic re-emissions, threshold fine-structure and tonal tinnitus. *Hear Res* 1980;2:233–52.
52. Norton SJ, Rubel EW. Active and passive ADP components in mammalian and avian ears. In: Dallos P, Geisler CD, Matthews JW, Ruggero MA, Steele CR, eds. *Mechanics and biophysics of hearing.* New York: Sperling-Verlag; 1990:219–26.
53. Whitehead ML, Lonsbury-Martin BL, Martin GK. Evidence for two discrete sources of $2f_1 - f_2$ distortion-product otoacoustic emission in rabbit: I. Differential dependence on stimulus parameters. *J Acoust Soc Am* 1992;91:1587–1607.
54. Martin GK, Lonsbury-Martin BL, Probst R, Coats AC. Acoustic distortion products in rabbit ear canal. II. Sites of origin revealed by suppression contours and pure-tone exposures. *Hear Res* 1987;28:191–208.
55. Siegel JH, Kim DO. Efferent neural control of cochlear mechanics? Olivocochlear bundle stimulation affects cochlear biomechanical nonlinearity. *Hear Res* 1982;6:171–82.
56. Arts HA, Norton SJ, Rubel EW. Influence of perilymphatic tetrodotoxin and calcium concentration on hair cell function. *ARO Abstracts* 1990;194 (abst.)
57. Kemp DT. Cochlear echoes—implications for noise-induced hearing loss. In: Hamernik RP, Henderson D, Salvi T, eds. *New perspectives in noise-induced hearing loss.* New York: Raven; 1982:189–207.
58. Lutman ME, Mason SM, Sheppard S, Gibbin KP. Differential diagnostic potential of otoacoustic emissions: a case study. *Audiology* 1989;28:205–10.
59. Ruggero MA, Rich NC. Furosemide alters organ of Corti mechanics: evidence for feedback of outer hair cells upon the basilar membrane. *J Neurosci* 1991;11:1057–67.
60. Kemp DT, Ryan S, Bray P. A guide to the effective use of otoacoustic emissions. *Ear Hear* 1990;11:93–105
61. Bonfils P, Avan P, Francois M, Marie P, Trotoux J, Narcy P. Clinical significance of otoacoustic emissions: a perspective. *Ear Hear* 1990;11:155–8.
62. Kemp DT. Evidence of mechanical nonlinearity and frequency selective wave amplification in the cochlea. *Arch Otorhinolaryngol* 1979;224:37–45.
63. Elberling C, Parbo J, Johnsen NJ, Bagi P. Evoked acoustic emission: clinical application. *Acta Otolaryngol* 1985;(Suppl 421):77–85.

64. Johnsen NJ, Bagi P, Elberling C. Evoked acoustic emissions from the human ear. III. Findings in neonates. *Scand Audiol* 1983;12:17–24.
65. Kemp DT, Bray P, Alexander L, Brown AM. Acoustic emission cochleography—practical aspects. *Scand Audiol* 1986;15(Suppl 25):71–95.
66. Probst R, Coats AC, Martin GK, Lonsbury-Martin BL. Spontaneous, click-, and toneburst-evoked otoacoustic emissions. *Hear Res* 1986;21:261–75.
67. Lonsbury-Martin BL, Martin GK. The clinical utility of distortion-product otoacoustic emissions. *Ear Hear* 1990;11:144–54.
68. Brown AM, Kemp DT. Suppressibility of the $2x_1-x_2$ stimulated acoustic emissions in gerbil and man. *Hear Res* 1984;13:29–37.
69. Harris FP, Glattke TJ. The use of suppression to determine the characteristics of otoacoustic emissions. *Semin Hear* 1992;13:67.
70. Gaskill SA, Brown AM. The behavior of the acoustic distortion product, $2x_1-x_2$, from the human ear and its relation to auditory sensitivity. *J Acoust Soc Am* 1990;88:821–39.
71. Harris FP, Lonsbury-Martin BL, Stagner BB, Coats AC, Martin GK. Acoustic distortion products in humans: Systematic changes in amplitude as a function of x_2/x_1 ratio. *J Acoust Soc Am* 1989;85:220–29.
72. Abdala C. Distortion product otoacoustic emission ($2f_1 - f_2$) amplitude as a function of f_2/f_1 frequency ratio and primary tone level separation in human adults and neonates. *J Acoust Soc Am* 1996;100(6);3726–40.
73. Probst R, Lonsbury-Martin BL, Martin GK. A review of otoacoustic emissions. *J Acoust Soc Am* 1991;89:2027–67.
74. Popelka GR, Osterhammel PA, Nielsen LH, Rasmussen AN. Growth of distortion product otoacoustic emissions with primary-tone level in humans. *Hear Res* 1993;71:12–22.
75. Owens JJ, Marcy J, McCoy MS, Lonsbury-Martin BL, Martin GK. Influence of otitis media on evoked otoacoustic emissions in children. *Semin Hear* 1992;13:53.
76. Sininger YS. Clinical applications of otoacoustic emissions. *Adv Otolaryngol Head Neck Surg* 1993;7:247–69.
77. Amedee RG. The effects of chronic otitis media with effusion on the measurement of transiently evoked otoacoustic emissions. *Laryngoscope* 1995;105:589–95.
78. Norton SJ, Stover LJ. Otoacoustic emissions: An emerging clinical tool. In: Katz J, ed. *Handbook of clinical audiology*. 4th ed. Baltimore: Williams & Wilkins; 1994:448–62.
79. Klein JO. Risk factors for otitis media in children. In: Kavanagh JF, ed. *Otitis media and child development*. Parkton: York; 1986:45–51.
80. Bargones JY, Burns EM. Suppression tuning curves for spontaneous otoacoustic emissions in infants and adults. *J Acoust Soc Am* 1988;83:1809–16.
81. Burns EM, Arehart KH, Campbell SL. Prevalence of Spontaneous Otoacoustic Emissions in Neonates. *ARO Abstracts* 1991;66 (abst.)
82. Strickland EA, Burns EM, Tubis A. Incidence of spontaneous otoacoustic emissions in children and infants. *J Acoust Soc Am* 1985;78:931–5.
83. Bilger RC, Matthies ML, Hammel DR, Demorest ME. Genetic implications of gender differences in the prevalence of spontaneous otoacoustic emissions. *J Speech Hear Res* 1990;33:418–32.
84. Martin GK, Probst R, Lonsbury-Martin BL. Otoacoustic emissions in human ears: normative findings. *Ear Hear* 1990;11:106.
85. Wier CC, Norton SJ, Kincaid GE. Spontaneous narrow-band otoacoustic signals emitted by human ears: a replication. *J Acoust Soc Am* 1984;76:1248–50.
86. Zurek PM. Spontaneous narrowband acoustic signals emitted by human ears. *J Acoust Soc Am* 1981;69:514–23.
87. Bright K, Glattke T. Spontaneous Otoacoustic emissions in normal listeners. In: Collins M, Glattke JJ, Harker LA, eds. *Sensorineural Hearing Loss: Mechanisms, Diagnosis and Treatment. The Reger Conference*. Iowa City: University of Iowa; 1984:201–8.
88. Bray P, Kemp DT. An advanced cochlear echo technique suitable for infant screening. *Br J Audiol* 1987;21:191–204.
89. Chuang SW, Gerber SE, Thornton ARD. Evoked otoacoustic emissions in preterm infants. *Int J Pediatr Otorhinolaryngol* 1993;26:39–45.
90. Lafreniere D, Jung MD, Smurzynski J, Leonard G, Kim DO, Sasek J. Distortion-product and click-evoked otoacoustic emissions in healthy newborns. *Arch Otolaryngol Head Neck Surg* 1991;117:1382–9.
91. Norton SJ, Widen JE. Evoked otoacoustic emissions in normal-hearing infants and children: emerging data and issues. *Ear Hear* 1990;11:121.
92. Smurzynski J. Longitudinal measurements of distortion-product and click-evoked otoacoustic emissions of preterm infants: preliminary results. *Ear Hear* 1994;15:210–33.
93. Stevens JC, Webb HD, Hutchinson J, Connell J, Smith MF, Buffin JT. Click evoked otoacoustic emissions in neonatal screening. *Ear Hear* 1990;11:128–33.
94. Abdala C, Sininger YS, Ekelid M, Zeng F-G. Distortion product otoacoustic emission suppression tuning curves in human adults. *Hearing Research* 98;1996:38–53.
95. Lasky R, Perlman J, Hecox K. Distortion-product otoacoustic emissions in human newborns and adults. *Ear Hear* 1992;13:430–41.
96. Prieve BA, Fitzgerald TS. Basic characteristics of COAEs and DPOAEs in infants and children. *ARO Abstracts* 1995;125 (abst.)
97. Smurzynski J, Jung MD, Lafreniere D, et al. Distortion-product and click-evoked otoacoustic emissions of preterm and full-term infants. *Ear Hear* 1993;14:258–74.
98. Prieve BA. Otoacoustic emissions in infants and children: basic characteristics and clinical application. *Semin Hear* 1992;13:37–52.
99. Popelka GR, Karzon RK, Arjmand EM. Growth of the $2f_1$-f_2 distortion product otoacoustic emission for low-level stimuli in human neonates. *Ear Hear* 1995;16:159–65.
100. Keefe DH, Bulen JC, Arehart KH, Burns EM. Ear-canal impedence and reflection coefficient in human infants and adults. *J Acoust Soc Am* 1993;94:2617–38.
101. Keefe DH, Bulen JC, Campbell SL, Burns EM. Pressure transfer function and absorption cross section from the diffuse field to the human infant ear canal. *J Acoust Soc Am* 1994;95:355–71.
102. Kruger B, Ruben RJ. The acoustic properties of the infant ear. *Acta Otolaryngol (Stockh)* 1987;103:578–85.
103. Saunders JC, Kaltenbach JA, Relkin EM. The structural and functional development of the outer and middle ear. In: Romand R, ed. *Development of auditory and vestibular systems*. New York: Academic; 1983:3–25.
104. Sininger YS, Abdala C. Auditory thresholds to click and tone-burst stimuli as measured by ABR in human neonates. *ARO Abstracts* 1995;136 (abst.)
105. Abdala C, Folsom RC. Frequency contribution to the click-evoked auditory brain-stem response in human adults and infants. *J Acoust Soc Am* 1995;97:2394–2404.
106. Bredberg G. Celluar pattern and nerve supply of the human organ of Corti. *Acta Otolaryng* 1968;(Suppl 236):6–135.
107. Lavigne-Rebillard M, Pujol R. Surface aspects of the developing human organ of Corti. *Acta Otolaryngol (Stockh)* 1987;(Suppl 436):43–50.
108. Lavigne-Rebillard M, Pujol R. Hair cell innervation in the fetal human cochlea. *Acta Otolaryngol (Stockh)* 1988;105:398–402.
109. Bonfils P, Uziel A. Clinical applications of evoked acoustic emissions: Results in normally hearing and hearing-impaired subjects. *Ann Otol Rhinol Laryngol* 1989;98:326–31.
110. Probst R, Lonsbury-Martin BL, Martin GK, Coats AC. Otoacoustic emissions in ears with hearing loss. *Am J Otolaryngol* 1987;8:73–81.
111. Bonfils P. Spontaneous otoacoustic emissions: clinical interest. *Laryngoscope* 1989;99:752–6.
112. Bonfils P, Uziel A, Pujol R. Screening for auditorty dysfunction in infants by evoked oto-acoustic emissions. *Arch Otolaryngol Head Neck Surg* 1988;114:887–90.
113. Rutten WLC. Evoked acoustic emissions from within normal and abnormal human ears: comparison with audiometric and electrocochleographic findings. *Hear Res* 1980;2:263–71.
114. Hinz M, Von Wedel H. Otoakustische Emissionen bei Patienten mit Hörsturz. *Arch Otorhinolaryngol* 1984;(Suppl II):128–30.
115. Harris FP. Distortion-product otoacoustic emissions in humans with high frequency sensorineural hearing loss. *J Speech Hear Res* 1990;33:594–600.
116. Spektor ZG, Leonard G, Kim DO, Jung MD, Smurzynski J. Otoacoustic emissions in normal and hearing-impaired children and normal adults. *Laryngoscope* 1991;101:965–74.
117. Kimberley BP, Hernadi I, Lee AM, Brown DK. Predicting pure tone thresholds in normal and hearing-impaired ears with distortion product emission and age. *Ear Hear* 1994;15:199–209.
118. Mills DM, Norton SJ, Rubel EW. Vulnerability and adaptation of

distortion produce otoacoustic emissions to endocochlear potential variation. *J Acoust Soc Am* 1993;94:2108–22.
119. Hotz MA, Harris FP, Probst R. Otoacoustic emissions: an approach for monitoring aminoglycoside-induced ototoxicity. *Laryngoscope* 1994;104:1130–34.
120. Long GR, Tubis A. Modification of spontaneous and evoked otoacoustic emissions and associated psychoacoustic microstructure by aspirin consumption. *J Acoust Soc Am* 1988;84:1343–53.
121. Wier CC, Pasanen EG, McFadden D. Partial dissociation of spontaneous otoacoustic emissions and distortion products during aspirin use in humans. *J Acoust Soc Am* 1988;84:230–7.
122. Brown AM, McDowell B, Forge A. Acoustic distortion products can be used to monitor the effects of chronic gentamicin treatment. *Hear Res* 1989;42:143–56.
123. Bonfils P, Avan P, Francois M, Trotoux J, Narcy P. Distortion-product otoacoustic emissions in neonates: normative data. *Acta Otolaryngol. (Stockh)* 1992;112:739–44.
124. White KR, Vohr BR, Behrens TR. Universal newborn hearing screening using transient evoked otoacoustic emissions: Results of the Rhode Island Hearing Assessment Project. *Semin Hear* 1993;14:18–29.
125. Bonfils P, Uziel A. Evoked otoacoustic emissions in patients with acoustic neuromas. *Am J Otol* 1988;9:412–17.
126. Prieve BA, Gorga MP, Neely ST. Otoacoustic emissions in an adult with severe hearing loss. *J Speech Hear Res* 1991;34:379–85.
127. Sininger YS, Hood LJ, Starr A, Berlin CI, Picton TW. Hearing loss due to auditory neuropathy. *Audiol Today* 1995;7:10–13.
128. Starr A, McPherson D, Patterson J, et al. Absence of both auditory evoked potentials and auditory percepts dependent on timing cues. *Brain* 1991;114:1157–80.

CHAPTER 10

Neonatal Hearing Screening

Early Identification

Jerry L. Northern and Stephen Epstein

Each year in the United States about 4,000 infants are born with profound deafness and another 37,000 infants are born with lesser degrees of hearing impairment. With an annual birth rate of 4,000,000 babies in the United States each year, the statistics suggest that 6 of every 1000 newborns will have a significant hearing loss. In fact, hearing impairment in children is 20 times more prevalent than other disorders such as phenylketonuria (PKU), sickle sell anemia, and hypothyrodism, which are mandated for screening at birth. It is reported to be ten times less expensive to identify one infant with hearing loss than to identify one infant with PKU, sickle cell anemia, or hypothyroidism (1).

Hearing is essential for the normal development of speech and language. Undetected hearing loss in an infant may have severe negative consequences on communication development and long-term impact on educational potential. The single most important factor responsible for the successful habilitation of a child with hearing impairment is the age at which special education is initiated. Children with hearing loss who receive early intervention to help develop their communication skills show significantly higher speech and language skills than do children with hearing impairment who do not receive intervention at an early age (2).

Critical period theory suggests that the development of language in a young child is dependent on appropriate auditory stimulation prior to 18 months of age. A baby who is deprived of language stimulation during this early period of life will likely never fully attain maximal language function (3).

J.L. Northern: Department of Otolaryngology, University of Colorado School of Medicine; and Head, Audiology Services, University Hospital Denver, Colorado 80262.

S. Epstein: Department of Otolaryngology—Head and Neck Surgery and Pediatrics, The George Washington University School of Medicine, Wheaton, Maryland 20902-2538.

Without adequate infant hearing-screening programs in the United States, children born with severe-to-profound hearing loss are often not identified until 24 months of age or later; some children with milder degrees of hearing loss may not be identified until they enter school at age 5 or 6 years of age. Unfortunately, the critical language developmental period for these children, when auditory input is so necessary to their receptive and expressive communication, has long passed.

Fortunately, the past few years has seen renewed attention from governmental agencies and professional societies addressed to reducing the age at which hearing loss is identified in children born in the United States. For example, in the early 1990s, the federal government conducted a review of national health care policy which resulted in a series of disease prevention objectives known as *Healthy People* 2000 (4). Included in this plan was a goal to reduce the average age at which children with significant hearing impairment would be identified by 12 months of age by the year 2000. The National Institutes of Health (NIH) attempted to resolve the problems of early identification of hearing loss through a Consensus Development Conference held in 1993 which recommended hearing screening of all infants (5). Infant hearing-screening guidelines undergo constant reevaluation and change as technology and medical sciences change. The recent recommendations for universal infant hearing screening proposed by the 1993 NIH Conference have yet to be widely implemented. None the less, many programs have undertaken the task of implementing universal screening. Within the next few years, new data from large mass screening programs, will be available for review.

The timing and location of the infant screening process is critical to program success. In today's health environment and the trend toward early discharge of new mothers and newborns within 8 to 12 hours following delivery, time is of the essence to screen the new baby's hearing. Many of today's births occur in rural and remote areas or in birthing clinics. Once the infant is out of the hospital's health-care system, many are lost to follow-up and do not return for hearing-screening. Thus, infant hearing screening programs must be planned and implemented with sufficient flexibility to meet the various geographic and economic situations to ensure that a practical majority of infants are provided hearing screening within the first 3 months of life.

Of course, the success of any screening program depends on the screening tools to have high test sensitivity (accuracy in the correct identification of those with the disorder) and high test specificity (accuracy in the correct identification of those without the disorder). In addition, the screening protocol must fulfill other criteria, such as being simple, efficient, safe, and cost effective. Infant hearing-screening programs should be administered and directed by qualified audiologists who often supervise trained technicians, volunteers, or both, who actually perform the tests with each infant. Consideration of cost effectiveness should not only include direct expenses related to the screening program, but reflect the cost savings due to early intervention. Early intervention may permit the child to be educated by mainstreaming into a normal classroom at significantly less expense than the requirement of a specialized self-contained classroom for children with hearing impairment or placement in residential schools for the deaf (6).

TECHNIQUES OF NEONATAL AND HEARING SCREENING

The earliest formal effort to screen the hearing of infants on a large scale in the United States was reported by Downs and Sterritt in 1964 (7). These researchers conducted a 1 year trial to screen the hearing of 17,000 infants born during one year in Denver, Colorado. Their test technique for infant hearing screening utilized a specially designed battery-operated device that emitted a sudden onset, narrowband noiseburst stimulus centered at 3,000 Hz, at 90 dB sound pressure level (SPL). The device was held 12 inches from the sleeping infant and trained observers noted the presence or absence of reflexive body movements (Moro response) immediately following presentation of the stimulus. Although their efforts identified nine profoundly deaf infants (approximately 1/1,700 live births), the behavioral testing technique utilized was fraught with high false-negative results and finally not generally accepted as a valid screening technique.

Other researchers attempted to modify the protocol for this behavioral observation technique during the next few years and to establish valid criteria based on scientific data collection. None the less, behavioral observation of auditory responses remains too subjective for general acceptance in mass infant hearing-screening programs. In fact, the 1994 Joint Committee on Infant Hearing concluded that behavioral measures cannot validly and reliably detect hearing loss of less than 30 dB HL in infants younger than 6 months of age (8).

Numerous innovative infant hearing-screening techniques have been developed and tested through the years in an effort to eliminate the subjective response scoring problems associated with behavioral observation testing. In particular, researchers have attempted to identify physiologic responses to sound stimuli that can be quantified to provide "objective" (i.e., nonsubjective) results.

Cardiac Response Audiometry

Schulman (9) utilized the unconditioned cardiac response, that is acceleration in heart rate, due to the onset of a narrowband noise stimulus of 34 dB SPL as an objective means to identify hearing loss in infants.

Crib-O-Gram

Simmons and Russ (10) developed the Crib-O-Gram, an ingenious automated system for detecting hearing loss in infants by use of a motion-sensitive transducer placed in the nursery crib. The system was a microprocessor-based program that automatically monitored the infant's movements prior to and following presentation of a narrowband stimulus from a transducer attached to the crib. The Crib-O-Gram was designed to turn itself on, perform the test, interpret the results, and turn itself off when the response paradigm indicated pass or failure of the infant to respond appropriately.

Auditory Response Cradle

The Auditory Response Cradle was developed in England in 1980 by Bennett (11). A more elaborate system than the Crib-O-Gram, the Auditory Response Cradle was designed to examine several infant motor responses following programmed auditory stimulus presentation. The device measured trunk and limb movements, the head-jerk startle reflex, and changes in respiration following presentation of an 85 dB SPL filtered noise stimulus presented to the infant through ear probes inserted into the external auditory canals.

Auditory Brainstem Response

The evoked auditory brainstem evoked response (ABR) has proven to be the most useful and valid technique for assessing hearing in infants. In this technique, developed in the late 1970s, minute physiologic electrical responses to sound are collected from the patient's head and passed through a summating-type computer. The result is a composite response of five to seven waves that reflect neural activity from the ascending auditory pathway. The ABR is noted for its strong replicability of waveform pattern and to be unaffected by the physiologic state of the patient. The response is generally easy to record with proper equipment and technique and is extremely sensitive to the presence of hearing impairment. Galambos and Hecox (12) were among the first to use the ABR technique to screen hearing in infants. The ABR technique has proven to be most efficient in the hearing screening of newborns because false positives are greatly reduced and false negatives are virtually eliminated. Murray, Javel, and Watson (13) and Hall, Kripal, and Hepp (14) provided extensive review and critique of large scale newborn hearing-screening programs based on ABR measurements. Cevette (15) reported data from Utah of newborn intensive care unit (NICU) programs employing ABR as the sole screening tool. In these programs the age of identification of hearing loss was reduced from 30 months to 16 months during a 4 year period.

Automated ABR

In recent years, the ABR test protocol was developed into specialized automated ABR instruments specifically designed for the hearing screening of infants. The automated ABR, Algo-1 screener (Natus Medical, Inc., Foster City, CA) (ALGO), is programmed to control many of the methodologic factors that influence the outcome of ABR test results (16). The ALGO is a battery-operated, microprocessor controlled device that uses a statistical model for objective ABR response detection and thereby eliminates the need for evaluation of ABR waveforms. Unfiltered clicks, used as auditory stimuli, are presented at 35 dB while the raw waveform data are analyzed and compared to a "normal" ABR template within the computer software. The automated ABR renders a Pass or Refer decision, which does not require professional interpretation. The advantages of automated ABR include cost savings, portability, specially designed artifact rejection algorithms to detect excessive environmental and physiologic noise, and simplicity of operation so that trained nonprofessional personnel can operate the equipment and screen the hearing of infants (17). Jacobson, Johnson, and Spahr (18) concluded that automated ABR systems provide a viable solution for neonatal auditory screening.

Otoacoustic Emissions

Otoacoustic emissions (OAE) are the most recent development to be considered as a physiologic response with potential for use in infant hearing screening programs. The OAE, first measured by Kemp of the United Kingdom, is a low-intensity, inaudible sound produced by vibratory motion of the outer hair cells in the cochlea (19). With use of specialized computer software with a miniature microphone and sound transducer sealed in the external auditory canal, evoked otoacoustic emissions (EOAE) can be recorded in 60 to 90 seconds. The EOAE response appears 5 msec following stimulation with acoustic clicks. The EOAE can be elicited from subjects with normal hearing in the mid-frequency test range, but are absent in patients with conductive hearing loss or sensorineural hearing loss greater than 35 dB HL. The development of EOAE as an objective, valid, and quick screening procedure holds considerable promise as an infant hearing-screening technique and may be the most efficient means to solve the problems of early identification of hearing loss in newborns (20).

At this time, ABR (including AGLO) and OAE are the most common methods used in the screening of hearing in infants. Ongoing experience, continued advances in technology, refinement of equipment, and further evaluation of testing protocols should improve the efficiency of these screening systems.

THE JOINT COMMITTEE ON INFANT HEARING

Infant hearing screening programs have been guided by an interdisciplinary group, the Joint Committee on Infant Hearing, for the past 25 years. The Committee, initially composed of representatives from three professional societies—the American Speech and Hearing Association, the American Academy of Pediatrics, and the American Academy of Otolaryngology, first convened in 1970. Following review of the limited data available on infant hearing screening, the Joint Committee issued a statement that additional research was needed before routine mass hearing screening of newborns could be recommended. The Joint Committee met again during 1971 and 1972 and established a list of indicators that would place a newborn at an increased likelihood for congenital deafness. The list, known as the High-Risk Factors for Deafness, included five medical indications that could be identified by parental interview or chart review (21):

1. History of hereditary childhood hearing impairment
2. Rubella or other nonbacterial intrauterine fetal infection
3. Defects of the ear, nose, or throat; malformed, low-set or absent pinnae; cleft lip or palate; any residual abnormality of the otorhinolaryngeal system
4. Birthweight less than 1,500 grams
5. Bilirubin level greater than 20 mg/100 ml serum

The Joint Committee on Infant Hearing met several more times in subsequent years, resulting in modification and revision of the original position statement. The 1974 Committee recommended the use of carefully conducted behavioral observation hearing screening of the infants at risk for deafness and called for additional research into protocol variables (22). During 1982, the Committee expanded the list of risk factors from five to seven by including bacterial meningitis and severe asphyxia (23).

The 1990 Joint Committee expanded the 1982 position statement considerably and divided the risk factors into a section for neonates (birth–29 days) and a section for infants (30 days–2 yr). Because of the high false-positive and false-negative rates still associated with behavioral observation screening, the 1990 Joint Committee recommended that the initial hearing screen be conducted with the ABR procedure.

TABLE 1. *Indicators associated with sensorineural and conductive hearing loss for use with neonates*

Family history of hereditary childhood sensorineural hearing loss
In utero infection, such as cytomegalovirus, rubella, syphilis, herpes, toxoplasmosis
Craniofacial anomalies, including morphological abnormalities of the pinna and ear canal
Birth weight less than 1,500 grams (3.3 lb)
Hyperbilirubinemia at a serum level requiring exchange transfusion
Ototoxic medications, including but not limited to the aminoglycosides, used in multiple courses or in combination with loop diuretics
Bacterial meningitis
Apgar scores of 0–4 at 1 min or 0–6 at 5 min
Mechanical ventilation lasting 5 days or longer
Stigmata or other findings associated with a syndrome known to include a sensorineural or conductive hearing loss

Neonate stage, birth through 28 days.
1994 Joint Committee on Infant Hearing Position Statement (8).

The position statement was brought into accord with the 1986 Education of the Handicapped Act Amendments (Public Law 99-457) by recommending specific habilitation steps for neonates and infants with congenital hearing impairment. The 1990 statement called attention to the need for additional data on cost, testing protocols, personnel, and follow-up services as needed for infant hearing-screening programs (24).

During the past decade, researchers have confirmed that the high-risk approach to infant hearing screening identifies only 50% of children with congenital deafness. Recognizing this fact, the recent 1994 Joint Committee on Infant Hearing, concerned about the inaccuracies of continued dependence on the high-risk register, endorsed the concept of universal detection of hearing loss in infants. The 1994 Joint Committee Position Statement maintained the importance of risk factors, now renamed indicators, for both neonates and infants (Tables 1 and 2). The 1994 Position Statement reflects concern about behavioral observation methods of infant screening, and points out that physiologic screening procedures outperform behavioral screening in infants younger than 6 months of age. Thus, the Joint Committee recommended that infant hearing-screening programs should employ ABR or OAE measurements. The 1994 Position Statement does not endorse any specific testing protocol, but recognizes that infant hearing-screening program procedures will vary by region, individual needs, and administrative structure (8).

UNIVERSAL DETECTION OF INFANTS WITH HEARING LOSS

In 1993 the NIH attempted to resolve the problems of early identification of hearing loss through a Consensus Development Conference. On the basis that the average age of identification of congenital hearing impairment in the United States was reported to be approximately 30 months and recognizing the limitations of the current dependence on the high-risk register as a means of detecting pediatric deafness, the Conference was called to develop a better approach to infant hearing screening. The Consensus Conference, after considering all available data and the testimony of numerous experts, recommended that universal infant hearing screening be undertaken with a two-stage protocol. The recommended universal procedure consisted of initial screening of all infants with OAE followed by ABR screening for infants who did not pass the OAE screening. This recommended protocol for universal infant hearing screening was considered a preliminary effort to gather a large-scale data-base and included plans to review the screening results at a later date.

Following the NIH Consensus Conference, a commentary published by Bess and Paradise (25) criticized the conclusions reached by the NIH panel of experts. The Bess-Paradise commentary acknowledged that the disorder of childhood deafness is important and associated with substantial morbidity and suffering. However, they questioned the rationale of a two-stage, national universal infant hearing-screening program as ill-considered and ill-advised on the basis of practicability, effectiveness, cost and harm-benefit ratio. Their commentary also challenged the effectiveness of early intervention for infants and young children with hearing loss.

Numerous supporters of universal infant hearing screening responded to the Bess-Paradise commentary (26). The respondents cited that sensorineural hearing impairment in infants is a serious condition that results in lifelong disability and that continued dependence on the high-risk registry approach would identify less than 50% of infants with significant hearing loss. The respondents also stated that valid techniques with acceptable sensitivity, specificity, and cost effectiveness are currently available. They also stressed that early intervention is essential for facilitating speech, language and cognitive skills, social-emotional development,

TABLE 2. *Indicators associated with sensorineural and conductive hearing loss for use with infants*

Parent/caregiver concern regarding hearing, speech, language, and/or developmental delay.
Bacterial meningitis and other infections associated with sensorineural hearing loss.
Head trauma associated with loss of consciousness or skull fracture.
Stigmata or other findings associated with a syndrome known to include a sensorineural and/or conductive hearing loss.
Ototoxic medications, including but not limited to chemotherapeutic agents or aminoglycosides, used in multiple courses or in combination with loop diuretics.
Recurrent or persistent otitis media with effusion for at least 3 months.

Infant stage, 29 days through 2 yr.
1994 Joint Committee on Infant Hearing Position Statement (8).

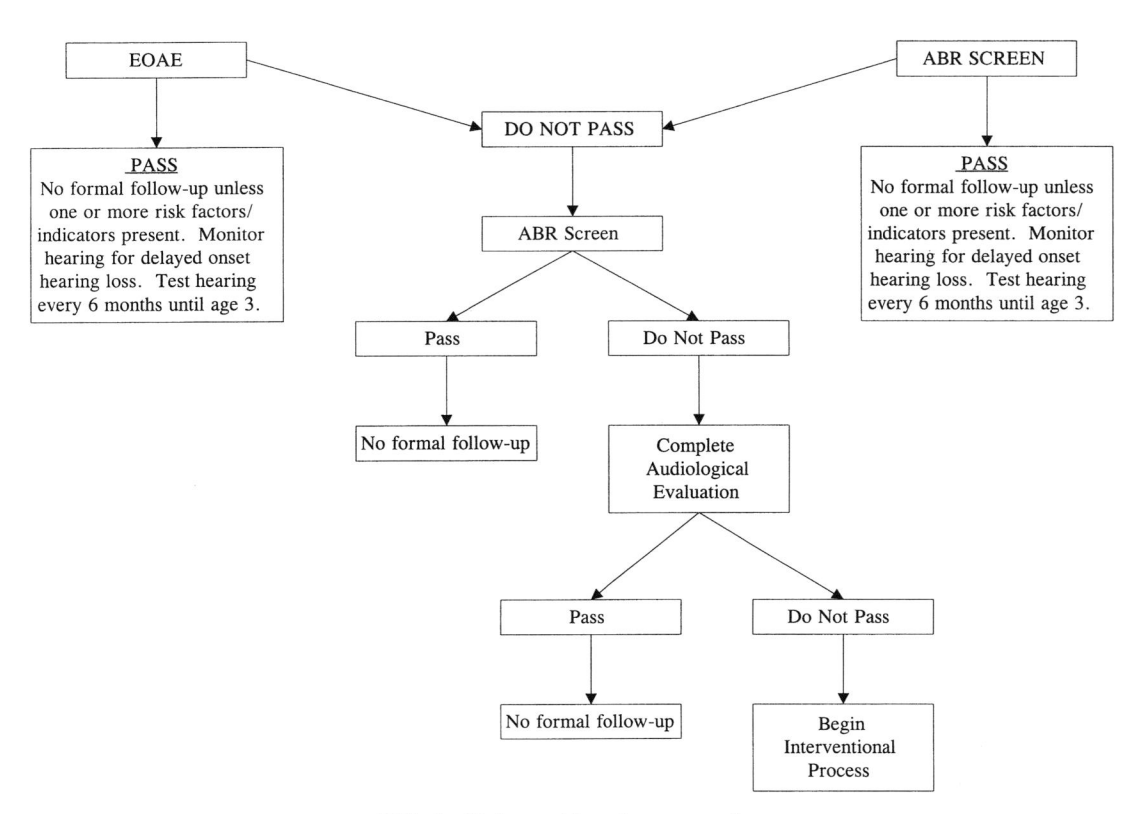

```
                    EOAE                                              ABR SCREEN
                    /  \                                                /      \
                   /    \         DO NOT PASS                          /        \
                  /      _____/          _____/          \
               PASS                    |                                       PASS
    No formal follow-up unless     ABR Screen                        No formal follow-up unless
    one or more risk factors/       /     \                          one or more risk factors/
    indicators present. Monitor    /       \                         indicators present. Monitor
    hearing for delayed onset    Pass    Do Not Pass                 hearing for delayed onset
    hearing loss. Test hearing    |         |                        hearing loss. Test hearing
    every 6 months until age 3.   |         |                        every 6 months until age 3.
                          No formal    Complete
                          follow-up    Audiological
                                       Evaluation
                                        /      \
                                      Pass    Do Not Pass
                                       |         |
                                  No formal    Begin
                                  follow-up    Interventional
                                               Process
```

FIG. 1. Universal hearing screening.

and academic achievement for hearing-impaired infants and young children.

To be sure, implementation of a national program for universal infant hearing screening will require ongoing and substantial professional commitment. To achieve success in screening the hearing of the 4,000,000 newborns annually in the United States will not be achieved easily or quickly. None the less, the NIH Consensus Statement and the 1994 Joint Committee on Infant Hearing Position Statement, both recommending universal detection of infants with impaired hearing, reflect the national interest in resolving the current problems of late identification of pediatric hearing disorders and will help move us toward better and improved methods for the early detection of hearing loss in infants (Fig. 1).

UNIVERSAL INFANT HEARING SCREENING PROGRAMS

The first statewide universal infant hearing-screening program was established in Rhode Island (27). This program was initiated as a research project to evaluate the feasibility of using EOAE as a technique for universal newborn hearing screening. Data were reported for 1,850 well-baby and NICU infants born during a 6-month period at the Women and Infants Hospital. From this cohort, 11 infants were identified with sensorineural hearing loss and an additional 37 newborns were identified with conductive hearing loss. The use of EOAE identified nearly twice as many hearing impaired infants with lesser degrees of hearing loss than would have been identified by the traditional high-risk registry as the screening procedure. The study reported a 5.9/1,000 prevalence in the general newborn population to have significant sensorineural hearing loss. Further, the EOAE testing procedure was accomplished in 3.3 minutes in sleeping infants. In comparing EOAE and ABR results in the same infants from the Rhode Island project, EOAE showed a sensitivity of 100% and specificity of 82%; ABR screening was reported to show sensitivity of 94% and specificity of 89%. The success of the pilot project conducted at the Women and Infants Hospital was subsequently used as the basis for the Rhode Island state legislature to mandate by law and regulate to be paid for by health insurance plans, that all newborns must be screened for hearing with EOAE.

A different model state program was initiated by the Colorado State Department of Health, which enlisted 20 hospitals and helped them establish within their facilities universal newborn hearing screening based primarily on the automated ABR technique. Although no state legislative mandate exists, the Health Department's Colorado Newborn Hearing Screening Project has monitored the births of about 37,000 newborns over a 2-year period. Based on the 21,000 babies (57%) of this total infant cohort who received a hearing screen prior to discharge, 1,500 (7%) were referred for additional audiometric evaluation. In this statewide sample of infants, 147 newborns had significant sensorineural or conductive hearing loss. These data reflect an incidence of bilateral or unilateral hearing losses of 1 in 256 (4/1000) births. No risk factors for deafness were presented in 57% of the hearing loss group, but 43% had associated risk indicators. According to V. Thomson of the Colorado Department of Health, Newborn Hearing Screening Program, Denver, Colorado (written communication, 1995) cost of testing every newborn with automatic audiometry ranged from $18 to $33 depending on the hospital's billing rate and the qualifications of the personnel involved in the testing program.

MEDICAL ASPECTS OF INFANT HEARING

A hearing impairment in an infant can develop in association with, or secondary to a genetic defect that is evident at birth or within the first few years of life. Congenital deafness accounts for approximately 25% of all childhood hearing impairment, and the remaining 75% of pediatric hearing loss is acquired sometime after birth. Within the congenital deafness classification, approximately 50% of the cases can be traced to familial inheritance; the remaining 50% are described as having unknown etiology. Approximately two thirds of patients with congenital deafness show no other organ system involvement (nonsyndromic). The remaining one third have congenital deafness in conjunction with other organ system abnormalities (syndromic) (28). Genetic inheritance for deafness can be identified in about 40% of patients as related to recessive gene transmission, 10% due to dominant gene transmission, and 3% due to a sex-linked gene (29). It is important to accurately identify the presence of a recognized syndrome because this may help to uncover occult anomalies or other related medical problems and predict the possibility of delayed or progressive hearing loss. Recognition of a syndrome is, of course, essential for genetic counseling of the family and the patient.

The diagnosis of hearing impairment in an infant or young child is a difficult task. Many primary care physicians have "never seen a pediatric patient with hearing loss" and place undue confidence in their ability to detect hearing impairment in infants and toddlers during routine physical examinations. Coplan, a developmental pediatrician, reviewed his case records of approximately 1,000 children seen during a 6 year period (30). He noted 46 children with permanent hearing loss. The mean age at diagnosis of profound congenital deafness was 24 months; lesser degrees of congenital deafness were not diagnosed until 48 months of age. Coplan advised that adherence to specific historical, physical, and developmental risk factors, regardless of the examiner's subjective impression of how well the child seems to hear, will help in achieving a timely diagnosis of hearing impairment.

Stein (31) described medical advances in the treatment and prevention of two leading causes of hearing loss in young children. These advances will likely reduce the number of pediatric cases of severe hearing impairment. The prevention of bacterial meningitis due to *Haemophilus influenzae* type b through universal immunization programs and the introduction of cephalosporin antibiotic and corticosteroid treatment of congenital toxoplasmosis represent important progress. As a result of these advances, however, there will be a corresponding increase in the unknown etiologies of congenital deafness. This situation presents a compelling argument in favor of universal hearing screening of infants.

A separate list of indicators that may be related to delayed onset of hearing loss or progressive hearing impairment is presented in Table 3. Physicians must also be aware of the presence of recurrent or persistent otitis media with effusion creating a conductive hearing loss—the most common cause of hearing loss in young children. Disorders of the eustachian tube anatomy and function can lead to problems, which if persistent, may lead to a conductive hearing loss. There is growing concern among professionals that mild hearing loss may result in substantive delay in the acquisition and use of language. Infants who demonstrate one or more of the indicators in the potential progressive hearing loss categories should have their hearing monitored at least every 6 months until the age of 3 years and at appropriate intervals thereafter.

TABLE 3. *Indicators for use with infants who require periodic monitoring of hearing*

Indicators of delayed-onset sensorineural hearing loss
Family history of hereditary childhood hearing loss
In utero infection, such as cytomegalovirus, rubella, syphilis, herpes, toxoplasmosis
Neurofibromatosis Type II and neurodegenerative disorders
Indicators of conductive hearing loss
Recurrent or persistent otitis media with effusion
Anatomic deformities and other disorders that affect eustachian tube function
Neurodegenerative disorders

Infant stage, 29 days through 3 yr.
1994 Joint Committee on Infant Hearing Position Statement (8).

FOLLOW-UP CARE AND EARLY INTERVENTION

An effective neonatal and infant hearing screening program requires the availability of appropriate follow-up care facilities and adequate early intervention services as required by the Individuals with Disabilities Education Act, (Part H), Public Law 102-119 (formerly Public Law 99-457). Optimal management of the young child with hearing impairment comes with the establishment of a multidisciplinary professional team. This team should include a physician with expertise in the diagnosis and management of early childhood otologic disorders and an audiologist with experience in assessing the hearing of infants and young children and in fitting amplification and assistive listening devices to pediatric patients. Other team members should include a speech-language pathologist, sign language specialist, qualified teacher of children with deafness and hearing impairment, or all three professionals. An individualized family service plan (IFSP) should be established within 45 days of referral. The IFSP should be based on the child's strengths and needs and be consistent with the family's resources, priorities, and cultural needs.

LEGISLATIVE MANDATES

There are no national legislative policies pertaining to the need of identification of hearing loss in infants and young children at the time of this writing. As part of the recent health-care reform movement in the United States, several major health bills have been introduced at the federal level to require universal screening of infant hearing. These bills have not been formally submitted for congressional consideration due to lack of funding and unclear policies regarding the hearing screening protocols.

On the individual state level, there are currently 18 states that have mandated statewide infant hearing screening requirements. An additional five states have established voluntary infant screening programs, and another 22 states report regional or hospital-based programs (Table 4). Most of the formalized state infant hearing-screening programs utilize the high-risk register approach at this time, but many are moving towards utilization of automated ABR and/or otoacoustic emissions as the primary screening technique (32).

SUMMARY

Hearing is essential for normal speech, language, and educational development in children. *Early* identification of a hearing loss in an infant or child followed by *early* intervention in the management of the hearing loss is necessary if the child is to develop speech and language and have the opportunity to be educated in a mainstream setting.

Early identification of hearing loss in children is dependent on a safe, cost-effective, and reliable hearing screening protocol. Various approaches to newborn and infant hearing screening have been attempted during the past 30 years. A major advancement in screening children for hearing loss has been the utilization of risk factors or indicators. Clinical trials and retrospective studies have shown that these risk factors or indicators fail to diagnose at least 50% of children born with a hearing loss. Because of these statistics the NIH Consensus Conference on Early Identification of Hearing Loss in Infants and Young Children and the Joint Committee on Infant Hearing 1994 Position Statement have, therefore, endorsed universal hearing screening for all newborns and infants.

Scientific research and technological advances have provided instrumentation that has the potential to screen all newborns and infants for hearing loss in a safe, reliable, and cost-effective manner. Continuing modification of these instruments and refinement of test protocols have improved the sensitivity, specificity and cost effectiveness of universal hearing screening protocols. Cost effectiveness must be measured not only in terms of the cost of each test per se but by the long-term savings benefits of early identification of the hearing loss. Any concerns or controversy that may exist in regard to the safety and reliability of universal hearing-screening should not act as a deterrent to the progress and implementation of newborn and infant hearing screening programs. Even though the current list of risk factors and indicators fails to detect at least 50% of these newborns, infants, and children born with a hearing loss, they still serve a purpose as a basis for identifying hearing loss in children, especially children born with syndromic and delayed-onset hearing loss. Paramount to any successful newborn and infant hearing screening program are the provisions by which all children identified with a hearing loss can be placed in interventional programs as soon as possible on the basis of family and cultural preferences.

TABLE 4. *State list of infant hearing impairment identification programs, by type*

Legislative Mandate (n = 18)	Individually Operated Programs (n = 22)
Arizona (2,3)	Alabama
California (2,3,4)	Delaware
Connecticut (3)	District of Columbia
Florida (2,3,4)	Idaho
Georgia (2,3)	Illinois
Hawaii (1)	Indiana
Kansas (2,3)	Iowa
Kentucky (2,3)	Maine
Louisiana (2,3,4)	Michigan
Maryland (2,3)	Minnesota
Massachusetts (2,3)	Mississippi
New Jersey (2,3)	Missouri
Ohio (2,3)	Montana
Oklahoma (2,3)	Nebraska
Rhode Island (1)	North Carolina
Virginia (2,3,4)	Pennsylvania
Washington (all birth defects)	South Carolina
West Virginia (2,3)	South Dakota
Statewide Programs (n = 5)	Texas
Arkansas (2,3,4)	Vermont
Colorado (3,4)	Wisconsin
North Dakota (2,3)	Wyoming
Oregon (2,3)	**Did Not Respond (n = 5)**
Utah (2,3,4)	Alaska
No Program (n = 1)	New Hampshire
Nevada	New Mexico
	New York
	Tennessee

1, screen all infants; 2, high-risk registry; 3, identify infants at risk (high-risk screening); 4, screen only high-risk infants.

REFERENCES

1. Johnson JL, Mauk GW, Takekawa KM, Simon PR, Sia CC, Blackwell PM. Implementing a statewide system of services for infants and toddlers with hearing disabilities. *Semin Hear* 1993;14:105.
2. Levitt H, McGarr NS, Geffner D. Development of language and communication skills in hearing-impaired children. Rockville, MD: Ameri-

can Speech-Language-Hearing Association 1987. ASHA Monograph no 26.
3. First LR, Palfrey JS. The infant or young child with developmental delay. *N Engl J Med* 1994;330:478.
4. *Healthy people 2000.* US Department of Health and Human Services, Public Health Service. Washington, DC: US Government Printing Office; 1990; DHHS publication no (PHS) 91-50213.
5. National Institutes of Health Consensus Statement. *Early identification of hearing impairment in infants and young children.* Bethesda, MD: NIH Office of Medical Applications of Research, 1993.
6. Northern JL, Hayes, D. Universal screening for infant hearing impairment: necessary, beneficial and justifiable. *Audiology Today* 1994;6: 14.
7. Downs MP, Sterritt GM. Identification audiometry for neonates: a preliminary report. *J Aud Res* 1964;4:69.
8. Joint Committee on Infant Hearing 1994 Position Statement. *Pediatrics* 1995;95:152.
9. Schulman C. Heart rate response habituation in high-risk premature infants. *Psychophysiology* 1970;6:690.
10. Simmons FB, Russ F. Automated newborn hearing screening, the Crib-O-Gram. *Arch Otolaryngol* 1974;100:1.
11. Bennett M. Trials with the auditory response cradle: headturns and startles as auditory responses in the neonate. *Br J Audio* 1980;14:122.
12. Galambos R, Hecox K. Clinical applications of the auditory brainstem response. *Otolaryngol Clin North Am* 1978;11:709.
13. Murray AD, Javel E, Watson CS. Prognostic value of auditory brainstem evoked response screening in newborn infants. *Am J Otolaryngol* 1985;6:120.
14. Hall JW III, Kripal JP, Hepp T. Newborn hearing screening with auditory brainstem response: measurement problems and solutions. *Semin Hear* 1988;9:15.
15. Cevette MJ: Auditory brainstem response testing in the intensive care unit. *Semin Hear* 1984;5:57.
16. Peters J. An automated infant screener using advanced evoked response technology. *Hear J* 1986;39:25.
17. Kileny PR. Algo-I automated infant hearing screener: preliminary results. *Semin Hear* 1987;8:15.
18. Jacobson J, Jacobson C, Spahr RC. Automated and conventional ABR screening techniques in high-risk infants. *J Am Acad Audiology* 1990; 1:187.
19. Kemp D. Stimulated acoustic emissions from within the human auditory system. *J Acoust Soc Am* 1978;64(5):1386.
20. Northern JL, Downs MP. *Hearing in children.* 4th ed. Baltimore: Williams & Wilkins; 1991:238.
21. Mencher GT. *Early identification of hearing loss.* Proceedings from the 1974 Nova Scotia Conference on Early Identification of Hearing Loss. Basel S. Karger; 1976.
22. American Speech-Language-Hearing Association. Supplementary statement of the Joint Committee on Infant Hearing Screening. *ASHA* 1974;16:160.
23. Joint Committee on Infant Hearing Position Statement. *Pediatrics* 1982;70:496.
24. Joint Committee on Infant Hearing 1990 Position Statement. *ASHA* 1991;33:3(Suppl 5).
25. Bess FH, Paradise JL. Universal screening for infant hearing: not simple, not risk-free, not necessary beneficial, and not presently justified. *Pediatrics* 1994;98:330.
26. Letters to the editor. *Pediatrics* 1994;94:948.
27. White K, Behrens T, eds. The Rhode Island hearing assessment project: implications for universal newborn screening. *Semin Hear* 1993;14:1.
28. Gorlin RJ, Toriello HV, Cohen MM. *Hereditary hearing loss and its syndromes.* New York: Oxford University Press; 1995.
29. Fraser GR. *The causes of profound deafness in childhood.* Baltimore: The Johns Hopkins University Press; 1976.
30. Coplan J. Deafness: ever heard of it? Delayed recognition of permanent hearing loss. *Pediatrics* 1987;79:206.
31. Stein L, Boyer KM. Progress in the prevention of hearing loss in infants. *Ear Hear* 1994;15:116.
32. Welsh R, Slater S. The state of infant hearing screening impairment programs. *ASHA* 1993;35:49.

CHAPTER 11

Assessment of Vestibular Function

David Foyt and William H. Slattery III

INITIAL EVALUATION

Proper assessment of vestibular function begins with a thorough neurotologic history and physical examination. This includes a complete otologic and full neurologic examination, including testing of cranial nerves, with an examination of the balance system. Audiologic and vestibular tests complement the physical examination. A judicious use of computed tomography (CT) or magnetic resonance imaging (MRI) may also be of help in selected cases. The neurotologic examination is much more difficult in children than in adults and must be tailored to the age and behavioral maturity of the child. By age 4 to 5, the examination of balance, coordination and vestibular testing can usually be performed as in an adult (1). Children under the age of 4 are more difficult to test and require additional time, patience, and special techniques. Technical difficulties in examining children of this age stem from their fear of strangers, insecurity in a foreign environment, and labile attention span. Neonates and infants are an even more challenging group to evaluate because their immature CNS is rapidly maturing and constantly changing. Only the assessment of primitive reflexes may be possible in this age group. The differential diagnosis of vertigo in children is quite varied and very different from that in adults (Fig. 1). Disorders that may be unique to children and uncommon in adults must be kept in mind throughout the evaluation.

The first step in the evaluation of a dizzy child is to obtain complete family and medical histories. The medical and family histories may be most efficiently obtained before the physician encounter by giving the patient and child a questionnaire that can be completed in the waiting room or at home (Fig. 2). The child may be more forthcoming and cooperative if the information is obtained in a place where the child feels safe and comfortable. A family history of hearing loss, vertigo, and otologic and neurologic diseases is elicited. A careful genetic history is obtained to help rule out inheritable syndromes. Many syndromes that affect the inner ear can present in a sporadically inherited manner or with incomplete expressivity and may, therefore, not be easily identifiable. Detailed information regarding the pregnancy and delivery of the child is obtained, including the type of delivery, complications of delivery, and postnatal course. The use of possible ototoxic medications, illicit drugs, cytomegalovirus, or alcohol during pregnancy is investigated as well as any prenatal infections such as measles, mumps, rubella, CMV or syphilis. Questions about previous otologic and neurosurgical diseases or surgeries, endocrine abnormalities such as diabetes or hypothyroidism, or any psychiatric problems with the child are relevant. The most common known cause of vertigo in children is otitis media (2). It is, therefore, important to obtain a complete account of current and past episodes of ear infections. A commonly missed but easily remedied source of vertigo in children is vision problems. Information regarding recent eye examinations or changes in eyeglass prescription needs to be obtained. Pediatric migraine and the closely related benign paroxysmal vertigo of childhood are also extremely common causes of vertigo in children (3). The child should, therefore, be asked about headache and nausea and vomiting preceding or following the vertiginous attacks.

After a thorough history is completed, a detailed chief complaint can be obtained. The time of initial onset, frequency, duration of vertigo, and associated symptoms, such as nausea and vomiting, tinnitus, and hearing loss, should be obtained from the child. The distinction between true vertigo and dizziness is an important one and should be elicited carefully from the child. Vertigo is an illusionary sense that either the environment or ones own body is revolving (4). Vertigo may or may not be due to a vestibular dysfunction. *Dizziness* is a nonspecific term used to describe a sensation of disorientation or altered sensorium. It is often equated erroneously to vertigo, even by adult patients. Young chil-

---

D. Foyt and W.H. Slattery III: House Ear Clinic and Department of Clinical Studies, House Ear Institute, Los Angeles, California 90057.

458 children

- Migrane 27.9%
- Paroxysmal Vertigo of Childhood 13.3%
- Recurrent Vestibulopathy 10.7%
- Psychiatric 6.8%
- Isolated ataxia with vertigo a central vestibular component
- Vestibular Neuronitis 4.8%
- Delayed Vertigo 4.8%
- BPPV 4.6%
- Temporal Bone Trauma 4.6%
- Meniere's Disease 2.6%
- Labyrinthitis 2.4%
- Other 17.5%

5535 adults

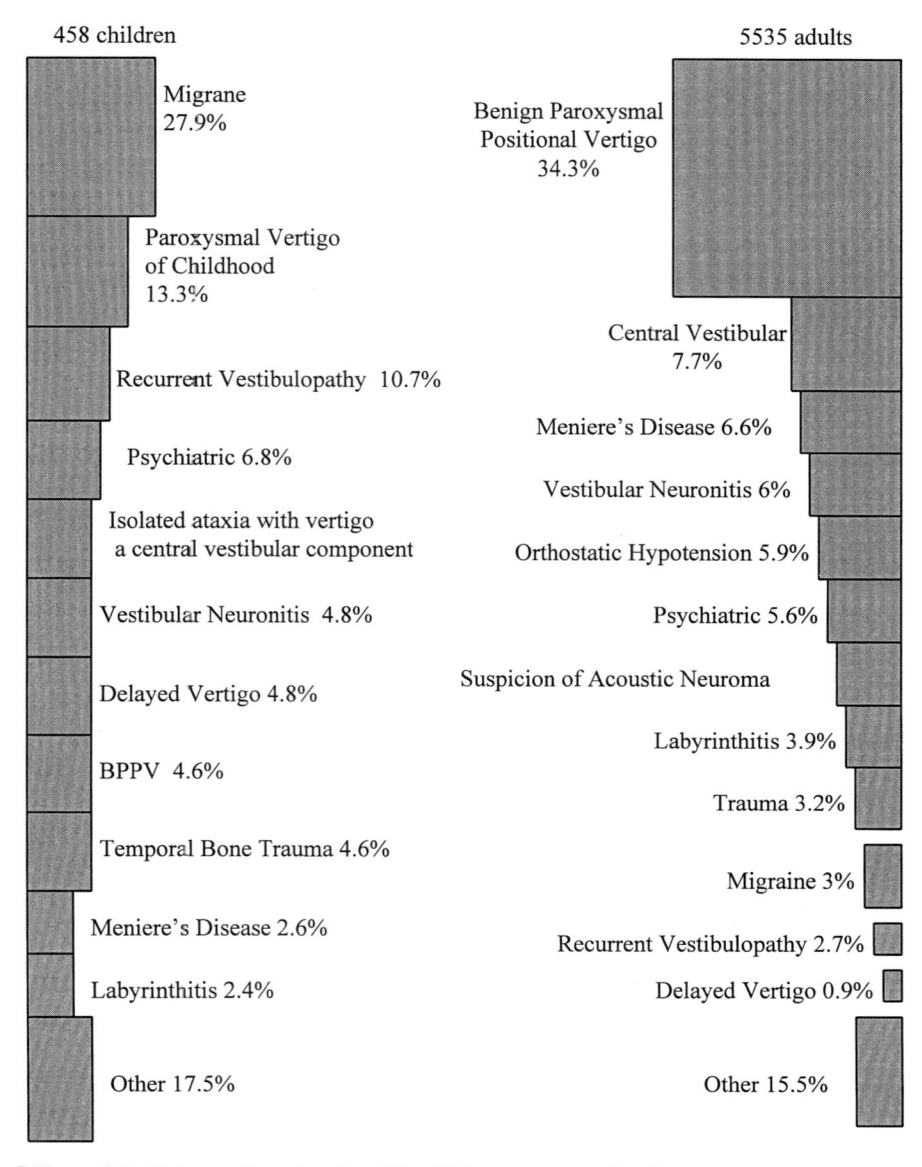

- Benign Paroxysmal Positional Vertigo 34.3%
- Central Vestibular 7.7%
- Meniere's Disease 6.6%
- Vestibular Neuronitis 6%
- Orthostatic Hypotension 5.9%
- Psychiatric 5.6%
- Suspicion of Acoustic Neuroma
- Labyrinthitis 3.9%
- Trauma 3.2%
- Migraine 3%
- Recurrent Vestibulopathy 2.7%
- Delayed Vertigo 0.9%
- Other 15.5%

FIG. 1. Differential etiology of vertigo in 453 children compared with 5,535 adults presenting with a complaint of vertigo. Translated by Fayad J from Toupet M, Toupet FN. Le vertige chez l enfant. Rev Prat (Paris) 1994;44:343.

dren may not have the verbal skills to describe their symptoms or make fine distinctions such as these. It is, however, important to have children describe their symptoms in their own words. Children will describe their symptoms in various manners relative to their age and maturity. An older child, for example, may be able to provide a clear distinction between true spinning vertigo and simply a dizzy sensation. A younger child may not be able to clearly describe symptoms or may use euphemisms. The input and help of a parent are important in these situations. The parent may be able to elaborate on the child's history with a more objective second-party observation, such as recent clumsiness, seizure activity, or altered levels of consciousness. The parent should be asked to record future episodes of vertigo including the duration, severity, and associated symptoms. The parents can also be instructed on how to examine the child for nystagmus during vertiginous attacks.

The method of conducting the physical examination must be tailored to the child's age and maturity. Of paramount importance is to gain the child's confidence by gently explaining each step in the examination process. It is impossible to perform an accurate neurotologic examination on a frightened or hysterical child. A general medical and otolaryngologic exam should first be performed, followed by a neurologic examination. A gross body survey may be done to look for any outward signs of genetic or developmental abnormalities. The heart and lungs should be examined. The presence of an upper respiratory infection may be the cause

DIZZINESS QUESTIONNAIRE

Name _____ Date _____

I When you are "dizzy" do you experience any of the following sensations? Please read the entire list first. Then circle (yes) or (no) to describe your feelings most accurately.

- Yes No 1. Lightheadedness or swimming sensation in the head.
- Yes No 2. Blacking out or loss of consciousness.
- Yes No 3. Tendency to fall: To the right?
- Yes No   To the left?
- Yes No   Forward?
- Yes No   Backward?
- Yes No 4. Objects spinning or turning around you.
- Yes No 5. Sensation that you are turning or spinning inside, with outside objects remaining stationary.
- Yes No 6. Sensation of the environment moving up and down while you walk.
- Yes No 7. Loss of balance when walking: Veering to the right?
- Yes No   Veering to the left?
- Yes No 8. Headache.
- Yes No 9. Nausea or vomiting.
- Yes No 10. Pressure in the head.
- Yes No 11. Palpitations, perspiration, shortness of breath, or a feeling of panic.

II Please Circle (yes) or (no) and fill in the blank spaces. **Answer all questions.**

1. My dizziness is:
- Yes No   Constant?
- Yes No   In attacks?

2. When did dizziness first occur? _____

3. If in attacks: How often? _____
   How long do they last? _____
   When was last attack? _____

- Yes No   Do you have any warning that the attack is about to start?
- Yes No   Do they occur at any particular time of day or night?
- Yes No   Are you completely free of dizziness between attacks?
- Yes No 4. Does change of position make you dizzy?
- Yes No 5. Do you have trouble walking in the dark?
- Yes No 6. When you are dizzy, must you support yourself when standing?

(Please turn page and finish questionnaire.)

FIG. 2. Dizziness questionnaire used by the House Ear Clinic, Inc. Modified from Busis, Acta Otolaryngol Suppl. 209, 1965. (From Sheehy JL. The Dizzy Patient. Arch Otolaryngol 1967;86:44.) *(continued)*

Yes	No	7. Do you know of any possible cause of your dizziness? What? _____	

8. Do you know of anything that will:

Yes	No	Stop your dizziness or make it better? _____
Yes	No	Make your dizziness worse? _____
Yes	No	Precipitate an attack? (Fatigue? Exertion? Hunger? Menstrual Period? Stress? Emotional Upset?)
Yes	No	9. Were you exposed to any irritating fumes, paints, etc., at the onset of dizziness?

10. **If you are allergic** to any medications, please list: _____

Yes	No	11. If you ever injured your head, were you unconscious?

12. **If you take any medications** regularly, for any reason, please list: _____

Yes	No	13. Do you use tobacco in any form? _____ How much? _____

III Do you have any of the following symptoms? Please circle (yes) or (no) and circle (ear) involved.

Yes	No	1. Difficulty in hearing?	Both ears	Right	Left
Yes	No	2. Noise in your ears?	Both ears	Right	Left
		Describe the noise _____			
Yes	No	Does noise change with dizziness? If so, how? _____			
Yes	No	3. Fullness or stuffiness in your ears?	Both ears	Right	Left
Yes	No	4. Pain in your ears?	Both ears	Right	Left
Yes	No	5. Discharge from your ears?	Both ears	Right	Left

IV Have you experienced any of the following symptoms? Please circle (yes) or (no) and circle if (constant) or if in (episodes).

Yes	No	1. Double vision, blurred vision or blindness.	Constant	In Episodes
Yes	No	2. Numbness of face.	Constant	In Episodes
Yes	No	3. Numbness of arms or legs.	Constant	In Episodes
Yes	No	4. Weakness in arms or legs.	Constant	In Episodes
Yes	No	5. Clumsiness of arms or legs.	Constant	In Episodes
Yes	No	6. Confusion or loss of consciousness.	Constant	In Episodes
Yes	No	7. Difficulty with speech.	Constant	In Episodes
Yes	No	8. Difficulty with swallowing.	Constant	In Episodes
Yes	No	9. Pain in the neck or shoulder.	Constant	In Episodes
Yes	No	10. Seasickness or car sickness.	Constant	In Episodes

FG220   rev. 8/94   rep. 5/95

FIG. 2. *Continued.*

of vertigo, presumably by the alteration of eustachian tube function. The ears should be examined with a pneumatic otoscope. Middle ear diseases, such as otitis media and eustachian tube dysfunction commonly produce vestibular symptoms in children and can be diagnosed easily. In a study of 154 children with surgically proven secretory otitis media, by Grace and Pfleiderer, 22% were found to have vestibular symptoms (5). It has also been theorized that negative middle ear pressure due to eustachian tube dysfunction can cause vestibular symptoms by displacement of the round window membrane (6). Tympanometry may be used if there is any question of tympanic membrane retraction or negative middle ear pressure. Vertigo and nystagmus during insufflation with the otoscope have their own clinical significance and are discussed later in the chapter. The nose should be examined for congestion and allergic rhinitis, because this may contribute to eustachian tube dysfunction and vertigo. Finally a full examination of the oropharynx, head, and neck is done to complete the otolaryngologic examination.

A full neurologic examination, including testing of cranial nerves, is an integral part of the evaluation. Occult or subtle neurologic deficits are often uncovered at this stage. Testing the olfactory nerve (CN 1) is difficult even in the adult population but can be grossly judged by history. A complaint of anosmia combined with a difficulty in tasting foods and recent weight loss may alert the physician to olfactory nerve deficits. Visual acuity (CN 2), however, can be readily measured in the clinic or office with a Snell chart. Extraocular motion (CN 3, 4, 6) can be measured easily by having the child follow a small toy to all four quadrants (Fig. 3). Facial sensation (CN 5) as well as assessment of the corneal blink reflex can be done with the sharp end or cotton end of a cotton-tipped applicator. Facial symmetry (CN 7) should be examined in both the stationary and grimacing positions. Gross auditory function (CN 8) can be examined with tuning forks or by simply whispering into the child's ear. A strong shoulder (CN 11) shrug can be elicited to measure spinal accessory nerve function. A positive gag reflex with midline tongue thrust (CN 9, 10, 12) completes the cranial nerve examination.

The cranial nerve examination should be followed by examination of deep tendon reflexes and gross motor strength in all four extremities. During the neurologic examination the physician should take note of any abnormality in the child's affect and behavior. A short mental status examination can even be performed. The child should be able to follow the physical examination in a manner that is appropriate to his or her age. A child with a blunted or inappropriate affect or one who behaves overemotionally may require psychiatric evaluation. The inability of the child to attend school or significant avoidance of everyday activities out of proportion to physical findings may be another clue that psychological factors are at play.

Balance refers to the ability of an individual to maintain a stable body position. Balance requires a synthesis of three sensory inputs: vision, somatosensation, and vestibular sensation. To maintain balance, two of the three systems must be intact. The basic principle behind balance testing rests in elucidating the relative importance of these three components to the patient's ability to maintain posture. During balance testing, one or more of the proprioceptive queues are removed and the patient is observed. Assessment of balance can be accomplished with the Romberg test, gait analysis, and tandem walking. In the standard Romberg test, the patient stands with feet together and arms crossed. The child is evaluated first with his or her eyes open and then closed. A positive test is characterized by uncontrollable falling when the eyes are closed. Instability or near-falling does not

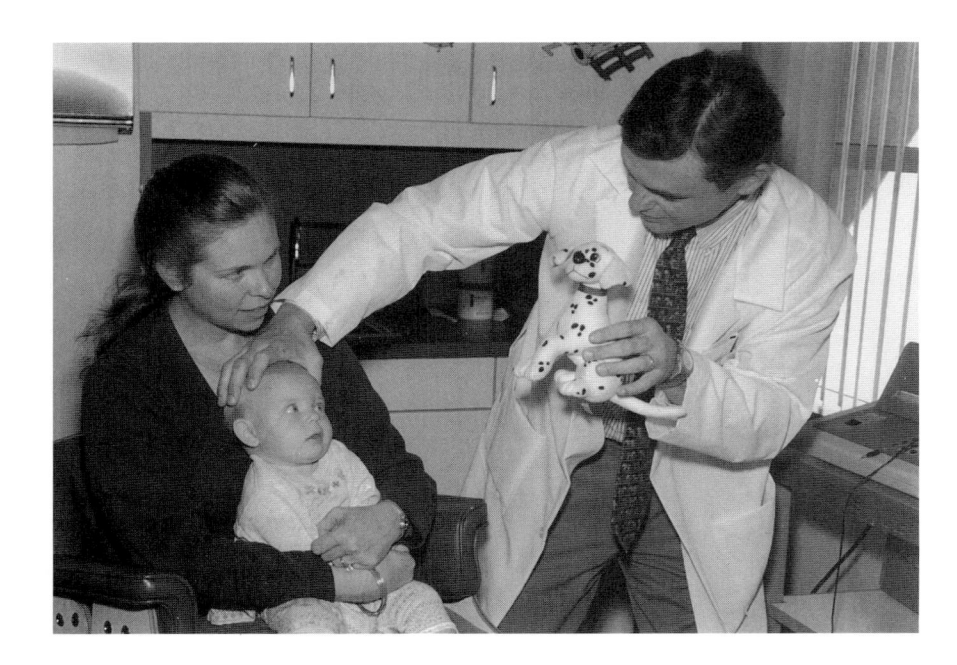

FIG. 3. Extraocular motion can be measured in infants by presenting a small toy to all four visual fields. Reprinted with permission of House Ear Institute.

constitute a positive result. A more demanding measure of balance is the tandem or sharpened Romberg. This is performed by standing with arms crossed and feet in the tandem position, as if walking a tightrope. An alternative technique to the tandem Romberg is to have the child stand on a foam pad during the test (7). This eliminates some of the proprioceptive queues and makes the test much more difficult. If the child falls after the eyes are closed, pathology is indicated. A positive test indicates that, when vision is removed, there is only one remaining properly functioning system: Either the vestibular or proprioceptive–cerebellar system is impaired. If the child does not have ataxia with eyes open, signifying a gross proprioceptive–cerebellar lesion, then one can assume a vestibular lesion. The child who cannot maintain equilibrium, even with eyes, open may have a severe uncompensated vestibular lesion or, more likely, a central or proprioceptive cause of the dysequilibrium.

Gait and tandem walking analysis can aid in the diagnosis of a vestibular lesion but is seldom localizing. The patient is asked to walk with a normal gait, followed by a heel-to-toe gait. A wide-based gait is seen in cerebellar dysfunction, while consistent falling to one side is characteristic of a vestibular or cerebellar dysfunction, often localized to that side. Other neurologic tests, such as past pointing and drift, may help suggest a more central pathology. Past pointing and drift are tested with the patient in the sitting position. The patient is asked to extend the arm and reach a small target positioned in front of the patient. A pathologic finding occurs if the patient repeatedly misses the target. Drift is measured with both of the patient's arms and hands extended in front, in the Superman position. The patient is instructed to hold the hands horizontally aligned while the eyes are kept closed. Drift of either arm away from horizontal is pathologic. Both past pointing and drift are measures of cerebellar dysfunction and may help steer the physician away from a diagnosis of vestibular dysfunction.

Not every child will be able to perform all the components of the neurotologic examination. Interpretation of performance should be tempered by the child's age. There are no clear-cut age-related standards regarding performance on balance and coordination tests because the rate of maturation of the nervous system varies among children. There are, however, certain age-related points of reference (8). While children of age 3 should be able to walk on their heels and toes, children below age 5 are not expected to walk in a straight line. Even 7-year-olds are allowed three near-falls while performing a 20-pace forward and backward walk. Most school-age children, however, should be able to hold a Romberg position for 15 seconds and a tandem Romberg for 6 seconds (9). The examination will also depend heavily on the child's relative emotional maturity and on the presence of any physical or psychiatric problems. Additional patience and perseverance are often required in these situations.

Examination of the infant requires special techniques. The infant's nervous system is in a rapid state of development and maturation through the first several years of life, and at times only rudimentary ''primitive'' reflexes can be elicited. By the age of 6 weeks, infants are able to follow an object in their visual field. Semicircular canal function may be tested by holding the infant or child at arms' length and spinning the child in a circle around the physician (Fig. 4). Newborns have an intact vestibulo-ocular reflex at birth and should display eye deviation upon angular acceleration. Infants up to 3 weeks of age may have a conjugate deviation of their eyes away from the direction of acceleration. This is called the doll's eye phenomenon. Normally, cortical inhibition of the vestibular nuclei suppresses this phenomenon in awake adults. In infants, it presence signifies a lack of

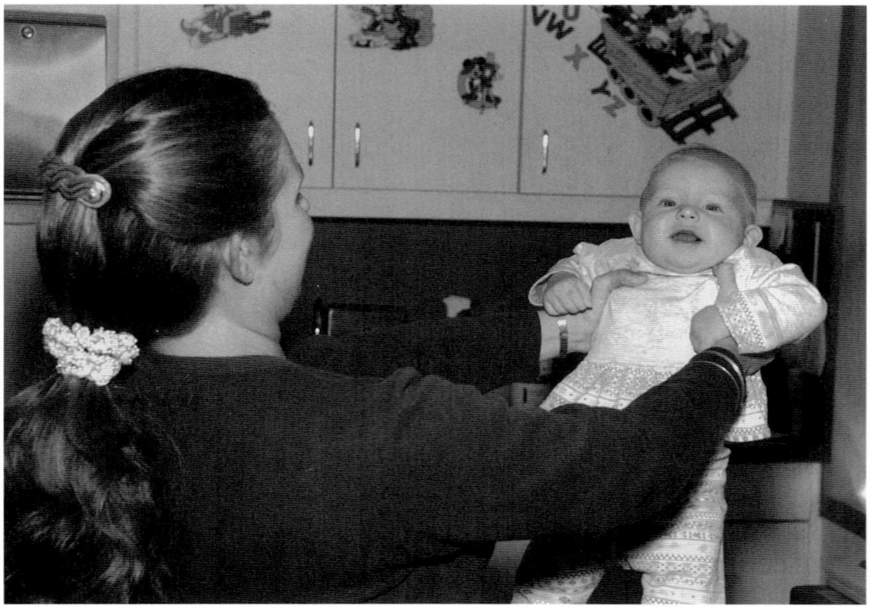

FIG. 4. An intact vestibulo-ocular reflex can be elicited by spinning the child in a circle and observing eye motion. Reprinted with permission of House Ear Institute.

maturation of the CNS. By 3 weeks of age, the saccadic eye movement system and cortical inhibitory pathways have developed enough so that older infants produce conjugate eye deviation toward the direction of acceleration as would an adult. In premature infants, the doll's eye phenomenon may persist for up to 3 months (1).

Infants display developmental reflexes that also can be tested (Table 1). These reflexes are more useful for following an infants neurologic development than directly testing vestibular function. These reflexes are not necessarily present in all children, but failure to outgrow any of these reflexes signifies serious neurologic deficits. Between birth and 4 months the infant displays righting and startle reflexes. The righting reflex is elicited by turning an infant's head to the side. The body should automatically turn with the head. If the body is restrained while the head is turned, the infant may assume a fencing position: The arm on the side that the head is turned is extended, while the contralateral arm is held in flexion. Soon after birth, the well-described Moro, or startle, reflex appears. Sudden stimulation by a loud noise or abrupt movement causes an abduction of the child's arm and fanning of the fingers. Auditory function as well as proprioceptive and vestibular function can be crudely tested with this reflex at a very early age. The startle reflex is ubiquitous in all children, and its absence is considered pathologic. By the sixth month of life, a rapid development of the nervous system has begun, with an integration of vestibular, visual, and proprioceptive inputs. A more coordinated righting reflex may be elicited at this age. If an infant is blindfolded, held upright, and then tilted, the head will right itself so that the eyes will maintain a horizontal position. The arm on the side of tilt should also extend, as if to break a fall. The parachute reflex involves holding the infant at arms' length and producing a vertical downward acceleration. The head should right itself to remain midline along the axis of the body. By 8 to 10 months, a hopping reflex may be elicited. The reflex is produced by holding the child by the torso and tilting the child backward and forward. The child should take a step in the direction of the tilt.

After a complete history and physical examination have been accomplished, formal audiologic examinations should be done. A full pure-tone audiogram with speech discrimination score may be performed on children as early as 3 years of age. Younger children require special audiologic techniques to obtain auditory thresholds. Finally, auditory brainstem response measurements may be performed on children that are unable to cooperate with formal audiologic testing. Because the auditory and vestibular components of the inner ear are intimately linked, a defect in one often parallels a deficit in the other. A hearing test is easily obtained, depending on the age of the child, and should be considered an integral part of a routine evaluation. An abnormal finding on audiometry may help localize a dysfunctional inner ear. Many congenital inner ear defects present with hearing loss either preceding or following vestibular dysfunction (10).

A hematological examination also should be done early in the work-up of vestibular dysfunction. Complete blood counts, serum glucose or glucose tolerance test, thyroid function tests, fluorescent treponemal antibody absorption, erythrocyte sedimentation rate, rheumatoid factor, and antinuclear antibody should be done if considered appropriate. The literature suggests that at least some types of endolymphatic hydrops may have an immune or autoimmune etiology (11). If there is any evidence that allergy may be contributing to the symptoms, an allergy work-up may be appropriate. This would include allergy testing and desensitization immunotherapy.

RADIOLOGICAL EVALUATION

If there are any questions of congenital ear or temporal bone malformations, trauma, or if a space-occupying lesion is suspected, radiologic imaging should be employed. Computed tomography is useful to visualize abnormalities of the labyrinth, middle ear, mastoid, and the petrous bone. An abnormally large vestibular aqueduct also known as large aqueduct syndrome, is an under-diagnosed source of labyrinthine dysfunction, which can present with or without sensorineural hearing loss (12). This abnormality is most easily demonstrated with thin-section CT imaging of the temporal bone. Erosion of the bone over a semicircular canal by cholesteatoma may also be seen with CT (Fig. 5). Any child with cholesteatoma and vertigo deserves imaging to rule out fistula. Congenital malformations that involve the bony inner ear, such as Mondini's dysphasia and Michel's aplasia, are readily seen with CT. The most common of the bony deformities, Mondini's dysphasia, often presents with sensorineural hearing loss and vestibular dysfunction at an early age. The characteristic fusion of the cochlear apical and middle turns can be visualized on CT (Fig. 6). Two of the most common inner ear malformations, Scheibe (cochleosaccular aplasia) and Alexander (aplasia of the cochlear duct with high-frequency hearing loss), are membranous malformations and cannot be seen on CT scan. Magnetic resonance imaging

TABLE 1. *Progression of developmental reflexes*

Age at first presentation	Reflex
24th week of gestation	Oculovestibular reflexes fully established
32nd week of gestation	Inner ear vestibular reflexes fully matured Moro reflex activated Doll's eye phenomenon present
0–6 mo	Neck-righting reflex Tonic neck reflex Moro reflex
6–18 mo	Body-righting reflex Parachute reflex Hopping reflex
3 yr	Child stands with broad base Child able to walk on heels and toes
5 yr	Child stands with narrow base Child able to walk in straight line

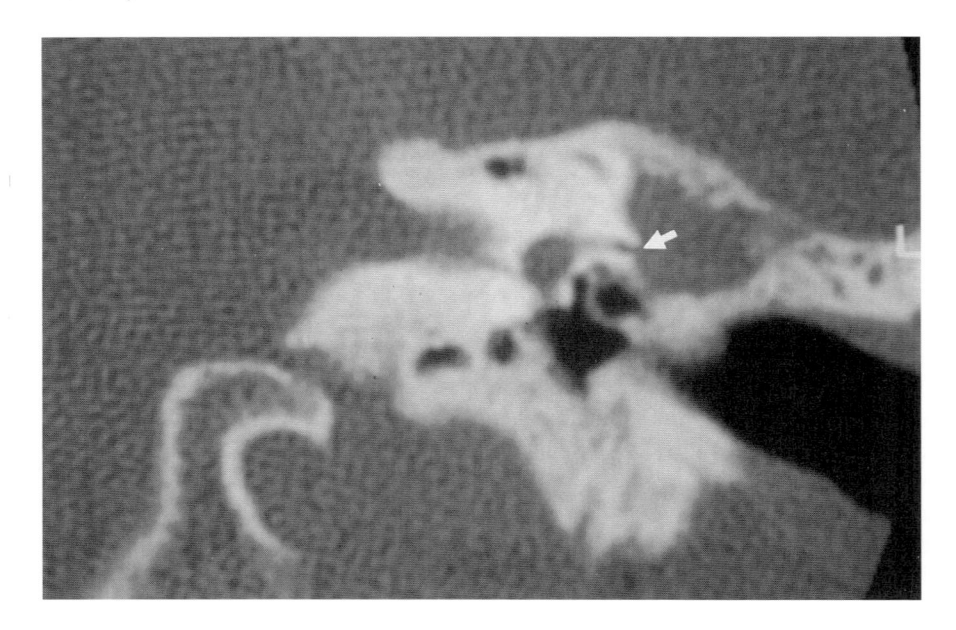

FIG. 5. Cholesteatoma can erode through the otic capsule into the inner ear, causing sensorineural hearing loss and vertigo. The lateral semicircular canal (*arrow*) is one of the most common sites of bone erosion. Reprinted with permission of House Ear Institute.

has yet to achieve the proper resolution to clearly visualize these membranous malformations. Definitive diagnosis may be possible only on postmortem histologic examination of the temporal bones.

Magnetic resonance imaging is most useful for high-resolution imaging of soft-tissue structures. Often, subtle soft-tissue changes, such as inflammation, can be seen. Magnetic resonance imaging of the temporal bone is most commonly obtained with intravenous contrast to visualize vestibular schwannomas. These tumors are exceedingly rare in the pediatric population. The only exception is in children with neurofibromatosis-2 (NF-2). This is an autosomal dominant inherited disorder that often occurs as a sporadic mutation. Acoustic neuromas present in a large majority of these patients as early as 10 years of age. Dysequilibrium may be the presenting symptom in these patients. If there is a family history of NF-2 or if the child presents with any stigmata of the disease, an MRI should be performed promptly. Similarly, MRI with contrast enhancement should be performed if there is any suspicion of a space-occupying lesion or other central nervous pathology such as multiple sclerosis (13). In a recent study of 400 children with vertigo presenting to an outpatient clinic, 3% had a primary CNS neoplasm (14). These children should never be misdiagnosed.

Cochleovestibular neuritis may be seen as an enhancement of the cochleovestibular nerve bundle on T2- and T1-weighted images with gadolinium (Fig. 7). Inflammatory labyrinthitis will show similarly enhancement of the vestibule on MRI in the acute phase. The enhancement usually disappears 6 months after resolution of symptoms (15).

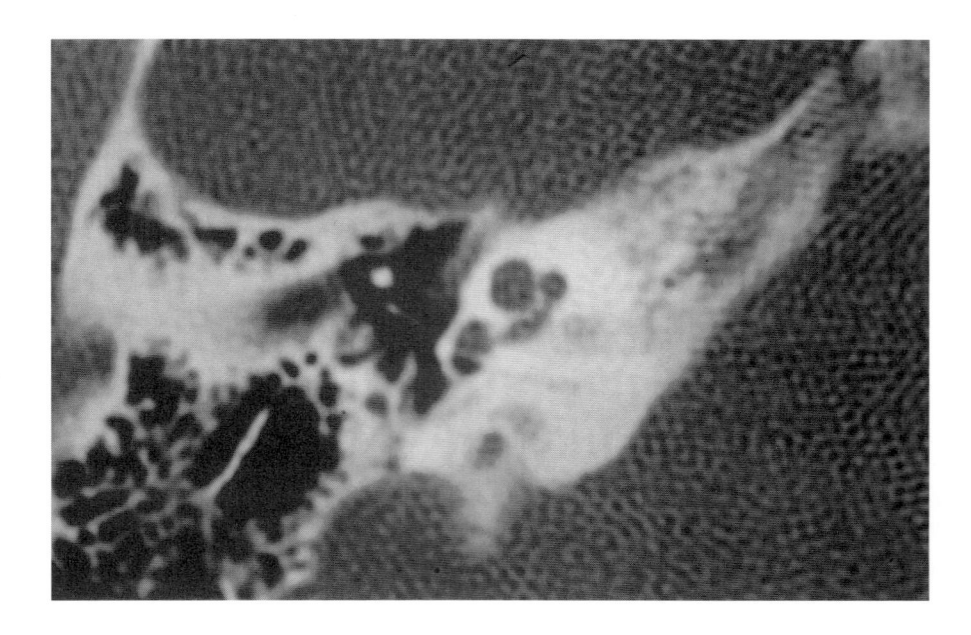

FIG. 6. A high-resolution CT scan with bone algorithm clearly shows the common cavity defect of Mondini dysplasia, which is caused by fusion of the cochlear apical and middle turns. Reprinted with permission of House Ear Institute.

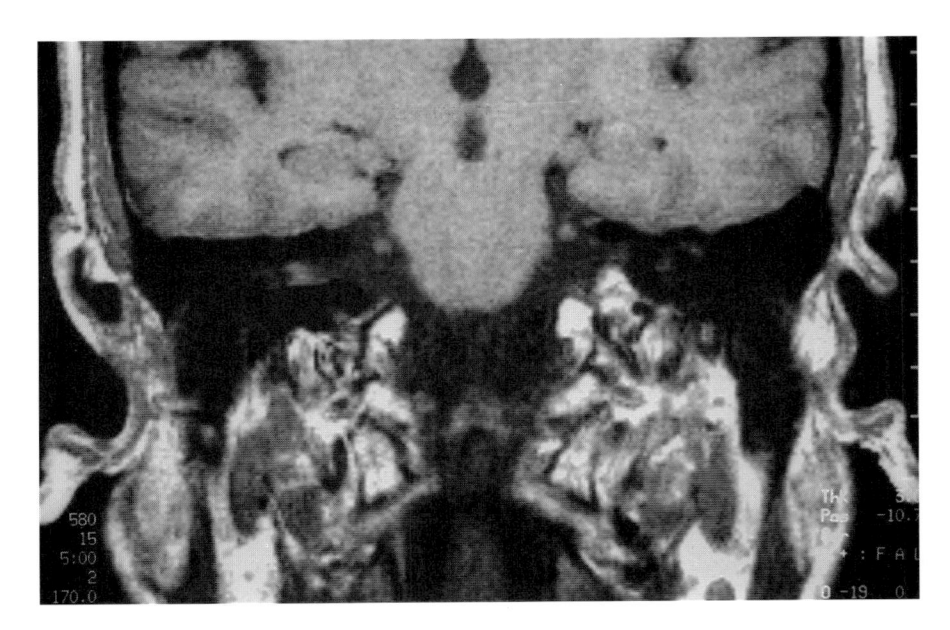

FIG. 7. T1-weighted image with contrast showing enhancement of cochleovestibular nerve in a young patient with sudden hearing loss after a viral upper respiratory infection. Reprinted with permission of House Ear Institute.

Trauma to the temporal bone is best evaluated with CT. Fractures through the labyrinth can be well visualized using bone window algorithms (Fig. 8). The technique is also particularly useful in visualizing the facial nerve and its relation to the fracture line. High-resolution MRI can demonstrate subacute bleeding within the labyrinth as a high signal on unenhanced T1 weighted images. Cerebrospinal fluid fistulae into the middle ear may be visualized on T2-weighted images (Fig. 9). Cerebrospinal fluid has a high signal intensity on T2, making it possible to visualize the CSF pathway through the fracture to the middle ear.

Other diagnostic modalities should be utilized as the clinical situation dictates. If a diagnosis of complex seizures is entertained, for example, an EEG may be considered along with a referral for complete neurologic evaluation (16).

TESTS OF VESTIBULAR FUNCTION

Vestibular testing is an integral part of the evaluation of a dizzy child. The goal of vestibular testing is first to document a peripheral (i.e., vestibular) source for the vertigo. As mentioned, the distinction between peripheral vestibular pathology and central pathology is a crucial branching point in the diagnostic algorithm. Each diagnosis has its own consequences and treatment modality, discussion of which is beyond the scope of this chapter. If a vestibular source of

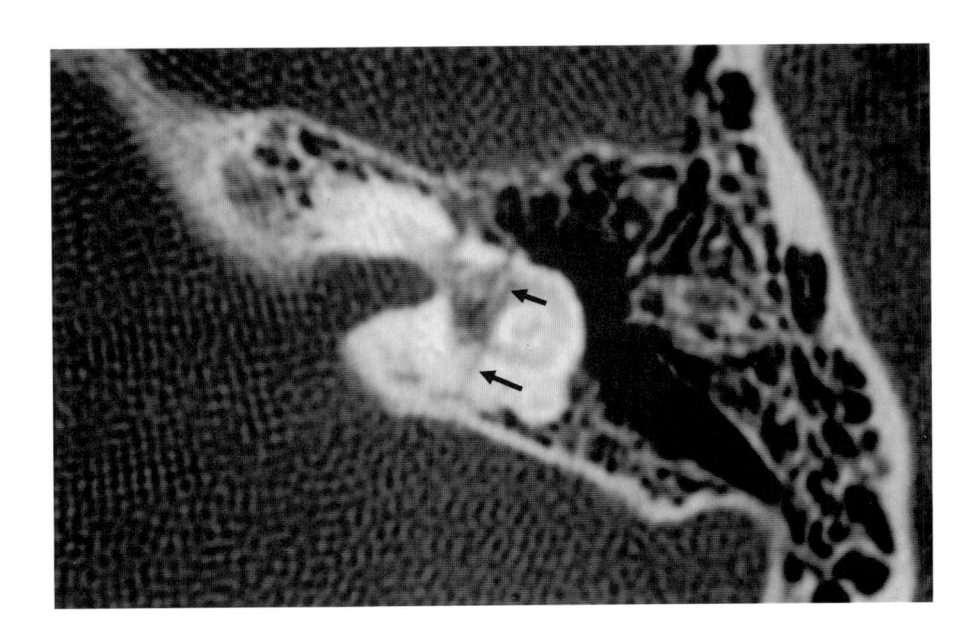

FIG. 8. Axial CT of temporal bone showing transverse temporal bone fracture (*arrows*) involving the vestibule. Reprinted with permission of House Ear Institute.

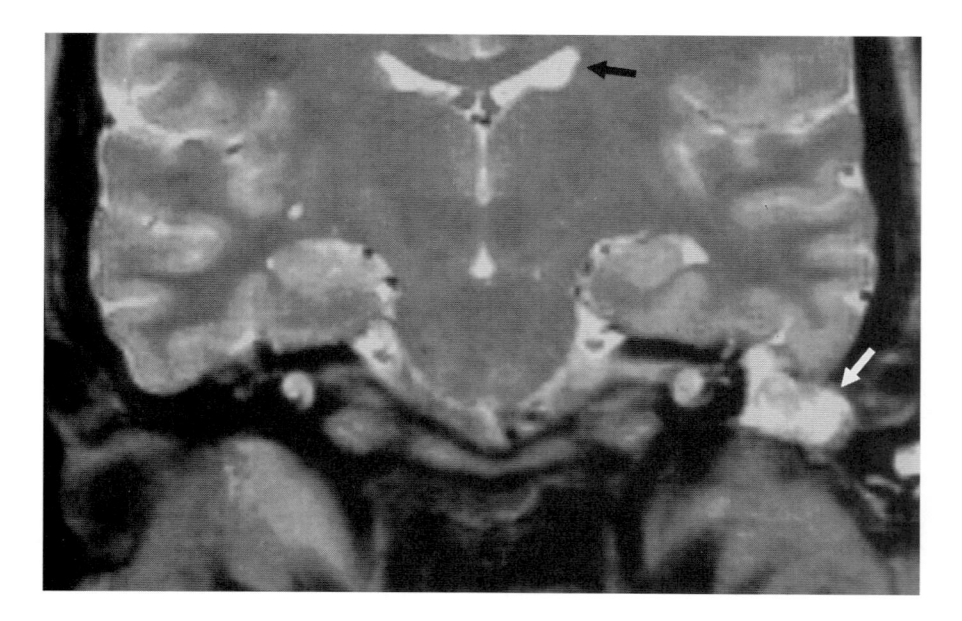

FIG. 9. Cerebrospinal fluid that appears bright on T2 weighted MRI is normal in the lateral ventricle. Cerebrospinal fluid leakage is clearly seen leaking into the middle ear cavity (*arrow*). Reprinted with permission of House Ear Institute.

the vertigo is discovered, the side of the dysfunctional labyrinth can then be deduced. More advanced vestibular testing can also be used to follow the progress of vestibular rehabilitation and is discussed later in the chapter.

Physiology

By school age, children are able to tolerate formal vestibular testing, much like adults. The various tests of vestibular function are firmly grounded in the anatomy and physiology of the human labyrinth. To gain an understanding of these tests, one must first review the basic anatomy and physiology of the vestibular system. The membranous labyrinth includes three semicircular canals situated at approximately right angles to one another, which function as sensors of angular acceleration of the head in three dimensions. The canals are sensitive only to head movements and are normally insensitive to gravitational forces. The other component of the membranous labyrinth is the saccule and utricle, which function as sensors of linear acceleration (gravity) but are seldom involved in vestibular testing. To a first-order approximation, each semicircular canal is hard-wired to its corresponding coplanar set of eye muscles (Fig. 10). The eyes are held in a midline position by tonic and equal activity from each canal. Stimulation or inhibition of a single canal causes an asymmetric relative hyperactivity of one labyrinth. This in turn causes a deviation of the eye toward the relatively hypoactive side, followed by a compensatory saccade in the opposite direction initiated by the reticular formation of the CNS. The basis for this phenomenon is the vestibulo-ocular reflex (VOR) arc. The VOR has a very short latency and normally functions to compensate for changes in head position, allowing images to remain relatively fixed on the retina while the head is moving. In the case of the lateral semicircular canal, for example, stimulation causes excitation of the ipsilateral medial rectus and contralateral lateral rectus while inhibiting the ipsilateral lateral rectus and contralateral medial rectus. A slow horizontal deviation to the contralateral ear in the plane of the canal occurs. A compensatory rapid correction (saccade) to counteract the deviation then occurs, mediated by the CNS. The direction of nystagmus is defined as the direction of the fast saccade phase. Due to eccentric insertion of the superior and inferior oblique muscles, eye motion is not always coplanar with the semicircular canal, explaining the oblique and rotational nystagmus that is often seen. This interaction between the semicircular canals, eye muscles, and CNS forms the basis of all vestibular testing. The VOR allows for a clinically objective measurement of vestibular function through the observation of eye motion and greatly aids in the assessment of patients with balance disorders.

Nystagmus can be divided into spontaneous and elicited. Spontaneous nystagmus can be observed passively and is a direct result of vestibular or central pathology. Nystagmus can also be elicited by various techniques that target sites within the labyrinth. In the following discussion, the most commonly used vestibular tests are explained.

Spontaneous Nystagmus

The simplest method of evaluating vestibular function is by direct observation of eye motion without labyrinthine stimulation. *Spontaneous nystagmus* refers to nystagmus observed with the patient sitting still, without external stimulation such as head tilt or caloric stimulation. This observation is a routine part of any neurotologic examination and can be done in the office with a patient of any age. Fine nystagmus is, however, often difficult to appreciate with the naked eye. This may be facilitated by the use of Frensel lenses. These glasses have 20-diopter lenses that eliminate visual

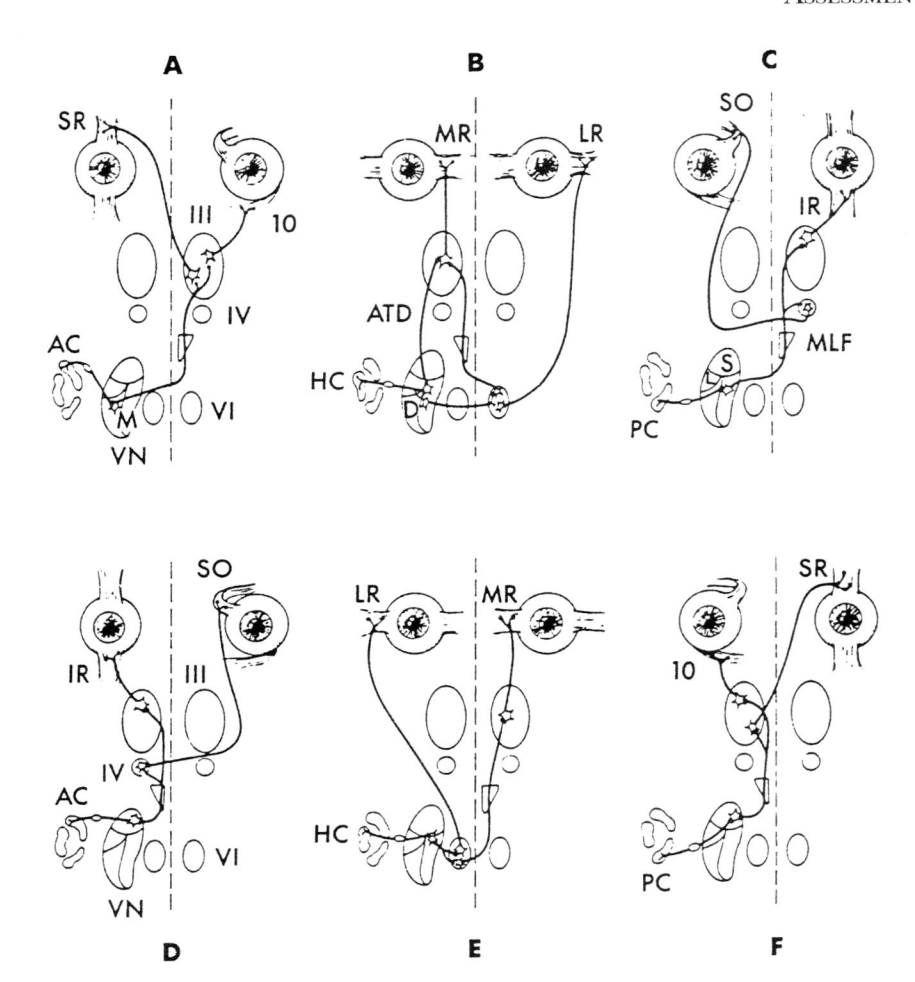

FIG. 10. (**A–C**) Excitatory and (**D–F**), inhibitory pathways between individual semicircular canals and eye muscles in cat. (Uchino et al., 1982; Uchino and Suzuki, 1983). *SR*, Superior rectus; *IO*, inferior oblique; *MR*, medial rectus; *LR*, lateral rectus; *SO*, superior oblique; *IR*, inferior rectus; *AC*, anterior canal; *HC*, horizontal canal; *PC*, posterior canal; *VN*, vestibular nuclei; *S*, superior vestibular nucleus; *D*, descending vestibular nucleus; *ATD*, ascending tract of Dieters; *VI*, abducens nucleus; *IV*, trochlear nucleus; *III*, oculomotor complex. From Baloh RW, Honrubia V. Clinical neurophysiology of the vestibular system, 2nd ed. Philadelphia: FA Davis, 1990.

fixation and magnify the patients eyes, resulting in easier visualization of nystagmus. In addition, these goggle-like glasses are illuminated by small bulbs that further facilitate the objective assessment of the eye movements. Despite continued refinements to this classic instrument, subtle eye movements are at times very difficult to appreciate and impossible to record objectively. Frensel lenses are nonetheless useful as an initial clinical evaluation of spontaneous and induced eye movements. Most commercial versions of these glasses are of adult size and cannot be fitted to children, thus limiting their use in the very young.

The pattern and character of the spontaneous nystagmus have both diagnostic and localizing value. Spontaneous nystagmus may result from an acute uncompensated imbalance in the vestibulo-ocular pathway. Damage with resultant paresis of one labyrinth results in spontaneous deviation of the eyes away from the lesion (slow component of nystagmus). The tonic vestibular input is no longer balanced by activity from the damaged side. This is followed by a fast saccade to the contralateral side. Pendular nystagmus without a fast or slow component is indicative of a congenital disorder, ocular disorder or multiple sclerosis. Central nervous system pathology often causes vertical, rotary, and anterior–posterior displacement nystagmus, which is seldom directly localizing. Nystagmus that occurs with far lateral gaze is called end-point nystagmus and is physiologic.

Post-Headshake Nystagmus

A simple office technique to induce nystagmus at any age is the head-shaking technique. The head is rotated back and forth at 2 Hz for 20 seconds (± 30 degree amplitude), after which the eyes are examined for nystagmus. The best results are obtained when Frensel lenses are used to better visualize the nystagmus and suppress fixation. The nystagmus is usually transient, lasting 5 to 20 seconds. The nystagmus often reverses direction and is associated with symptoms of dizziness, dysequilibrium, and vertigo. The phenomenon presumably represents an asymmetry of the vestibulo-ocular pathway. Head-shaking nystagmus is seen in 34% to 90% of patients with unilateral vestibulopathy (17). The utility of this test is limited to being only a gross assessment of vestibular symmetry that can be done easily in the office. No localizing or lateralizing information can be derived from this test. Extreme care and prudent judgment must be exercised with this technique in the evaluation of smaller children. Children with Down syndrome are prone to atlanto-occipital dislocation and should not be subjected to the maneuver.

Labyrinthine Fistula Test

The fistula test is performed by insufflating air into the external auditory canal with a pneumatic otoscope while observing eye motion. This can be performed with the pneumatic otoscope during the initial physical examination of the child. On positive pressure insufflation, conjugate deviation of the eyes toward the opposite side, followed by a fast component of nystagmus toward the affected side, is observed with a positive fistula test. Negative pressure causes the opposite effect. The labyrinthine fistula test should always be performed in a patient with a perforated tympanic membrane and vertigo. A positive fistula test in the setting of chronic suppurative otitis media implies the presence of a lateral semicircular canal or otic capsule erosion down to the endosteum of the labyrinthine cavity. In this situation, alterations in air pressure through a perforated tympanic membrane place direct pressure on the sensitive labyrinth, causing symptoms. For the test to be positive, however, the involved vestibule must be viable. It should also be noted that a positive fistula test with an intact tympanic membrane also may be encountered in patients who have had fenestration or stapedectomy operations, and in patients with Meniere's disease, traumatic or spontaneous perilymph fistulae, and/or otosyphilis (18). There are several theories regarding the pathophysiology of a positive fistula test in these diseases. The leading theory is that the endolymphatic hydrops in Meniere's disease and otosyphilis causes the saccule to dilate and come into contact with the stapes footplate. Pressure on the ossicular chain from insufflation may thus be transmitted directly to the vestibule. An abnormally mobile stapes footplate or a softening of the bone over the lateral semicircular canal in syphilis has also been implicated as a possible cause, but convincing evidence is lacking.

An uncommon clinical manifestation of labyrinthine fistula or severe endolymphatic hydrops is the Tullio phenomenon. In such cases, the patient experiences vertigo by the sudden application of a loud sound to the affected ear. To display a true Tullio phenomenon, the patient must have a fistula of the lateral semicircular canal and an intact conducting mechanism to the inner ear, including intact tympanic membrane and ossicular chain. This combination of findings is, however, quite rare.

POSITIONAL TESTS

Positional testing is done easily in a clinical office setting where a bed, bench, or reclining chair is available. Testing should be done with the child's eyes open wearing Frensel lenses, so that the eyes may be observed for nystagmus; or it may be done with electro-oculography for objective measurement of eye movement. The Hallpike maneuver

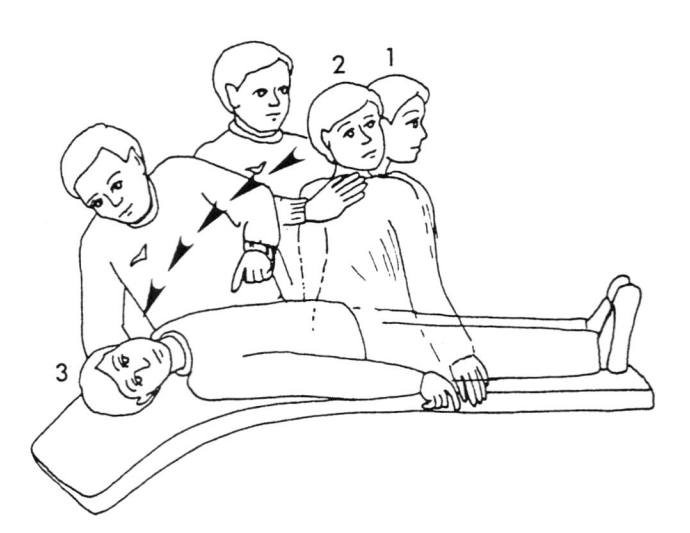

FIG. 11. Dix-Hallpike test for benign paroxysmal positional vertigo (BPPV). While patient is in a sitting position, the head is first turned to the side and then the patient is moved into a supine position with the head slightly below the horizontal plane of the body. This maneuver should be performed with the head turned initially toward the side of the suspected lesion. From Cyr DG, Harker LA. Vestibular Function Tests. In: Cummings CW, Fredrickson JM, Krause CJ, Harker LA, Schuller DE, eds. Otolaryngology—Head and Neck Surgery. 2nd ed. St. Louis, MO: Mosby-Yearbook, 1993:2652.

(Fig. 11) as described by Dix and Hallpike (19) is used as a test for benign paroxysmal positional vertigo (19). The subject is seated with the feet on an examining table so that, if supine, the head would hang over the edge of the table. The head is held by the examiner, while the subject is suddenly placed in the supine position with the head hanging slightly over the edge of the table and rotated laterally toward the examiner. The examiner bends down with the subject and observes the eyes for positional nystagmus for at least 20 seconds. After the nystagmus has ceased the patient is suddenly sat upright and the eyes are again observed for nystagmus. The test is repeated with the head turned in the opposite lateral direction. Two types of abnormal responses may be seen. Static positional nystagmus remains as long as the position is held, although it may fluctuate in frequency and amplitude. It may be in the same direction in all positions or change directions in different positions. Direction-fixed static positional nystagmus or direction-changing nystagmus can be associated with peripheral or central disorders. Benign paroxysmal positional nystagmus is the classic response to the Hallpike maneuver. After the head is placed in the head-hanging left, center, or right, there is a latent period of 5 to 10 seconds. The characteristic nystagmus is rotary (torsional). The vertigo and nystagmus usually have an intense onset and attenuate in approximately 20 to 30 seconds. This is always accompanied by vertigo, and its direction does not change. On repeating the test, the subsequent responses progressively fatigue, and the nystagmus may not appear at all after two or three repetitions of the Hallpike maneuver. (The pathophysiology is discussed further Chapter 28).

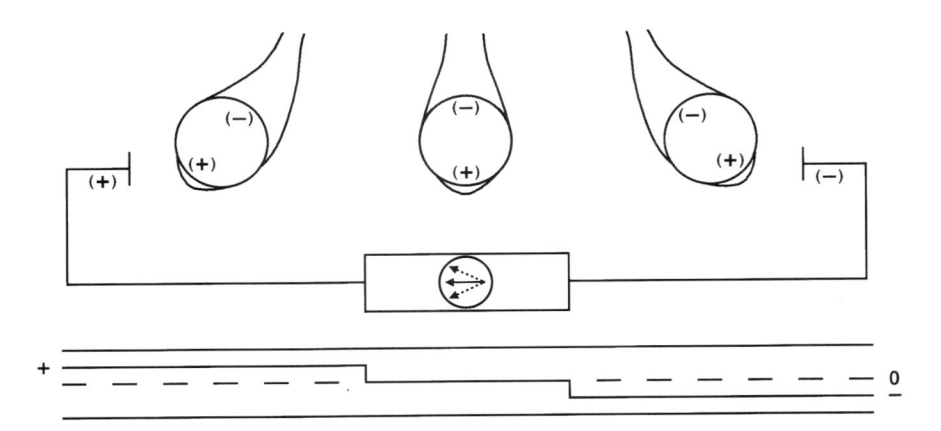

FIG. 12. Principle of EOG. Two active electrodes placed on either side of the globe measure shifts in the corneoretinal potential. This signal is amplified and recorded on moving recorder paper or on a computer screen. Reprinted with permission of House Ear Institute.

OBJECTIVE MEASUREMENT OF VESTIBULAR FUNCTION

The most widely applied methods of objectively studying vestibular function are electronystagmography (ENG), rotary testing, and posturography. Investigational methods such as otolith function tests, stimulation of the vestibular nerve with a galvanic current, and high-frequency vestibular autorotation tests are beyond the scope of this chapter and are not discussed here (for review, see Baloh and Honrubia [20]).

To quantitatively assess nystagmus, one must have a method of precisely measuring eye position and motion. Electro-oculography (EOG) an objective method of monitoring eye movements, has been widely used in the diagnostic evaluation of patients with vertigo, dizziness, or unsteadiness. The principle of EOG is based on the fact that there are steady dc potentials (corneal-retinal potentials) between the cornea and pigmented retina of each eye (Fig. 12). The cornea retains a positive potential relative to the retina. This potential creates an electrical field in the front of the head that rotates as the eyes rotate in their orbits. Rotation of this electrical field produces a change in the voltage between electrodes that are attached to the skin on either side of the eyes. Horizontal eye position is monitored by electrodes placed on the patient's temples. Vertical eye position is monitored by electrodes placed above and below each of the patient's eyes. An electrode placed near the eye becomes more positive as the eye rotates toward it and less positive as the eye rotates away. In this way, eye position and motion can be monitored precisely. This technique, however, senses eye motion in the horizontal and vertical planes only. It is insensitive to rotational or torsional eye movements, that are commonly seen in many types of nystagmus. Newer techniques using infrared video monitoring can detect these torsional eye movements and are gaining in popularity (21). The infrared video system can be easily adapted for use with small children (Fig. 13).

Electronystagmography

The gold standard of vestibular function tests is ENG. The ENG test battery generally consists of seven tests. Four of the tests primarily assess vestibular function, although they sometimes reveal nonvestibular eye movement abnormalities as well: (a) The bithermal caloric test is designed primarily to detect unilateral lesions of the labyrinth or vestibular nerve; (b) the gaze test is designed to detect nystagmus induced by eccentric gaze; (c) the positional test is designed to determine if different head positions induce or modify

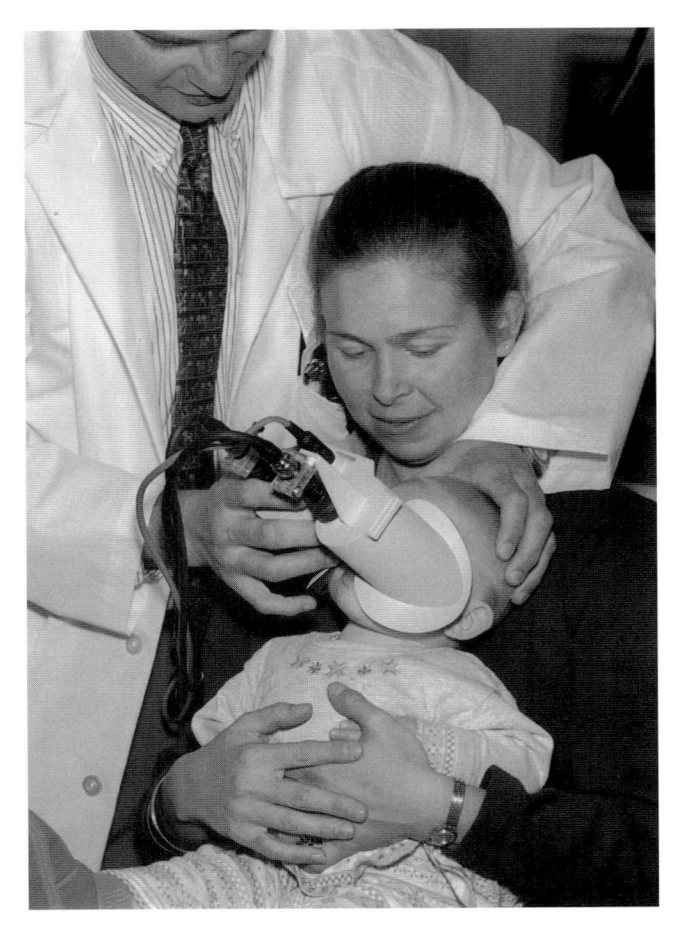

FIG. 13. The infrared video system can detect rotary, vertical, and horizontal nystagmus. The instrument may be used on small children. Reprinted with permission of House Ear Institute.

nystagmus; and (d) the Hallpike maneuver is designed to provoke a nystagmus response in patients with benign positional vertigo. The remaining three tests assess eye movement function independent of the peripheral vestibular system: (a) the saccade test is designed to detect disorders of the saccade eye movement control system, and (6) the tracking test and (c) the optokinetic test are both designed to detect disorders of the pursuit eye movement control system. Saccade and pursuit eye movements are tested routinely because abnormalities are occasionally detected in patients complaining of balance difficulty but are usually due to central pathology. Electronystagmography has been computerized, which permits efficient storage, retrieval, and analysis of eye movement data. In addition, computerized ENG allows rapid and sophisticated analysis of saccade, tracking, and caloric test data.

The clinician should be facile with traditional ENG analysis. Eye movements are usually recorded on polygraph paper that is moving at a known constant velocity. A marking pen charts the position of the eyes during the test as either upward or downward deflections. By convention, a horizontal eye movement to the left is recorded as a downward deflection, and movement to the right as an upward deflection. Fast eye deviations (saccades) are identifiable as the line deflection with the greater slope. The ENG measurement must first be calibrated so that a standard angle of eye deviation is reflected by a known amplitude of marker deflection. Calibration is accomplished by having the patient fixate on targets at known angles within their visual field. The position of a 20-degree eye deviation, for example, is then marked on the polygraph paper. Once this relationship is established, the velocity, amplitude, and direction of nystagmus can be calculated.

Bithermal Caloric Test

The bithermal caloric test is best suited for identifying unilateral lesions of the peripheral vestibular system because it permits the examiner to stimulate each ear separately. Other vestibular tests, such as rotation testing, necessarily involve simultaneous stimulation of both labyrinths and, therefore, may mask abnormal responses from one labyrinth by normal responses from the opposite ear.

The caloric test is performed with the patient supine and the head elevated 30 degrees. This is done to place the lateral semicircular canal into the vertical plane. Each of the patient's ears is then irrigated with water that is either 7° above (44°) or 7° below (30°) body temperature for 40 seconds. Eye motion is then recorded.

The caloric test uses warm or cold water to create a temperature gradient within the lateral semicircular canal by convection through the middle ear and temporal bone. This induces an endolymphatic flow caused by a thermally induced difference in endolymphatic specific gravity. In the lateral canal, water above body temperature causes ampullopetal flow, causing the cupola to deviate toward the utricle,

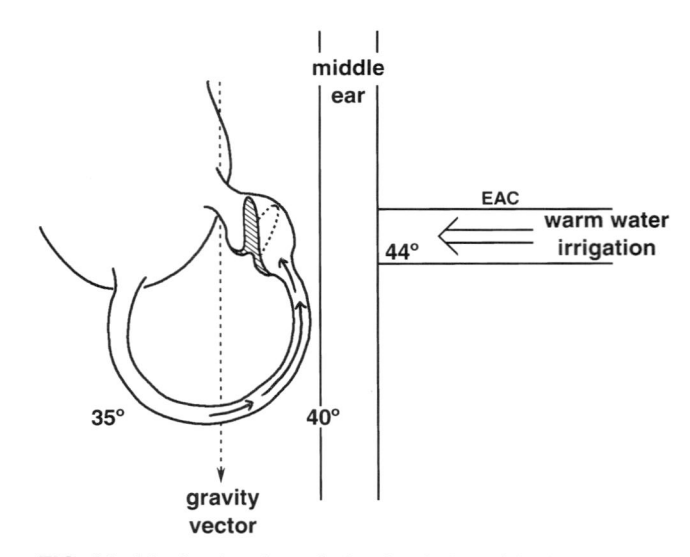

FIG. 14. Mechanism for caloric stimulation of the lateral semicircular canal. The patient's head is positioned so that the lateral canal is parallel to gravity. A thermal gradient is then created across the temporal bone with warm or cold water irrigation. Warm water (44°) causes ampullopetal flow. Reprinted with permission of House Ear Institute.

thus causing nerve stimulation (Fig. 14). Initially, stimulation first causes deviation of the eyes away from the side, followed by a compensatory saccade, as mentioned previously. The lateral canal develops the largest temperature gradient because it is the most exposed of the canals in the middle ear and closest to the external auditory canal. The bithermal caloric test is, therefore exclusively a test of the integrity of the horizontal semicircular canals and their afferent pathways.

Alternative thermal stimulation methods are available for use in patients who have perforations of their tympanic membranes to avoid injury and contamination of the middle ear. A closed-loop system can be used that comprises a small balloon placed deep into the ear canal, which can be inflated with warm or cold water. Alternatively, cold or warm air stimulation also can be used. Abnormal responses are recorded and calculated as either canal paresis (hypofunction) or directional preponderance (relative hyperfunction). The labyrinth that is hypoactive is usually the involved side of a vestibular lesion. Relative to adults, children normally have classically induced nystagmus that is dysrhythmic and of wider amplitude and slower onset (22). Longer periods of caloric-induced nystagmus are usually associated with central lesions.

Caloric stimuli are uncalibrated; that is, stimulus strength varies from person to person depending on the size and shape of the external ear canal and other uncontrollable variables. However, the basic assumption of the caloric test is that for a given individual, the two ears receive equal caloric stimuli. If both ears are normal, they should produce responses of approximately equal intensity. Therefore, the strengths of the caloric responses of the two ears are compared. Although the bithermal caloric test is highly sensitive to unilateral peripheral vestibular lesions, it is relatively insensitive to bilateral lesions, because the caloric stimulus is uncalibrated. However, rotational testing is sensitive to detection of bilateral peripheral lesions and is discussed later.

Gaze Test

The eye movements are monitored as the patient fixates while gazing 30° rightward, 30° leftward, 30° upward, and 30° downward. Young, normal individuals rarely have any nystagmus at all while fixating at any of these gaze positions, but many elderly individuals have end-point nystagmus. This nystagmus is always faint with centripetal slow phases that generally are of equal intensity on rightward and leftward gazes.

The gaze test detects many types of nystagmus of both vestibular and nonvestibular origin. For example, upbeat nystagmus occurs most commonly as a result of medullary lesions involving vertical vestibular pathways (23). Medulloblastoma in children may present with such upbeating nystagmus. Other types of central nystagmus seen in the gaze test are described by Leigh and Zee (24). The gaze test also may detect spontaneous nystagmus caused by a unilateral vestibular lesion, although spontaneous nystagmus is better appreciated during the positional test without visual fixation.

Positional Test

The purpose of the positional test is to determine if different head positions induce or modify vestibular nystagmus. The patient's eye movements are monitored with the head in at least four positions: sitting, supine, right ear down, and left ear down. Some examiners also test the patient in the head-hanging position. Eye movements are monitored in each position, both with visual fixation at center gaze and without visual fixation. Some forms of nystagmus are suppressed if the patient voluntarily or unconsciously fixates on an object. This is called *fixation inhibition of nystagmus* and can be overcome by closing the patient's eye or using Frensel glasses. The examiner usually asks the patient to perform a mental task, such as mental arithmetic, when testing with visual fixation denied to maintain mental alertness. This avoids suppression of the nystagmus.

A common abnormality seen in the positional test is spontaneous nystagmus. This is seen after a unilateral insult, creating a tonic vestibular asymmetry. After acute injury, the nystagmus is ablative, with the fast component directed away from the affected ear. With peripheral lesions, it is suppressed by visual fixation, and often suppression is so strong that spontaneous nystagmus is abolished by fixation. If fixation suppression is poor, spontaneous nystagmus is an indication of a CNS lesion.

Hallpike Maneuver

The patient is subjected to the Hallpike maneuver, as described in a previous section. The characteristic eye movements associated with paroxysmal positional nystagmus can be appreciated readily by visual observation of the patient wearing Frensel lenses in a darkened room. Electro-oculography, as mentioned previously, is insensitive to the torsional component of the nystagmus but does record the horizontal and vertical components. Infrared video monitoring may help to visualize the rotational nystagmus that is seen in benign paroxysmal positional vertigo.

Saccade Test

The purpose of the saccade test is to detect abnormalities of saccadic eye movement. The horizontal eye movements are monitored as the patient visually fixates on a computer-controlled visual target that is oscillating in the horizontal plane in an unpredictable sequence. The complete sequence consists of approximately 80 target jumps (40 to the right and 40 to the left), with amplitudes ranging from 5° to 25°. After testing, the computer deletes invalid eye movement data, then calculates three values—peak velocity, accuracy, and latency for each saccade—and plots these data in graphic form.

Patients may show abnormalities on any of these three measures. Abnormally slow saccades bilaterally are characteristic of many central degenerative and metabolic diseases. Patients also may show abnormalities of saccade accuracy, making saccades that are too small or too large, indicating a lesion of the cerebellar vermis. Abnormally long saccade latencies also may be present that are associated with lesions of the frontoparietal cortex. A thorough review of saccade abnormalities and their localizing value can be found in the textbook authored by Leigh and Zee (24).

Pursuit Tests

Two tests of pursuit, smooth pursuit and the optokinetic test, are commonly performed in the ENG examination. The smooth pursuit tracking test is often performed by monitoring the patient's horizontal eye movements as they follow a computer-controlled visual target moving in the horizontal plane. The target moves back and forth, following a sinusoidal waveform at frequencies of 0.2 to 0.7 Hz. After testing, the computer deletes invalid eye movement data and interpolated saccades, differentiates the eye position signal, calculates the gain of eye velocity with respect to target velocity separately for rightward and leftward tracking at each target frequency, and plots these data. Normal individuals are able to follow the target smoothly in both directions at all target frequencies.

In the optokinetic test, the patient's horizontal eye movements are monitored as they follow a series of visual targets rotating first to the right and then to the left. Clinically, optokinetic nystagmus (OKN) may be induced by having the subject watch a rotating drum with vertically oriented stripes. The fast component will be in the direction opposite to the drum motion. (This stimulus provokes nystagmus with slow phases in the direction of target motion periodically interrupted by fast phases in the opposite direction.) Optokinetic nystagmus is normally equal bilaterally, and its suppression on one side is a valuable localizing sign for lesions in the parietal occipital region, brainstem, and cerebellum. In these cases, an impairment in OKN occurs when the stimulus moves toward the damaged side. The optokinetic test, like the smooth pursuit tracking test, is a test of pursuit eye movement pathways, and the results of the tracking and optokinetic tests agree if task difficulty is the same. In normal individuals, the velocities of nystagmus slow phases approximately match target velocity for both rightward and leftward moving targets.

Rotation Tests

Quantitative rotational testing of vestibular function is based on the VOR of both ears measured together. Rotational testing usually involves positioning the patient so that the rotational axis is vertical and passes through the center of the head, thus stimulating only the horizontal semicircular canals. Horizontal eye movements are monitored using EOG, as in ENG testing. Rotational testing of the horizontal semicircular canal offers several advantages over caloric testing: (a) Multiple graded stimuli can be applied in a relatively short period of time; (b) it is well tolerated by patients; and (c) in contrast to caloric testing, rotational stimulus to the horizontal semicircular canals is unrelated to physical characteristics of the external auditory canal or middle ear. All aspects of rotation testing including stimulus generation, response measurement, and data analysis, are currently computer controlled.

The most frequently performed rotational test uses a sinusoidal stimulus. The patient is seated in a chair mounted on a servo-controlled torque motor enclosed within a light-proof, sound-attenuated booth. The patient's head is tilted 30° forward so that the horizontal semicircular canals are in the plane of rotation. The patient is tested in total darkness with eyes open while performing mental arithmetic in order to maintain mental alertness. Sinusoidal oscillation around the vertical axis is performed at several different frequencies. The precise test protocol varies between laboratories, but common oscillation frequencies are 0.0125 to 1.6 Hz, with peak angular velocities of 15 to 120 degrees/sec (27). The patient undergoes multiple cycles of oscillation at each frequency. Eye motion is recorded electronically and the velocity and direction of the slow component of nystagmus is calculated. The velocity of the slow component (response) is then plotted in relation to the corresponding chair rotational velocity (stimulus). In normal subjects, the relationship between the magnitude of the response and stimulus should be constant and symmetrical for each cycle of rotation. In acute or uncompensated unilateral vestibular lesions, this relationship changes. Patients with unilateral vestibular paresis display an asymmetric response to rotary stimuli because of the difference in excitation and inhibition with ampullopetal and ampullofugal stimulation of the respective semicircular canals.

Rotational testing is most ideally suited for testing patients with bilateral peripheral lesions, because both labyrinths are stimulated simultaneously and the degree of remaining function can be quantified accurately. Caloric testing is relatively insensitive to symmetric vestibular hypofunction because one labyrinth is evaluated relative to the other. Also, the variance in eye motion associated with a normal rotary response is less than that associated with caloric responses. This is because rotary testing is not influenced by physical variables such as external auditory canal anatomy, as mentioned previously. For these reasons, rotary testing is much more sensitive to small variations in bilateral vestibular dysfunction. Because bilateral vestibular hypofunction can be identified earlier using rotary stimuli than calorics, rotary testing can be useful in detecting early ototoxic effects of medications that may not be identified by caloric tests.

The major disadvantage of rotational tests is that no directional or localizing information can be derived because both labyrinths are stimulated simultaneously. An impression of unilateral weakness, however, can be made by comparing the intensity of nystagmus in one direction with the other direction. The instrumentation for the formal rotational test is quite expensive and elaborate, preventing its use in everyday clinical practice.

Computerized Dynamic Posturography

Computerized dynamic posturography is a new test modality that determines the relative importance of the various sensory inputs: vision, vestibular sensation, and proprioception (25). The patient is asked to stand on a special pressure-sensitive platform (Fig. 15). Sensors on the platform detect small fluctuations in foot pressure, which are created by the patient while attempting to maintain balance. The platform is constructed on a gimbal mechanism to allow free-pitch motion. It can alternatively be locked into place to create a stable perch. The platform is also mechanized and able to forcefully pitch the patient forward and backward. During testing, strain gauges measure the patient's reaction times and forces applied to the platform as the patient attempts to maintain balance. In addition, a colored background is placed in front of the patient. The background is designed to be able to move either independently of or with the posturography platform. This allows the examiner to provide either stabile or a sway-referenced visual input. By providing distorted or incorrect visual sensory information, the patient is forced to rely on vestibular inputs to maintain balance. In this way, one can add, remove, or isolate the various balance sensory components (Fig. 16) (26).

The dynamic posturography test battery consists of six sensory conditions, termed the *sensory organization test* (Table 2). They increase in difficulty as one ascends the scale. The six test conditions include (1) platform stable, with eyes open and a stable visual surround; (2) platform stable, with eyes closed; (3) platform stable, with eyes open and a moving visual surround; (4) platform moving, with eyes open and a stationary visual surround; (5) platform moving, with eyes closed; and (6) platform moving, with eyes open and a moving visual surround. Patients who have difficulty with conditions 5 and 6 are said to exhibit a vestibular pattern (27). In these conditions, the patient has had two of the three sensory queues to maintain balance removed and is forced to rely on the vestibular end organs to stay upright. The 5, 6 pattern implies recent uncompensated unilateral peripheral vestibular damage or bilateral peripheral vestibular deficits. Difficulty with condition 4 as well as 5 & 6 (4, 5, 6 pattern) implies a difficulty in using visual information as well to maintain balance. This pattern has been identified with more severe peripheral vestibular deficits. It has also been reported to be common in the geriatric population. Posturography has been useful in identifying functional vestibular problems. An *aphysiologic pattern* is typically seen in malingering patients. The patient will seem to do very poorly on even the easiest conditions at the beginning. As the test difficulty increases, performance remains stable or even improves (28,29). Wide variations in performance from one test run to another also suggest malingering.

The clinical usefulness of dynamic posturography is still under debate. Posturography does not provide localizing, or even lateralizing, information as to the site of lesion. It does, however, provide a functional measure of a patient's ability to use various sensory inputs to maintain balance. The test can also aid in the choice of rehabilitation therapy as well as follow a patient's progress through therapy (30).

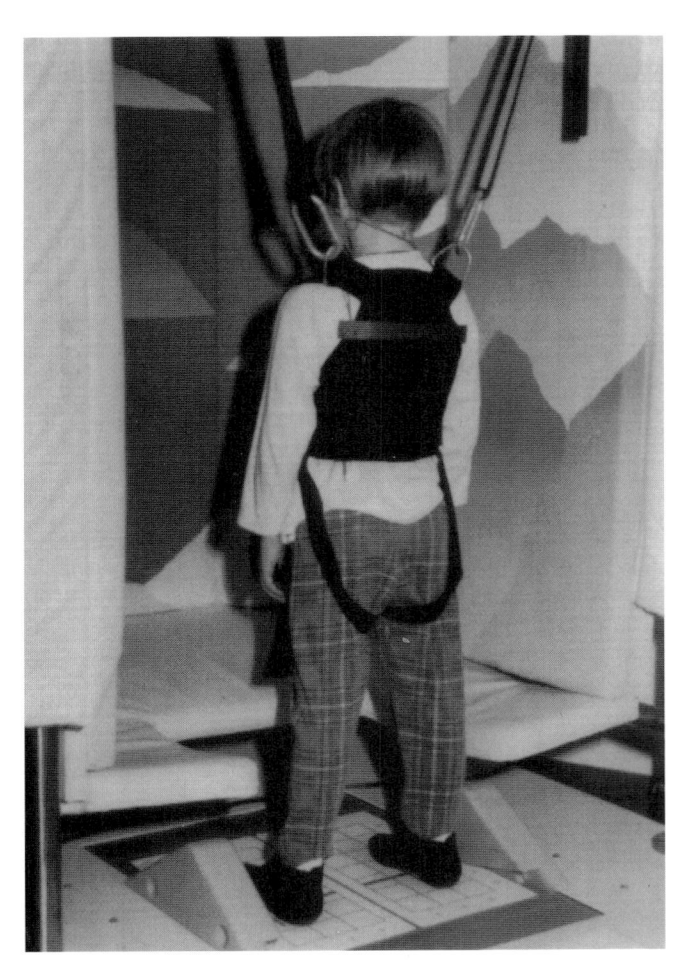

FIG. 15. Equi test posturography system. The child stands on a platform surrounded by a colored background. The platform and background are able to move together or independently. Pressure sensors on the platform detect the patient's sway. Note the safety harness for preventing injury to the child should a fall occur. From NeuroCom International, Inc., Clackamas, OR.

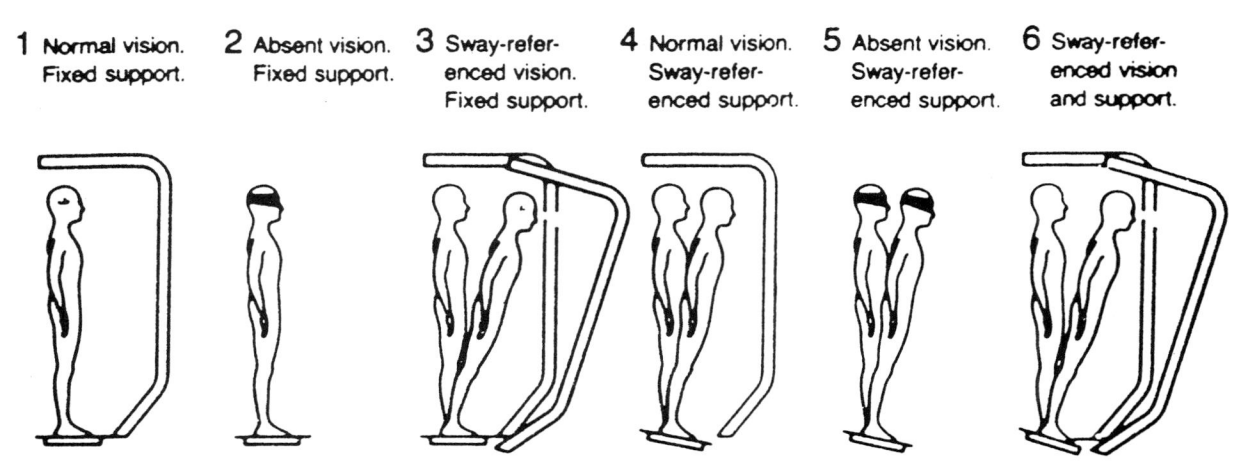

FIG. 16. Six conditions of the sensory organization test for computerized dynamic posturography. (From NeuroCom International, Inc., Clackamas, OR.)

TABLE 2. *Sensory inputs presented to the subject during various posturography test conditions*

Testing conditions	Sensory inputs		
	Vision	Somatosensory	Vestibular
1. Eyes open, platform stable, visual field stable	Present	Present	Present
2. Eyes closed, platform stable	Absent	Present	Present
3. Eyes open, platform stable, visual field moved	Absent	Present	Present
4. Eyes open, platform moving, visual field stable	Present	Absent	Present
5. Eyes closed, platform moving	Absent	Absent	Present
6. Eyes open, platform moving, visual field moved	Absent	Absent	Present

SUMMARY

Evaluation of a vertiginous child can be a very difficult and time-consuming undertaking. Children require special skills and techniques combined with a great deal of patience and cannot simply be treated as little adults. Language and emotional maturity barriers exist that one does not have to deal with routinely in adults. An accurate history or physical examination may not always be obtainable from a young child. The physician may be forced to rely on the parent's interpretation of the problem, which may or may not be accurate. Auditory and vestibular testing is limited by the patients ability to comply with the testing. The physician must gather all possible information from both the parents and child, while keeping in perspective the limitations of that information. As with adult patients, a firm diagnosis and simple treatment are not always possible. Referral for complete neurologic evaluation or for genetic counseling may sometimes be required. If an isolated vestibular deficit is responsible for the symptoms, the family and child can be reassured that accommodation will probably proceed quickly. In general, a restrained, conservative approach is most appropriate.

REFERENCES

1. Busis SN, Busis BA. The neurologic examination. In: Jackler RK, Brackman DE., eds. *Neurotology.* St. Louis, MO: Mosby; 1994.
2. Bower CM, Cotton RT. The spectrum of vertigo in children. *Arch Otolaryngol Head Neck Surg* 1995;121:911.
3. Abu-Arafeh I, Russell G. Paroxysmal vertigo as a migraine equivalent in children: a population based study. *Cephalaglia* 1995;15:22.
4. *Dorland's Medical Dictionary,* 28th ed., WB Saunders; 1994.
5. Grace ARH, Pfleiderer AG. Dysequilibrium and otitis media with effusion: what is the association? *J Laryngol Otol* 1990;104(9):682.
6. Golz A, Westerman ST, Gilbert LM, Joachims HZ, Netzer A. The effect of middle ear effusion on the vestibular labyrinth. *J Laryngol Otol* 1991;105:987.
7. Weber PC, Cass SP. The clinical assessment of postural stability. *Am J Otol* 1993;14:566.
8. David RB. *Pediatric neurology for the clinician.* Norwalk, CT: Appleton & Lange; 1992.
9. Eviatar L. Vertigo. In: Swaiman KF, ed. *Pediatric neurology.* St. Louis, MO: CV Mosby, 1989:249.
10. Gorin RJ. Genetic hearing loss associated with eye disorders. In: Gorlin RJ, Toriello HV, Cohen MM, eds. *Hereditary hearing loss and its syndromes.* New York: Oxford University Press; 1995.
11. Derebery MJ, Rao VS, Siglock TJ, Linthicum FH, Nelson RA. Ménière's disease: an immune complex-mediated illness? *Laryngoscope* 1991;101:225.
12. Schessel DA, Nedzelski JM. Presentation of large vestibular aqueduct syndrome to a dizziness unit. *J of Otol* 1992;21(4):265.
13. Bellet PS, Benton C, Matt BH, Myer CM. The evaluation of the ear canal, middle ear, temporal bone, and cerebellopontine angle masses in infants, children, and adolescents. *Adv Pediatr* 1992;39:167.
14. Toupet M, Toupet F. Vertigo in children. *Rev Prat* (France) 1944;44(3):343.
15. Vignaud J, Marsot-Dupuch K, Pharaboz C, Derosier C, Cordoliani Y. Imaging of the vestibule. *Otolaryngol Head Neck Surg* 1995;112:36.
16. Murphy JV, Dehkharghani F. Diagnosis of childhood seizure disorders. *Epilepsia* 1994;35 Suppl 2:7.
17. Panosian MS, Paige GD. Nystagmus and postural instability after headshake in patients with vestibular dysfunction. *Otolaryngol Head Neck Surg;* 112:399.
18. Smith ME, Canalis RF. Otologic manifestations of AIDS: the otosyphilis connection. *Laryngoscope* 1989;99:365.
19. Baloh RW. Approach to the evaluation of the dizzy patient. *Otolaryngol Head Neck Surg* 1995;112:3.
20. Baloh RW, Honrubia V. *Clinical neurophysiology of the vestibular system.* Philadelphia: F.A. Davis, 1990.
21. Di Scenna AO, Das V, Zivotofsky AZ, Seidman SH, Leifg RJ. Evaluation of a video tracking device for measurement of horizontal and vertical eye rotations during locomotion. *J Neurosci Methods* 1995;58(1–2):89.
22. Busis SN. Vertigo. In: Bluestone CD, Stool CE, Kenna MK, eds. *Pediatric otolaryngology.* 3rd ed. Philadelphia: WB Saunders; 1996.
23. Fisher A, Gresty M, Chambers BR, Rudge P. Primary position upbeating nystagmus: a variety of central positional nystagmus. *Brain* 1983;106:949.
24. Leigh RJ, Zee DS. *The neurology of eye movements,* 2nd ed. Philadelphia, F.A. Davis.
25. Furman JM. Role of posturography in the management of vestibular patients. *Otolaryngol Head Neck Surg* 1995;112:8.
26. Voorhees R. The role of dynamic posturography in neurotologic diagnosis. *Laryngoscope* 1989;99:995.
27. Goebel J, Paige G. Posturography following rotation: a model of postural control during vestibular dysfunction. *Otolaryngol Head Neck Surg* 1990;102:722.
28. Cyr D, Moore G, Moller C. Clinical application of computerized dynamic posturography. *Ear Nose Throat J* 1988;67(suppl):36.
29. Dickins J, Cyr D, Grahm S, Winston M, Sanford M. Clinical significance of type 5 patterns in platform posturography. *Otolaryngol Head Neck Surg* 1992;107:1.
30. Shepard N. Talian S, Smith-Wheelock M, Raj A. Vestibular and balance rehabilitation therapy. *Ann Otol Rhinol Laryngol* 1993;102:198.

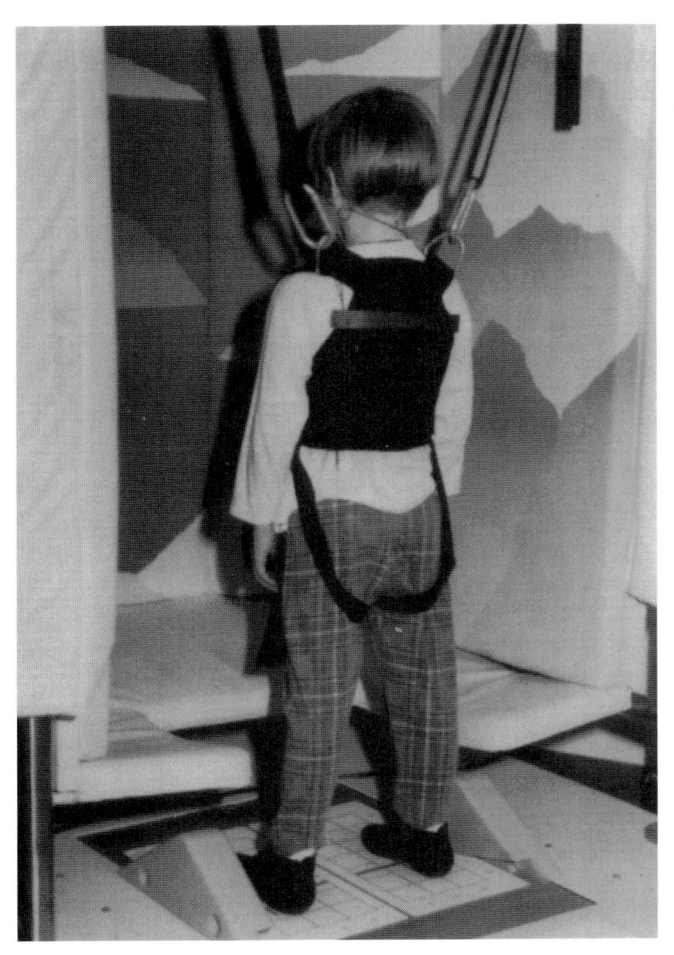

FIG. 15. Equi test posturography system. The child stands on a platform surrounded by a colored background. The platform and background are able to move together or independently. Pressure sensors on the platform detect the patient's sway. Note the safety harness for preventing injury to the child should a fall occur. From NeuroCom International, Inc., Clackamas, OR.

The dynamic posturography test battery consists of six sensory conditions, termed the *sensory organization test* (Table 2). They increase in difficulty as one ascends the scale. The six test conditions include (1) platform stable, with eyes open and a stable visual surround; (2) platform stable, with eyes closed; (3) platform stable, with eyes open and a moving visual surround; (4) platform moving, with eyes open and a stationary visual surround; (5) platform moving, with eyes closed; and (6) platform moving, with eyes open and a moving visual surround. Patients who have difficulty with conditions 5 and 6 are said to exhibit a vestibular pattern (27). In these conditions, the patient has had two of the three sensory queues to maintain balance removed and is forced to rely on the vestibular end organs to stay upright. The 5, 6 pattern implies recent uncompensated unilateral peripheral vestibular damage or bilateral peripheral vestibular deficits. Difficulty with condition 4 as well as 5 & 6 (4, 5, 6 pattern) implies a difficulty in using visual information as well to maintain balance. This pattern has been identified with more severe peripheral vestibular deficits. It has also been reported to be common in the geriatric population. Posturography has been useful in identifying functional vestibular problems. An *aphysiologic pattern* is typically seen in malingering patients. The patient will seem to do very poorly on even the easiest conditions at the beginning. As the test difficulty increases, performance remains stable or even improves (28,29). Wide variations in performance from one test run to another also suggest malingering.

The clinical usefulness of dynamic posturography is still under debate. Posturography does not provide localizing, or even lateralizing, information as to the site of lesion. It does, however, provide a functional measure of a patient's ability to use various sensory inputs to maintain balance. The test can also aid in the choice of rehabilitation therapy as well as follow a patient's progress through therapy (30).

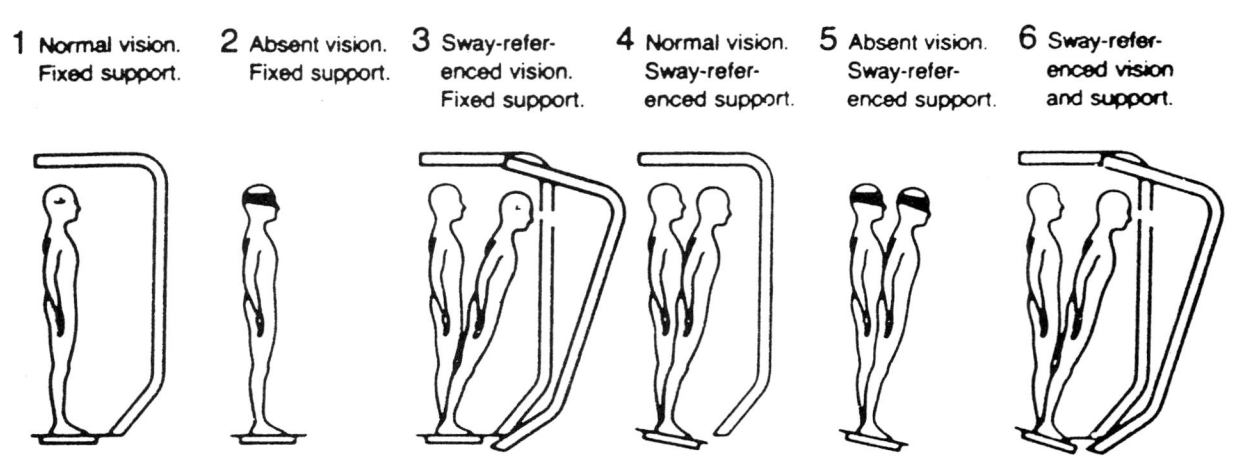

FIG. 16. Six conditions of the sensory organization test for computerized dynamic posturography. (From NeuroCom International, Inc., Clackamas, OR.)

TABLE 2. *Sensory inputs presented to the subject during various posturography test conditions*

Testing conditions	Sensory inputs		
	Vision	Somatosensory	Vestibular
1. Eyes open, platform stable, visual field stable	Present	Present	Present
2. Eyes closed, platform stable	Absent	Present	Present
3. Eyes open, platform stable, visual field moved	Absent	Present	Present
4. Eyes open, platform moving, visual field stable	Present	Absent	Present
5. Eyes closed, platform moving	Absent	Absent	Present
6. Eyes open, platform moving, visual field moved	Absent	Absent	Present

SUMMARY

Evaluation of a vertiginous child can be a very difficult and time-consuming undertaking. Children require special skills and techniques combined with a great deal of patience and cannot simply be treated as little adults. Language and emotional maturity barriers exist that one does not have to deal with routinely in adults. An accurate history or physical examination may not always be obtainable from a young child. The physician may be forced to rely on the parent's interpretation of the problem, which may or may not be accurate. Auditory and vestibular testing is limited by the patients ability to comply with the testing. The physician must gather all possible information from both the parents and child, while keeping in perspective the limitations of that information. As with adult patients, a firm diagnosis and simple treatment are not always possible. Referral for complete neurologic evaluation or for genetic counseling may sometimes be required. If an isolated vestibular deficit is responsible for the symptoms, the family and child can be reassured that accommodation will probably proceed quickly. In general, a restrained, conservative approach is most appropriate.

REFERENCES

1. Busis SN, Busis BA. The neurologic examination. In: Jackler RK, Brackman DE., eds. *Neurotology.* St. Louis, MO: Mosby; 1994.
2. Bower CM, Cotton RT. The spectrum of vertigo in children. *Arch Otolaryngol Head Neck Surg* 1995;121:911.
3. Abu-Arafeh I, Russell G. Paroxysmal vertigo as a migraine equivalent in children: a population based study. *Cephalaglia* 1995;15:22.
4. *Dorland's Medical Dictionary,* 28th ed., WB Saunders; 1994.
5. Grace ARH, Pfleiderer AG. Dysequilibrium and otitis media with effusion: what is the association? *J Laryngol Otol* 1990;104(9):682.
6. Golz A, Westerman ST, Gilbert LM, Joachims HZ, Netzer A. The effect of middle ear effusion on the vestibular labyrinth. *J Laryngol Otol* 1991;105:987.
7. Weber PC, Cass SP. The clinical assessment of postural stability. *Am J Otol* 1993;14:566.
8. David RB. *Pediatric neurology for the clinician.* Norwalk, CT: Appleton & Lange; 1992.
9. Eviatar L. Vertigo. In: Swaiman KF, ed. *Pediatric neurology.* St. Louis, MO: CV Mosby, 1989:249.
10. Gorin RJ. Genetic hearing loss associated with eye disorders. In: Gorlin RJ, Toriello HV, Cohen MM, eds. *Hereditary hearing loss and its syndromes.* New York: Oxford University Press; 1995.
11. Derebery MJ, Rao VS, Siglock TJ, Linthicum FH, Nelson RA. Ménière's disease: an immune complex-mediated illness? *Laryngoscope* 1991;101:225.
12. Schessel DA, Nedzelski JM. Presentation of large vestibular aqueduct syndrome to a dizziness unit. *J of Otol* 1992;21(4):265.
13. Bellet PS, Benton C, Matt BH, Myer CM. The evaluation of the ear canal, middle ear, temporal bone, and cerebellopontine angle masses in infants, children, and adolescents. *Adv Pediatr* 1992;39:167.
14. Toupet M, Toupet F. Vertigo in children. *Rev Prat* (France) 1944; 44(3):343.
15. Vignaud J, Marsot-Dupuch K, Pharaboz C, Derosier C, Cordoliani Y. Imaging of the vestibule. *Otolaryngol Head Neck Surg* 1995;112:36.
16. Murphy JV, Dehkharghani F. Diagnosis of childhood seizure disorders. *Epilepsia* 1994;35 Suppl 2:7.
17. Panosian MS, Paige GD. Nystagmus and postural instability after headshake in patients with vestibular dysfunction. *Otolaryngol Head Neck Surg;* 112:399.
18. Smith ME, Canalis RF. Otologic manifestations of AIDS: the otosyphilis connection. *Laryngoscope* 1989;99:365.
19. Baloh RW. Approach to the evaluation of the dizzy patient. *Otolaryngol Head Neck Surg* 1995;112:3.
20. Baloh RW, Honrubia V. *Clinical neurophysiology of the vestibular system.* Philadelphia: F.A. Davis, 1990.
21. Di Scenna AO, Das V, Zivotofsky AZ, Seidman SH, Leifg RJ. Evaluation of a video tracking device for measurement of horizontal and vertical eye rotations during locomotion. *J Neurosci Methods* 1995; 58(1–2):89.
22. Busis SN. Vertigo. In: Bluestone CD, Stool CE, Kenna MK, eds. *Pediatric otolaryngology.* 3rd ed. Philadelphia: WB Saunders; 1996.
23. Fisher A, Gresty M, Chambers BR, Rudge P. Primary position upbeating nystagmus: a variety of central positional nystagmus. *Brain* 1983;106:949.
24. Leigh RJ, Zee DS. *The neurology of eye movements,* 2nd ed. Philadelphia, F.A. Davis.
25. Furman JM. Role of posturography in the management of vestibular patients. *Otolaryngol Head Neck Surg* 1995;112:8.
26. Voorhees R. The role of dynamic posturography in neurotologic diagnosis. *Laryngoscope* 1989;99:995.
27. Goebel J, Paige G. Posturography following rotation: a model of postural control during vestibular dysfunction. *Otolaryngol Head Neck Surg* 1990;102:722.
28. Cyr D, Moore G, Moller C. Clinical application of computerized dynamic posturography. *Ear Nose Throat J* 1988;67(suppl):36.
29. Dickins J, Cyr D, Grahm S, Winston M, Sanford M. Clinical significance of type 5 patterns in platform posturography. *Otolaryngol Head Neck Surg* 1992;107:1.
30. Shepard N. Talian S, Smith-Wheelock M, Raj A. Vestibular and balance rehabilitation therapy. *Ann Otol Rhinol Laryngol* 1993;102:198.

CHAPTER 12

Radiology of the Temporal Bone

Congenital Abnormalities

Peter D. Phelps and Gilbert Vézina

The major advances in computerized imaging that have occurred in the past few years have found many applications in pediatric otolaryngology. The principles of technique that apply to imaging in adults apply equally to the demonstration of head and neck lesions in infants and children. Optimal spatial and density resolution with the lowest possible level of patient irradiation and freedom from movement artifacts must be achieved. Limitation of the dose of radiation is particularly important in this age group, and minimal patient movement is hard to obtain.

The middle and inner ears are fully developed at birth, but the temporomandibular joint, external auditory canal (EAC), and mastoid process are not. Postnatal changes in the temporal bone consist of growth and pneumatization of the mastoid process and alteration in the shape of the tympanic ring. Prior to full ossification of the petrous pyramid, the dense bone of the labyrinthine capsule can be clearly identified by plain mastoid views, thus enabling gross developmental abnormalities to be identified without the need for sectional imaging (Fig. 1). In the middle ear, the ossicles can be shown and, in the neonate, even marrow spaces within them. The mastoid antrum is fully developed at birth but further pneumatization posteriorly occurs only during the first decade of life with the development of the mastoid process. It is not yet clear how much the variable extent of this pneumatization is due to genetic factors or to interference by disease processes such as otitis media. Plain (x-ray) lateral oblique mastoid views show the extent of pneumatization (Fig. 2), which some surgeons prefer for preoperative assessment. Pneumatization can also be assessed by plain skull views, but x-ray examinations are rarely indicated, are inferior to computed tomography (CT) and are no substitute for adequate clinical assessment of the eardrum in inflammatory ear disease.

Computed tomography is now the imaging investigation of choice in most cases because of short scan times, excellent bone detail, and better outlining of soft tissue abnormalities. Only from the point of view of tissue characterization has CT been disappointing and measurements of x-ray attenuation have only a very limited role, for example, for bone dysplasias such as otosclerosis. Careful consideration must always be given to the amount of radiation, especially to the eyes, which should be kept clear of the direct beam whenever possible.

Absence of radiation and some tissue characterization make magnetic resonance imaging (MRI) best for the pediatric age group, although difficulties may occur when there is need for sedation or general anesthesia. Lack of signal from bone is both a disadvantage and advantage. Because both air and cortical bone appear black on MRI they cannot be distinguished. Generally speaking, MRI does not demonstrate the middle-ear cleft unless it is filled with fluid. Although absence of bony landmarks is therefore a problem, it does mean that soft-tissue entities and both normal and pathologic fluids are demonstrated clearly. New MRI techniques such as fast spin echo (FSE) and three-dimensional Fourier transform (3DFT) allow thinner sections to be obtained with high spatial resolution that gives bone detail comparable with that from high-resolution CT. Magnetic resonance angiography MRA using the phase contrast or time of flight techniques is improving rapidly and replacing conventional angiography in many situations.

P.D. Phelps: Department of Radiology, The Royal National Throat, Nose, and Ear Hospital NHS Trust, London WCIX 8DA, United Kingdom.

G. Vézina: Department of Diagnostic Imaging and Radiology, Children's National Medical Center, Washington, DC 20008.

COMPUTED TOMOGRAPHY

The basic examination of the petrous temporal bone consists of contiguous axial and coronal sections 1.5 mm or less

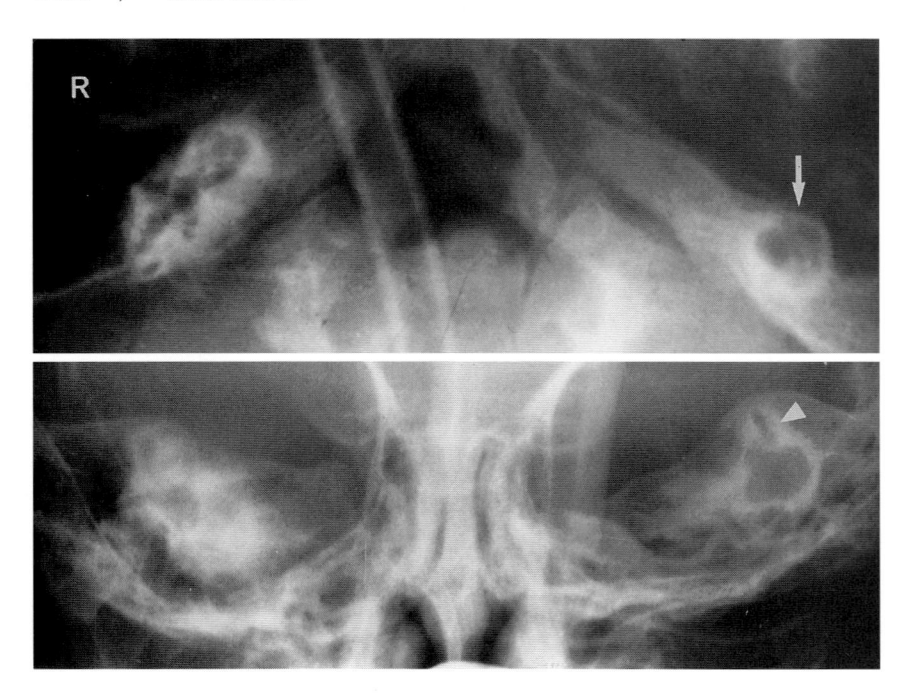

FIG. 1. Plain film views of the petrous temporal bones of a child basal view (*above*) and perorbital (*below*) show a normal labyrinth on the right but on the left a severe deformity consisting of a sac (*arrow*) with endolymphatic appendage (*arrowhead*).

thick at 30 degrees to the anthropological baseline parallel to the roof of the orbit defined on a lateral scout view (Fig. 3). This is to limit the radiation dose to the eye, because although some slices pass through the orbit, the center of the globe is not in the direct x-ray beam. The sections are viewed on a wide window setting of 4,000 Hounsfield units. If greater detail is required, for instance, for the oval window or incudostapedial joint region, then 1-mm sections are necessary. To optimize resolution, individual sides are reformatted to a 10-cm field of view, a 512×512 pixel matrix.

Sections in the axial plane (Fig. 4) start just below the external auditory meatus and show the basal turn of cochlea and round window niche. These sections best show the internal auditory meatus (IAM) and the vestibular aqueduct (VA). The head of the malleus and the body and short process of the incus are also shown at the level of the vestibule.

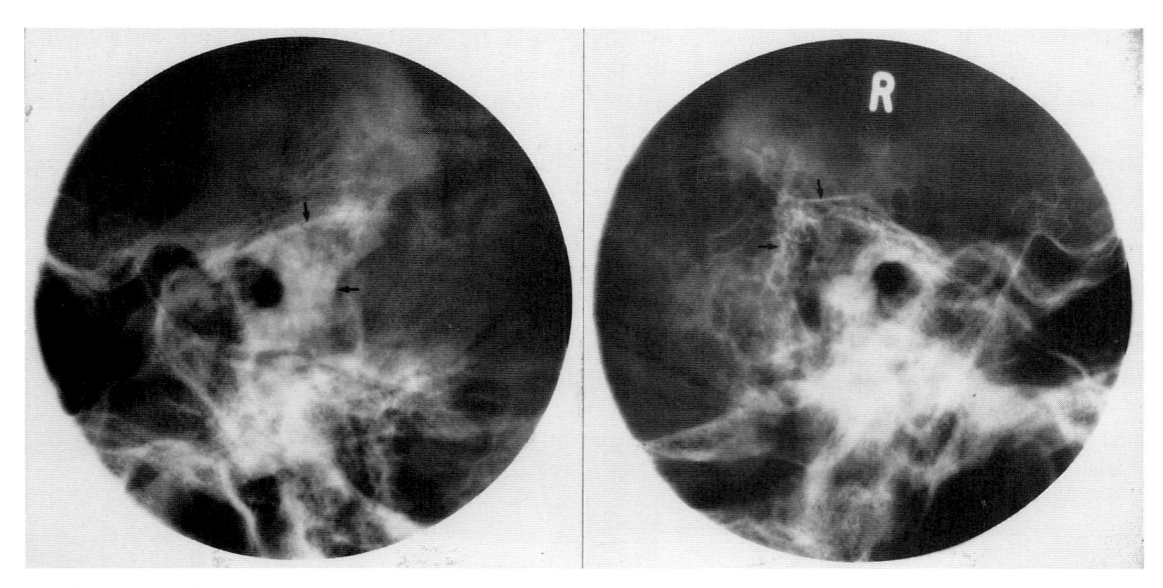

FIG. 2. Plain lateral oblique mastoid views showing full pneumatization (*right*) but poor pneumatization (*left*). The arrows point to the dural place and sigmoid sinus plate.

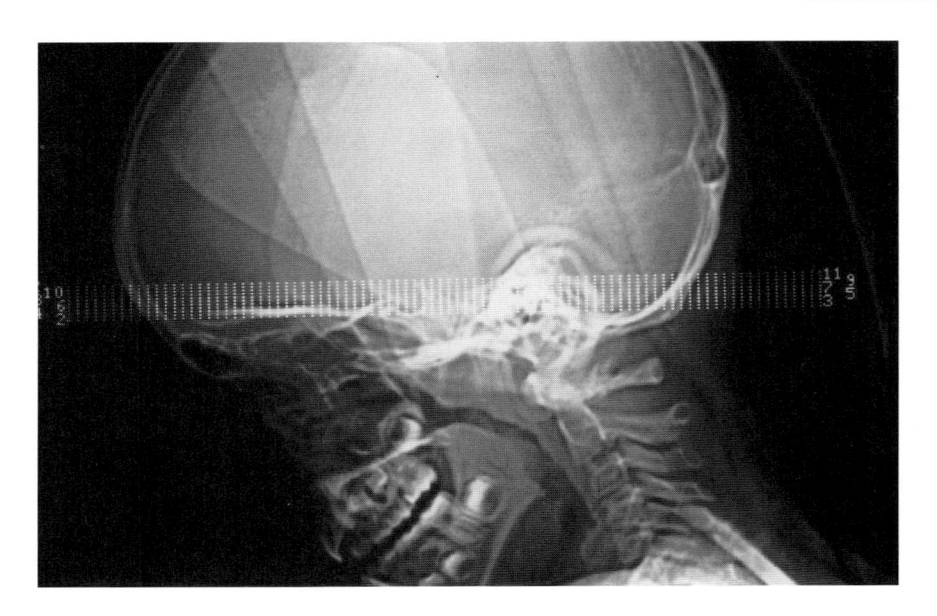

FIG. 3. Lateral scout view showing the scan planes for an axial CT examination.

The three parts of the facial nerve canal can be identified, although the axial plane is least satisfactory for the descending portion, which is seen in cross section behind the pyramidal eminence. The small muscles of the middle ear, the tensor tympani in front and the stapedius posteriorly, are best shown in the axial plane with the stapes between them (Fig. 5).

Coronal Sections

Coronal sections are obtained in head-hanging or chin-up position. Sections 1.5 mm or less thick are obtained as near as possible in the coronal plane aided by gantry tilt. The radiation dose to the eyes from coronal sections is very low because the eyes are not in the x-ray beam.

The eight most important coronal sections are shown in Fig. 6. They begin at the level of the carotid canal and curl of the central bony spiral of the cochlea. The malleus is well shown at this level. Further back, the section at the level of the vestibule shows the internal auditory meatus as well as the stapes and oval window. Further back still, at the most prominent part of the lateral semicircular canal, the pyramidal eminence is shown between facial recess and sinus tympani. The descending facial canal and jugular fossa are assessed, and the examination finishes at the posterior semicircular canal, although further sections may be necessary to show the mastoid antrum and air cells.

Examinations with Contrast

Examinations using CT with contrast are now rarely performed because of the availability of MRI, but they may be necessary to view intracranial or extracranial complications of suppurative ear disease, such as extradural or brain abscess.

Reformatted Images

These can be obtained from multiple thin contiguous axial sections. Reformatted images can be made in any plane but the quality is always inferior to a direct examination and depends on two factors: (a) the number, thickness, and overlap of individual sections and therefore the amount of raw data available for the reconstruction process; and (b) absolute immobility of the patient while the sections are being obtained. Reformatted images in the sagittal plane are helpful to assess a large vestibular aqueduct (see below).

Three-dimensional Scanning

Three-dimensional (3-D) CT is a relatively new imaging facility available for radiology and has come about due to the advanced capabilities of computer systems. From a series of two-dimensional CT scan slices it is now possible to obtain 3-D reconstructions. This can be achieved by manipulating the data obtained from a 2-D study with use of specific 3-D software computer program.

The full advantages of this imaging technique are not yet fully explored; however, it has proved to be particularly useful for facial reconstructions due to trauma or to congenital deformities. Only recently has 3-D CT been used to investigate other more specific anatomy, namely the petrous bone.

The scanning parameters in the 2-D plane have a major influence on the quality of the resultant 3-D image, including spatial resolution and contrast. An important factor to be taken into consideration when using 3-D is the slice thickness and the bed increment of the original study. Obviously, the thinner the slice thickness, the greater the resolution of the 3-D image, but this level of resolution comes at a cost—namely, a possible increase in the radiation dose to the patient because the total number of scans in any one

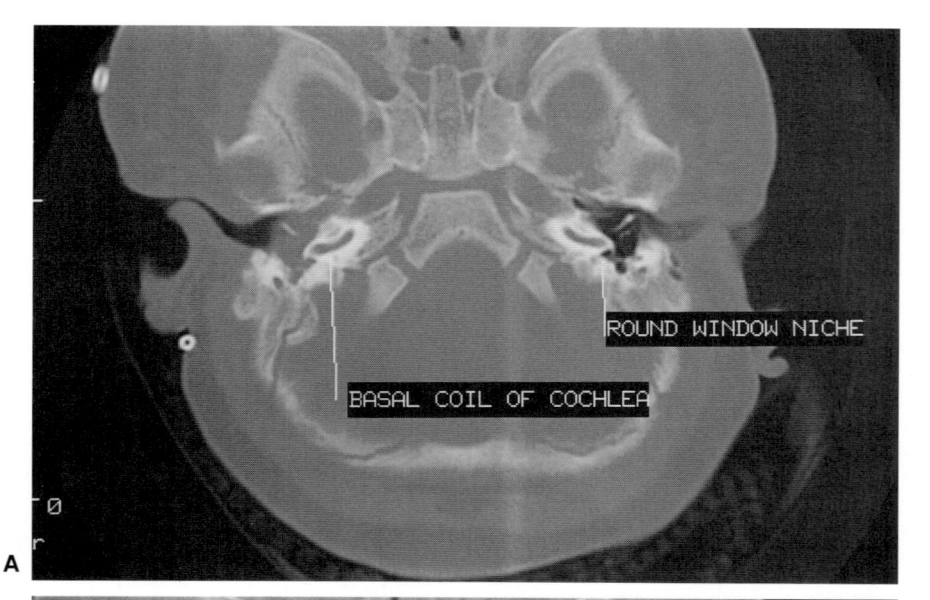

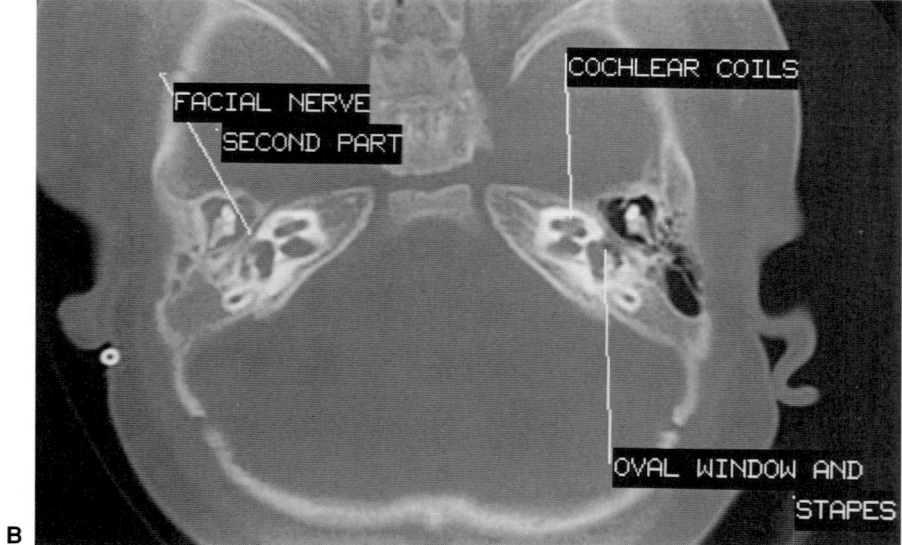

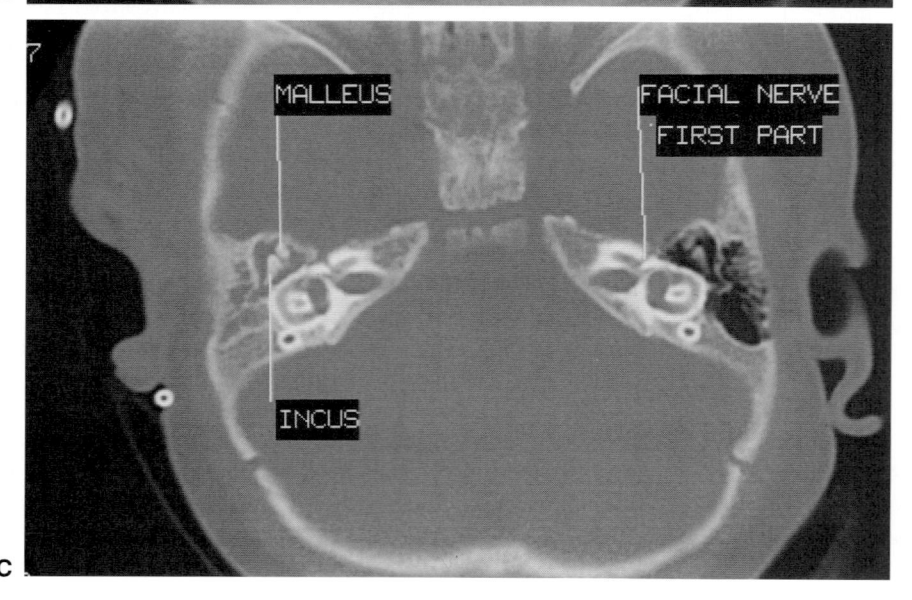

FIG. 4. Four axial CT sections of the petrous temporal bones of a child with the two sides at slightly different levels. The sections are: mid-modiolar section showing the individual coils of the cochlea and incudostapedial region; the section through the vestibule and loop of the lateral semicircular canal, and then the superior and posterior semicircular canals at right angles to each other.

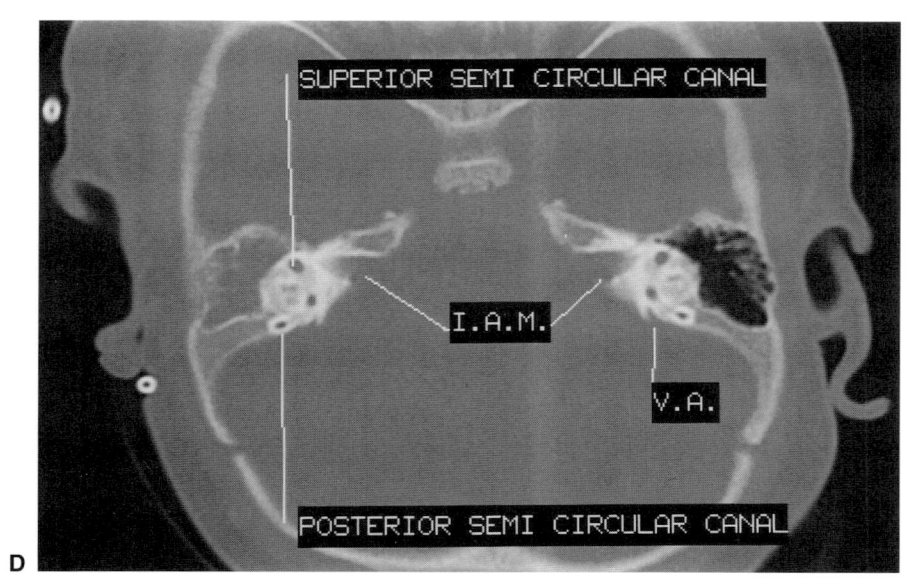

FIG. 4. *Continued.*

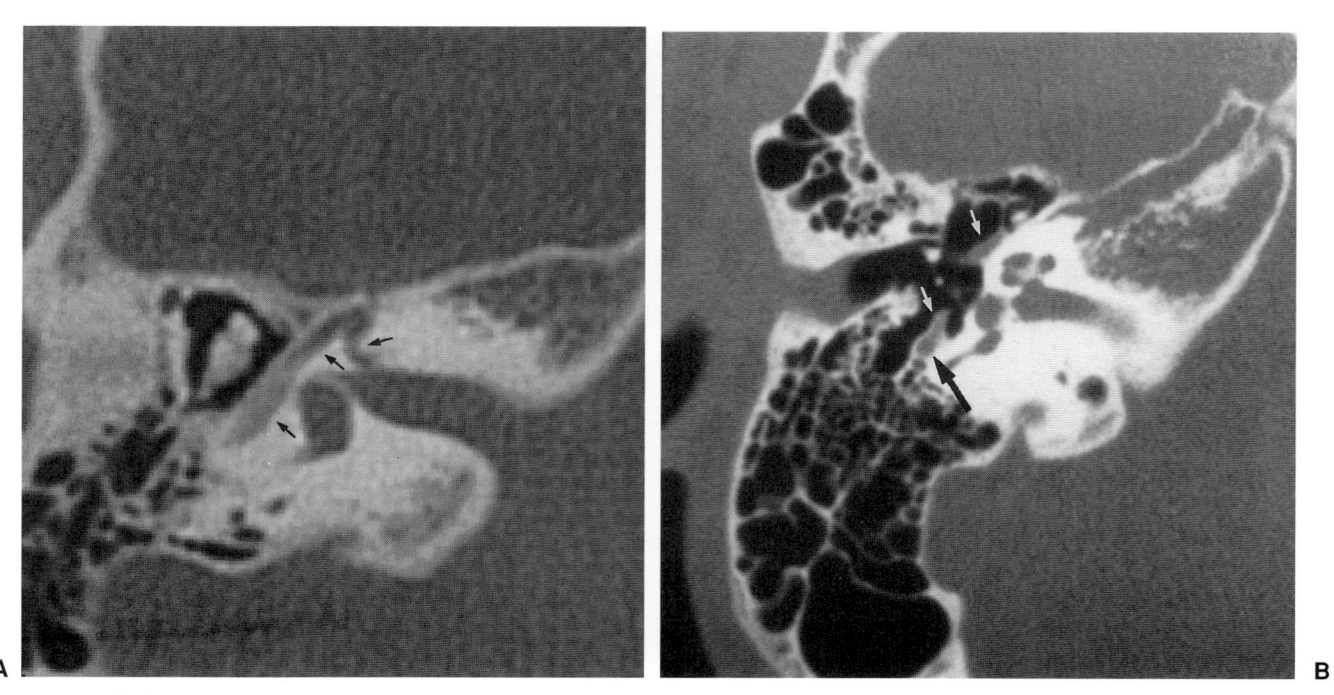

FIG. 5. A: Axial CT scan showing the first and second parts of the facial nerve canal (*black arrows*). **B:** Axial scan showing the third descending part of the facial canal (*black arrow*) as well as the two small muscles of the middle ear cavity (*white arrows*) with the crura of the stapes between them.

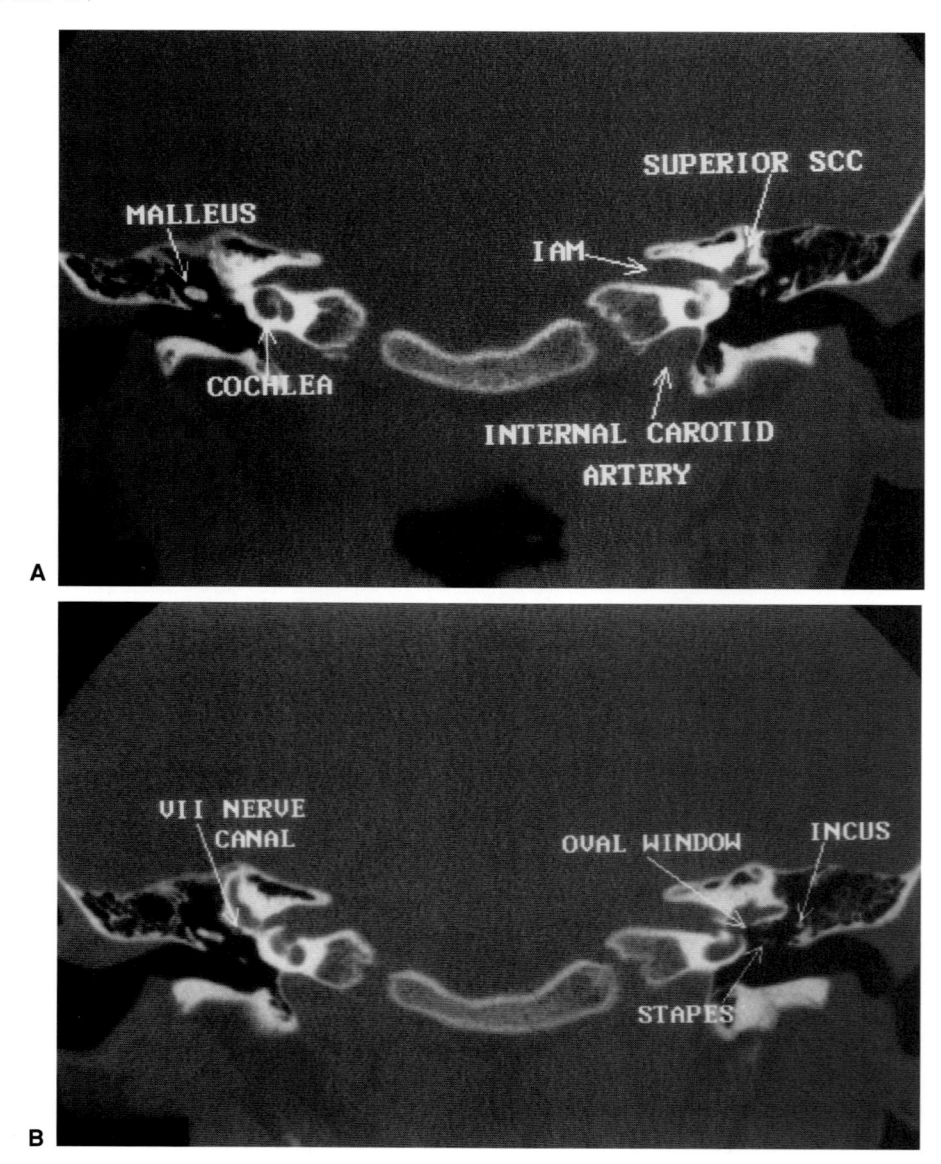

FIG. 6. Four CT sections (**A–D**) in the coronal plane with the two sides at slightly different levels in each section. *(continued)*

plane is increased. However, this may eliminate scanning in both axial and coronal positions if other reconstructions are to be obtained. Patient movement must be avoided; good radiographic techniques must be employed to avoid degradation in quality due to movement. Scanning parameters, such as zoom factor must not be altered while the scans are being done because such alterations cannot usually be compensated for by the software package. Thus, it is important to know whether 3-D will be helpful. For a typical 3-D reconstruction, approximately 20 to 30 slices are required to gain a good 3-D image. Depending on the software, magnification plus rotation functions and other manipulations, as cutting planes, can be executed relatively easily to provide further useful information.

It is also possible to undertake 3-D images selecting different tissue parameters such as bone or soft tissue. The region of interest and tissue type are defined by the obtained CT scan slices and entered into the 3-D software program. Recently, spiral CT imaging with a slice thickness of 1 mm and a reconstruction interval of 0.2 mm have been used for multiplanar and 3-D surface-reconstruction images.

MAGNETIC RESONANCE IMAGING

In the early days of MRI, it soon became apparent that this imaging was better than CT for the investigation of the posterior cranial fossa because of better soft-tissue differentiation, multiplanar capability, and freedom from beam-hardening artifacts. However, because air and bone give essentially no magnetic resonance signal the normal middle

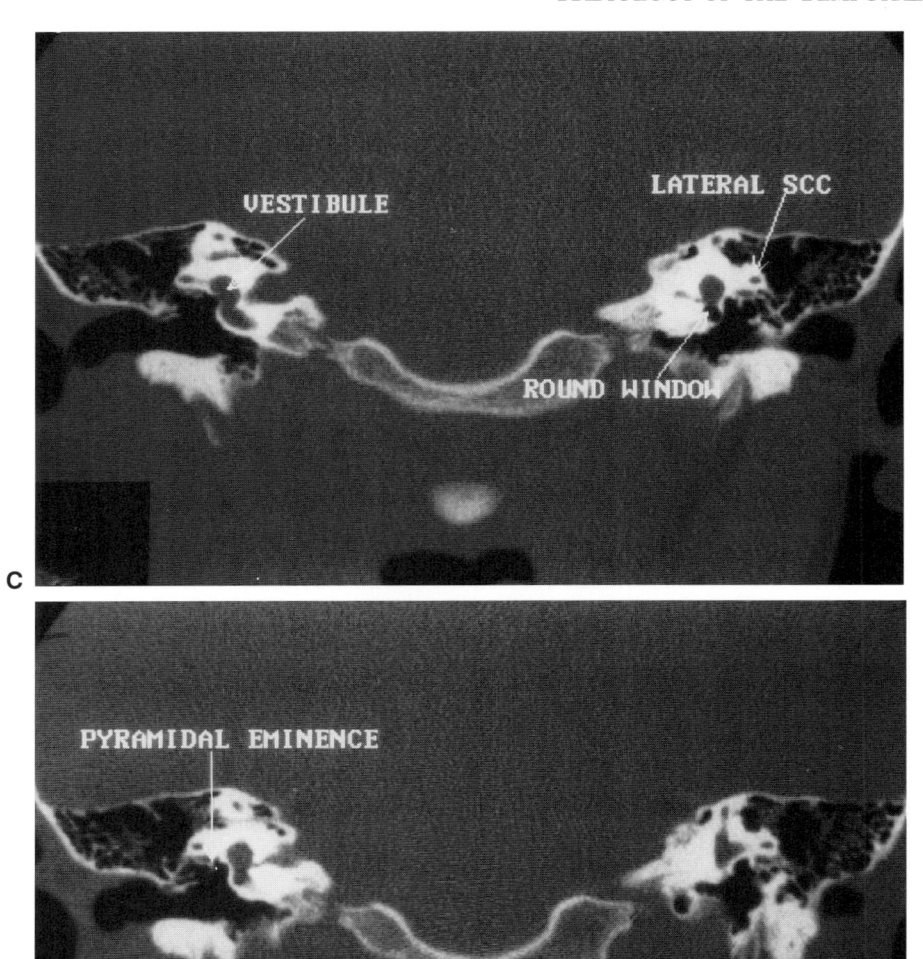

FIG. 6. *Continued.*

ear is not depicted adequately. The fluids of the labyrinth give high signal on T2-weighted sequences, and nerves in the internal auditory meatus and cerebellopontine angle can be seen as well as the facial nerve in its whole length—the nerve itself is shown as opposed to the facial-nerve canal defined by CT.

The original MRI examinations used T1-weighted spin echo sequences showing intermediate signal from the nerves and fluids in the inner ear and high signal from the marrow fat in the petrous apex. The routine precontrast T1-weighted images provide sharp depiction of the fatty and fascial planes of the deep neck and skull base. By providing clear definition of these planes, a pathologic process can easily be detected as an infiltrating lesion extending into and distorting these normal anatomic boundaries. A T2-weighted spin echo sequence takes longer but shows the fluids in the inner ear and the cerebrospinal fluid as high signal. The contrast-enhancing agent Gadolinium diethylenetriamine pentaacetic acid (DTPA) revolutionized the demonstration of tumors such as acoustic neuromas, which are clearly depicted when large or small. Use of gadolinium DTPA is now known to show almost any inflammatory lesion probably related to increased vascularity. Thus increased signal intensity, usually of the tympanic portion of the facial nerve, is shown after administration of gadolinium DTPA in Bell's palsy (Fig. 7). Enhancement has also been shown to occur in the cochlea, vestibule, or both in cases of altered inner ear function, such as those assumed to be caused by labyrinthitis (Fig. 8) (1).

New Imaging Techniques

New imaging techniques have been described recently.

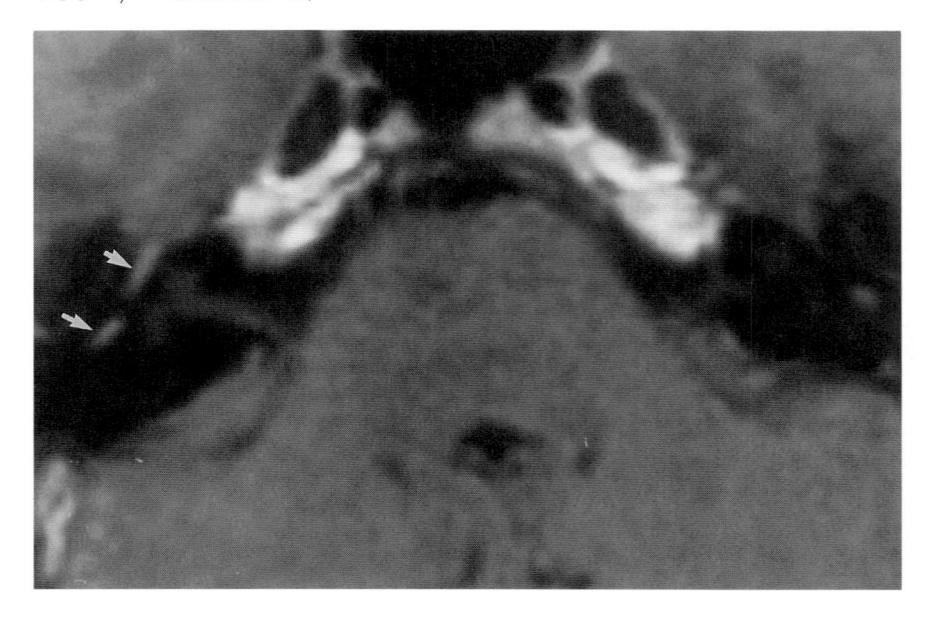

FIG. 7. Axial T1-weighted MRI through the temporal bones and posterior cranial fossa. Intravenous gadolinium DTPA has been given, and high signal from the second part of the facial nerve (*arrows*) is shown on one side.

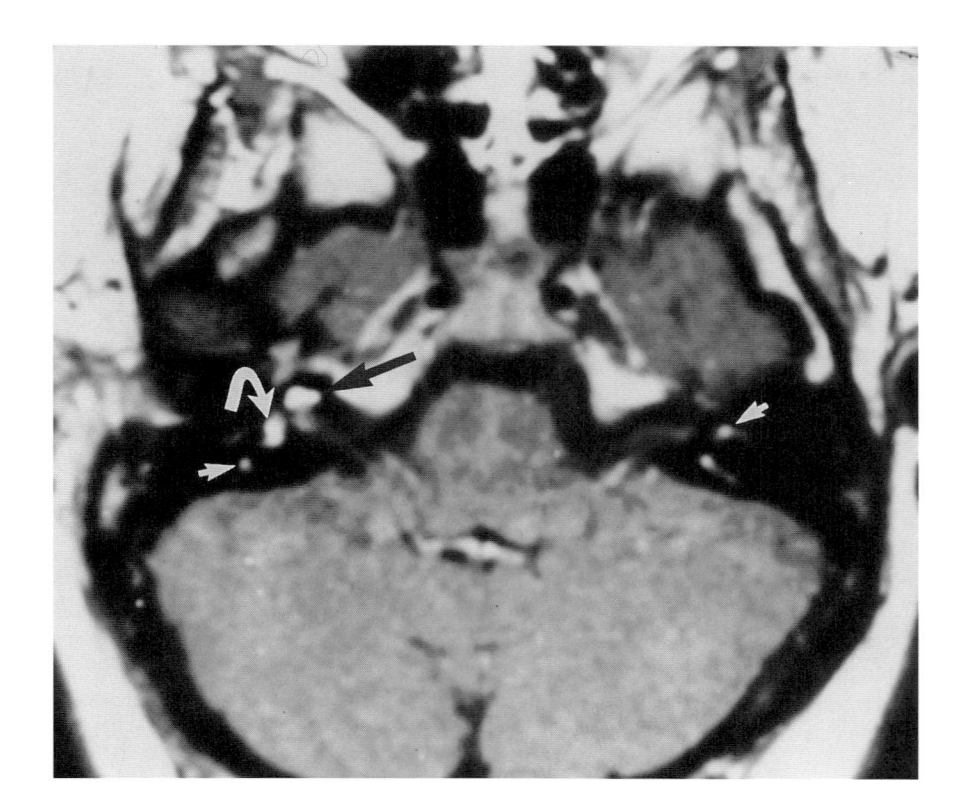

FIG. 8. Viral labyrinthitis in a 13-year-old girl. Abnormal enhancement is seen in the right cochlea (*long arrow*), the right vestibule (*curved arrow*), and the left semicircular canals (*short bilateral arrows*) on the gadolinium-enhanced axial T1-weighted MRI.

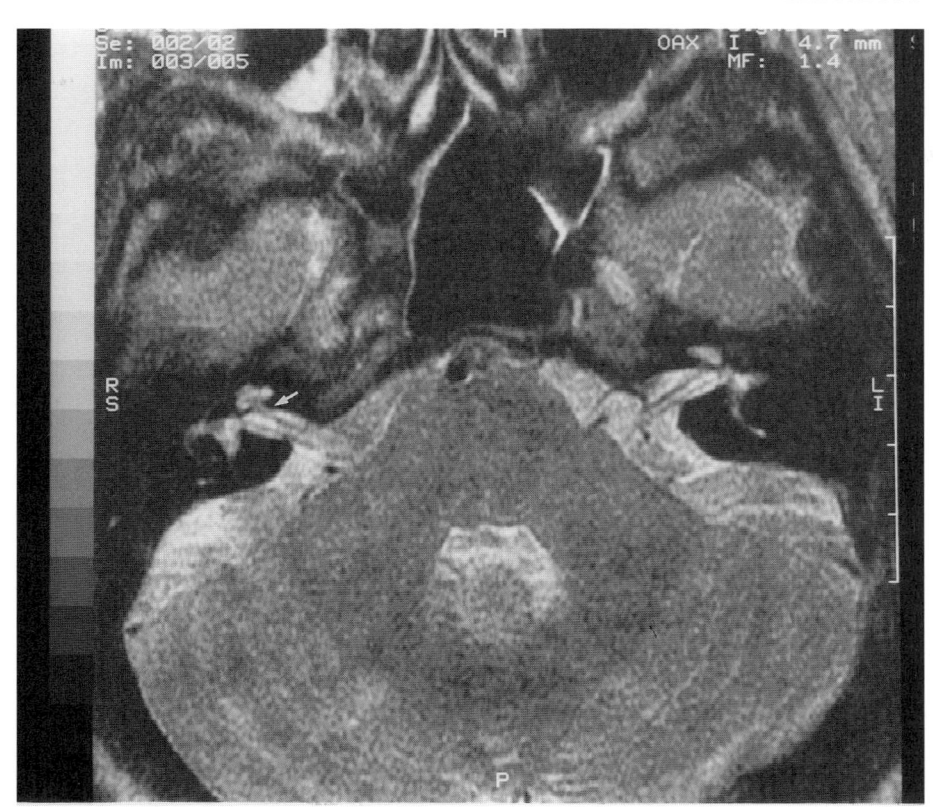

FIG. 9. Axial fast spin echo image shows clearly the nerves in the internal auditory meatus on both sides surrounded by high signal cerebrospinal fluid. The arrow points to the cochlear nerve and spiral ganglion in the base of the modiolus of the cochlea.

Fast Spin Echo

Fast spin echo is a new fast scanning method that uses spin echoes and altered k-space (collection of raw data) filling. It is designed to provide more conventional spin echo-type contrast in shorter times by the use of repetitive refocusing 180-degree radio frequency pulses, which means that 8 to 32 times as much k-space can be filled compared with a traditional spin echo in which one line of k-space is generally completed per resolution time (TR). Each echo is acquired with a different phase encode gradient. The total acquisition time is greatly reduced with FSE, thus enabling a greater number of phase encoding steps to be made. The matrix size can therefore be increased to provide improved spatial resolution and still maintain an acceptable examination time. Thus the latest MRI equipment can give image detail almost on a par with that of CT, 2 mm or less thick sections and good contrast between bone, soft tissues, and fluids of the inner ear. The normal cranial nerves in the internal auditory meatus are clearly seen surrounded by the high signal cerebrospinal fluid (Fig. 9).

Gradient Echo Imaging

The usual 90-degree pulse of the spin echo sequence provides the highest signal as long as the longitudinal magnetization has almost completely recovered. If shorter TR values are used, the signal becomes weaker, but better signal-to-noise ratios can be achieved per unit time with use of pulse flip angles less than 90 degrees. This is known as gradient echo because the echoes are generated by gradient reversal instead of the subsequent 180-degree pulse used in spin echo imaging. The contrast of gradient echo images is adjusted by varying the flip angle and the echo time (TE). The ability to use shorter TR makes thin sliced 3-D volume practical and although the presentation of 3-D data is usually in 2-D slices, 3-D pictures can be made by postprocessing (Fig. 10) (2).

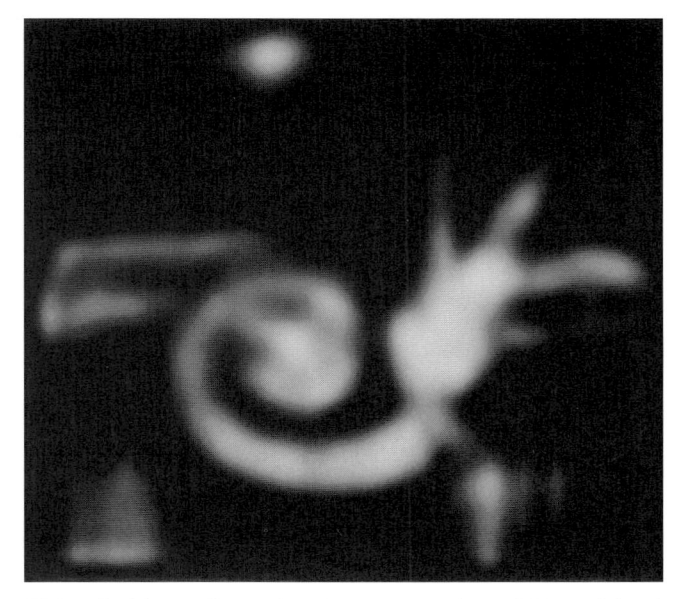

FIG. 10. Three-dimensional reconstruction of T2-weighted MRI of the labyrinth. Courtesy of Dr. D. Doyon, CHU Bicetre, Paris, France.

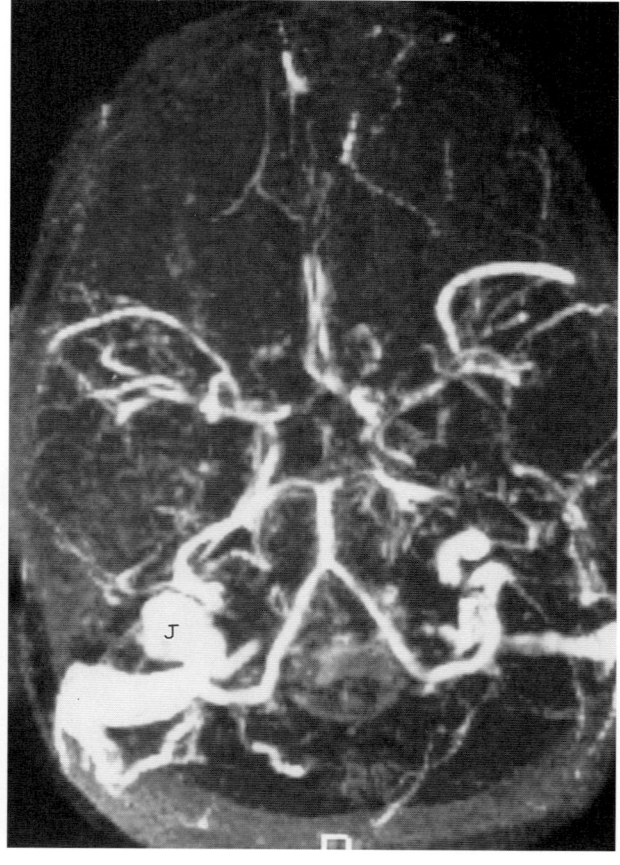

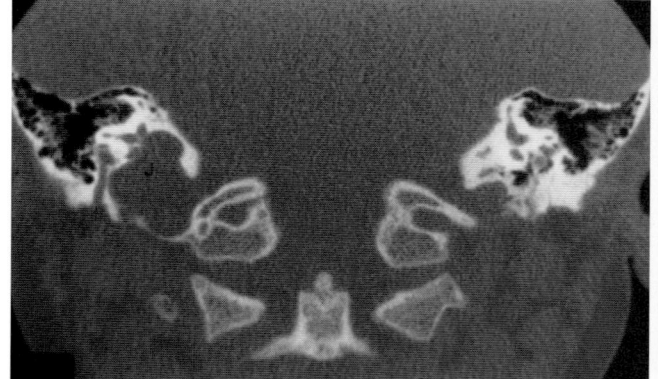

FIG. 11. **A:** Coronal CT scan showing a large jugular bulb (*J*) close to the descending facial nerve canal (*arrow*). **B:** Venous MR angiogram showing the intracranial venous system confirming the large jugular bulb (*J*). From Good et al. (3). Previously reported in the Journal of Laryngology and Otology and reproduced with permission.

Fat Suppressed Imaging

The short tau inversion recovery sequence (STIR) was the first imaging protocol to demonstrate satisfactorily a lesion obscured by high signal from surrounding fat. Although this is not a problem in the cranial cavity, lesions in the orbit or below the skull base can be shown better if the signal from fat is suppressed. A specific time to inversion (TI) (approximately 100–160 msec, depending on field strength) is chosen in a way that fat will be at its nil point and will not show a significant signal. Unfortunately, STIR can also suppress gadolinium-enhanced signal and thus may not be beneficial with enhancing agents. The best method of fat suppression when gadolinium has been used consists of a selective presaturation radiofrequency (RF) pulse at the resonant frequency of fat. The fat signal can thereby be selectively removed and dispersed by a following crusher gradient. A major advantage of contrast-enhanced fat suppression imaging is improved lesion conspicuity. By suppressing fat signal, an enhancing lesion is more easily detected against a background of low-signal-intensity fat. The main disadvantages of chemical shift fat suppression are the artifacts produced by bulk and the magnetic susceptibility effects (for an explanation of these phenomena and how they can be overcome a more technical book should be consulted).

Magnetic Resonance Angiography

Magnetic resonance angiography is a new technique that is rapidly replacing conventional angiography. It employs flowing blood as a physiologic contrast medium, is a noninvasive technique with no risks for the patient, and can be added to routine MRI study.

Arterial MRA can be accomplished with time of flight or phase contrast sequence. Large and medium-sized arteries can be demonstrated, but evaluation of the type and extent of vascular pathology may be upset by altered (nonlaminar) blood flow. Arterial MRA has limited use in evaluation of smaller-sized vessels (e.g., tumoral vascularity such as that in glomus tumors); catheter angiography is still the modality of choice in this circumstance.

Venous MRA requires the employment of sequential flow compensated sequences due to the slow blood flow in veins. Venous MRA are optimized by employment of an additional RF saturation pulse below the imaging slices minimizing signal from arterial blood flow. Venous MRA can demonstrate the intracranial venous sinus system and has replaced catheter venography (Fig. 11). The images in Fig. 11 are from a 4-year-old child who presented with left-sided sensorineural hearing loss (SNLH) as the only abnormality. Routine CT imaging revealed the large left jugular fossa, which was smoothly outlined and seemed to be a normal variant. However, the progressive nature of the loss was worrying and MRI seemed to rule out an expansile space occupying lesion. As expected, the T1-weighted MRI scan showed no signal in this location because the bone of the jugular fossa and flowing blood in the jugular bulb contributed no signal. Venous MRA successfully showed the large jugular bulb and sigmoid sinus (3).

IMAGING CHILDREN WITH HEARING LOSS

Appropriate imaging of children with hearing loss depends on knowledge of the clinical examination and audiometric analysis. Probably any child with unexplained SNHL or deafness needs imaging of the petrous temporal bones to exclude a structural abnormality of the inner ear. Noncontrast high-resolution CT is the imaging modality of choice for evaluation of most children with hearing loss (sensorineural, mixed or conductive). Enhanced MRI is indicated for documented acute hearing loss or for patients in whom coexistent cranial nerve or central nervous system pathology is suspected.

Otic Capsule Dysplasias

Otic capsule dysplasias are identified in approximately 20% of children with sensorineural hearing loss, and include a variable group of malformations caused by arrested development of the otic capsule during the first trimester of gestation (4,5).

The *enlarged vestibular aqueduct* (EVA) is the most common congenital cause for sensorineural hearing loss shown by imaging (6). The EVA is best demonstrated in the axial plane or with sagittal reconstructions (Fig. 12). On the basis of various assessments of the normal range of the caliber of the VA (initially by polytomography), any VA wider than 1.5 mm at the midpoint of the postisthmic segment or halfway between the external aperture and the common crus is considered enlarged. To assess the size of a visible VA, the semicircular canals can be used as an internal measurement reference; any VA larger than the semicircular canals should be viewed with suspicion and measured.

An enlarged VA occurs bilaterally in approximately 30% of patients, and may have associated abnormalities of the vestibule, semicircular canals, or cochlea. Patients with EVA present with either progressive or stable SNHL (7). The relationship between EVA and SNHL is not well understood.

In 1791 Mondini described a case of cochlear hypoplasia

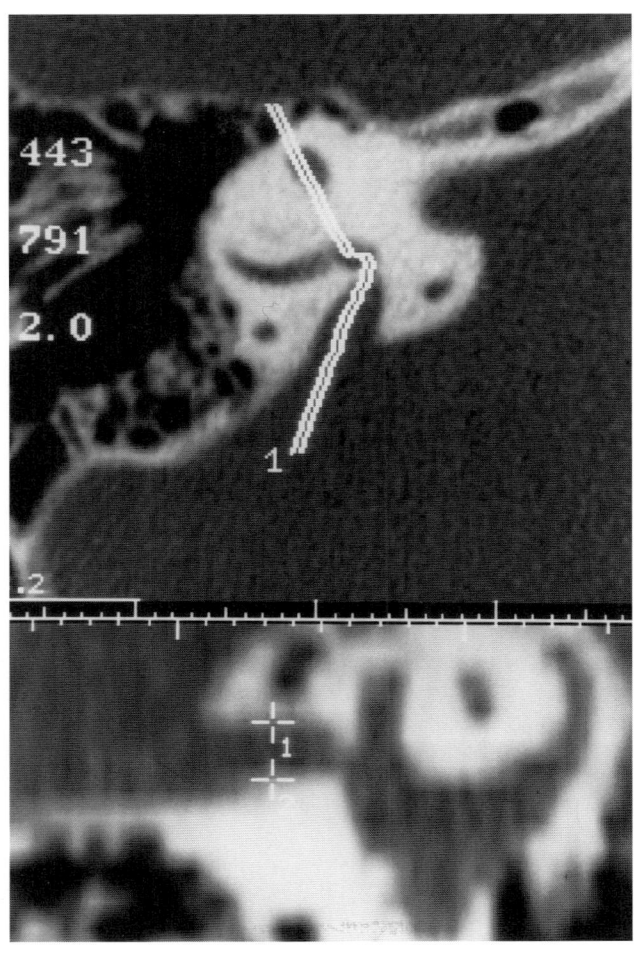

FIG. 12. Axial CT section (*above*) showing a large vestibular aqueduct and the plane (*1*) for which the sagittal reformatting is made. The reformatted image (*below*) shows the large vestibular aqueduct and its measurement of 2.0 mm at the midpoint of the descending limb (*1*).

associated with a large vestibular aqueduct (8). The true *Mondini malformation* of the cochlea consists of a normal basal turn and a distal sac or common cavity. It is due to an insult at 7 weeks of fetal age and is the second most common imaging finding in children with SNHL (5). It is usually associated with progressive and perhaps fluctuant deafness but not complete anacusis. Because the basal turn of the cochlea is not enlarged, there is no risk of a cerebrospinal fistula. Such patients are therefore candidates for cochlear implantation and MRI can be a useful adjunct to CT for confirming the presence of the cochlear nerve (Fig. 13).

More severe degrees of cochlear dysplasia produce a spectrum of increasingly anomalous cochlea, with widening of the basal turn, and ultimately the appearance of a common cavity lesion. The common cavity lesion with a direct connection between the subarachnoid space in the internal auditory meatus and the perilymph-endolymph space of the cavity was first described by Cook in 1838. This is a most important inner ear deformity because it carries a very real risk of meningitis, cerebrospinal fistula, or both (Fig. 14)

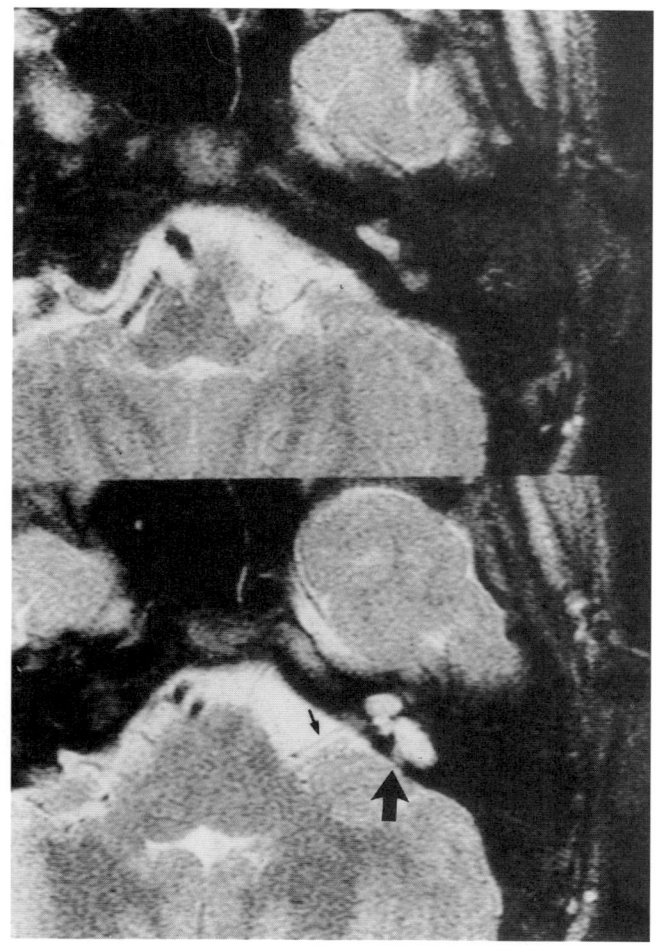

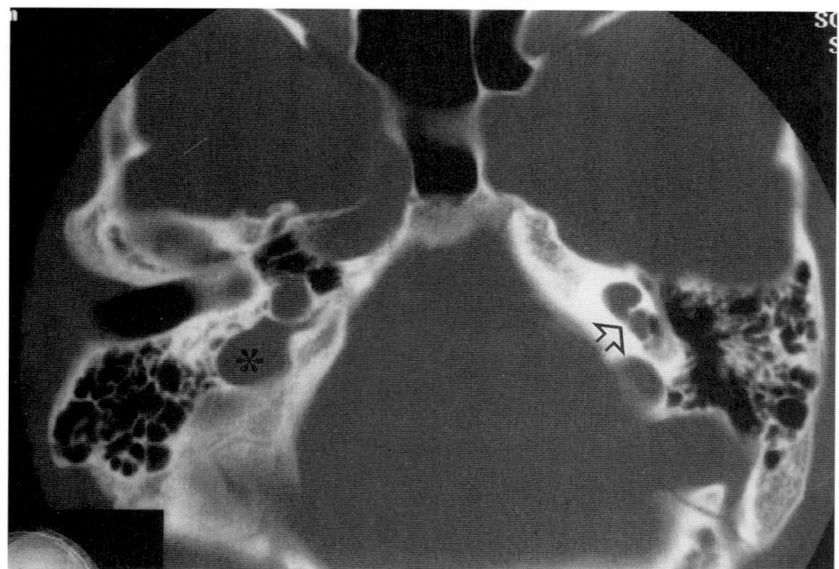

FIG. 13. A: True axial fast spin echo T2-weighted sections showing a normal basal turn of cochlear (*above*) and (*below*) a distal sac, dilated vestibule, and a large vestibular aqueduct (*large arrow*). The small arrow points to the cochlear nerve. **B:** The equivalent axial CT section showing the normal basal turn of the Mondini deformity (*open arrow*). On the other side is a more severe deformity consisting of a simple sac in front of the jugular fossa (∗).

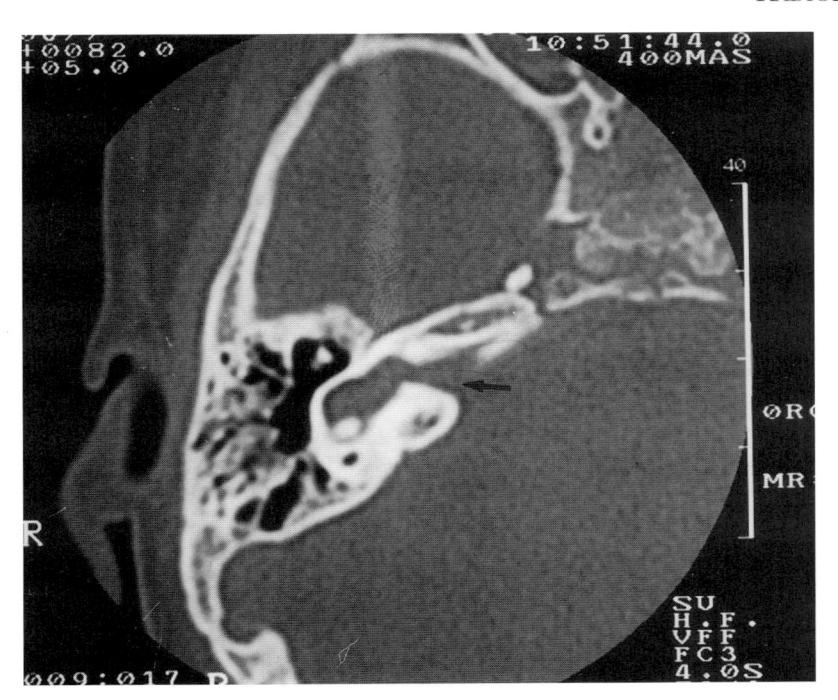

FIG. 14. Axial CT of a common cavity lesion of the inner ear open to the subarachnoid space of the posterior cranial fossa (arrow). This child had recurrent attacks of meningitis. Courtesy of Professor Hans Bergstedt, Karolinska Sjukhuest, Stockholm, Sweden.

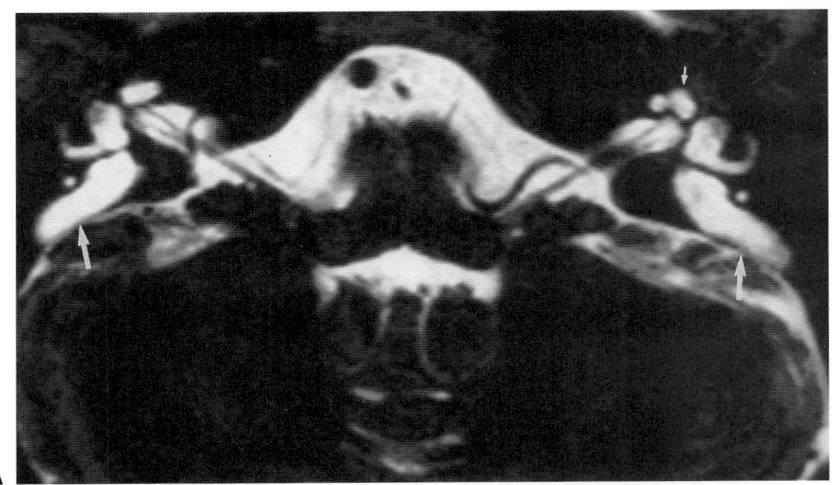

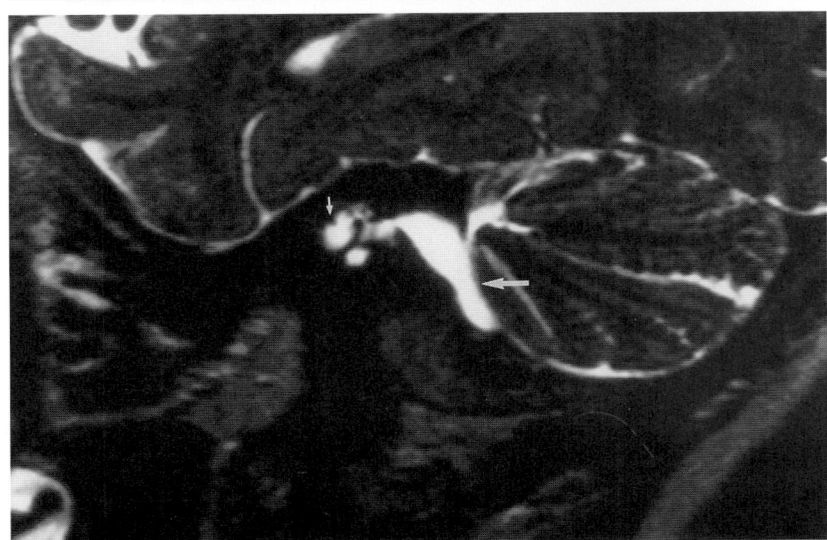

FIG. 15. A: Axial images. **B:** sagittal images of a case of Pendred syndrome with Mondini cochlea (short arrows) and greatly enlarged endolymphatic sac and ducts (long arrows). The nerves in the internal auditory canals are normal.

(9). Patients with widened basal turn of the cochlea can also develop perilymphatic fistulas caused by absence or defects in the stapes foot plate, which may allow for otorrhoea, rhinorrhea, or recurrent meningitis (10). Various anomalies of the vestibule, VA, and semicircular canals may be associated with cochlear dysplasias (Fig. 15).

The *Michel deformity* results from arrested development (at approximately 4 weeks of gestational age) of the labyrinth, resulting in cochlear and vestibular aplasia and profound SNHL that is often bilateral. Imaging reveals absence of the inner ear structures, one or multiple cystic cavities, and small (hypoplastic) internal auditory canals (Fig. 16). The middle-ear cavity is expanded due to the missing cochlea; this petrous bone maldevelopment (namely, a concave medial wall) is useful in differentiating the Michel anomaly from a heavily mineralized labyrinth as a result of labyrinthitis obliterans-ossificans (5). *X-linked SNHL* presents in young men with profound mixed or sensorineural hearing loss. The imaging hallmark is an enlarged, bulbus internal auditory canal, typically bilateral. This abnormality causes perilymphatic hydrops due to a fistulous connection between the internal auditory canal and the base of the cochlea. Widening of the proximal facial nerve canal, enlargement of the VA, and hypoplasia of the cochlear base may also be seen (11).

The most common congenital abnormality causing conductive deafness is stapes ankylosis with fixation of the footplace in the oval window (12). Unfortunately, stapes fixation cannot be predicted reliably by imaging alone, and the next most common cause of congenital conductive loss, namely minor discontinuities (Fig. 17) or fixations in the incudostapedial region, is difficult to predict radiologically especially if there is soft-tissue opacification adjacent to the minor bony deformities, which produces soft-tissue silhouetting of the images. Such cases can only be assessed adequately and treated appropriately by exploratory tympanotomy. A persistent and stable air or bone gap on the audiogram is the basic requirement for such a strategy.

Stenosis and complete atresia of the oval window are less common and produce conductive or mixed hearing loss. The oval window is best identified on the coronal CT image showing the vestibule, opposite the falciform crest of the internal auditory canal (see Fig. 6B). With aplasia of the oval window, the horizontal portion of the facial nerve canal can be located inferior and medial to its usual course (Fig. 18). The stapes is present within the middle ear but in an abnormal position.

Other Etiologies of Pediatric SNHL

If a high-resolution CT fails to reveal anomalies of the temporal bone in a child with SNHL, an MRI examination should be considered in the appropriate setting. A list of the causes of pediatric SNHL is presented in Table 1; most of these conditions are either more easily or exclusively diagnosed with MRI.

Labyrinthitis is most commonly viral in ethology. Bacterial infection from the middle ear or meninges and autoimmune disorders can also cause labyrinthitis. The imaging hallmark is labyrinthine enhancement on postgadolinium

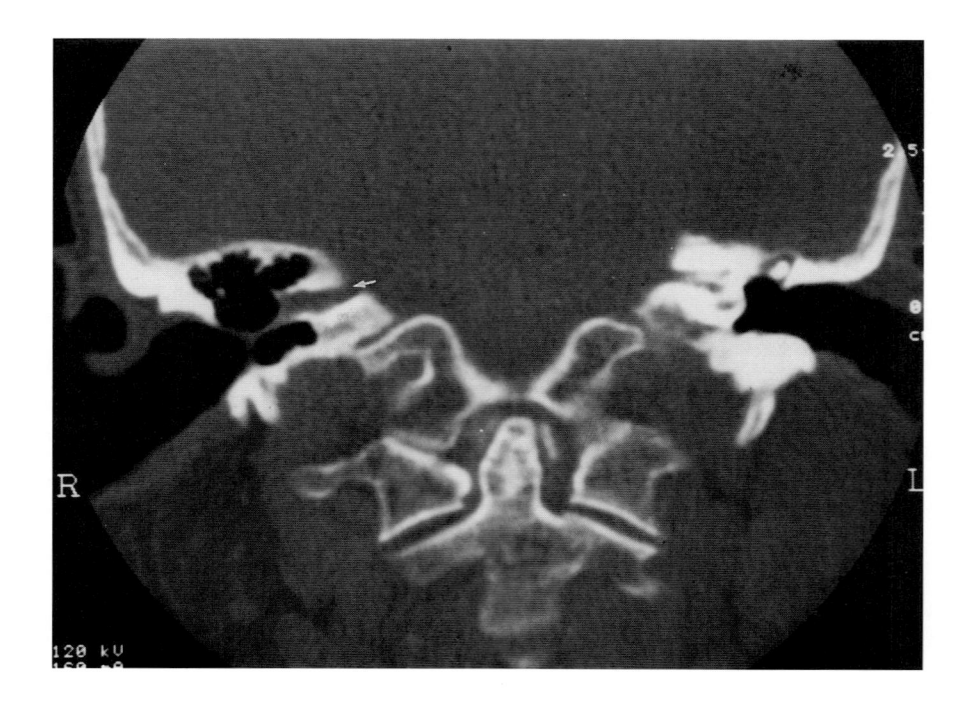

FIG. 16. Coronal CT demonstrates absence of the labyrinth on the right (Michel defect); only the internal auditory meatus is present.

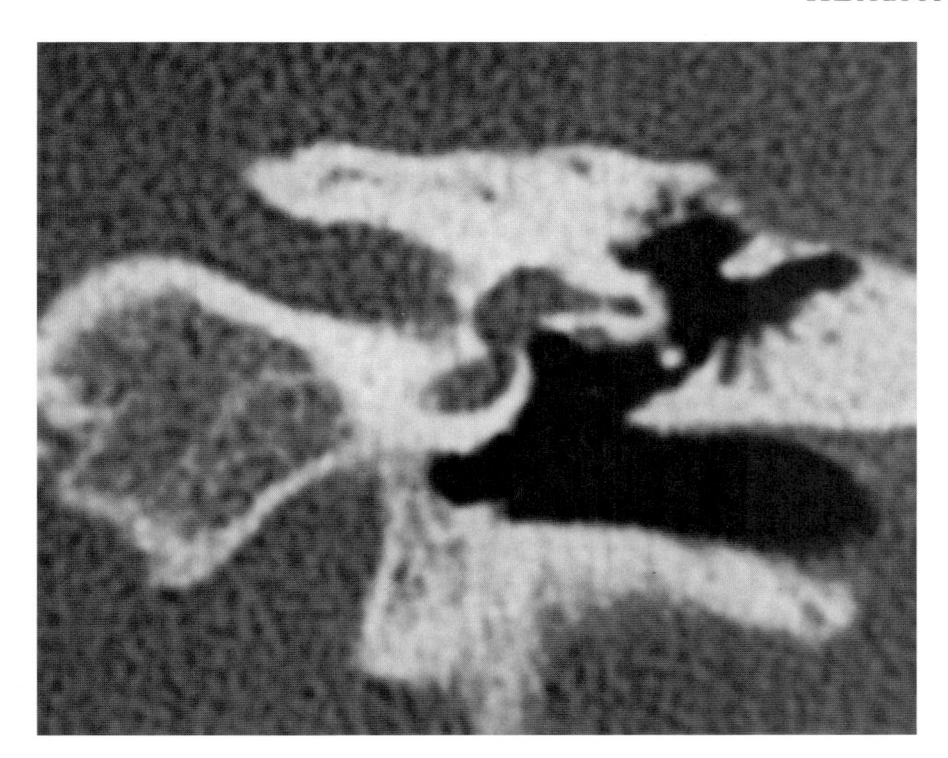

FIG. 17. Coronal CT scan at the level of the oval window showing just a remnant of the body of the incus and no evidence of long process of incus or stapes.

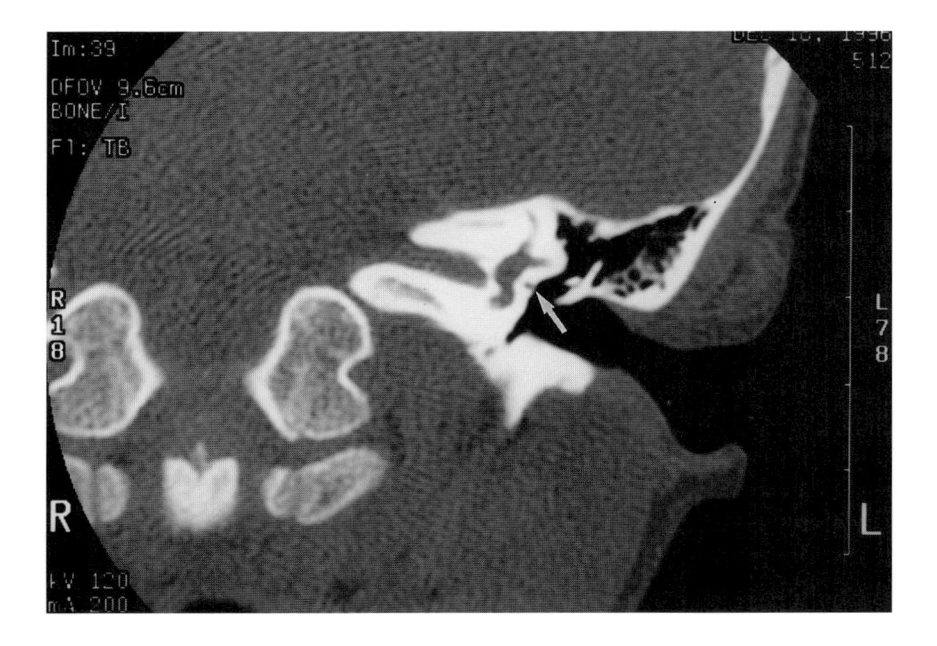

FIG. 18. Coronal CT scan at the level of the vestibule reveals absence of the oval window. The facial nerve is positioned in the expected location of the oval window (*arrow*).

TABLE 1. *Pediatric sensorineural hearing loss*

Labyrinth
  Otic capsule dysplasia
  Labyrinthitis (acute)
  Labyrinthine hemorrhage
  Labyrinthitis ossificans
  Labyrinthine masses
  Otosclerosis
Internal auditory canal
  Primary
    Acoustic neuroma
    Arteriovenous malformation
    Hemangioma
    Acoustic neuritis
    Lipoma
  Secondary
    Direct extension (from temporal bone, cerebellopontine angle, labyrinth)
    Metastases
    Leptomeningeal disorders (leukemia, lymphoma)
Central nervous system
  Brainstem glioma
  Dysmyelination (e.g., peroxisomal disorders)
  Demyelination (multiple sclerosis)
  Infarction
  Bilateral temporal lobe disease (cortical dysplasia, infarction)

T1-weighted MRI (Fig. 8) (1). Both labyrinthine inflammation and hemorrhage can lead to obliteration of the fluid spaces of the labyrinth. Membranous obliteration is identified as foci of signal void within the normally fluid-filled spaces of the labyrinth on T2-weighted MRI. The fibrosing process can ultimately lead to ossification of the labyrinth—labyrinthitis obliterans (Fig. 19).

Primary masses of the labyrinth are extremely rare in children. Masses within the internal auditory canal (either primary or secondary to extension from adjacent meningeal, cerebellar or temporal bone tumors) are often accompanied by unilateral SNHL. Due to early decussation of cochlear nerve fibers in the upper medulla, more central lesions are less likely to cause hearing loss and are more difficult to localize. However, patients with coexistent bilateral temporal lobe, or multifocal diffuse brain stem disorders can have bilateral SNHL.

CONCLUSION

Unlike the situation in the adult, congenital abnormalities of the temporal bone are the most common abnormalities detected by x-ray in children with SNHL. High-resolution CT is still the first imaging modality used in the majority of cases. With resolution improving, MRI studies are increasingly performed. In many cases, MRI is likely to replace CT as the imaging modality of choice in evaluation in children with SNHL, once the resolution and the reliability of CT in defining anomalies of the temporal bones are matched by MRI.

CT remains the preferred modality in cases of mixed or conductive hearing loss due to its superior delineation of the anatomy of the ossicles and the oval and round windows. If a middle-ear mass is demonstrated on CT and intracranial extension is suspected, MRI provides better resolution of the intracranial structures.

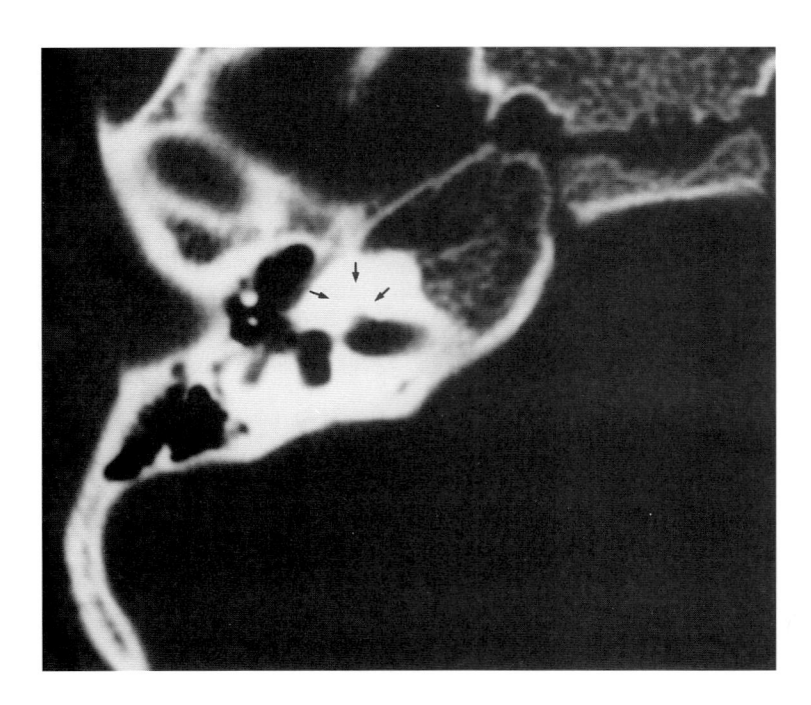

FIG. 19. Labyrinthitis ossificans in a 4-year-old girl with a history of pneumococcal meningitis at age 8 months. Axial CT shows obliterative calcification of the cochlea (*arrows*). Note that the medial wall of the middle ear retains a normal convex border (compare with Michel defect, Fig. 16).

REFERENCES

1. Mark AS, Seltzer S, Nelson-Drake J, Chapman JC, Fitzgerald DC, Gulya AJ. Labyrinthine enhancement on Gadolinium-enhanced magnetic resonance imaging in sudden deafness and vertigo: correlation with audiologic and electronystagmographic studies. *Ann Otol Rhinol Laryngol* 1992;101:459.
2. Casselman JW, Kuhweide R, Deimling M, Ampe W, Dehaene I, Meeus L. Constructive interference in steady stage-3DFT MR imaging of the inner ear and cerebellopontine angle. *AJNR* 1993;14:48.
3. Good CD, Phelps PD, Lim DP. Radiology in Focus. Case report: Greatly enlarged jugular fossa with progressive sensorineural hearing loss. *J Laryngol Otol* 1995;109:350–352.
4. Weissman JL. Hearing Loss. *Radiology* 1996;199:593–611.
5. Fisher NA, Curtin HD. Radiology of congenital hearing loss. *Otolaryngol Clin North Am* 1994;27:511–531.
6. Valvassori GE, Clemis JD. Large vestibular aqueduct syndrome. *Laryngoscope* 1978;88:723–738.
7. Zalzal GH, Tomaski SM, Vezina LG, Bjornsti P, Grundfast KM. Enlarged vestibular aqueduct and sensorineural hearing loss in childhood. *Arch Otolaryngol Head Neck Surg* 1995;121:23–28
8. Phelps PD. Historical article: Ear dysplasia after Mondini. *J Laryngol Otol* 1994;108:461–465
9. Phelps PD. Michaels L. The common cavity congenital deformity of the inner ear. An important precursor of meningitis described in 1838. *J Otol Rhinol Laryngol* 1995;57:228–331.
10. Phelps PD, King A, Michaels L. Cochlear dysplasia and meningitis. *Am J Otol* 1994;15:551—557.
11. Phelps PD, Reardon W, Pembrey M, Bellman S, Luxom L. X-linked deafness, stapes gushers and a distinctive defect of the inner ear. *Neuroradiology* 1991;33:326–330.
12. Teunissen EB, Cremers CWRJ. Classification of congenital middle ear anomalies. *Ann Otol Rhinol Laryngol* 1993;102:606–612.

PART III
Congenital Abnormalities

CHAPTER 13

Congenital Anomalies of the Inner Ear

P. Gerard Reilly, Anil K. Lalwani, and Robert K. Jackler

An understanding of the nature of malformations of the inner ear requires familiarity with its normal embryologic development. At about the fourth week of gestation, the otocyst develops from an invagination of the ectoderm and then separates from it to become a discrete structure. It then branches and coils to form the membranous labyrinth. Chondrofication and then ossification occur in the second trimester to form the bony capsule of the inner ear. The sensory epithelium of the primordial inner ear develops from the lining cells of the membranous labyrinth. Maturation of the sensory epithelium continues throughout the second trimester of pregnancy. Development of the inner ear is essentially complete by the 26th week of gestation, although maturation of the sensory epithelium continues for some time.

Knowledge of the temporal sequence of inner ear development allows a better appreciation of the types of abnormalities that may be encountered in clinical practice.

Abnormalities of the inner ear can arise as a result of

1. Aplasia or dysplasia of sensory epithelium
2. Failure of the labyrinth to divide and coil properly
3. Deficiencies of the bony framework

Abnormalities of the inner ear can be divided into those in which the membranous labyrinth is abnormal but the bony capsule is normal, or those in which both are abnormal. At present, only the latter can be characterized with certainty during life becuase abnormalities of the membranous labyrinth alone cannot be seen by computed tomography (CT) scanning. Therefore, it is difficult to determine the exact incidence of different types of abnormality. However, newer techniques, such as constructive interference in steady-state three-dimensional fourier transformation magnetic resonance imaging (3DFT MR), allow fast and detailed imaging of inner ear structures and may be able to allow three-dimensional membranous labyrinth reconstructions (1). This may help in a more complete diagnosis of abnormalities limited to the membranous labyrinth. Despite these uncertainties, it can be assumed that all children who present with congenital sensorineural hearing impairment would have abnormalities of their inner ears if they could be examined histopathologically, unless there is a purely central cause for their hearing impairment.

Several attempts have been made at classification of inner ear malformation. Most rely on historical descriptions and eponyms and are complicated and difficult to remember. Jackler, Luxford and House (2) devised a classification of inner ear abnormalities according to the site and type of defect (Table 1). This involves dividing defects into those in which only the membranous labyrinth is affected from those in which both bony and membranous labyrinths are abnormal. This distinction will remain useful until membranous labyrinthine abnormalities can be diagnosed with certainty by radiologic imaging.

It is difficult to be certain of the exact incidence of different types of inner ear abnormalities, but overall about 1 in 1,000 children are born with a significant degree of sensorineural hearing impairment (3). Brown (4) analyzed several sets of data and concluded that about 25% of childhood hearing loss could be attributed to identifiable prenatal or postnatal disease or trauma, 18% to undiagnosed disease or genetic factors, 15% to autosomal dominant genes, 40% to autosomal recessive genes, and 2% to sex-linked genes. As has already been stated, only those patients whose abnormalities include bony malformations can currently be fully diagnosed with certainty, because only these will be amenable to diagnosis by radiologic imaging.

The causes of inner ear malformation stem from defects in development. Most occur in the first trimester of pregnancy during formation of the membranous labyrinth. This may occur as a result of inborn genetic abnormalities or teratogenic influences. Inborn genetic defects can be autosomal dominant or recessive and may be of incomplete penetrance and variable expression. Just under 2% are X-linked (5).

A.K. Lalwani and R.K. Jackler: Department of Otolaryngology—Head and Neck Surgery, University of California, San Francisco, California 94143.
P.G. Reilly: York District Hospital, York YO 3 7HE, United Kingdom.

TABLE 1. *A classification of congenital malformations of the inner ear*

I. Malformations limited to the membranous labyrinth
   A. Complete membranous labyrinthine dysplasia
   B. Limited membranous labyrinthine dysplasia
      i. Cochleosaccular dysplasia (Scheibe)
      ii. Cochlear basal turn dysplasia (Alexander)
II. Malformations of the osseous and membranous labyrinths
   A. Complete labyrinthine aplasia (Michel)
   B. Cochlear anomalies
      i. Cochlear aplasia
      ii. Cochlear hypoplasia
      iii. Incomplete partition (Mondini)
      iv. Common cavity
   C. Labyrinthine anomalies
      i. Semicircular canal dysplasia
      ii. Semicircular canal aplasia
   D. Aqueductal anomalies
      i. Enlargement of the vestibular aqueduct
      ii. Enlargement of the cochlear aqueduct
   E. Abnormalities of the internal auditory canal
      i. Narrow internal auditory canal
      ii. Wide internal auditory canal

From Jackler RK, Luxford WM, House WF. Congenital malformations of the inner ear: a classification based on organogenesis. *Laryngoscope* 1987;97(Suppl 40):2.

There has been much interest in the genetics of hearing loss, especially because there are several useful animal models. Comparison of the available genetic maps of mouse and human indicate the presence of a number of conserved linkage groups where gene content and order are preserved (6). These conserved linkage groups allow identification of mouse homologous genes in mouse and humans, providing access to new mouse models of human genetic disease (7). They also allow the identification of genes mapped in humans that may be candidates for mouse mutations or, alternatively, the identification of gene sequences mapped in the mouse that may be candidates for human disease mutations. An example is the *splotch* (sp) mouse mutation, which has abnormalities in the Pax-3 gene (8). The human homologue of this is Waardenburg's syndrome type 1, which has a mutation in the PAX-3 gene located at chromosome 2q37.

Steel and Bock (9) have proposed a classification for inner ear abnormalities based on animals with hereditary inner ear defects. They describe three groups:

1. Morphogenetic abnormalities, involving gross structural deformities of the labyrinth
2. Neuroepithelial abnormalities, in which there appears to be a primary Organ of Corti defect and Reissner's membrane remains in its normal position
3. Cochleosaccular abnormalities, showing collapse of Reissner's membrane and restriction of vestibular abnormalities to the saccule.

Genetic abnormalities may result in isolated cochlear defects or defects of the whole labyrinth. In addition, there may be variable expression in each ear such that there may be a difference in severity of a defect between right and left ears or one ear may even be normal. Any may be associated with other abnormalities and recognizable as syndromes (10,11). During the period of inner ear organogenesis, several teratogenic influences may cause abnormalities. These include infection (e.g., cytomegalovirus, toxoplasmosis, and rubella), radiation exposure, and drugs (e.g., thalidomide) (12). During the third trimester of pregnancy, the inner ear is susceptible to other teratogenic influences, such as aminoglycoside antibiotics, which have been shown to cause hair cell damage (13).

MALFORMATIONS LIMITED TO THE MEMBRANOUS LABYRINTH

These defects account for about 90% of causes of congenital sensorineural deafness. The severity varies from dysplasia, affecting only part of the inner ear, to conditions affecting the whole cochlea, saccule, utricle, and semicircular canals.

Complete Membranous Labyrinthine Dysplasia (Bing Siebenmann)

This defect is rare. It was first reported by Siebenmann and Bing in 1907. It may be associated with cardiac abnormalities. It can be recognized in the Jervell and Lange-Nielson syndrome and in Usher's syndrome (14).

Limited Membranous Labyrinthine Dysplasia

Cochleosaccular Dysplasia (Scheibe)

This was first described by Scheibe in 1892. It represents the most common inner ear abnormality resulting in hearing impairment and occurs in the phylogenetically newer part of the inner ear. It is inherited as an autosomal recessive trait and is found in diseases such as Usher's syndrome. The gene for this defect has been located to chromosome 1q32. Histologic examination shows partial or complete aplasia of the organ of Corti and collapse of the cochlear duct; Reissner's membrane may be adherent to the limbus. The stria vascularis is degenerated, and there may be colloidal inclusions present within it. The stria vascularis may have areas of dysplasia together with areas of hyperplasia and gross deformity. There is a great deal of variation in the cochlear changes; aplasia may be severe in the basal turn but normal in the remainder of the cochlea or may be severe throughout. The wall of the saccule is normally collapsed and seen to be lying on an atrophic sensory epithelium and deformed otolithic membrane. The semicircular canals and utricle are usually normal (15,16). Cochleosaccular dysplasia can be found in several animal models and is often associated with white spotting of the hair (e.g., deaf white cat, Dalmatian dogs, and several mouse mutants). This white spotting may be due to mutations that affect migratory melanocytes, which have their origin in the neural crest. Melanocyte-like cells are present in the stria vascularis, and their function may be affected by similar mutations, although abnormalities of pigmentation per se are not necessarily associated with inner ear anomalies. If this were the case, albinism would be associated with hearing impairment, and this is clearly not so (8,9).

Cochlear Basal Turn Dysplasia (Alexander)

This abnormality was first described in 1904. The inner ear apart from the basal turn of the cochlea remains normal. This condition may be related to familial high-frequency sensorineural hearing loss. There is often sufficient low-frequency hearing to allow good benefit to be gained from amplification.

MALFORMATIONS OF BOTH MEMBRANOUS AND OSSEOUS LABYRINTHS

These types of abnormality have deformations of the otic capsule and so are amenable to radiologic imaging (Fig. 1). There is a wide spectrum of severity of hearing disability among these patients. Some are completely deaf, but most retain some hearing into adult life. However, it is common for there to be a slowly progressive hearing loss, and there are often sudden decrements in hearing that may be associated with minimal head trauma. It is presumed that there may be latent weaknesses in Reissner's membrane or in the osseous spiral lamina; defects here will allow mixture of endolymph and perilymph, thus altering endocochlear potentials and so adversely affecting hair cell function.

Radiologic examination of patients with observable inner ear abnormalities shows a wide variation in morphologic appearances (2,17,18)). The cochlea, semicircular canals, and vestibular apparatus may be affected either in combination or individually.

Examination of abnormal inner ears shows an appearance similar to that seen in the fetal inner ear. It can be assumed that most congenital inner ear abnormalities occur as a result of cessation of normal development. In general, the earlier arrest of development occurs, the more abnormal the inner ear and the more severe the hearing loss (Fig. 2).

Complete Labyrinthine Aplasia (Michel)

Michel described a case of this exceedingly rare defect in 1863, although it was first described by Saissy in 1819 (19). There is complete absence of inner ear structures and, therefore, total deafness. It is likely that there is developmental arrest very early in gestation before the formation of an otocyst. This defect has been seen to occur in association with thalidomide exposure and anencephaly (12,15).

Cochlear Abnormalities

Cochlear Aplasia

There is complete absence of the cochlea. There are only semicircular canals (which are usually deformed) and a vestibule present. No auditory function is possible.

Cochlear Hypoplasia

This results from an arrest in development about the sixth week of gestation. The cochlea is imperfectly formed and usually consists of only a small bud about 1 to 3 mm in diameter protruding from the vestibule (Fig. 3). There may be associated abnormalities of the remnant of the cochlea. Auditory function is variable and may be relatively good, considering the very small size of the cochlea.

Incomplete Partition

This defect, also known as the Mondini defect, occurs when arrest of development occurs at the seventh week of gestation. This is the most common type of cochlear malformation and accounts for over 50% of all cochlear deformities (2). Radiologic examination shows that the cochlea is smaller than normal (5–6 mm in vertical height instead of a normal height of 8–10 mm) and may be seen to possess fewer turns than normal, although it is difficult to determine the number of turns accurately, even on high-definition CT scanning. The interscalar septum is partially or completely absent (Fig. 4). The level of development of the organ of Corti is variable, and the neuronal population varies. The severity of hearing loss varies considerably from one patient to another, from normal hearing to profound deafness. Semicircular canal deformities may accompany the incomplete partition abnormality in about 20% of cases.

Common Cavity

In this anomaly, the cochlea and vestibule are confluent and form an ovoid space visible on CT scanning. Care must be taken to differentiate a common cavity defect from dysplasia of the lateral canal: A common cavity lies predominately anterior to the internal auditory meatus on axial CT scan, whereas a dysplastic lateral canal lies posterior to it. Histologic examination shows an ovoid cystic smooth-walled cavity that contains a primitive primordium of the membranous labyrinth. There may be recognizable segments of the organ of Corti. The neuronal population is normally sparse or absent. Hearing is usually poor.

LABYRINTHINE ABNORMALITIES

Semicircular Canal Dysplasia

Dysplasia of the lateral semicircular canal is a common malformation and is often associated with cochlear malfor-

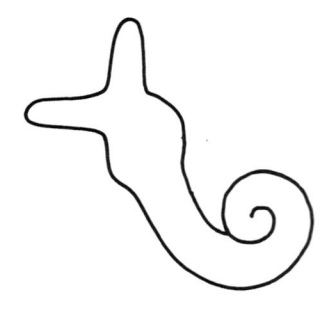

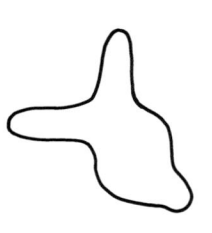

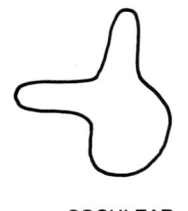

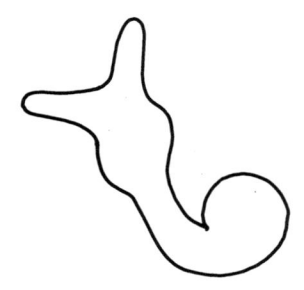

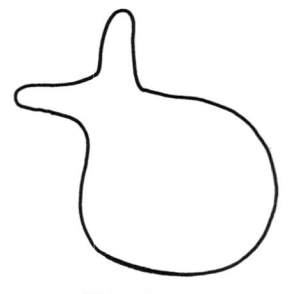

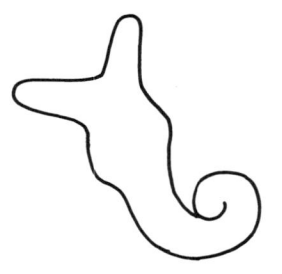

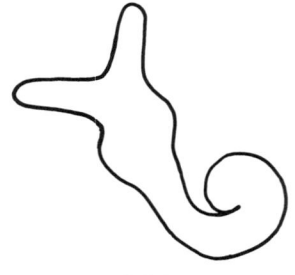

FIG. 1. Cochlear malformations. From Jackler RK, Luxford WM, House WF. Congenital malformations of the inner ear: a classification based on organogenesis. *Laryngoscope* 1987;97 (Suppl 40):2.

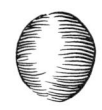

4th WEEK
COMMON CAVITY

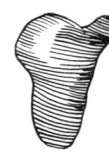

5th WEEK
COCHLEAR AGENESIS

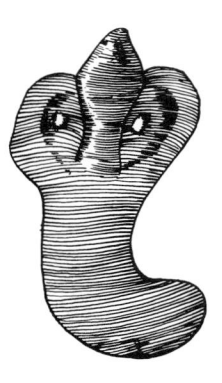

6th WEEK (early)
COCHLEAR HYPOPLASIA

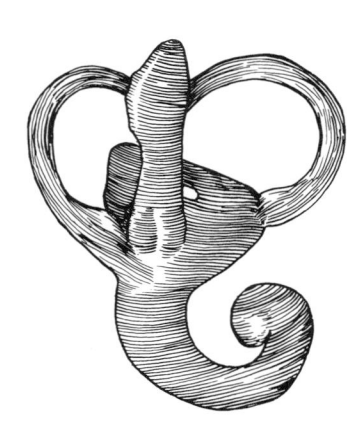

6th WEEK (late)
COCHLEAR HYPOPLASIA

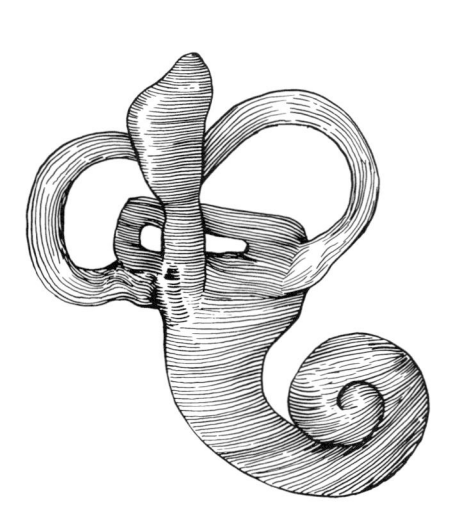

7th WEEK
INCOMPLETE PARTITION
(classical Mondini's)

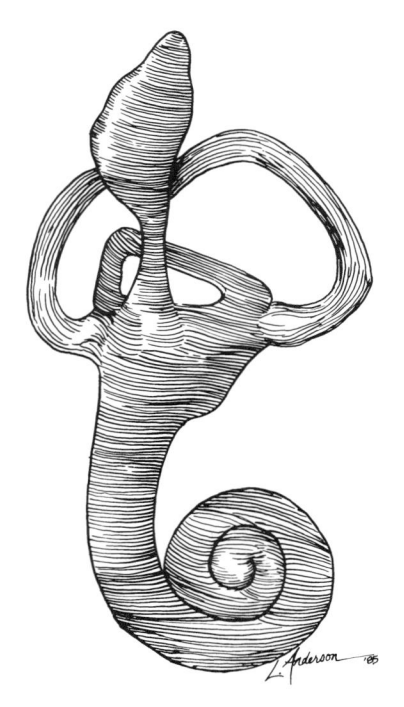

8th WEEK
NORMAL DEVELOPMENT

FIG. 2. Embryogenesis of cochlear malformations. From Jackler RK, Luxford WM, House WF. Congenital malformations of the inner ear: a classification based on organogenesis. *Laryngoscope* 1987; 97(Suppl 40):2.

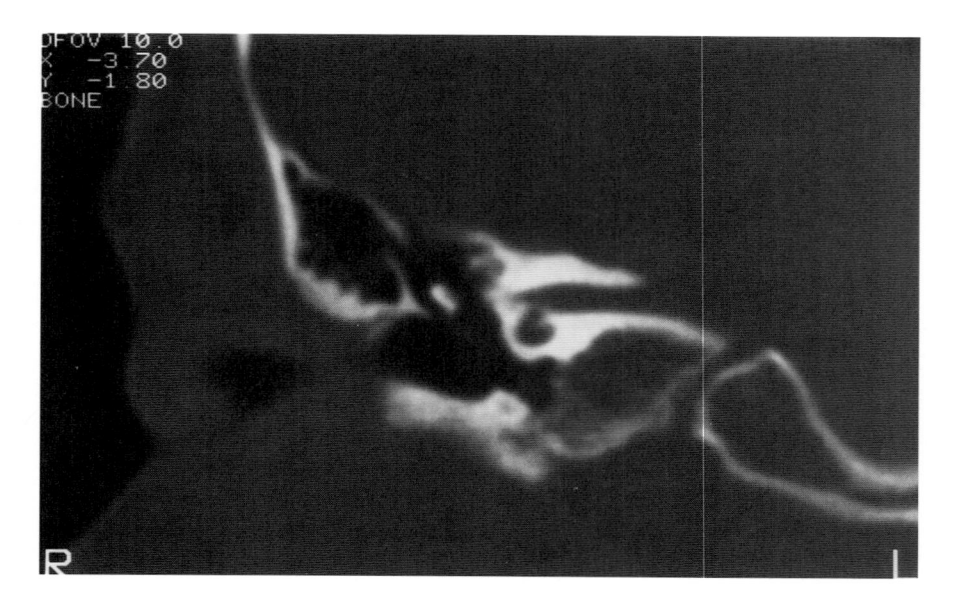

FIG. 3. Cochlear hypoplasia on coronal CT scan. The cochlea consists of only a small bud off of the vestibule. From Jackler RK. Congenital malformations of the inner ear. In: Cummings CW, Fredrickson JM, Harker LA, Krause CJ, Schuller DE, eds. Otolaryngology—Head and Neck Surgery. Vol. 4. *Ear and Cranial Base.* 2nd ed. St. Louis: Mosby Year Book; 1993:2761.

mation, although it also may occur as an isolated malformation (Fig. 5). The lateral semicircular canal is most commonly affected, probably because it develops at an earlier stage of gestation than the posterior or superior canals (Fig. 6). The typical appearance of lateral semicircular canal dysplasia is of a short, broad, cystic space that is continuous with the vestibule. If caloric responses are tested, there is usually evidence of reduced or absent function. If malformation is limited to the vestibular system, hearing may be normal.

Semicircular Canal Aplasia

This is much less common than semicircular canal dysplasia and is usually associated with cochlear abnormalities. It is presumed to arise as a consequence of failure in development of the vestibular anlage before the sixth week of gestation.

AQUEDUCTAL ABNORMALITIES

Enlargement of the Vestibular Aqueduct

The normal diameter of the vestibular aqueduct, when measured halfway between the common crus and its external aperture is between 0.4 and 1.0 mm. It is said to be enlarged when its diameter exceeds 2.0 mm (Fig. 7). Histologic examination of an enlarged vestibular aqueduct shows a lack of vascularity and rugosity, which is thought to be essential for normal function.

It has been shown that enlargement of the vestibular aqueduct is the most common radiographically detectable abnormality of the inner ear (20). High-definition CT scanning of

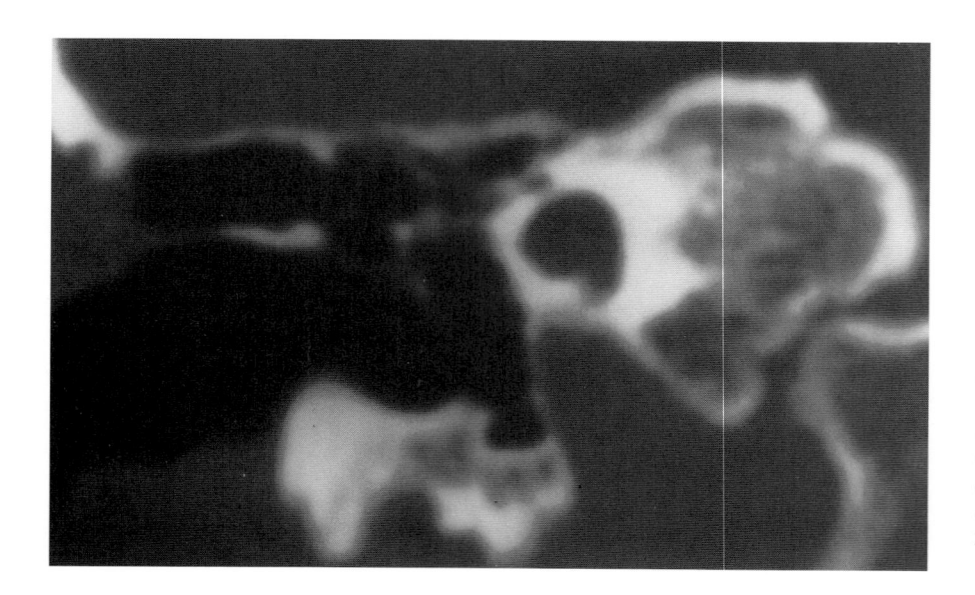

FIG. 4. Incomplete partition on coronal CT scan. Note the absence of an interscalar septum. From Jackler RK. Congenital malformations of the inner ear. In: Cummings CW, Fredrickson JM, Harker LA, Krause CJ, Schuller DE, eds. Otolaryngology—Head and Neck Surgery. Vol. 4. *Ear and cranial base.* 2nd ed. St. Louis: Mosby Year Book; 1993:2761.

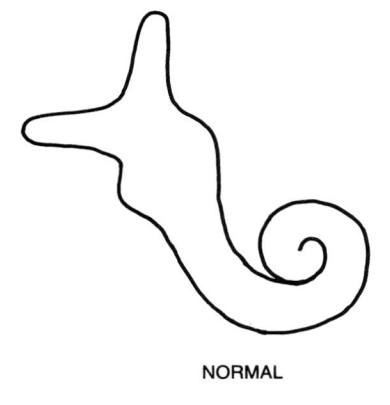

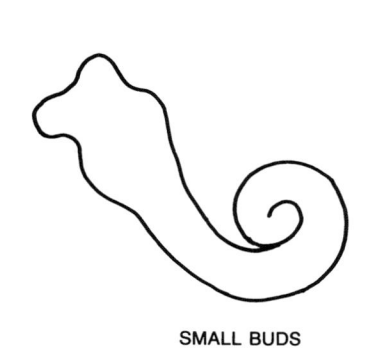

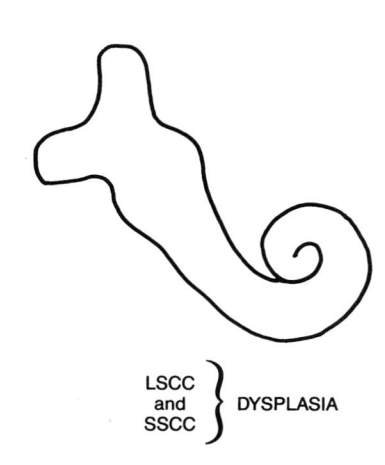

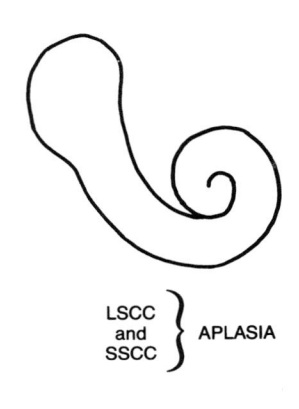

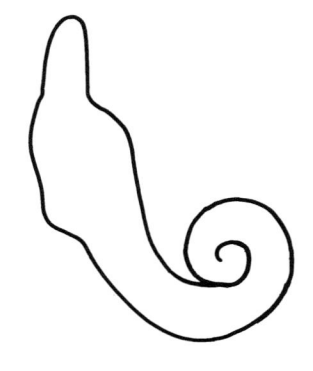

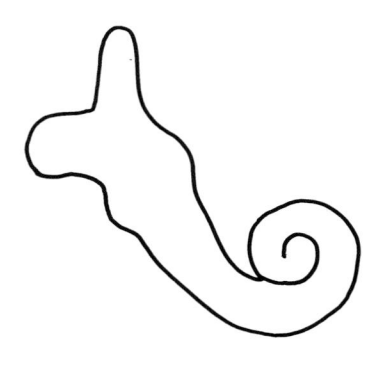

FIG. 5. Semicircular canal malformations. From Jackler RK, Luxford WM, House WF. Congenital malformations of the inner ear: a classification based on organogenesis. *Laryngoscope* 1987;97(Suppl 40):2.

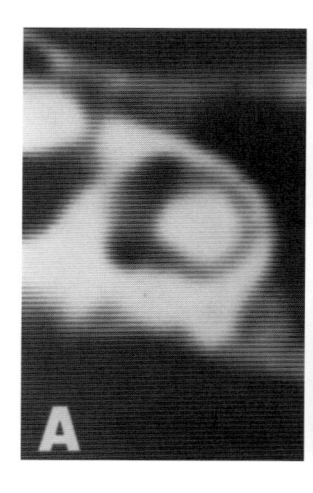

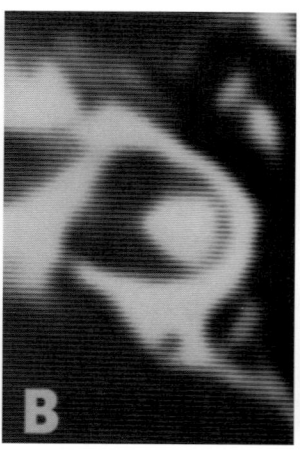

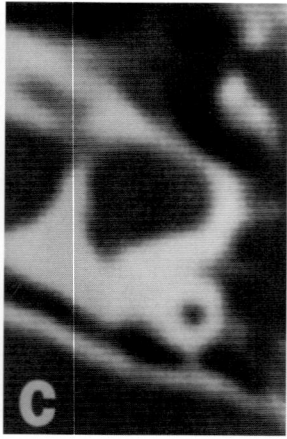

FIG. 6. Lateral semicircular canal dysplasia on axial CT scan. The normal appearance (**A**) should be contrasted with mild (**B**) and complete dysplasia (**C**). These images illustrate how semicircular canal dysplasia may arise from a failure of adhesion of the central region of the vestibular evagination during development. From Jackler RK, Luxford WM, House WF. Congenital malformations of the inner ear: a classification based on organogenesis. *Laryngoscope* 1987; 97(Suppl 40):2.

this anomaly shows a vestibular aqueduct that is shortened and broader than usual. This is in accordance with the appearance to be expected from a study of the embryologic development of the vestibular aqueduct that shows that it begins as a short wide pouch that elongates and narrows. Vestibular aqueduct abnormalities may accompany cochlear and semicircular canal abnormalities and are often seen in conjunction with the Mondini deformity.

Children born with the large vestibular aqueduct syndrome usually have normal or mildly impaired hearing, which gradually deteriorates during childhood and early adult life. At least 40% will develop profound sensorineural hearing loss. A case of large vestibular aqueduct syndrome associated with stapes fixation has been reported (21).

Enlargement of the Cochlear Aqueduct

In the past, there were several reports of enlargement of the cochlear aqueduct. However, most cases presented show a wide, medial, funnel-shaped opening into the posterior fossa, with no evidence of widening of the remainder of the aqueduct. Flow through a tube is dependent on the cross-sectional area of its narrowest part, and so a wide medial end is of no real consequence. Currently, there are no convincing reports of demonstrably wide cochlear aqueducts throughout the lateral and intermediate portions (22).

ABNORMALITIES OF THE INTERNAL AUDITORY MEATUS

The internal auditory meatus (IAM) is very rarely absent altogether, except after prenatal thalidomide exposure. Therefore, abnormalities are limited to widening or narrowing of the meatus.

Wide Internal Auditory Meatus

A wide IAM, up to 10 mm, is usually of no significance unless there is other evidence to suggest neurofibromatosis or unless there is an associated stapes fixation. In the latter case, stapes surgery may be associated with a "gusher," particularly if the IAM is widened at the lateral end. In cases of congenital fixation of the stapes, a CT scan showing the IAM should be obtained prior to consideration of surgery (21).

Narrow Internal Auditory Meatus

This defect may indicate absence of the eighth cranial nerve. Facial nerve function is usually normal, even in the

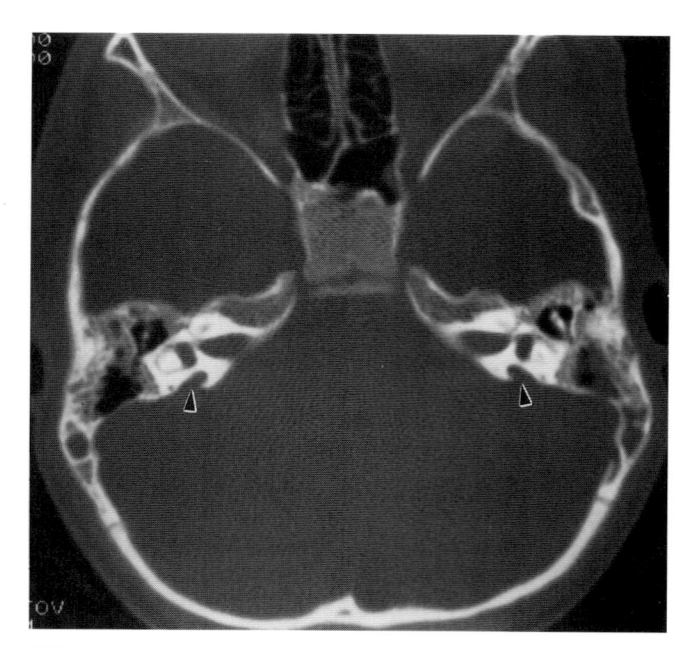

FIG. 7. Bilateral enlargements of the vestibular aqueducts (*arrows*) on axial CT scan. From Jackler RK. Congenital malformations of the inner ear. In: Cummings CW, Fredrickson JM, Harker LA, Krause CJ, Schuller DE, eds. Otolaryngology—Head and Neck Surgery. Vol. 4. *Ear and cranial base*. 2nd ed. St. Louis: Mosby Year Book; 1993:2764.

absence of an IAM of normal diameter. Narrowing of the IAM can occur in fibrous dysplasia affecting the skull.

EVALUATION OF CONGENITAL ANOMALIES

High-resolution CT scanning of the temporal bones is recommended in the investigation of a child suspected of having congenital malformation of the inner ear. Axial views with 1-mm cuts with 0.5-mm overlap are recommended to obtain sufficient detail of the relevant structures (23). T2-weighted magnetic resonance imaging scans are superior to CT in evaluating cochlear patency and should be obtained if cochlear implantation is being considered. A new technique using constructive interference in steady-state 3DFT MR imaging has been able to give fast and detailed imaging of inner ear structures and may be able to allow three-dimensional membranous labyrinth reconstructions. Also, narrowing and obliteration of the endolymph spaces can be detected with this technique (1).

MANAGEMENT OF THE DYSPLASTIC INNER EAR

The goals of management of the patient with congenital malformations of the inner ear are similar to those in other types of sensorineural hearing loss; to arrest further loss of function and to provide rehabilitation to limit the disability with appropriate amplification and ancillary services. Unfortunately there is little that can be done to alter the progression of sensorineural hearing loss that is due to congenital malformation. Short courses of high-dose steroids may be given in an attempt to limit sudden decrements in hearing thresholds, but there is little evidence to support the efficacy of this. It is wise to discourage contact sports and activities such as scuba diving and parachuting, which may lead to barometric trauma.

It has been suggested that endolymphatic sac surgery is useful in preventing further deterioration of hearing thresholds in patients with Mondini s dysplasia (24). However, Jackler et al. (25), after evaluation of a series of 40 patients, concluded that endolymphatic sac surgery for the purposes of hearing stabilization in patients with congenital anomalies of the inner ear was ineffective and even led to further immediate deterioration in the hearing in 30%.

Congenitally malformed inner ears may be associated with CSF leakage (26), and thus development of meningitis is a very real possibility. Parents of children with inner ear anomalies should be instructed in the early symptoms and signs of meningitis, so that should they occur, they can seek immediate consultation and appropriate investigation if necessary. Consideration also should be given to immunization against common organisms implicated in meningitis.

The possibility of presence of a perilymph fistula should be considered in children with malformed inner ears when there is a sudden deterioration in hearing following a definite event of head trauma or barometric trauma. Even in this relatively clear case, however, the results of surgical exploration directed at closing a fistula have been disappointing (27).

For auditory rehabilitation, hearing aids of appropriate amplification should be provided to allow maximum benefit to be obtained from residual hearing. Amplification should be implemented as soon as possible following diagnosis.

Patients who are not adequately rehabilitated with hearing aids should be considered for cochlear implantation. There are theoretical considerations that suggest that cochlear implants may not be as effective in this group of patients, compared with those who had a normal inner ear at birth. Cochlear implantation for auditory rehabilitation relies on the presence of the cochlear nerve population, even in the absence of hair cells. The normal human spiral ganglion cell count is between 25,000 and 30,000. In congenitally malformed ears, the cell counts are markedly reduced. Schmidt (28) studied eight congenitally dysplastic ears and found cell counts between 7,677 and 16,110 (average, 11,478). Ears that were deaf due to otosclerosis or ototoxicity or sudden hearing loss had counts between 18,000 and 22,000 (29). It can be seen that although congenitally dysplastic ears can be electrically stimulated, the results may not be expected to be as good in terms of speech discrimination compared with other forms of sensory deafness. However, the critical number of neurons necessary for successful cochlear implantation cannot be defined. Further, commercially manufactured, multichannel electrodes are designed to fit a cochlea of normal morphology: The dysplastic cochlea may not allow optimal electrode positioning and may allow stimulation of the facial nerve at current levels lower than the threshold for auditory perception.

In contrast to expectations, it is interesting to find that good results have been obtained in cochlear implantation in congenitally dysplastic ears. Miyamoto et al. (30) reported the case of a profoundly deaf boy with congenital deafness as a result of Mondini's dysplasia. Cochlear implantation allowed auditory stimulation at thresholds that were comparable to those of pediatric subjects deafened by other causes. Jackler, Luxford, and House (31) reported results of five ears in four patients with congenitally malformed inner ears who had had cochlear implants. They found that four out of five ears had an auditory response to stimulation by the implant at the same level as ears deafened by other disorders. However, one of these patients had an auditory response to stimulation that also caused facial stimulation; this precluded use of the implant. The one patient who failed to show an auditory response had a very narrow IAM on CT scan which suggested a rudimentary or absent audiovestibular nerve. Tucci et al. (32) reported results of six patients with cochlear malformations who underwent cochlear implantation. They found that it was possible to activate at least ten electrodes in the array and that all patients displayed improved performance after implantation.

The only absolute contraindications to cochlear implantation in congenitally dysplastic ears are complete cochlear aplasia or absence of the auditory nerve. Both of these conditions can be diagnosed with the aid of CT. The diameter of the internal auditory canal should be measured on CT. A diameter of less than 3 mm is a strong, adverse predictor of adequate neural population (33) and, therefore, would be a relatively strong contraindication for cochlear implantation.

REFERENCES

1. Casselman JW, Kuhweide R, Deimling M, Ampe W, Dehaene I, Meeus L. Constructive interference in steady state-3DFT MR imaging of the inner ear and cerebellopontine angle. *Am J Neuroradiol* 1993;14:47.
2. Jackler RK, Luxford WM, House WF. Congenital malformations of the inner ear: a classification based on organogenesis. *Laryngoscope* 1987;97(Suppl 40):2.
3. Haggard MP, Pullen CR. Staffing and structure for pediatric audiology services in hospital and community units. *Br J Audiol* 1989;23:99.
4. Brown KS. The genetics of childhood deafness. In: McConnel F, Ward PH, eds. *Deafness in childhood.* Nashville: Vanderbilt University Press; 1967:177.
5. Fraser GR. Sex-linked recessive congenital deafness and the excess of males in profound childhood deafness. *Ann Hum Genet* 1965;29:171.
6. Brown SD. Integrating maps of the mouse genome. *Curr Op Genet Dev* 1994;4:389.
7. Nadeau JH, Davisson MT, Doolittle DP, et al. Comparative map for mice and humans. *Mamm Genome* 1992;3:480.
8. Steel KP, Brown DM. Genes and deafness. *Top Genet* 1994;10:428.
9. Steel KP, Bock GR. Hereditary inner-ear abnormalities in animals. Relationships with human abnormalities. *Arch Otolaryngol* 1983;109:22.
10. Beighton P, Sellars S. *Genetics and otology* London: Churchill Livingstone, 1982.
11. Konigsmark BW, Gorlin RJ. *Genetic and metabolic deafness.* Philadelphia: WB Saunders; 1976.
12. Jorgensen MB, Kristensen HK. Thalidomide induced aplasia of the inner ear. *J Laryngol Otol* 1964;78:1095.
13. Raphael Y, Fein A, Nebel L. Transplacental kanamycin ototoxicity in the guinea pig. *Arch Otolaryngol* 1983;238:45.
14. Friedmann I, Fraser GR, Froggat P. Pathology of the inner ear in the cardio-auditory syndrome of Jervill and Lange-Nielsen. *J Laryngol* 1966;80:451.
15. Lindsay JR. Profound childhood deafness: inner ear pathology. *Ann Otol Rhinol Laryngol* 1973;83(Suppl 15):1.
16. Schuknecht HF. *Pathology of the ear.* Cambridge, MA: Harvard University Press; 1993:177.
17. Phelps PD, Lloyd GAS. Radiological investigation of congenital deafness. In: *Radiology of the ear.* Oxford: Blackwell Scientific; 1983:26.
18. Phelps PD. Mondini and pseudo-Mondini [Editorial]. *Clin Otolaryngol* 1990;15:99.
19. Phelps PD. Ear dysplasia after Mondini. *J Laryngol Otol* 1994;108:461.
20. Jackler RK, De La Cruz A. The large vestibular aqueduct syndrome. *Laryngoscope* 1989;99:1238.
21. Shirazi A, Fenton JE, Fagan PA. Large vestibular aqueduct syndrome and stapes fixation. *J Laryngol Otol* 1994;108:989.
22. Jackler RK, Hwang PH. Enlargement of the cochlear aqueduct: fact or fiction? *Otolaryngol Head Neck Surg* 1993;109:14.
23. Jackler RK, Dillon WP. Computed tomography and magnetic resonance imaging of the inner ear. *Otolaryngol Head Neck Surg* 1988;99:494.
24. Goin DW, Rasband RW, Mischke RE. Endolymphatic sac surgery in Mondini's dysplasia: a report of 16 cases. *Laryngoscope* 1984;94:343.
25. Jackler RK, Luxford WM, Brackmann DE, Monsell EM. Endolymphatic sac surgery in congenital malformations of the inner ear. *Laryngoscope* 1988;98:698.
26. Phelps PD. Congenital cerebrospinal fluid fistulae of the petrous temporal bone. *Clin Otolaryngol* 1986;11:79.
27. Pappas DG, Simpson LC, Godwin GH. Perilymphatic fistula in children with preexisting sensorineural hearing loss. *Laryngoscope* 1988;98:507.
28. Schmidt JM. Cochlear neuronal populations in developmental defects of the inner ear: implications for cochlear implantation. *Acta Otolaryngol* 1985;99:14.
29. Nadol JB, Young YS, Glynn RJ. Survival of spiral ganglion cells in profound sensorineural deafness: its implications for cochlear implantation. *Ann Otol Rhinol Laryngol* 1989;98:411.
30. Miyamoto RT, Robbins AM, Myres WA, Pope ML. Cochlear implantation in the Mondini inner ear malformation. *Am J Otol* 1986;7:258.
31. Jackler RK, Luxford WM, House WF. Congenital malformations of the inner ear: sound detection with cochlear implant in five ears of four children with congenital malformations of the cochlea. *Laryngoscope* 1987;97(Suppl 40):15.
32. Tucci DL, Telian SA, Zimmerman-Phillips S, Zwolan TA, Kileny PR. Cochlear implantation in patients with cochlear malformations. *Arch Otolaryngol Head Neck Surg* 1995;121:833.
33. Shelton C, Luxford WM, Tonokawa LL, Lo WW, House WF. The narrow internal auditory canal in children: a contraindication to cochlear implants. *Otolaryngol Head Neck Surg* 1989;100:227.

CHAPTER 14

Skull-Base Abnormalities

Todd T. Kingdom, Steven W. Cheung, and Anil K. Lalwani

CRANIOCERVICAL JUNCTION ABNORMALITIES

The first anatomical descriptions of craniocervical junction (CCJ) abnormalities were reported in the early part of the 19th century. Autopsy findings stimulated clinical interest, but confirmation of the diagnosis was lacking until postmortem examination. The 20th century brought rapid advances in neuroradiologic capabilities and refinements in microsurgical technique. Postmortem reports have been replaced by clinical and radiologic studies of abnormalities and correlated with intraoperative findings. Through these profound advances, the skull-base surgeon now has access to whole new vistas. The CCJ is one such area.

The CCJ encompasses the foramen magnum and the first two cervical vertebral levels. Elaborate osseoligamentous relationships provide critical mechanical stability to this region and allow for remarkably complex movements. Disturbance of these relationships, either surgically or as a consequence of disease, render the CCJ incompetent and lead to neurologic compromise. Abnormalities of the CCJ comprise a variety of congenital malformations, acquired deformities, and neoplastic processes that produce symptoms related to compression of nervous and vascular structures at the cervicomedullary junction. Compromise of the cervicomedullary junction results in a multiplicity of symptoms and signs that may present as brainstem and cervical myelopathy, cranial nerve and cervical root dysfunction, and alteration of blood supply to these structures (1). Pathology of the CCJ in the pediatric age group is more commonly congenital or developmental in origin; however, neoplastic diseases of the skull base must also be considered in a discussion of the histopathology of this region (2).

The neurotologist frequently plays an important role in the evaluation and management of patients with CCJ abnormalities. Tinnitus, vertigo, hearing loss, and cranial nerve deficits are commonly seen in this patient group. A number of surgical approaches have been developed to access the pathology of this region. A complete understanding of the anatomy and pathophysiology of disease processes involving the CCJ is critical for successful therapy. The pathophysiology of the CCJ syndromes include direct compression on neural tissue at the foramen magnum, traction injury to lower cranial and upper cervical nerves, and compression of blood flow to the cervicomedullary junction.

Congenital and Developmental Malformations

Congenital and developmental anomalies comprise the majority of CCJ malformations. Anomalies can be broadly grouped into neural or osseous malformations. Impingement on the neuroaxis can be anterior, posterior, or a combination of both. Consequently, there is variability in clinical presentation.

Chiari Malformations

The most common neural malformation of the CCJ are the Chiari malformations. These malformations constitute a group of posterior fossa congenital herniation syndromes. Four types of hindbrain malformation have been described. In type I, commonly seen in adults, there is downward herniation of the cerebellar tonsils through the foramen magnum. In type II, also known as the Arnold-Chiari malformation, the cerebellar vermis projects through the foramen magnum and the lower pons and medulla are caudally displaced (Fig. 1). A portion of the fourth ventricle extends into the spinal canal and is commonly associated with myelomeningocele and hydrocephalus. In type III, herniation of the

---

T.T. Kingdom: Department of Otolaryngology—Head and Neck Surgery, Emory University School or Medicine, Atlanta, Georgia 30322.

S.W. Cheung and A.K. Lalwani: Department of Otolaryngology—Head and Neck Surgery, University of California at San Francisco, San Francisco, California 94143.

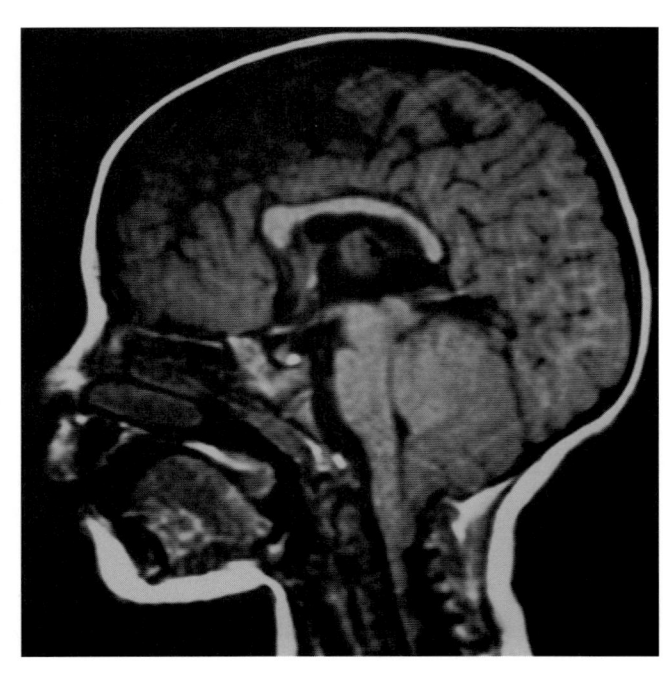

FIG. 1. Sagittal MRI of a Chiari II malformation in a 3-month-old child. The cerebellar vermis is projecting through the foramen magnum. A syrinx of the cervical spinal cord is also present.

cerebellum occurs through a wide rachischisis of the upper cervical spine and is accompanied by a meningocele. The most severe malformation, type IV, is sometimes considered a variant of the Dandy-Walker syndrome and represents cerebellar hypoplasia (3,4).

Types II, III, and IV usually present in childhood with florid symptoms due to the occurrence of associated spinal dysraphism. Type II is the most common malformation and usually manifests in the first few months of life. It is commonly associated with spina bifida, hydrocephalus, and myelomeningocele. Levy, Mason, and Hahn (5) analyzed 127 adult cases of Arnold-Chiari malformation and found the most common symptoms were headaches (65%), sensory changes (50%), ataxia (43%), and upper-extremity weakness (29%). Physical findings among this group revealed hyperreflexia (52%), nystagmus (47%), upper-extremity weakness (33%), and lower-cranial-nerve dysfunction (26%) to be most frequent. In 1984, Emery and Fearon (6) reviewed 71 children with vocal cord palsy, 8 (11%) of which were secondary to Arnold-Chiari malformation. The average age at diagnosis was 9.5 months and in none of the patients was laryngeal dysfunction the sole presenting symptom; all patients had associated myelomeningocele.

In contrast, type I malformations are more difficult to diagnose with the signs and symptoms often delayed until young adulthood. The majority of patients will present in their fourth to sixth decades with an average duration of symptoms of 9 years (4). Rydell and Pulec analyzed 130 cases of Chiari I malformation and found that 20% had auditory or vestibular symptoms (7). Progressive hearing loss, tinnitus, vertigo, and ataxia are the most frequent complaints in this population (4,7–9). The trigeminal nerve is the most commonly affected cranial nerve in patients with Chiari I malformation, though deficits involving cranial nerves VII through XII have been described (4,7,10,11). Dyste and Menezes (12) reviewed 50 patients with Chiari malformations (41 type I) who did not have associated myelomeningocele and found that 24% of patients presented with both ataxia and nystagmus. Interestingly, vertigo was present in only 8% and tinnitus in 2%. The most common symptoms were extremity weakness (60%), pain (54%), and parasthesias (34%).

Several theories have been developed to explain the etiology of the Chiari malformations. Most theories center on hemodynamic perturbations, which tend to inferiorly displace the contents of the posterior fossa. In 1959, Gardner presented his theory based on differential cerebrospinal fluid (CSF) production where production in the ventricles is greater than in the fourth ventricle, resulting in eventual herniation (13). Related theories focus on abnormalities in CSF resorption (14,15). Hemodynamic theories have also been used to explain the association of syringomyelia with the Chiari malformations (16). Despite the many theories proposed, the presence of associated developmental defects seen with the Chiari malformations argues for a defect in neural development as a possible unifying etiology.

Most cases of Chairi malformation are amenable to posterior fossa decompression by suboccipital craniectomy and C-1–C-2 laminectomy. In cases of anterior impingement or progression of symptoms after posterior approaches, transoral decompression may be beneficial (17). In their review of the literature (18 series, 648 patients), Levy, Mason, and Hahn found that 46% of cases improved, 32% were unchanged, and 28% progressed after surgical intervention (5). Operative 3mortality was 3%. Shunting of the syrinx, when present, was not clearly shown to impact on outcome.

Basilar Invagination

The terms basilar invagination, basilar impression, and platybasia are often used interchangeably. They are not synonymous and require definition. Basilar invagination is an upward migration of the vertebral column into the skull base with impingement of the upper spinal cord and lower brainstem. This condition is a congenital abnormality often associated with other systemic or developmental anomalies of the CCJ (1,18–21). In addition, there is an increased incidence of neural dysgenesis with basilar invagination. The most common neural anomalies are the Arnold-Chiari malformations or syringohydromyelia, which may have associated basilar invagination in 25 to 35% of cases (1).

Basilar impression refers to secondary or acquired forms of basilar invagination and is due to softening of bone at the skull base resulting in cervicomedullary compression. It is characterized by invagination at the skull base as a consequence of diseases such as Paget's disease, osteogenesis imperfecta, osteomalacia, rickets, hyperparathyroidism, Hurler syndrome, osteomyelitis, osteoporosis, neurofibromatosis, and rheumatoid arthritis(1,20,22–24). Platybasia refers only to an abnormal obtuse basal angle formed by the clivus and anterior skull base planes. This angle is of anthropologic significance only. There are no symptoms or signs that can be attributed to platybasia.

The radiologic diagnosis of basilar invagination-impression is based on pathologic alterations of the CCJ with use of x-rays, polytomography, computed tomography (CT), and magnetic resonance imaging (MRI). Multiple reference lines have been described to identify basilar invagination on the lateral radiographic projections (Fig. 2). Chamberlain's line is defined by a straight line drawn from the hard palate to the posterior lip of the foramen magnum. It is considered abnormal for the tip of the odontoid process to project more than 2.5 mm above this line (25). McRae's line, defined as the line drawn from the anterior to the posterior margins of the foramen magnum, should not be crossed by the odontoid tip in normal circumstances (26). Wackenheim's clival line is drawn along the posterior surface of the clivus on the lateral projection; the odontoid process normally lies anterior and inferior to this line (27).

Synostoses (Segmentation Abnormalities)

Failure of segmentation between the skull base and the first cervical vertebra or between the upper cervical vertebral bodies constitute a rare group of osseous anomalies which may produce cervicomedullary compression. The estimated incidence of segmentation abnormalities in the general population is 0.25% to 1%. Atlanto-occipital fusion has been referred to as assimilation or occipitalization of the atlas. The bony fusion can be partial and involve only the skull and the posterior arch of the atlas, the anterior arch of the atlas and clivus, or the lateral atlanto-occipital joints with absence of the articulating space. In the case of total assimilation, all three anomalies are present. Other reported anomalies associated with atlanto-occipital assimilation include absent or bifid atlantal arches, odontoid anomalies, accessory occipital vertebrae, and free lateral atlantal mass (20,28). Neurologic symptoms are absent in the majority of cases. McRae and Barnum reviewed 25 cases of atlanto-occipital fusion and found 18 patients had associated C-2–C-3 fusion with progressive atlantoaxial instability (29). In symptomatic cases, there is gradual posterior subluxation of the odontoid with progressive cervicomedullary compromise. Symptoms become evident in the third or fourth decade, often following minor trauma to the CCJ (1,20). Common complaints include suboccipital headache, stiff neck, and torticollis. Left untreated, ataxia, progressive spastic quadriparesis, and lower cranial neuropathies ensue.

Atlantoaxial fusions are rare and are typically associated with other cervical spine abnormalities, such as the Klippel-Feil syndrome. The incidence of Klippel-Feil syndrome is estimated to be 1 in 42,000 individuals. The classic triad of the syndrome includes a low posterior hairline, short neck, and limitation of neck movement (30). The complete triad is present in only 50% of patients. Multiple bone abnormalities such as atlanto-occipital fusion, atlantoaxial fusion, hemivertebra, spina bifida occulta, and scoliosis have been associated with the Klippel-Feil syndrome. The most common anomaly is fusion of one or two cervical interspaces with atlanto-occipital fusion.

Atlantoaxial Dislocation and Instability

Dislocation or instability of the atlantoaxial joint may be classified as either congenital or acquired. The stability of

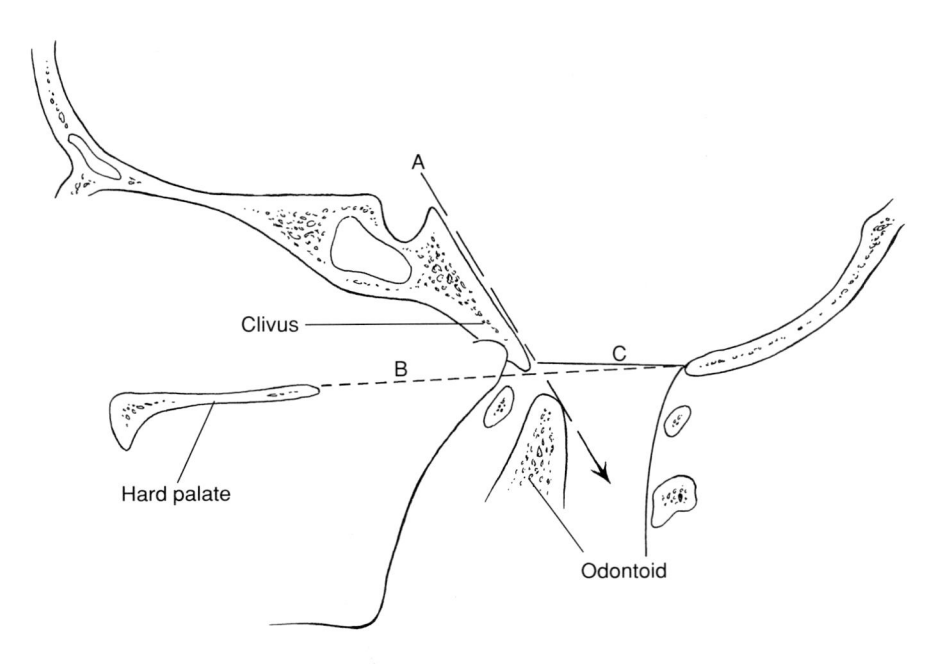

FIG. 2. Lateral craniometry of the craniocervical junction with points of reference. **A:** Wackenheim clivus canal line. **B:** Chamberlain line. **C:** McRae line. Adapted with permission from Van-Gilder et al. (1).

the first and second cervical vertebra depends on the integrity of the odontoid process, the anterior arch of the atlas, the transverse ligaments, the alar ligaments, and the accessory ligaments. If any of these relationships are abnormal, atlantoaxial instability (dislocation) may occur. Joint instability is documented by flexion-extension lateral cervical radiographs; 5 mm of motion or spacing between the odontoid process and the anterior arch of the atlas is strongly suggestive of instability (31). The normal atlanto-dens interval in adults is less than 3 mm and in children is believed to be less than 4 mm (32,33). Chronic instability and subluxation, regardless of etiology, may lead to formation of granulation tissue and ultimately compression of the cervicomedullary junction with progressive neurologic compromise.

Congenital atlantoaxial instability may arise from laxity of the transverse ligaments, abnormalities of the odontoid process, or atlanto-occipital fusion. Several conditions have been associated with atlantoaxial instability and include: Down syndrome, congenital scoliosis, osteogenesis imperfecta, type I neurofibromatosis, Morquio syndrome, Klippel-Feil syndrome, Hurler syndrome, achondroplasia, and odontoid dysplasias. Symptoms typically manifest in adulthood and are rare before the age of 20. Signs and symptoms in children with atlantoaxial instability are variable and may include generalized weakness, syncope, tetraplegia, torticollis, and dysesthesia (1,3,34).

Acquired forms of atlantoaxial instability or dislocation include traumatic etiologies, rheumatoid arthritis, and ankylosing spondylitis. Inflammatory conditions of the head and neck have also been associated with spontaneous atlantoaxial dislocation in children. Dally, in 1875, published an early case of nontraumatic atlantoaxial dislocation secondary to pharyngeal infection (35). Numerous related reports of atlantoaxial instability have since followed. Atlantoaxial instability has been associated with upper respiratory infection, mastoiditis, parotitis, pharyngotonsillitis, tuberculosis, and cervical adenitis (1). The clinical syndrome of torticollis due to dislocation of the atlas following an acute infectious process of the head and neck was redefined by Grisel in 1930 and DesFosses several years later (36,37). These authors proposed that dislocation was due to contraction of the occipital musculature following regional lymphadenitis secondary to a nasopharyngeal process. The current accepted theory is joint capsule distension and ligament laxity secondary to an inflammatory effusion. The lymphatic drainage of the CCJ is the upper cervical lymph-node chain, which also drains the nasopharynx. Thus, retrograde spread of an inflammatory process from a nasopharyngeal source is possible with secondary involvement of the atlantoaxial joint. This is perhaps the most common etiology for acquired atlantoaxial dislocation in children. The prognosis for recovery is excellent if treated early and adequately. Appropriately directed antibiotics combined with cervical immobilization is usually all that is required in uncomplicated cases.

Anomalies of the Odontoid Process

Three types of odontoid malformations have been described in the literature (38–40). Agenesis of the odontoid is an uncommon anomaly characterized by complete absence of the odontoid process. Hypoplasia of the odontoid is characterized by a shortened odontoid process with its superior extent typically at the level of the atlantoaxial articulation. The os odontoideum malformation, the most common anomaly of the odontoid, is characterized by a smooth-bordered, round ossicle of bone separated from the axis (Fig. 3). If the bone is located where the normal odontoid would be, it is said to be orthotopic; if the bone is located near the base of the occiput, it is referred to as dystopic. Possible etiologies for the os odontoideum malformation include congenital, traumatic, or vascular causes although the exact nature of the condition remains unclear.

All three conditions typically manifest as instability of the atlantoaxial junction with cervicomedullary compromise. In practical terms, distinguishing aplasia, hypoplasia, and os odontoideum is of limited value. The incidence of odontoid anomalies is uncertain and the presence of such an abnormality is often discovered on routine radiographic examination following head and neck trauma (40). Odontoid anomalies are particularly more common in individuals with Down syndrome, the Kippel-Feil syndrome, and certain skeletal and spondyloepiphyseal dysplasias. These patients live a precarious existence with the specter of minor trauma triggering symptoms, which may range from transient paresis to severe myelopathy. Most authors agree that surgical stabilization

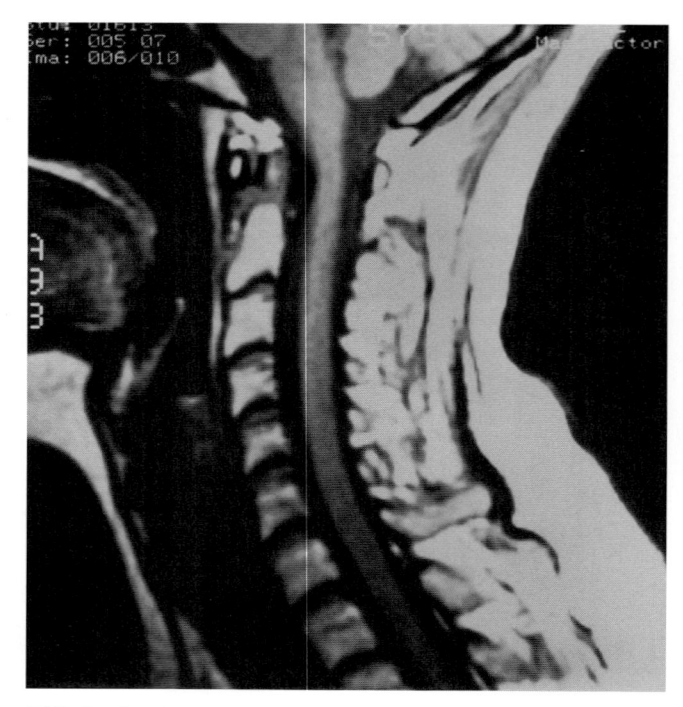

FIG. 3. Sagittal MRI demonstrating an os odontoideum malformation. The patient presented with atlantoaxial instability and cervical myelopathy.

procedures are required when radiographic evidence of instability exists or in the face of persistent signs and symptoms of cervicomedullary compression (1,3,34).

Down Syndrome

The child with Down syndrome deserves special attention because these children frequently require otolaryngologic procedures and are at increased risk for cervical spine injury. The incidence of radiographic atlantoaxial instability is significant, ranging from 15% to 20%; although the incidence of neurologic compromise as a result may be less than 1% (21,41,42). Pueshel et al. studied 236 children with Down syndrome and found 40 cases of atlantoaxial instability; 7 presented with neurologic deficits (43). Odontoid anomalies are common in the Down's patient and may approach an incidence of 35% (1) These underlying osseoligamentous abnormalities lead to CCJ instability. The natural history of the atlantoaxial instability in the Down syndrome child appears to be chronic and progressive instability with an ever present predisposition for neural compromise. Serial examinations are recommended (21). However, some prospective studies suggest that progression to symptomatic disease is uncommon (44). Nevertheless, the CCJ in children with Down syndrome is at risk for injury during procedures that require neck hyperextension, such as adenotonsillectomy, head rotation, or positioning for otologic procedures. Despite the paucity of data on the role of screening cervical spine x-rays for detecting atlantoaxial instability in the asymptomatic patient, many practitioners proceed with screening radiographic evaluation before elective otolaryngologic procedures (42,44).

Rheumatoid Arthritis

Rheumatoid arthritis of the cervical spine was reported by Garrod in 1890 and now is recognized to affect nearly 90% of adult patients (24). The incidence of cervical spine involvement in the pediatric population is less well defined. The most common abnormality seen in cervical rheumatoid arthritis is subluxation of the atlantoaxial joint. Atlantoaxial subluxation is initiated by loss of tensile strength and stretching of the transverse ligament due to destructive inflammatory changes from the rheumatoid disease and to secondary changes from the underlying vasculitis. The chronic inflammatory process leads to erosion of bone, growth of granulation tissue, and destruction of the synovial joints throughout the CCJ. These collective changes lead to instability and compression of the cervicomedullary junction. Skull-base changes can be visualized radiographically and include atlantoaxial subluxation, basilar impression (cranial settling), and rheumatoid granulation or inflammatory pannus. Symptomatic cervical rheumatoid arthritis has been described in children; however, it appears to be a rare occurrence (2).

Clinical Presentation

Pathology of CCJ is diverse in its clinical presentation. The clinical diagnosis of a CCJ lesion may be difficult to make for several reasons. No single symptom or neurologic finding is pathognomonic. A lesion below the medulla yet above the cervical plexus produces no cranial nerve or radicular findings to help localize the level of involvement. Patients with junction lesions often have a fluctuating course, mimicking multiple sclerosis or brainstem neoplasms. The symptoms usually begin insidiously, progress slowly, and may present an array of falsely localizing signs. An antecedent history of trauma may be a common triggering event (45)

Menezes and colleagues at the University of Iowa have reported an extensive experience evaluating and treating patients with CCJ disorders. Over 1,300 symptomatic patients with CCJ abnormalities have been evaluated by this group (46). VanGilder, Menezes, and Dolan (1) compiled the neurologic deficits seen in 219 patients with lesions of the CCJ based on the University of Iowa neurosurgical experience (Table 1). Myelopathy, seen in 202 of 219 patients, was the most common neurologic deficit. The severity of the myelopathy is variable and may present as different degrees of weakness in the upper and lower extremities. The most common symptom, suboccipital pain, was present in 181 of 219 patients. The pain is described as beginning in the suboccipital region and radiating to the vertex of the skull in the distribution of the greater occipital nerve.

The neurotologic manifestations of CCJ abnormalities have been recognized by several authors and perhaps are under appreciated in clinical practice. VanGilder, Menezes,

TABLE 1. *Neurologic deficits in 219 patients with craniocervical junction abnormalities*

Deficit	Number of patients
Motor myelopathy	
Quadriparesis	148
Paraparesis	40
Monoparesis	7
Hemiparesis	4
Triparesis	3
Brainstem dysfunction	
Nystagmus	35
Ataxia	19
Dysmetria	17
Apnea	13
Facial diplegia	4
Cranial nerve dysfunction	
Hearing loss	52
Dysphagia	31
Soft palate paralysis	27
Trapezius weakness	22
Tongue atrophy	3
Vascular symptoms	
Vertigo	37
Syncope	16

Adapted with permission from VanGilder et al. (1).

```
                    REDUCIBLE           IRREDUCIBLE
                       │                     │
                      ┌┴┐              ┌─────┴─────┐
                      │ │           VENTRAL      DORSAL
                      │ │              │           │
              Immobilization  Posterior  Transoral   Posterior
                              Fusion    Decompression Decompression
                                         ┌───┴───┐      │
                                      Stable  Unstable  Stable
                                                │
                                          Posterior Fusion
```

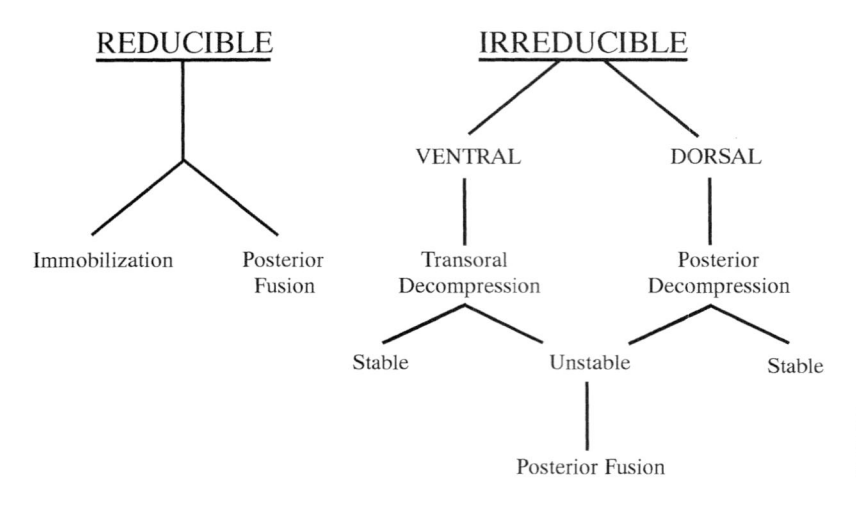

FIG. 4. Systematic approach to the management of craniocervical abnormalities. Adapted with permission from VanGilder et al. (1).

and Dolan (1) reported hearing loss in 24% of patients, thus documenting this as the most common cranial nerve deficit. Kumar et al. (47) discussed the role of neurotologic testing in this patient group and identified gaze nystagmus, vertical down-beating nystagmus, and vestibular decruitment as signs suggestive of a CCJ lesion. Other common electronystagmography abnormalities include impairment of smooth pursuit and fixation suppression (3). Elies and Plester (48) examined 180 patients with nonspecific dizziness and unilateral hearing loss and found 32 cases with CCJ malformations. Chiari malformations have associated audiovestibular findings in 20% of patients, and the Klippel-Feil syndrome has a 30% incidence of sensorineural hearing loss (3,4,7).

Management

The management of symptomatic CCJ abnormalities can be divided into patients with reducible pathology and patients with irreducible pathology (Fig. 4) (1). Radiographic studies are obtained to demonstrate not only the anatomical but also the pathophysiologic characteristics of the CCJ. Thus, the factors influencing specific treatment should be determined by plain x-rays, pleuridirectional tomography, thin-section high-resolution CT, and MRI in the axial, coronal, and sagittal planes. Flexion and extension dynamic views are obtained in the midsagittal plane. Cervical traction via an MRI-compatible halo can be used to determine the reducibility of the lesion (46). Although MRI has simplified the radiologic evaluation of the CCJ and has become the most commonly used modality, each technique has important features and may provide complementary information in the assessment of these patients (49–51).

When radiologic evaluation identifies a reducible lesion, initial realignment and immobilization is typically obtained by using as much as 15 pounds of skeletal traction in a halo vest. Patients with persistent instability require posterior stabilization by use of autogenous bone grafting, typically combined with rigid mechanical fixation (1,46,52).

Patients with irreducible lesions require surgical decompression of the cervicomedullary junction. An anterior approach, typically transoral, is utilized when compression is ventral and a posterior approach used when dorsal encroachment is present. The goals of operative management of CCJ anomalies should include: (a) decompression of the neural structures compromised by the soft tissue or bony abnormality, (b) stabilization of the joints subjected to abnormal movements that cause secondary compression of the neuroaxis, and (c) reestablishment of normal patterns of CSF circulation.

Historically, the surgical treatment of irreducible ventral pathology of the CCJ consisted of posterior decompression via posterior or posterolateral approaches. The morbidity and mortality associated with these routes for ventrally placed lesions were inordinately high in the setting of restricted surgical exposure (17). Subsequently, surgical approaches based on an understanding of the CCJ dynamics, site of compression on neural elements, and the stability of the CCJ have been developed and include anterior midline, anterolateral, and lateral approaches (Table 2) (45,53). de Oliveira, Rhoton, and Peace reviewed the surgical anatomy and surgical approaches to the CCJ based on cadaveric dissections (54). (The interested reader is referred to this exhaustive work for further detail into this topic.)

TABLE 2. *Surgical approaches to the craniocervical junction*

Anterior approaches
Transoral-transpharyngeal
Transsphenoethmoidal
Transoral-transmandibular
Subfrontal-transbasal
Anterolateral approaches
Transcervical-extrapharyngeal
Lateral
Infratemporal fossa
Extreme lateral
Posterior approaches
Suboccipital

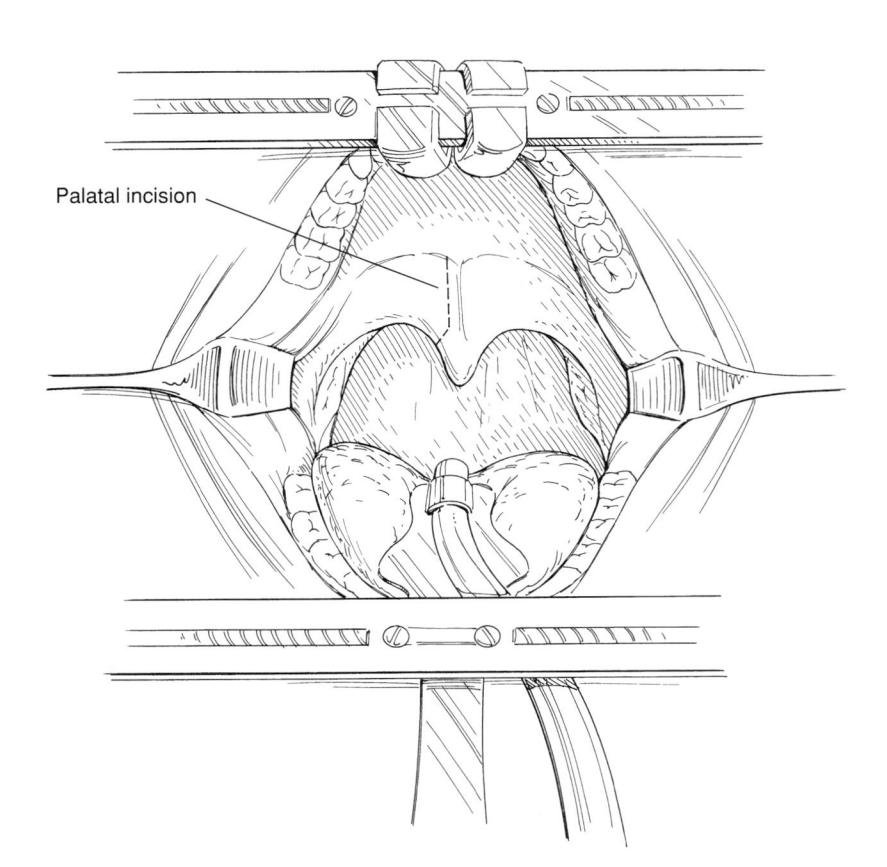

FIG. 5. Oral retractor in place for exposure of the oropharynx. Dashed line marks the incision used for splitting the soft palate.

The transoral-transpharyngeal approach is the most direct route to ventral pathology of the CCJ. The main indication for this approach is irreducible extradural ventral pathology compressing the cervicomedullary junction. This may be osseous, inflammatory, or neoplastic. With increasing utilization, the transoral-transpharyngeal approach has proved to be a reliable, technically sound method for gaining anterior extradural exposure to the CCJ (17,46,53,55,56). The operative highlights are outlined in Figs. 5 through 10. This technique allows for 1.5 to 2.0 cm of exposure lateral to the clivus midline and from the inferior clivus to C-3 in the vertical dimension (Fig. 11). Complications of this approach may include palatal or pharyngeal wound dehiscence, CSF leakage, tongue edema, meningitis, and velopharyngeal insufficiency (46). Menezes reviewed his experience with 76 children undergoing the transoral-transpharyngeal approach for irreducible ventral lesions of the CCJ and found this route to be safe, reliable, and technically simple (17,46). There were no reported deaths and the only morbidity was pharyngeal dehiscence in two patients.

The transsphenoethmoidal approach provides access to the sella turcica and upper clivus. Modifications of this approach allow exposure more laterally and inferiorly; however, lesions below the clivus are often accessible only when the transsphenoethmoidal approach is combined with other approaches (17,57). The anterolateral approaches provide improved access to ventral lesions via an extrapharyngeal route but place several neurovascular structures at risk with limited exposure of the clivus and craniocervical border (17,58,59). The lateral approaches are typically reserved for neoplasms extending lateral and posterior to the CCJ (60). The primary indication for the extreme lateral approach is anteriorly situated tumors that straddle the CCJ (61).

Postoperative craniocervical instability after surgical decompression is an important consideration. The occipitoatlantoaxial junction is a single functional unit stabilized by ligamentous attachments between the occiput and axis. Wide excision of these osseoligamentous components increases the risk of instability. The majority of patients undergoing transoral-transpharyngeal decompression require posterior stabilization. Menezes found that 158 of 188 (84%) required stabilization after transoral odontoidectomy and Di Lorenzo reported a similar experience with 22 of 25 (88%) requiring stabilization (17,52). Children have the potential to regenerate new bone if the transverse ligaments and the odontoid periosteum are not compromised during the transoral resection, thus possibly avoiding the need for posterior stabilization (62). Menezes reported 66 of 76 (89%) of children demonstrated instability after transoral ventral decompression (17).

OSTEODYSTROPHIES OF THE TEMPORAL BONE

Osteodystrophies of the posterolateral skull base affect upon the patency of neurovascular foramina that span across

218 / CHAPTER 14

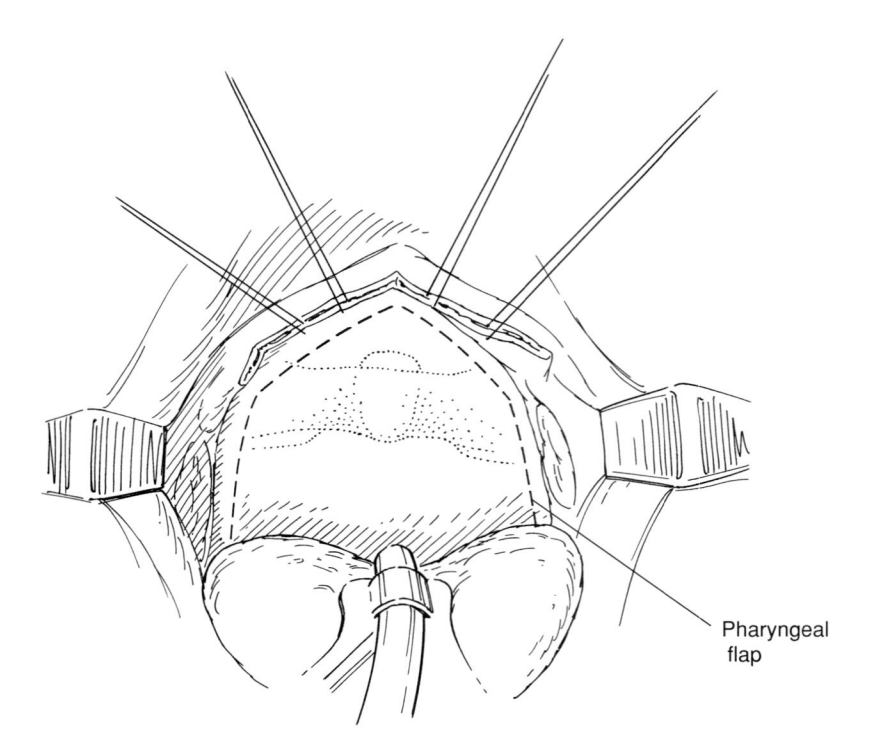

FIG. 6. With the soft palate split and retracted, exposure to the posterior pharyngeal wall is obtained. An inferiorly based U-shaped pharyngeal flap is outlined.

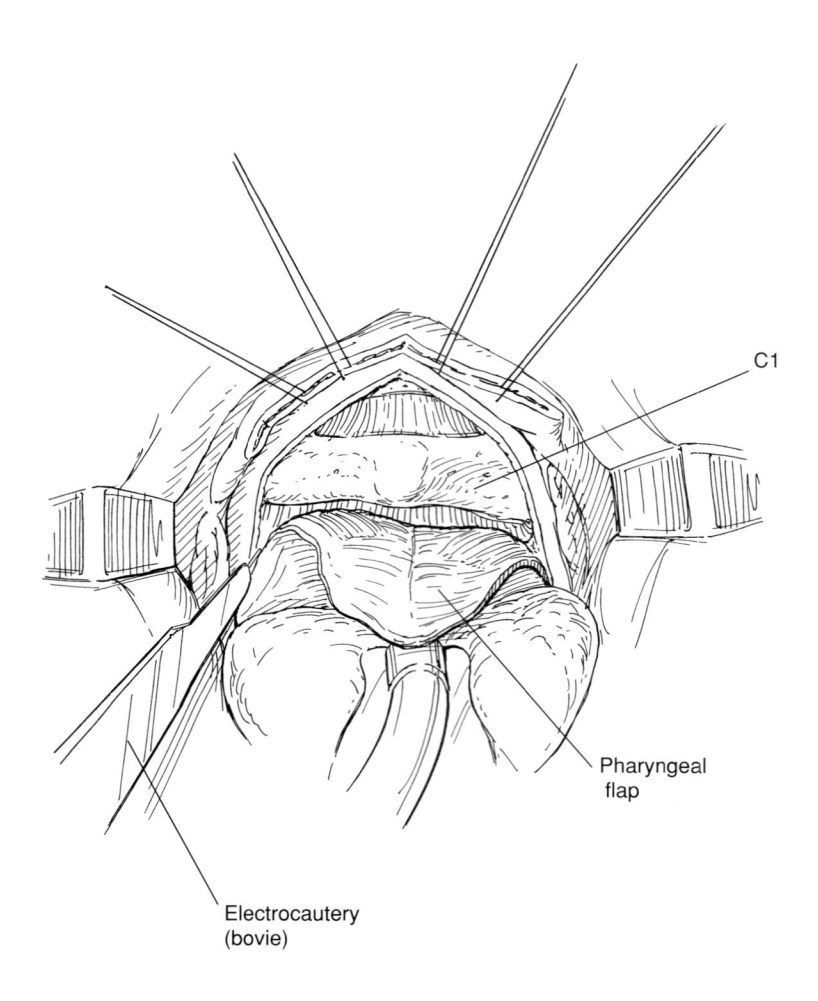

FIG. 7. Pharyngeal mucosa, pharyngeal constrictor musculature, and longus coli musculature are elevated as a single myomucosal flap.

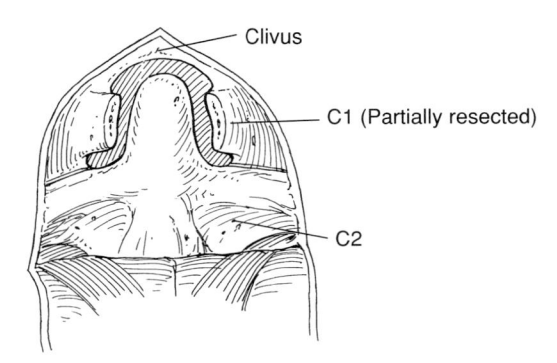

FIG. 8. The inferior clivus, arch of C-1, odontoid, and body of C-2 are in view. Removal of these structures, as indicated by the disease process, with a high-speed drill provides bony decompression and affords exposure to the cervicomedullary junction.

the cranial base, intratemporal canals and cavities, and biomechanical properties of the affected bone. In the pediatric population, fibrous dysplasia, the osteopetroses, and osteogenesis imperfecta are commonly encountered osteodystrophies.

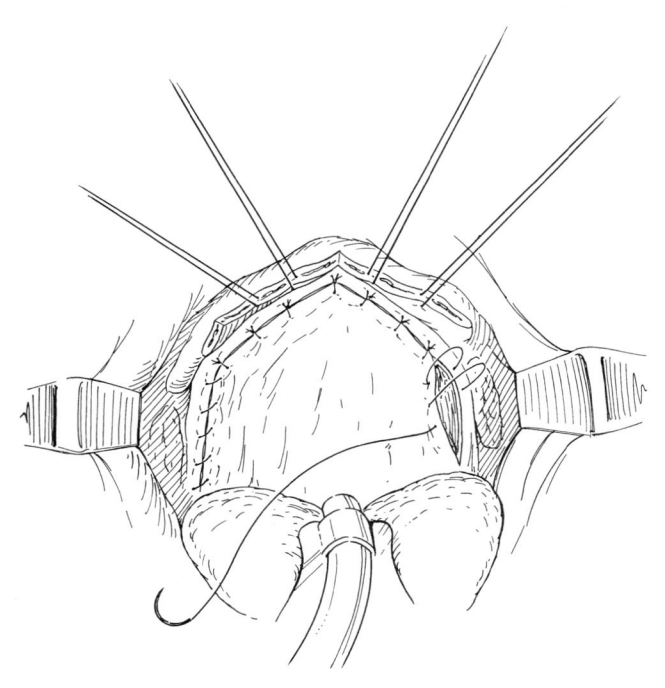

FIG. 10. Meticulous water-tight closure of the pharyngeal mucosa with absorbable suture material. The palate is approximated in three layers.

Fibrous Dysplasia

Fibrous dysplasia encompasses 7% of all benign bone tumors (63). It is a fibro-osseous disorder of unknown etiology that is driven by a proliferative medullary process that erodes surrounding cortical bone into a thin shell. The replaced bone

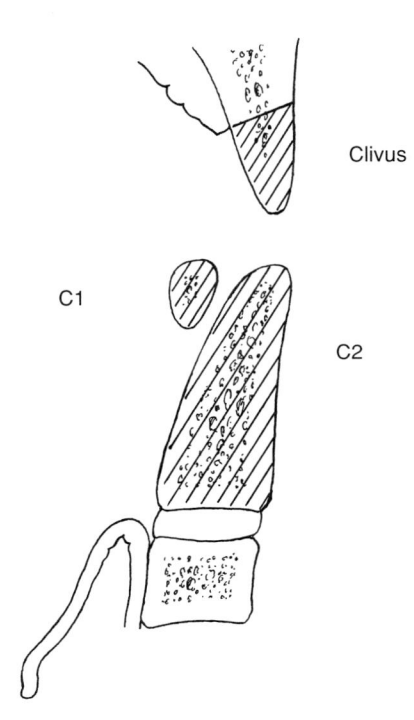

FIG. 9. Sagittal view identifying bony structures *(shaded areas)* which can be removed via this route.

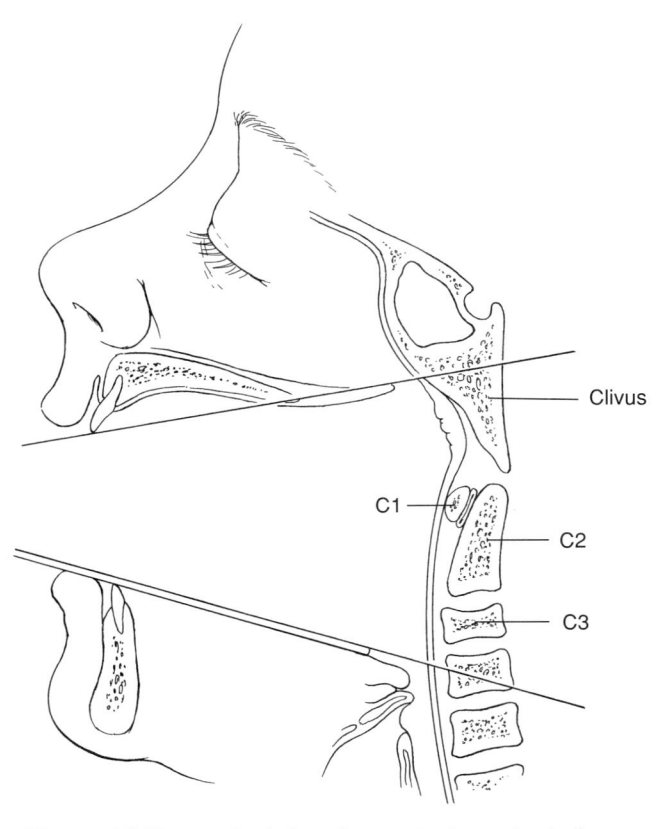

FIG. 11. Midline sagittal view demonstrating extent of exposure of the craniocervical junction using the transoral-transpharyngeal approach after splitting of the soft palate; inferior clivus to anterior body of C-3.

is weak and subject to fracture. In monostotic disease (70% of patients), there is a single bony lesion (64). In polyostotic disease (30% of patients), multiple sites are involved. Craniofacial involvement is relatively uncommon in monostotic fibrous dysplasia, but rises to 50% to 100% in the polyostotic variety (65). A special case that affects the pediatric population is the McCune-Albright syndrome (66,67). This disorder primarily affects girls and is characterized by polyostotic fibrous dysplasia, cutaneous hyperpigmentation, endocrinopathy, and, occasionally, precocious puberty.

The most common clinical manifestations of temporal bone fibrous dysplasia are stenosis of the external auditory canal and swelling of the postauricular region due to expansion of proliferative bone in the tympanic ring and mastoid cortex, respectively (68,69) (Fig. 12A). Not unlike congenital atresias of the external auditory meatus, a number of complications arising from entrapped cholesteatoma have been reported. Chronic infection, ossicular chain fixation and destruction, and fallopian canal erosion are problems reported with intratemporal entrapped squamous epithelium (68–73). Hearing loss is largely conductive and may affect 30% to 57% of patients with temporal bone fibrous dysplasia (68,69). Sensorineural hearing loss is rare, but may occur in cases of aggressive cholesteatoma eroding the otic capsule or, possibly, secondary to internal auditory canal stenosis. The facial nerve is at risk for injury by erosive cholesteatoma, undrained infection and fallopian canal stenosis (68,74).

On plain x-rays and CT, three patterns are seen with fibrous dysplasia. The "ground glass" pattern refers to homogeneous sclerosis associated with bony expansion (see Fig. 12B) (75,76). Another appearance is the pagetoid pattern, in which areas of radiolucency are admixed with regions of irregular sclerosis. In the cystic pattern, ovoid radiolucencies are surrounded by sclerotic borders.

Management of skull-base fibrous dysplasis should include clinical monitoring to assess for external auditory meatus stenosis, cranial neuropathy, and malignant transformation. Sarcomatous degeneration of fibrous dysplasia has been estimated to be 0.4% in monostotic and polyostotic disease and 4% in the McCune-Albright syndrome (77). Pain, swelling, and radiographic evidence of bony destruction are clinical signs of sarcomatous degeneration (68). When sarcomatous degeneration occurs, the prognosis is poor. Mean survival time is 3.4 years (78–80). Because of the concern of added risk for malignant transformation with radiotherapy, this modality of treatment for fibrous dysplasia should be avoided.

The vast majority of surgical procedures for treatment of temporal bone fibrous dysplasia is focused on the creation of an adequate external auditory canal. Radical resection of all fibrodysplastic bone is not necessary for this largely benign disease. Surgical recontouring procedures are commonly successful in short-term follow-up, but they are plagued by restenosis because the biology of the underlying fibrodysplastic process is uncontrolled. An elongated exter-

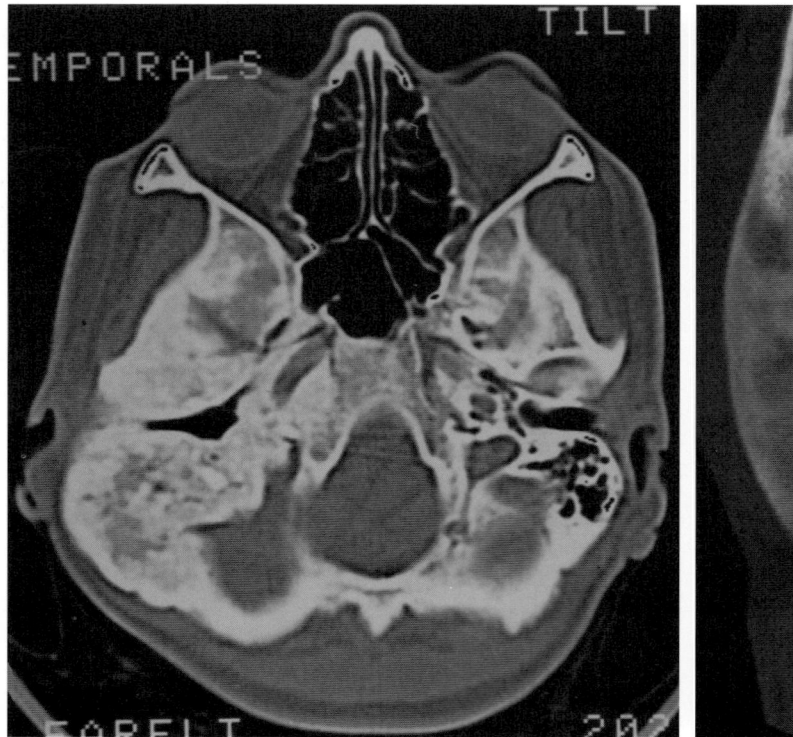

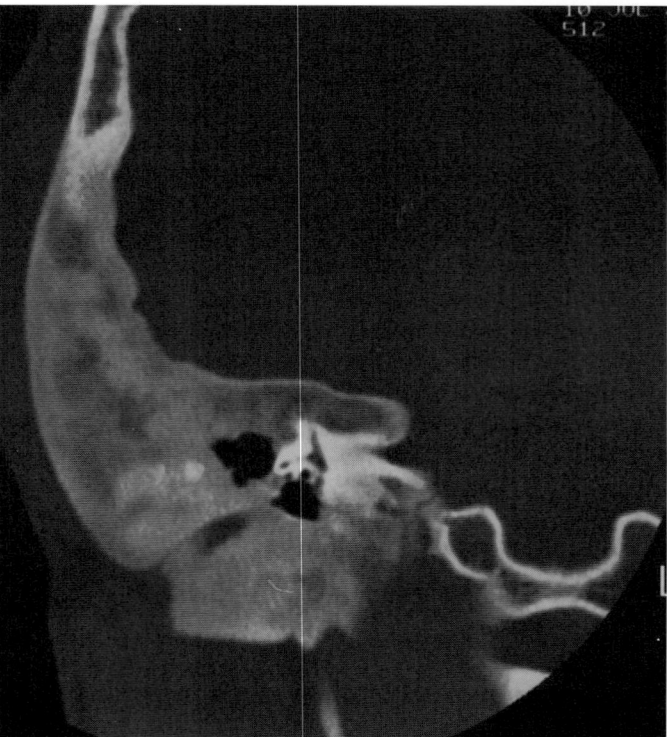

FIG. 12. Fibrous dysplasia. **A:** Axial CT scan shows extensive temporal bone involvement with narrowing of the external auditory canal. **B:** Coronal CT view demonstrating ground glass appearance.

nal auditory canal may be encountered at the time of surgery. Care should be taken to create a wide opening. Skin grafts and stents may be helpful to produce a sustained result (68,71,73,81).

Osteopetroses

The osteopetroses are a group of related metabolic bone disorders characterized by diffuse, dense sclerosis and faulty bone remodeling. A primary defect in osteoclast function has been postulated as an important contributing factor in its genesis (82–85). The osteopetrotic bone is immature, chalklike in appearance and brittle. Hence, the names *chalk disease* and *marble bone* disease have been affixed to this disease. Despite its thickened appearance, the immature bone is at risk for easy fracture because it is weak to certain dimensions of mechanical deformation. Clinically, the categorization of the osteopetroses into two types have been useful. In the congenita or lethal form, inheritance is autosomal recessive. These children succumb to hemorrhage, anemia, or overwhelming infection because medullary bony overgrowth results in obliteration of the marrow (86,87). In the tarda (adult) form, inheritance is mostly autosomal dominant but sometimes autosomal recessive. Also known as Albers-Schönberg disease, the adult benign form is often diagnosed on routine x-rays and has a variable clinical course.

Clinical presentation of the osteopetroses are manifestations of symptomatic neural canal and foramina stenosis, and middle-ear cleft encroachment by proliferative bone. In one series, Johnston et al (88) reviewed 50 reported cases and found optic atrophy (78%), hearing loss (22%) and facial palsy (10%) to be significant features. Temporal bone histologic studies support epitympanic crowding and ossicular chain infiltration by osteopetrotic bone as the bases of conductive hearing loss (89,90). Ophthalmic and facial nerve injury probably results from foraminal stenosis.

Plain x-ray and CT radiography of osteopetrosis will demonstrate diffuse chalky sclerosis and thickening of the cranial vault. With high-resolution temporal bone CT, stenosis of neural canals and foramina, encroachment of pneumatic spaces, and infiltration of the ossicles by osteopetrotic bone can be accurately evaluated.

Treatment of conductive hearing loss in osteopetrosis is largely the fitting of appropriate amplification devices. The dampened efficiency of the ossicular chain system is the result of bony fixation within the middle-ear cleft and mass loading of the ossicles by infiltrative osteopetrotic bone. The stapes has been reported to be malformed, and the footplate and round window obliterated by dysplastic bone. In view of the ongoing underlying process and possible technical pitfalls during ossiculoplasty, strong consideration should be given for primary amplification in the remediation of hearing loss encountered in osteopetrosis (91–95).

Facial-nerve dysfunction in osteopetrosis may be recurrent in nature. Partial recovery between events with worsening facial function after each episode is not uncommon. A number of reports support the role of transmastoid-subtemporal total facial nerve decompression (87,91,96,97). Surgical treatment appears beneficial in the treatment of facial-nerve dysfunction due to canal stenosis. When surgery is undertaken, it is important to ensure complete decompression of all possible skip segments of stenosis along the entire fallopian canal.

Osteogenesis Imperfecta

Osteogenesis imperfecta encompasses a group of connective tissue disorders that render variable defects in bone metabolism. Overall, there is a high rate of bone turnover, with the deposition of immature, osteopenic bone that is weak and fragile (98). Recurrent fractures are common in osteogenesis imperfecta. A classification scheme was introduced by Sillence, Senn, and Danks (99) on the basis of genetic and clinical criteria. Type I, autosomal dominant, is mild and manifested by blue sclerae and early hearing loss. The triad of fragile bones, blue sclerae and hearing loss was described by Van der Hoeve and de Kleyn in 1918. Type II, autosomal dominant or recessive, is uniformly lethal. Type III, autosomal recessive, is marked by progressive skeletal deformities with extreme fragility of bones and very short stature. Type IV, autosomal dominant, is intermediate between types I and III and exhibits skeletal fragility with moderately short stature (100).

By far, the most common clinical otologic problem associated with osteogenesis imperfecta is hearing loss. In a review of 201 patients with osteogenesis imperfecta, Pederson (101) found hearing loss in half the subjects. The nature of the hearing loss was mixed in 54%, conductive in 24%, sensorineural in 16%, and complete in 6% of patients. The onset of hearing loss was noted between the second and third decades of life in the majority of patients studied. Audiometrically, hearing loss in osteogenesis imperfecta may be indistinguishable from otosclerosis. Another problem associated with osteogenesis imperfecta is facial-nerve dysfunction. This is, however, an uncommon finding. The cause of facial dysfunction in osteogenesis imperfecta is attributed to exuberant dysplastic bone in and around the otic capsule, causing damage to the facial nerve in the labyrinthine and tympanic segments (102).

Osteogenesis imperfecta temporal bone CT findings may be indistinguishable from those found in otosclerosis (103–105). In both cases, an excrescent promontory mass may protrude from the oval window niche (106,107). Retrofenestral involvement manifests as a band of cochlear lucency around the cochlea; it is also known as the "double ring" sign. There may be extensive endochondral demineralization of the otic capsule in advanced cochlear otosclerosis. However, distinguishing imaging features of osteogenesis imperfecta are diffuse resorptive changes in large areas of the otic capsule and proliferative undermineralized bone that impinges on the fallopian canal (104).

The treatment of conductive hearing loss in osteogenesis imperfecta is the same as that for otosclerosis. A number of studies support the role stapedectomy in its management (108,109). Long- and short-term results appear favorable with stapes surgery. A precautionary note is warranted during exploratory tympanotomy for conductive hearing loss in osteogenesis imperfecta. The scutum may be brittle, incus susceptible to fracture, and footplate easily mobilized (110). Use of the laser for footplate manipulation and a noncrimping stapes prostheses may be advantageous in these cases.

Facial-nerve paralysis secondary to proliferative dysplastic encroachment of the fallopian canal can be managed with a cable graft to bypass areas infiltrated by disease. When there is facial weakness and imaging evidence of fallopian canal encroachment by disease, decompression may be indicated. No definitive study has been reported to address this issue specifically.

TEMPORAL BONE ENCEPHALOCELES

An encephalocele is the presence of cranial contents beyond the normal confines of the skull (112,113). The term broadly includes meningocele (herniation of meninges and cerebrospinal fluid), encephalomeningocele (herniation of brain and meninges) and hydroencephalomeningocele (herniation of cranial ventricles, brain, and meninges). The incidence of encephalocele has been estimated to be 1 in 3,000 to 10,000 live births. Cranial encephaloceles most commonly arise in the occiput due to a defect in membranous ossification. However, there are regional differences with regard to the dominant site of the encephalocele. Although the occipital encephaloceles account for 80% to 90% of all encephaloceles in the Western Hemisphere, occipital and frontobasal locations are equally common in the Eastern Hemisphere (including Southeast Asia and Africa). The cranial base is a distinctly uncommon location for encephaloceles. Only 5% of lesions occur at this site; in this category, the middle fossa is most common location (114).

Temporal bone encephaloceles are uncommon. Fewer than 150 cases have been reported in the past 40 years (115–121). They are characterized by herniation of meninges, brain tissue, or both into the cavities of the temporal bone (Fig. 13). Also known as an endaural encephalocele, the aberrant tissue usually arises from middle cranial fossa, rarely from the posterior cranial fossa (122,123). Iurato, Ettorre, and Selvini (118) in 1989 reviewed 139 cases of mastoid and middle-ear encephaloceles and found that 59% occurred as a complication of mastoid surgery; an additional 21% were spontaneous or idiopathic; 9% were a complication of chronic otitis media or chronic mastoiditis, and 9% followed trauma.

Pathogenesis

Spontaneous temporal bone encephaloceles can be divided into two categories: congenital or idiopathic. Knowledge of the embryology of the temporal bone is necessary to understand how a congenital encephalocele may arise. The squamous portion of the temporal bone arises from the membranous bone of the root of the zygomatic process and begins intramembranous ossification from one ossification center around the eighth week of fetal life. The tympanic part of the temporal bone is derived from membranous bone and ossification begins around the ninth to tenth week of fetal development; at birth, it is an incomplete ring that is open superiorly. The petrous portion of the temporal bone, first preformed in cartilage, begins ossification from front to back during the sixth month of fetal life at 14 separate ossification centers. The mastoid portion of the temporal bone arises from the dorsal aspect of the petrous bone and does not begin ossification until 25 to 30 weeks of gestation (124). Analogous to occipital encephaloceles, disturbance in the normal ossification of the temporal bones, especially the squamous and petrous portions, may lead to the formation of congenital encephaloceles.

Nontraumatic or spontaneous encephaloceles presenting late in life, without a history of surgery, trauma, or chronic ear infection, have been reported. Age at presentation ranges from 6 to 72 years with a mean age of 50 years and a 12 to 15 male to female ratio (115). Several theories regarding the etiology of spontaneous encephaloceles have been proposed and include bony defects of the floor of the middle fossa and the presence of temporal bone arachnoid granulations. The presence of multiple tegmental defects along the floor of the middle fossa has been reported by several authors. The incidence of such bone defects has been reported to range from 20% to 34% (115,125–128). Bilateral and multiple defects appear to be common.

Aberrant arachnoid granulations may a factor in the formation of encephaloceles and cerebrospinal fluid fistulae. Normally arachnoid granulations protrude into the lumen of venous structures and are involved in resorption of cerebrospinal fluid. The incidence of arachnoid granulations along the temporal floor has been estimated to be 22%; the incidence approaches 9% for the surface of the posterior fossa (129). When arachnoid granulations enlarge, adjacent bone is eroded and absorbed. Radiologically, these lesions appear as small, rounded defects in the bony middle or posterior fossa plate. Arachnoid granulations greater than 3 mm^2 appear to have a greater propensity to erode into the mastoid–air-cell system (130).

Mastoid surgery for chronic ear infection is the most common cause of temporal bone encephalocele. The prevalence has increased in recent times due to increased frequency of revision mastoid surgery (131). The pathogenesis of encephalocele formation following mastoid surgery is well described. Dural exposure due to tegmental dehiscence at the time of mastoid surgery is insufficient to cause brain herniation; the dura is able to support brain over large bony defects. Dural tear or incompetence at the site of bony defect is a prerequisite for herniation of intracranial tissue (132). Dedo and Sooy (133) noted that brain herniation may occur

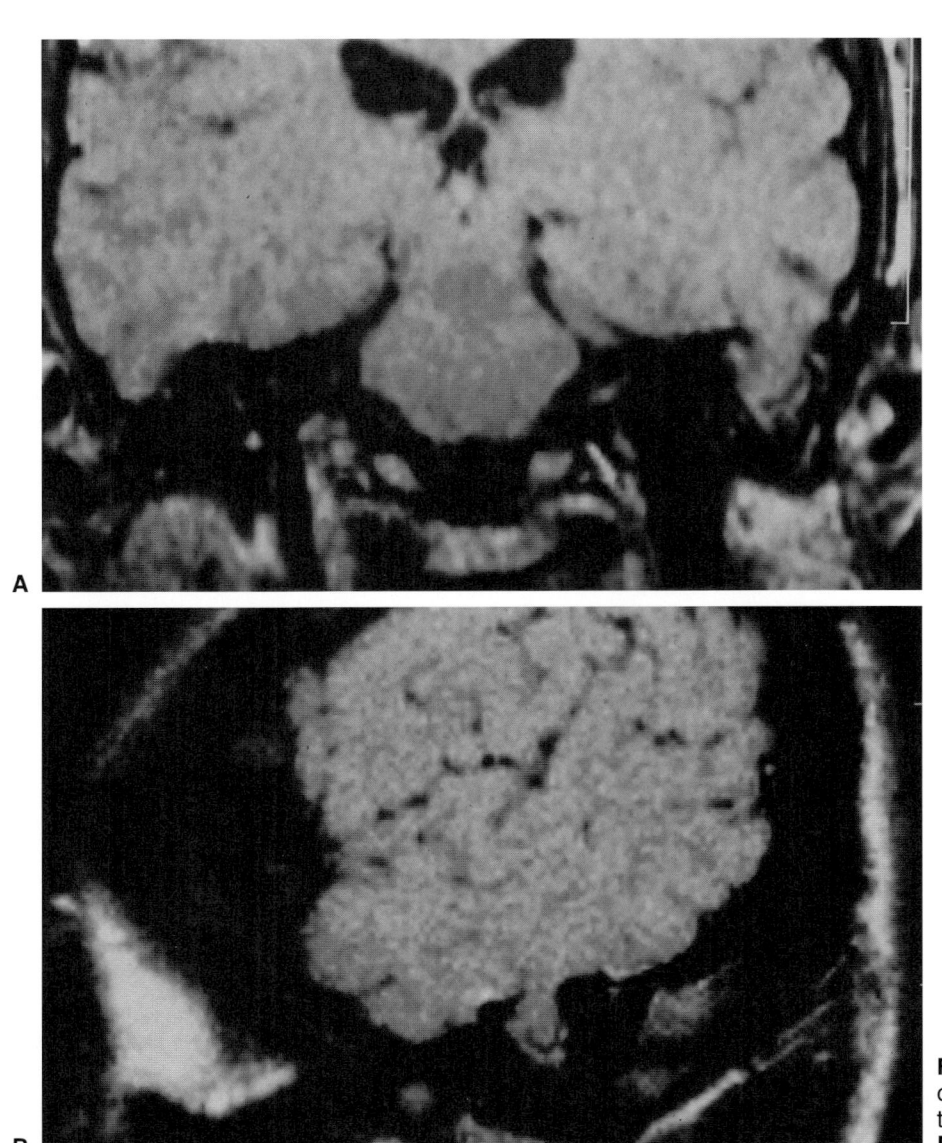

FIG. 13. Temporal bone encephalocele. **A:** Coronal MRI demonstrating soft tissue herniating into left mastoid cavity. **B:** Sagittal MRI view.

through a dural defect as small as 2 mm. The encephalocele may develop within weeks or after many years following surgery. Other etiologies include skull base trauma and cholesteatoma, although they appear to be less frequent.

Clinical Presentation

Clinical findings include intermittent or continuous CSF otorrhea or rhinorrhea, CSF masquerading as serous otitis media, conductive hearing loss, recurrent meningitis, headache, and, rarely, a mass behind the tympanic membrane (134,135). Some unusual findings include expressive aphasia, temporal lobe seizures, and facial-nerve weakness (136–138). History of ear surgery, chronic otitis media, cholesteatoma, and trauma should be elicited.

Serous-appearing middle-ear effusion on otoscopy or clear otorrhea following myringotomy is a common presenting clinical finding. Lesions of the temporal floor are usually associated with recurrent or transient CSF leaks. The CSF fistula opens with rise in the intracranial pressure and is intermittently closed by the weight of the overlying temporal lobe. Unlike the middle fossa floor, CSF drainage into the mastoid from posterior fossa plate defects are often continuous and profuse because they lack gravitational sealing of the fistula by intracranial contents. In patients presenting with suspected CSF otorrhea or rhinorrhea, evaluation of the fluid for glucose, protein, and chloride is useful in confirming the diagnosis of CSF leak. A glucose level 60% of the serum value, protein concentration of less than 200 mg/dl, and chloride greater than the serum concentration (normal serum value 99–107 mmol/L) is suggestive of CSF leak. A more contemporary technique for evaluation is the β_2-transferrin assay (139). β_2-transferrin, produced by the neuraminidase activity in the brain, is found only in CSF and can be detected in quantities as small as 1 μL. Therefore, definitive diagnosis of CSF otorhinorrhea can be made even in the presence of contaminating nasal mucous, saliva, or blood.

A bluish grey mass in the external auditory canal, mastoid cavity, or behind an intact tympanic membrane may be seen on otoscopic examination (135,140,141). The mass is soft to touch, pedunculated or sessile, and is characteristically pulsatile. The mass increases in size and is less pulsatile following maneuvers that raise intracranial pressure. Audiologic evaluation usually reveals a conductive hearing loss most likely caused by CSF in the middle ear or mass effect of herniated brain on the ossicles.

The abnormal communication between the tympanic cleft and the cranial cavity serves as a route for retrograde spread of infection from the ear, resulting in meningitis or brain abscess. Ferguson et al. (126) reported that 36% of the 33 patients in their series with tegmen or posterior fossa defects developed meningitis; it was the presenting symptom in 24% of their patients. Tension pneumocephalus is an unusual presentation of temporal bone encephalocele (142). Air enters the cranial cavity via the bony defect, dural defect, or both when the extracranial pressure exceeds the intracranial pressure and is unable to escape due to one-way valve effect of the herniating tissue. As a result, the patient may present with focal neurologic signs, seizures, and progressive neurologic deterioration. Isolated case reports of iatrogenic tension pneumocephalus following insufflation of air in the external auditory canal in patients with bony defects in the temporal bone have been reported (143,144).

Histologically, the herniated brain tissue has extensive gliosis, degenerative changes, and chronic inflammation. Macrophages are the predominant inflammatory cells. The surface of the encephalocele may be covered either with middle ear mucosa or modified glial cells (117,145).

Radiology

Plain x-rays and polytomography have been replaced by CT and MRI. High-resolution CT scans in the coronal and axial planes are needed to define defects. Although CT is ideally suited to study osseous anatomy of the temporal bone, it is limited in its ability to distinguish between a variety of soft tissue densities. CT with intrathecal administration of contrast agent may be useful to identify the location of a clinically suspicious CSF fistula.

MRI is far superior in delineating the nature of soft tissue and is required to differentiate herniated brain from fluid, cholesteatoma, cholesterol granuloma, and other lesions (146). In addition, the availability of images in multiple planes with MRI is of significant value in precise characterization of the anatomic defect. When CT suggests a tegmen defect, high-resolution MRI with 3-mm sections should be performed. MRI is ideal for determining the integrity of the overlying dura. Distortion of the gyri resulting from herniating temporal lobe into the temporal bone ("tear-drop" sign) on coronal CT or MRI strongly suggests an encephalocele (145).

Surgical Treatment

The temporal bone encephalocele can be repaired via a transmastoid approach, middle fossa craniotomy, or by a combined transmastoid-middle fossa procedure. The transmastoid approach is ideal for small lesions involving the tegmen tympani, tegmen mastoideum, or posterior fossa defects (122,131,133,140,147–149). In the transmastoid approach, the herniated glial tissue is amputated with bipolar cautery and the tegmen defect is repaired with bone or composite cartilage-perichondrium graft. The mastoid cavity is obliterated with temporalis muscle or the Palva flap to reinforce the closure. The transmastoid approach allows visualization of the middle and posterior fossa plates as well as direct access to the middle ear. Depending on the status of the patient's hearing, lesions of the petrous apex may be reached via the subcochlear or transcochlear approach.

The middle fossa approach is ideal for larger encephaloceles without ossicular involvement, allowing excellent exposure of the temporal floor. In patients with serviceable hearing, the middle fossa approach is also preferred for anteromedial defects, to reach the petrous apex. The repair of the dural defect can be performed extradurally, intradurally, or both. Dura should be reconstituted with a thick connective-tissue graft, such as temporalis fascia, pericranium, and fascia lata. The osseous defect is best repaired with a bone or cartilage graft. The bone graft may be obtained by harvesting the inner table of the middle fossa craniotomy bone flap. The superior portion of the temporalis muscle should be rotated to provide vascular covering for this free bone graft and to provide an additional tissue layer between the cranium and the mastoid cavity. Thus, there is a three-layer repair of the tegmen defect with a free temporalis fascia graft placed intradurally, the inner table of the middle fossa craniotomy bone flap placed extradurally along the middle fossa floor, and an inferiorly based temporalis muscle flap placed between the dura and the bone graft. This technique is uniformly effective in the treatment of temporal bone encephalocele. The disadvantages of the middle fossa approach are directly related to the craniotomy and the temporal lobe retraction. Vascular injury can result in venous infarction of the temporal lobe.

For large encephaloceles that impinge on the ossicles, the combined transmastoid-middle fossa approach is indicated to address the conductive mechanism of the middle ear (132,141,150–153). The transmastoid component provides the additional exposure needed to permit atraumatic dissection of the herniated brain tissue from the ossicular chain (145). The combined transmastoid-middle fossa approach provides excellent exposure from above and below, is highly reliable, and is associated with low risk of recurrence. It is the method of choice of many surgeons for repair of temporal bone encephalocele.

TUMORS OF THE PEDIATRIC SKULL BASE

Tumors of the skull base are rare in the pediatric population. In most instances, however, many of the standard innovative skull-base approaches for extirpation can be applied with few modifications (154). Radiologic imaging for diagnostic evaluation is similar to that used for adult patients. Multimodality techniques are the foundation for complete evaluation preoperatively.

Juvenile Nasopharyngeal Angiofibroma

Juvenile nasopharyngeal angiofibroma (JNA) is a rare, histologically benign, vascular tumor arising in the nasopharynx. This tumor affects adolescent boys almost exclusively, with a mean age of 17 years at presentation (155). It is locally aggressive, spreading along natural tissue planes and foramina of the skull base. JNA originates at the roof of the posterior-superior nasal vault or nasopharynx, specifically at the superior margin of the sphenopalatine foramen. Classic presentation includes recurrent epistaxis and nasal obstruction. Less commonly, patients complain of headache, otalgia, facial deformity, and middle-ear symptoms secondary to eustachian tube dysfunction.

The tumor begins its growth at the posterior-superior aspect of the nasal cavity and eventually fills the nasopharynx. Lateral extension occurs through the sphenopalatine foramen into the pterygopalatine fossa and subsequently into the infratemporal fossa. Superior extension via the foramina of the skull base may lead to intracranial involvement (156). These tumors are typically localized to the nasopharynx; however, intracranial invasion has been reported to be as high as 36% (157). A basic understanding of the unique growth characteristics of JNA has lead to the development of several classification schemes based on the anatomic location of the tumor at diagnosis (156,158–160).

High-resolution thin-section axial and coronal CT as well as multiplanar-gadopentatate dimeglumine (gadolinium-DTPA)-enhanced MRI scans are performed to demonstrate the bony and soft-tissue extension of the tumor and to delineate the anatomic location precisely. The MRI appearance of JNA is said to be pathognomonic and has obviated the need for biopsy in the majority of cases (161). Selective angiography can be performed by means of a digital subtraction technique, which provides excellent resolution, although is rarely necessary for diagnosis. Preoperative angiography for embolization of feeding vessels is helpful in minimizing blood loss during resection (156,161,162). The primary role of angiography is not for diagnosis but for preoperative embolization.

Surgical resection and radiation therapy are the treatments of choice for this tumor. Because of the potential long-term risks of radiation therapy for an adolescent, most otolaryngologists advocate surgical extirpation as the primary mode of treatment. Radiation therapy is typically reserved for residual disease, unresectable tumor, or evidence of inaccessible recurrent growth. However, some centers argue that radiotherapy should be used as primary treatment for all JNAs (163). Controversy still exists as how to best manage lesions with intracranial extension. Increased mortality, tumor recurrence, and operative complications have been associated with the management of JNAs with intracranial extension (164,165). Some have argued that patients with intracranial disease should be considered unresectable and treated with radiation therapy (155). Complete surgical excision via a combined neurosurgic-otolaryngologic approach, however, has been advocated by many authors as safe and effective in a single stage (157,162,166). It appears that both surgical resection and radiation therapy have definite roles in specific situations; curative rates of approximately 80% have been reported for both treatment modalities (157,167,168).

Craniopharyngioma

Craniopharyngiomas are benign congenital neoplasms that account for approximately 3% of all intracranial tumors and most likely arise from remnants of Rathke's pouch (154). Approximately 30% to 40% of craniopharyngiomas are found in patients younger than 15 years of age. It is the most common supratentorial intracranial tumor of childhood and the mean age at diagnosis is 8 years (169). Children with craniopharyngioma most commonly present with headaches, visual disturbances, and endocrine disorders. Although the radiologic findings of a cyst, calcification, and contrast enhancement on CT are practically diagnostic for craniopharyngioma, MRI has evolved to become the neuroimaging study of choice for preoperative and postoperative assessment because it provides superior tissue discrimination (170).

Controversy continues to surround the most appropriate management strategy for this neoplasm. Two general philosophies have evolved: subtotal resection with adjuvant radiotherapy and radical resection with gross total removal of disease. Advocates for subtotal resection combined with radiotherapy argue that this approach offers fewer tumor recurrences and less neurologic, endocrinologic, and psychological morbidity (171–173). However, other investigators feel advanced microsurgical technique and refinement of neuroimaging modalities in selected cases permits radical surgical resection with improved control rates and acceptable morbidity (169,174,175). Postoperative complications are common and include multiple endocrinopathies, visual disturbances, and cranial nerve deficits. Regardless of the approach chosen, recurrence rates range from 10% to 65% (157).

Meningioma

Meningiomas are rare in the pediatric population with an incidence of approximately 2 in 100,000. Although meningiomas comprise nearly 20% of all brain neoplasms, they constitute only 1% to 4% of all primary brain tumors in children and adolescents (176,177). One series demonstrated that 24% of children presenting with meningiomas have neurofibromatosis (178). The most commonly reported locations of meningiomas are parasagittal-falcine, sphenoid ridge-middle fossa, convexity, olfactory-suprasellar, optic canal-orbital, and posterior fossa (179). Meningiomas of the skull base appear to be more unusual in childhood. Doty et al. (177) found only three skull-base tumors in their review of 13 cases of pediatric meningioma. Perilongo et al. (179) reported 4 of 20 pediatric patients had skull-base involvement: one temporal bone, one orbital, and two optic nerve tumors. Surgical excision in symptomatic cases is preferred when tumors are deemed resectable. The role of radiation therapy in the treatment of childhood meningiomas is not well defined. In adults, radiotherapy is commonly used postoperatively after incomplete resection, recurrence of symptoms, and on the basis of histologic grade. Given the potential deleterious affects of radiotherapy on the developing brain, this modality is generally reserved as a treatment of last resort in children with inoperable or recurrent tumors not amenable to surgical resection (176,179). Chemotherapy has no proven role in the treatment of these tumors. Survival rates for children with meningiomas have historically been poorer than those for adults, primarily because in children there is a greater incidence of malignant change, tumors are larger, and there is a propensity for unusual locations (188).

Chordoma

Chordomas are rare neoplasms thought to arise from remnants of the primitive notochord. Chordomas are particularly rare in patients younger than 30 years of age. The peak incidence for these neoplasms is in the fourth to sixth decade of life. Approximately 50% of chordomas occur in the sacrococcygeal region, 35% occur at the base of skull (clival, spheno-occipital), and the remaining 15% can be found involving the cervical vertebrae (Fig. 14). Several studies have suggested a cranial or skull base predominance of chordoma in the pediatric population (180). Headache, cranial nerve dysfunction (especially abducens and hypoglossal nerve palsies), dysphagia, ataxia, nasal obstruction, and visual complaints are common signs and symptoms (180,181).

Chordomas are histologically benign, slow growing, locally invasive tumors. Their growth characteristic is one of relentless extension and recurrence. Gross total resection is the primary goal. In practice, surgical extirpation is often limited by restricted access and proximity of vital structures. This often leads to incomplete resection and a high rate of local recurrence. Historically, adjuvant radiotherapy has not significantly impacted on locoregional control due to the presumed radioresistance of the tumor. Recent experience, however, has supported the use of postoperative charge particle radiotherapy (proton beam) for chordomas (182). Five-year survival approaches 82% with this combined approach. Commonly used surgical approaches for clival chordomas include the transoral-transpharyngeal and transsphenoethoidal routes (56,57). These techniques may be combined with a lateral approach for more extensive disease, often in staged resections (60).

ACKNOWLEDGMENT

The figures appearing in this chapter demonstrating the transoral surgical technique were based on and adapted from

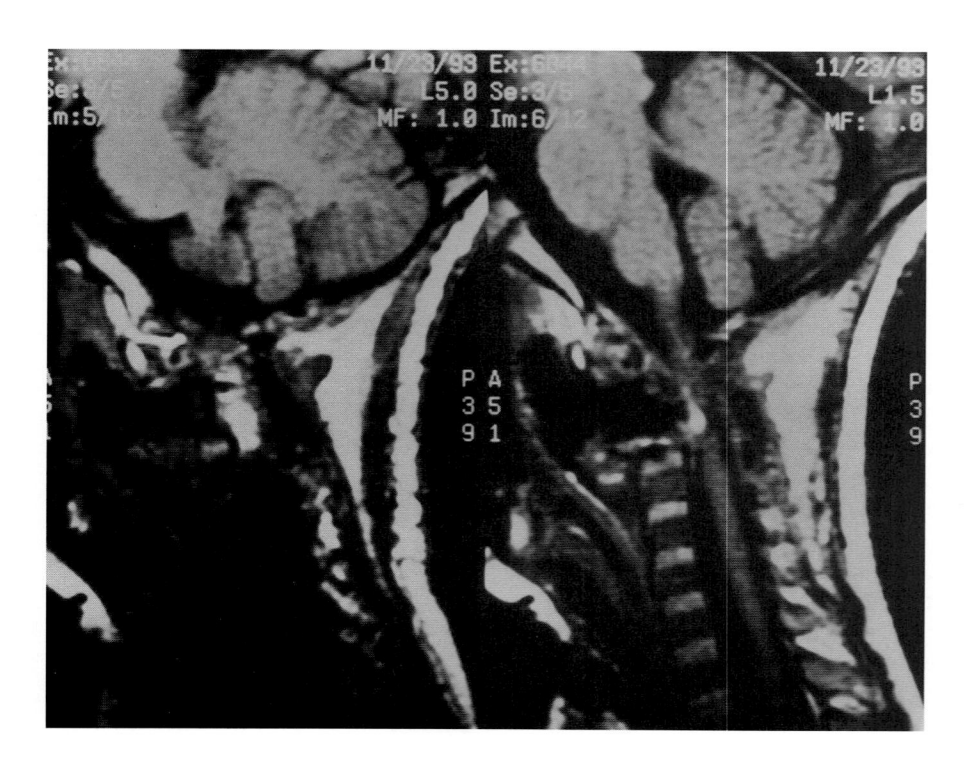

FIG. 14. Cervical chordoma. Sagittal T1-weighted MRI shows destructive lesion of C-1–C-2 in a 4-year-old patient presenting with quadriparesis. Successful resection and decompression was achieved via a transoral-transpharyngeal approach.

118. Iurato S, Ettorre GC, Selvini C. Brain herniation into the middle ear: two idiopathic cases treated by a combined intracranial-mastoid approach. *Laryngoscope* 1989;99:950.
119. Robson AK, Jones AJ, Slack RW. CSF otorrhoea secondary to a tegmen defect. *J Laryngol Otol* 1989;103:980.
120. Thompson JW. Transmastoid encephaloceles. A case report. *Int J Pediatr Otorhinolaryngol* 1988;15:179.
121. Williams DC. Encephalocele of the middle ear. *J Laryngol Otol* 1986;100:471.
122. Kamerer DB, Caparosa RJ. Temporal bone encephalocele—diagnosis and treatment. *Laryngoscope* 1982;92(8 Pt 1):878.
123. Ramanikanth TV, Smith MC, Ramamoorthy R, Ramalingam KK. Postauricular cerebellar encephalocoele secondary to chronic suppurative otitis media and mastoid surgery. *J Laryngol Otol* 1990;104(12):982.
124. Virapongse C, Shapiro R, Sarwar M, Bhimani S, Crelin ES. Computed tomography in the study of the development of the skull base: 1. Normal morphology. *J Comput Assist Tomo* 1985;9:85.
125. Ahern C, Thulen CA. Lethal intracraial complication following inflation of the external auditory canal in treatment of serous otitis media and due to defects in the petrous bone. *Acta Otolaryngol (Stockh)* 1965;60:407.
126. Ferguson BJ, Wilkins RH, Hudson W, Farmer J Jr. Spontaneous CSF otorrhea from tegmen and posterior fossa defects. *Laryngoscope* 1986;96:635.
127. Kapur TR, Bangash W. Tegmental and petromastoid defects in the temporal bone. *J Laryngol Otol* 1986;100:1129.
128. Lang DV. Macroscopic bony deficiency of the tegmen tympani in adult temporal bones. *J Laryngol Otol* 1983;97:685.
129. Gacek RR. Evaluation and management of temporal bone arachnoid granulations. *Arch Otolaryngol Head Neck Surg* 1992;118:327.
130. Gacek RR. Arachnoid granulation cerebrospinal otorrhea. *Ann Otol Rhinol Laryngol* 1990;99:854.
131. Neely JG, Kuhn JR. Diagnosis and treatment of iatrogenic cerebrospinal fluid leak and brain herniation during or following mastoidectomy. *Laryngoscope* 1985;95:1299.
132. Ramsden RT, Latif A, Lye RH, Dutton JE. Endaural cerebral hernia. *J Laryngol Otol* 1985;99:643.
133. Dedo HH, Sooy FA. Endaural brain hernia (encephalocele): diagnosis and treatment. *Laryngoscope* 1970;80:1090.
134. Jahrsdoerfer RA, Richtsmeier WJ, Cantrell RW. Spontaneous CSF otorrhea. *Arch Otolaryngol* 1981;107:257.
135. Lalwani AK, Jackler RJ. Endaural encephalocele. *Otolaryngol Head Neck Surg* 1992;106:309.
136. Hyson M, Andermann F, Olivier A, Melanson D. Occult encephaloceles and temporal lobe epilepsy: developmental and acquired lesions in the middle fossa. *Neurology* 1984;34:363.
137. Leblanc R, Tampieri D, Robitaille Y, Olivier A, Andermann F, Sherwin A. Developmental anterobasal temporal encephalocele and temporal lobe epilepsy. *J Neurosurg* 1991;74:933.
138. Uri N, Shupak A, Greenberg E, Kelner J. Congenital middle ear encephalocele initially seen with facial paresis. *Head Neck* 1991;13:62.
139. Oberascher G. A modern concept of cerebrospinal fluid diagnosis in oto- and rhinorrhea. *Rhinology* 1988;26:89.
140. Dedo HH, Sooy FA. Endaural encephalocele and cerebrospinal fluid otorrhea. *Ann Otol Rhinol Laryngol* 1970;79:168.
141. Feenstra L, Sanna M, Zini C, Gamoletti R, Delogu P. Surgical treatment of brain herniation into the middle ear and mastoid. *Am J Otol* 1985;6:311.
142. Cartwright MJ, Eisenberg MB. Tension pneumocephalus associated with rupture of a middle fossa encephalocele. *J Neurosurg* 1992;76:292.
143. Fairman HD, Brown NJ, Hallpike CS. Air embolism as a complication of inflation of the tympanum through the external auditory meatus. *Acta Otolaryngol* 1968;66:65.
144. Fisnes KA. Lethal intracranial complication following air insufflation with a pneumatic otoscope. *Acta Otolaryngol* 1973;75:436.
145. Lalwani AK, Jackler RK, Harsh GR IV, Butt FYS. Bilateral temporal bone encephaloceles following cranial irradiation. *J Neurosurg* 1993;79:596.
146. Kaseff LG, Seidenwurm DJ, Nieberding PH, Nissen AJ, Remley KR, Dillon W. Magnetic resonance imaging of brain herniation into the middle ear. *Am J Otol* 1992;13:74.
147. Bartels L, Luk LJ, Balis G, Bald C. Endaural brain hernia: repair using mastoid cortical bone. *Am J Otol* 1985;Suppl:121.
148. Fernandez-Blasini N, Longo R. Surgical correction of dural herniation into the mastoid cavity. *Laryngoscope* 1977;87:1841.
149. Neely JG, Neblett CR, Rose JE. Diagnosis and treatment of spontaneous cerebrospinal fluid otorrhea. *Laryngoscope* 1982;92:609.
150. Bowes AK, Wiet RJ, Monsell EM, Hahn YS, O'Connor CA. Brain herniation and space-occupying lesions eroding the tegmen tympani. *Laryngoscope* 1987;97:1172.
151. Glasscock ME, Dickins JR, Jackson CG, Wiet RJ, Feenstra L. Surgical management of brain tissue herniation into the middle ear and mastoid. *Laryngoscope* 1979;89:1743.
152. Graham MD. Surgical management of dura and temporal lobe herniation into the radical mastoid cavity. *Laryngoscope* 1982;92:329.
153. Kemink JL, Graham MD, Kartush JM. Spontaneous encephalocele of the temporal bone. *Arch Otolaryngol Head Neck Surg* 1986;112:558.
154. Kennedy JD, Haines SJ. Review of skull base surgery approaches: with special reference to pediatric patients. *J Neurooncol* 1994;20:291.
155. Economou TS, Abemayor E, Ward PH. Juvenile nasopharyngeal angiofibroma: an update of the UCLA experience, 1960-1985. *Laryngoscope* 1988;98:170.
156. Shaw C, Fisch U. Benign tumors of the infratemporal and pterygopalatine fossae. In: Jackler RK, Brackman DE, eds. *Neurotology*. St. Louis: Mosby-Year Book; 1994:1069.
157. Jafek BW, Krekorian EA, Kirsch WM, Wood RP. Juvenile nasopharyngeal angiofibroma: management of intracranial extension. *Head Neck Surg* 1979;2:119.
158. Chandler JR, Goulding R, Moskowitz L, Quencer RM. Nasopharyngeal angiofibromas: staging and management. *Ann Otol Rhinol Laryngol* 1984;93:322
159. Johns ME, MacLeod RM, Cantrell RW. Estrogen receptors in nasopharyngeal angiofibromas. *Laryngoscope* 1980;90:628.
160. Sessions RB, Bryan RN, Naclerio RM, Alford BR. Radiographic staging of juvenile angiofibroma. *Head Neck Surg* 1981;3:279.
161. Shah MV, Haines SJ. Pediatric skull, skull base, and meningeal tumors. *Neurosurg Clin N Am* 1992;3:893.
162. Deschler DG, Kaplan MJ, Boles R. Treatment of large juvenile nasopharyngeal angiofibromas. *Otolaryngol Head Neck Surg* 1992;106:278.
163. Cummings BJ. Relative risk factors in the treatment of juvenile nasopharyngeal angiofibroma. *Head Neck Surg* 1980;3:21.
164. Neel HB III, Whicker JH, Devine KD, Weiland LH. Juvenile angiofibroma: review of 120 cases. *Am J Surg* 1973;126:547.
165. Krekorian EA, Kato R. Surgical management of nasopharyngeal angiofibroma with intracranial extension. *Laryngoscope* 1977;87:154.
166. Close LG, Schafer SD, Mickey BE, Manning SC. Surgical management of nasopharyngeal angiofibroma involving the cavernous sinus. *Arch Otolaryngol Head Neck Surg* 1989;115:1091.
167. Wiatrak BJ, Koopmann CF, Turrisi AT. Radiation therapy as an alternative to surgery in the management of intracranial juvenile nasopharyngeal angiofibroma. *Int J Pediatr Otorhinolaryngol* 1993;28:51.
168. Cummings BJ, Blend R, Keane T, et al. Primary radiation therapy for juvenile nasopharyngeal angiofibromas. *Laryngoscope* 1984;94:1599.
169. Tomita T, McLone DG. Radical resections of childhood craniopharyngiomas. *Pediatr Neurosurg* 1993;19:6.
170. Pusey E, Kortman KE, Flanningan BD, Tsuruda J, Bradley WG. MR of craniopharyngiomas, tumor delineation and characterization. *AJR* 1987;149:383.
171. Regine WF, Kramer S. Pediatric craniopharyngiomas: long term results of combined treatment with surgery and radiation. *Int J Radiat Oncol Biol Phys* 1992;24:611.
172. Fischer EG, Welch K, Shillito J, Winston KR, Tarbell NJ. Craniopharyngiomas in children. Long term effects of conservative surgical procedures combined with radiation therapy. *J Neurosurg* 1990;73:534.
173. Baskin DS, Wilson CB. Surgical management of craniopharyngiomas. *J Neurosurg* 1986;65:22.
174. Yasargil MG, Curcic M, Kis M, et al. Total removal of craniopharyngiomas. Approaches and long-term results in 144 patients. *J Neurosurg* 1990;73:3.
175. Al-Mefty O, Hassounah M, Weaver P, et al. Microsurgery for giant craniopharyngiomas in children. *Neurosurgery* 1985;17:585.
176. Drake JM, Hendrick EB, Becker LE, et al. Intracranial meningiomas in children. *Pediatr Neurosci* 1985;12:134.

177. Doty JR, Schut L, Bruce DA, Sutton LN. Intracranial meningiomas in childhood and adolescence. *Prog Exp Tumor Res* 1987;30:247.
178. Deen HG Jr, Scheithauer BW, Ebersold MJ. Clinical and pathological study of meningiomas of the first two decades of life. *Prog Exp Tumor Res* 1987;30:255.
179. Perilongo G, Sutton LN, Goldwein JW, et al. Childhood meningiomas. Experience in the modern era. *Pediatr Neurosurg* 1992;18:16.
180. Wold LE, Laws ER. Cranial chordomas in children and young adults. *J Neurosurg* 1983;59:1043.
181. Sen CN, Sekhar LN, Schramm VL, Janecka IP. Chordoma and chondrosarcoma of the cranial base: an 8-year experience. *Neurosurgery* 1989;25:931.
182. Austin-Seymour M, Munzenrider J, Goiten M, et al. Fractioned proton radiation therapy of chordoma and low-grade chondrosarcoma of the base of the skull. *J Neurosurg* 1989;70:13.

PART IV
Infectious and Inflammatory Disorders

CHAPTER 15

Otitis Media

A Spectrum of Diseases

Charles D. Bluestone

Otitis media is the most common diagnosis of patients who make office visits to physicians in the United States. This finding was reported by the National Center for Health Statistics, which also found that this diagnosis had increased from about 10 million visits in 1975 to 25 million in 1990 (1); most likely, even more patients have the diagnosis today (Fig. 1). As reported by the Center, the annual visit rate for children under the age of 2 years statistically increased by 224% during the period of the study, and significant increases occurred in older children but not as dramatically. In Boston, a survey of about 17,000 office visits during the first year of life revealed that otitis media was the diagnosis in approximately one third of visits for illness and one fifth of all office visits (2). A recent report estimated that over $5 billion is spent annually for the care of otitis media in the United States (3). Of the estimated 120 million prescriptions written for oral antimicrobial agents each year in the United States, over one fourth are for the treatment of otitis media (4). Myringotomy with insertion of tympanostomy tubes is the most common surgical procedure performed in children for which a general anesthetic is required, and tonsillectomy and adenoidectomy are still the most common major surgical procedures performed in children, many of which are for the prevention of otitis media.

Otitis media can be classified into otitis media without effusion, acute otitis media, persistent middle-ear effusion that frequently follows an attack of acute otitis media, otitis media with effusion that is relatively asymptomatic, and associated conditions, such as eustachian tube dysfunction and atelectasis of the tympanic membrane–middle ear (Table 1).

Otitis media can occur without an effusion that is visualized through the tympanic membrane, but this is just an early stage of acute otitis media that can precede the stage of effusion. The intratemporal complications and sequelae of otitis media (and certain related conditions) include hearing loss, perforation of the tympanic membrane, chronic suppurative otitis media, retraction pocket and cholesteatoma, adhesive otitis media, tympanosclerosis, ossicular fixation and erosion, mastoiditis, petrositis, labyrinthitis, facial paralysis, and eczymatoid external otitis. In this chapter, the features of this spectrum of diseases are described.

OTITIS MEDIA WITHOUT EFFUSION

Otitis media can occur without effusion. In an early stage of disease, only inflammation of the middle-ear mucous membrane (i.e., mucositis) and tympanic membrane is present, without any evidence of a middle-ear effusion. Typically, the tympanic membrane are inflamed, as visualized with the pneumatic otoscope, which has been termed *myringitis*. The membrane is usually opaque and there is relatively normal mobility to applied positive and negative pressure. Blebs or bullae may be present when the disease is acute. However, what appears to be a bulla of the tympanic membrane may be only bulging of the pars flaccida or posterosuperior quadrant due to positive middle-ear pressure, or there is an effusion in the middle ear. Otitis media without effusion is usually present in the early stages of acute otitis media but also may be found in the stage of resolution of acute otitis media, or even may be present for a prolonged time (i.e., subacute or chronic) without any signs or symptoms of acute infection. Evidence for the existence of this type of otitis media has been provided by the examination of histopathologic specimens of the temporal bone. The absence of a middle-ear effusion when a myringotomy is per-

---

C.D. Bluestone: Department of Otolaryngology, University of Pittsburgh School of Medicine; and Department of Pediatric Otolaryngology, Children's Hospital of Pittsburgh, Pittsburgh, Pennsylvania 15213.

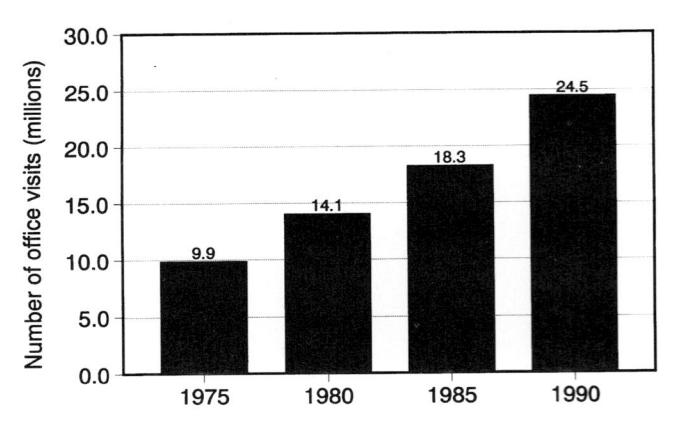

FIG. 1. Office visits with the principal diagnosis of otitis media in the United States. Modified with permission from Schappert (1).

formed in the presence of otitis media has provided clinical proof that this condition exists in certain cases. In infants and children, acute otitis media without effusion is usually caused by the same organisms that are isolated from acute otitis media, in which an effusion is present and a middle-ear aspirate can be cultured; studies have been performed on patients in which saline is instilled through the site of a tympanocentesis or myringotomy into the middle ear and the aspirate is then cultured. However, in the older patients, *Mycoplasma pneumoniae* has been recovered from the middle ear. Also, the disease may be encountered when a child has a tympanostomy tube in place and has an acute onset of otalgia and fever, but there is no evidence of otorrhea or even significant changes in the tympanic membrane, except for a small area of erythema in the inferior quadrants.

ACUTE OTITIS MEDIA

Acute otitis media is present most frequently in infants. In a study from Pittsburgh of 198 newborns who were followed prospectively at monthly intervals to their second birthday, Casselbrant and associates (5) reported the cumulative incidence of acute otitis media to be about 43% and the average rate of episodes to be approximately 86%. Similar findings were reported from Boston, in which infants had an average of 1.2 and 1.1 episodes per year of acute otitis media (6). The study also showed that 46% of children had three or more episodes of acute otitis media by 3 years of age, and 16% had six or more.

In addition to young age as a risk for acute otitis media, the infection is more common in boys than girls, and in children from selected racial groups (e.g., Native Americans, and American and Canadian Eskimos), and there is a familial predisposition. When the first episode occurs in the first 6 months of life, the infant is more likely to have recurrent disease than those babies who do not have an early onset of acute otitis media. Children with anatomic defects, such as cleft palate, or congenital or acquired immunologic deficiencies (e.g., agammaglobulinemia, chronic granulomatous disease, acquired immunodeficiency syndrome) are at risk for recurrent episodes. Even though not systematically studied and reported, upper respiratory tract allergy is considered a risk factor for otitis media. Exposure to smoke in the household has been associated with increased incidence of acute otitis media and increased duration of middle-ear effusion (7). Breast feeding has been identified as an important factor in prevention of respiratory infections in general, including otitis media. Teele and colleagues (6) reported that breast feeding for 3 months or more was associated with decreased risk for acute middle-ear infections and recurrent episodes in the first year of life. Paradise, Elster, and Tan (8) reported that infants with cleft palate appeared to be protected by breast milk rather than other modes of feeding. There is a seasonal incidence of acute otitis media that parallels the seasonal variations of respiratory tract infections; the summer months usually are associated with a decrease in incidence. Crowded living conditions, poor sanitation, and inadequate medical care have been associated with acute and recurrent middle-ear infections. In a study from Great Britain, significantly more episodes of acute attacks were identified in children who slept prone (9).

Of all the risk factors, probably the most important is day care. Children in a public day-care facility have a fivefold increase in otitis media at age 2 years compared with children in home care (10). Children in group day-care centers had a sevenfold increase in myringotomy and tube insertion by year 2 compared with children in home care, which could not be attributed to variations in health-care delivery (11). It is likely that the increase in day-care attendance during

TABLE 1. *Classification of otitis media and its complications and sequelae*

Otitis media without effusion
Acute otitis media
Otitis media with effusion
Eustachian tube dysfunction
Atelectasis of tympanic membrane—middle ear
Intratemporal complications and sequelae
    Hearing loss
    Perforation of tympanic membrane
    Chronic suppurative otitis media
    Cholesteatoma and retraction pocket
    Adhesive otitis media
    Tympanosclerosis
    Ossicular discontinuity and fixation
    Mastoiditis
    Petrositis
    Labyrinthitis
    Facial paralysis
    Cholesterol granuloma
    Infectious eczematoid dermatitis
Intracranial complications
    Meningitis
    Extradural abscess
    Subdural empyema
    Focal otitis encephalitis
    Brain abscess
    Lateral sinus thrombosis
    Otitis hydrocephalus

the past two decades has been the most responsible for the dramatic rise in the disease in infants and young children.

Diagnosis

The rapid, brief onset of signs and symptoms of infection in the middle ear is termed acute *otitis media*. Synonyms such as *acute suppurative* or *purulent otitis media* are acceptable. One or more of the following are present: otalgia (or pulling of the ear by the infant), fever, or irritability of recent onset. The tympanic membrane is full or bulging, opaque, and has limited mobility (or none) to pneumatic otoscopy, all of which are indicative of a middle-ear effusion. The acute onset of ear pain, fever, and a purulent discharge (otorrhea) through a perforation of the tympanic membrane (or tympanostomy tube) is also evidence of acute otitis media.

When the diagnosis of acute otitis media is in doubt or when determination of the etiologic agent is desirable, aspiration of the middle ear should be performed by the clinician; if he or she is not skilled in this procedure, the patient can be referred to an otolaryngologist (12). With the emergence of resistant bacterial organisms causing otitis media, (e.g., beta-lactamase-producing *Haemophilus influenzae* and *Moraxella catarrhalis,* and the more recent troublesome rise in penicillin-(as well as multidrug)-resistant pneumococcus (13,14) tympanocentesis is an evermore important diagnostic procedure. Indications for tympanocentesis (or myringotomy) include the following:

1. Otitis media in patients who have severe otalgia, are seriously ill, or appear toxic
2. Unsatisfactory response to antimicrobial therapy
3. Onset of otitis media in a child who is receiving appropriate and adequate antimicrobial therapy
4. Otitis media associated with a confirmed or potential suppurative complication
5. Otitis media in a newborn infant, a sick neonate, or an immunologically deficient patient, any of whom might harbor an unusual organism (15).

Unfortunately, nasopharyngeal cultures do not accurately identify the causative organism in children with acute otitis media.

Microbiology

Effective treatment of acute otitis media in infants, children, and adults should be based on a knowledge of the bacterial etiology. Figure 2 shows the distribution of bacteria from middle-ear aspirates isolated from 1980 to 1989 at our Otitis Media Research Center (16). *Streptococcus pneumoniae* was the predominant pathogen cultured (35%) from aspirates of patients who had acute otitis media during this 10-year period; however, this rate significantly increased from 29% in 1980 to 44% in 1989 (Fig. 3). *H. influenzae* was the second most common pathogen isolated in acute ear infections (23). Prior to 1980, the incidence of *M. catarrhalis* was less than 10%, but is now present in 14% of acute effusions. Group A beta-hemolytic streptococcus, *Staphylococcus aureus,* anaerobic bacteria, and viruses were infrequently cultured from middle-ear aspirates of these children.

Figure 4 shows that the percentage of *H. influenzae* (primarily nontypable in otitis media) that are beta-lactamase-producing is now more than 30% in the Pittsburgh area. This percentage increased during the 1980s, as has that for *M. catarrhalis*. Currently, most, if not all, strains of *M. catarrhalis* produce beta-lactamase.

Penicillin-resistant *S. pneumoniae* has been isolated from the middle ear at an increasing rate during the past several years in the United States (13,14). Mason and colleagues (17) reported that the middle ear was the most common site at which resistant pneumococcus was isolated at their children's hospital in Houston. Reichler and coworkers (18) re-

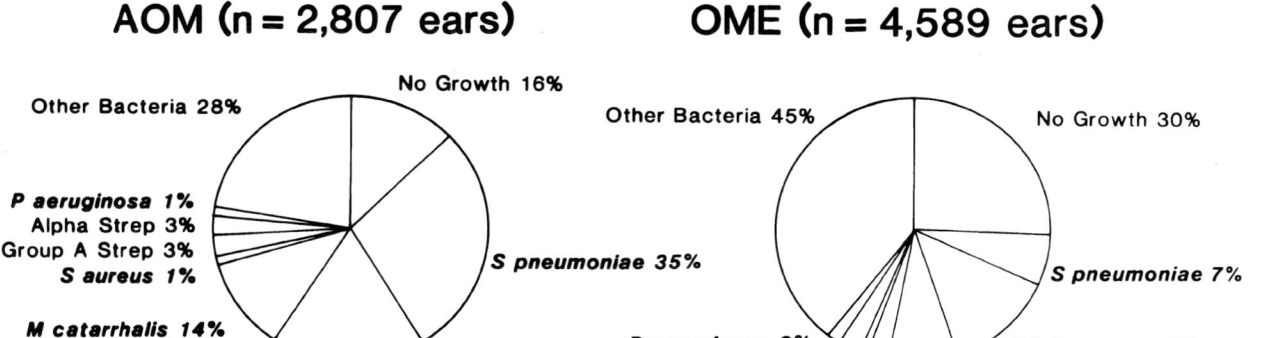

AOM (n = 2,807 ears)

Other Bacteria 28%
No Growth 16%
P aeruginosa 1%
Alpha Strep 3%
Group A Strep 3%
S aureus 1%
M catarrhalis 14%
S pneumoniae 35%
H influenzae 23%

OME (n = 4,589 ears)

Other Bacteria 45%
No Growth 30%
S pneumoniae 7%
H influenzae 15%
M catarrhalis 10%
P aeruginosa 2%
Alpha Strep 3%
Group A Strep 1%
S aureus 3%

FIG. 2. Comparison of bacteria from middle ear aspirates obtained by tympanocentesis in infants and children with acute otitis media or otitis media with effusion, the latter immediately prior to insertion of tympanostomy tubes. Totals may add up to more than 100% due to the presence of multiple pathogens. From Bluestone CD, Stephenson JS, Martin LM. Ten-year review of otitis media pathogens. *Pediatr Infect Dis J* 1992;11:S7.

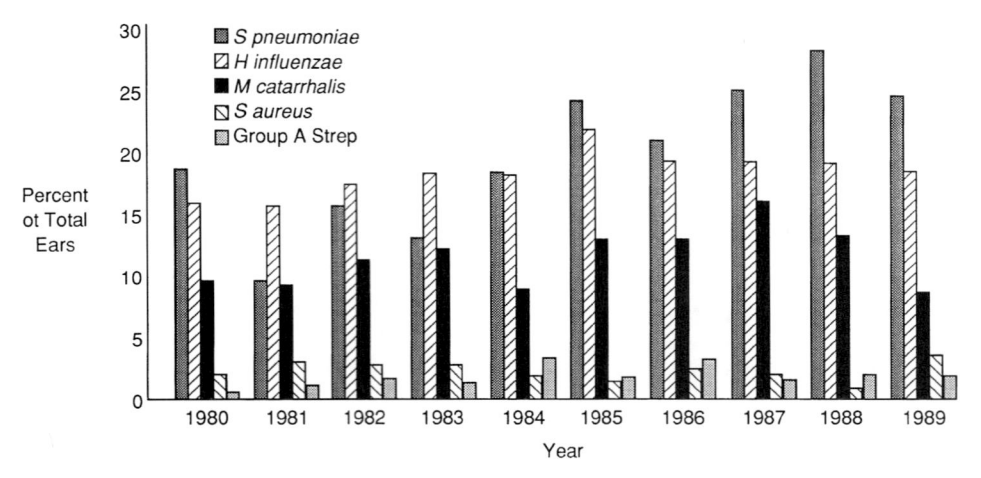

FIG. 3. Frequency of the most common pathogens causing acute otitis media during the 1980s. From Bluestone CD, Stephenson JS, Martin LM. Ten-year review of otitis media pathogens. *Pediatr Infect Dis J* 1992;11:S7.

ported a high rate of nasopharyngeal carriage of resistant pneumococcus in children attending a day-care center in Ohio, which was attributed the use of antimicrobial treatment and prophylaxis for otitis media. Figure 5 shows that the rate of these resistant organisms has increased at the Children's Hospital of Pittsburgh from 12% in 1988 to 31% in 1994, and highly resistant pneumococci are now more common than intermediate resistant strains.

With the relatively recent emergence of resistant bacterial organisms causing otitis media, such as beta-lactamase-producing *H. influenzae* and *M. catarrhalis,* and the more recent troublesome rise in penicillin-and multidrug-resistant pneumococcus, tympanocentesis should be considered in patients who are seriously ill or appear toxic or in those children and adults who fail to rapidly improve on appropriate and adequate antimicrobial therapy (19). The change in the incidence of these pathogens and the increasing emergence of beta-lactamase-producing organisms has an important impact on the management of acute otitis media.

Acute Otorrhea

It is not uncommon for an episode of acute otitis media to be associated with a spontaneous perforation of the tympanic membrane, which results in otorrhea. Unfortunately, there are few studies in children that have adequately studied the microbiology of the acute otorrhea due to improper technique of obtaining the culture; that is, the investigators have not cleaned the external auditory canal and aspirated the middle ear contents through the perforation, but have simply

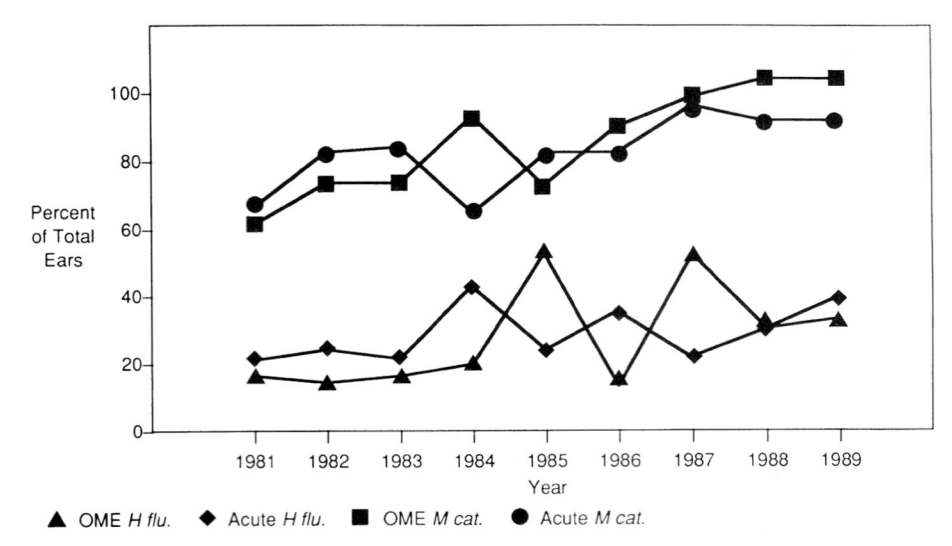

FIG. 4. Percent beta-lactamase-producing *H. influenzae* and *M. catarrhalis* in acute otitis media (AOM) and otitis media with effusion (OME) (1981 and 1989). From Bluestone CD, Stephenson JS, Martin LM. Ten-year review of otitis media pathogens. *Pediatr Infect Dis J* 1992;11:S7.

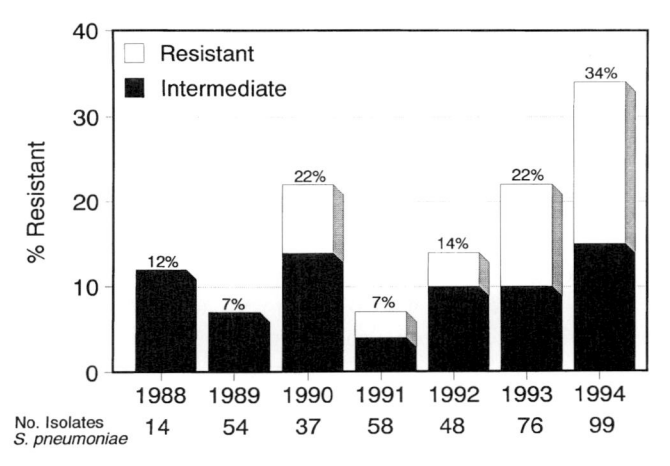

FIG. 5. Resistance of *S. pneumoniae* to penicillin G at Children's Hospital of Pittsburgh. Breakpoint for susceptibility for penicillin is less than 0.1 μg/ml. Isolates tested by broth microdilation using Mueller-Hinton medium containing 2% lysed sheep blood. Courtesy of R. Wadowsky, Children's Hospital of Pittsburgh, unpublished data.

taken a culture from the external canal, which can be potentially contaminated with organisms from the canal, such as S. aureus and Pseudomonas. However, there is a report on the microbiology of acute otorrhea that occurs when there is a tympanostomy tube in place. Mandel, Casselbrant, and Kurs-Lasky (20) reported that infants and young children who had acute onset of otorrhea through a tympanostomy tube usually had the common organisms that cause acute otitis media when the tympanic membrane is intact, whereas, in older children, especially in the summer, the predominant organism was frequently Pseudomonas, presumably due to contamination of the middle ear during swimming (Fig. 6).

PERSISTENT MIDDLE-EAR EFFUSION

Following an episode of acute otitis media, an effusion may persist despite initial treatment of the episode. The effusion is usually asymptomatic in most children. The diagnostic criteria are similar to those described when otitis media with effusion is present (see discussion in next section). Persistence of middle-ear effusion for weeks to months after onset of acute otitis media was frequent in Boston children (6): Seventy percent of children still had effusion at 2 weeks, 40% had effusion at 1 month, 20% had effusion at 2 months, and 10% had effusion at 3 months. Similar results of persistent middle-ear effusion after an episode of acute otitis media have been noted in studies from other centers, except for the study by Kaleida and coworkers (21). They included recurrent acute otitis media in their study, which occurred in 50% of subjects during the following 3 months, and the point prevalence of middle-ear effusion ranged between about 40% at 30 days and 23% at 90 days after the onset of the initial attack. The conclusion from these studies is that persistent middle-ear effusion that frequently follows an attack of acute otitis media usually clears without further treatment (22).

The microbiology of middle-ear effusions that persist in children who have been treated with antimicrobial agents for acute otitis media and who are asymptomatic has not been formally studied; however, the bacteria are probably similar to those described when children have otitis media with effusion.

OTITIS MEDIA WITH EFFUSION

Relatively asymptomatic middle ear effusion has many synonyms (e.g., *secretory, nonsuppurative,* or *serous otitis media*), but the most commonly used term is *otitis media with effusion.* The duration (not the severity) of the effusion can be classified as acute (<3 wk), subacute (3 wk–3 mo), or chronic (>3 mo). Otitis media with effusion also is commonly present in infants and children who attend a day-care center. In Pittsburgh children 2 to 6 years of age, observed monthly over a 2-year period in a day-care center, approximately 50% had one or more episodes that were usually associated with an upper respiratory tract infection; however, the study also revealed that two thirds of the episodes spontaneously cleared within a month (23). In a similar study of 126 school children aged 5 to 12 years, the incidence of otitis media with effusion was found to be much lower in children 6 years of age and older (24). In many children, the duration of effusion may be as short as 1 or several days. Thus, relatively asymptomatic otitis media with effusion is relatively frequent in healthy children but usually resolves without medical or surgical intervention, and the incidence decreases after age 5 years. Past studies reported that African American children had a lower incidence of middle ear disease than white children, but a relatively recent study from Pittsburgh, in which both African American and white infants were prospectively followed from birth to 2 years of age, found no difference in the incidence of either acute otitis media or otitis media with effusion (5).

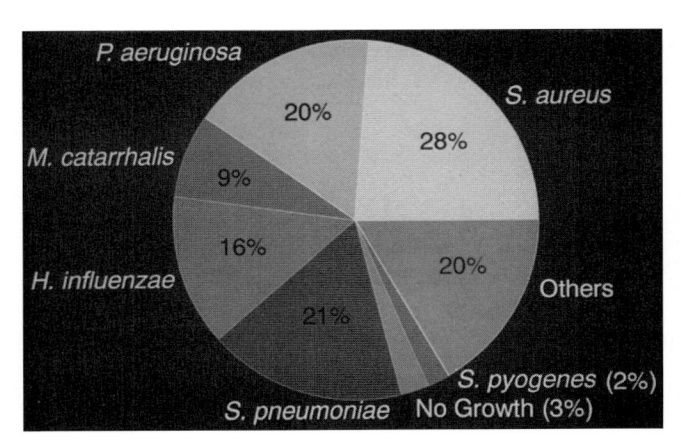

FIG. 6. Bacteriology of 176 episodes of acute otorrhea in 109 children (194 ears) with tympanostomy tubes at Children's Hospital of Pittsburgh. From Mandel et al., *Ann Otol Rhinol Laryngol* 1994;103:713.

Diagnosis

Otitis media with effusion usually occurs in association with an upper respiratory tract viral infection, but the child usually does not have any symptoms referable to the ears. Pneumatic otoscopy frequently reveals either a retracted or concave tympanic membrane, the mobility of which is limited or absent. However, fullness or even bulging may be visualized. In addition, an air-fluid level or bubbles, or both, may be observed through a translucent tympanic membrane. The most important distinction between this type of disease and acute otitis media is that the signs and symptoms of acute infection are lacking in otitis media with effusion (e.g., otalgia, fever), but hearing loss is usually present in both conditions.

Microbiology

For decades, otitis media with effusion was assumed to be sterile, because several reports described unsuccessful attempts to culture bacteria; however, studies reported during the past 15 years identified bacteria by means of smears and cultures. A study was conducted in Pittsburgh by Riding and coworkers (25) of 179 children aged 1 to 16 years who had chronic middle ear effusions. Of 179 ears, bacteria were cultured from 86 (48%) chronic middle ear effusions. Bacteria were present in serous and mucoid effusions as well as the purulent type.

More recent findings from our center (Fig. 7) show that in middle ear aspirates from ears with chronic otitis media with effusion, about two thirds had bacteria isolated; of the one third that were considered to be pathogens, the most common bacteria were *H. influenzae*, *M. catarrhalis*, and *S. pneumoniae*, which are the common pathogens found in middle ear aspirates from children with acute otitis media. In addition, *Staphylococcus epidermidis* was cultured from many middle ears when it was not cultured from the external canal of the same ear. (A culture preceded sterilization and tympanocentesis.) Beta-lactamase activity was similar to that reported for isolates from ears with acute otitis media; anaerobic bacteria were also isolated in about 10%

Post and colleagues (26) found that 78% of middle ear effusions had evidence of the three major organisms (i.e., *H. influenzae*, *M. catarrhalis*, and *S. pneumoniae*) by polymerase chain reaction, whereas only 28% of the aspirates were culture-positive. The investigators postulated that bacteria may have a larger role in the inflammatory process than previously believed.

EUSTACHIAN TUBE DYSFUNCTION AND ATELECTASIS OF THE MIDDLE EAR

Otitis media is usually the result of dysfunction of the eustachian tube. However, abnormal function of the eustachian tube may cause otologic symptoms without an apparent effusion. The tympanic membrane may have a normal appearance and mobility may be unimpaired when tested with a pneumatic otoscope or by tympanometry. Two types of eustachian tube dysfunction can be present: obstruction or abnormal patency (see Chapter 2).

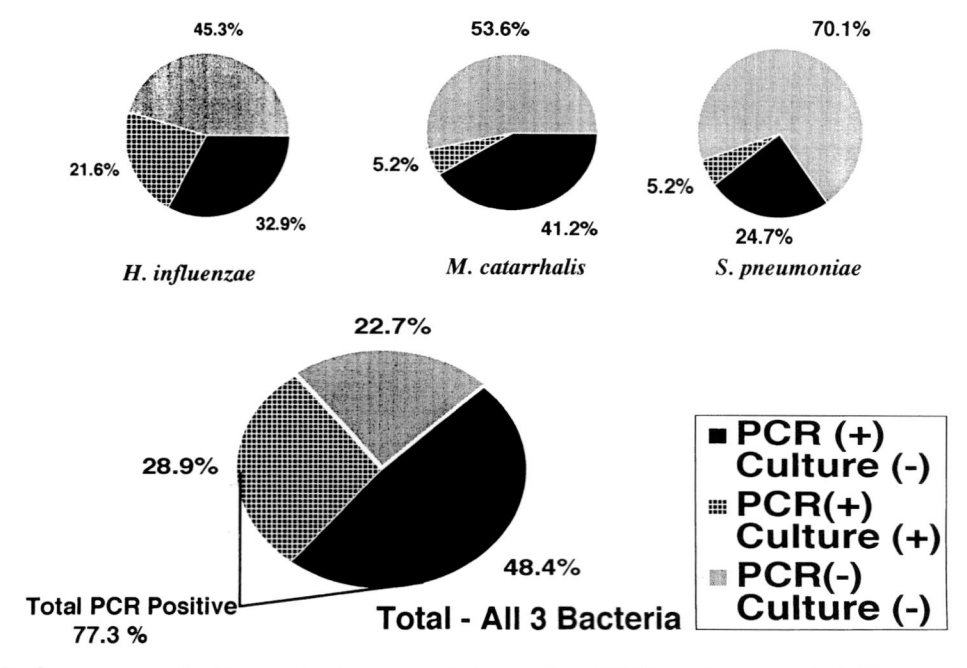

FIG. 7. Comparison of culture and polymerase chain reaction *(PCR)* results from 97 middle ear effusions from children analyzed for *H. influenzae*, *M. catarrhalis*, and *S. pneumoniae*. Adapted from Post JC, Preston RA, Aul JJ, et al. Molecular analysis of bacterial pathogens in otitis media with effusion. *JAMA* 1995;273(20):1598.

The eustachian tube may be obstructed, which can be due to either an anatomic obstruction (such as can occur when there is infection or allergy), or a failure of the opening mechanism of the tube (i.e., functional obstruction), or both, but no effusion is present. The tube periodically opens (i.e., dilates) to equalize the gas pressure in the middle ear cavity (i.e., to ventilate the middle ear) but at less frequent intervals than normal; in this case high negative intratympanic pressure may be present for relatively long but transient periods. This type of intermittent middle ear pressure regulation may cause periods of otalgia, a feeling of fullness or pressure, hearing loss, popping and snapping noises, tinnitus, and even vertigo. If the condition is present only during an acute upper respiratory tract infection, medical treatment should be directed toward relief of the nasal congestion. If the symptoms are of a chronic nature, a search for an underlying cause should be attempted, and, if found, appropriate management should be instituted.

Eustachian tube dysfunction also can be caused by abnormal patency. In its extreme form, the hyperpatent eustachian tube is open even at rest (i.e., patulous). Lesser degrees of abnormal patency result in a semipatulous eustachian tube that is closed at rest but has low tubal resistance to airflow in comparison with the normal tube. A patulous eustachian tube may be caused by abnormal tube geometry or a decrease in extramural pressure, such as occurs as a result of weight loss or, possibly, mural or intraluminal changes. These latter conditions may be seen when the extracellular fluid is altered by medical treatment of another, unrelated condition. Interruption of the innervation of the tensor veli palatini muscle has also been shown to be a cause of a hyperpatent eustachian tube (27).

Patulous eustachian tube may occur in adolescents and adults but is less common in children. The patient frequently complains of hearing his or her own breathing in the ear or of autophony. Otoscopic examination reveals a tympanic membrane that moves medially on inspiration and laterally on expiration; the movement can be exaggerated with forced respiration. The condition is relieved when the patient is recumbent, because extramural pressure in the eustachian tube is increased by paratubal venous engorgement in this position. The patient should therefore be examined in the sitting position. The diagnosis can also be made by measuring the impedance of the middle ear (28). A tympanogram is obtained while the patient is breathing normally, and a second one is obtained while the patient holds his or her breath. Fluctuation in the tympanometric line should coincide with breathing. The fluctuation can be exaggerated by asking the patient to occlude one nostril and close the mouth during forced inspiration and expiration, or by performing the Toynbee or Valsalva maneuver.

Atelectasis of the tympanic membrane–middle ear can be acute or chronic, localized or generalized, and mild or severe and may or may not be associated with abnormal negative pressure. Retraction of the tympanic membrane may be attributable to the presence of high negative pressure. On the other hand, a flaccid, atelectatic tympanic membrane may not be associated with high negative intratympanic pressure: The abnormal negative pressure may have been the original cause of such a condition of the membrane but may no longer be present. Localized atelectasis or a retraction pocket may be seen in the area of a healed perforation or at the site where a tympanostomy tube had been inserted (atrophic scar or dimeric membrane). A retraction pocket in the posterosuperior portion of the pars tensa or a pars flaccida retraction pocket is more frequently associated with the development of more serious sequelae (ossicular discontinuity or cholesteatoma) than is a retraction pocket in other areas of the tympanic membrane. These variations should be kept in mind when deciding how to manage atelectasis. When atelectasis is progressive and high negative pressure is present, eustachian tube obstruction is present. The obstruction can be either anatomic or due to failure of tubal opening, or both.

CHRONIC SUPPURATIVE OTITIS MEDIA

Chronic suppurative otitis media is a stage of ear disease in which there is chronic infection of the middle ear and mastoid and in which a "central" perforation of the tympanic membrane (or a patent tympanostomy tube) and discharge (otorrhea) are present. Mastoiditis is invariably a part of the pathologic process. The condition has been called *chronic otitis media,* but this term can be confused with chronic otitis media *with effusion,* which is not characterized by perforation. It is also called *chronic suppurative otitis media and mastoiditis, chronic purulent otitis media,* and *chronic otomastoiditis.* The most descriptive term is *chronic otitis media with perforation, discharge, and mastoiditis,* but this is not common usage. When a cholesteatoma is also present, the term *chronic suppurative otitis media with cholesteatoma* is used; however, an acquired aural cholesteatoma does not have to be associated with chronic suppurative otitis media.

Microbiology

Chronic suppurative otitis media develops from a chronic bacterial infection; however, the bacteria that caused the initial episode of acute otitis media with perforation and otorrhea may not be those that are isolated from the chronic discharge when there is chronic infection in the middle ear and mastoid. Thus, the antimicrobial therapy recommended for acute otitis media may not be effective for most cases of chronic suppurative otitis media (29). The microbiology of chronic suppurative otitis media without cholesteatoma in children has been reported by Kenna, and coworkers (30). From the 51 ear cultures obtained from 36 children, 23 microbiologic species were isolated. One organism was isolated from 18 ears, two from 20 ears, three from three ears, four from four ears, and five from two ears. The most common bacterial species isolated was *Pseudomonas aeruginosa,* which was present in 34 ears (67%) and was the only isolate in 16 ears (31%). Of the 15 children who had bilateral otorrhea, 11 (73%) had the same organism(s) identified in both middle ears: seven children had *P. aeruginosa* isolated, four had *S. aureus,* and one each had *S. epidermidis, Candida albicans,* and diphtheroids.

The bacteriology of chronic suppurative otitis media with cholesteatoma in children has been reported (31,32). The most common aerobic microbiologic organisms isolated were *P. aeruginosa* and *S. aureus,* and the most frequent anaerobic organisms were *Bacteroides, Peptostreptococcus,* and *Peptococcus* species (31,33). It is important to make the distinction between chronic suppurative otitis media with and without cholesteatoma, because tympanomastoid surgery is indicated when cholesteatoma is present, whereas medical management *may* be effective when it is not.

REFERENCES

1. Schappert SM. Office visits for otitis media: United States, 1975–90. *Vital Health Stat* (of the Centers for Disease Control/National Center for Health Statistics) 1992;214:1.
2. Teele DW, Klein JO, Rosner B, et al. Middle ear disease and the practice of pediatrics. Burden during the first five years of life. *JAMA* 1983;249(8):1026.
3. Gates GA. Cost effectiveness considerations in otitis media treatment. Abstracts of the Sixth International Symposium on Recent Advances in Otitis Media. Fort Lauderdale, FL, June 4–8, 1995:4.
4. Nelson WL, Kuritsky JN, Kennedy DL, et al. Outpatient pediatric antibiotic use in the U.S.: trends and therapy for otitis media, 1977–1986. Program and Abstracts of the 27th Interscience Conference on Antimicrobial Agents and Chemotherapy. Washington, DC: American Society for Microbiology, 1987.
5. Casselbrant ML, Mandel EM, Kurs-Lasky M, Rockette HE, Bluestone CD. Otitis media in a population of black American and white American infants, 0–2 years of age. *Int J Pediatr Otorhinolaryngol* 1995;33:1.
6. Teele DW, Klein JO, Rosner BA, and the Greater Boston Otitis Media Study Group. Epidemiology of otitis media during the first seven years of life in children in Greater Boston: a prospective, cohort study. *J Infect Dis* 1989;160:83.
7. Etzel RA, Pattishall EN, Haley NJ, Fletcher RH, Henderson FW. Passive smoking and middle ear effusion among children in day care. *Pediatrics* 1992;90:228.
8. Paradise JL, Elster BA, Tan L. Evidence in infants with cleft palate that breast milk protects against otitis media. *Pediatrics* 1994;94:853.
9. Gannon MM, Haggard MP, Golding J, Fleming P. Sleeping position—a new environmental risk factor for otitis media? Abstracts of the Sixth International Symposium on Recent Advances in Otitis Media. Fort Lauderdale, FL, June 4–8, 1995:24.
10. Henderson FW, Giebink GS. Otitis media among children in day care: epidemiology and pathogenesis. *Rev Infect Dis* 1986;8:533.
11. Wald ER, Dashefsky B, Byers C, Guerra N, Taylor F. Frequency and severity of infections in day care. *J Pediatr* 1988;112:540.
12. Bluestone CD, Klein JO. *Otitis media in infants and children.* 2nd ed. Philadelphia: WB Saunders; 1995.
13. Spika JS, Facklam RR, Plikaytis BD, Oxtoby MJ. Antimicrobial resistance of Streptococcus pneumoniae in the United States, 1979–1987. The pneumococcal surveillance working group. *J Infect Dis* 1991;163:1273.
14. Welby PL, Keller DS, Cromien JL, Tebas P, Storch GA. Resistance to penicillin and non-beta-lactam antibiotics of Streptococcus pneumoniae at a children's hospital. *Pediatr Infect Dis J* 1994;13:281.
15. Bluestone CD, Klein JO. Otitis media, atelectasis, and eustachian tube dysfunction. In: Bluestone CD, Stool SE, Kenna MA, eds. *Pediatric otolaryngology.* 3rd ed. Philadelphia: WB Saunders; 1996.
16. Bluestone CD, Stephenson JS, Martin LM. Ten-year review of otitis media pathogens. *Pediatr Infect Dis J* 1992;11:S7.
17. Mason EO Jr, Kaplan SL, Lamberth LB, Tillman J. Increased rate of isolation of penicillin-resistant Streptococcus pneumoniae in a children's hospital and in vitro susceptibilities to antibiotics of potential therapeutic use. *Antimicrob Agents Chemother* 1992;36:1703.
18. Reichler MR, Allphin AA, Breiman RF, et al. The spread of multiple resistant Streptococcus pneumoniae at a day-care center in Ohio. *J Infect Dis* 1992;166:1346.
19. Bluestone CD, Klein JO. The appropriateness of tympanostomy tubes for children. *JAMA* 1995;273(9):697.
20. Mandel EM, Casselbrant ML, Kurs-Lasky M. Acute otorrhea: bacteriology of a common complication of tympanostomy tubes. *Ann Otol Rhinol Laryngol* 1994;103:713.
21. Kaleida PH, Bluestone CD, Rockette HE, et al. Amoxicillin-clavulanate potassium compared with cefaclor for acute otitis media in infants and children. *Pediatr Infect Dis J* 1987;6:265.
22. Stool SE, Berg AO, Carney CJ, et al. Otitis Media with Effusion in Young Children. Clinical Practice Guideline No. 12. AHCPR Pub No. 94-0622. Rockville, MD: Agency for Health Care Policy and Research, Public Health Service, U.S. Department of Health and Human Services, July 1994.
23. Casselbrant ML, Brostoff LM, Cantekin EI, et al. Otitis media with effusion in preschool children. *Laryngoscope* 1985;95:428.
24. Casselbrant ML, Brostoff LM, Cantekin EI, Ashoff VM, Bluestone CD. Otitis media in children in the United States. In: Sade J, ed. *Proceedings of the International Conference on Acute and Secretory Otitis Media.* Amsterdam: Kugler; 1986:161.
25. Riding KH, Bluestone CD, Michaels RH, et al. Microbiology of recurrent and chronic otitis media with effusion. *J Pediatr* 1978;93:739.
26. Post JC, Preston RA, Aul JJ, et al. Molecular analysis of bacterial pathogens in otitis media with effusion. *JAMA* 1995;273:1598.
27. Perlman HB. The eustachian tube: abnormal patency and normal physiologic state. *Arch Otolaryngol* 1939;30:212.
28. Bluestone CD. Diagnosis of chronic otitis media with effusion: description, otoscopy, acoustic impedance measurements, and assessment of hearing. *Pediatr Infect Dis* 1982;1:S38–72.
29. Dohar JE, Kenna MA, Wadowsky RM. Therapeutic implications in the treatment of aural Pseudomonas infections based on in vitro susceptibility patterns. *Arch Otolaryngol Head Neck Surg* 1995;121:1022.
30. Kenna MA, Bluestone CD, Reilly JS, Lusk RP. Medical management of chronic suppurative otitis media with cholesteatoma in children. *Laryngoscope* 1986;96:146.
31. Harker LA, Koontz FP. Bacteriology of cholesteatoma: clinical significance. *Trans Pa Acad Ophthalmol Otolaryngol* 1977;84:683.
32. Brook I. Aerobic and anaerobic bacteriology of cholesteatoma. *Laryngoscope* 1981;91:250.
33. Jokipii AMM, Karma P, Ojala K, et al. Anaerobic bacteria in chronic otitis media. *Arch Otolaryngol* 1977;103:278.

CHAPTER 16

Adenoidectomy in the Management of Otitis Media in Children

George A. Gates

Management of otitis media is a major part of the practice of pediatric otolaryngology. Considerable controversy exists regarding optimal therapy for otitis media, and treatment guidelines vary widely. The annual health care expenditure in the United States for treatment of otitis media, which is estimated at around $5 billion (1), has prompted considerable scrutiny of current treatment practices. In the ongoing national effort to lower treatment costs for otitis media, patients and their families often appear to be caught between the policies of cost-oriented health management administrators and the recommendations of patient-oriented physicians. It is hoped that an evidence-based incremental treatment plan would offer optimal effectiveness at reasonable cost.

Unresolved questions about the management of otitis media in children include: (a) Do all cases of acute otitis media need medical therapy? (b) What is the best agent to use? (c) When is surgery indicated? and (c) What is the best procedure? This chapter addresses the evidence related to these questions to provide a rational basis for selecting therapy.

The recently introduced Guidelines for Management of Chronic Otitis Media with Effusion in Young Children by the Agency for Health Care Policy and Research (AHCPR) has generated much attention (2). Although the guidelines have much to recommend them, they are focused on a small subset of the otitis media problem, children 3 years of age and younger who are not experiencing episodes of acute otitis media. This chapter also addresses management for children of all ages with otitis media.

Terminology

Otitis media with effusion (OME) is used herein as a label for an infectious, inflammatory condition of the middle ear associated with liquid effusion medial to an intact tympanic membrane. Acute otitis media with effusion (AOME) is characterized by pain and redness of the tympanic membrane in addition to effusion. Pain and fever are more evident in younger children and may be absent in older children. Redness of the tympanic membrane without middle-ear effusion (MEE) is called acute myringitis and is often mistaken for AOME.

Chronic OME (COME) refers to an accumulation of inflammatory liquid in the middle-ear cleft without other signs of inflammation. Effusions resulting from barotrauma, skull fracture, or cerebrospinal fluid otorrhea are not included in this category. Many, if not most, chronic effusions result from unresolved AOME. This has been called persistent OME; a new term, otitis media with persistent effusion, which has recently been suggested by Berman (3), is appealing. Because it is not clinically possible to distinguish a persistent effusion from COME, it is appropriate to label all cases of OME lasting more than 30 days as well as chronic effusions of unknown duration as COME. Although 30 days is the usual time distinction between an acute effusion and a chronic one, this is an arbitrary, albeit necessary, distinction to make. Indeed, these terms may prove to be stages of the same pathophysiologic condition.

In this chapter, OME is used as a general term for inflammatory effusions of any duration. Because it is not possible to distinguish the etiology of an effusion on the basis of its physical characteristics (i.e., serous, mucoid, purulent), OME includes all types of inflammatory effusions. Although the effusion may vary from serous to purulent to mucoid from patient to patient or in the same patient at different times, the underlying pathologic disorder is the same.

Secretory otitis media implies an hyperplastic condition of the middle ear mucosa that produces MEE on an ongoing basis; this term has had a specific implication of a noninfectious etiology. More recently, however, secretory otitis

---

G. A. Gates: Department of Otolaryngology—Head and Neck Surgery; Virginia Merrill Bloedel Hearing Research Center, University of Washington, Seattle, Washington 98195.

media is being used interchangeably with COME to indicate an asymptomatic (i.e., painless) middle-ear effusion. These terms are used synonymously in this chapter.

Risk Factors

That susceptibility to OME is an inherited trait is a highly plausible assumption, given the number of otitis-prone families. Whether susceptibility is mediated through defects in the immune system, in the biologic structure of the middle ear and eustachian tube, or both is not easy to determine. Socioeconomic factors, such as overcrowding, poor diet, and lack of health care, may also contribute to the development of otitis media. Certain ethnic groups, notably Native Americans, have a high prevalence of OME, presumably due to differences in the anatomy of their eustachian tube and skull base (4). Other risk factors include male gender, bottle feeding, and position of feeding (children fed while supine are at greater risk for OME than are children held upright) (5). Cigarette smoking in the home appears to be a risk factor for OME (6). Children in day care have more OME than do children reared at home because of endemic upper respiratory infections (URI) in groups. Similarly, children in the early school grades have an increased frequency of OME. It has been well established that antecedent URI is a major risk factor for OME (7).

Effect of Otitis Media with Effusion on the Child

Recurrent acute illness is often associated with considerable morbidity from fever, malaise, pain, anorexia, and inadequate sleep. In children, the associated symptoms may produce behavioral changes such as poor attention span, and irritability and may lead to social isolation, thus resulting in impaired learning and poor socialization. In addition to the disruptive effects on the child's behavior, OME produces a mild to moderate conductive hearing loss due to the middle-ear effusion. Such hearing losses may impair communication and create additional difficulties in interpersonal relations, affect the development of speech and language skills, and, perhaps, retard intellectual achievement (8,9). A further problem is the impact of sickness on family dynamics. Time lost from work or social activities due to illness of a child may impose additional hardships on intrafamily relationships. In addition, the otitis-prone child is often perceived as being unhealthy, which affects his or her relations within the family. These considerations contribute significantly to the quality of life in families with frequent episodes of OME.

PATHOPHYSIOLOGY

Acute Otitis Media with Effusion

Acute OME is an inflammatory disorder induced by microorganisms in the middle ear. The principal route of bacterial entry into the middle ear appears to be from reflux of infected secretions from the nasopharynx through the eustachian tube. Three factors appear to enhance bacterial reflux into the middle ear: bacterial colonization of the nasopharynx, incompetence of the protective function of the eustachian tube, and a pressure differential between the middle ear and the nasopharynx.

Acute OME is a sequel of URI (10). Viral rhinitis breaks down mucosal barriers that prevent bacterial adherence and growth in both the nose and nasopharynx. In addition, swelling of the adenoids and nasal mucosa alters the aerodynamics of the upper airway. Pathogenic bacteria appear in the nasopharynx following an URI and are the same as bacteria cultured from middle-ear effusions, namely *Streptococcus pneumoniae* and *Haemophilus influenzae* (11). Pillsbury et al. (12) demonstrated higher bacterial colony counts in the adenoids of children with recurrent otitis media than in those undergoing adenoidectomy for adenoid hypertrophy without otitis media. Thus, it appears that the adenoid may be the source of the microorganisms that infect the middle ear.

Eustachian tube dysfunction is generally believed to be an underlying cause of OME. However, controversy remains about the nature of the dysfunction and whether it precedes or follows OME. The eustachian tube has three functions: protection of the middle ear, clearance of middle-ear secretions, and equalization of pressure between the nose and middle-ear. The child's eustachian tube is short, horizontal, and composed of relatively flaccid cartilage; its protective function of the middle-ear is less effective, and retrograde reflux of nasopharyngeal secretions may occur (13).

Clearance results mainly from ciliary action. It is presumed that ciliary function of the middle ear and eustachian tube mucosa is impaired during AOM, fluid accumulates because of ciliary paralysis, and clearance of fluid follows recovery of ciliary function. However, thick, viscous fluid may occlude the tube secondarily because of its rheologic properties. Pressure equalization is normally mediated by tubal opening from contraction of the tensor veli palatini muscle in response to stimuli mediated by the tympanic plexus (14).

The third factor in the genesis of acute OME–pressure differential may result a negative pressure in the middle ear or positive pressure in the nasopharynx. Obstruction of the nose secondary to viral rhinitis may result in the equivalent of the Toynbee maneuver during swallowing. Because most upper respiratory infections result in nasal obstruction, normal swallowing during URI may increase the nasopharyngeal pressure, which opens the tube and tends to push secretions earward. Nose blowing also increases nasopharyngeal pressures. Sniffing is a common symptom of URI and it is known to produce negative middle-ear pressure, which may facilitate reflux process by creating a negative pressure differential that would pull on any material entering the eustachian tube (15).

Chronic Otitis Media with Effusion

The current concept of the pathogenesis of chronic OME is that it is a frequent sequel of acute otitis media and is due to goblet-cell hyperplasia and hypersecretion. Some have held that chronic OME is a primary disorder of multiple etiologies resulting in eustachian tube dysfunction. However, the Greater Boston Collaborative Otitis Media Study demonstrated persistent effusion following an acute OME for 1 month in 40% of patients for 2 months in 20% and for 3 months or longer in 10% of patients (16). Further support comes from the work of many other investigators who have demonstrated pathogenic bacteria in the fluid obtained from the middle ears of children with chronic OME. Clinical studies of OME in young children also support an infectious etiology (17). Eustachian tube dysfunction has long been held to result sequentially in underaeration of the middle ear, negative middle-ear pressure, and hypoxia and hypercapnia of the mucosa. These, in turn, are thought to lead to the hypersecretory state of the middle ear. However, recent work has indicated that the normal middle-ear gas is hypoxic and hypercapnic in relation to inspired air (18) and that eustachian tube obstruction, per se, does not result in severe negative middle-ear pressure (19). Thus, the available evidence supports the theory that the secretory changes in the middle ear in cases of chronic OME are the histologic sequelae of chronic infection rather than a separate pathologic disorder.

There is growing acceptance of the theory that the majority of cases of chronic OME begin as acute infection of the middle ear, that postinflammatory alterations in the middle-ear mucosa and eustachian tube lead to persistence of effusion, and that obstruction of the eustachian tube is secondary to the infection rather than the cause. This theory appears to satisfactorily explain the clinical phenomena of OME.

ANTIBIOTIC TREATMENT

Acute Otitis Media with Effusion

Clearance of an acute episode of OME usually follows control of the infecting organism through immunologic means. It is well known that AOME clears more rapidly and with fewer complications when an antimicrobial agent is used during the acute stage. The majority of cases are due to aerobic organisms, with *S. pneumoniae*, *H. influenzae*, and *Moracella (Branhamella) catarrhalis* being the most frequent offenders (in order). Routine culture of the middle-ear contents is not done in practice. Given that about 20% of cases of AOME have negative cultures, there is uncertain knowledge about the causative agent in these cases (virus, anerobes) or whether the wrong diagnosis was made. In many European countries antimicrobial agents are withheld pending spontaneous resolution, which is not uncommon (20). Children are often given analgesics and antipyretics, and antimicrobials are started if the infection persists after several days or if the tympanic membrane ruptures.

Chronic OME was virtually unknown before antimicrobial therapy became available in the 1940s. Whether this was the result of the widespread use of antibiotics or better diagnostic methods is moot. However, there may be some reality in the assertion that antimicrobial therapy predisposes to persistent effusion because the incidence of nonhealing perforations from AOME is clearly lower than that in the preantibiotic era. Such perforations permit prolonged drainage of the ear, which prevents chronic OME. This hypothesis is not a justification to withhold antimicrobial agents in AOME.

The usual therapy in the United States is amoxicillin for 10 days. Although shorter courses are probably adequate, the evidence is incomplete. The principal reasons for use of an antimicrobial are to lower the risk of meningitis in babies and shorten the duration of symptoms. Current practice conventions suggest that treatment with another agent is indicated when symptoms fail to resolve promptly or if fluid persists in the middle ear. These conventions should be studied in more detail because in some cases fever is due to a systemic viral infection and the redness of the tympanic membrane in a crying infant is mistakenly used as evidence of AOME. In such cases, lack of effusion in the middle ear should be considered as clinical evidence against a diagnosis of AOME and a second antimicrobial agent would, therefore, not be indicated. Further, presence of effusion even as long as 3 months after an episode of AOME is not unusual and is not, in itself, an indication for a second or later round of antimicrobial therapy. If the clinician is concerned about lack of response of a bacterial AOME to the agent used, culture of the middle ear via tympanocentesis is a time-honored method for clarifying the pathogenesis of the signs and symptoms.

Alternative agents are the third-generation cephalosporins, the combination of sulfizoxasole and erythromycin (Pediazole), and the trimethoprim sulfas. Doses should be based on body weight.

Recurrent Acute Otitis Media with Effusion

Referrals from primary care physicians to otolaryngologists for surgical therapy for patients with AOME usually fall into two groups: patients with recurrent AOME and patients with intractable AOME. In the first instance, the goal of treatment is to prevent new episodes of AOME through medical and surgical prophylaxis; and in the second, to use surgical drainage of the middle ear to stop a prolonged episode of symptomatic AOME that has resisted medical therapy. In each instance, persistent effusion may be present.

For children with recurrent AOME, prevention of additional episodes is the therapeutic goal. Gebhart (21) was the first to demonstrate a reduction in the number of new episodes of AOME following the insertion of tympanostomy tubes (TT). Subsequently, TT placement has become the primary surgical prophylaxis against recurrent AOME as well as the principal method for prolonged drainage of the middle ear.

Although adenoidectomy has been found to be of value in the treatment of COME, Paradise et al. (22) also found a significant reduction in the incidence of AOME in the first year following adenoidectomy (but not in the second year). However, a formal study of adenoidectomy in the management of recurrent AOME has not been done; thus, extrapolation of the results of studies done for COME may or may not be appropriate. Nonetheless, adenoidectomy is a logical surgical treatment for surgical prophylaxis against recurrent AOME, particularly for patients with persistent effusion as well as recurrent infection. Adenoidectomy has been shown to be a safe procedure for children older than 18 months (23).

Chronic Otitis Media with Effusion

Antimicrobial Therapy

Although Mandel et al. (24) demonstrated a small effect of antimicrobial therapy in COME, the effectiveness is reduced as the number of treatments increases. It is a common experience to see children with persistent OME who have received four or more courses of antimicrobials in a 3-month period. For these children, additional antimicrobial therapy is futile. Rosenfeld and Post demonstrated through a meta-analysis that the benefit of antimicrobial therapy in COME is marginal (25).

Corticosteroid Therapy

Short-term corticosteroid therapy has been studied, with conflicting results. Schwartz, Puglese, and Schwartz (26) found otoscopic improvement in the treated subjects, whereas Lambert et al. (27) found no difference in outcomes between the corticosteroid group and the control group. Rosenfeld et al. (28) performed a meta-analysis of the published studies and found that the odds ratio for clearance was 3.6 in children treated with steroids. However, the long-term benefit of corticosteroid therapy has yet to be determined as well as the risks of corticosteroid therapy compared with short-term control of effusion. The AHCPR guideline (2) did not recommend steroid therapy, with or without an antimicrobial for OME.

SURGICAL THERAPY

OME is the most common indication for a surgical procedure in children. Surgical therapy is recommended only when medical therapy fails. Thus, medical and surgical therapy are sequential, not alternative. During the past decade, several prospective, randomized clinical trials have validated the efficacy of surgical therapy of OME. The goals of surgical therapy are correction of the underlying pathophysiologic condition, if possible; prevention of recurrence of OME; and remediation of symptoms, primarily hearing loss. If inadequate ventilation of the middle ear is the principal problem, insertion of tympanostomy tubes (TT) is the treatment of choice. If infection of the middle ear from reflux of nasopharyngeal organisms is the chief problem, adenoidectomy is the treatment of choice. In most cases of chronic OME, both conditions exist concurrently and, thus, the combined operation is indicated.

Insertion of Tympanostomy Tubes

Use of tympanostomy tubes (TT) was popularized by Armstrong (29); and insertion of TT is the most common operation performed in children. The TT serve as an artificial eustachian tube to ventilate the middle ear and equalize the middle-ear pressure to atmospheric. Middle-ear clearance is also aided because negative pressure cannot occur from the piston effect as the bolus of thick fluid is propelled into the eustachian tube by ciliary action. The greater efficacy of TT in OME as opposed to simple drainage by myringotomy has been established (30).

The finding that the time to recurrence of OME after myringotomy is the same as that after extrusion of TT (31) suggests that ventilation of the middle ear provides palliation of the symptoms of OME rather than correcting the underlying problem. Therefore using TT that remain in place for long durations is a logical choice.

The major differences among the multitude of tubes that are available relate to lumen size, length, and retention time. In general, the short grommet tubes extrude sooner than the long, T-shaped tubes. The larger the bore of the tube and the longer it stays in place, the more likely persistent perforation of the tympanic membrane. Perforation has occurred after myringotomy as often as after insertion of TT using short-term grommets (31). Long-term tubes have a greater perforation rate but also greater freedom from OME during their soujourn. Closure of persistent perforations is easily accomplished with a fat-graft myringoplasty done as an outpatient procedure (32).

Adenoidectomy

Adenoidectomy was once the primary surgical treatment of children with OME. During the 1960s and 70s, adenoidectomy was performed far less often because of the popularity of TT and because several studies, which would be considered flawed by today's standards, failed to show a significant effect of adenoidectomy on outcome. Three separate, prospective, randomized clinical trials have shown that adenoidectomy significantly reduces morbidity from chronic OME (22,31,33). These studies have demonstrated that (a) adenoidectomy is an effective treatment for patients with OME and (b) that the effect is independent of the size of the adenoid.

Given (a) that in the San Antonio study (31) children receiving adenoidectomy had a significant reduction in morbidity as compared to those who did not have their adenoids removed; (b) if adenoidectomy were done, the outcome was similar regardless of whether a TT was used; and (c) there is a very low rate of complications from adenoidectomy and only a modest additional cost to do TT insertion, an argument can be made to perform adenoidectomy and myringotomy—with or without TT insertion—as the primary procedure for chronic OME in children age 4 years and older (34). Paradise and Bluestone (35) argued that adenoidectomy, being slightly riskier and more expensive than TT insertion, should be reserved for recurrent cases.

The AHCPR guideline (2) stated that adenoidectomy was not effective in children under the age of 4 years. This conclusion was reached because the AHCPR guideline pertains specifically to children through 3 years of age. However, adenoidectomy has been shown to benefit children 4 to 8 years of age (31). The AHCPR guideline might have been more accurate if a statement had been included acknowledging the paucity of data addressing efficacy of the adenoidectomy in children less than 4 years of age, while also noting that lack of evidence of efficacy is not evidence of lack of efficacy. Given the high cost of clinical trials and the diminishing funding of clinical research, there will probably be no new evidence in the foreseeable future. Therefore, one must make recommendations on the basis of available evidence. The study by Paradise et al. (22), which was not cited by the AHCPR report, showed that the effect of adenoidectomy did not differ by age (about one third of the children were younger than 4 years of age). Common knowledge indicates that there is little physiologic difference between a 3-year-old and a 4-year-old child. The effect of adenoidectomy was greater for the younger children in the San Antonio study (31). Therefore, one could make the case that high-risk children should have adenoidectomy at a younger age to accrue the greatest benefit. As mentioned earlier, adenoidectomy in children older than 18 months has been shown to be a safe procedure (23).

Certainly, these arguments are logical, but they are untested; the reader will have to decide this matter in his or her own practice according to local costs and practice guidelines. Two important, parallel misconceptions still appear to influence clinical decisions about adenoidectomy by some physicians. The first is that adenoidectomy is indicated for OME if the adenoids are enlarged; the second is that the enlarged adenoids must be pathologic. All three clinical trials on adenoidectomy (23,31,33) showed that the size of the adenoid is irrelevant to outcome. Adenoid hyperplasia is a reaction of the healthy adenoid to antigenic stimulation, but the chronically infected adenoid, which is associated with otitis media (36) is small because it is unable to mount an immune response. The decision for adenoidectomy should, therefore, be made on the basis of the severity and persistence of the middle-ear disease, not on the size of the adenoid. Until direct methods for evaluating adenoid pathology are found, it is well to remember that the status of the middle ear may indirectly indicate the status of the adenoid in children with histories of OME and that the AHCPR report (2) noted that adenoidectomy for specific pathology was an exception to their guideline. If one accepts the premise that adenoid infection is a risk factor for OME—as I believe it is—it follows logically that treatment of patients with severe otitis media that has failed medical therapy should include treatment of the adenoid disease.

Patient Selection for Surgical Therapy

Ultimate control of OME depends on growth of the skull and eustachian tube and the maturation of the immune system. The goals of treatment are reduction in the number of episodes of OME and relief of the conductive hearing loss, especially during the key developmental periods for language and education. Specific objectives are removal of effusion, prolonged drainage of the middle ear, and elimination of a septic focus in the nasopharynx.

Therapy for OME differs by the age of the patient and whether the process is acute or chronic. Because antimicrobial therapy is the standard of treatment for AOME in the United States but a controversial issue in Europe (20), patients with occasional, isolated episodes of AOME do not generally come to the attention of the otolaryngologist. Therefore, only recurrent or chronic cases are considered in the United States.

Recurrent Acute Otitis Media with Effusion

Children with recurrent AOME may exhibit normal middle-ear examinations in between episodes, but some children retain effusion and could therefore also be categorized as having COME. The chief goal for those who clear between episodes is preventing new episodes of infection. Although medical prophylaxis has been used for more than 20 years (37), overreliance on long-term treatment with low-dose antimicrobial therapy appears to be a contributing factor to the emergence of resistant strains of *S. pneumoniae*. Therefore, surgical prophylaxis is being considered more frequently (38). Depending on the child's age, TT, adenoidectomy, or both may be recommended.

Insertion of TT is recommended for infants and children who are under the age of 18 months and who fail medical therapy regardless of whether there is residual fluid in the middle ear. In otitis-prone children age 18 months and older, I recommend adenoidectomy in addition to TT insertion. If the child is in the older range of the AOME group (i.e., 3 yrs or older) and the middle ears are containing air, adenoidectomy and myringotomy without TT is preferred in selected cases. This treatment cannot be recommended for all children with recurrent AOME because the efficacy of adenoidectomy for prevention of AOME has not been rigorously studied. However, the reduction in new episodes of AOME noted by Paradise et al. (22) in the first year after adenoidectomy and the beneficial effect of adenoidectomy in treatment of children with chronic OME justify the study of this indication for adenoidectomy in children with recurrent AOM.

Chronic Otitis Media with Effusion

Earlier principles of treatment for COME were based on the theory that secretory otitis media was primarily due to eustachian tube obstruction and that ventilation of the middle ear was both necessary and a sufficient treatment. It now appears that ventilation of the middle ear via TT bypasses the problem but does not correct the underlying disorder; adenoidectomy appears to modify the underlying pathophysiology. Gates et al. (31) compared adenoidectomy (and myringotomy) with TT and found no significant differences in the outcome variables, including hearing. Further, it was demonstrated that outcome after adenoidectomy did not vary with the size of the adenoids. Although adenoidectomy and myringotomy with or without TT insertion is a more expensive and slightly riskier procedure than is TT insertion, it has fewer relapses and is equally cost effective (1).

Selecting patients for adenoidectomy should be done on the basis of the severity of their middle ear disease. The presence of infection of the adenoid as seen with a transnasal fiberscope supports a consideration of adenoidectomy; however, in many patients, the infectious nature of the process is not obvious to clinical inspection but is evident on histologic examination. Parents should be made aware of the risks and benefits of adenoidectomy. If adenoidectomy is chosen, bilateral myringotomy and suction evacuation of the middle ear is always done. Insertion of tubes is an option often exercised when the effusion is mucoid in nature.

Preoperative Evaluation and Patient Counseling

The indication for surgery for recurrent AOME is failure of medical therapy either to clear the middle ear or to prevent recurrences. However, the criteria for failure vary among specialists. Many authorities accept 4 episodes of AOME in 6 months as a minimum. A more recent addition to this criterion is failure of medical prophylaxis; that is, a breakthrough episode of OME while receiving prolonged antimicrobial therapy. Many children with recurrent episodes of AOME also retain middle-ear effusion in between episodes and thus also carry a diagnosis of chronic OME. In these situations, the prudent physician should act according to the diagnosis with the more serious implications.

The indication for surgery for COME is failure of medical therapy to clear middle-ear effusion and restore hearing to normal levels within a reasonable time. Although controversy remains as to what constitutes a reasonable time, most clinicians and parents agree that if an effusion has not cleared in 3 months with adequate (three courses) antimicrobial therapy, the effusion is truly persistent, should be removed, and additional steps should be taken (TT insertion, adenoidectomy, or both) to prevent recurrence. In children with documented learning difficulties and bilateral conductive hearing loss, a case can be made to proceed with surgery after 60 days. It is helpful to note that the time criterion is used as an index of the likelihood of spontaneous resolution; many effusions clear within 90 days, and surgery should not be performed in such self-limited cases. Once an effusion has persisted for 90 days, it is likely that it may persist for months or even years. Maw (39) noted an average of duration of effusion in the untreated ear of 7.8 years. In such a circumstance, there is little doubt that correction of the hearing loss should be done to avoid developmental delays. Although the evidence that mild to moderate conductive hearing loss causes developmental delays is inconsistent, it is clear that hearing loss occurs in many patients; it seems prudent, therefore, to prevent the problem rather than to seek remedial education after the fact.

Documentation

Current cost-containment strategies by third-party-payors have led to increasing scrutiny of the indications for surgical treatment of OME. A variety of schemes have been developed to verify the history, physical findings, and prior treatment. The criteria for precertification vary among the payors in spite of widely circulated indications used by otolaryngologists. As a result, an increasing burden is placed on the staff of the surgeon's office to collect the additional information beyond that needed for patient care. A written summary from the referring pediatrician fulfills the documentation requirements of most payors.

Demonstration of an enlarged adenoid has been the classic indication for adenoidectomy. Now that it is known that the size of the adenoid is not related to outcome, basing the decision on adenoid size is no longer justified. Children being considered for adenoidectomy should be free of defects of the soft palate. The most insidious problem is submucous cleft of the soft palate, which can be suspected by a bifid uvula, a bluish white band (zona pellucida) in the midline of the palate where the muscles are absent, absence of a spine on the posterior edge of the hard palate, and a groove in the posterior surface of the soft palate seen on fiberoptic nasopharyngoscopy.

Counseling

Three aspects of surgical therapy for OME should be stressed: (a) benefits, (b) limitations, and (c) complications.

Benefits

The chief benefits are improved hearing and a reduction in the number of subsequent episodes of OME. Additional benefits are a reduction in the secondary problems of illness (behavior, time lost from work, etc). The cost effectiveness of surgical therapy for COME has been shown to be high (1).

Limitations

Parents are advised that surgical therapy for OME is generally not curative, but it does correct hearing loss and generally reduces the number and severity of subsequent episodes. TT correct conductive hearing loss as long as they remain open and in place. However, when the tube extrude, many children experience recurrent OME. Adenoidectomy removes a source of infection from the nasopharynx and is associated with a reduction in the number of new episodes. Removal of adenoids often improves sleep and decreases mouth breathing. However, if mouth breathing is an established pattern, the child may still breathe through the mouth, even with a patent nasal airway.

Complications

Purulent otorrhea is a frequent problem with TT, requiring oral and topical antimicrobial agents for control, and water precautions (keeping the ears dry) for prevention. Perforation of the tympanic membrane occurs in 1% to 15% of patients, depending on the size of the tube, the number of intercurrent infections, and the duration of intubation. Recurrence of effusion is not uncommon after extrusion or removal of TT. Adenoidectomy requires treatment for hemorrhage in about 1 patient in 250 (0.4%); transfusion has not been necessary in my practice, although this remains a theoretic risk. Temporary incompetence of velopharyngeal closure occurs in less than 5% of patients, principally in those with very large adenoids. Permanent velopharyngeal insufficiency is rare and seldom occurs in the absence of a submucous cleft palate. Regrowth of the adenoids is uncommon, and repeat adenoidectomy has never been necessary in my practice.

Technical Considerations

Insertion of Tympanostomy Tubes

Sterilization of the external auditory canal is not routinely done because of the low rate of infection and the lack of efficacy. Thorough cleaning of the canal is important for visualization of the tympanic membrane and for postoperative care. Postoperative use of topical antimicrobial drops is controversial because of contradictory evidence from several studies (40). They are generally deemed useful in younger children and in patients with purulent or mucoid effusion. However, the magnitude of the effect of these agents is small because infection in the control group is low. The ototoxicity of these preparations precludes their use in situations in which absorption through the round window membrane is possible, such as in ears with normal middle-ear mucosa. In patients who have thickened mucosa, the risk of absorption appears to be low, but a few episodes of sensorineural loss and vestibular loss in humans from this use have been documented. Unfortunately, there are no nonototoxic agents currently approved for topical prophylaxis; further, it should be noted that the manufacturer's recommendations specifically exclude patients with a perforated tympanic membrane. Quinolone antibiotics, which are noncochleotoxic, are now available in a topical ophthalmic solution. Although they are not approved for otic use by the Food and Drug Administration, topical quinolone solutions are approved and are used in other countries to treat otorrhea.

Choice of TT is dictated by the surgeon's experience and the treatment goals. The choice of tubes available is staggering in number and variety. However, direct comparison of tubes by using a prospective randomized study design with stratification by important risk factors has not been done. The discussions may be reduced to three considerations: duration of intubation, risk of water contamination, and ease of removal. For short-term intubation (e.g., as with placement for severe acute otitis media), a short grommet is a logical choice. For long-term intubation (e.g., for an 11-mo-old child in day care and who has had eight documented episodes of AOM, persistent effusion, a strong family history of otitis media, and smoking in the family) long-stemmed TT may be a better choice. Short, wide-bore TT compared to the long-shafted TT offer little resistance to water entry into the middle ear. In addition, long TT can be easily removed in the office, whereas removal of short grommet TT with rigid flanges may require a general anesthetic.

The risk of otorrhea and permanent perforation increases with the duration of the intubation. However, the risk of recurrent effusion appears to lessen as the duration of intubation increases. Thus, there is a trade-off between effectiveness and complications. I discuss with the parents the possibility of a permanent perforation rate of 15% that might be expected with long-stemmed TT staying for 5 years versus 5 years of freedom from effusion and the 90% closure rates of such perforations with an outpatient fat-graft myringoplasty. In my mind, the 15% perforation rate, which is lower than the 34% reoperation rate with grommets, is acceptable. However, it is important to involve the parents in such discussions so that they understand the implications of the choices available to them.

Adenoidectomy

Adenoid curettes are available in several sizes and configurations. Those with an angulated handle are easier to use than those with a straight handle. A 10 Fr catheter is used to retract the soft palate. Laryngeal mirrors of several sizes permit inspection of the nasopharynx by using a headlight or a binocular microscope as a light source. A malleable suction cautery may be used to control bleeding.

Technical Details

Myringotomy and Insertion of Tympanostomy Tubes

Myringotomy is usually done at the beginning of the procedure. After cleaning the patient's ear canal of debris, I make a curved anteroinferior incision paralleling the annulus fibrosis. Care is taken to avoid separating the epithelium from the fibrous layer because this predisposes to tympanosclerosis. The fluid is removed with a 5 Fr cannula, or if the fluid is very mucoid, a 7 Fr cannula. If TT is to be inserted, I prefer modified TT with shorter wings and stem. It is important to position TT so that the lumen may be inspected postoperatively and suctioned as needed.

Adenoidectomy

The patient is given a general anesthetic and the airway ensured by endotracheal intubation. The middle ears are aspirated through a myringotomy incision (see above). The patient is placed in the Rose position with the neck extended over a rolled sheet. A mouth gag is inserted and the soft palate is retracted with a catheter. The adenoid is excised with curved curettes of various sizes and shapes with use of a large mirror and either a headlight or the operating microscope to inspect the nasopharynx to ensure completeness of removal. Care must be taken to avoid injury to the prevertebral fascia and muscles, which may cause excessive bleeding. Curved biting forceps are useful to remove tissue not accessible by the curette. The basket adenotome is seldom used because its curved shape may promote incomplete removal.

Bleeding usually stops promptly; pressure applied for a few minutes via sponges in the nasopharynx appears to assist the process, as does irrigation with saline at room temperature. Suction electrocautery permits precise coagulation of bleeding vessels and avoids the risk of stenosis from indiscriminate field cauterization.

The goal of the surgery is complete removal of the midline adenoid pad to achieve smooth reepithelialization of the nasopharynx. Curettage of the tissue in the fossa of Rosenmüller is not done for fear of formation of scar tissue and contracture that might contribute to eustachian tube reflux. Care must be taken to avoid direct injury to the eustachian tube, which might result in stenosis. Inadequate removal of adenoid tissue may be avoided by careful inspection of the nasopharynx with a mirror.

Postoperative Care

A cotton ball is inserted into the ear canal to absorb any drainage; the cotton may be changed by the parents as often as necessary. For patients with mucoid or mucopurulent effusion, a topical solution of polymicrobial and corticosteroid is used twice daily for 5 days or until the drainage ceases. A postoperative office visit is made between the 10th and 14th days to assure that the tube is properly positioned and that the infection is under control. This provides an additional opportunity for counseling regarding water protection.

Following adenoidectomy, mild ear pain is common. Acetaminophen is prescribed for pain control. The child is able to eat normally as soon as nausea from the anesthetic has subsided. Transient nasal speech may occur in a small percentage of patients, but frank regurgitation of liquids through the nose is rare. These transient sequelae may occur after removal of a large adenoid mass. Palatal and pharyngal wall compensation occurs quickly. Permanent voice change is highly unusual.

Periodic Follow-Up Visits

The modified TT, which are slightly shorter than the original Goode TT (41), are favored because they remain in situ for several years. The child should be examined at 6-month intervals to assure tubal patency, freedom from infection, and proper position of the tube. These tubes are well tolerated. Occasionally granulation tissue forms around the base of the tube; this situation usually responds well to use of the same topical solution used postoperatively.

Parents are instructed to treat any episode of otorrhea with the same topical drops and, if otorrhea continues for more than 48 hours, to obtain an oral antimicrobial agent effective against β-lactamase-producing organisms from the primary care physician. If the discharge fails to resolve promptly with this regimen, the child should be seen in the office for cleaning of the canal, softening any debris in the tube (if necessary) with hydrogen peroxide and opening the tube by gentle suctioning, and culture for identification and antimicrobial sensitivity. Repeated office cleaning and continued use of topical drops usually suffices. If not, the tube is removed in the operating room, and the middle ear is inspected and cultured. If the middle ear looks healthy, the tube is replaced; if there is significant inflammation, the tube is removed and medical treatment is continued. Rarely, a resistant organism occurs and that situation may require intravenous antimicrobial therapy, either at home (with visiting nurse support) or in the hospital. The choice of agent depends on the sensitivity of the organism. In most cases, a resistant *Pseudomonas* sp. is found. With home intravenous therapy becoming available in many cities, the prolonged used of intravenous antipseudomonal agents becomes practical.

COMPLICATIONS AND MANAGEMENT

Tympanostomy Tubes

Otorrhea

The most prevalent sequel of TT is purulent otorrhea. In young children, the organisms recovered are often the same organisms of AOME. Oral antimicrobial therapy may be effective. In older children, *Pseudomonas* sp. are usually grown. Some cases of otorrhea are due to water contamination of the ear; others are the result of AOME. Treatment is the same: a topical polymicrobial-steroid solution, an oral antibiotic agent for younger children, and, if the otorrhea continues, suction cleaning of the ear in the otologist's office. Fortunately, most episodes clear promptly. On rare occasions, an unusual organism may the cause. Therefore, in recalcitrant cases, the tube is removed, culture of the middle ear is taken, a new tube is inserted, and topical therapy is continued. For situations that fail to clear, tube removal is the next step. If the otorrhea continues, mastoidectomy with tympanoplasty is done. Fortunately, the need for this procedure is uncommon.

Persistent Perforation

In from 1% to 15% of patients, the tympanic membrane fails to heal following tube removal or extrusion. If the child is older, it may be possible to close the perforation with cautery to the edges with trichloroacetic acid and patching with a patch of adhesive strip. More often, however, the standard treatment, after the ear is dry, is to perform a fat-graft myringoplasty. This procedure offers an uncomplicated and effective remedy that can be performed on an outpatient basis.

Adenoidectomy

The most common complication of adenoidectomy is postoperative bleeding. However, the incidence is low—of 250 cases done by 13 surgeons, only one child required operative treatment for bleeding and none needed or received blood transfusion (31). Helmus, Grin, and Westfall (42) noted that only 4 in 1000 (0.4%) patients bled after outpatient adenoidectomy and that all instances occurred in the first 6 postoperative hours and were managed without transfusion.

Other less common complications include nasopharyngeal stenosis and velopharyngeal incompetence (VPI). Stenosis results from excessive tissue destruction, such as might occur from excessive use of the electrocautery, excessive curettage of the fossa of Rosenmüller, and removal of the lateral pharyngeal bands. Transient velopharyngeal insufficiency may occur after removal of a large adenoid but resolves quickly in the majority of cases. Persistent VPI is the most feared complication because it requires either a prosthesis or a secondary procedure (pharyngeal flap) for correction. The majority of cases are due to a undetected submucous cleft palate. Preoperative evaluation with fiberoptic nasopharyngoscopy is useful in detecting an occult posterior submucous cleft.

REFERENCES

1. Gates GA. Cost-effectiveness considerations in treatment of OME. *Otolaryngol Head Neck Surg* 1995.
2. Stool SE, Berg AO, Carney CT, et al. Otitis media with effusion in young children. Rockville MD: Agency for Health Care Policy and Research, Public Health Service, U.S. Department of Health and Human Services; 1994:192–208. Clinical Practice Guideline, no. 12. AHCPR publication no. 94-0622.
3. Berman S. Otitis media in children. *N Engl J Med* 332:1560–1565.
4. Doyle WJ. *A functiono-anatomic description of eustachian tube vector relations in four ethnic populations an osteology study.* [Dissertation]. Pittsburgh, PA: University of Pittsburgh, 1977.
5. Bluestone CD, Klein JO. *Otitis media in children.* 2nd ed. Philadelphia: WB Saunders; 1995.
6. Kraemer JM, Richardson MA, Weiss NS, et al. Risk factors for persistent middle-ear effusions: otitis media, catarrh, cigarette smoke exposure, and atopy. *JAMA* 1983;249:1022–1025.
7. Henderson FW, Collier AM, Sanyal MA, et al. A longitudinal study of respiratory viruses and bacteria in the etiology of acute otitis media with effusion. *N Engl J Med* 1982;306:1377–1383.
8. Klein JO, Teele DW, Mannos R, et al. Otitis media with effusion during the first three years of life and development of speech and language. In: Lim DJ, Bluestone CD, Klein JO, Nelson JD, eds. *Recent advances in otitis media with effusion.* Philadelphia: BC Decker; 1984:332–335.
9. Hubbard TW, Paradise JL, McWilliams BJ, et al. Consequences of unremitting middle-ear disease in early life: otologic, audiologic, and developmental findings in children with cleft palate. *N Engl J Med* 1985;312:1529–1534.
10. Giebink GS, Payne EE, Mills EL, et al. Experimental otitis media due to *Streptococcus pneumoniae:* immunopathogenic response in the chinchilla. *J Infect Dis* 1976;134:595–604.
11. Howie VM, Ploussard JH. Simultaneous nasopharyngeal and middle ear exudate cultures in otitis media. *Pediatr Digest* 1971;13:31–35.
12. Pillsbury HC III, Kveton JF, Sasaki CT, Frazier W. Quantitative bacteriology in adenoid tissue. *Otolaryngol Head Neck Surg* 1981;89:355–363.
13. Bluestone CD, Paradise JL, Beery QC. Physiology of the eustachian tube in the pathogenesis and management of middle ear effusions. *Laryngoscope* 1972;82:1654–1670.
14. Eden AR, Laitman JT, Gannon PJ. Mechanisms of middle ear aeration: anatomic and physiologic evidence in primates. *Laryngoscope* 1990;100:67–75.
15. Aschan G, Ekvall L, Magnusson B: Reverse aspiratory middle ear disease: a neglected pathogenic principle. In: Munker G, Arnold W, eds: *Physiology and pathophysiology of eustachian tube and middle ear.* New York: Thieme-Stratton; 1980:90–96.
16. Teele DW, Klein JO, Rosner BA. Epidemiology of acute otitis media in children. *Ann Otol Rhinol Laryngol* 1980;89(Suppl 68):5–6.
17. Stangerup SE, Tos M. The etiologic role of acute suppurative otitis media in chronic secretory otitis media. *Am J Otolaryngol* 1985;6:126–131.
18. Segal J, Ostfeld E, Yinon J, et al. Mass spectrometric analysis of composition in the guinea pig middle ear-mastoid system. In: Lim OJ, Bluestone CD, Klein JO, Nelson JD, eds. *Recent advances in otitis media with effusion.* Philadelphia: BC Decker, 1983:68–70.
19. Cantekin EI, Doyle WJ, Phillips DC, Bluestone CD. Gas absorption in the middle ear. *Ann Otol Rhinol Laryngol* 1980;69 (Suppl 68):71–75.
20. van Buchem FL, Peetes MF, van't Hof MA. Acute otitis media: a new treatment strategy. *Br Med J (Clin Res Ed)* 1985;290:1033–1037.
21. Gebhart DE: Tympanostomy tubes in the otitis media prone child. *Laryngoscope* 1981;91:849–866.
22. Paradise JL, Bluestone CD, Rogers KD, et al. Efficacy of adenoidectomy for recurrent otitis media in children previously treated with tympanostomy-tube placement. *JAMA* 1990;263:2066–2073.
23. Gates GA, Muntz H, Gaylis B. Adenoidectomy. *Ann Otol Rhinol Laryngol* 1992(Suppl 155):24–32.
24. Mandel EM, Rockette HE, Bluestone CD, Paradise JL, Nozza RJ. Efficacy of amoxicillin with and without decongestant-antihistamine for otitis media with effusion in children. *N Engl J Med* 1987;316:432–437.
25. Rosenfeld RM, Post JC. Meta-analysis of antibiotics for treatment of otitis media with effusion. *Otolaryngol Head Neck Surg* 1992;106:378–386.
26. Schwartz RH, Puglese J, Schwartz DM. Use of a short course of prednisone for treating middle ear effusion: a double-blind crossover study. *Ann Otol Rhinol Laryngol* 1980(Suppl 68):296–300.
27. Lambert PR. Oral steroid therapy for chronic middle ear effusion: a double-blind crossover study. *Otolaryngol Head Neck Surg* 1986;95:193–199.
28. Rosenfeld RM, Mandel EM, Bluestone CD. Systemic steroids for otitis media with effusion in children. *Arch Otolaryngol Head Neck Surg* 1991;117:984–989.
29. Armstrong BW. A new treatment for chronic secretory otitis media. *Arch Otolaryngol* 1954;69:653–654.
30. Mandel EM, Bluestone CD, Paradise JL. Myringotomy with and without tympanostomy tube insertion in the treatment of chronic otitis media with effusion. *Arch Otolaryngol Head Neck Surg* 1989;115:1217–1224.
31. Gates GA, Avery CA, Prihoda TJ, Cooper JC. Effectiveness of adenoidectomy and tympanostomy tubes in the treatment of chronic otitis media with effusion. *N Engl J Med* 1987;317:1444–1451.
32. Gross C, Bessila M, Lazar RH, et al. Adipose plug myringoplasty: An alternative to formal myringoplasty techniques in children. *Otolaryngol Head Neck Surg* 1989;101:617–620.
33. Maw AR. Chronic otitis media with effusion (glue ear) and adenotonsillectomy: a prospective randomized controlled study. *BMJ* 1983;287:1586–1588.
34. Gates GA, Avery CA, Prihoda TJ, Cooper JC Jr [Letter]. Adenoidectomy and chronic otitis media. *N Engl J Med* 1988;318:1470–1471.
35. Paradise JL, Bluestone CD [Letter]. Adenoidectomy and chronic otitis media. *N Engl J Med* 1988;318:1470.
36. Brodsky L, Koch RJ. Bacteriology and immunology of normal and diseased adenoids in children. *Arch Otolaryngol Head Neck Surg* 1993;119:821–829.
37. Maynard JE, Fleshman JK, Tschopp CR. Otitis media in Alaskan Es-

kimo children: prospective evaluation of chemoprophylaxis. *JAMA* 1972;219:597–599.
38. Bluestone CD, Klein JO. Clinical practice guideline on otitis media with effusion in young children: strengths and weaknesses. *Otolaryngol Head Neck Surg* 1995;112:507–511.
39. Maw R. *Glue ear in childhood*. Cambridge: Cambridge University Press; 1995.
40. Garcia P, Gates GA. The effect of topical antibiotic prophylaxis upon post-tympanostomy otorrhea: a meta-analysis. *Ann Otol Rhinol Laryngol* 1992;103:54–58.
41. Goode RL. T tube for middle ear ventilation. *Arch Otolaryngol* 1973;97:402–403.
42. Helmus C, Grin M, Westfall R. Same-day stay adenotonsillectomy. *Laryngoscope* 1990;100:593–596.

CHAPTER 17

Complications of Otitis Media

William H. Slattery III and John W. House

Acute otitis media is a common problem of childhood, accounting for many physician visits by children. The incidence of chronic otitis media has decreased in recent years due to the use of antibiotics and the aggressive treatment of otitis media with effusion with myringotomy and tubes. Complications of acute otitis media, otitis media with effusion, and chronic otitis media are rare but if undiagnosed or untreated, result in permanent disability and death. Prior to the introduction of antibiotics, intracranial complications occurred in 2.3% of all cases of otitis media (1). The introduction of antimicrobial agents and new surgical techniques have led to a decrease in the complication rate to 0.15% to 0.04% (2,3).

Otitis media, by definition, involves inflammation of the middle ear space. Complications of otitis media occur when the inflammatory process extends into adjacent anatomic areas. The acute phase of otitis media is characterized by the classic inflammatory response, which includes edema of the lamina propria, a dilation and increased permeability of capillaries, and a polymorphonuclear leukocyte infiltration. Otitis media with effusion results from an increase in the number of ciliated and goblet cells within the middle ear mucosa. Mixed populations of inflammatory cells and polymorphonuclear and mononuclear leukocytes are seen in the middle ear at this time. The increase in goblet cells and inflammatory cells tends to increase the mucoid effusion found in the middle ear space. Chronic otitis media results when the inflammatory process causes a permanent alteration in the middle ear mucosa. An increased number of polynuclear cells, such as macrophages, lymphocytes, and plasma cells are found within the middle ear mucosa. Granulation tissue results when inflammatory mediators and growth factors are produced by activated mononuclear cells.

When granulation tissue is in contact with bone, it may cause an intense inflammation of the adjacent bone and result in bone absorption (4).

The temporal bone contains many air-containing spaces lined with mucosa: the middle ear, mastoid, and petrous apex. Infections in the middle ear may travel via pneumatization to the aerated regions and structures that are in proximity to the middle ear space. An episode of otitis media will frequently result in purulent fluid filling the adjacent pneumatized areas, causing inflammation of the mucosa in these areas. Inflammation of the mucosa in these adjacent areas does not necessarily indicate true infection. During an episode of otitis media, computed tomography (CT) and magnetic resonance imaging (MRI) scans will typically demonstrate fluid or inflammation of the mucosa in these adjacent areas. Complications of otitis media occur when the structures outside the normally lined mucosa are involved (i.e., bone, nerve, labyrinth, and dura). This may occur as the infection spreads through the lamina propria of the mucosa to involve adjacent structures. The infection also may spread by direct extension in an area where mucosa has been denuded or by local hematogenous spread.

Mastoiditis, facial paralysis, serous labyrinthitis, and meningitis are examples of these pathologic processes. Unfortunately, patients still present with these life-threatening complications despite the widespread use of antibiotics. It is postulated that antibiotics may suppress the most common early symptoms seen with these complications, and this may allow the disease process to progress until late symptoms present. The scarcity of these rare disorders may lower the index of suspicion if clinicians have never experienced a patient with them. A high index of suspicion is required to diagnose these disorders early in the course of the disease process when only subtle signs may be present.

This chapter reviews the intratemporal and intracranial complications associated with otitis media. The presenting symptoms, diagnostic decisions, and treatment options for each complication is discussed. It is hoped that expertise gained from this chapter will allow clinicians to adequately

---

W.H. Slattery III: House Ear Clinic and Department of Clinical Studies, House Ear Institute, Los Angeles, California 90057-9927; Department of Otolaryngology, University of Southern California, Los Angeles, California 90057.

J.W. House: House Ear Institute and House Ear Clinic, Los Angeles, California 90057.

diagnose and treat these potentially life-threatening disorders.

CONDUCTIVE HEARING LOSS

A mild-to-moderate conductive hearing loss of approximately 15 to 40 dB is found in almost every child with otitis media. Fria, Cantekin, and Eichler (5) found a mean speech reception threshold in children of 22.7 dB hearing level and a speech awareness threshold (SAT) of 24.6 dB in infants (5). This conductive hearing loss is usually reversible once the fluid clears. While the hearing loss is usually reversible, irreversible changes may occur in the middle ear mucosa due to the presence of the infection. The most common sequela is tympanosclerosis, but the development of adhesive otitis media and/or cholesteatoma also may occur.

Children with some air in the middle ear have a better threshold than those with a completely fluid-filled middle ear. The conductive hearing loss associated with otitis media may be fluctuant, remain stable, or alternate with periods of normal hearing. However, the long-term effects of the conductive hearing loss associated with otitis media are not known. Several studies have demonstrated that children with a sensorineural hearing loss have decreased verbal skills and maladjusted behavior patterns.

It is believed that the longer the duration of a conductive hearing loss, the greater the impact on acquisition of speech and language skills. Otitis media also may affect language acquisition if the conductive hearing loss is present during a time of critical language acquisition and perception growth. A 1-month-old infant with normal language development is capable of speech sound discrimination. By 6 weeks of age, the infant is able to differentiate human voices from environmental sounds. Babbling normally occurs at 5 to 6 months, and by 18 months the child is able to put words together into sentences. By 4 years of age, a child with normal language development will have a vocabulary that is near completion (6).

The agency for Health Care Policy and Research convened the otitis media guideline panel in July 1994. The panel found there was inadequate evidence at that time to determine the short-term and long-term effects of conductive hearing loss on development of speech and language skills and behavior in young children with otitis media. This group did find a trend toward the association of otitis media with effusion that occurs early in life with abnormal speech and language development in young children. They also found a weak association between early otitis media and delays in expressive language development and behavior in older children (greater than 4 yrs) (7).

The effect of a unilateral conductive hearing loss due to otitis media has not been well studied. A mild conductive hearing loss in a child with an only-hearing ear may cause significant problems with communication. A unilateral conductive hearing loss will create difficulty with sound localization and auditory discrimination in background noise. It is our recommendation that these children are treated aggressively to restore the hearing to the baseline level. Children with a preexisting sensorineural loss will also experience much greater effects from the conductive hearing loss than children with no sensorineural loss. These children are already at risk for a speech and language developmental delay and, therefore, the conductive hearing loss should be treated aggressively.

TYMPANIC MEMBRANE PERFORATION

Tympanic membrane perforations may occur as a complication of either acute otitis media or otitis media with effusion. The perforation usually occurs in the pars tensa of the tympanic membrane and may occur in any quadrant of the pars tensa. The perforation is usually secondary to increased pressure from purulence in the middle ear space. It also may be associated with changes in atmospheric pressure, such as occurs in flight. Children with otitis media are at increased risk when changes in barometric pressure occur. Acute perforations will usually heal without incident. If they do not heal, however, a chronic perforation results. The perforation may also prevent other more serious complications because it allows the purulence to drain from the middle ear space and the infection to resolve. Perforations result not only from otitis media, but also from treatment of otitis media (i.e., myringotomy and tube placement).

Certain ethnic groups are more prone to tympanic membrane perforations associated with acute otitis media. The Alaskan Native and Native American populations have tympanic membrane perforation with almost every episode of otitis media. The reason for this association is unknown, yet theories abound regarding the host immune system, structural abnormality, versus the difference in virulence of the bacterial organisms.

The treatment for acute otitis media or otitis media with effusion in association with a tympanic membrane perforation is the same treatment as if the perforation were not present. Drainage of the middle ear fluid is termed *otorrhea*. Culture of this material is rarely indicated because the bacteria that cause tympanic membrane perforations associated with otitis media are the same organisms that cause otitis media in general. However, a culture should be considered if (a) an infection persists despite the use of appropriate antibiotics; (b) a complication associated with otitis media is present (i.e., mastoiditis, petrousitis); (c) the child is immunodeficient or has other coexisting serious medical conditions, or (d) the child appears seriously ill from otitis media or is toxic. A culture should be taken from the middle ear space, with aspiration through the tympanic membrane perforation after material is removed from the external auditory canal. This technique will prevent contamination that may occur in the external auditory canal secondarily to the acute process.

Drainage from an acute perforation may cause a secondary dermatitis of the external auditory canal or pinna. A patient or parent should be instructed to clean this area daily with a cotton ball. The cotton can be rolled into a long shaft and used to clean the external auditory canal. The patient and parent should be cautioned against the use of cotton tip applicators. These may cause abrasions of the ear canal, additional tympanic membrane perforations, and ossicular discontinuity if the child moves while the parent is cleaning the ear. Ototopical preparation may be used when dermatitis is present or when coexisting external otitis has developed.

Usually, conservative antibiotic treatment of otitis media with acute perforation will allow the infection to resolve. The tympanic membrane will usually heal spontaneously within 1 to 2 weeks of onset. Occasionally, otitis media with effusion may occur after the tympanic membrane has healed, and this must be treated as discussed in another chapter of this book.

Perforations that persist are usually the result of squamous epithelium fusing with the middle ear epithelium on the undersurface of the tympanic membrane. The timing of treatment for this perforation is determined based on the size of the perforation, the associated hearing loss, and the overall health status of the child. The child and parents are cautioned to prevent water from getting into the middle ear space through the perforation. The risk of future otitis media in children treated with tympanoplasty must be considered when discussing the timing of surgery. The tympanic membrane perforation will provide ventilation of the middle ear space similar to the role of tympanostomy tubes. Monitoring of the perforation may be considered in the otitis-prone child. Conservative management of this type may be considered until the child's risk of otitis media has resolved and surgical repair can be performed. The tympanic membrane may also cause a conductive hearing loss and possible chronic drainage. The best predictor for determining timing of surgical intervention is the status of the opposite ear, which will give a good indication of the functional status of the eustachian tube in the child. When the opposite ear has no further evidence of otitis media and it appears that the child has outgrown the episodes of otitis media, surgical intervention may be considered. The surgical techniques for tympanoplasty are discussed in a later chapter.

TYMPANOSCLEROSIS

Tympanosclerosis is a pathologic process in which degeneration of collagenous fibrous tissues occurs. Thickening of this homogenous hyaline mass may occur, and occasionally the deposition of extracellular calcium and phosphate crystals may occur (Fig. 1). This may involve the submucosal connective tissue layer of the middle ear mucosa or the middle fibrous layer of the tympanic membrane. When tympanosclerosis is confined only to the tympanic membrane, it is referred to as myringosclerosis. The clinical presentation of tympanosclerosis may vary depending on the location and degree of tympanosclerosis present. This may be completely asymptomatic, or it may cause a significant conductive hearing loss due to the loss of elasticity of the tympanic membrane or the loss of mobility of the ossicular chain (Fig. 2).

The most common site for tympanosclerotic plaques is on the tympanic membrane. Most commonly this involves the anterior and posterior inferior quadrants. The central tympanic membrane is most commonly affected, as opposed to the more peripheral locations (8). Tympanosclerosis also may involve other sites of the middle ear space, but it rarely involves the mastoid. Small tympanosclerotic plaques may cause significant hearing loss if they occur in an area that fixes the ossicles. Common areas for ossicular fixation include the oval window with stapedius fixation, epitympanic

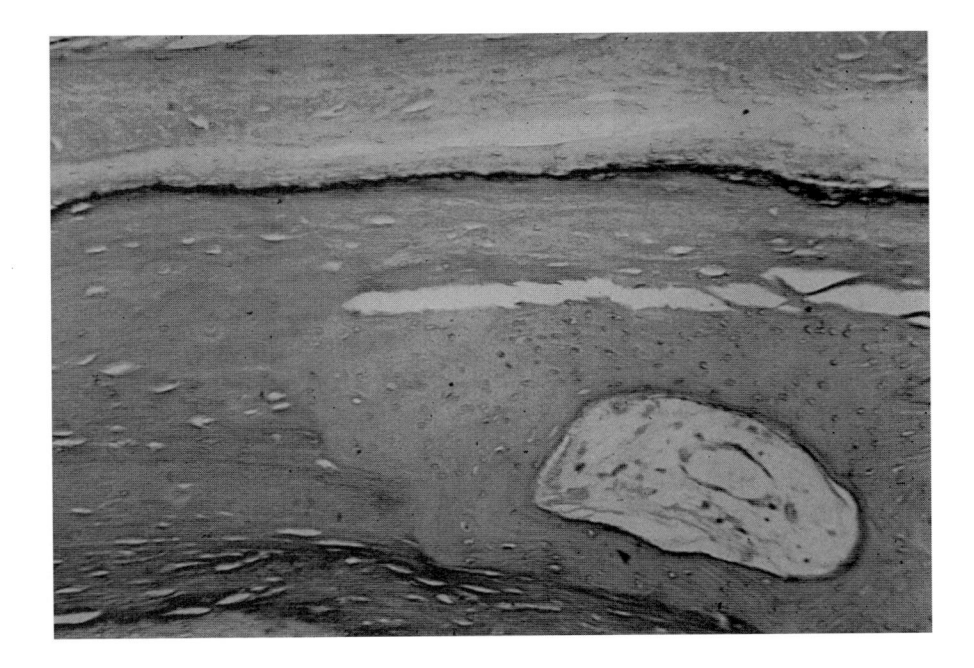

FIG. 1. Tympanosclerosis of the tympanic membrane. Fibroblast proliferation thickens the tympanic membrane. An area of ossification or new bone formation is seen within the fibrous tissue. Reprinted with permission of House Ear Institute.

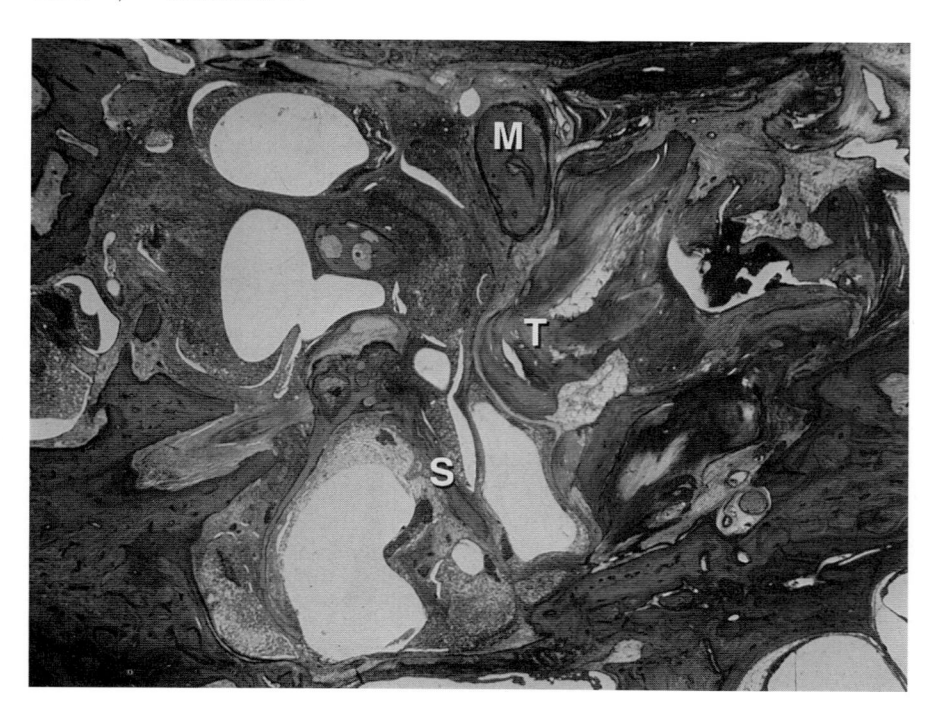

FIG. 2. Tympanosclerosis of the middle ear. This case demonstrates extensive tympanosclerosis (*T*) of the middle ear space with fibrous changes throughout the middle ear space. The tympanosclerosis surrounds the malleus (*M*) and stapes (*s*). Areas of chronic inflammation are seen. Reprinted with permission of House Ear Institute.

tympanosclerotic plaques that cause fixation of the incus–malleus complex, tensor tympani tympanosclerosis in which the tendon becomes fixed, and tympanosclerosis involving the anterior mallear ligament, which occurs anterior to the malleus. Tympanosclerosis may occur at any age; however, middle ear tympanosclerosis is more common in adults. Tos, Bonding, and Paulsen (9) found a 5% to 7% incidence of tympanosclerosis in all children at the ages of 5 to 6. Tympanosclerosis is believed to occur in approximately 10% of cases of otitis media (10).

The etiology of tympanosclerosis is unknown. A possible immune response reaction has been proposed, as has a theory that hyaluronidase produced by streptococci may incite the tympanosclerotic process. The use of ventilation tubes increases the incidence of tympanosclerosis. This risk is increased the longer the tube is present. The reason for this association is not known (10). The histopathology of tympanosclerosis reveals interlacing bundles of normal collagen fibers with the appearance of calcium. It is thought that fibroblasts overproduce the collagen, which results in the thickened plaques.

The treatment of tympanosclerosis is indicated if a conductive hearing loss is present. If an individual is asymptomatic, no treatment is necessary. We recommend removing the tympanosclerotic plaque whenever tympanic membrane grafting is performed. The treatment of tympanosclerosis for ossicular fixation is determined by the location(s) of the plaque(s). When performing tympanoplasty, the incudostapedial joint is separated, and mobility of the malleus–incus complex is assessed separately from the stapes. Removal of the plaque is associated with a high risk of recurrence, especially in the epitympanum. We prefer ossicloplasty with a partial ossicular prosthesis or an incus interposition and malleus head removal if this is indicated. Tympanosclerosis that involves the stapes may result in small or large plaques. If the stapedius tendon is involved, cutting the tendon will result in mobility of the stapes. A small focus of tympanosclerosis may be removed from the oval window area, resulting in stapes mobility. When a large focus of tympanosclerosis is present, the surgeon must recognize that the annular ligament is usually not involved, and normally the footplate is mobile underneath the tympanosclerotic plaque. Either piecemeal removal of the plaque fixing the stapes or a stapedectomy may be performed. The use of a hearing aid should be discussed with children and parents in all cases prior to performing surgery for a conductive hearing loss.

CHOLESTEATOMA

Cholesteatoma is the presence of keratinizing squamous epithelium in the middle ear or in a pneumatized portion of the temporal bone. Acquired cholesteatomas result from otitis media when retraction of the tympanic membrane occurs due to a functional obstruction of the eustachian tube. Acquired cholesteatomas may also occur from ingrowth of epithelium that migrates through a tympanic membrane perforation. Negative middle ear pressure may cause the tympanic membrane to lose its elasticity and become flaccid. A retraction pocket forms and continues to enlarge with persistent negative middle ear pressure. The retraction usually begins in the posterior portion of the pars tensa. Retraction of the pars flaccida is sometimes referred to as an attic perforation. This is not a true perforation, but the otoscopic examination only allows the clinician to visualize the neck of the retraction pocket, which may appear to be a perforation. The retracted tympanic membrane becomes fixed or fused with surrounding ossicles and bone. Bone resorption may occur due to the pressure of the enlarging mass or secondary to collagenase production, allowing the retraction pocket to enlarge. Bone resorption of the ossicles may result in ossicular discontinuity and a conductive hearing loss.

The treatment for a shallow retraction pocket is typically a myringotomy and tube. This allows resolution of the negative middle ear pressure and may allow the tympanic membrane to return to its normal position. A cholesteatoma requires surgical treatment. This is discussed in Chapters 19, 20.

CHOLESTEROL GRANULOMA

Cholesterol granulomas may result from otitis media. Idiopathic hemotympanum is a variant of otitis media with effusion in which a thick motor oil fluid accumulates within the middle ear space. This fluid is an accumulation of middle ear secretions and the breakdown of RBCs. Cholesterol crystals and granulation tissue may be found in the middle ear space (Fig. 3). Cholesterol granuloma has also been described as idiopathic hemotympanum, because a bluish dark tint is seen behind the ear drum. The differential diagnosis of a blue tympanic membrane must also include a high jugular bulb, a glomus tumor, or an aberrant carotid artery.

Typically, this condition does not respond to medical therapy, and surgical treatment is required. A myringotomy and tube rarely result in resolution of the thick brown fluid. Cholesterol granulomas of the petrous apex are usually cured with adequate ventilation. For the disease to be controlled, tympanomastoidectomy is typically required for cholesterol granulomas of the middle ear and mastoid. Long-term middle ear ventilation is usually required until adequate aeration of the middle ear space and mastoid will allow the pathologic process to resolve.

ADHESIVE OTITIS MEDIA

Adhesive otitis media is considered a late stage of otitis media. This usually begins with an atelectatic flaccid ear drum that results from persistent eustachian tube dysfunction. The normal aerated middle ear space becomes obliterated with fibrous tissue, allowing scarring of the middle ear mucosa to the inner surface of the tympanic membrane. The tympanic membrane may wrap around ossicles and can occasionally cause ossicular discontinuity, most commonly due to erosion of the long process of the incus. The entire tympanic membrane is usually observed with otoscopy to have a cellophane "shrink wrap" appearance (Fig. 4). Retraction pockets into the epitympanic space may occur whenever the fibrous tissue fixes the tympanic membrane.

Adhesive otitis media may present asymptomatically, with only a mild conductive hearing loss. In this situation, the tympanic membrane usually appears adherent to the middle ear mucosa and ossicles, but no retractions are present. The tympanic membrane may wrap around the incus and stapes. Occasionally, otitis media with effusion produces a severe retraction and atelectasis of the tympanic membrane, creating a clinical appearance similar to that of adhesive otitis media. Myringotomy and tympanostomy tube should be considered in all cases, because this may reverse the pathologic process. Unfortunately, once fibrous tissue has obliterated the middle ear space, the tympanostomy tube is no longer an option.

Children that present with adhesive otitis media, a minimum conductive hearing loss, and no retraction pockets may be managed conservatively. Water precautions are indicated. The ear requires frequent evaluations to ensure no retraction pockets or further progression of the disease process. A hearing aid may be considered in those with a significant hearing loss.

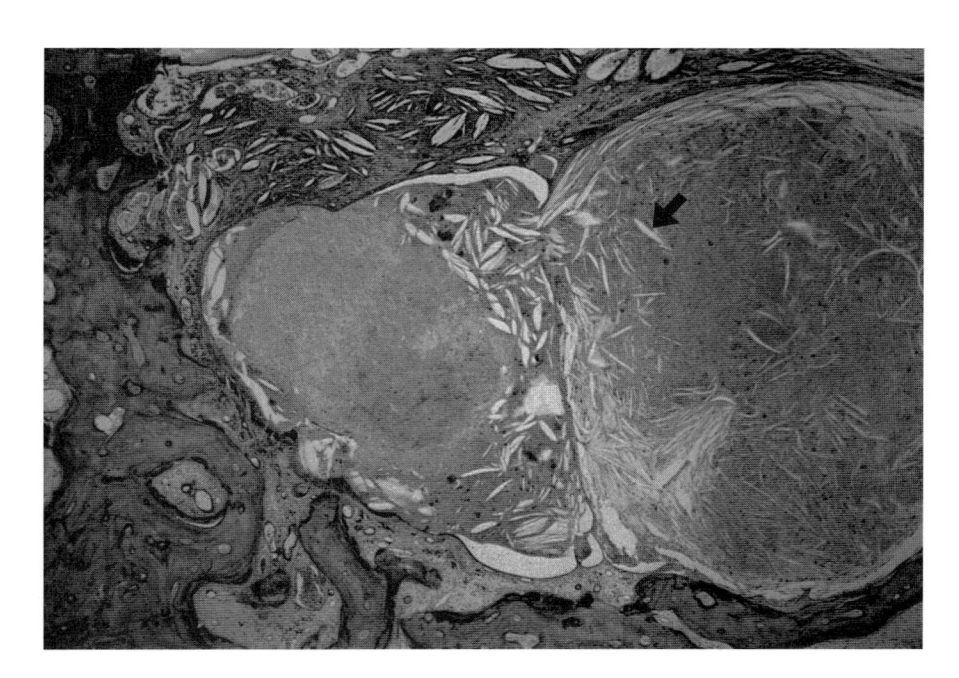

FIG. 3. Cholesterol granuloma. Large cholesterol granuloma filling the mastoid with cholesterol clefts (arrow) in a substrate of chronic granulation tissue with numerous multinucleated foreign body giant cells. Reprinted with permission of House Ear Institute.

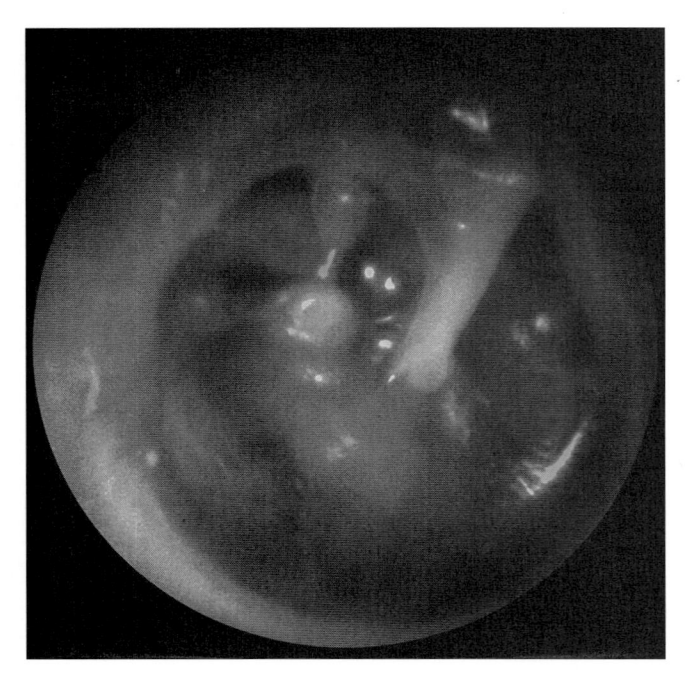

FIG. 4. Adhesive otitis media. The cellophane-wrapped tympanic membrane has completely collapsed surrounding the ossicles, with no middle ear space present. Reprinted with permission of House Ear Institute.

Children that present with a retraction pocket or a significant conductive hearing loss due to ossicular erosion require surgical intervention. This will usually require a two-stage procedure due to the significant amount of fibrosis within the middle ear space. Thick silastic is placed in the middle ear space to allow the middle ear mucosa to repopulate. A single-stage procedure usually results in recurrent fibrosis or retraction of the tympanic membrane against the denuded middle ear space.

FACIAL PARALYSIS

Facial paralysis may occur as a result of acute or chronic otitis media. The facial nerve travels through the long course of the fallopian canal, winding throughout areas of the temporal bone. This may explain its involvement with otitis media. The course through the middle ear space, especially if areas of congenital dehiscence exist, makes it particularly vulnerable to paralysis. The facial nerve may be involved with the pathologic process of otitis media by direct extension of the inflammatory process, pressure from a pathologic process (i.e., cholesteatoma or granulation tissue), or toxic effects of the inflammatory process, causing vascular stenosis and venous thrombosis. These processes may cause edema of the nerve, resulting in neuropraxia, which is similar to the pathologic course of Bell s palsy.

Coalescent bone erosion that occurs in mastoiditis may erode the bone surrounding the fallopian canal. The suppurative process may involve the facial nerve directly or indirectly. In chronic otitis media, bone erosion may occur from polyps, granulation tissue, or cholesteatomas. Cholesteatomas may infiltrate the fallopian canal and compress the facial nerve within the bony canal. This pressure may cause occlusion of the blood supply to the facial nerve.

The diagnosis of facial palsy requires a high index of suspicion because children can maintain good facial tone in the presence of facial nerve paralysis. Any child that presents with a facial paralysis in the presence of acute otitis media should have a CT scan to rule out coalescence within the mastoid.

The treatment of facial paralysis associated with acute otitis media includes a large myringotomy and tube, with culture of the middle ear aspirate. In older, cooperative children, this may be performed without general anesthesia. Broad-spectrum intravenous antibiotics should be administered. In many cases, the facial paralysis will improve within 24 hours postoperatively. The increased pressure in the middle ear space contributes to the neuropraxia, but once this is relieved, facial paralysis improves. If the infection fails to resolve or the facial paralysis persists, further surgical intervention should be considered. Electrical testing is required at this point to determine if denervation has occurred in cases of complete paralysis. A simple mastoidectomy should be performed to treat the osteitis that is involving the fallopian canal. Decompression of the nerve in the acute inflammatory process must be approached with caution because granulation tissue can involve the perineurium. Therefore, careful blunt dissection along the course of the facial nerve is recommended when removing granulation tissue.

The results of conservative therapy for facial paralysis seen with acute otitis media are usually excellent. Even if mastoidectomy is required, the results are usually good. The results in chronic otitis media are usually related to the length of time the paralysis is present prior to surgical intervention. Acute paralysis that is treated immediately will usually resolve with good results.

Facial nerve paralysis that presents with chronic otitis media or cholesteatoma warrants immediate surgical intervention. The cholesteatoma must be carefully removed from the area of facial nerve involvement. The facial nerve should be decompressed proximally and distally to the area of dehiscence. This allows visualization, to ensure that all cholesteatoma has been removed, and that no cholesteatoma invaded the fallopian canal. This also allows decompression for swelling, which should be performed until healthy nerve is encountered.

LABYRINTHITIS

Labyrinthitis may result when the infectious process or toxic mediators of otitis media with effusion have reached the cochlea or vestibular system. This is usually thought to occur via the oval or round window, although congenital defects in the labyrinthine bone also may be responsible. Schuknecht (11) described three types of labyrinthitis: serous labyrinthitis, otogenic suppurative labyrinthitis, and meningitic suppurative labyrinthitis.

Serous labyrinthitis occurs when the inner ear fluid systems become irritated due to bacterial toxins. This may result in different degrees of hearing loss and vertigo. The hearing loss with otitis media and labyrinthitis is usually mixed, because the middle ear fluid results in a conductive component. When the inner ear fluid irritation is mild, the sensorineural loss usually resolves without permanent damage. When severe, the toxic effects may cause permanent damage to the hair cells, resulting in a permanent sensorineural hearing loss.

Suppurative labyrinthitis results from direct bacterial invasion of the inner ear. This usually leads to severe hearing loss and vertigo, with the hearing loss often permanent. New bone formation may occur as a result of the osteogenic process within the inner ear (Fig. 5). In acute otitis media, the bacterial invasion usually occurs through the round or oval window, similar to the bacterial toxins entry into the labyrinth seen in serous labyrinthitis. Chronic otitis media may result in direct extension of the infectious process into the inner ear as a result of bone destruction. Cholesteatoma invasion into the inner ear may allow bacteria to enter into the inner ear, resulting in suppurative labyrinthitis. Later stages of suppurative labyrinthitis may result in an intracranial complication.

Meningococcal suppurative labyrinthitis results when the labyrinth is invaded by bacteria from the CSF or meninges. This is typically not a complication of otitis media.

The incidence of labyrinthitis associated with acute otitis media is unknown. Because the toxins reach the round window affecting the basal turn of the cochlea, the resulting hearing loss would be localized to the high frequencies. Margolis et al. (12) tested high frequency hearing in children with a history of acute otitis media and a matched control group. The children who had suffered acute otitis media demonstrated a high-frequency loss as compared with the control. Sensorineural hearing loss occurs in 1% of children with otitis media with effusion (13). The incidence of serous labyrinthitis is believed to be higher when bullous myringitis occurs, but the mechanism for this is not understood (14). Paparella, Goycoolea, and Meyerhoff (15) found that children with chronic otitis media had a higher incidence of sensorineural hearing loss.

The diagnosis of labyrinthitis can be made only if bone conduction testing is performed in the presence of otitis media. Unfortunately, this is not usually performed and the sensorineural hearing loss may not be detected until after the episode of otitis media has resolved. Bone conduction testing is recommended whenever audiometric studies are performed in any individual with otitis media.

Corticosteroids should be considered as adjuvant therapy for otitis media associated with labyrinthitis. The corticosteroids may hinder the inflammation associated with bacterial toxins. Myringotomy and tubes should be performed in children that have evidence of serous labyrinthitis associated with otitis media. A culture of the fluid is performed and initial antimicrobial therapy is started and directed towards *Staphylococcus pneumoniae, Haemophilus influenzae,* and *Branhamella catarrhalis*. The symptoms should resolve with medical treatment.

Suppurative labyrinthitis associated with chronic otitis media requires surgical intervention and antibiotic therapy. The disease is treated by removing the inciting process: cholesteatoma, granulation tissue, or osteitis. The surgeon must use extreme caution when removing this material because a labyrinthine fistula may be present (Fig. 6).

The child with no hearing or vestibular function should

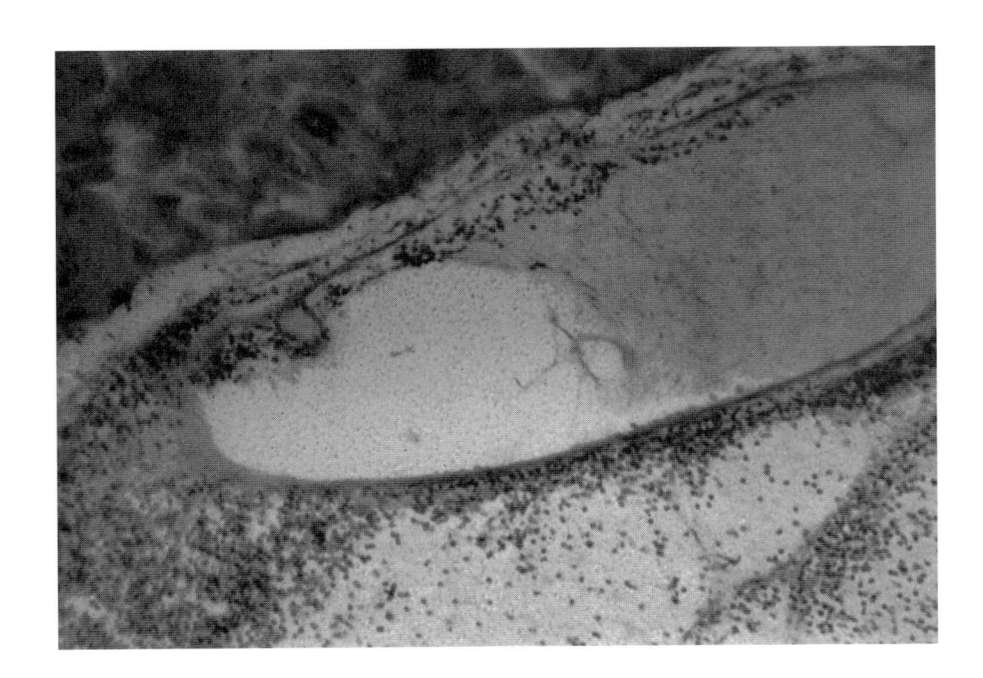

FIG. 5. Suppurative labyrinthitis. Multiple small inflammatory cells or lymphocytes are seen throughout the semicircular canal. The majority of the lymphocytes are found in the endolymphatic spaces. Reprinted with permission of House Ear Institute.

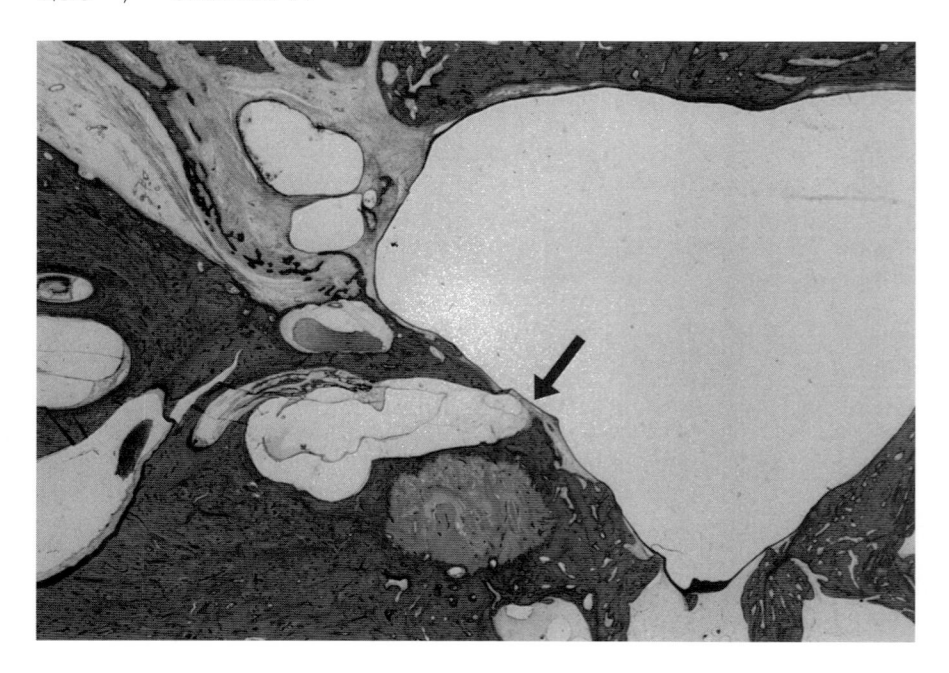

FIG. 6. Labyrinthine fistula. Arrow demonstrates cholesteatoma extending into the mastoid and eroding the bone over the horizontal semicircular canal. Squamous epithelium is adherent to the endosteum of the semicircular canal. Reprinted with permission of House Ear Institute.

have a labyrinthectomy performed at the time of a cholesteatoma removal. Persistent dizziness as a result of suppurative labyrinthitis may also require a labyrinthectomy to control the dizziness.

ACUTE MASTOIDITIS

The incidence of mastoiditis has decreased with the use of antibiotics to treat acute otitis media. A brief review of acute mastoiditis is included in this chapter, although a more thorough discussion is described in Chapter 18. All children with otitis media will have fluid within the mastoid. Mastoiditis occurs when the inflammatory process passes through the mucosal-lined air cells and involves the bone. A subperiosteal abscess may occur as the infection breaks through the cortex of the mastoid. Enzymes produced by the inflammatory process may cause bone resorption of the trabeculated bone within the mastoid cortex. This makes the pneumatized airspaces appear to coalesce, and a mastoid empyema occurs. The organisms responsible for acute mastoiditis are similar to those responsible for acute otitis media.

Acute mastoiditis may occur in association with acute otitis media. It also may occur after a partially treated acute otitis media or secondary to inadequate treatment, in which case the middle ear has cleared but the osteitis in the mastoid persists. The child will usually present with redness over the mastoid, postauricular swelling, and mastoid tenderness, and the pinna is displaced anteriorly (Fig. 7). Symptoms of otitis media, including hearing loss, fever, and otalgia, are present with mastoiditis. However, the child may appear more toxic. Extreme swelling in the postauricular area with flux indicates a subperiosteal abscess. Needle aspiration of this area will confirm the presence of purulence.

A CT scan is helpful to determine the extent of abscess formation and to confirm the presence of a subperiosteal abscess. A CT also may demonstrate loss of septa between the normally pneumatized air cells. When acute mastoiditis is suspected, contrast enhancement is recommended when performing a CT to help evaluate for other intratemporal or intracranial complications.

The treatment of acute coalescent mastoiditis is surgical. A simple mastoidectomy must be performed to reestablish communication of the mastoid air cells to the middle ear space. A myringotomy and tube is inserted to allow aeration

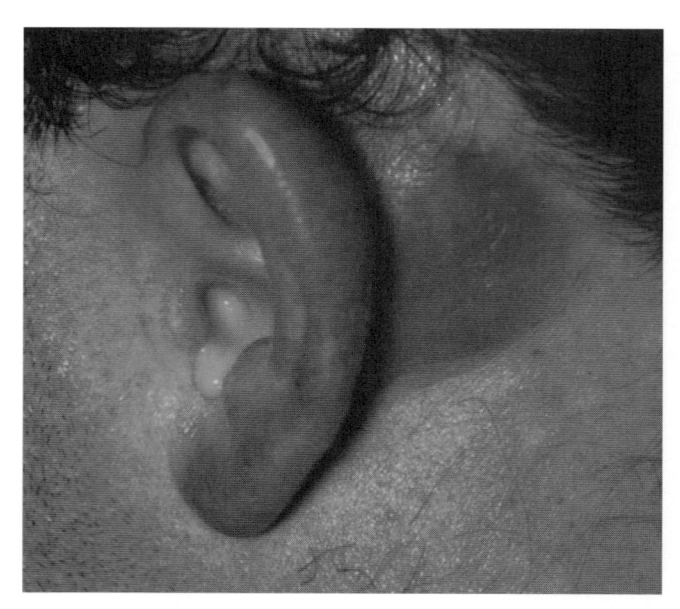

FIG. 7. Acute mastoiditis with purulent otorrhea and postauricular swelling. This individual had a subperiosteal abscess associated with the mastoiditis. Reprinted with permission of House Ear Institute.

of the middle ear space and drainage of purulent material. Cultures should be obtained and an appropriate intravenous antibiotic administered. All mastoid air cells should be exonerated to allow complete aeration. Failure to remove all air cells may result in pockets of subclinical infection that may be masked with antibiotics. These air cells may result in persistent infection or may cause other latent complications.

PETROUSITIS

Petrousitis, a rare complication of otitis media, occurs when the inflammatory process extends to the pneumatized petrous apex air cells. The petrous apex is not well pneumatized in most individuals, but inflammation may occur in the marrow spaces. Schuknecht (11) described an acute and chronic petrousitis. The pathology of acute petrousitis is similar to acute coalescent mastoiditis, in which osteitis of the bone trabecular system occurs. This may result in bone destruction and abscess formation. Chronic petrousitis is usually associated with chronic otitis media. Bone resorption and new bone formation may occur. The osteitis of the bone or bone marrow spaces may occur, creating a low-grade infection. Intracranial complications are common with petrousitis due to the proximity of the petrous apex to important adjacent structures. The organisms responsible for acute petrousitis are similar to those responsible for acute otitis media and acute mastoiditis. Organisms responsible for chronic petrousitis are those organisms associated with chronic otitis media, specifically *Pseudomonas* and *Proteus*. The characteristic clinical presentation is that of pain in the retro-orbital area. A deep ear pain also may occur, depending on the exact location of the infection. The classic symptoms of Gradenigo's syndrome include retro-orbital pain, abducent paralysis (cranial nerve VI), and ipsilateral otitis media. The full triad may or may not be present, based on the extent of the infection. Persistent discharge after radical mastoidectomy may be the sign of chronic petrousitis (16). A CT scan will demonstrate coalescence and osteitis of the petrous apex. Osteitis of the labyrinthine bone is uncommon due to the dense nature of this bone. A high index of suspicion is important to swiftly make this diagnosis.

The treatment of petrousitis is surgical. Other infections must be treated concurrently. Treatment includes myringotomy and tympanostomy tube placement for drainage of the middle ear infection. A culture is obtained from the middle ear fluid, as described earlier. Coexisting mastoiditis is treated with mastoidectomy, as described previously. The treatment of petrousitis requires drainage of the abscess cavity and permanent aeration of the area. There are a variety of different approaches for reaching the petrous apex. Different pneumatization patterns are seen in multiple temporal bones. The surgical approach is based on the pneumatization patterns demonstrated by the high-resolution CT scan. The infracochlear approach has been utilized most extensively for the approach to the petrous apex (17). The middle fossa approach provides access to the petrous apex; however, permanent aeration of the petrous apex is difficult with this approach. Concurrent intravenous antibiotics are required to treat the infection and prevent other complications.

MENINGITIS

Meningitis results from inflammation of the meninges, with a corresponding infection of the CSF. Meningitis is the most common intracranial complication associated with otitis media. Meningitis most commonly occurs in children less than 5 years of age. Otogenic meningitis may follow either an acute or chronic episode of otitis media. There are three mechanisms by which meningitis may occur as a result of otitis media. The predominant mechanism is thought to occur from bacteremia and a hematogenous spread of the infecting organisms to the meninges. This may occur from a generalized bacteremia or through local thrombophlebitis of temporal bone veins. Inflammation also may occur as a result of direct spread of the infection from the middle ear space to the meninges. This may occur in areas where there is a bony dehiscence of the dura. This also may occur along preformed tissue planes, such as the subarcuate artery, or along the soft tissue of the petrous–squamous suture line. A third mechanism of spread is through the inner ear. The bacteria may penetrate the round window membrane and pass into the CSF through the modiolus. This has been proposed as a more common etiology than previously thought. Recurrent meningitis associated with otitis media and/or acute meningitis that occurs simultaneously with acute otitis media may demonstrate abnormalities of the inner ear. Such abnormalities of the inner ear are more likely to allow a transcochlear transmission of bacteria. Abnormalities of the inner ear may be identified with high-resolution CT scanning. Meningitis associated with chronic otitis media occurs most commonly by either a direct spread of the infection or a transcochlear route. The transcochlear route occurs with labyrinthine fistula and when there is evidence of bacterial labyrinthitis. The most common organisms associated with otogenic meningitis associated with adhesive otitis media are *Streptococcus pneumoniae* and *H. influenzae*.

Fever, headache, nuchal rigidity, and irritability are common clinical signs in children with meningitis. This may progress to nausea, vomiting, photophobia, confusion, and ultimately coma. The physician may find an irritable child in the early stages of the infection, and the child may become more somnolent as the infection progresses. The neck may be stiff, and the child may have abnormal signs associated with movement of the meninges. Brudzinski's sign is abnormal when flexion of the neck results in flexion of the hip and knee. A contralateral sign occurs with meningitis when passive flexion of one lower limb by an examiner causes a similar involuntary movement in the opposite lower limb. Kernig's sign is present with meningitis when the thigh is flexed and the patient is unable to extend the leg completely. Both of these signs are abnormal when inflammation of the meninges is present. A lumbar puncture may determine if meningitis is present and allows for the causative organisms to be determined by culture. The CSF protein level is increased, and there is a corresponding decrease in the glucose level. Polymorphic mononuclear cells are present in the face of an acute infection. Other complications associated with otitis media also may be present in the face of meningitis. Increased intracranial pressure may be present as a result of other intracranial otitis media complications. A CT or MRI scan should be obtained to rule out any coexisting intracranial complication prior to performing a lumbar puncture. This allows identification of a space-occupying lesion and prevents temporal lobe herniation during the spinal tap, which may result from increased intracranial pressure.

Otogenic meningitis requires intensive medical therapy for the meningitis and properly timed surgical intervention for the initial otogenic process. Treatment of meningitis requires intravenous antibiotics of subsequent duration to ensure the infection has been completely eradicated. Intravenous steroids may be added to decrease the risk of sensorineural hearing loss and brain dysfunction. The initial lumbar puncture will direct antibody therapy. Subsequent lumbar punctures are required to monitor the progress of the therapy.

A myringotomy with tympanocentesis for cultures should be performed on all children that present with acute otitis media and meningitis. Depending on the child's mental status, general anesthesia may not be required. If recurrent otitis media or otitis media with effusion was present prior to the meningitis episode, insertion of grommet tubes should be considered once the child is able to tolerate general anesthesia. Children that present with otogenic meningitis from an inner ear abnormality should undergo surgery once the meningitis is treated, to prevent a relapse.

A perilymphatic fistula may occur in children with abnormal cochleas and be responsible for the entrance of bacteria from the middle ear to the labyrinth. If no hearing is present in the ear, the stapes may be removed and muscle packed into the vestibule to prevent future episodes of meningitis. The surgeon must expect a CSF leak during this procedure; therefore, a small hole is placed in the stapes prior to removing it to determine if this will occur. If free flow of CSF occurs, the stapes should not be removed, and muscle should be packed around the stapes and round window after the mucosa in these areas has been roughened to allow the muscle to seal. This usually results in resolution of the meningitic episodes from acute otitis media.

Otogenic meningitis from mastoiditis is treated initially with a myringotomy and tympanocentesis for culture. The treatment, described earlier, is performed once the patient is able to tolerate general anesthesia and should be performed as soon as possible. The CT with contrast will aid in identifying other intracranial complications that may be associated with acute mastoiditis. This may include the subtle identification of a subdural abscess.

Chronic otitis media associated with otitic meningitis requires antibiotics effective against organisms associated with chronic otitis media: *Pseudomonas aeruginosa* and *Staphylococcus aureus*. These infections usually occur as a result of direct invasion. This may occur as a result of bone destruction and infection next to the dura or from invasion of the labyrinth with bacteria, such as occurs with labyrinthine fistula. Ceftazadime is usually required to cover *P. aeruginosa,* and nafcillin is considered for staphylococcal control. Once the patient is able to withstand general anesthesia, surgery is performed to remove the infected tissue. As with mastoiditis, other intracranial and intratemporal bone complications must be considered or ruled out by CT scanning. During surgery, dural granulation tissue must be removed and the dura checked for small perforations that may have allowed bacterial entry into the CSF. Bone must be removed over the dura and inspected directly to rule out small subdural abscesses. Small holes in the dura may be plugged with muscle. This usually controls the CSF leakage. Aggressive surgical intervention is usually required for otogenic meningitis associated with chronic otitis media.

SIGMOID SINUS THROMBOSIS

Sigmoid sinus thrombosis or lateral sinus thrombosis is a rare intracranial complication associated with otitis media. This is more commonly associated with chronic otitis media and may occur in association with intracranial or intratemporal complications of otitis media. Rarely, thrombosis occurs as a result of surgical intervention during routine mastoid surgery if the sigmoid sinus is exposed or compressed for any period of time.

Thrombosis within small venules of the mastoid may propagate into the sigmoid sinus and be responsible for thrombosis. Granulation tissue over the sinus may cause inflammation of the intima of the sinus, increasing the coagulable state and thus causing thrombus formation. Lateral sinus occlusion may cause an increase in intracranial pressure. Infection of the thrombus clot may occur, and intraluminal abscess formation may be a late result. Progression of the thrombus or abscess may lead to occlusion of the inferior petrosal sinus, cavernous sinus, jugular bulb, or transverse sinus. Jugular foramen occlusion may cause jugular foramen syndrome with cranial nerves IX, X, and XI being involved.

The classic clinical symptoms of lateral sinus thrombosis include picket fence fever. The fever is thought to be the result of bacteremia that occurs as a result of the infected sinus. Between the fever spikes, the patient is alert and feels well. The fever spikes are associated with chills and profuse sweating and may occur every 24 hours. Griesinger's sign is pain over the ipsilateral mastoid caused by occlusion of the mastoid emissary vein. Antibiotics may mask the symptomatology, and a more indolent course may occur. This may include a low-grade fever, with a vague nonlocalizing headache. It may progress to symptoms similar to those of otic hydrocephalus, which will be discussed later.

The diagnosis of lateral sinus thrombosis requires a high index of suspicion. This entity should be considered when

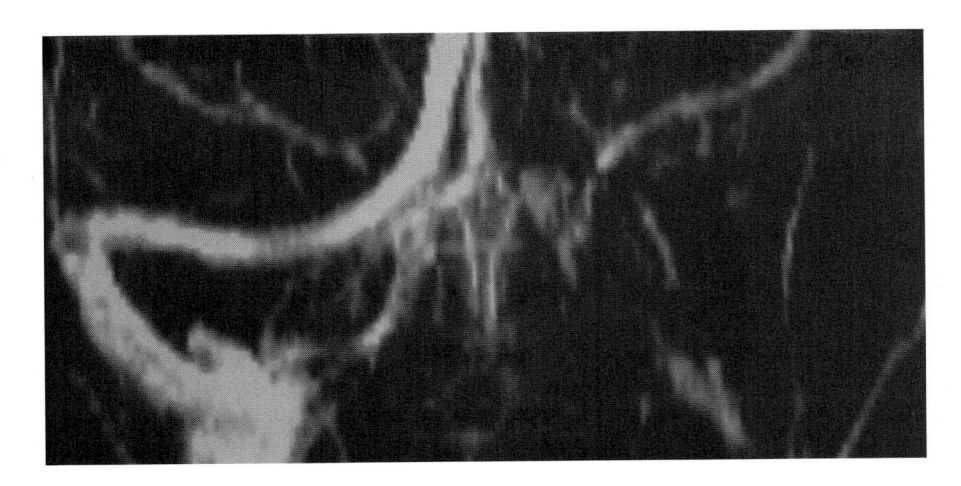

FIG. 8. Sigmoid sinus thrombosis. Magnetic resonance venogram demonstrates filling of the right transverse and sigmoid sinus. Absence of blood flow in the left sigmoid sinus is due to thrombosis. Reprinted with permission of House Ear Institute.

any other intracranial complications occur. The diagnosis may be confirmed with imaging studies. Radionuclide scans may detect septic pulmonary emboli and reveal venous sinus asymmetry, which is suggestive of thrombosis. The reliability of radionuclide scans is unknown in diagnosing lateral sinus thrombosis. However, systemic complications are detected with this study.

Computed tomography may not be able to determine the presence of a sigmoid sinus thrombosis. These studies require thin cuts with a concentrated contrast medium injected and special window settings. A routine CT may miss sigmoid sinus thrombosis and, therefore, is not recommended as the initial study.

Magnetic resonance imaging is considered the technique of choice for identifying lateral sinus thrombosis (Fig. 8). A high-intensity signal on both T1- and T2-weighted images is indicative of a venous thrombosis. Low-flow states also may cause a bright intraluminal signal, and, therefore, an MR angiogram may be required to determine the exact status of flow intraluminally. The enhancement is increased when compared with the opposite side. The use of contrast material will enhance the intensity seen on T1-weighted images. Magnetic resonance imaging also is useful in determining other intracranial complications that frequently occur with lateral sinus thrombosis.

The goal for treatment of lateral sinus thrombosis is to clear the infection and, hopefully, restore bloodflow while decreasing the risk of embolization. The underlying pathology must first be treated. The treatment of aseptic lateral sinus thrombosis is dependent on the patient's clinical symptoms. Initially, medical therapy with anticoagulation agents may be considered if the patient is only minimally symptomatic. If other pathology is present or the symptoms progress, surgical intervention is warranted. Mastoid exploration and treatment of any underlying cholesteatoma or chronic otitis within the temporal bone are first required. The bony plate covering the sigmoid sinus is first removed. Palpation of the sigmoid sinus may be deceptive because an early thrombus may have a soft clot. Palpation also is contraindicated because it may cause septic emboli. Needle aspiration is first performed to determine if blood flow is present. If blood flow is present, Avitene (MedChem Products, Inc. Woburn, Ma.) or Gelfoam (Upjohn Co., Kalamazoo, Mich.) may be placed over the puncture site and the wound closed. If no blood is aspirated, the sinus is opened and the thrombus or granulation tissue is removed. Prior to opening the sinus, the sinus is occluded both proximal and distal to the area of thrombus formation, with Surgicel (Johnson & Johnson, Arlington, Tx.) placed extraluminally between the dura of the sinus and the overlying bone to occlude the sinus. A vertical incision is then created and the thrombus aspirated. The Surgicel occluding the sinus is removed to ensure blood flow has been reestablished and all thrombi are removed. This first occurs inferiorly and then superiorly. Jugular vein ligation is rarely indicated unless septic emboli have occurred. If ligation is required, the jugular vein is ligated above the common facial vein. If granulation tissue is present, this should be removed until normal dura is seen. Septic lateral sinus thrombosis requires emergency surgery and broad-spectrum antibiotics.

EXTRADURAL ABSCESS

An extradural abscess results when purulent fluid collects between the dura and bone of the temporal bone. This most commonly occurs as a result of direct bone erosion next to the dura during the infectious process. Extradural abscesses also may occur as a result of thrombophlebitis of small venules or by spread of infection in preformed tissue planes. The size of the abscess is limited in the posterior fossa because the dura of the posterior fossa is tightly adherent to the internal auditory canal, subarcuate fossa, and the sigmoid sinus.

Patients may present with signs of otitis media and an associated headache. The headache may be localized over the region of the abscess. It is common, however, for the patient to be completely asymptomatic from the infection.

The diagnosis of an extradural abscess is usually made with a contrast-enhanced CT scan or an MRI (Fig. 9). These studies are important when an extradural abscess is suspected, to rule out coexisting brain abscess. A lumbar punc-

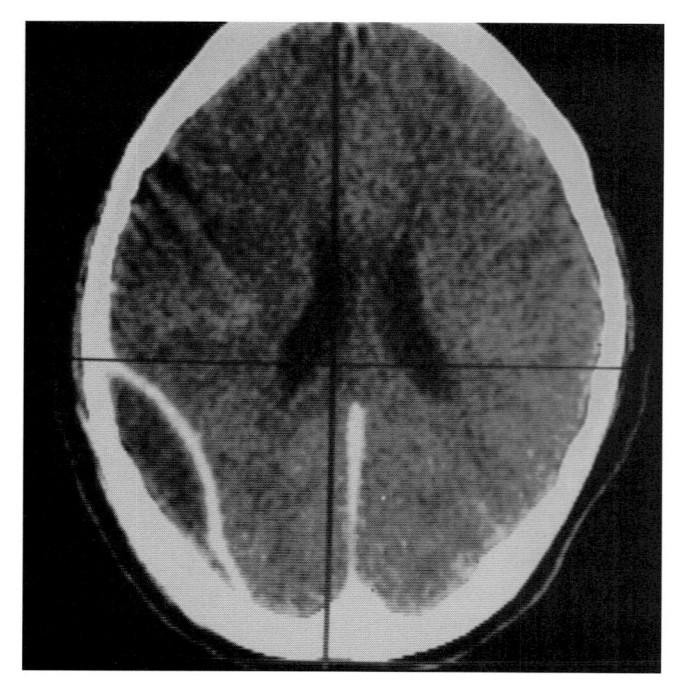

FIG. 9. Epidural abscess. Enhancing subdural abscess from chronic mastoiditis is seen in the left parietal occipital region. Reprinted with permission of House Ear Institute.

ture may reveal normal CSF chemistries. Extradural abscesses rarely produce a mass effect.

Extradural abscesses require appropriate antimicrobial therapy to prevent intradural complication. Surgical treatment of an extradural abscess requires removal of the bone adjacent to the abscess area to allow the drainage of abscess material into the mastoid cavity. Granulation tissue is uncovered, exposing the infected dura until normal dura is seen, ensuring that no remaining abscess or fluid collection is present. During the removal of granulation tissue, it is important to avoid piercing the inflamed dura because a resultant CSF leak may occur. Any corresponding cholesteatoma must be treated appropriately. Small cholesteatomas may be removed completely. A cholesteatoma matrix from large cholesteatomas may be left on the dura, because this is commonly very adherent to the dura. In a large mastoid cavity, a meatoplasty must be created to ensure adequate drainage.

BRAIN ABSCESS

A brain abscess may occur with an episode of acute otitis media or chronic otitis media. It can occur at the time of the infection or up to a month following the infection. The purulent abscess is surrounded by a zone of encephalitis. This space-occupying lesion may produce a mass effect. Brain abscesses usually result from perivascular extension of an infection or may occur by retrograde thrombosis. If the abscess persists for 5 to 6 weeks, a fibrous capsule is formed, surrounding the abscess. As the advancing area of acute inflammation expands, brain destruction occurs. The location of the brain abscess is usually in close proximity to the area of the temporal bone affected by otitis media, typically in the temporal lobe and cerebellar regions. The temporal lobe abscess is more common than a cerebellar abscess. Herniation of the temporal lobe may occur as a late result of the mass effect, or overwhelming sepsis may occur if the abscess ruptures into the ventricular system.

Presenting symptoms of a brain abscess may include fever, a severe headache, nausea, vomiting, seizure, or mental status changes. The diagnosis is made with CT or MRI. A ring-enhancing mass within the parenchyma of the brain is seen on these studies (Fig. 10). A lumbar puncture is contraindicated due to the risk of herniation from the mass effect. Cerebrospinal fluid studies may be normal in the presence of brain abscess.

Mixed infections predominate with brain abscess (18). Aerobic gram-positive cocci, such as *streptococcus* and *staphylococcus,* are the most common aerobic organisms involved in brain abscesses. *Proteus* species are the most common gram-negative bacilli, and anaerobic organisms also may be found (19).

A patient with a brain abscess is initially placed on broad-

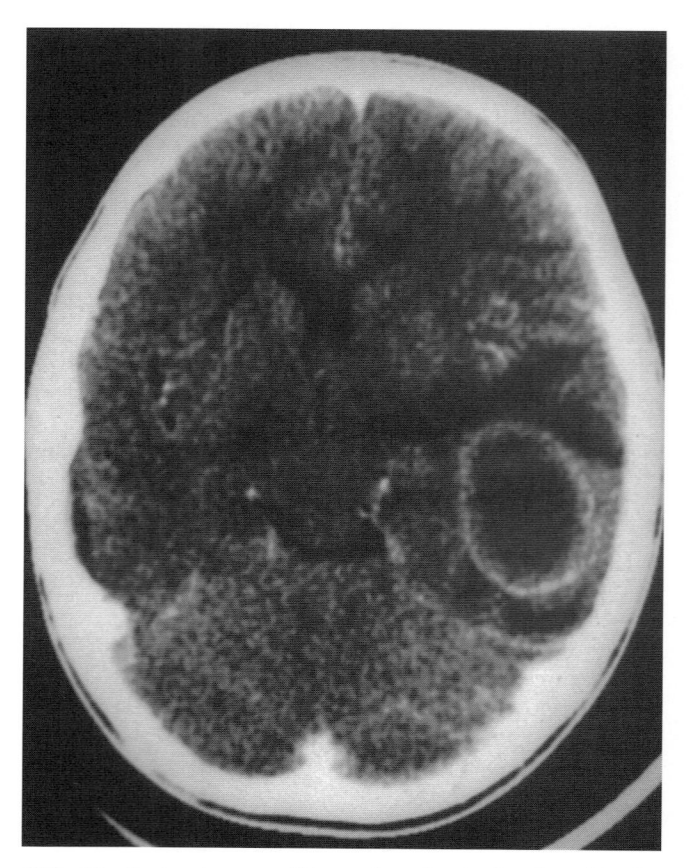

FIG. 10. Brain abscess. Ring-enhancing lesion found in the temporal area as a result of chronic otitis media. Treatment is aimed at draining the abscess and adminstration of intravenous antibiotics. Reprinted with permission of House Ear Institute.

spectrum systemic antibiotics covering the organisms just described. Intravenous steroids are used to help decrease surrounding brain inflammation and decrease the risk of permanent brain damage. The abscess is drained as soon as the patient is able to withstand general anesthesia. The procedure is performed through a clean field when otitis media is present. A formal craniotomy may be performed with drainage of the abscess cavity, or aspiration of the abscess may be performed through a burr hole. There is no need to remove the abscess wall because this may cause further brain damage. The purulent material must be removed to prevent brain destruction. Aspiration may need to be repeated because fluid may recur with this technique. The underlying mastoid disease is then treated, with timing dependent on the clinical situation.

OTIC HYDROCEPHALUS

Otic hydrocephalus may result as a complication of otitis media. This condition presents when an increase in intracranial pressure occurs despite signs of hydrocephalus evident on imaging studies (i.e., normal ventricular size). This is believed to be associated with lateral sinus thrombosis that results in a decreased absorption in the arachnoid granulation secondary to a decreased bloodflow (20). Thus, the decreased absorption of CSF results in an increased intracranial pressure. This may be seen as a complication of otitis media and is also seen following other neurotologic procedures when sigmoid sinus thrombosis occurs.

The presenting symptoms of otic hydrocephalus mimic those found with increased intracranial pressure, including headache, vomiting, and pappilledema. A unilateral or bilateral sixth nerve palsy may occur, with resultant blurred vision. Severe pappilledema may lead to optic atrophy and blindness. The diagnosis is made when the presenting signs are consistent with otic hydrocephalus, as described, and the CT and MRI scans do not demonstrate evidence of increased intracranial pressure. A lateral sinus thrombosis may be visualized. A lumbar puncture will demonstrate elevated opening pressures. The CSF pressure may be over 300 mm Hg.

The treatment of acute otic hydrocephalus includes treatment of the underlying ear disease. This would include a mastoidectomy for mastoiditis or associated lateral sinus thrombosis. (Treatment of lateral sinus thrombosis was discussed earlier.) The increased intracranial pressure must be reduced, and acetazolamide is commonly used for this purpose. Other diuretics, such as Lasix or mannitol, also may be used. The increased intracranial pressure may take weeks to months to completely return to normal. A long-term otic hydrocephalus rarely occurs. Visual fields should be monitored, because visual field changes occur prior to changes in visual acuity with increased intracranial pressure. This may require ventricular peritoneal shunting. The prevention of blindness from this disorder is imperative.

CONCLUSION

Despite antibiotics, complications from otitis media still occur. It is important for the clinician to recognize these life-threatening disease processes early in order to provide prompt and appropriate treatment. Currently, discussions regarding the treatment of otitis media include limiting antibiotics to reduce the risk of superinfection. Equal concern must be devoted to avoiding more serious complications, which may result from withholding necessary medical intervention.

REFERENCES

1. Turner AL, Reynolds FE. *Intracranial pyogenic diseases.* Edinburgh: Oliver & Boyd; 1931.
2. Jeanes A. Otogenic intracranial suppuration. *J Laryngol* 1962;76:388.
3. Palva T, Virtanen H, Mäkinen J. Acute and latent mastoiditis in children. *J Laryngol Otol* 1985;99:127.
4. Wright CG, Meyerhoff WL. Pathology of otitis media. *Ann Otol Rhinol Laryngol* 1994;103(Suppl 163):24.
5. Fria TJ, Cantekin EI, Eichler JA. Hearing acuity of children with otitis media with effusion. *Arch Otolaryngol* 1985;111:10.
6. Menyuk P. Effects of hearing loss on language acquisition in the babbling stage. In: Jaffee BF, ed. *Hearing loss in children.* Baltimore: University Park Press; 1977:621.
7. Stool SE, Berg AO, Berman S, et al. *Otitis media with effusion in young children.* Clinical Practice Guideline; Number 12. AHCPR Publication No. 94-0622. Rockville, MD: U.S. Agency for Health Care Policy and Research, Public Health Service, Department of Health and Human Services, 1994.
8. Bhaya MH, Schachern PA, Morizono T, Paparella MM. Pathogenesis of tympanosclerosis. *Otolaryngol Head Neck Surg* 1993;109:413.
9. Tos M, Bonding P, Poulsen G. Tympanosclerosis of the drum in secretory otitis after insertion of grommets. A prospective, comparative study. *J Laryngol Otol* 1983;97:489.
10. Gibb AG, Pang YT. Current considerations in the etiology and diagnosis of tympanosclerosis. *Eur Arch Otorhinolaryngol* 1994;251:439.
11. Schuknecht HF. *Pathology of the ear.* 2nd ed. Philadelphia: Lea & Febiger; 1993:211.
12. Margolis RH, Hunter LL, Rykken JR, Giebink GS. Effects of otitis media on extended high-frequency hearing in children. *Ann Otol Rhinol Laryngol* 1993;102:1.
13. Harada T, Yamasoba T, Yagi M. Sensorineural hearing loss associated with otitis media with effusion. *ORL* 1992;54:61.
14. Hariri MA. Sensorineural hearing loss in bullous myringitis. A prospective study of eighteen patients. *Clin Otolaryngol* 1990;15:351.
15. Paparella MM, Goycoolea MV, Meyerhoff WL. Inner ear pathology and otitis media. A review. *Ann Otol Rhinol Laryngol* 1980;89(Suppl 68):249.
16. Shambaugh GH Jr. *Surgery of the ear.* 2nd ed. Philadelphia: WB Saunders; 1967.
17. Giddings NA, Brackmann DE, Kwartler JA. Transcanal infracochlear approach to the petrous apex. *Otolaryngol Head Neck Surg* 1991;104:29.
18. Ayyagari A, Pancholi VK, Kak VK, et al. Bacteriological spectrum of brain abscess with special reference to anaerobic bacteria. *Indian J Med Res* 1983;77:182.
19. Neely JG. Complications of temporal bone infection. In: Cummings CW, ed. *Otolaryngology head and neck surgery.* St. Louis: Mosby; 1986:2988.
20. Symmonds CP. Hydrocephalic and focal cerebral symptoms in relation to thrombophlebitis of the dural sinus and cerebral veins. *Brain* 1937;60:531.

CHAPTER 18

Acute Mastoiditis

Nikolas H. Blevins and Anil K. Lalwani

The term *acute mastoiditis* (AM) incorporates a spectrum of suppurative complications of acute otitis media. Because there is a continuum of disease severity and clinical presentation, the actual definition of this disease often remains unclear. The mastoid–air-cell system is normally continuous with the middle-ear cleft via the additus ad antrum and is therefore involved in the vast majority of uncomplicated cases of acute otitis media (acute tympanomastoiditis) (AOM). Histopathologic studies have confirmed that acute mastoiditis, strictly defined as an inflammation of the mastoid air cell mucosa, is present from the first day of an AOM (1). Therefore, AOM is in fact an acute tympanomastoiditis, and the term acute mastoiditis could theoretically be applied in every case of uncomplicated otitis.

Such definition of acute mastoiditis, however, is not clinically useful, especially because there exists an acute infectious disease of the mastoid largely independent of the middle-ear cleft, which requires therapy beyond that needed for common AOM. The term acute mastoiditis has therefore historically referred to the suppurative extension of AOM in which not only the mucosa of the mastoid air cells is involved, but also its periosteum, bone, or both. It is useful to subdivide AM into two categories on the basis of whether the bone of the mastoid is involved (2). These categories are (a) AM with periosteitis and (b) coalescent AM (AM with osteitis). This distinction has important clinical ramifications in determining the best course of treatment. A variation, classified as subacute mastoiditis, also exits, characterized by a protracted time course and a paucity of clinical symptoms. The definitions used in this chapter are shown in Table 1; one should remember that the definitions are still an attempt to subdivide a spectrum of disease.

N.H. Blevins: Department of Otolaryngology—Head and Neck Surgery, Tufts University School of Medicine, New England Medical Center, Boston, Massachusetts 02111.

A.K. Lalwani: Department of Otolaryngology—Head and Neck Surgery, University of California at San Francisco, San Francisco, California 94117.

The incidence of acute mastoiditis has sharply declined since the introduction of antibiotics for the treatment of otitis media (3–10). Before the introduction of antibiotics, acute mastoiditis was the most common suppurative complication of AOM, diagnosed in as much as 25% to 50% of cases (3). Its frequency and multiple serious complications, including high mortality, prompted surgical intervention in as much as 20% of all cases of AOM (11). After the introduction of sulfonamide in 1935 and penicillin in 1944, the incidence of AM dropped to 3% to 6% with an 86% reduction of mortality (11,12). The incidence continued to decline as antibiotics became more effective and widely used. Palva reported a 0.4% incidence of AM of all AOM in 1959, but with a 0.004% incidence in the 1980s (13). Another series from 1986 estimated an incidence of 0.02% of all AOM in Sweden (14). Despite these encouraging statistics, AM still persists. Some authors have noted a recent increase in its occurrence and have suggested that reduced or inappropriate antibiotic treatment for AOM may be partly responsible for this trend (9,10,15,16).

PATHOPHYSIOLOGY AND EPIDEMIOLOGY

Pathophysiology

AM is the result of the inoculation of the mastoid–air-cell system from AOM, and subsequent anatomic isolation of the infected mastoid from the middle-ear, allowing the mastoid infection to progress independent of the middle ear component. The stages of the development and progression of AM may be summarized as follows: (a) AOM, (b) attic blockade, (c) AM with periosteitis, (d) coalescent AM, and (e) extension.

Acute Tympanomastoiditis

The development of AM begins with AOM (Fig. 1). Because the mastoid antrum and air cells are normally continuous with the middle ear cleft through the additus ad antrum, infection can freely spread from the middle ear to the mas-

TABLE 1. *Definitions*

Acute mastoiditis—Rapidly progressive (usually <2 weeks) suppurative complication of acute otitis media with infection of the mastoid involving periosteum and/or bone presenting with erythema, tenderness, and edema of the retroauricular soft tissues
  Acute mastoiditis with periosteitis—Infection of the periosteum of the mastoid and overlying soft tissues without osteitis
  Acute coalescent mastoiditis (acute mastoiditis with osteitis, surgical mastoiditis)—Osteitis of the mastoid with bone destruction
Subacute mastoiditis (masked mastoiditis, silent mastoiditis, latent mastoiditis)—Slowly evolving (usually >2 weeks) infection of the mastoid with mild clinical symptoms which may progress to involve periosteum and/or bone
Chronic mastoiditis (chronic otitis media)—Long-standing (>2 months) infection involving the middle ear and mastoid with tympanic-membrane perforation and otorrhea

toid air cells, producing the common acute tympanomastoiditis. At this stage, the mucosa is hyperemic and edematous. Mucopurulent material collects in both the mastoid air cells and the middle-ear cleft. In most cases, when the purulence is allowed to drain from the middle ear either through the eustachian tube or through a tympanic-membrane perforation, even untreated AOM abates at this stage.

Attic Blockade

During the course of the infection, the normal anatomic continuity between the antrum and the middle ear may be lost, producing attic blockade (Fig. 2). If separation occurs, mucopurulent material in the mastoid may be left undrained despite the normal egress of pus from the middle ear though the eustachian tube or tympanic-membrane perforation. In this case, otoscopy of the middle-ear space may be largely unrevealing of the persistent disease in the mastoid. The obstruction may be secondary to reversible mucosal edema, and antibiotic therapy may be sufficient to reestablish the drainage pathway.

With prolonged or severe infection, the anatomic alterations causing the blockage may be refractory to routine medical intervention (17,18). Granulation tissue may form after about 1 week of low-grade inflammation, causing loculation of regions of the air-cell system or complete separation of the mastoid air cells from the middle ear cleft. The mucosa may also become thickened by an organized fibrinous exudate and adhesion formation. Glandular hypertrophy leads to further obstruction by causing mucosal thickening and increasing the volume of mucoid exudate. In addition, osteoneogenesis is stimulated by infection. The resultant hypertrophic and sclerotic bone may contribute to the deformation of normal drainage pathways.

Acute Mastoiditis with Periosteitis

An undrained collection of pus in the mastoid may then spread infection to involve the periosteum overlying the mastoid bone (Fig. 3). This probably occurs though venous pathways and accounts for the physical findings of retroauricular pain, swelling, and induration. Periosteitis should be differentiated from the more severe subperiosteal abscess, which results from the contiguous spread of purulence through the mastoid cortex, because AM with periosteitis does not necessarily require surgical therapy. However, if left inadequately treated, AM with periosteitis may progress to coalescent mastoiditis.

Coalescent Mastoiditis

If mastoid purulence remains undrained, the infection can spread to the bone itself, resulting in coalescent mastoiditis

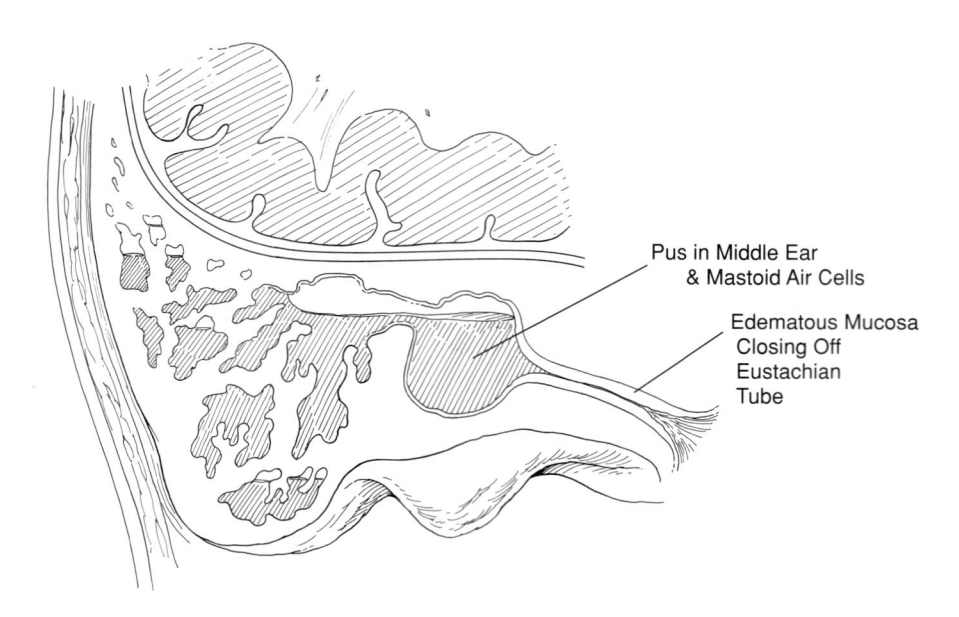

FIG. 1. Acute otitis media.

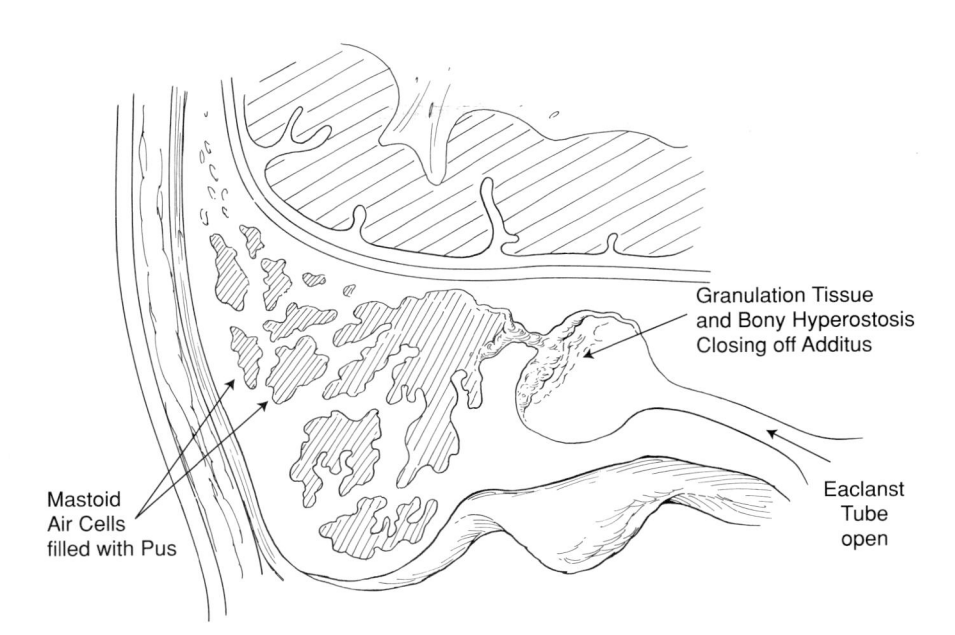

FIG. 2. Attic blockade.

or AM with osteitis (Fig. 4). Pus under pressure can cause necrosis and demineralization of the bony trabeculae of the mastoid–air-cell system. The resultant bony resorption then leads to a coalescence of the mastoid abscess. This situation requires surgery to reestablish the drainage and aeration pathways for resolution.

Extension

Once osteitis has been established, the loss of bony architecture expands until the abscess can drain (Fig. 5). This may occur in several described directions: (a) laterally through the cortex of the mastoid process, resulting in a subperiosteal abscess, which is the most common finding; (b) medially though the petrous air cells resulting in petrositis, with possible involvement of the labyrinth, facial nerve, or both; (c) anteriorly into the middle ear, which may spontaneously reestablish a drainage pathway allowing resolution. (d) inferiorly through the mastoid tip medial to the digastric muscle and dissecting into the upper neck, forming a Bezold's abscess (Fig. 6). (e) posteriorly to result in occipital calvarial osteomyelitis or dural sinus thrombophlebitis; (f) intracranially, resulting in epidural abscess, subdural empyema, or meningitis.

Epidemiology

Children of any age may develop AM, although the majority are younger than 10 years old. Recent reports have demonstrated a trend towards a greater percentage occurring in

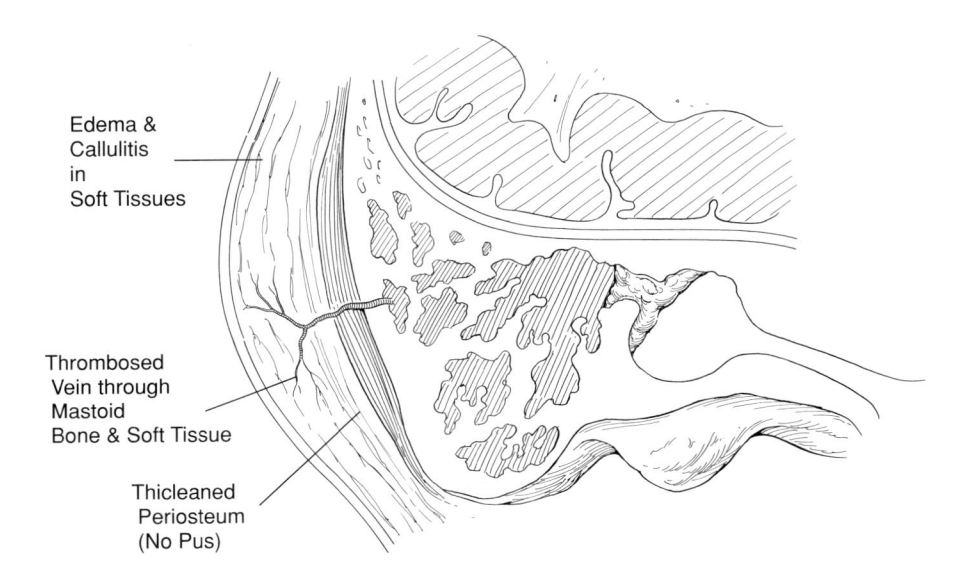

FIG. 3. Acute mastoiditis with periosteitis.

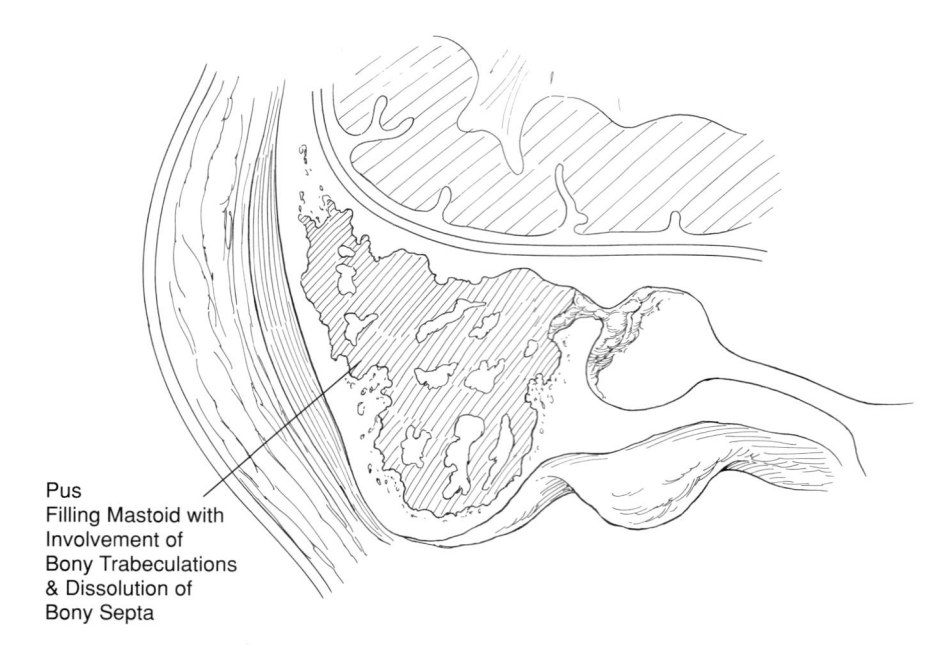

Pus Filling Mastoid with Involvement of Bony Trabeculations & Dissolution of Bony Septa

FIG. 4. Coalescent mastoiditis.

infancy, with as many as 60% of patients being younger than 24 months old (6,16,19). At birth, only a single air cell, the mastoid antrum, is present. Additional mastoid pneumatization develops predominantly during the next 2 years, although further development may continue throughout life. As a result of this incomplete pneumatization, only a small percentage of cases of AM were found in the first year of life. In 1891, St. John Roosa reported only 2 of 93 cases to occur in infants (20). Similar findings exist in countries in which antibiotics are not readily available. A review from Nigeria in 1985 found no infants in 42 cases of AM (21).

In 1984, Scott and Jackler proposed that the use of antibiotics has been more effective in reducing the incidence of AM in older children than it has in infants, thus producing a relative increase in frequency of AM in the first year of life. This may be secondary to the relative difficulty of diagnosing AOM in infancy. The narrow nature of the external canal may impede otoscopy, and the nonspecific symptoms from otitis in this age group may prevent the efficacious use of antibiotics (18).

Patients with AM are usually healthy and without significant otologic history. The majority of patients with AM have

Epidural Abscess

Subperiosteal Abscess

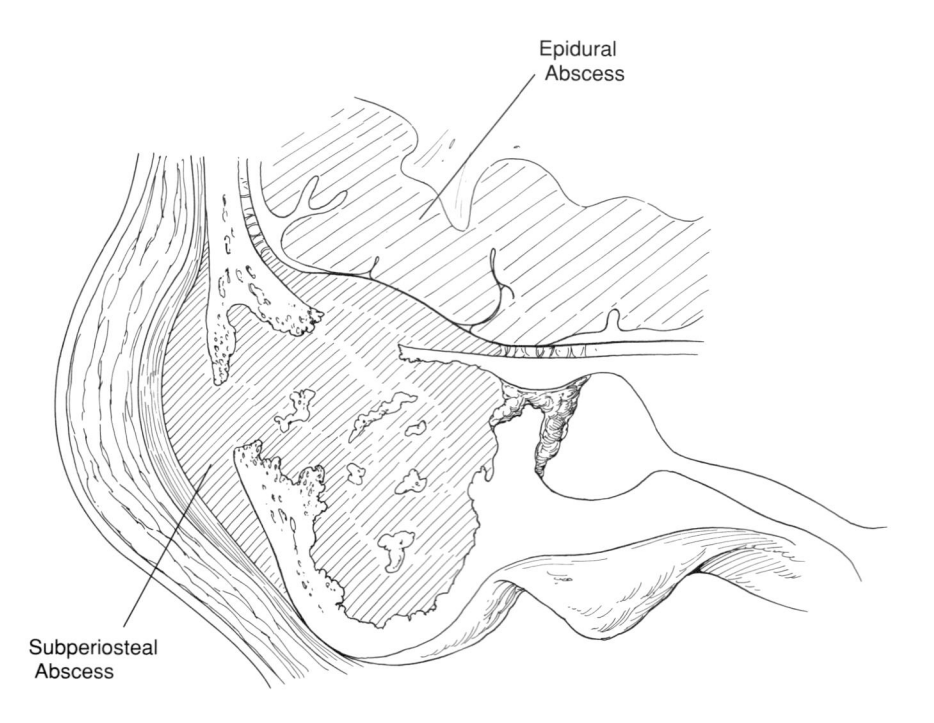

FIG. 5. Extension.

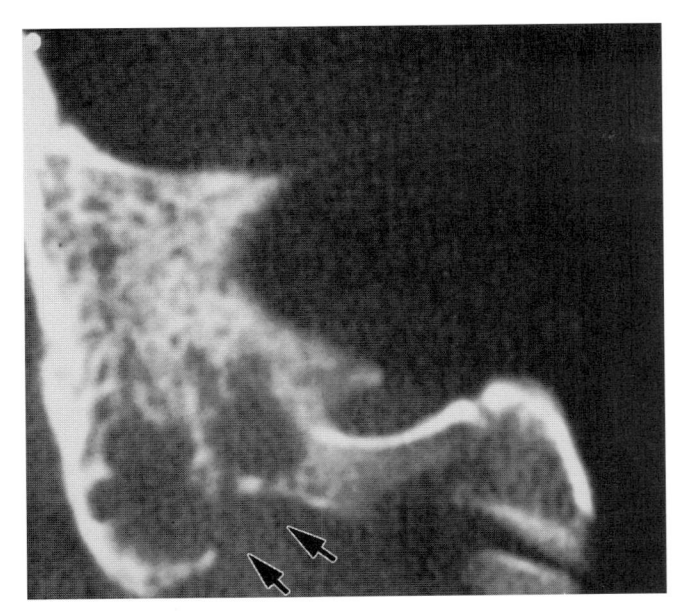

FIG. 6. Bezold's abscess. Coronal CT of a patient with otitis media that has extended into the upper neck, resulting in a Bezold's abscess. The cortex of the medial mastoid tip is eroded (*arrows*) and purulence has spread medial to the digastric muscle into the neck.

had no previously documented episodes of AOM. Recent reviews suggest that more than 75% have no history of otitis (9,16,19,22). However, in countries in which rapid administration of antibiotics for otitis is not the rule, the majority of AM is seen complicating long-standing chronic otitis media (21). The incidence of AM appears to be more common in boys, with the reported male to female ratios from 1:1 to 3.5:1 (14,16,19,21). Bilateral AM has been reported, but is quite rare (10,16).

The likelihood that a child has received antibiotics prior to presentation with AM is dependent on the characteristics of the population surveyed and the availability of antibiotic therapy. Several recent reviews indicate that as many as 36% to 72% of cases of AM developed despite previous antibiotic treatment (9,14,19,22,23). It has been suggested that previous treatment with antibiotics may be responsible for a relative increase in the incidence of subacute (masked) mastoiditis (24). Symptoms evolve slowly and are often minimal, although the risk for serious neurologic complications remains high. The initial treatment may suppress systemic toxicity and otologic symptoms while reducing middle-ear inflammation significantly to prevent spontaneous rupture and drainage of middle-ear purulence. If there is an isolated collection of purulence in the mastoid secondary to loculation or attic blockade or if early osteitis is present, antibiotic concentrations may be insufficient to eradicate the mastoid component of the infection. However, the correlation between the chronicity of the mastoiditis and previous treatment has not been definitively established, because both the classic and subacute forms can occur regardless of prior antibiotic administration (10,19,25). It appears that the strength of an individual's immune system relative to the virulence of the pathogens also plays a significant role in the development of the disease process (24,26,27). At surgery, these patients may have chronic inflammatory changes with granulation tissue within the mastoid air cells, or coalescence of bony septations and mature abscess formation (10,19).

Microbiology

The most common pathogens responsible for AM are listed in Table 2. These data are derived from a number of case series (6,9,14,19,23). The cultures are often of mixed pathogens. The responsible flora are similar, although not identical to the spectrum of bacteria known to frequently cause AOM. *Streptococcus pneumoniae* remains the most commonly found pathogen, followed by *S. pyogenes, Staphylococcus aureus,* and *Haemophilus influenzae.* Anaerobes such as *Bacteroides* and *Peptostreptococcus,* and gram-negative bacilli such as *Pseudomonas, Klebsiella, Escherichia coli,* and *Proteus* species are also represented. Patients previously treated with antimicrobials are less likely to show growth on bacterial cultures (14). The bacterial spectrum of AM has changed significantly since the widespread use of antibiotics for otitis media. *S. pyogenes,* for example, which formerly accounted for about half the cases of AOM, is now is responsible for less than 20% (28). In one study, patients previously treated with antibiotics and who had positive cultures yielded no *Streptococcus* species, but more than 70% of those previously untreated grew at least one of the pathogens (14). This is likely an indication of the efficacy of most antibiotic regiments against these bacteria. In one study, *S. pyogenes* was found to be the most prevalent organism. This brought into question the initial use of trimethoprim-sulfamethoxazole antibiotics for AOM in this population, because this combination is often ineffective against this organism (7).

H. influenzae is rarely found in AM in contrast to its incidence in AOM in children and adults, which may approach

TABLE 2. *Microbiology of acute mastoiditis*

Organism	Approximate incidence (%)
No growth	(20–30)
Streptococcus pneumoniae	(15–40)
Streptococcus pyogenes	(10–20)
Staphylococcus aureus	(5–15)
Haemophilus influenzae	(5–15)
Anaerobes (*Bacteroides, Peptostreptococcus*)	(<10)
Gram-negative bacilli (*Proteus, Pseudomonas, Escherichia coli, Klebsiella*)	(<10)

Table shows the most prevalent pathogens responsible for AM on the basis of combined findings of a number of clinical series (6,9,14,19,23).

25% (29,30). The low incidence in AM does not seem to be secondary to antibiotic resistance or use of vaccine for haemophilus (19,31). One possible explanation is that *H. influenzae* has a relatively low tendency towards bone invasion which may be necessary in the pathogenesis of AM (6). Conversely, *Staph. aureus* is a much more common pathogen in AM (about 10%) than it is in pediatric AOM (about 1%) (29). Similar reasoning may explain this discrepancy, given that *Staph. aureus* has a tendency toward invasion of bone and is a common pathogen in osteomyelitis elsewhere in the body. Conventional doses of antibiotics sufficient to eradicate common AOM may not achieve therapeutic concentrations in bone. Therefore, bacteria that can establish osteitis early are more likely to progress into suppurative complications.

Gram-negative bacilli and anaerobes are more likely to be responsible for subacute form of mastoiditis (2,24). Gram-negative bacilli are also known to be a more common cause of AOM in infants than in older children (32), and so their presence should be especially considered in the very young. Although gram-negative bacilli appear more commonly in patients previously treated with antibiotics, they can also cause AM in untreated groups. The presence of anaerobic pathogens may be related to an increased risk of intracranial complications resulting from clinically silent mastoiditis (9,33).

Immunocompromised Host

The incidence of AM in immunocompromised children, such as those with congenital deficiencies, transplants, or acquired immunodeficiency syndrome (AIDS) is not currently known. The immunocompromised child does not figure prominently into series of AM in the literature. Although immunocompromised children with AM have been reported (10), the majority of patients are otherwise healthy. Therefore, AM by itself is not an indication of an impaired immune system. However, AIDS is known to increase a child s risk for acute and chronic otitis media (34,35) and has also been shown to alter the histopathologic structure of the middle ear and mastoid system in adults, showing the presence of granulation tissue and chronic inflammatory changes which could effectively alter the normal drainage pattern (36). In addition, human immunodeficiency virus (HIV)-infected children appear to be at greater risk from *S. pneumoniae* infections, a common pathogen in AM (37). All these findings tend to suggest that HIV-infected children are at greater risk for the development of AM, however, this remains to be shown. Debilitated patients and those with diabetes appear to be at greater risk for the subacute form of mastoiditis (24,26,27).

Although the majority of infections in the immunocompromised are caused by routine pathogens, all cases of otitis in the immunocompromised patient must raise suspicion for unusual organisms. *Mycobacterium,* fungus, and *Pneumocystis carinii* may all cause otitis the immunocompromised child, and appropriate stains and cultures should be done. In addition, the differential diagnosis of a postauricular mass must be broadened to include additional neoplastic processes commonly seen in this population (e.g., lymphoma, Kaposi's sarcoma).

CLINICAL MANIFESTATIONS AND DIAGNOSIS

The classic presentation of AM involves the development of retroauricular pain, erythema, and a protruding pinna shortly following an episode of an upper respiratory infection with AOM (Fig. 7). However, the presentation is highly variable. Signs of AM usually occur 10 to 14 days before presentation, and weeks may pass before the diagnosis of AM is made (10,19,23). Significantly shorter periods may also be found, with symptoms developing within days. Many children present with AM as the first sign of ear disease. Therefore, the lack of a distinct upper respiratory infection or AOM prodrome does not exclude the diagnosis of AM (7,10,23). Furthermore, the majority of children with AM have no antecedent history of otologic disease (9,16,19,22). Nonspecific symptoms such as otalgia, headache, rhinorrhea, and hearing loss are common. A low-grade fever is often present.

Otoscopy generally shows evidence of AOM with a purulent effusion. A tympanic-membrane perforation with purulent drainage, causing the accumulation of pus and debris in the external auditory canal, may be present in a minority of children. Careful cleaning of the ear should be performed with the aid of a microscope. There may be edema or sagging of the posterosuperior external auditory canal from periosteal thickening adjacent to the additus. Occasionally, the

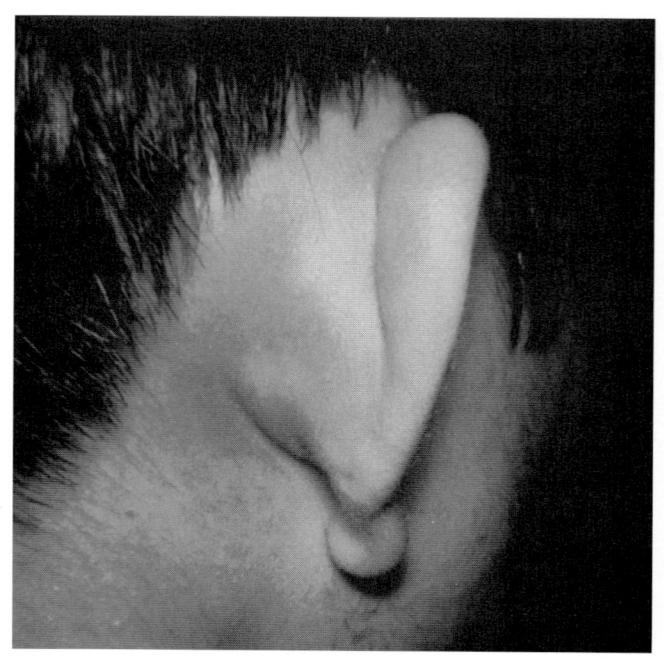

FIG. 7. Acute mastoiditis.

middle ear is free from signs of infection despite the presence of AM. This occurs in patients in whom the additus ad antrum has been blocked by edematous mucosa or granulation tissue. In this setting, the middle-ear component of the infection may resolve because the space is drained through a functioning eustachian tube, loculated pus remains in the mastoid cavity. Therefore, a relatively normal-appearing middle ear does not exclude the possibility of acute mastoiditis.

The soft tissue overlying the mastoid is tender, red, and thickened, causing the classic inferolateral displacement of the pinna (see Fig. 6). This may be secondary to either soft-tissue edema in AM with periosteitis, or the accumulation of frank pus in the subperiosteal space as is often seen in coalescent mastoiditis. The differentiation between the two conditions can be difficult on clinical grounds alone, although occasionally fluctuance or a draining fistula may be present. In the presence of equivocal physical findings, a temporal computed tomography (CT) scan of the bone can aid differentiation. In the physical examination one should meticulously search for the extension of an abscess into the surrounding soft tissues. The upper neck should be examined for the presence of a Bezold abscess (pus deep to the sternocleidomastoid muscle secondary to erosion of the mastoid tip bone). Additional adjacent soft-tissue abscesses may be present, and draining fistulas may occasionally be encountered.

A complete neurologic examination should be performed for evidence of intracranial and intratemporal suppurative complications. The presence of meningeal signs, suggestive of meningeal irritation, should be evaluated, with appropriate radiologic imaging followed by lumbar puncture. A complete cranial nerve examination should be performed. Cranial nerve VI may be involved if the infection has spread to the petrous apex (Gradenigo syndrome). Cranial nerve VII may be weak if the process has involved the fallopian canal. If possible, auditory function should be assessed with the Weber test, Rinne test, and formal audiometry. A conductive loss is expected if middle-ear effusion exists. A sensorineural deficit may be indicative of labyrinthitis and direct spread of infection into the inner ear. In this case, vertigo and nystagmus may also be prominent findings.

Hematologic studies can be abnormal, although they are not specific for AM. White blood cell (WBC) counts are often mildly elevated, ranging from normal to about 30,000/ μl. The mean is approximately 15,000 μl (14,19). About half the patients have an erythrocyte sedimentation rate greater than 30 mm/hr (9).

Appropriate cultures should be obtained as soon as possible in cases of suspected AM. In draining ears, care should be taken to obtain a representative specimen by first cleaning the ear of accumulated purulent debris and then obtaining a fresh sample of the drainage at the perforation site with a thin cotton swab. If the tympanic membrane is intact, culture should be obtained through tympanocentesis or at the time of myringotomy under sterile conditions. The advantage of tympanocentesis is that it allows the cultures to be sent early so that antibiotics may be begun while the child is undergoing evaluation for general anesthesia. The use of blood cultures has been found to be of low yield, and is probably not needed unless the patient is septic (9). A postauricular aspirate of the subperiosteal space has been advocated to obtain cultures (7,22). All culture specimens should be handled appropriately for anaerobic cultures and transported promptly to maximize the yield of potential anaerobic pathogens.

Subacute Mastoiditis

Patients with subacute mastoiditis display a significantly different clinical picture than do those with classic AM. Subacute mastoiditis is a more slowly evolving variant of mastoiditis. It has alternatively been called "silent," "masked," or "latent" mastoiditis because of the paucity of clinical symptoms (7,10,24,25,38). Subacute mastoiditis represents a more indolent infection, developing over weeks or months, and associated with minimal otologic symptoms. It may develop from a recurrent or refractory otitis media. Pain, mastoid erythema, and protrusion of the pinna are usually absent. In fact, the development of a regional suppurative complication may be the first indication of the presence of mastoid disease (24,19,39). One review found an association between intractable infantile diarrhea and subacute mastoiditis, although the mechanism of this association remains unclear (40).

Radiology

Radiographic evaluation is useful to demonstrate both the nature of local disease in the mastoid, and the extension of infection to adjacent regions. Plain x-rays may show mastoid cloudiness from the presence of fluid or soft tissue within the air space (19,24). Bone demineralization and coalescence in the presence of osteitis may also be seen on x-ray. Although mastoid films are generally sensitive to the presence of mastoid disease, they may be normal despite the classic clinical appearance of AM (6,9,19,22). At present, the use of x-ray has largely been replaced by CT scanning, which is both more sensitive and specific for alterations in mastoid bone and air cells.

High-resolution CT images in both axial and coronal planes remain the standard for imaging mastoid bony architecture. Intravenous contrast should be used to clarify the presence of local suppurative extension. In the early stages of acute mastoiditis, as in AOM, the mastoid–air-cell system is opacified by either soft tissue or an effusion. As the process spreads to the overlying mastoid periosteum (AM with periosteitis), soft tissue edema and enhancement of the mastoid periosteum may be evident. As the disease progresses to coalescent mastoiditis, decalcification of bony trabeculae may be seen, with loss of normal septations. Loss of the mastoid cortex is evident along with an adjacent purulent collection in cases of coalescent mastoiditis with subperiosteal abscess. In cases of long-standing infection, sclerosis of the mastoid bone with obliteration of normal air-cell spaces may be evident secondary to a hypertrophic inflammatory reaction. Additional local extension of infection, whether intratemporal (e.g., petrous apecitis) or intracranial (e.g., epidural abscess), may also be seen in an enhanced CT series.

Magnetic resonance imaging (MRI) does not define bony anatomy as well as does CT scanning; thus it is not the modality of choice to define the extent of local disease in AM. However, MRI with gadolinium enhancement is more sensitive in detecting subtle soft-tissue alterations from infection and is thus better in identifying early intracranial suppurative complications. Therefore, an enhanced MRI of the head and skull base should be performed whenever intracranial extension is clinically suspected.

Differential Diagnosis

Postauricular swelling in children may be secondary to eosinophilic granuloma, rhabdomyosarcoma, and branchial cleft anomalies (41,42). Atypical infections, such as tuberculosis, may also produce similar symptoms even in immunocompetent individuals. Appropriate skin testing should be pursued in populations at risk for exposure to such pathogens.

MANAGEMENT

The goals for management of AM include the resolution of middle ear and mastoid disease, the preservation of a normally functioning and aerated ear, and most important, the prevention of potentially serious neurologic complications. The treatment armamentarium includes intravenous antibiotics, myringotomy, and simple mastoidectomy and drainage. The degree to which these options are used remains controversial, although it is reasonable to modify the therapy on the basis of the individual patient's clinical picture. It is worth noting that the clinician should be concerned with prevention of AM by timely use of appropriate antibiotics for suppurative otitis media. In addition, the need for patient compliance with the full course of treatment should be stressed to prevent future episodes of AM.

Antibiotic Choice

Once the diagnosis of AM has been made, hospital admission with administration of an appropriate intravenous antibiotic remains central in the treatment. Treatment should not be delayed, although it is preferable that cultures be sent first to maximize the yield of the responsible pathogen. The agent used should be specific for bacteria commonly found in AM and should be directed by culture results as soon as they are available. Pending the return of culture information, an initial antibiotic such as cefuroxime, which adequately covers most likely pathogens, is a sound choice. Intravenous antibiotics should be continued until significant clinical improvement is apparent (usually 3–4 days), and then the child should be switched to oral antimicrobials. Oral antibiotics should be continued for a total treatment period of about 3 weeks.

Surgery

The indications and timing for surgery in AM remains the topic of some debate. Myringotomy should be performed in all cases of AM associated with an intact tympanic membrane. A ventilating tube may be placed to ensure continued patency. The tube provides aeration of the middle-ear cleft and, potentially, the mastoid air cells once the anatomic continuity of the additus is restored. Myringotomy yields material for culture. If the diagnosis of AM with periosteitis is made clinically and there is no bone destruction or intracranial or intratemporal extensions on radiographic evaluation, intravenous antibiotics combined with myringotomy are often sufficient therapy. The patient must be observed closely to assess the possible progression to coalescent mastoiditis and abscess formation. Clinical improvement is expected in the first 24 to 48 hours of treatment. Cortical mastoidectomy and surgical drainage is reserved for patients in whom symptoms fail to resolve in a timely manner.

Coalescent Mastoiditis

In contrast to AM with periosteitis, coalescent mastoiditis is an indication for immediate surgical intervention. It has often been referred to as "surgical mastoiditis," appropriately stating the need for open drainage and debridement. This is the case once bony destruction has been confirmed on CT imaging, even in the absence of a subperiosteal fluid collection. Emergent surgery should be considered to prevent additional morbidity and should be undertaken as soon as the child is medically stable for the administration of general anesthesia. If a subperiosteal abscess is present, it is drained through the postauricular incision. Dissection of the postauricular tissues must be undertaken with great care because the facial nerve, which is normally superficial in children, is at risk in the presence of bone resorption from osteitis. A complete cortical mastoidectomy should be performed, and infected material sent for culture. The antrum should be carefully inspected, and any obstructing granulation tissue or adhesions should be carefully removed to reestablish the normal drainage pathway. The wound is then closed over a passive drain placed in the mastoidectomy defect. Tympanostomy with tube insertion should also be performed concurrently to provide for prolonged drainage and aeration of the middle-ear cleft.

The presence of a suppurative intracranial complication is also an indication for surgery. In this case, evaluation and planning for the approach and timing of surgery should be undertaken in conjunction with a neurological surgeon. The mastoid procedure may have to wait until a more life-threatening abscess is drained. In the case of a contiguous spread of pus from the temporal bone, the intracranial drainage procedure may be undertaken concurrently with the mastoidectomy.

CONTROVERSOAL ASPECTS OF MANAGEMENT

A trial of antibiotics and myringotomy without mastoidectomy for AM with periosteitis is controversial. Those who advocate this approach cite evidence suggesting that the majority of these patients improve without the need for mastoidectomy (6,9,18,23,43). Patients who do not improve within 48 hours may then be surgically treated without subjecting them to additional risk for morbidity. Others advocate immediate surgical drainage with mastoidectomy even in the absence of coalescent mastoiditis or abscess formation (10,13,16,44), believing that the risk-benefit ratio favors early surgery and that small subperiosteal abscesses may be missed on physical examination. In one series, a subperiosteal abscess was missed in 6 of 9 patients undergoing surgery (16). However, the risk of missing a subclinical abscess is decreased if physical examination is augmented by a CT scan, as is the likelihood of diagnosing bony resorption (18).

Similar arguments apply if the diagnosis of subacute mastoiditis is made in the absence of suppurative complications. Simple mastoidectomy in this case has been advocated by some (38), and others have reasonable argued for myringotomy for drainage and culture purposes, with continued use of culture-specific antibiotics (2). Mastoidectomy is then reserved for persistent disease or patients showing developing evidence of osteitis. Tubes may be reserved for children with a history of recurrent otitis. It has been suggested that early tympanostomy tubes may be protective against the eventual development of AM and its complications, although this is not proven (19).

COMPLICATIONS

Once osteitis is established, infection may spread to adjacent structures in a number of ways, including direct extension through bony erosion, thrombophlebitis, hematogenous spread, or tracking along preformed pathways such as the internal auditory canal, the greater superficial petrosal nerve, the fallopian canal, and the temporal bone suture lines. The spread of infection from AM to adjacent regions remains a significant risk. Neurologic suppurative complications such as meningitis, epidural abscess, subdural empyema, cerebritis, brain abscess, dural sinus thrombophlebitis, hydrocephalus, facial-nerve paralysis, petrous apicitis with Gradenigo syndrome, and death have been documented (6,9,10,14,16,19,24,45). In addition, purulence may track into the soft tissues of the head and neck and produce abscesses, such as subperiosteal mastoid abscess or a Bezold's abscess deep to the sternocleidomastoid muscle.

Despite the dramatic drop in the incidence of AM since the usage of antibiotics, the same cannot be said for the rate of neurologic complications once AM has occurred. Zoller reported an incidence of 11.5% complications including meningitis, brain abscess, and death in 444 patients with AM between the years of 1937 and 1945 (45). In the years 1955 to 1979, Ginsburg reported a similar incidence of complications of 12% in 57 patients with AM (6). Ogle reported that 20% (6 of 30) of patients with AM from 1973 to 1984 manifested neurologic complications, including meningitis, facial palsy, subdural empyema, and brain abscess (9). In contrast, Prellner reported no complications in any of 22 patients (14), and Faye-Lund found only one complication in 27 patients (10).

The clinician must remember that subacute mastoiditis may present with neurologic complications in previously healthy individuals without overt evidence of otologic disease. There are numerous reports in the literature, of a child brought to medical attention for a neurologic complication, and, after complete work-up, silent mastoiditis is discovered radiographically and confirmed at the time of surgery (9,19,24).

Illustrative Cases

Case History 1

A previously healthy 6-month-old child presented in the emergency room with a 2-week history of low-grade fever. Left-sided otitis media was diagnosed by otoscopy, although the right side was obscured by debris. A small right-sided postauricular swelling was noted but was thought to be secondary to trauma. The child was treated with a course of oral ampicillin. Two days later, the fever persisted and the child became increasingly irritable, prompting presentation to the otolaryngology department.

The right postauricular swelling had increased, causing the auricle to protrude. The right ear was cleaned of debris, and a bulging erythematous tympanic membrane was noted. Myringotomy yielded purulent material that later grew *Staph. aureus*. A CT scan showed opacification of the right middle ear and mastoid air cells with erosion of the mastoid outer cortex (Fig. 8). The WBC count on admission was $10.9 \times 10^3/\mu l$.

The diagnosis of coalescent mastoiditis was made, and a simple mastoidectomy was performed. The antrum was filled with abundant granulation tissue extending through the mastoid cortex. A Penrose drain was left to drain the antrum for 2 days. Bilateral ventilation tubes were placed to drain purulent material. Intravenous cefuroxime was administered for 3 days. The child was then discharged with an oral course of cephradine. There were no long-term sequellae.

Case History 2

An otherwise healthy 3-month-old girl presented to the emergency room with a 4-day history of post auricular ery-

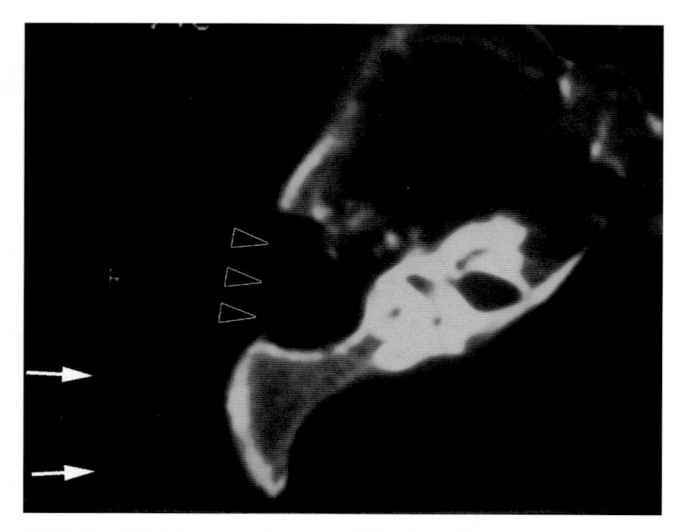

FIG. 8. Axial temporal bone CT of coalescent mastoiditis (Case History 1). Note the marked postauricular swelling (*white arrows*) and the erosion of the outer mastoid cortex (*black arrows*). At surgery, the mastoid cavity contained purulent debris.

thema and irritability. The tissue over the right mastoid was noted to be tender and warm. The pinna was protruding and inferiorly displaced. The tympanic membrane was somewhat injected although the middle ear cavity appeared aerated. The girl was afebrile and had a WBC count of $11.5 \times 10^3/\mu l$.

Intravenous cefuroxime was begun, and CT scan was obtained, (Fig. 9). revealing a right-sided mastoiditis with osteitis. A focal subperiosteal abscess was present adjacent to the antrum. Myrigotomy failed to produce drainage. A simple mastoidectomy was performed with placement of a ventilation tube. The mastoid, filled with granulation tissue and pus, was drained with a Penrose drain for 2 days. Cultures failed to reveal a causative pathogen. The child was given a 3-day course of intravenous antibiotics and was discharged home. She continued to receive oral amoxicillin/clavulanic acid. Recovery was uneventful.

Case History 3

An 11-month-old girl was admitted with right-sided postauricular edema and erythema. Two weeks prior, she had had an upper respiratory infection with purulent nasal discharge that had since largely resolved. On admission, the child was febrile with a temperature of 38.9°C, and her WBC count was $13.1 \times 10^3/\mu l$. The pinna was mildly displaced laterally, and the right tympanic membrane was dull and bulging.

An x-ray of the mastoid revealed opacification of the right mastoid, although no bony destruction was noted. Tympanocentesis yielded purulence that grew *Staph. epidermidis*. Intravenous nafcillin was begun, and a myringotomy with ventilation tube placement was performed. The child showed rapid clinical improvement, and no further surgical intervention was required. The child was discharged on hospital day 3, with a course of oral amoxicillin. Despite future episodes of otitis media, no further complications were encountered.

SUMMARY AND CONCLUSIONS

Although the incidence of AM has dropped significantly in the age of antibiotics, it continues to produce significant morbidity as a complication of AOM. The process develops when infection from otitis media becomes loculated in the mastoid–air-cell system and is prevented from draining through the normal routes. The disease may be subdivided into AM with periosteitis, in which the mucosa and periosteum of the mastoid is involved, and coalescent AM, in which mastoid osteitis is also present. Both conditions generally present with retroauricular swelling and tenderness following an episode of AOM. A variant of mastoiditis, subacute mastoiditis, follows a more indolent course but retains the potential for producing life-threatening complications.

An understanding of the pathophysiology and natural history of mastoiditis is essential for the clinician to fully evaluate and treat the numerous manifestations of this process. A complete physical examination, supplemented by appropriate radiologic data establishes the extent of the disease. Admission, culture-specific intravenous antibiotics, and myringotomy are appropriate measures throughout the spectrum of AM. In cases of coalescent AM, intracranial complications, abscess formation, or lack of timely symptomatic improvement, a cortical mastoidectomy for debridement and drainage is also indicated. Vigilance must be maintained for the

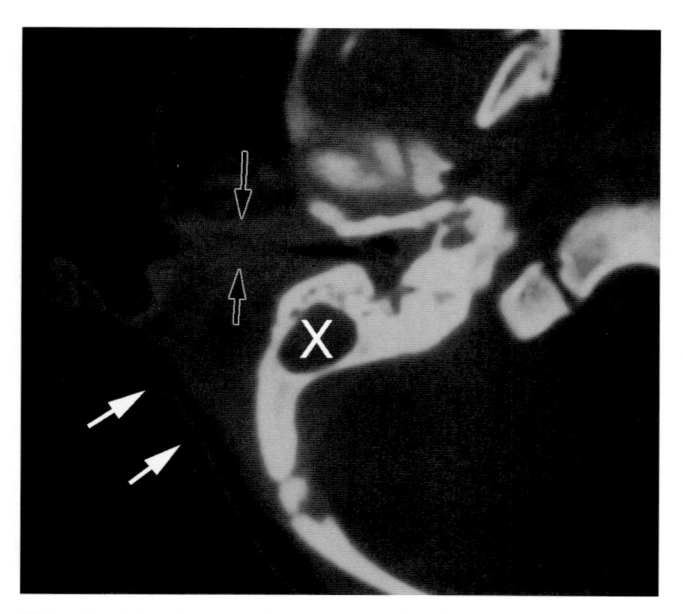

FIG. 9. Axial temporal bone CT of subperiosteal abscess (Case 2). Note the postauricular swelling with anterior displacement of the pinna (*white arrows*), and the edema causing marked narrowing of the external auditory canal (*black arrows*). The mastoid antrum (*x*) is filled with purulent debris; however, the outer cortex of the mastoid has remained intact.

early recognition and treatment of frequent serious intracranial complications.

ACKNOWLEDGMENT

The authors acknowledge Dr. Timothy Scott and Dr. Robert Jackler for allowing the use of their case presentations and radiographic images (18).3

REFERENCES

1. Freidman I. The pathology of otitis media. *J Clin Pathol* 1956;9:229.
2. Bluestone CD, Stool SE. *Pediatric otolaryngology.* Philadelphia: WB Saunders;1983:546–552.
3. Mygind H. Subperiosteal abscess of the mastoid region. *Ann Otol Rhinol Laryngol* 1910;19:254–265.
4. Palva T, Pulkinen K. Mastoiditis. *J Laryngol Otol* 1959;73:573–588.
5. Sorensen H. Antibiotics in suppurative otitis media. *Otolaryngol Clin North Am* 1977;10:45–50.
6. Ginsburg CM, Rudoy R, Nelson JD. Acute mastoiditis in infants and children. *Clin Pediatr* 1980;19:549–553.
7. Hawkins DB, Dru D, House JW, Clark RW. Acute mastoiditis in children: a review of 54 cases. *Laryngoscope* 1983;93:568–572.
8. Herwig SR. Acute pediatric otomastoiditis: a review. *Mil Med* 1984;149:216–218.
9. Ogle JW, Lauer BA. Acute mastoiditis. *Am J Dis Child* 1986;140:1178–1182.
10. Faye-Lund H. Acute and latent mastoiditis. *J Laryngol Otol* 1989;103:1158–1160.
11. Neilsen JC. *Studies of the aetiology of acute otitis media.* Copenhagen: E. Munksgard; 1945.
12. Goodale RL, Montgomery WW. Dangers inherent in the non-surgical concept of acute otitis media. *Ann Otol Rhinol Laryngol* 1955;64:181–191.
13. Palva T, Virtanen H, Mäkinen J. Acute and latent mastoiditis in children. *J Laryngol Otol* 1985;99:127–136.
14. Prellner D, Rydel R. Acute mastoiditis. *Acta Otolaryngol (Stockh)* 1986;1002:52–56.
15. Rubin JS, Wei WI. Acute mastoiditis: a review of 34 patients. *Laryngoscope* 1985;95:963–965.
16. Hoppe JE, Köster S, Bootz F, Niethammer D. Acute mastoiditis—relevant once again. *Infection* 1994;22:178–182.
17. Senturia B, Carr CD, Ahlvin RC. Middle ear effusions: pathologic changes of the mucoperiosteum in the experimental animal. *Ann Otol Rhinol Laryngol* 1962;71:632–647.
18. Scott TA, Jackler RK. Acute mastoiditis in infancy: a sequella of unrecognized acute otitis media. *Otolaryngol Head Neck Surg* 1989;101:683–687.
19. Luntz M, Keren G, Nusem S, Kronberg J. Acute mastoiditis—revisited. *Ear Nose Throat J* 1994;73:648–654.
20. St. John Roosa DB. *Diseases of the ear.* New York: William Wood; 1891:526–535.
21. Odetoyinbo O. The changing pattern of mastoid abscess. *J Laryngol Otol* 1985;99:1081–1084.
22. Holt GR, Young WC. Acute coalescent mastoiditis. *Otolaryngol Head Neck Surg* 1981;89:317–321.
23. Rosen A, Ophir D, Marshak G. Acute coalescent mastoiditis. *Otolaryngol Head Neck Surg* 1981;89:317–321.
24. Holt GR, Gates GA. Masked mastoiditis. *Laryngoscope* 1983;93:1034–1037.
25. Goodhill V. *Ear diseases, deafness, and dizziness.* New York: Harper and Row; 1979:345.
26. Farrior JB. Acute suppurative mastoiditis in geriatrics. *Laryngoscope* 1942;52:688–696.
27. Badrawy R, Abou-Bieh A, Taha A. Masked diabetic mastoiditis. *J Otolaryngol Otol* 1975;89:815–821.
28. Qvarnberg Y. Acute otitis media. A prospective clinical study of myringotomy and antimicrobial treatment. *Acta Otolaryngol (Stockh)* 1981;(Suppl. 375).
29. Bluestone CD, Stephenson JS, Martin LM. Ten year review of otitis media pathogens. *Pediatr Infec Dis J* 1992;11:7–11.
30. Celin SE, Bluestone CD, Stephenon JS, et al. Bacteriology of acute otitis media in adults. *JAMA* 1991;226:2249–2252.
31. Faden H, Bernstein J, Brodsky L, et al. Effect of prior antibiotic treatment on middle ear disease in children. *Ann Otol Rhinol Layngol* 1992;101:87-910.
32. Pestalozza G. Otitis media in newborn infants. *Int J Pediatr Otorhinolaryngol* 1984;8:109–124.
33. Moloy PJ. Anaerobic mastoiditis: a report of two cases with complications. *Laryngoscope* 1983;92:1311–1315.
34. Williams MA. Head and neck findings in pediatric acquired immune deficiency syndrome. *Laryngoscope* 1987;97:713–716.
35. Barnett ED, Klein JO, Pelton SI, Luginbuhl LM. Otitis Media in children born to human immunodeficiency virus-infected mothers. *Ped Infect Dis J* 1992;11:360–364.
36. Chandrasekhar SS, Siverls V, Sekhar HK. Histopathologic and ultrastructural changes in the temporal bones of HIV-infected human adults. *Am J Otol* 1992;13:207–214.
37. Gesner M, Desiderio D, Kim m, Kaul A, Lawrence R, Chandwani S, Pollack H, Rigaud M, Krasinski K, Borkowsky W. Streptococcus pneumoniae in human immunodeficiency virus type 1-infected children. *Ped Infect Dis J* 1994;13:697–703.
38. Mawson SR, Lundman H. *Diseases of the ear: a textbook of otology.* Chicago: Year Book Medical; 1979:378–380.
39. Ronis BJ, Ronis ML, Liebman EP. Acute Mastoiditis as seen today. *Ear Nose Throat J* 1968;47:502–507.
40. DeSousa JS, DaSilva A, DaCosta RV. Intractable diarrhea of infancy and latent otomastoiditis. *Arch Dis Child* 1980;55:937–940.
41. Dehner LP, Chen TK. Primary tumors of the external and middle ear. *Arch Otolaryngol* 1978;104:399–403.
42. Shelby JH, Sweet RM. Eosinophilic granuloma of the temporal bone: medical and surgical management in the pediatric patient. *South Med J* 1983;76:65–70.
43. Nadal D, Herrmann P, Baumann A, Fanconi A. Acute mastoiditis: clinical, microbiological, and therapeutic aspects. *Eur J Pediatr* 1990;149:560–564.
44. Pfaltz CR, Griesemer C. Complications of acute middle ear infections. *Ann Otol Rhinol Laryngol* 1986;93(Suppl 112):133–137.
45. Zoller H. Acute mastoiditis and its complications: a changing trend. *South Med J* 1972;65:477–80.

PART V

Cholesteatoma

CHAPTER 19

Congenital Cholesteatoma

Jacob Friedberg

In 1830, Korner became the first to hypothesize that the aural lesion, later to become known as cholesteatoma (1), might be of congenital origin (Fig. 1). In 1854, von Remak (2) suggested that these growths might be due to congenital epithelial cell rests. Since then, various names (3) have been proposed including primary cholesteatoma (from Greek *chole* [bile] + *stear* [tallow, suet]), true or cholesteatoma verum, primary epidermoid, and genuine cholesteatoma, as well as margaritoma (from Greek *margarites* [a pearl] (Fig. 2), steatoma, and keratoma (from Greek *keratos* [horn]). Both the nomenclature and the pathogenesis of this entity have been a source of debate, controversy, and argument ever since.

There has always been a wide-ranging level of detraction or support for a congenital origin of middle ear cholesteatoma. In the latter category, Cawthorne (4) in 1963 was able to believe that the deep-seated petrous cholesteatoma auris was always of congenital origin, and on occasion, so was the more superficial attic cholesteatoma. He went so far as to suggest, as had Diamant (5), McKenzie (6), and Toglia et al. (7) that all cholesteatomas might be congenital and that the growth came before the infection. Mawson (8), on the other hand, while acknowledging the possibility of a congenital origin, felt that its presentation in the middle ear was likely the result of extension from the temporal bone subsequently resulting in infection.

In 1936, R.W. Teed (9) had recognized an epithelial thickening of ectodermal, origin which developed in close relationship to the geniculate ganglion at the dorsal end of the first pharyngeal cleft, in the upper mesotympanum, medial to the neck of the malleus. He believed that under most circumstances, this structure involuted, but in those rare instances when it persisted, its continued growth could give rise to what would later present as a cholesteatoma. Such a congenital cholesteatoma developed not from some aberrant or anomalous epithelium but from a normally occurring structure. Although referred to from time to time in the literature (10), it was largely overlooked until the work of Michaels (11) in 1986.

H.P. House (12) is generally credited with reporting the first bona fide case of congenital cholesteatoma of the middle ear behind an intact tympanic membrane (in 1953). The patient was a 26-year-old woman, with only a 3-year history and a lesion measuring just 4 mm in diameter in the incudostapedial region. This would not be considered a typical case in today's clinical experience.

In 1959, Sheehy (13) reported two cases of cholesteatoma occurring behind an intact tympanic membrane, both of which would be acceptable by contemporary criteria. His second patient was 25 years old at the time of presentation with a facial palsy. Radiography undertaken about 7 months after the onset of paralysis demonstrated extensive bone destruction, and subsequent mastoid surgery confirmed a massive cholesteatoma that may very well have been a quarter century in the making. There was no significant history to suggest other than a congenital origin. Radiography, which was critical in the management of this case, was not then the readily utilized instrument that it is today. Sheehy emphasized the need for temporal bone radiography in any case of apparently idiopathic facial nerve paralysis.

Derlacki and Clemis (14) can be credited with legitimizing congenital cholesteatoma. In 1965, they simplified the classification into petrous pyramid, mastoid, and tympanic types. They presented criteria for the diagnosis of middle ear congenital cholesteatoma, described an initial series of ten patients with this condition, and rightly pointed out that once the cholesteatoma had breached the tympanic membrane or become secondarily infected, it would be impossible to assume a congenital origin with any degree of certainty. Even in hindsight, the diagnosis can be supported in at least six or seven of their patients. In 1968, Derlacki, Harrison, and Clemis (15) presented seven further patients, all of whom were children under 13 years of age. A congenital etiology to these cholesteatomas was much easier to accept than in some presented in their previous paper.

J. Friedberg: Department of Otolaryngology, University of Toronto, Hospital for Sick Children, Toronto, Ontario M5G 1X8 Canada.

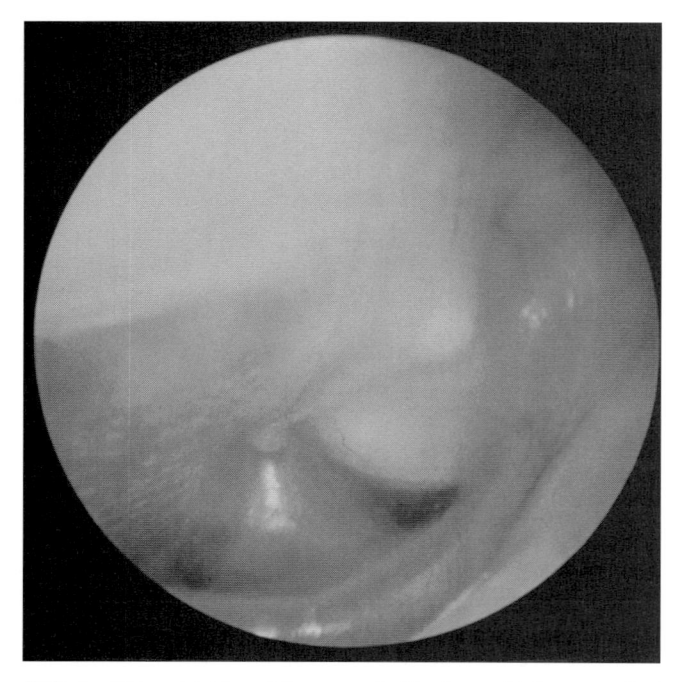

FIG. 1. This smooth, white, rounded lesion, which presented in the anterosuperior quadrant of the left middle ear in a 22-month-old boy, is typical of what today would be accepted as a congenital cholesteatoma. Reproduced, with permission, courtesy of *The Laryngoscope.*

Peron and Schuknecht (16), reviewing congenital cholesteatomas in 1975, considered the probability of epithelial rests as a source of some cholesteatomas but felt that once they had become infected, the true pathogenesis would be impossible to determine. The following year, A. Palva (17), in a review of 66 cases of cholesteatoma in children under 16 years of age, did not even consider the possibility of a congenital etiology. The features of rapid, expansile growth, filling the middle ear and extending into what was usually a well-pneumatized mastoid, system were attributed to the presumed greater growth potential of cholesteatoma in children as compared with adults (18,19). These features could equally have been interpreted as being compatible with the expected course of a congenital middle ear cholesteatoma readily and rapidly expanding into a normally cellular mastoid bone.

In 1980, House and Sheehy (20) reviewed 41 patients who presented with cholesteatoma behind an intact tympanic membrane. They felt that many of these lesions were congenital in origin and recommended elective reexploration because of the high rate of residual disease. In 1989, Sculerati and Bluestone (21), in a discussion of the pathogenesis of cholesteatoma, felt that a diagnosis of congenital cholesteatoma was essentially a diagnosis of exclusion, because one could never completely rule out the possibility of a prior significant infection, perforation, or injury. Finally, in 1990, T. Palva (22) in a review of the pathogenesis of cholesteatoma, while recognizing the likely role of the epidermoid formation described by Teed (9) and Michaels (11,23,24) as a source for the classic anterosuperior lesion presenting in childhood, still considered this to be a rare condition.

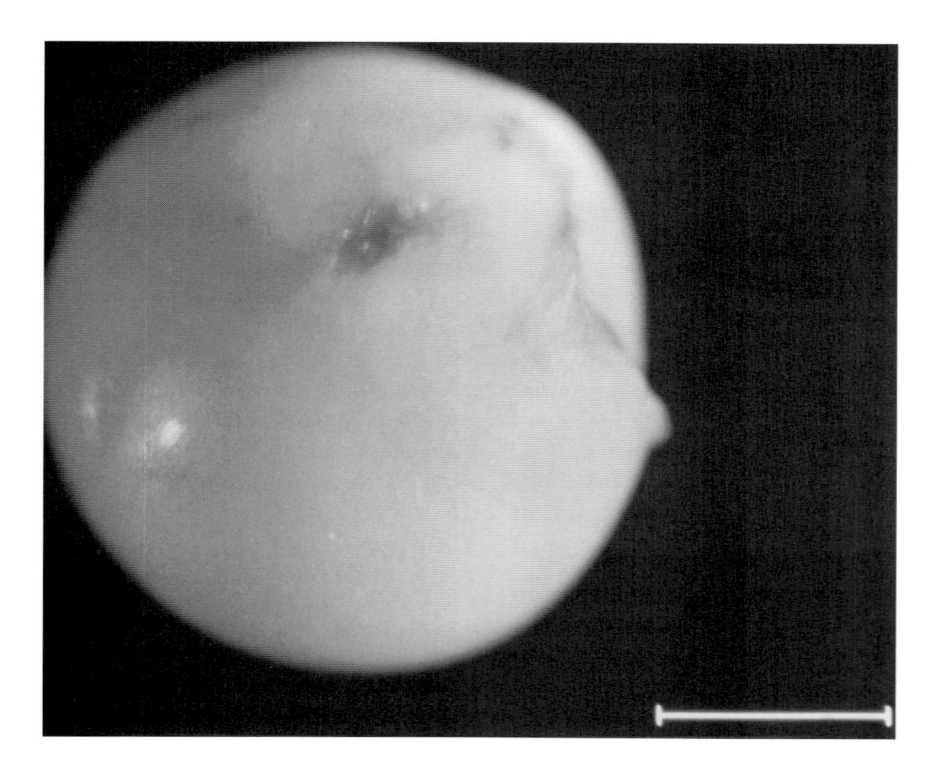

FIG. 2. The name *pearl* is well deserved, at least for the smaller lesions. Note the thin investing mucosal layer, which was incised during removal. Scale = 1 mm. Reproduced, with permission, courtesy of *The Laryngoscope.*

CHANGING INCIDENCE: REAL OR APPARENT

There has been a dramatic decrease in the incidence of acquired cholesteatoma in recent years, at least in developed countries. Over the same period there has been an apparent increase in the reported incidence of congenital cholesteatoma (25–32). In 1925, Nager (33) considered the possibility of congenital cholesteatoma but that its incidence was so rare as to be of no practical importance. Fifty years later, various authors were reporting a 2% to 4 % incidence (25, 35,36). In 1983, Schwartz et al. (37) felt that 18% of cholesteatomas treated by their group were of congenital origin, while Parisier et al. (38), in 1989, with perhaps even more rigid diagnostic criteria, recognized 24% of all cholesteatomas occurring in patients under 18 years of age to be of congenital origin.

This opinion was not universally held. In 1990, Schuring et al. (39), in a review of 354 patients with cholesteatoma, which included 38 children under 9 years of age, did not even consider the possibility of a congenital origin. The authors did recognize a relatively greater incidence of pars tensa cholesteatomas, which were associated with a higher rate of recurrence and ossicular damage in children than in adults.

The introduction and acceptance of the operating microscope has been the keystone of modern otology. Holmgren (40) is credited with the introduction in 1923 of what was originally a modified dissecting microscope for otosclerosis surgery. Cawthorne soon applied the operating microscope to facial nerve surgery. By 1940, Simpson-Hall, in Edinburgh, had firmly established the use of the operating microscope in fenestration surgery for otosclerosis, and at about the same, time Shambaugh instituted its similar use in North America. The operating microscope truly came into its own with the introduction of stapedectomy in 1956 by Shea (41). This was a significant step forward (42) from "the hook probe and magnifying glass" approach to diagnosis, as reported earlier by Nager (33). It was not until the mid 1970s, however, that the operating microscope became commonplace, although not universal, in the clinical setting. It is still seldom available to non-otologists.

Halogen lighting for otoscopy was first introduced in 1973 and by 1975 was well established as the standard. It provided approximately three times the brightness of comparable conventional incandescent bulbs. This consistently bright light coupled with alkaline batteries or rechargeable handpieces, the popularization of pneumatic otoscopy, and routine hearing screening tests permitted the appreciation of tympanic membrane detail and color as never before. In a creditable number of instances, the diagnosis of congenital cholesteatoma, or at least the detection of a "lesion" behind the tympanic membrane, has been made by the referring pediatrician or general practitioner with the help of these instruments (28).

It is possible that in past years many of these lesions were spontaneously aborted as a result of acute suppurative otitis media with rupture of the tympanic membrane and subsequent extrusion of middle contents, including a weakly attached (Fig. 3) epithelial remnant. Spontaneous tympanic membrane rupture and protracted otorrhea are far less common occurrences now due to the widespread use of antibiotics, both acutely and prophylactically. This condition may have been self-curing in some patients. One might speculate that antibiotics are indirectly responsible for this "new" disease. Some lesions may have been unknowingly removed by aspiration of the middle ear at the time of insertion of a ventilating tube (28). The increased incidence of congenital cholesteatoma may be both real and apparent.

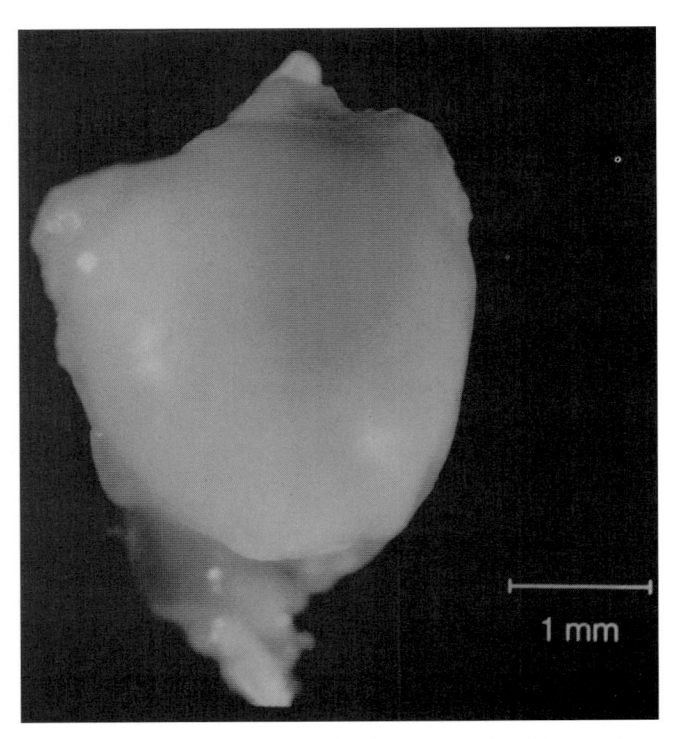

FIG. 3. This lesion was attached to the neck of the malleus by a delicate mucous membrane and became freely mobilized after minimal surgical manipulation. The stalk did not contain any epidermoid tissue. Separation across this stalk assured a complete removal. Reproduced, with permission, courtesy of *The Laryngoscope*.

BILATERAL CONGENITAL CHOLESTEATOMA

Bilateral lesions (Fig. 4) are rare, affecting approximately 3% of congenital cholesteatoma patients (28,32,43–49). The finding of nearly identical lesions in each ear gives further support to a congenital etiology from similar epithelial rests. These lesions need not present at the same time, and long-term follow-up should always include careful scrutiny of the "normal" ear.

IMPLANTATION, METAPLASIA, AND EPITHELIAL MIGRATION

A preexisting history of otitis media does not preclude a diagnosis of congenital cholesteatoma, nor should a history

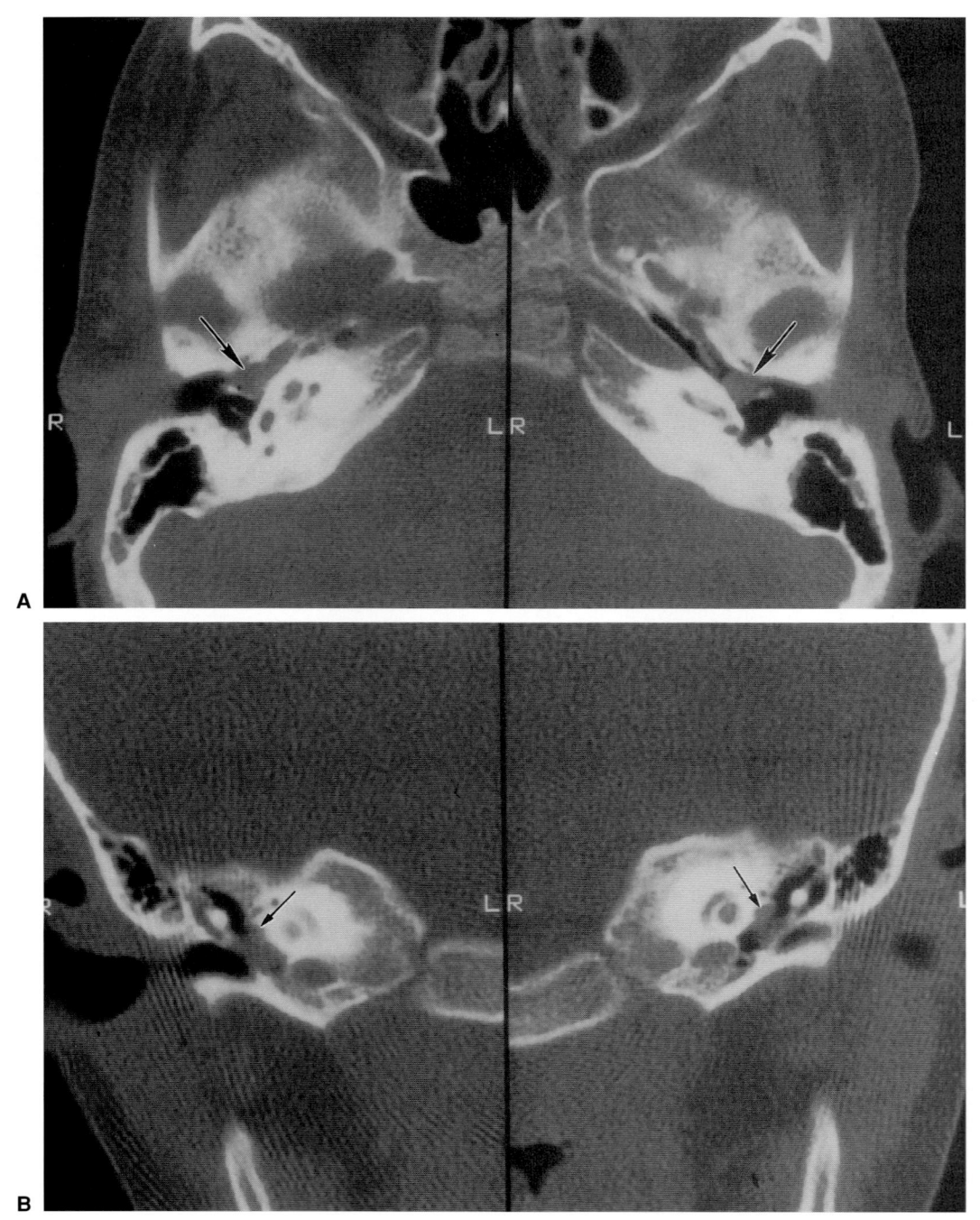

FIG. 4. A, B: This 35-month-old boy presented with bilateral, almost symmetrical, anterior mesotympanic congenital cholesteatomas *(long arows)*. Both lesions were located anterior to the handle of malleus occluding the eustachian tube and inferior to the tensor tympani *(short arrows)*. Approximately 3% of patients with congenital cholesteatoma may have a similar lesion in each ear, but they may not present at the same time. Careful follow-up for the apparently normal ear is advised in all patients with congenital cholesteatoma.

of insertion of a ventilating tube, but, the possibility of an implantation epidermoid cyst secondary to such surgery can never be ruled out completely; however, such a complication would appear to be extremely rare (28,46,50).

Sade, Babiacki, and Pinkus (35) demonstrated that squamous metaplasia of the middle ear mucosa was present in 40% of cases of simple chronic otitis media. Rarely, keratinization could also be present and a possible source of cholesteatoma developing behind an intact tympanic membrane. This has not been a widely accepted concept and would not explain the remarkable consistency of location and presentation of the typical congenital cholesteatoma.

Aimi (51) suggested that under normal circumstances the tympanic ring inhibited or restricted ingrowth of ectoderm from the external canal into the middle ear. Should this mechanism fail, migration of keratinizing epithelium into the middle ear might result in the formation of a congenital cholesteatoma.

EMBRYONIC CELL REST

In 1922, Cushing (52) suggested, as had von Remak (44) in 1854, that many of the cholesteatomas reported by otologists were likely true dermoids originating from epidermal rests laid down in the temporal bone during embryologic development of the ear. He even went so far as to suggest that the cholesteatoma itself was primary rather than secondary to the otitis media. Teed (9), as previously noted, described just such an embryologic entity in 1925. Subsequent temporal bone studies (53,54) failed to demonstrate histologic evidence of embryonic cell rests. This should have been anticipated if under normal circumstance these cell rests were expected to atrophy and disappear, but such negative observations argued against an embryonic cell rest theory of origin.

Sanna and Zini (36) suggested that congenital middle ear cholesteatoma arose from epidermal cells trapped in the posterior mesotympanum during embryonic development, because that was the most common site of presentation they had observed.

Levenson et al. (29,55), while supporting a congenital origin, were concerned by the apparent increase in frequency since the introduction of effective antibiotics. They proposed that the epidermal rest described by Teed, instead of undergoing its usual involution, might, as a result of inflammatory irritation, give rise to a keratin-producing cyst, which, if expanded laterally, would appear as an acquired cholesteatoma or, if medially, a petrous cholesteatoma later in life.

In 1986, Michaels (11) demonstrated the embryologic presence of an epidermoid formation in the anterosuperior middle ear mucosa. This formation could be recognized in a fetus of only 5 or 6 weeks of gestation (24) in as many as 54% of specimens and apparently involuted by 33 weeks. It was located on the lateral wall of the tympanic cavity just below the level of the pars flaccida. The epithelium was stratified squamous and in some instances, keratinizing. Although the epidermoid formation was very close to the external auditory canal early in gestation, at no point was any continuity demonstrable (51). He suggested, as had Teed, that this was a normal structure that usually underwent involution but if persistent, could give rise to a primary (congenital) cholesteatoma located in the anterosuperior part of the tympanic cavity. This epidermoid body corresponded to the structure Teed (9) had described in a 22-week fetus. The presence of such a structure obviated the need to invoke a metaplastic mechanism for the development of a cholesteatoma behind an intact tympanic membrane. Wang, Hawkes, and Kwok (56) confirmed the presence of this epidermoid formation but only in 17% of specimens, none of which demonstrated any keratinization.

It appeared at the distal end of the eustachian tube even before the development of the middle ear space. Michaels suggested that this structure might serve as an organizer in the subsequent development of the middle ear and tympanic membrane. Although prepared to accept this epidermoid formation as a source of the small anterosuperior congenital cholesteatoma, he was less certain of its role in the development of a larger lesion, which might fill the middle ear.

He noted that while most of the resulting lesions would be of the "closed" type (i.e., cystic), some would be "open" (i.e., presenting as a sheet or a plaque) (30,57). The margins of this open type of congenital cholesteatoma might be more difficult to define at surgery, and theoretically one would expect a higher incidence of recurrence in such patients.

Meyerhoff and Truelson (58), in a discussion of the staging of cholesteatoma, recognized congenital cholesteatoma as resulting in the middle ear from a nidus of trapped squamous epithelium, presumably present prenatally. As well they defined a "tertiary acquired cholesteatoma" as having developed behind an otherwise normal tympanic membrane from a traumatic implantation or as the result of a preceding middle ear infection, as promoted by Ruedi (59). In the absence of a clear history of penetrating or explosive injury, such a distinction would be impossible.

The embryonic middle ear epidermoid formation, as described by Teed (9), Michaels (11,23,24,31), and Wang, Hawke, and Kwok (56), provides an entirely satisfactory source for congenital middle ear cholesteatoma. McGill et al. (30) noted that until one could demonstrate the presence a middle ear cholesteatoma at some point between 33 weeks of gestation, when this epidermoid body normally involuted and when it became clinically manifest as a typical middle ear lesion, conclusive proof that this was indeed the source of congenital cholesteatoma would be lacking.

CLINICAL PRESENTATION

Cholesteatoma in general is more common in males (60). Congenital cholesteatoma is also predominantly a male disease, with a near 3:1 preponderance in the more contemporary reports (25,28,37,46,55). The mean age of presentation is about 4.5 years (3,28,37,38).

The characteristic appearance of the classical antero-superior congenital cholesteatoma (Figs. 1, 12) is diagnostic; however, this is the area of the tympanic membrane least likely to be well visualized, and a minority are diagnosed by the primary care physician. Most present to the otolaryngologist as refractory otitis media or some other unidentified abnormality of the tympanic membrane. A surprising number may not be recognized even by the otolaryngologist until the time of myringotomy (28).

The incidence of otitis media and the frequency of ventilating tube insertion in this group of patients is much the same as in the general population (28). Pain or discharge is not a feature until late in the disease, and hearing loss may be assocated with middle ear effusion secondary to eustachian tube occlusion or from ossicular erosion. Unilateral hearing loss, if otherwise asymptomatic, is not a symptom about which young children complain. A diagnosis of congenital cholesteatoma should be considered in any isolated conductive hearing loss (46,61).

Symptoms may be minimal until the lesion has achieved a substantial size, the so-called giant cholesteatoma (28,62). Some authors consider such a cholesteatoma to simply be more aggressive in children (3,63) while others (55) are reluctant to consider such lesions as being congenital in origin, and in these cases one can never truly rule out the possibility of posttraumatic implantation or significant infection. Nevertheless, there are patients (28) who have presented with unilateral hearing loss, a massive lesion with extensive erosion, yet emphatically deny any known infection or injury and radiographically demonstrate normal mastoid development and aeration of the contralateral temporal bone. These lesions may have been a long time in the making and were simply missed until the diagnosis was unavoidable.

FACIAL PARALYSIS

Facial palsy was a common presentation in past (4,43,64), but is much less so today (28). Jefferson and Smalley (10) speculated that the origin of petromastoid cholesteatomas presenting with progressive facial palsy could best be explained by the existence of a congenital epithelial rest deep to the tympanic membrane rather than by ingrowth through a perforation. They pointed out that the epithelial mass described by Teed (9) was closely related to the geniculate ganglion of the facial nerve and suggested that this might explain the facial palsy as the presenting symptom in their patients.

Cawthorne and Griffith (65) reported nine cases of congenital cholesteatoma that presented with progressive facial palsy and were believed to be of petrous origin. Believing that the earliest symptom was almost invariably related to the facial nerve, they assumed that the cholesteatoma had reached the middle ear by lateral extension. Cawthorne (4) subsequently reported on several more patients who had presented with facial palsy, including two young children (of unstated age) with widespread cholesteatoma in cellular mastoids, which he recognized as an unusual finding. Cannoni et al. (64) suggested, as had Fisch (66), that these petromastoid congenital cholesteatomas originated at the level of the facial nerve ganglion.

Hough (34) observed that in 20% to 30% of patients, there was a congenital dehiscence of the facial canal in the region of the oval window. This could account for the development of a facial palsy, even in the presence of a comparatively small cholesteatoma with minimal or perhaps no inflammation. Brosnan (43) reported three patients with apparent congenital cholesteatoma. Each had an intact tympanic membrane, a bony dehiscence over the posterior segment of the facial nerve, and a hypotympanum free of disease. All three were uninfected at the time of operation.

AGE, LOCATION, AND OSSICULAR INVOLVEMENT

The mean age of presentation, as reported in more contemporary reviews, is about about 4.5 years (28,30,32,48). This is certainly younger than in earlier reports (14,15,18,20,26) and is likely the result of increased clinical awareness and may reflect more stringent diagnostic criteria. The majority of these lesions present in the anterosuperior mesotympanum (8,25,28,29,30,38,48,55,57,67). Its middle ear relations would consist of the eustachian tube anteriorly, the tensor tympani, its tendon and related mucosal folds superiorly, the malleus immediately posteriorly, and the tympanic membrane laterally (Fig. 5).

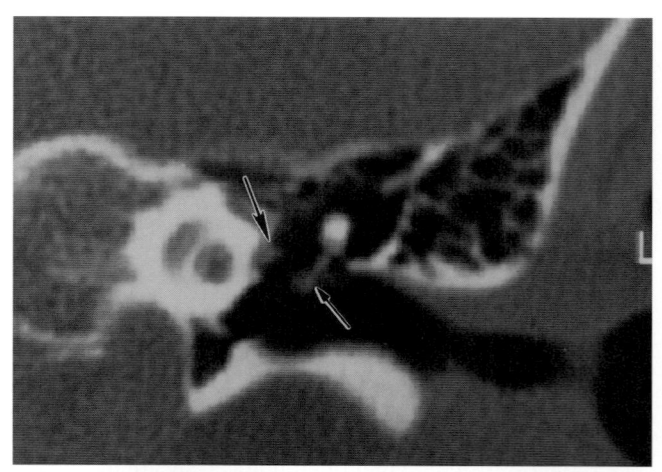

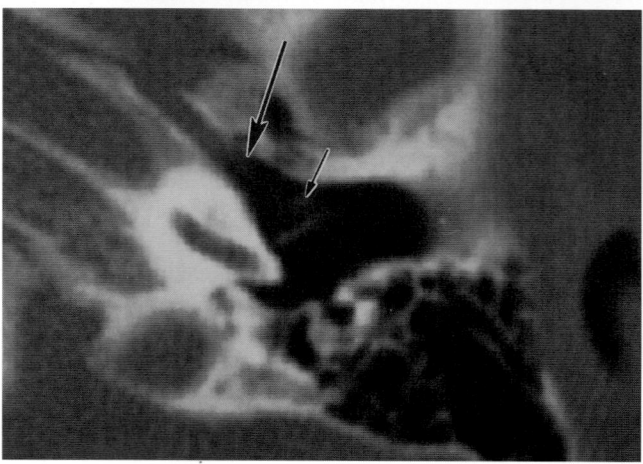

FIG. 5. A, B: This 1.5-mm anterosuperior lesion in a 25-month-old was immediately adjacent and anterior to the neck of the malleus *(small arrow)*. It was just below the tendon of tensor tympani *(long arrow)* and well away from the medial wall of the middle ear. Although situated at the mouth of the eustachian tube *(extra-long arrow)*, it was too small to cause obstructive complications.

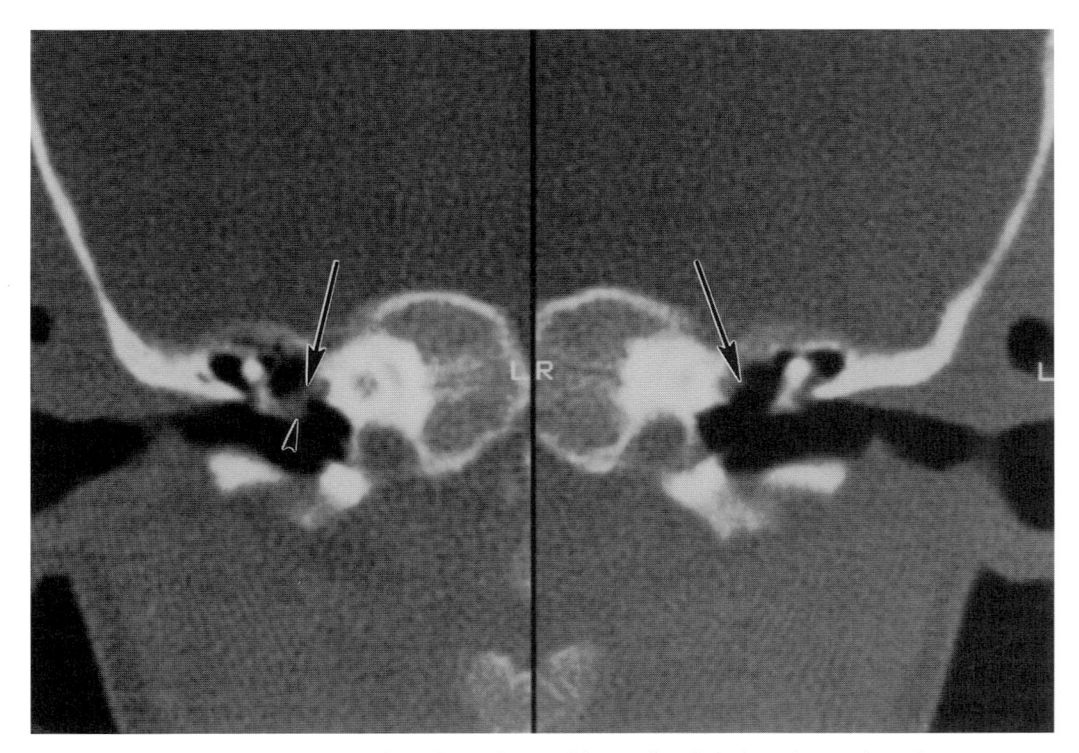

FIG. 6. This still small lesion *(arrowhead)* was located immediately below the tendon of tensor tympani *(long arrow)*. This fortuitous arrangement may explain the tendency of congenital cholesteatoma to be confined to the middle ear until relatively advanced.

Initially, its growth is confined to the middle ear below the tympanic isthmus, presumably restricted by the adjacent structures. Early on, the only significant complication is otitis media with effusion secondary to eustachian tube occlusion (see Fig. 12). There should be no ossicular erosion, and any conductive hearing loss is readily reversible. Indeed, a conductive hearing loss in the absence of an effusion indicates ossicular involvement in spite of the clinical picture (25). By the time the affected child is 4 or 5 years of age, the cholesteatoma will begin to extend into the posterior mesotympanum, with increasing risk of erosion of the incus and, to a lesser degree, of the stapes. By age 6 or 7, the cholesteatoma will usually have extended beyond the mesotympanum into the attic and antrum, with inevitable ossicular involvement (28,30,38,44,47); although, there have been cases of extensive mesotympanic cholesteatoma presenting in infants as young as 3 months of age (37).

At the time of presentation the cholesteatoma is usually confined to a part of the mesotympanum (Fig. 6), most often anterosuperiorly; nevertheless, as many as one fourth of the patients present with widespread mesotympanic involvement, and a similar number with extension beyond the mesotympanum (28). The degree of involvement is directly related to age.

SITE OF PRESENTATION

There are good embryologic data available (9,11,23, 24,32,56) that demonstrate the presence of an ectodermal body at this anterosuperior site, which, if persistent, could give rise to a cholesteatoma. This does not explain the presentation of a significant, albeit fewer, number of cases elsewhere in the middle ear (28) (Fig. 7). No comparable ectodermal rest has thus far been demonstrated elsewhere in the middle ear space (68).

Parisier et al. (38) felt that this particular formation did not explain those lesions presenting in the posterosuperior mesotympanum and suggested that perhaps a second such body might be present in that area. Wang, Hawkins, and Kwok (56) demonstrated that the epidermoid body in some specimens consisted of two and even three distinct structures adjacent to one another, but no such embryologic structure has been demonstrated remote from this location (68).

Several authors (18,28,69) have commented on how tenuously these pearls may be attached and the ease with which they could become mobile during the course of surgical removal (see Fig. 3). This ready mobilization may account for the apparent "migration" reported in a 4-month-old boy who was found to have bilateral middle ear lesions recognized during a routine examination (49). The lesions were initially noted to be located anteroinferiorly, but by the time of surgery, one was found to be anterosuperior. It is possible that the anterosuperior site may be the only one at which a congenital cholesteatoma normally develops, but as a result of relatively minor trauma, it may become dislodged and reimplant elsewhere in the middle ear space. The posterosuperior quadrant, by

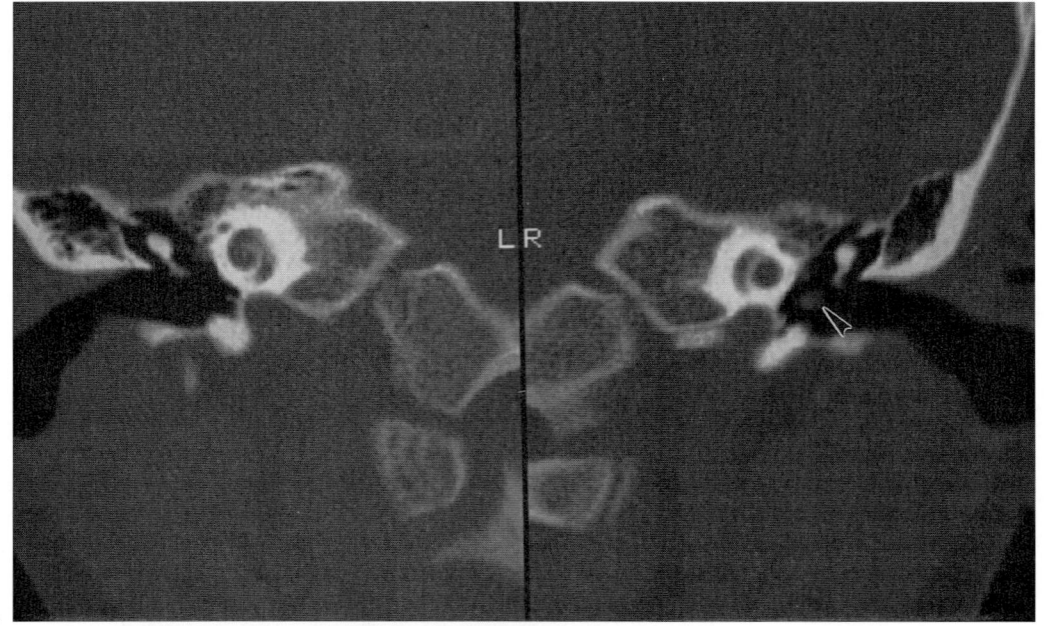

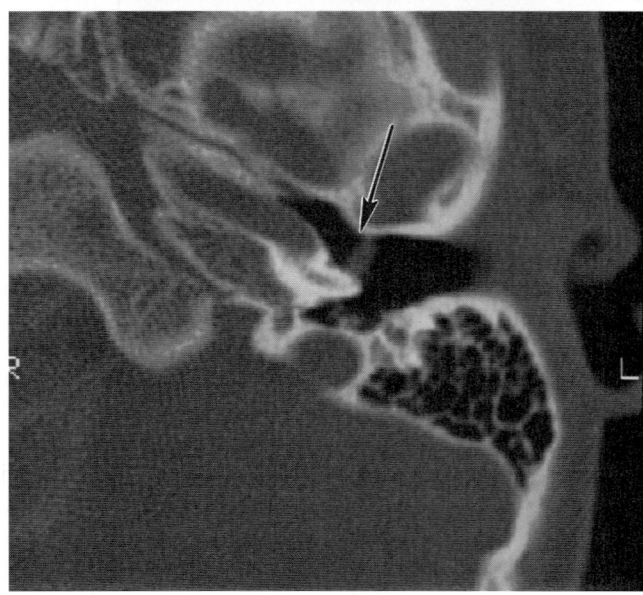

FIG. 7. A, B: This 49-month-old boy presented initially with acute otitis media. When his effusion had resolved, he was found to have a lesion anteromedial to the umbo *(arrowhead)* of the malleus as opposed to the more common site anterior to its neck. It was immediately opposite the mouth of the eustachian tube *(arrow)*.

virtue of its shallowness, its complex mucosal folds, and conjunction of ossicles, may simply be a favored spot in which to become ensnared and, thus, the second most common site of presentation.

HEARING

Hearing level is clearly related to ossicular chain integrity and that in turn a function of patient age and the degree to which the cholesteatoma has extended beyond the anterosuperior middle ear quadrant (28). Hearing ought to be normal (30) in those patients whose lesion is restricted to the anterosuperior quadrant, unless a middle ear effusion is present. If not, the cholesteatoma must have extended posteriorly with involvement of the stapes superstructure and/or the lenticular process of the incus; however, even with ossicular erosion, the hearing may be normal, because the cholesteatoma may serve to complete the ossicular chain (Fig. 8). If any posterior extension is present or suspected, the patient or, more appropriately, the parents should be forewarned of this possibility and that the hearing might be significantly poorer postoperatively.

DIFFERENTIAL DIAGNOSIS

The majority of white lesions developing behind an intact tympanic membrane are either cholesteatoma, congenital or acquired, or bony, such as an osteoma arising from the pro-

In the preoperative assessment of the typical congenital cholesteatoma, one is primarily interested in the precise location and size of a lesion, which may be only a few millimeters in diameter. High-resolution (CT) can resolve overlapping 1.5-mm sections (71,73) and is able to identify minute areas of bone erosion, as seen in ossicular involvement or facial nerve exposure (Figs. 10, 11).

Phelps and Wright (74) noted that although bony erosion could be well defined by CT, the cholesteatoma itself could not be differentiated from some other soft-tissue density or from a middle ear effusion. Thus, if an acute otitis media or serous otitis happened to be present at the time of the study, the true extent of the lesion could not be appreciated, although the presence or absence of bone erosion might be recognized. In view of the relative frequency of acute otitis media in this age group, they recommended that the patient's ear be examined immediately prior to any radiographic studies.

Although cholesteatoma may be distinguished from cholesterol granuloma, granulation tissue or serous effusion by magnetic resonance imaging (74,75), this modality is of limited value, because these features are frequently found associated with many middle ear or mastoid conditions. Although gadolinium enhancement can demonstrate the increased vascularity of the associated granulation tissue of infection or inflammation, bone erosion cannot be appreciated.

MANAGEMENT

The management of middle ear cholesteatoma is prompt surgical removal. Complete resection and preservation of hearing can almost always be expected while the cholesteatoma is confined to the anterosuperior mesotympanum. With posterior extension, ossicular involvement and hearing loss is the rule. Once the cholesteatoma has extended beyond the middle ear and into what is most often a well-developed and aerated mastoid bone, it may appear even more aggressive than an acquired lesion. This process is related directly to patient age and the functional outcome related directly to the age of diagnosis and intervention (28). There is no role for observation except in postoperative follow-up. A wide range of surgical procedures has been advocated for the management of congenital cholesteatoma, from simple myringotomy and removal to radical mastoidectomy, and open versus closed techniques with and without staged second-look surgery (39,76).

MYRINGOTOMY

Not infrequently, the diagnosis of congenital cholesteatoma has been made at myringotomy for insertion of a ventilating tube (28) and it can be tempting to proceed with removal via the myringotomy incision. This can be an effective procedure and the entire lesion removed, at least in the smaller lesions, because attachment to the lateral aspect of

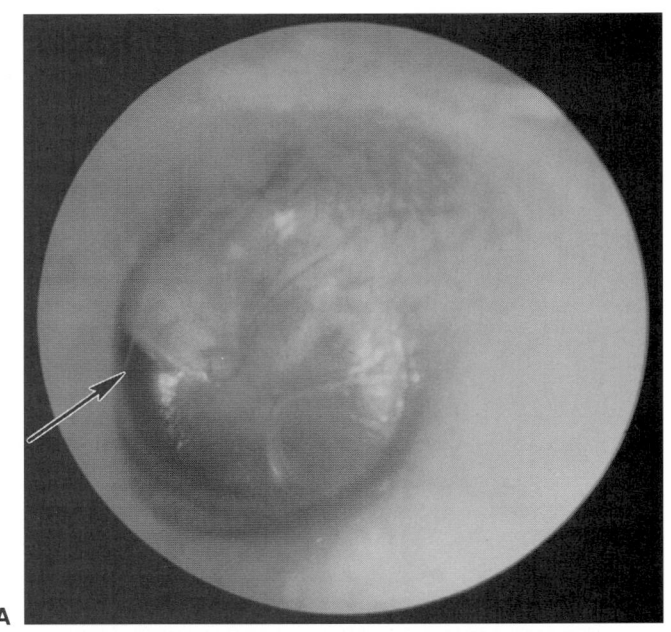

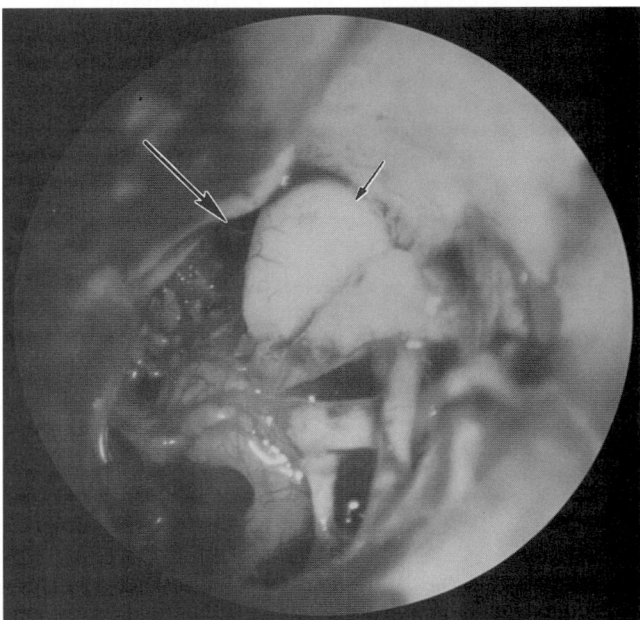

FIG. 12. A: This patient presented with a left-sided acute otitis media, which was likely secondary to occlusion of the eustachian tube by the congenital cholesteatoma. The anterosuperior lesion was not recognized until the effusion had largely resolved. Its relationship to the eustachian tube orifice *(long arrow)* could be seen through the intact tympanic membrane. **B:** The lesion was approached via a postauricular incision with complete elevation of the tympanic membrane in continuity with the external canal skin. This approach provided complete exposure of the middle ear, confirming the location and extent of the cholesteatoma *(small arrow).* It was confined to the anterosuperior mesotympanum, lightly attached by mucosa only to the neck of the malleus. The ossicles were otherwise not involved.

the middle ear is by a tenuous mucosal stalk and not by the cholesteatoma matrix itself (see Fig. 3).

Biopsy, piecemeal removal, or tube insertion should be avoided for fear of seeding or the formation of middle ear adhesions. Removal via a formal, perhaps extended, tympanotomy should be carried out unless the lesion is so small (e.g., 1–2 mm) in diameter that it can be lifted out in toto through the myringotomy. The size of the lesion is much more likely to be clinically underestimated, rather than overestimated and the cholesteatoma may be multiloculated. Wide visualization of the middle ear is recommended.

TYMPANOTOMY

The majority of lesions located in the anterior mesotympanum may be adequately approached and removed through a conventional or extended inferiorly based tympanotomy (77). Those involving the posterior mesotympanum may require some form of atticotomy or mastoidectomy for complete access and removal; however, a significant number of posterior and even some extensive mesotympanic congenital cholesteatomas may also be adequately visualized and resected using an extended tympanotomy approach, in which the tympanic membrane can be completely separated from the ossicles and the middle ear widely exposed.

In small children or those with particularly narrow external canals, a tympanotomy may be carried out via a postauricular incision in which the tympanic membrane is completely elevated from the ossicles while still attached to the external canal skin. This approach exposes the entire middle ear (Fig. 12). Visualization is unparalleled, allowing for easy removal of cholesteatoma and reconstruction, as indicated.

The usual rules of chronic middle ear surgery need not necessarily apply in congenital cholesteatoma. There is usually little reaction or adhesion between the middle ear mucosa and the adjacent cholesteatoma matrix in these patients. The mucosa appears normal (36) and there is usually a discrete plane of separation between the mucosa surrounding the cholesteatoma and that lining the middle ear or enveloping the ossicles (Fig. 13) as opposed to the usual findings in chronic middle ear disease where inflammatory changes are extensive and normal middle ear mucosa deficient or absent (28). This plane may be obliterated to some degree if there have been frequent infections, if the lesion has been biopsied, or if a ventilating tube has been inserted. It is entirely apppropriate to approach any of these lesions via an extended tympanotomy, even in the presence of eustachian tube occlusion, middle ear effusion, or facial palsy, provided there is no evidence of gross bony erosion (Fig. 14) in the epitympanum or mastoid on CT (28). This approach can always be extended into an atticotomy or mastoidectomy in those cases in which a tympanotomy alone does not allow adequate access.

Stabilization and healing of the tympanic membrane is rapid when the middle ear has been exposed via this postauricular tympanotomy approach and the external canal epithelium unbreached. Within a few weeks it should appear normal, and the hearing will be optimized.

MASTOIDECTOMY

In the absence of obvious mastoid involvement, it is reasonable to assume that the cholesteatoma is still confined within the middle ear and attic, even if the cell system is filled with effusion. Once the cholesteatoma has extended superiorly to the tympanic isthmus (i.e., into the epitympanum, the attic, or beyond), complete removal is unlikely via a conventional tympanotomy, and some form of atticotomy or modified mastoidectomy must be utilized.

Because these children usually have had relatively little or even no middle ear inflammation, their mastoid bones

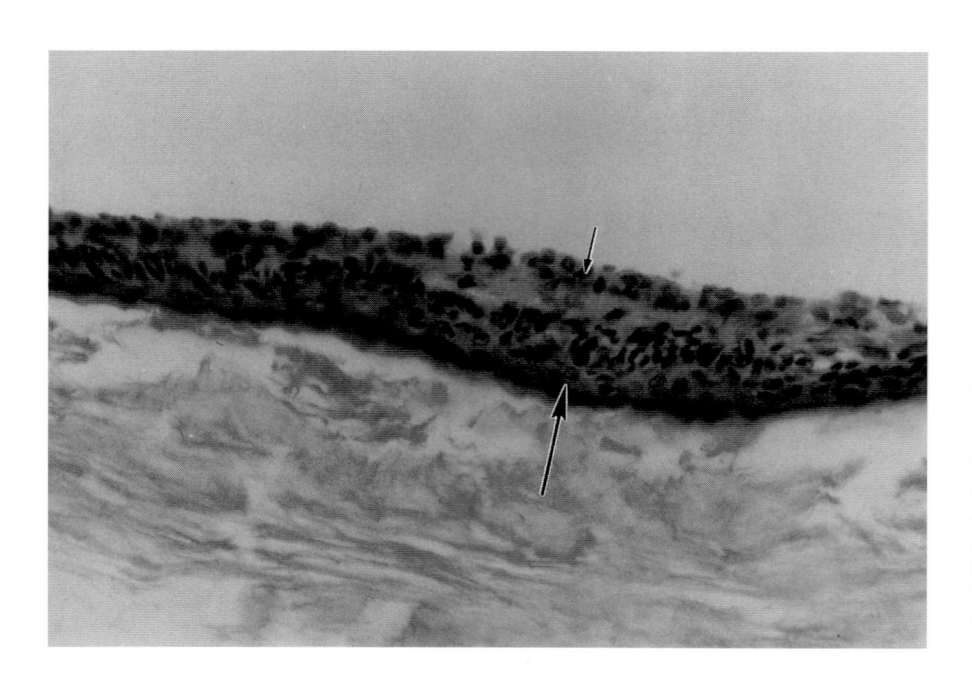

FIG. 13. The wall of the congenital cholesteatoma consists of two discrete layers: an outer mucosal layer *(small arrow),* which allows for a clean surgical separation from the adjacent middle ear mucosal lining, and an inner layer of stratified keratinizing squamous epithelium *(long arrow),* which sheds keratin centripetally into the lesion. With repeated infection and inflammation, the mucosal layer will be lost, as will be the plane of separation.

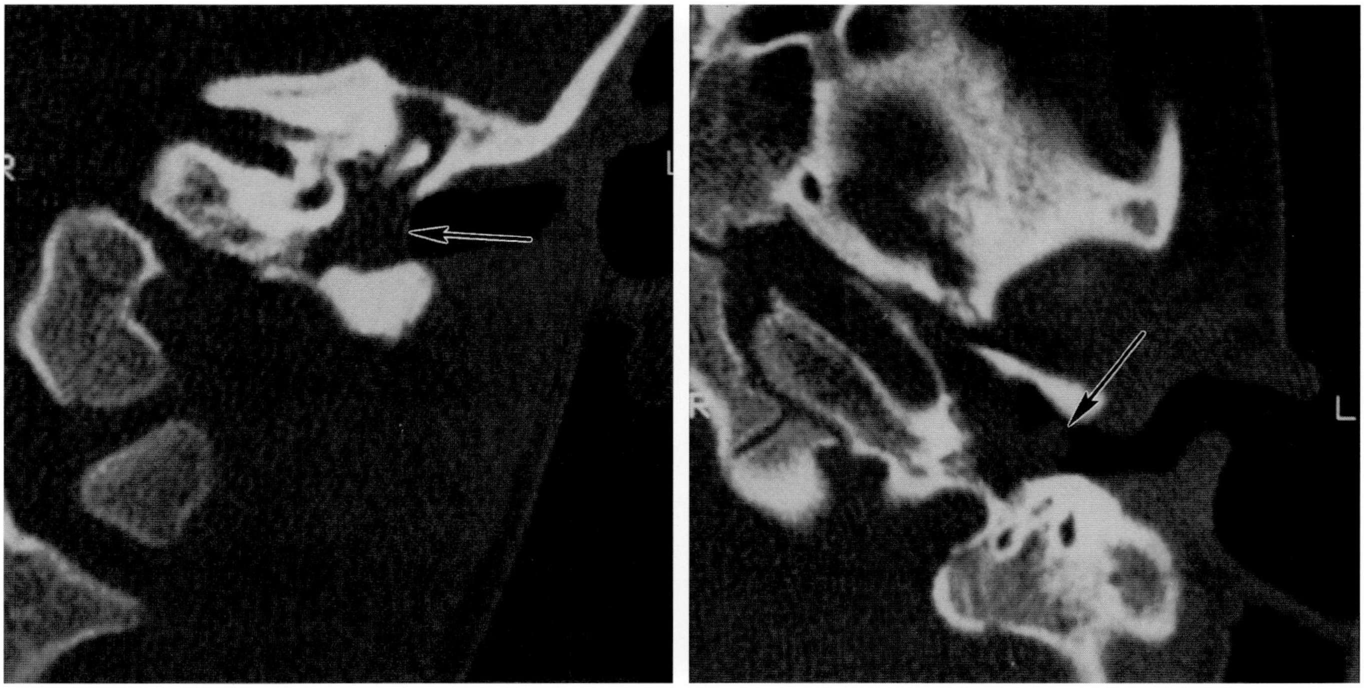

FIG. 14. A, B: This large congenital cholesteatoma was prolapsing the tympanic membrane (arrow) and filling the middle ear. The degree of mastoid involvement was unclear because of effusion. Because there was no bony erosion apparent on CT, the lesion was approached via a tympanotomy. At surgery, minimal erosion of the long process was found, but the ossicular chain was in continuity and there was a clean plane of separation between the cholesteatoma and the middle ear mucosa. Complete removal and preservation of hearing was possible. Reproduced, with permission, courtesy of The Laryngoscope.

tend to be well pneumatized. Cholesteatoma in children has long been recognized as being more extensive than in adults, faster growing, and frequently with widespread involvement. This appreciation stimulated the introduction and promotion of intact canal wall procedures. In spite of the significant recurrence rates (18,48,76) the use of closed procedures has been well supported (18,20,36,47) in order to avoid a problematic mastoid cavity and facilitate middle ear reconstruction. Surgery can be initiated as a tympanotomy, extended into an atticotomy or mastoidectomy if necessary, and bony resection carried out only to the limits of the cholesteatoma, usually leaving a very small, carefree cavity. A complete mastoidectomy with its need for frequent toilet should, if at all possible, be avoided.

There is probably little role for a classical radical mastoidectomy. Even with the most extensive congenital cholesteatoma, there will still be some tympanic membrane remnant, the hypotympanum almost always clear and the eustachian tube functional. As a minimum, some form of cavum minor can be fashioned and expected to heal.

Widespread involvement of the mastoid bone is highly unlikely before the age of 4 or 5 years, emphasizing the importance of early diagnosis and intervention (28,44).

REEXPLORATION AND RECURRENCE

Routine reexploration is not necessary in those patients whose disease was sharply circumscribed and confined to the anterior mesotympanum. Any recurrence in this group will be limited, at least initially, to the middle ear and easily detected transtympanically on clinical follow-up. A second look need not be undertaken unless there is obvious recurrent disease, there is an unexplained deterioration in hearing, or there is a serious concern about the adequacy of the initial surgery. Recurrent disease can usually be managed by repeat tympanotomy, and subsequent mastoidectomy, open or closed, should rarely be required (28,30,76).

Because of the recognized high rate of recurrence, routine reexploration between 6 and 12 months post-operatively has been recommended (32,48,78,79) for those patients whose disease extended into the antrum or mastoid. Multiple revisions may be required in patients with extensive disease whose posterior canal has been left intact (76).

It is recommended (28) that follow-up for those patients with initial disease limited to the middle ear be no less than 24 months. Those patients who required some form of modified mastoidectomy and are likely to need ongoing care should be followed indefinitely.

SUMMARY

A congenital cholesteatoma, as initially defined by Derlacki and Clemis (14), was one that arose from an embryonal inclusion of squamous epithelium of undifferentiated tissue in the middle ear and developed behind an intact tympanic membrane. There could be no history of otitis media. Derlacki (18,26) was subsequently prepared to accept this diagnosis in the presence of a perforation if a history of otitis media were lacking. It is, however, the rare child who was had no otitis media; indeed, most have had two or more episodes by 3 years of age (80).

Levenson et al. (29,55,67) felt that a history of prior bouts of otitis media was not grounds for exclusion. The pars flaccida and pars tensa had to be normal and there could be no history of otorrhea or perforation and no prior otologic surgical procedures. Patients with canal atresia and those with intramembranous or giant cholesteatomas were also excluded.

An acute perforation with or without otorrhea is a common sequela to acute otitis media and in some children is associated with virtually every episode, while in others, it may go unrecognized by the patient's parents yet be readily apparent on clinical examination. It would be difficult if not impossible to assume that any patient presenting with an otherwise "classical" congenital cholesteatoma had never had such a perforation.

The exclusion of patients with a history of an otologic surgical procedure has some validity. The possibility of an implantation epidermoid, particularly following a myringotomy and tube insertion, is real but would appear to be exceedingly rare (28,46).

Regardless of which criteria one accepts for a cholesteatoma to be considered congenital in origin, there will always be clinicians for whom this is an unacceptable diagnosis, and there will always be lesions that do not quite fit the usual strict criteria and yet are clearly not typical of so-called primary acquired or secondary acquired cholesteatomas. The possibility of metaplasia or posttraumatic implantation can never be categorically ruled out, nor can it be assured that any past episodes of otitis media, no matter how few or mild, have been insignificant.

Nevertheless, there is a group of young patients, primarily male, whose disease presents most frequently within the first 4 or 5 years of life, behind a currently intact tympanic membrane and in whom there is no obvious history of trauma or major ear infection. The mastoid cell systems are most often symmetrically well developed and aerated. Retraction pockets of either the attic or mesotympanum are not a feature, and the eustachian tube is apparently functional. These lesions are usually unilocular and restricted to the middle ear, presenting anterosuperiorly in the majority of cases.

At surgery, there may be few if any gross inflammatory changes or adhesions, and the cholesteatoma can usually be cleanly separated from the ossicles and middle ear recesses, preserving a normal mucosal lining. This is so unlike the situation found in the usual case of cholesteatoma associated with chronic suppurative otitis media. The surgical management of such patients is determined more by these physical attributes than by the pathogenesis (20,28,81).

When the diagnosis is early, ideally before 3 or 4 years of age, and the cholesteatoma confined to the anterosuperior quadrant of the middle ear, one can expect curative removal and the preservation of normal hearing. Even when the middle ear appears to be completely filled with cholesteatoma, an extended tympanotomy is still a worthwhile and often adequate approach. If the diagnosis is missed until the disease has spread beyond the middle ear and into what is likely a well-pneumatized mastoid bone, the ossicles will most assuredly have been eroded, and some form of mastoidectomy and rehabilitation will be required.

ACKNOWLEDGMENTS

The author wishes to thank Dr. Michael W. Hawke for his invaluable help in obtaining the clinical photographs used in this chapter and Mr. Gordon Sloan who has been of long-standing support in the development of a radiographic photo-library from which these examples were taken.

REFERENCES

1. Muller J. Von der geschichteten perlmutterglanzenden Fettgeschwulst, Cholesteatoma. In: Uber den feineren Bau und die Formen der krankhaften Geschwulste. Berlin: Reimer; 1838:50.
2. Critchley M, Ferguson F. The cerebrospinal epidermoids (cholesteatomata). *Brain* 1928;51:334.
3. Jahn AF. Cholesteatoma: what is it, how did it get there, and how do we get rid of it? *Otolaryngol Clin North Amer* 1989;22:847–857.
4. Cawthorne T. Congenital cholesteatoma. *Arch of Otolaryngol* 1963;78:40–44.
5. Diamant M. Anatomical etiological factors in chronic middle ear discharge. *Ann Otol* 1957;46:380–389.
6. McKenzie D. Pathogeny of aural cholesteatoma. *J Laryngol Otol* 1931;46:163–189.
7. Toglia JU, Netsky MG, Alexander E. Epithelial (epidermoid) tumours of the cranium. *J Neurosurg* 1965;23:384–393.
8. Mawson SR. Diseases of the ear. City: Edward Arnold; 1963:293.
9. Teed RW. Cholesteatoma verum tympani (its relationship to the first epibranchial placode). *Arch Otolaryngol* 1936;24:455–474.
10. Jefferson G, Smalley AA. Progressive palsy produced by intratemporal epidermoids. *J Laryngol* 1938;5:417–442.
11. Michaels L. An epidermoid formation in the developing middle ear: possible source of cholesteatoma. *J Otolaryngol* 1986;15:169–174.
12. House HP. An apparent primary cholesteatoma case report. *Laryngoscope* 1953;63:712–713.
13. Sheehy JL. True cholesteatoma. *Arch Otolaryngol* 1959;69:57–60.
14. Derlacki EL, Clemis JD. Congenital cholesteatoma of the middle ear and mastoid. *Ann Otol Rhinol Laryngol* 1965;74:706–727.
15. Derlacki EL, Harrison WH, Clemis JD. Congenital cholesteatoma of the middle ear and mastoid: a second report presenting seven additional cases. *Laryngoscope* 1968;78:1050–1078.
16. Peron DL, Schuknecht HF. Congenital cholesteatoma with other anomalies. *Arch Otolaryngol* 1975;101:498–505.
17. Palva A, Pekka P, Karja J. Cholesteatoma in children. *Arch Otolaryngol* 1977;103:74–77.
18. Derlacki EL. Congenital cholesteatoma of the middle ear and mastoid: a third report. *Arch Otolaryngol* 1973;97:177–182.
19. Schuknecht HF. Pathology of the ear. Cambridge, MA: Harvard University Press; 1974.
20. House JW, Sheehy JL. Cholesteatoma with intact tympanic membrane: a report of 41 cases. *Laryngoscope* 1980;90:70–76.
21. Sculerati N, Bluestone CD. Pathogenesis of cholesteatoma. *Otolaryngol Clin North Am* 1989;22:859–868.
22. Palva T. The pathogenesis and treatment of cholesteatoma. *Acta Otolaryngol (Stockh)* 1990;109:323–330.
23. Michaels L. Evolution of the epidermoid formation and its role in the development of the middle ear and tympanic membrane during the first trimester. *Otolaryngol* 1988;17:22–28.
24. Michaels L. Origin of congenital cholesteatoma from a normally occur-

ring epidermoid rest in the developing middle ear. *Int J Pediatr Otorhinolaryngol* 1988;15:51–65.
25. Chen JM, Schloss MD, Manoukian JJ, Shapiro RS. Congenital cholesteatoma of the middle ear in children. *J Otolaryngol* 1989;18:44–48.
26. Derlacki EL. Congenital cholesteatoma today. *Am J Otol* 1985;6:19–21.
27. Fernandez C, Lindsay JR, Moskowitz M. Some observations on the pathogenesis of middle ear cholesteatoma. *Arch Otolaryngol* 1959;68:537–546.
28. Friedberg J. Congenital cholesteatoma. *Laryngoscope* 1994;104(3 pt 2):1–24.
29. Levenson MJ, Michaels L, Parisier SC. Congenital cholesteatomas of the middle ear in children: origin and management. *Otolaryngol Clin North Amer* 1989;22:941–954.
30. McGill TJ, Merchant S, Healy GB, Friedman EM. Congenital cholesteatoma of the middle ear in children: a clinical and histopathological report. *Laryngoscope* 1991;101:606–613.
31. Michaels L. Biology of cholesteatoma. *Otolaryngol Clin North Am* 1989;22:869–881.
32. Parisier SC, Weiss MH. Recidivism in congenital cholesteatoma surgery. *Ear Nose Throat J* 1991;70:362–364.
33. Nager FR. The cholesteatoma of the middle ear—its etiology, pathogenesis, diagnosis and therapy. *Ann Otol Rhinol Laryngol* 1925;34:1249–1258.
34. Hough TJVB. Congenital malformations of the middle ear. *Arch Otolaryngol* 1963;78:335–343.
35. Sade J, Babiacki A, Pinkus G. The metaplastic and congenital origin of cholesteatoma. *Acta Otolaryngol* 1983;96:119–129.
36. Sanna M, Zini C. Congenital cholesteatoma of the middle ear: a report of 11 cases. *Am J Otol* 1984;5:368–378.
37. Schwartz RH, Grundfast KM, McAveney WJ, Merida MA, Feldman B. Congenital middle ear cholesteatoma. *Am J Dis Child* 1983;137:501–503.
38. Parisier SC, Levenson MJ, Edelstein DR, Bindra GS, et al. Management of congenital cholesteatomas. *Am J Otol* 1989;10:121–123.
39. Schuring AG, Lippy WH, Rizer FM, Schuring LT. Staging for colesteatoma in the child, adolescent, and adult. *Ann Otol Rhinol Laryngol* 1990;99:256–260.
40. Holmgren G. Some experiences in surgery for otosclerosis. *Acta Otolaryngol* 1923;5:1923.
41. Shea JJ. Fenestration of the oval window. *Ann Otol Rhinol Laryngol* 1958;67:932.
42. Smith R, Moran WB. Tympanic membrane keratoma (cholesteatoma) in children with no prior otologic surgery. *Laryngoscope* 1976;86:237–245.
43. Brosnan ML. Primary cholesteatomas of the temporal bone. *Arch Otolaryngol Head Neck Surg* 1967;86:29–32.
44. Curtis AW. Congenital middle ear cholesteatoma: two unusual cases and a review of the literature. *Laryngoscope* 1979;89:1159–1165.
45. Fedok FG, Bellissimo JB, Wiegand DA. Bilateral congenital aural cholesteatoma. *Otolaryngol Head Neck Surg* 1990;103:1028–1030.
46. Paparrella MM, Rybak L. Congenital cholesteatoma. *Otolaryngol Clin North Am* 1978;11:113–120.
47. Rizer FM, Luxford WM. The management of congenital cholesteatoma: surgical results of 42 cases. *Laryngoscope* 1988;98:254–256.
48. Schwartz RH, Grundfast KM, Feldman B, Linde RE, Hermansen KL. Cholesteatoma medial to an intact tympanic membrane in 34 young children. *Pediatrics* 1984;74:236–240.
49. Wang R, Zubick HH, Vernick DM, Strome M. Bilateral congenital middle Ear cholesteatomas. *Laryngoscope* 1984;94:1461–1463.
50. Herdman R, Wright JLW. Grommets and cholesteatoma in children. *J Laryngol Otol* 1988;102:1000–1002.
51. Aimi K. Role of the tympanic ring in the pathogenesis of congenital cholesteatoma. *Laryngoscope* 1983;93:1140–1146.
52. Cushing H. A large epidermal cholesteatoma of the parieto-temporal region deforming the left hemisphere without cerebral symptoms. *Surg Gynec Obstet* 1922;34:557–567.
53. Friedmann I. Congenital cholesteatoma. In: *Pathology of the ear.* Oxford: Blackwell Scientific; 1974:99–103.
54. Ruedi L. Cholesteatoma of the Attic. *J Laryngol* 1958;72:593–609.
55. Levenson MJ, Michaels L, Parisier SC, et al. Congenital cholesteatomas in children: an embryologic correlation. *Laryngoscope* 1988;98:949–955.
56. Wang R, Hawke M, Kwok R. The epidermoid formation (Michaels' structure) in the developing middle ear. *J Otolaryngol* 1987;16:327–330.
57. Cohen D. Locations of primary cholesteatoma. *Am J Otol* 1987;8:61–65.
58. Meyerhoff WL, Truelson J. Cholesteatoma staging. *Laryngoscope* 1986;96:935–939.
59. Ruedi L. Cholesteatoma formation in the middle ear in animal experiments. *Acta Otolaryngol* 1959;50:233–242.
60. Cody DTR. The definition of cholesteatoma. In: McCabe B, Sade J, Abramson M, eds. *Cholesteatoma: first international conference.* Birmingham: Aesculapius; 1977:6
61. Reilly PG. Congenital cholesteatoma presenting as a post-auricular mass. *J Laryngol Otol* 1989;103:1069–1070.
62. Borgstein J, Martin F, Soda A. Giant congenital cholesteatoma. *Ann Otol Rhinol Laryngol* 1992;102(8 pt 1):646–647.
63. Jahnke V. Clinical, pathological and therapeutic aspects of cholesteatoma in children. In: Sade J, ed. Cholesteatoma and mastoiod surgery. Amsterdam: Kugler; 1982:25–28.
64. Cannoni M, Pech A, Fuchs S, Zanaret M, et al. Congenital cholesteatoma of the petrous bone. Etiopathogenic discussions apropos of 11 cases. *Rev Laryngol Otol Rhinol* 1989;110(1):33–42.
65. Cawthorne T, Griffith A. Primary cholesteatoma of the temporal bone. *Arch of Otolaryngol* 1961;73:252–260.
66. Fisch U. Congenital cholesteatoma of the supra-labyrinthic region. *Clin Otolarygol* 1978;3:369–376.
67. Levenson MJ, Parisier SC, Chute P, Wenig S, Juarbe C. A review of twenty congenital cholesteatomas of the middle ear in children. *Otolaryngol Head Neck Surg* 1986;94:560–569.
68. Huang TS, Lee FP. Congenital cholesteatoma: a review of twelve cases. *Am J Otolaryngol* 1994;15:276–281.
69. Brownlie Smith A. Congenital cholesteatoma. *J Laryngol Otol* 1975;82:1049–1051.
70. Moriarty B, Rutka J. Middle ear masses: the importance of color and location. *Can J Diagn* 1990;7:81–95.
71. Swartz JD. Cholesteatomas of the middle ear: diagnosis, etiology, and complications. *Radiol Clin North Am* 1984;22:15–35.
72. Buckingham RA, Valvassori GE. Tomographic evaluation of 88 cholesteatomas the middle ear and mastoid. *Otolaryngol Clin North Amer* 1973;6:363–378.
73. Mafee MF, Aimi K, Valvassori GE. Computed tomography in the diagnosis of primary tumors of the petrous bone. *Laryngoscope* 1984;94:1423–1430.
74. Phelps PD, Wright A. Imaging cholesteatoma. *Clin Radiol* 1990;41:156–162.
75. Valvassori GE. Diagnosis of retrocochlear and central vestibular disease by magnetic resonance imaging. *Ann Otol Rhinol Laryngol* 1988;97:19–22.
76. Doyle KJ, Luxford WM. Congenital aural cholesteatoma: results of surgery in 60 cases. *Laryngoscope* 1995;105:263–267.
77. Grundfast KM, Thomsen JR, Barber CS. The inferiorly based superior tympanomeatal flap for removal of congenital cholesteatoma. *Laryngoscope* 1990;100:1341–1343.
78. Gray JD; The treatment of cholesteatoma in children. *Proc Roy Soc Med* 1964;57:769–771.
79. Smyth GD. Postoperative cholesteatoma. In: McCabe BF, Abramson M, Sade J. eds. First International Conference on Cholesteatoma. Birmingham: Aesculapius; 1977:355–362.
80. Teele DW, Klein JO, Rosner B. Epidemiology of otitis media during the first seven years of life in children in greater Boston: a prospective, cohort study. *J Infect Dis* 1989;160:83–94.
81. Laskiewicz B, Chalstrey S, Gatland DJ, Jones N, Michaels L. Congenital cholesteatoma *J Laryngol Otol* 1991;105:995–998.

Chapter 20

Acquired Cholesteatoma

Simon C. Parisier, Adam J. Cohen, Bryan A. Selkin, and Jin C. Han

Historically, suppurative ear disease and its complications were greatly feared because they frequently resulted in prolonged illnesses and death. The introduction of antibiotics, which were very effective therapy for acute otitis media, changed the course of otology. Prior to 1940 the otologist was preoccupied with reducing the significant mortality and morbidity associated with ear infections. If one could surgically make an ear safe, the intervention was considered successful. The fact that the ear continued to drain or that the hearing was reduced was acceptable. Shortly after World War II, as antibiotics became widely available, the dreaded life-threatening complications of acute otitis media and the need for ear surgery to treat them were greatly reduced. In the 1950s, the binocular, operating microscope was perfected so that it provided both magnification and illumination. Innovative otologists, freed from the overwhelming concern with otologic infections, generated the microsurgical era. The operating microscope, first used to perform fenestration surgery for otosclerosis, was applied for hearing reconstruction. At present, the foci of the otologic surgeon are ''chronic'' ears, especially those with cholesteatoma and the emergence of acute otitis media caused by the resistant organisms that is refractory to antibiotic therapy. Both these conditions are associated with similar complications.

In the past 25 years, many otologic surgeons have made the avoidance of the mastoid cavity a primary goal of ear surgery (1). Prior to the mid-1950s many otologists operating with surgical tools that are now considered primitive feared that they might cause facial paralysis, injure the inner ear, or damage intracranial structures. To avoid complications, a conscious attempt was made by some surgeons not to come ''too close'' to the facial nerve, the oral window, or other critical structures even if doing so meant leaving residual disease. Even today, in spite of significant technological advances, the poorly trained or inexperienced otorhinolaryngologist avoids using the facial nerve as a key surgical landmark. Fear of harming the patient has led to the utilization of limited techniques aimed at making the ear ''safe'' by exteriorizing the disease without striving for its total removal. Consequently, many inadequately treated patients were troubled postoperatively by persistent or recurrent disease and drainage from poorly healed, difficult-to-clean mastoid cavities.

Influenced by these problems, skillful otologic surgeons condemned techniques that created a mastoid cavity. Purposefully using the facial nerve as a key surgical landmark, innovative operative procedures that avoided a mastoid recess were developed. Consequently, canal wall up (CWU) techniques became very popular and were used to treat the majority of cases of chronic mastoiditis caused by cholesteatoma. Otologic surgeons prided themselves in their technical ability to preserve the posterior canal wall regardless of the adequacy of eustachian tube function, the extent of the disease, or the anatomic limitations imposed by the sized of the mastoid. It would seem that otologic surgeons had become preoccupied with preserving the posterior canal wall as an end in itself, even if that compromised the results, as evidenced by the significant rate of recidivism. At present, the pendulum seems to be swinging back to a more realistic position. The surgical management of patients with chronic mastoiditis caused by cholesteatoma should be individualized; the best operative procedure should be selected for a given patient regardless of whether that procedure is a canal-wall-up or canal-wall-down (CWD) procedure.

This chapter reviews the complications caused by cholesteatoma and the relationship of adhesive otitis media to acquired cholesteatoma. The chapter also reviews specific operative technique and the results achieved using this method of management. Some underlying controversies regarding acquired pediatric cholesteatoma are also discussed.

S.C. Parisier and B.A. Selkin: Department of Otolaryngology—Head and Neck Surgery, Manhattan Ear, Eye, and Throat Hospital, Cornell University Medical Center, New York, New York 10021.
A.J. Cohen: Internal Medicine, Staten Island University Hospital, New York, New York 10128.
J.C. Han: Department of Otorhinolaryngology, Manhattan Eye, Ear, and Throat Hospital, New York, New York 10021.

CLASSIFICATION OF CHOLESTEATOMA

Cholesteatoma is keratinizing squamous epithelium that grows within the temporal bone. It exhibits unrestrained proliferation, erodes bone, can be highly destructive if not fully removed, and has a tendency to grow back. The process does not grow in a continuous linear fashion. Generally, its growth is stimulated by infection, inflammation, and pressure produced by retained keratin. Cytokines, lymphokines, and growth factors are involved in its aggressiveness. Cholesteatomas may remain clinically dormant for extended periods of time or they may grow insidiously, producing symptoms only when their erosion causes a significant complication.

Cholesteatoma can be classified into several clinical categories according to how they originated: congenital, primary or secondarily acquired, and recidivistic/iatrogenic (regrowth after surgery). Regardless of origin, they have a similar histologic appearance and pathologic tendencies. Because choleteatoma is a destructive process, it has the capability to cause life-threatening and crippling complications (2). The most common symptom is a conductive hearing loss produced by ossicular destruction (Fig. 1). Involvement of the facial nerve may cause a disfiguring paralysis. Extension through the bony covering of the semicircular canal induces vertigo, and progression into the fluid-filled membranous labyrinth results in a serous or purulent labyrinthitis and neurosensory hearing loss. Untreated, meningitis may occur when the labyrinthine infection spreads through existing communications from the perilymphatic into the cerebrospinal fluid spaces. A cholesteatoma may erode

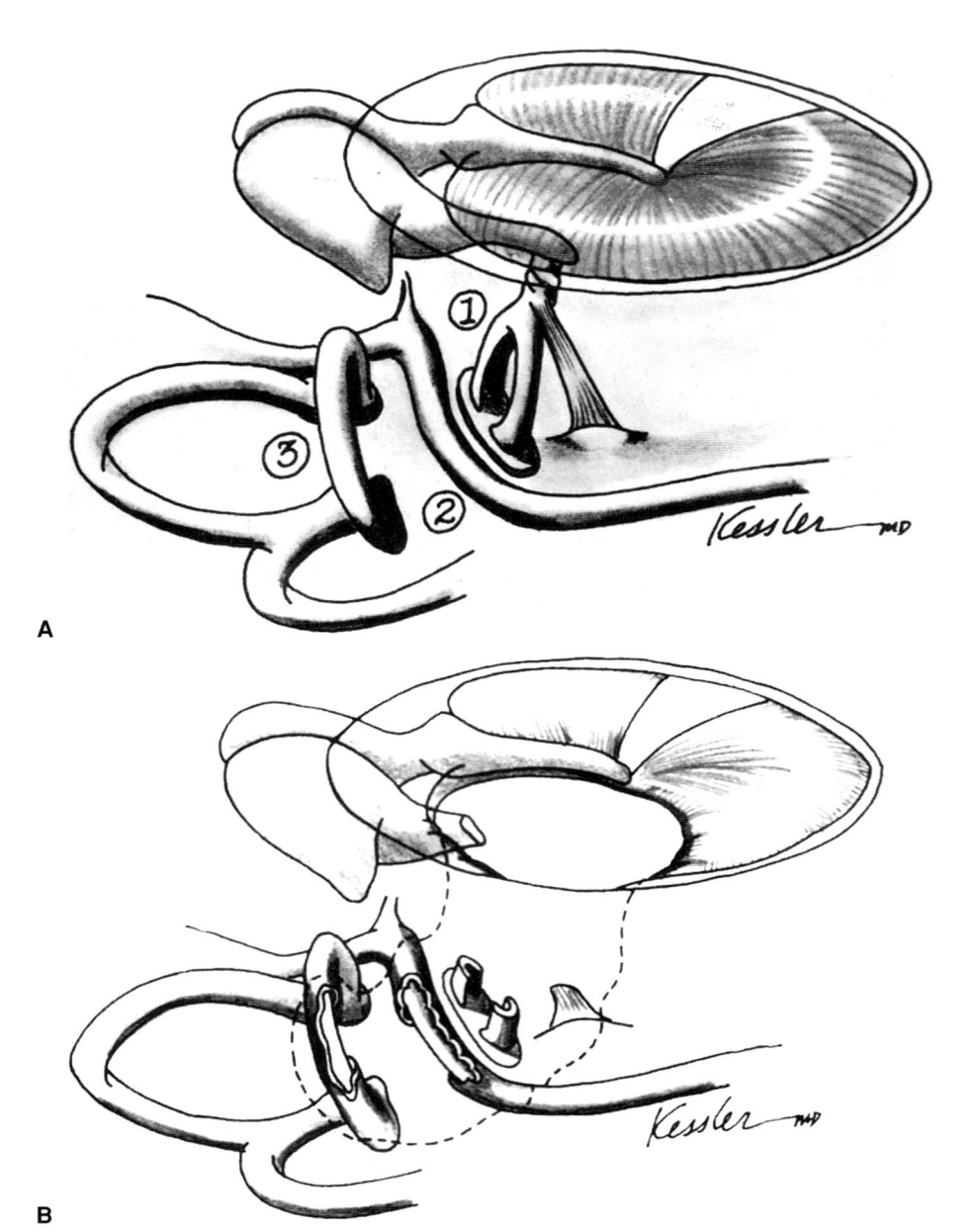

FIG. 1. A: Structures within the temporal bone that are vulnerable to cholesteatoma (1) ossicular chain, (2) facial nerve, and (3) semicircular canals. **B:** The most common complications caused by cholesteatoma (stippled lines) are erosion of the incus and stapes, facial nerve involvement, and semicircular canal fistula.

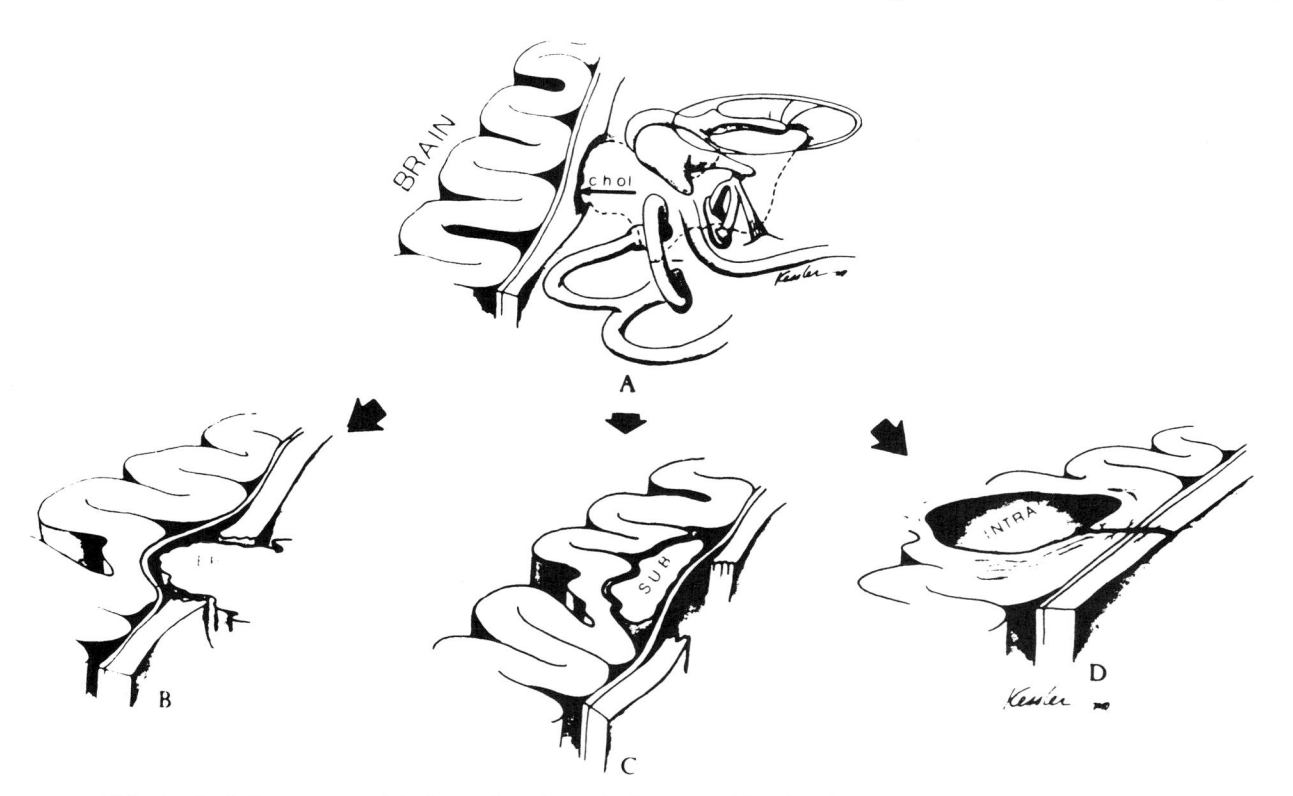

FIG. 2. A cholesteatoma (chol) eroding through the mastoid to involve dura **(A)**, causing an epidural (EPI) abscess **(B)**. Spread of infection through dura can produce a subdural (SUB) abscess **(C)**. Phlebitis of small vessels can lead to the formation of an intracerebral (INTRA) abscess **(D)**.

either through the mastoid tegmen, exposing the temporal lobe dura, or through the medial wall, exposing the posterior fossa dura. Extension of the infection intracranially can lead to the development of an epidural, subdural, or intracerebral abscess (or a combination of these types of abscess) (Fig. 2).

Alternatively, the infection can extend to involve the central nervous system by phlebitic involvement of the emissary vessels traversing through the temporal bone into adjacent meningeal structures. Lateral sinus involvement results when erosion within the mastoid exposes this venous structure, leading to thrombus formation within its lumen (Fig. 3). Bacterial infection of the intraluminal clot can produce a lateral sinus phlebitis and septicemia. Otic hydrocephalus occurs when venous obstruction interferes with the blood return from the brain or when the mechanisms for the reabsorption of cerebrospinal fluid are prevented from functioning effectively. Although effective control of acute otitis media with antibiotic therapy has almost eradicated coalescent mastoiditis, chronic mastoids due to cholesteatoma and the otitic complications are still commonly encountered.

Primary Acquired Cholesteatoma

Clinically, the most common type of cholesteatoma encountered arises because of an existing eustachian tube dysfunction (Fig. 4). Persistent negative middle-ear pressure causes the tympanic membrane to become retracted. The superior or posterior (or both) portions of the tympanic membrane become invaginated into the attic area of the mastoid or extend medial to the scutum posteriorly to produce a skin-lined retraction pocket. Keratin accumulating with in this retraction pocket forms an epithelial-lined cyst that gradually enlarges and erodes the surrounding bone. This process, a primary acquired cholesteatoma, results from an invagination of a portion of the intact, skin-lined, retracted tympanic membrane into the mastoid. The term is appropriate because it implies that the condition is not secondary to a previous tympanic-membrane perforation.

Retraction Pockets

The differentiation of a tympanic-membrane retraction pocket from a primary acquired cholesteatoma can present a clinical dilemma. Retraction pockets usually involve the pars flaccida or the posterior portion of the pars tensa, or both. Shallow, wide-mouthed, skin-lined invagination of the pars flaccida superior to the lateral malleus process are frequently observed; when asymptomatic, this condition can generally be ignored. However, when a patient has a history of recurrent otorrhea or has hearing loss, the possibility should be considered that only the tip of the cholesteatomatous iceberg is being visualized.

Retractions of the posterior-superior pars tensa can be

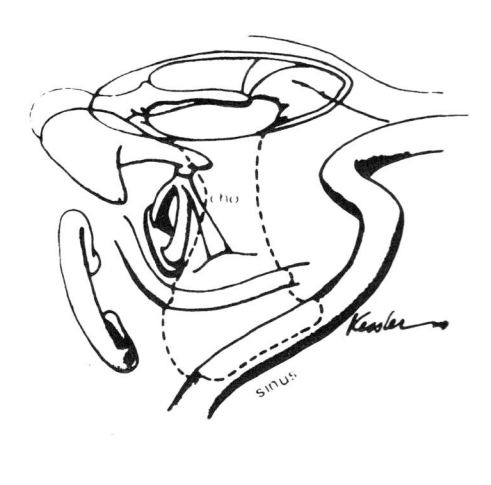

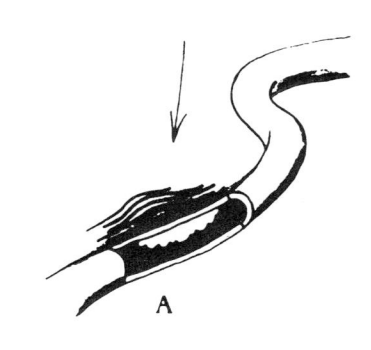

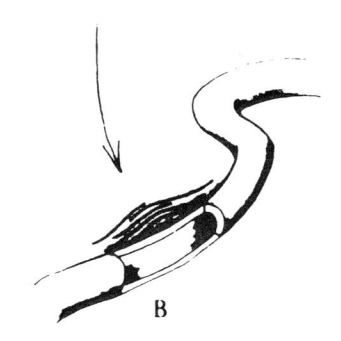

FIG. 3. The cholesteatoma (chol) can erode to expose the lateral sinus, producing either a lateral sinus phlebitis **(A)** or progress to an occlusion thrombosis **(B)** of the lumen.

classified into two clinical forms: mobile retraction pockets and fixed retraction pockets. Pneumatic otoscopy is very useful in differentiating the two types. When a negative pressure is created in the external canal, the mobile retraction pocket, which is not adherent to any underlying ear structures, balloons out, giving the affected portion of the tympanic membrane a dome-like appearance. A retraction pocket that has become adherent to the long process of the incus, the stapes, the sinus tympani, or the round window niche is not mobilized with pneumatic otoscopy. Occasionally, when a child who appears to have a fixed retraction pocket undergoes general anesthesia, nitrous oxide fills the middle-ear space and the invaginated tympanic membrane balloons out, indicating that the retraction pocket is actually mobile. Insertion of middle-ear ventilation tubes in ears with mobile retraction pockets frequently results in reexpansion of the middle-ear space. When the retraction pocket is fixed, pressure-equalizing tubes are unlikely to mobilize the retraction, but they may prevent progression to a cholesteatoma. To accomplish this goal, the tubes must be left in place continuously until, with the child's growth, the anticipated improvement in eustachian tube function is realized, and the middle ear becomes aerated.

Another important characteristic of a retraction pocket is the depth of its extension. Has a pars flaccida retraction eroded into the epitympanic spaces to become a cholesteatoma that involves the mastoid attic? Does it retain keratin? Is a posterior tympanic membrane retraction that extends medial to the scutum shallow and therefore benign? On otomicroscopy, can its end be reached with a right-angle probe? If the retraction is shallow, it may be a self-limiting process that is not progressive. Alternatively, the retraction may represent the neck of a flask-shaped, large multilobulated cholesteatoma that extends into mastoid and thus requires surgery. Middle-ear cholesteatomas may form when retractions of an atrophic pars tensa extends into the sinus tympanic round window niche areas. With time, budlike keratinizing extensions grow into the adjacent hypotympanic air cells inferior to the cochlea. Alternatively, growth may occur posteriorly, medial to the vertical portion of the facial nerve. When these extensions retain keratin, they develop into erosive middle-ear cholesteatomas and present formidable surgical challenges. In an attempt to prevent these developments, which technically are difficult to eradicate, early excision of the atrophic retraction pockets with primary grafting had been recommended. However, if this procedure is carried out in a young child with persistent eustachian tube dysfunction, atelectatic changes may recur, and the insertion of a ventilation tube may be required. Early eardrum reconstruction of retracted ear drums is controversial.

When is a retraction pocket considered to be a small cholesteatoma? This question is difficult to answer authoritatively and opinions vary among otologists. Three criteria are helpful indications that the process is a cholesteatoma. One is the presence of retained keratin in an inaccessible area from which the debris cannot be removed, even when an operating microscope is used. Second is evidence of bone destruction. Third is the recurrent formation of granulation tissue and otorrhea in the area of the retraction pocket.

Computed tomography (CT) can be a very valuable adjunct for differentiating a retraction pocket from a cholesteatoma. A CT scan can frequently demonstrate the extent of soft tissue ingrowth and the presence of bone destruction. However, interpretation of the CT scan in many cases may be confused by the coexistence of middle-ear effusion, which is frequently present in children. The fluid images as opacification of the middle ear and mastoid, which may mask signifi-

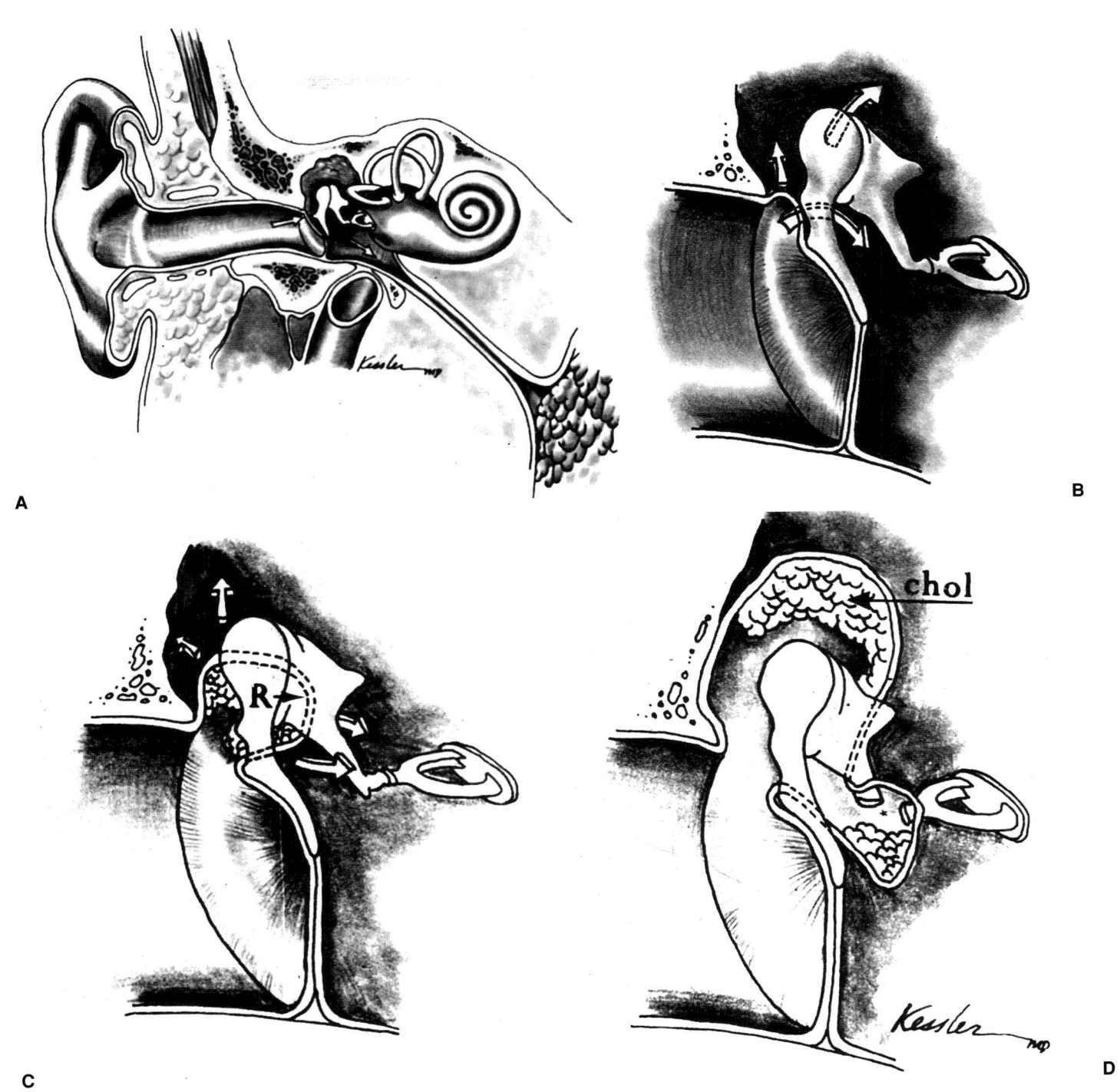

FIG. 4. A and **B:** Inadequate eustachian tube function results in a negative middle-ear pressure (NEG pp). **C:** Over time, the pars flaccida forms a retraction pocket (R). **D:** Retention of keratin and erosion of bone signifies evolution of the process to a cholesteatoma (chol).

cant soft-tissue disease or, conversely, can mimic extensive cholesteatomatous involvement. When a CT scan is obtained in a child who has middle-ear effusion, eliminating the fluid before performing the study by using either medical (i.e., antibiotics) or surgical (i.e., myringotomy and tube) therapy is helpful.

Will a retraction pocket progress to become a cholesteatoma? One cannot assume that all retractions of the tympanic membrane evolve into more extensive disease and eventuate into cholesteatoma. Some patients with significant fixed retraction pockets have been observed to have stable conditions when followed over many years. Conversely, in others, the retraction pockets progress and evolve into extensive cholesteatomas.

Secondary Acquired Cholesteatoma

A second mechanism for the formation of cholesteatoma is the ingrowth of keratinizing epithelium into the middle ear through a preexisting defect in the tympanic membrane (Fig. 5). When a perforation involves loss of the tympanic fibrous annulus because of trauma or infection, it is termed a marginal perforation. In such cases, canal wall skin can extend into the middle-ear cleft and migrate into the mastoid area, forming a secondary acquired cholesteatoma.

Keratinizing squamous epithelium can gain access from the tympanic membrane into the middle-ear cleft in several other ways. For instance, when a patient with an adhesive otitis media develops an ear infection, a perforation may occur (Fig. 6). The squamous epithelium adherent to the middle ear mucosa can become isolated from the tympanic membrane. Over time, the keratinizing epithelium grows in the middle ear and extends into the mastoid and eventually a cholesteatoma develops. If the original perforation heals, the cholesteatoma presents as a whitish mass behind an intact tympanic membrane, mimicking a congenital cholesteatoma. Injuries to the ear can also tear and implode the tympanic membrane, producing a flap that gets folded back through the perforation and becomes adherent to the middle-ear mucosal surface of the tympanic membrane (Fig. 7). Growth of this keratinizing tissue results in epidermization of the middle ear surface of the tympanic membrane with the formation of a cholesteatoma. Canal wall skin can also become trapped within bony fragments following a temporal bone fracture. Over time, growth of the skin within the healed fracture produces a destructive cholesteatoma.

Recidivistic/Iatrogenic Cholesteatoma

Recidivism is a term used to indicate regrowth of cholesteatoma that occurs after an initial surgical attempt to eradicate it. There are two common forms of recidivistic cholesteatoma, which have different pathophysiologic origins. One type of recidivism is seen in residual cholesteatomas, which arise when keratinizing epithelium is incompletely removed from a diseased ear and grows back over time (Fig. 8). A residual cholesteatoma reflects the surgeon's inability to remove every bit of cholesteatoma. The retained keratinizing epithelium cells proliferates over time and forms a residual cholesteatoma. Generally, residual cholesteatomas develop within 36 months after the initial procedure. However, it appears that the retained keratinizing squamous epithelial cells occasionally can remain dormant for a period of time before their growth produces recognizable disease.

A second type of recidivism is seen in recurrent cholesteatomas, which have a different pathophysiology. Recurrent cholesteatomas arise in ears in which the surgeon has preserved the posterior canal wall and a mastoid air space (Fig 9). Recurrence is related to inadequate eustachian tubal function. When the posterior canal wall is preserved (CWU technique), the middle ear and mastoid must be ventilated. Air must pass from the eustachian tube through the middle-ear cleft into the mastoid. When ventilation is inadequate, negative pressure that causes a retraction of the tympanic membrane develops, forming a pocket or sac within which keratin debris is retained. Over time, as the debris accumulates, it

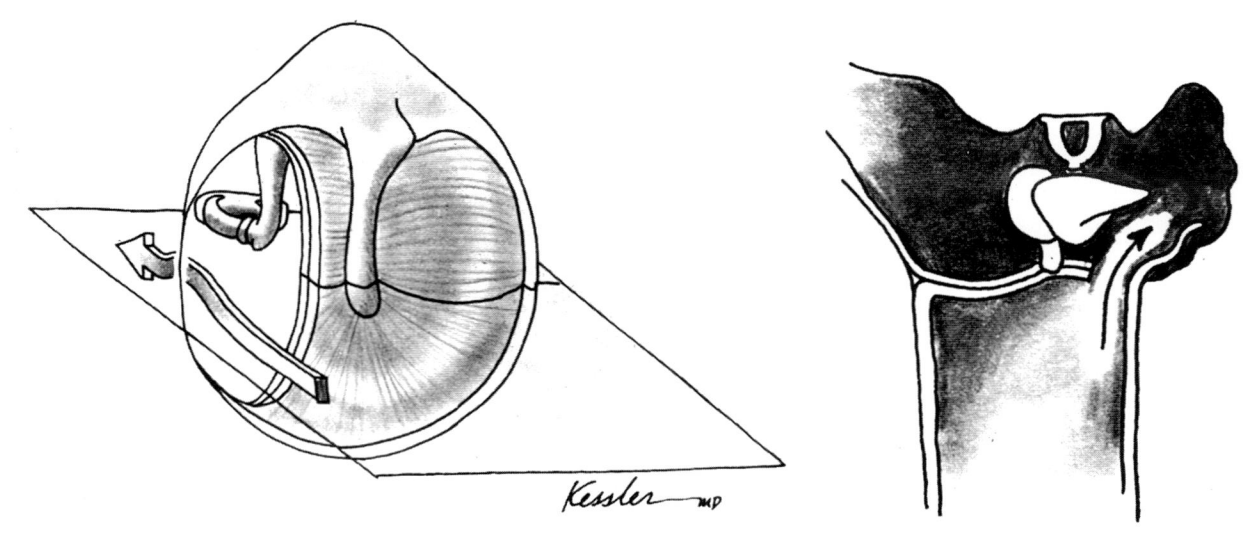

FIG. 5. A and **B:** Marginal perforation occurs in an area of the tympanic membrane that is devoid of a fibrous annulus. **B:** A cholesteatoma forms when keratinizing squamous epithelium from the canal wall skin extends unimpeded through the tympanic membrane defect (*arrow*) to replace middle ear and mastoid mucosa.

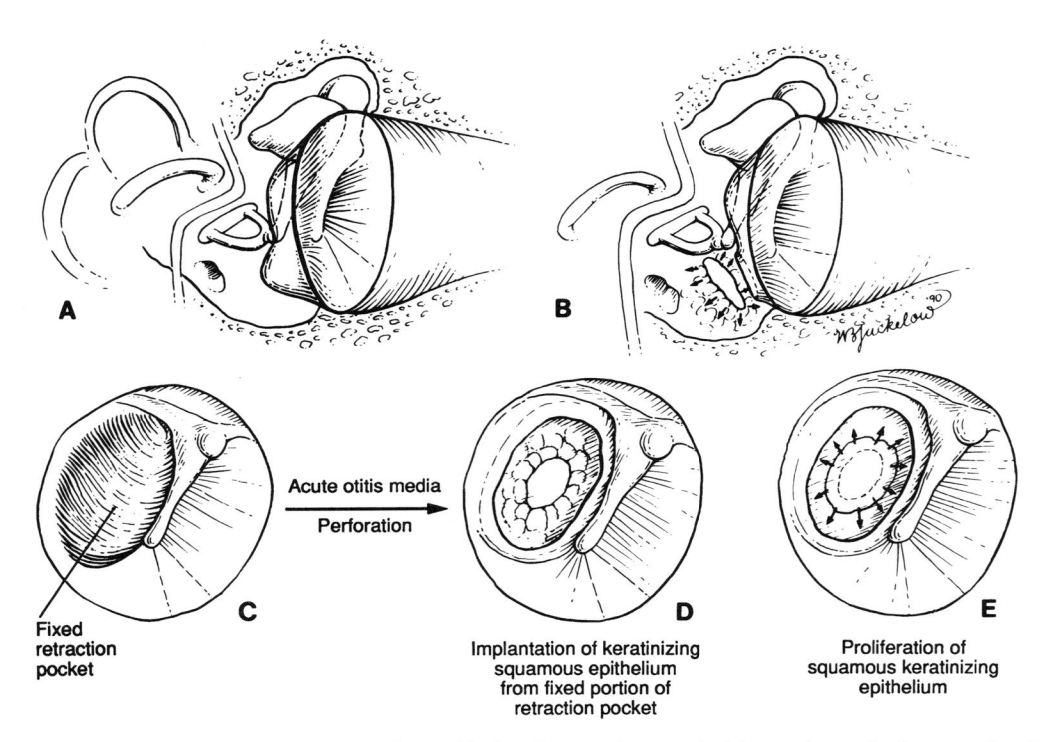

FIG. 6. A: Acute otitis media in a patient with fixed retraction pocket (*arrow*) results in a perforation. **B:** The squamous epithelium (se) adherent to the middle ear mucosa becomes isolated from the tympanic membrane. **C:** Growth of this island of keratinizing epithelium can result in a secondary acquired cholesteatoma.

grows and extends into the mastoid or retracts into sinus tympanic, thereby becoming a recurrent cholesteatoma. This second type of regrowth may develop many years after the initial surgery. For example, an individual who had a CWU mastoidectomy for cholesteatoma initially does well. Years later, the patient develops sinusitis or rhinitis. The nasal problem adversely affects the eustachian tubal function and interferes with proper middle-ear mastoid ventilation. As a result, many years after the original operation, a retraction pocket extending into the mastoid develops and forms a recurrent cholesteatoma. An advantage of CWD procedures is that the ears do not develop recurrent cholesteatomas. Because the procedure collapses the mastoid to become part of the enlarged external canal, the presence of a mastoid that requires aeration is eliminated.

DIAGNOSIS

Children with cholesteatoma usually have a history that includes recurrent episodes of foul-smelling otorrhea and a hearing loss (2). The ear drainage usually reflects acute infectious exacerbations arising in chronically involved bone and soft tissue. The hearing loss is caused by ossicular disruption or, less frequently, by labyrinthine involvement. However, hearing may be normal when the ossicular chain is intact. Alternatively, despite ossicular chain disruption, in some patients the hearing remains normal because the cholesteatoma acts as a columella to conduct sound from the surface of the tympanic membrane to the stapes remnant. Pain is not a common complaint, though it may occur when the ear becomes acutely infected, mimicking an external otitis. Persistent, localized, boring pain in the postauricular or temporal area may be a more ominous symptom reflecting underlying dural inflammation, and indicating an impending central nervous system complication that requires aggressive treatment. Indications of labyrinthine involvement are the onset of vertigo or a positive fistula sign (i.e., transient vertigo produced when pressure applied to the ear canal is transmitted directly to the membranous labyrinthine structures because the protective bony capsule has been eroded). Facial spasms, paresis, and paralysis indicate facial nerve involvement. Symptoms of meningitis, posterior fossa irritation, septicemia, or increased intracranial pressure in a child with a draining ear must be assumed to be related to the otitic process until proven otherwise.

A child presenting with a significant ear problem should be evaluated with an operating microscope. A cholesteatoma usually presents with aural polyps or granulation tissue that originates either in a perforation or in a tympanic membrane marginal retraction. Keratin debris accumulates within the defect. When present, debris should be gently removed and the existing pathologic conditions defined. Most children can be successfully examined if they are forewarned that the suctioning will be noisy and will make them feel as if they

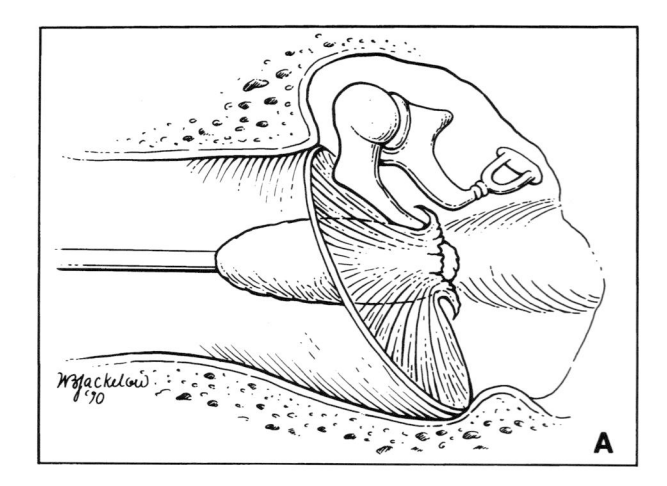

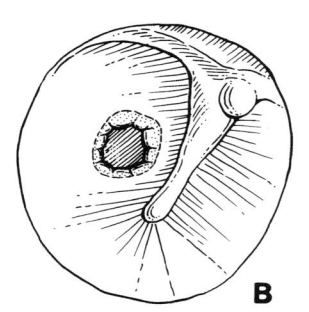

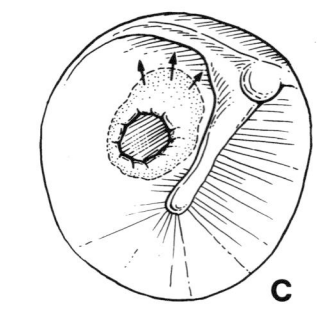

FIG. 7. A: Trauma to the ear produces an implosive force. **B:** A torn flap becomes folded on to the undersurface of the tympanic membrane. **C:** The keratinizing squamous epithelium extends on the medial surface of the tympanic membrane (*arrows*), producing a secondary acquired cholesteatoma.

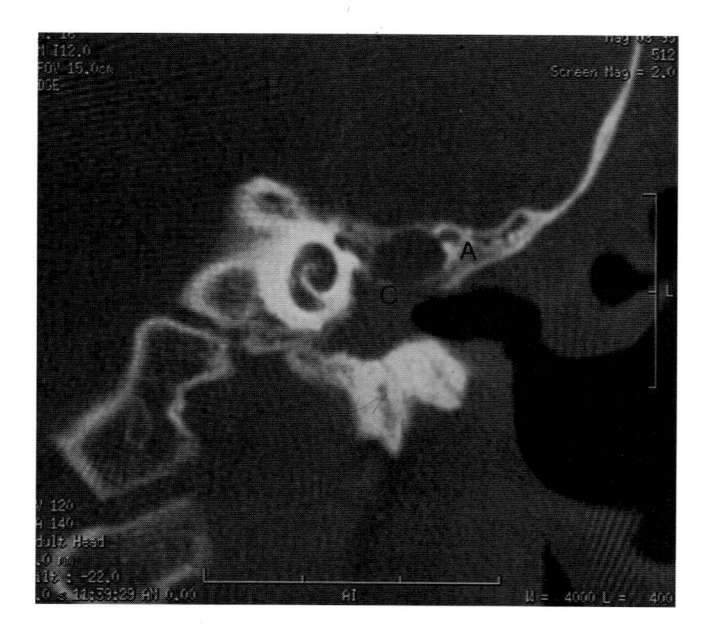

FIG. 8. Saggital CT of temporal bone at post-operative CWD mastoidectomy. Residual cholesteatoma (C) and opacified air cells that were not exenterated at the intitial operation (A). The contained cholesterol granulomatous disease produced mucoid otorrhea.

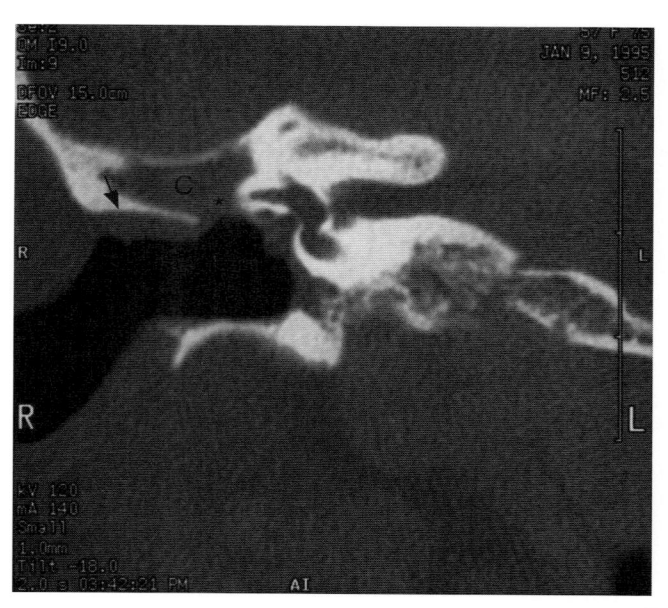

FIG. 9. Saggital CT of temporal bone at post-operative CWU mastoidectomy. Recurrent cholesteatoma filling the mastoid cavity (C) and facial recess opening.

are on a merry-go-round. Introducing the instruments to be used as the "doctor's toys" and allowing the child to hold the instruments may allay the child's fear.

Audiometric evaluation provides a quantitative determination of hearing and is also a useful diagnostic test to help assess the destructive effect of the cholesteatoma. Even in young children, hearing can be tested with behavioral and play audiometry, though the examination may provide only a general assessment of auditory function. Commonly, a conductive hearing loss is observed. The presence for a sensory loss may indicate extension of the disease process into the inner ear. When such a labyrinthine involvement has occurred, vertigo may be a prominent clinical symptom.

Use of CT with thin (1½ mm) section overlapping techniques in both coronal and sagittal planes produces elegant images of the temporal bone. However, when the clinical diagnosis of a cholesteatoma has been firmly made and intracranial complications are not suspected, this sophisticated test may not be necessary. It is a costly examination that exposes the child to a small but significant amount of radiation. Because the patient must not move during the study, young children frequently must be sedated or occasionally, given a general anesthetic. Therefore CT should be performed only to obtain specific information.

A CT scan is informative in cases of recidivism because it reveals the extent of the previous surgery and can reveal the presence of dehiscenses in the tegmen, lateral sinus, or posterior fossa. It may indicate the extent of recurrent and residual cholesteatomas. Unfortunately, it may be difficult radiologically to differentiate pathologic soft-tissue disease and bone erosion from surgically induced scar tissue and bony defects.

Patients in whom complications are suspected should undergo CT. Labyrinthine fistulas can be clearly defined and their size determined preoperatively. Areas of facial nerve involvement are more difficult to pinpoint, especially when the horizontal and intralabyrinthine segments are involved. Suspected intracranial complications are best imaged with contrast-enhanced CT, which demonstrates pathologic changes within the temporal bone of the brain. In selected patients with intracranial involvement, magnetic resonance imaging (MRI) may be necessary to better delineate the existing abnormalities or to sequentially follow up the progression of intracranial pathologic conditions of soft tissue.

A CT scan of the temporal bone, although frequently helpful in demonstrating abnormalities, is not diagnostically infallible. The quality of a study can vary, depending on the radiologist's interest and experience as well as the quality of the equipment available. Technically poor studies may be less useful than plain x-rays of the mastoid. Radiographic imaging provides useful information that must be interpreted intelligently. Ultimately, the diagnosis of cholesteatoma has been, and remains, an otologic clinical conclusion.

Plain x-rays of the mastoid are of limited use, but because x-rays require that the patient not move for only short increments of time, in children they may be easier to obtain than CT scans. X-rays are relatively inexpensive and remain useful in delineating the mastoid size and its degree of pneumatization. This information is helpful preoperatively in selecting a specific surgical approach for the removal of a cholesteatoma.

PREOPERATIVE MANAGEMENT

Young children with significant tympanic membrane retraction should be treated aggressively to try to arrest progression of the retraction (2). The presence of developmental soft palate defects that are frequently associated with eustachian tube dysfunction should be detected. Adenoidectomy should be considered, especially in a child with nasal airway obstruction and sinusitis. When allergy is suspected, appropriate diagnostic studies should be obtained and if allergy is indicated, treatment provided.

It is generally accepted that in most children eustachian tube function improves with age until full growth and sexual maturity are reached. In young children with significantly retracted tympanic membranes, long-term, persistent ventilation of the middle-ear space over time might prevent progression of the atelectatic changes to cholesteatoma. For these patients, "T"-type tubes, modified by trimming the length of the middle-ear flanges, are highly effective. The tubes are inserted anteriorly where a residual air space is present. Admittedly, a small percentage of children in whom the tubes have remained in place for 2 years or longer develop perforations of the tympanic membrane. The longer the tubes have stayed in place, especially in ears with thin, atrophic, retracted tympanic membranes, the greater the incidence of residual perforations after the tubes are withdrawn.

When long-term ventilation has been required, it has not been uncommon for the tubes to remain in place and to function for 5 years or longer. Interestingly, one can view the presence of a perforation that develops from the ventilating tube as beneficial because it provides persistent middle-ear ventilation in the problem ears.

Tubes that spontaneously extrude in 6 to 9 months are not effective when long-term ventilation is required. Replacement of the tubes generally requires frequent general anesthesia. Reconstruction of an atelectatic ear in which the tympanic membrane is adherent to the promontory (and which may be associated with a cholesteatoma) is a difficult surgical challenge. However, the operative repair of a tympanic-membrane perforation with an aerated middle-ear cleft is generally successful. Consequently, a tympanic-membrane perforation caused by a ventilating tube that has provided long-term middle-ear aeration may be an acceptable strategy in children with compromised middle-ear aeration.

The child with a significant retraction pocket should be examined periodically. Sequential CT scans may be useful in detecting progression of the disease process. In fully grown teenagers in whom eustachian tube function has improved, reconstruction of the middle ear and tympanic membrane should be considered.

The keratin desquamation and retention characteristic of cholesteatoma is excacerbated when water gets into the affected ear during bathing and swimming or when otorrhea develops in association with an upper respiratory infection. Increased keratin retention clinically seems to be associated with cholesteatomatous activation, which results in bone erosion and invasion of surrounding structures. Furthermore, the moist desquamated material is a good growth medium for bacteria, whose proliferation produces infections that in turn stimulate cholesteatomatous activity and expansion.

Examination of a chronically draining ear generally reveals granulation tissue within the retraction pocket and may involve the adjacent canal wall skin. Characteristically, the drainage is foul smelling. Cultures frequently grow out *Proteus, Pseudomonas,* and fungi as well as other organisms. However, in these chronically wet ears, one must question whether organisms cultured from the drainage in the external canal are an overgrowth or whether they represent the true pathogens.

Generally, with office treatment, the ear can be returned to a dry state. An operating microscope should be used to meticulously clean out any crusts, exudate, and keratin that have accumulated within a retraction pocket and when a perforation is present from the middle-ear space. Crusts that obscure retractions may be difficult to remove at the initial visit. Granulation tissue should be debrided and the underlying vascular base neatly cauterized because persistence of pyogenic granuloma-like growths ensures that the ear will continue to drain. In wet ears, topical otic or ophthamological preparations are prescribed for 2 weeks or longer. In addition, an adequate course of a broad-spectrum systemic antibiotic, not inactivated by penicillinase-producing organ-

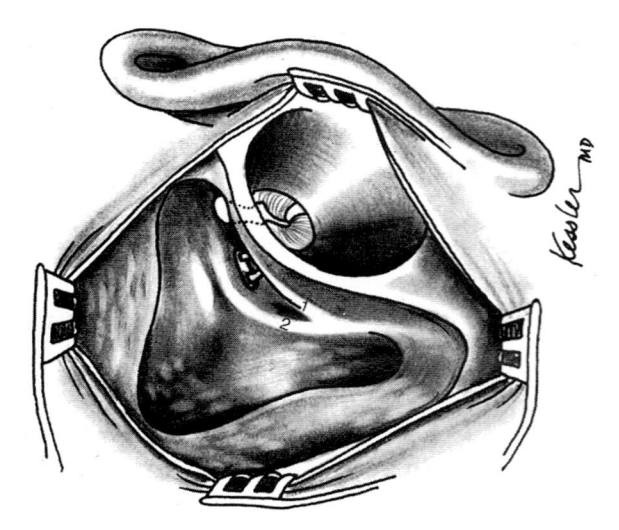

FIG. 10. CWU technique. A mastoidectomy has been performed in which the canal wall has been preserved. The posterior middle ear has been entered by drilling between the chorda tympani (1) and facial nerve (2).

isms, is prescribed for 14 days and occasionally longer. The goal of office treatment is twofold. First, elimination of acute changes allow an accurate assessment of the existing pathologic conditions. Second, when surgery is to be performed, the reduction of inflammatory vascularity minimizes intraoperative bleeding, and thereby facilitates microscopic ear surgery.

OPERATIVE MANAGEMENT

The primary goal of the surgical treatment of chronic mastoiditis due to cholesteatoma is its complete eradication to provide the patient with a safe, dry ear. This can be accomplished by meticulously removing all of the cholesteatoma, diseased bone, granulation tissue, and irreversibly diseased mucosa. An important but secondary goal is to improve or preserve hearing acuity by reconstructing the tympanic membrane and the ossicular mechanism to restore an aerated middle-ear cleft. An additional goal is to minimized the need for long term care of the operated ear and eliminate concern about getting water in the ear when bathing and swimming.

Types of Mastoid Operations

The procedures used for treating cholesteatoma may be divided into two broad categories (3). One is CWU technique in which an air-containing mastoid and an external ear canal are preserved (Fig. 10). Examples of canal wall up procedures are the atticotomy (with and without mastoidectomy) and a mastoidectomy with a facial recess approach (i.e., posterior tympanotomy). The second category is comprised of CWD techniques (Fig. 11) in which the posterior canal wall is removed and the mastoid marsupialized into the enlarged ear canal, to form a common cavity (hence the term "open technique" because the mastoid recess can be examined otoscopically). Use of this tecnique eliminates the need to aerate the canal wall via the middle-ear cleft. Historically, canal wall down techniques were termed radical and modified radical mastoidectomies. By today's standards, however, these techniques are hardly radical.

The assessment of eustachian tubal function is key to selecting the appropriate procedure. If tubal function is inadequate, CWU procedures are foredoomed to failure. Three clinical indicators have been identified as useful for assessing eustachian tubal function in patients undergoing surgery for cholesteatoma. One is the appearance of the pars tensa. A normal pars tensa suggests that the eustachian tube effectively ventilates the middle ear cleft and therefore might

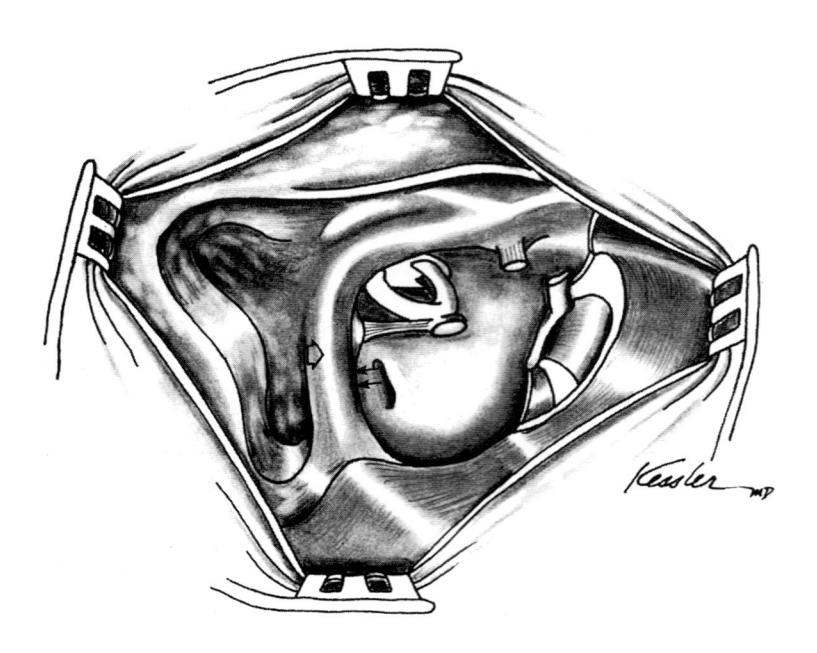

FIG. 11. CWD technique. The posterior canal wall has been lowered to the vertical facial nerve (*open arrow*). The mastoid is marsupialized into the external ear canal. All accessible air cells have been meticulously exenterated. Skelatinizing the vertical portion of the facial nerve unroofs the sinus tympani (*solid double arrows*).

function adequately enough to aerate the mastoid and support a CWU procedure. The presence of middle-ear effusion behind an otherwise normal pars tensa represents a "grey" area. It may indicate that tubal function will be inadequate to ventilate the mastoid if the canal wall is preserved. In some instances, however, the eustachian tube dysfunction is caused by correctable abnormalities such as inflammatory mucosal changes, occlusion of the middle ear tubal aperture by a prolapse of the cholesteatoma or a synechial band. In these situations, a CWU procedure may be considered. However, observation of a severely retracted pars tensa suggests that the patient has had inadequate eustachian tubal function and is a poor candidate for a CWU procedure.

The second clinically useful indicator of eustachian tubal function is mastoid cellular development. The presence of a large pneumatized temporal bone, especially if aerated, suggests good eustachian tubal function and encourages consideration of a CWU procedure. The observation of fluid or cholesterol granulomatous disease in a well-developed cellular mastoid indicates a failure of aeration, which may be caused by a localized attic antral block and can be surgically corrected to permit CWU surgery. However, when middle-ear mucosal abnormalities are diffuse and extend to involve the mastoid, the existing eustachian tube dysfunction may not be correctable. A contracted sclerotic mastoid is factor that would encourage a CWD procedure. In these ears, the mastoid bowl that results from the CWD procedure is small and relatively easy to clean.

The third clinical clue used to assess eustachian tubal ventilation is the status of the middle-ear mucosa. Normal, thin, translucent middle-ear mucosa indicates that middle-ear cleft ventilation has been normal and is a good indicator that CWU surgery can be successfully carried out. Hyperplastic, polypoid, irreversibly diseased middle-ear mucosa or adhesive-type changes in which squamous epithelium lines the promontory suggest that eustachian tube function has been compromised. The latter findings indicate that a CWD procedure should be considered.

When the patient has extensive disease in a small sclerotic mastoid, a CWD technique is routinely performed. Also, in patients with pneumatized mastoids and who have extensive disease, CWD may be required to obtain better operative exposure. Postoperatively, the patient is left with a mastoid recess that will have to be examined and cleaned through the external canal. Thus, as an integral part of the surgery, a meatoplasty to enlarge the canal opening is performed. The decision whether to preserve the canal wall or to lower it is frequently made during the operative procedure. An accurate understanding of the extent of cholesteatomatous involvement relative to the anatomic configuration of the patient's mastoid in conjunction with the clinical assessment of eustachian tubal ventilation allows the surgeon to select the best technique for each patient.

The facial nerve should routinely be identified when one performs either CWU or CWD procedures. When the posterior canal wall is lowered, it should be taken down to the level of the vertical facial nerve, which is routinely visualized through the thinned overlying bony covering. Definitive identification of the nerve reduces the risk of inadvertently damaging it and causing facial paralysis, a complication of mastoid surgery. When one performs CWD surgery, all accessible air cells that communicate with the antrum must be meticulously exenterated. If these isolated air cells are not drilled out, there is a propensity for them to become problematic. Deprived of ventilation, they develop mucosal disease and produce troublesome postoperative otorrhea, an undesirable complication. It is critical during the course of chronic ear surgery, that the stapes remains intact. Nevertheless, occasionally when one removes disease from the oval window or round window area, the perilymphatic spaces may be entered inadvertently. Thus, it is advisable to postpone working in these critical areas until all other areas have been cleaned out and drilling with irrigation has been completed. Although labyrinthine fistulas are unusual in children, they occasionally occur (4). Generally, complete removal of the matrix from the fistula site is attempted in these patients. When the fistula is small, the squamous epithelium can be peeled off without violating the perilymph space. However, if the fistula is large the epithelium may be densely adherent. In these patients, leaving a small patch of uninflamed matrix, rather than risk violating the inner ear structures may be preferable.

The optimal treatment for pediatric cholesteatoma remains a highly debated issue (5–10). Proponents of intact canal wall techniques claim that this procedure produces better functional results than do open cavity procedures and that the procedure is associated with a lower incidence of postoperative otorrhea. Those in favor of open-cavity techniques point to the high rate of recidivism that has been reported following intact canal wall procedures. The high recidivistic rate is the basis of the "second-look" operation commonly employed to verify eradication of cholesteatoma after intact canal wall surgery. Some surgeons treat each cholesteatoma individually, assessing anatomic and clinical factors both preoperatively and intraoperatively to determine the type of surgery that will best control the patient's disease.

Review of Cases

Ideal surgical management of pediatric cholesteatoma can become evident only by assessing the results of many clinical studies. Our goal is not to settle a controversy regarding the optimum treatment of pediatric cholesteatoma but to report the results of a retrospective analysis of our own relatively large series of pediatric patients who underwent single-stage surgery for cholesteatoma. Specific issues addressed in our review are the efficacy of CWU and CWD surgery and the feasibility of single-stage management of pediatric cholesteatoma. Parameters examined in the review of cases are recidivism, hearing, and postoperative cavity status.

Hospital records, office charts, operative reports, and audiometric studies of 209 children (216 ears) with cholestea-

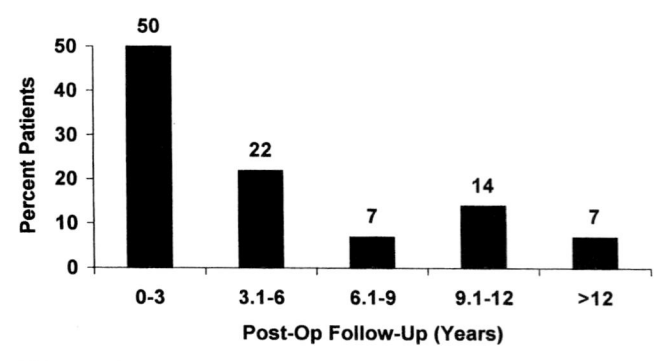

FIG. 12. Length of follow-up following surgery for cholesteatoma.

toma and who were operated on by Parisier from 1970 to 1994 were retrospectively reviewed and analyzed. All patients were 18 years or younger with average age of at the time of surgery of 8.6 years. There were 141 (65%) boys, and 75 (35%) girls. One hundred eleven (51%) cases involved the right ear and 105 (49%) involved the left ear. There were seven cases of bilateral cholesteatoma. The length of follow-up for the patients in this series is presented in Fig. 12.

The cholesteatomas were divided into four categories. There were 74 (34%) congenital cholesteatomas resulting from embryonic keratinizing squamous epithelial remnants in the middle ear or mastoid. Eighty-seven (40%) of the cholesteatomas were classified as primary acquired resulting from an invagination of a portion of the intact skin-lined retracted tympanic membrane into the mastoid. There were 21 (10%) secondary acquired cholesteatomas in which skin grew through a tympanic membrane perforation into the middle ear and mastoid. Finally, 34 (16%) of the cholesteatomas were the result of previously unsuccessful surgery; it was therefore not possible to classify the original type of cholesteatoma. Each case was treated with a single-stage procedure, as shown in Table 1. A CWD technique was utilized in 104 (48%) cases and a CWU technique was employed in 112 (52%) cases. Included in this latter group were patients who underwent a tympanotomy approach for small cholesteatomas confined to the middle ear space. This procedure was most frequently used for small congenital cholesteatomas.

In 161 (75%) cases, a primary ossicular reconstruction was performed as part of the surgical procedure. No reconstruction was performed in the remainder of cases, either because the ossicular chain was intact or (infrequently) because the reconstruction was staged. Autograft cartilage obtained from the floor of the ear canal or an autograft ossicle was positioned on the ossicular remnant to reconstruct the sound transmission mechanism. In rare instances, alloplastic total or partial ossicular replacement prostheses were used.

Postoperatively, patients were reexamined every 4 months for the first 2 years, then every 6 months until 5 years after surgery, and then later once a year or as needed, depending on accumulation of debris in the cavity.

Results of Surgery

All patients who developed recidivistic (residual or recurrent) disease after the primary operation were noted. In addition to recording the date at which recidivism was definitively diagnosed, a distinction was made between recurrent and residual disease. The type of surgery used for the revision operation was also recorded.

Survival was defined as the interval from the date of initial diagnosis of cholesteatoma to the date of last follow-up or the date of diagnosis of recidivism, whichever occurred first. Survival analysis was performed using the Kaplan-Meier method. The log rank test was used for the comparison of survival distributions. It was more useful to report results as rates of recidivism than as rates of survival.

Postoperative aural discharge was used as an indicator of cavity status. Specifically, objective assessment of the mastoid–middle-ear region was performed to determine the number of moist cavities following each type of surgery.

Preoperative and postoperative audiometric data included air and bone conduction at 500, 1,000, 2,000, and 4,000 Hz, speech reception threshold (SRT), and speech discrimination (SD). The post-operative period was divided into immediate postoperative, which extended to 9 months from the date of surgery, and subsequent intervals of approximately 2 to 3 years to each patient's most recent hearing test. Air conduction and bone conduction assessment was facilitated by the calculation of a pure-tone average encompassing the respective air and bone conductions at 500, 1000, and 2000 Hz. This calculation allowed subsequent calculation of an air-bone gap (ABG) by subtracting the bone conduction pure-tone average (BCPTA) from the air conduction pure-tone average (ACPTA). The comparison of hearing test results from the preoperative period through different phases of the postoperative period was conducted though the use of repeated measures analysis of variance (RMANOVA) and Student's T tests. Therapeutic efficiency curves were used to show the changes in ABG following each type of surgery. The curves show the distribution of hearing changes following surgery plotted in 10-dB increments, which creates a curve with a normal distribution of data and facilitates comparison of surgical results both within the series at hand and with the reported results of other series.

TABLE 1. *Pediatric cholesteatoma profile and treatment*

	CWU	CWD	Total no. (%)
Congenital	60	14	74 (34)
Acquired	39	69	108 (50)
Recidivistic	13	21	34 (16)
Total	112 (52%)	104 (48%)	216

TABLE 2. *Pediatric residual cholesteatoma*

	CWU	CWD	Total no. (%)
Congenital	5	1	6 (38)
Acquired	1	7	8 (44)
Recidivistic	0	9	3 (18)
Total	6 (35%)	11 (65%)	17

Recidivism

There were 25 patients who reached the endpoint of recidivism. One patient developed two recidivistic lesions, both in the form of residual cholesteatoma. The first lesion became apparent 3 years postoperatively, and the second one presented 11 years after the initial surgery. On the survival curves, this patient was treated as having had only one residual lesion. The incidence of residual and recurrent cholesteatoma by type of surgery and by type of cholesteatoma, is summarized in Tables 2 and 3. For all patients combined, the 5- and 10-year rates of recidivism were $13 +/- 6\%$ and $22 +/- 10\%$ respectively (Fig. 13). In terms of type of surgery, the 5- and 10-year survival rates for CWD surgery were $14 +/- 8\%$ and $14 +/- 8\%$, respectively (Fig. 14). For CWU techniques, the rates were $12 +/- 8\%$ and $34 +/- 22\%$, respectively. The difference in recidivism between the two techniques was not statistically significant. With regard to the type of revision surgery performed, eight patients who had originally been operated on with a CWU technique developed a recurrent cholesteatoma, and all underwent a CWD procedure during the revision.

Cavity Status

On physical examination, a total of 24 (11%) patients were found to have postoperative otorrhea. Specifically, 10 (9%) patients in the CWU group and 14 (13%) patients in the canal wall down group experienced postoperative aural discharge.

Hearing

Audiometric data were available for 198 cases. In 18 young children, audiometric evaluations consisted of sound detection thresholds in a free-field test situation. Difficulty in testing subsets of younger children precluded obtaining complete audiometric data. No patients were profoundly deaf prior to or following surgery. When the hearing data

TABLE 3. *Pediatric recurrent cholesteatoma*

	CWU	CWD	Total no. (%)
Congenital	5	0	5 (62)
Acquired	1	0	1 (13)
Recidivistic	2	0	2 (25)
Total	8 (100%)	0 (0%)	8

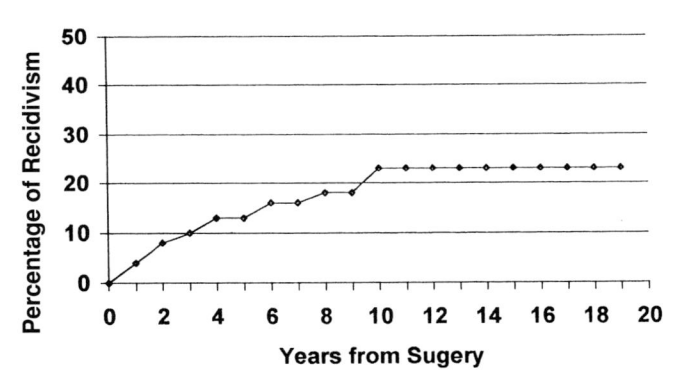

FIG. 13. Overall time to recidivism.

were analyzed separately according to use of CWD and CWD procedures, there were no significant changes from the preoperative to postoperative period in either group. Of importance, CWU patients exhibited significantly better values than did CWD patients at both intervals in terms of ACPTA ($p < .05$), BCPTA ($p < .05$), ABG ($p < .05$), and SRT ($p < .05$) (Tables 4,5). The immediate postoperative audiometric data were compared with the audiometric data obtained at consecutive intervals of 2 to 3 years and the final audiogram available for each patient. There were no statistically significant changes over time ($p > .05$).

Of the 198 cases analyzed, 161 (81%) involved a primary ossicular reconstruction. Thirty-seven (19%) of the cases analyzed involved either an intact ossicular chain or, more infrequently, a staged hearing reconstruction and were therefore omitted from this analysis. When the subgroup of cases with ossicular reconstructions was analyzed by the type of mastoidectomy performed, it was observed that CWD cases showed a statistically significant deterioration in BCPTA from 6.7 dB to 9.6 dB ($p < .05$) and a statistically significant improvement in ABG from 37.5 dB to 33.3 dB ($p < .05$) when the preoperative to postoperative results were compared there were no significant changes in ACPTA, SRT, and SD. The CWU cases in this subgroup did not show any significant changes in this time interval. Figure 15 shows the "therapeutic efficiency" in terms of changes in ABG of both canal wall up and canal wall down surgery performed with a primary ossicular reconstruction.

INTERPRETATION AND SIGNIFICANCE OF ANALYSES

The main goal of surgery for cholesteatoma is to ensure the patient of a disease-free ear. Functional results and all other factors should always be secondary to the attempt to prevent recidivism. No surgery can be considered to be truly effective if it is associated with a high risk of an adverse outcome, regardless of the other benefits it may offer to the patient.

When one examines the efficacy of surgery for cholesteatoma, the reporting of rates of recidivism needs to be addressed. A true rate consists of a numerator, a denominator,

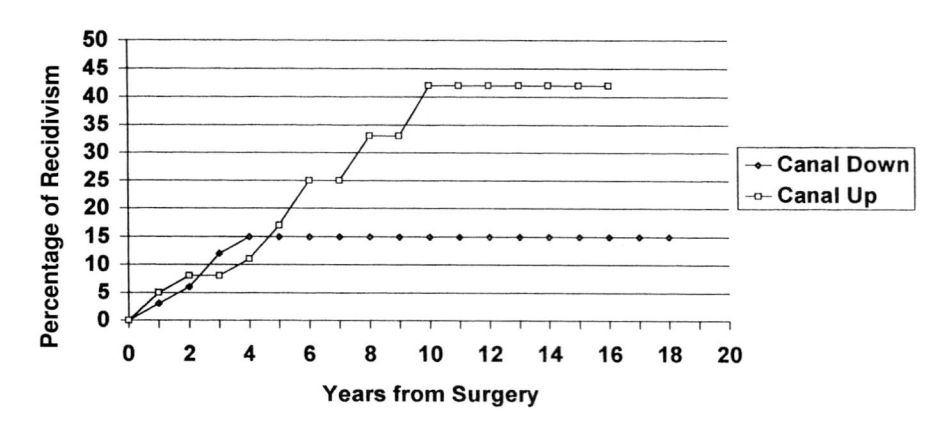

FIG. 14. Time to recidivism, by type of surgery.

TABLE 4. *Pediatric audiometric results for CWU cases with primary ossicular reconstruction*

	ACPTA (n = 70)	BCPTA (n = 60)	SRT (n = 69)	SD (n = 61)	ABG (n = 60)
Preoperative	32.6	6.6	31.3	95.2	27.8
Postoperative	31.4	7.0	29.1	95.1	25.4
p (two-tailed)	>.05	>.05	>.05	>.05	>.05

Results presented in dB.
ABG, air-bone gap; ACPTA, air conduction pure-tone average; BCPTA, bone conduction pure-tone average; SD, speech discrimination; SRT, speech reception threshold.

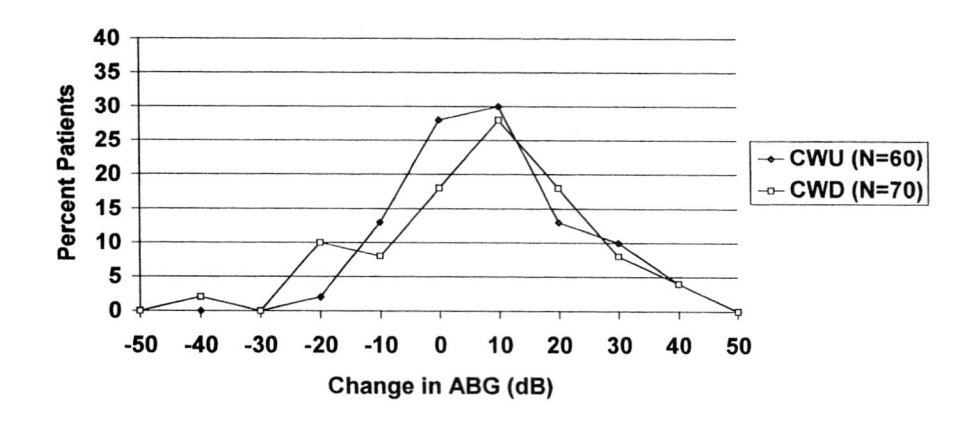

FIG. 15. Changes in bone air gap comparing canal wall up and canal wall down procedures.

TABLE 5. *Pediatric audiometric results for CWD caes with primary ossicular reconstruction*

	ACPTA (n = 83)	BCPTA (n = 70)	SRT (n = 82)	SD (n = 70)	ABG (n = 70)
Preoperative	44.0	6.7	41.2	94.3	37.5
Postoperative	42.0	9.6	39.2	95.9	33.3
p (two-tailed)	>.05	<.05*	>.05	>.05	>.05*

Results presented in dB.
ABG, air-bone gap; ACPTA, air conduction pure-tone average; BCPTA, bone conduction pure-tone average; SD, speech discrimination; SRT, speech reception threshold.
* p is significant.

and the specified time in which events occurred (11). However most surgeons report the total incidence or recidivism in the series analyzed, not the true rate. There are certain disadvantages in reporting results in this manner. For one thing, the overall incidence of recidivism depends on the length of follow-up of the population being studied, and the length of follow-up is different for each series analyzed. Studies with a relatively short length of follow-up may underestimate the true incidence of recidivism. By using survival analysis and reporting rates of recidivism at exact postoperatively periods, surgeons can more accurately compare results. Moreover, the results are less biased due to the ability to include all patients, regardless of length of follow-up, in the analysis.

The results of our analysis show that there is no statistically significant difference between CWU and CWD techniques in terms of recidivism. However, a trend suggesting that CWD surgery produces better long-term results was observed. In this group of patients, CWU procedures were performed only in patients assessed to have adequate eustachian tubal function. There was a trend towards a higher rate of postoperatively recidivism with intact canal wall surgery after 5 years. This trend may be due to cases of recurrent cholesteatoma that occurred following CWU procedures in spite of the clinical selection method for deciding when the posterior canal could be preserved for a given patient. The data suggest that ears with cholesteatoma treated with CWU procedures could develop recurrent disease long after the initial operative procedure and might be related to nasal and paranasal sinus diseases and their effect on eustachian tubal function or to intrinsic tubal dysfunction.

A number of published reports use survival analysis to report rates of recidivism for pediatric cholesteatoma. Rosenberg, Moura, and Bluestone (12) using the Kaplan-Meier method reported a recidivistic rate of 57% at 5 years postoperatively. Lau and Tos (13) approximated the rates that would have been achieved with survival analysis and reported a 5 year recidivistic rate of 16%. In both series, the status of the canal wall was reported as being not significantly related to the rate of recidivism.

One main argument against CWD techniques is that the creation of an open cavity leads to a high frequency of bothersome postoperative otorrhea. This problem can be largely eliminated by exenterating all accessible air cells. When mucosal lined mastoid air cells are isolated from their normal physiologic aeration, hyperplasia of the mucus-producing glands and cholesterol granulomatous changes occur, which produce excess moisture and result in a wet cavity. Also, grafting the eardrum and mastoid bowl with temporalis fascia and areolar connective-tissue enhances primary healing. In this analysis, patients with open cavities were not greatly inconvenienced. More than 85% of patients with open cavities in this series have maintained dry ears. Patients with open cavities were routinely advised to take precautionary measures such as the use of ear plugs in situations exposing the operated ear to water. These patients were also instructed to have the affected ear cleaned out two to three times a year. The findings are similar to those of Tos (9) and of Schmidt (14), who reported incidences of postoperative otorrhea following open cavity procedures as 16% and 7%, respectively, in their series of pediatric cholesteatoma cases. Therefore, the assumption that open cavities lead to disturbing otorrhea seems to be unfounded. It appears that the problems associated with CWD mastoid operations are related more to inadequate surgery than to the technique itself.

The functional results of CWU surgery were compared to resuls of CWD surgery. Overall, the analysis showed no statistically significant differences in hearing acuity for preoperative and postoperative results. The only significant changes noted were a small significant improvement in ABG and a slight but significant deterioration in BCPTA in patients who received CWD surgery involving a primary ossicular reconstruction. Notably, CWU patients had significantly better values both preoperatively and postoperatively for four of the five parameters used in the analysis which implies that CWU patients who have CWU surgery have less extensive disease and a better prognosis to begin with. Therefore, the claim that there are superior auditory results following intact canal wall techniques is confounded by disease severity; in reality, the type of mastoidectomy performed does not substantially affect hearing.

As pointed out previously, functional results are secondary to the attempt to maintain a safe, healthy ear. Nevertheless, hearing is crucial for speech and language development in children. The results obtained in this series using a single-stage tympanoplasty as part of the operative procedure in nearly all patients who needed ossicular reconstruction compare favorably with the results of other reported series. Therefore, the results agree with Schuknecht (15) who stated that "Every effort should be made to eliminate disease and maximize hearing results at the first operation." Hough (15) follows a similar philosophy and pointed out that "With a philosophy of a planned second-stage procedure, these patients might be denied the opportunity to have had success with the first operation, thus requiring a needless second procedure."

Considering all primary operations and revision operations for recidivism, the patients in this series needed an average of 1.1 operations to control their disease. In all but one patient, the revision operation was effective in eradicating the recidivistic lesion. Had staging been used, the mean number of operations per patient would have been at least two. Therefore, it is important to examine the need for a "second-look" operation in controlling the patient's disease. Smyth (16) found that more than 10% of patients with negative findings during a second-look performed as part of an intact canal wall procedure subsequently developed recurrent cholesteatoma as late as 8 years after surgery. Similarly, Sanna (17) reported a recurrence rate of 12% in a series of 91 patients followed for a minimum of 5 years after a second-look was performed as part of a CWU procedure. Such incidences of recidivism following two-stage surgery are similar to the rates in this series for single-stage surgery. All in all, two-stage surgery seems to be no more effective than single-stage surgery in achieving the primary goal of cholesteatoma management: permanent eradication of disease.

There is concern that allowing disease to become manifest clinically (as opposed to aggressively trying to validate its absence) condemns patients to more advanced pathology. In our series of patients, who were methodically examined by the operating surgeon postoperatively, there were no serious complications of recidivistic cholesteatoma. Austin (18) and Hirsch, Kamerer, and Doshi (19), other advocates of single-stage surgery, similarly reported no serious, life-threatening complications of clinically apparent recidivistic disease in their series of 251 and 118 patients, respectively. Smyth (20) has suggested that the squamous pearls commonly discovered during a second-look operation are of theoretical, not practical concern. Smyth found the incidence of squamous pearls found during a second-look operation to be much higher than the rate of residual disease that manifested clinically. The pathophysiology that underlies the eventual development of such pearls into overt cholesteatoma or the regression of such pearls is not well understood.

It appears that patients undergoing two-stage procedures have a similar incidence of recidivism to that of patients undergoing a single-stage procedure. This finding is important because there are financial, geographic, and patient-compliance issues associated with the two-stage treatment of cholesteatoma. Moreover, there are risks associated with the second operation itself, including complications of anesthesia and the small but still present risk of sensorineural hearing loss. Finally, the patient or his or her guardian may not fully comprehend the extent of the surgical procedure at the time that permission for a staged operation is given.

The alternatives to a second-look procedure are long-term office follow-up with microear examinations to detect either residual or recurrent disease. In selected cases, postoperative sequential CT scans in children suspected of possibly having occult cholesteatomatous regrowth have been useful. Alternatively, it has been suggested that fiberoptic endoscopy might be useful in assessing the middle ear for residual disease (21).

CONCLUSIONS

Results of analyses in the series described here show that there is no statistically significant difference in recidivism or in auditory results following either an intact canal wall procedure or open-cavity procedures. Postoperative otorrhea following open-cavity techniques occurred very infrequently. The low rate of recidivism is attributed to careful selection of operative technique for each patient. The rates of recidivism following single-stage surgery are equivalent, and in some instances lower than rates reported following staged surgery. No serious complications occurred in patients who developed recidivistic cholesteatoma postoperatively. Therefore, single-stage surgery (incorporating both the primary procedure and an ossicular reconstruction as required) with thoughtful selection of an operative procedure that incorporates clinical assessment of eustachian tubal function is recommended. The patients should be routinely followed postoperatively with microscopic ear exams, and sequential CT scans should be done for patients suspected of having regrowth of their disease.

REFERENCES

1. Parisier SC. Managment of cholesteatoma. *Otolaryngol Clin North Am* 1989;22:927.
2. Parisier SC, Weiss MH, Edelstein DR. Treatment of cholesteatoma. *Adv Otorhinolaryngol* 1993;5:107.
3. Parisier SC, Weiss MH. Canal wall up or canal wall down—that is the question. In: Sade J, ed. *The eustachian tube, clinical aspects.* 1991 Amsterdam: Kugler Ann Ghedini; 1991:339.
4. Parisier SC, Edelstein DR, Han JC, Weiss MH. Management of laryrinthine fistulas caused by cholesteatoma. *Otolaryngol Head Neck Surg* 1991;104:110.
5. Abramson M. Open or closed tympanomastoidectomy for cholesteatoma in children. *Am J Otol* 1985;6:167–169.
6. Abramson M, Lachenbruch PA, McCabe BF. Results of conservative surgery for middle ear cholesteatoma. *Laryngoscope* 1977;87:1281–1287.
7. Glasscock ME, Dickins JRE, Wiet R. Cholesteatoma in children. *Laryngoscope* 1981;91:1743–1753.
8. Palva A, Karma P, Karja J. Cholesteatoma in children. *Arch Otolaryngol* 1977;103:74–77.
9. Tos M. Treatment of cholesteatoma in children: a long term study of results. *Am J Otol* 1983;4:189–197.
10. Sheehy JL, Brackmann DE, Graham MD. Cholesteatoma surgery: residual and recurrent disease. A review of 1,024 cases. *Ann Otol Rhinol Laryngol* 1977;88:451–463.
11. Last JM, ed. *A dictionary of epidemiology.* 2nd ed. New York: Oxford University Press; 1988.
12. Rosenfeld RM, Moura RL, Bluestone CD. Predictors of residual-recurrent cholesteatoma in children. *Arch Otolaryngol Head Neck Surg* 1992;118:384–391.
13. Lau T, Tos M. Cholesteatoma in children. recurrence related to observation period. *Am J Otolaryngol* 1987;8:364–375.
14. Schmid H, Dort JC, Fisch U. Long-term results of treatment for children's cholesteatoma. *Am J Otol* 1991;12:83–87.
15. Sheehy JL, Shelton C. Tympanoplasty.to stage or not to stage. *Otolaryngol Head Neck Surg* 1991;104:399–407.
16. Smyth GDL. Surgical treatment of cholesteatoma: The role of staging closed operations. *Ann Otol Rhinol Laryngol* 1988;97:667–669.
17. Sanna M, Zini C, Scandellari R, et al. Residual and recurrent cholesteatoma in closed tympanoplasty. *Am J Otol* 1984;5:277–282.
18. Austin DF. Single-stage surgery for cholesteatoma: an actuarial analysis. *Am J Otol* 1989;10:419–425.
19. Hirsch BE, Kamerer DB, Doshi S. Single-stage management of cholesteatoma. *Otolaryngol Head Neck Surg* 1992;106:351–354.
20. Smyth GDL. Cholesteatoma surgery: the influence of the canal wall. *Laryngoscope* 1985;95:92–96.
21. Rosenberg S, Silverstein H, Gordon M, et al. *Endoscopy in otology and neurotology.* Paper presented to the American Neurotology Society, Los Angeles, CA, April 18, 1993.

PART VI
Hearing Disorders

CHAPTER 21

Nonsyndromic Hereditary Hearing Impairment

Umang Khetarpal and Anil K. Lalwani

Hearing loss is the most common form of sensory impairment. Wilson (1) estimated that in 1985 as many as 70 million people across the world had a hearing loss of 55 dB or more. It has been estimated that there are 12 million hearing-impaired individuals and 2 million deaf individuals in the United States (2). In the earlier decades of this century, congenital and childhood loss from genetic and nongenetic causes, especially infections, comprised a large proportion of hearing loss in the population. However, as the population has aged in overdeveloped, developed, and developing countries, the prevalence of late-onset hearing loss appears to be increasing, especially that of hearing loss associated with aging and noise trauma. Sensorineural hearing loss (SNHL) was considered a diagnostic and therapeutic dilemma. However, recent exciting innovations and discoveries in the fields of acoustical physics and electronic engineering, molecular biology, and computational genetics, combined with rapid technologic advances in computer software and chemistry, have made possible the investigation of the etiologic basis of these hearing losses and restoration of these hearing losses in part by sophisticated hearing aids, assistive listening devices, and cochlear implants. Additionally, the mapping of and identification of genes for mouse models for human hereditary hearing loss holds great promise in the identification of genetic basis for these diseases. The era of organ-targeted gene therapies and substitution of defective protein with normal protein appears very much in sight for certain life-threatening disorders. It would only seem logical to apply these emerging technologies in the restoration, prevention or rehabilitation of genetic and "nongenetic" hearing losses. Because nonsyndromic (SNHL) is seen so often in clinical practice by both the otolaryngologist and audiologist, these recent discoveries emphasize the need for genetic history taking and audiometric analysis of relatives or sibling when a genetic hearing loss is suspected. The era of molecular biology promises to unravel the mysteries of auditory and vestibular processing and of hearing loss and vestibulopathies. Hopefully, this new information will permit newer and more efficacious treatment in the future.

BRIEF HISTORY OF GENETIC HEARING LOSS

References to genetic diseases have been made in older Hindu texts dating back to about 2500 B.C. In fact, in the *Rig Veda,* one of the classic texts of Hindus, it has been stated that "intermarriage within the family or caste is not progressive" due to suspected higher incidence of diseases. In the Western literature, both autosomal dominant and recessive hearing losses had been described by the seventeenth century (3,4). The role of parental consanguinity in recessive hearing loss had been alluded to by Wilde (5) (1853) and later by Hartmann (6) (1880). Politzer (7) emphasized that the most frequent causes of congenital hearing losses are hereditary. Bel (8) and Fay (9) both conducted studies involving the study of deaf-mutes and deaf marriages in the United States. The latter found that the incidence of deaf offspring in matings involving deaf individuals were 9% for deaf × deaf matings, 25% for congenitally deaf × congenitally deaf and 13.5% for deaf × hearing matings. Bell's philosophy on prevention of intermarriage of the deaf and elimination of segregated schools for the deaf struck a chord with the then-eugenics movement and later in Nazi Germany. The disparaging effects of such philosophies were far reaching and continue to exist in one form or another, especially the emphasis on intensive oral education. However, the inclusion of Sign Language in the media news and other programming is a step forward in bringing deaf individuals into the mainstream. Current efforts by some

---

U. Khetarpal: Department of Otolaryngology—Head, Neck, and Craniofacial Surgery, SUNY Health Science Center, Syracuse, New York 13210-2399.
A.K. Lalwani: Department of Otolaryngology—Head and Neck Surgery, University of California, San Francisco, California 94143.

members of the deaf community are focused on educating people to accept Sign Language as a fundamental language and on deaf rights. Although problems concerning delineation of types of hearing loss into separate entities versus "lumping" into similar entities will continue, it appears that more than 175 types of syndromic and nonsyndromic hereditary hearing losses exist that may be due to mutations in different genes (10). For some of these, the genetic mutations have been identified and for some others, the genes mapped. The application of information obtained from these recent and future advances will need to be monitored carefully so that discrimination at the work place, in schools, or otherwise does not take place. Given this backdrop the foresight of the Human Genome Project, which allocated almost 5% of its budget on ethical issues that may be generated by detection of many thousands of genetic mutations and polymorphisms that determine and predispose to diseases, should be praised.

EPIDEMIOLOGY

Hereditary SNHL has been estimated to occur in more than 27 in 1,000 persons (11). Profound childhood SNHL has an incidence ranging from 4 to per 1,000 births in developed countries, with an estimated prevalence of 1 in 1,000 births being genetic (12–19). Estimates drawn from studies of hearing-impaired populations and others indicate that in at least 33 to 50%, the likely etiology is genetic and possibly a single gene mutation (12,19–21). It is estimated that as many as 5% of school-age children have unilateral and/or mild-to-moderate hearing loss, representing a potentially reversible cause of learning difficulty (12). About 25% to 33% of childhood SNHL is considered to result from environmental or "nongenetic" causes, while the remaining 25% to 33% are sporadic hearing losses for which the etiology is not determined (19,21). It is possible that a majority of hearing losses in the latter group also may be genetic. In addition to congenital or early/adult-onset SNHL, high-frequency progressive hearing loss, or presbycusis, is believed to occur as a part of the normal aging process. By the age of 65 years, there is a one in six chance of having a functionally significant hearing loss, and by the age of 80 years, hearing impairment of a significant degree involves nearly half of the population (22). Recent evidence indicates a genetic basis for hearing loss associated with aminoglycoside toxicity and aging. Additionally, it is increasingly speculated that the underlying predisposition for middle ear and inner ear infections is genetic. While nongenetic causes continue to play an important role in auditory sensory impairment, it is likely that the underlying predisposing genetic factors will be identified in the forthcoming years.

In many cases, hereditary hearing loss is associated with systemic abnormalities such as ectodermal, craniofacial, skeletal, or ocular dysplasias; nephropathies; neuropathies; and/or inborn errors of metabolism, which therefore occur as a syndrome. Although more than 175 identifiable hearing-loss syndromes have been described (10,23), a small percentage of them account for the bulk of these disorders. For example, Waardenburg's and Usher's syndromes are estimated to acount for about 2% to 3% and 1% of childhood SNHL, respectively. Overall, among known hereditary hearing loss, at least 15% to 30% are syndromic (19). While syndromic hearing loss can be distinguished because of its association with other systemic features, nonsyndromic hearing loss occurs in absence of association with any other clinically detectable systemic manifestation. These hearing losses may be inherited in simple mendelian fashion, mitochondrially, or by complex inheritance patterns, such as digenic, polygenic, or combinations of mitochondrial and mendelian inheritances. It is generally believed that approximately 77%, 22%, and 1% to 2% of genetic hearing loss in childhood is transmitted recessively, dominantly, or by sex-linked inheritance, respectively (22). Mitochondrial inheritance is considered to contribute to less than 1% of all genetic hearing losses. Proctor (11) has further estimated that the incidence of autosomal dominant SNHL without any associated abnormalities is about 1 in 40,000. Marres and Cremers (24) have estimated that 1 in 4,000 children is affected with autosomal recessive profound SNHL.

INHERITANCE PATTERNS

It is well known that there is tremendous heterogeneity in genetic conditions (25). One way in which this heterogeneity manifests in hereditary hearing loss is by different inheritance patterns. These include chromosomal abnormalities, simple monogenic mendelian inheritance, mitochondrial inheritance and multifactorial inheritance patterns. (These have been described in an earlier chapter.) The characteristic features of two additional types that have relevance to hearing loss are described next.

Digenic Inheritance

Digenic, or two-gene inheritance was recently identified in some patients with autosomal dominant retinitis pigmentosa (26). In this entity, mutations in two genes involved in the same cell-signaling pathway were found to be responsible for the disease. No other disease of digenic inheritance has been documented. A form of digenic inheritance (two-locus biallelic recessive model without sporadic cases) has been postulated by Majumder, Ramesh, and Chinnappan (15) for autosomal recessive congenital nonsyndromic SNHL. However, this requires corroboration by linkage analysis and gene localization and has not been borne out by studies on recessive deafness that have been mapped so far. Another impact of this latter model, if proven true, is a marked reduction in recurrence risks.

Digenomic Inheritance

This term is proposed here for diseases that are determined by a gene in the nuclear genome and mitochondrial genomic mutation or deletion participating as cofactors in the causation of the disease. Although mitochondrial mutations have been described in such disease, nuclear genomic mutations that play a role remain to be identified. These diseases include specific type of diabetes and deafness (27,28) and autosomal dominant external ophthalmoplegia (29). More recently, a gene locus on chromosome 10 appears to predispose the mitochondrial genome to deletions in the case of autosomal dominant external ophthalmoplegia (29). The postulation for a digenomic inheritance is made if many members of a family harbor homoplasmic mitochondrial mutations but not all are affected. A second predisposing nuclear genomic gene is then suspected and sought by linkage analysis.

CLASSIFICATION

Nonsyndromic hereditary hearing loss (NHHL) can be classified by the inheritance pattern. Within this classification, audiometric, vestibular, and radiologic characteristics define subtypes of NHHL (Table 1). A classification encompassing genetic and audiometric criteria was first described by Konigsmark and Gorlin in 1976 (30) and has recently been modified by Gorlin, Torrielo, and Cohen (10). This latter classification is possible because hearing loss can be represented as a quantitative and frequency-dependent trait. Audiometric features taken into consideration for classification are laterality, severity, progression, frequency affected at onset, age at onset, and type of hearing loss. In addition to these, the inclusion of further subtypes based on the presence or absence of vestibular symptoms, results of the vestibular test battery, and temporal bone findings have been proposed (31–33). The lack of vestibular data in many of these subtypes of hearing loss indicates that this classification will undergo further revisions as these data continue to be accumulated. Additionally, the refinement of vestibular findings expressed in a reliable, quantitative manner in terms of frequencies affected and caloric responsiveness, along with cheaper costs of vestibular tests, may allow further refinement in this classification. Furthermore, subtypes in this classification have been proposed on the basis of differing slopes of hearing loss seen in different families (34,35) and on the basis of progression (phasic vs gradual) (36). A review of the literature indicates that audiometric slopes and type of progression vary tremendously within families and with respect to ages studied. However, this area is clearly worthy of pursuit (discussion follows). There is compelling evidence that radiographic criteria (abnormality of the inner ear on computed tomography [CT] scans) should be included in the classification of X-linked hearing loss (see later discussion).

More important, however, is that the validity of Konigsmark and Gorlin's classification (modified by Gorlin, Torrielo, and Chohen [10]), using the specific objective parameters described previously, needs to be corroborated by further studies and by demonstration that these different hearing losses are a result of mutations in different genes and not the result of stochastic variations or allelic heterogeneity within the same gene. Recent evidence from four craniosystosis syndromes—Apert's, Crouzon's, Pfeiffer's, and Jackson-Weiss—all clinically distinguishable syndromes, are a case in point. All four syndromes have been found to be due to mutations in the fibroblast growth factor receptor 2 (FGFR2) gene (37–39). In fact, identical mutations were found in some Pfeiffer's and Crouzon's syndrome patients (38) while Apert's and Crouzon's syndromes are allelic for FGFR2 mutations. It appears that their differences might be related to specific mutations within the gene. These findings suggest that "lumping" certain syndromes based on a predominant phenotype may have advantages over "splitting" them on the basis of other minor phenotypes. However, in nonsyndromic SNHL subtypes, there is some evidence to suggest the occurrence of genetic heterogeneity. For example, in autosomal dominant, low-frequency hearing loss, in many families the gene for this disorder does not map to

TABLE 1. *Clinical criteria adopted for classifying nonsyndromic hereditary hearing loss*

Parameter	Subtype
Inheritance pattern	Autosomal dominant, autosomal recessive, X-linked dominant, X-linked recessive, mitochondrial, digenic, digenomic
Audiometric features	
Type	Sensorineural, mixed, conductive
Age at onset	Congenital, noncongenital (early vs. late)
Frequency affected at onset	Low, mid, high
Laterality	Unilateral, bilateral (follow-up is necessary)
Severity (?)	Mild to moderate, severe to profound
Progression	Nonprogressive, progressive (slow vs. rapid)
Audiometric slope (?)	Steep, gradual
Vestibular features	
Symptoms	Absent, present (vertigo, ataxia, clumsy in dark)
Tests (caloric, OPK, rotation testing, posturography)	Normal, abnormal
Radiographic features	Normal, abnormal (Mondini's deafness, Michel's deafness, bulbous IAC, absent cribrose areas)

OPK—optokinetic test; IAC—internal auditory canal.
Modified from Grundfast and Lalwani, *ENT Journal*, 71:479–493, 1992, with permission.

5q31. For X-linked congenital SNHL, genes have been mapped to Xp21.2 and Xq21.1. In X-linked hearing loss, inclusion of radiologic evidence of abnormality or normality on the basis of thin sections of temporal bone by high-resolution CT scanning appear to be valuable for the purposes of gene localization (see following discussion). We hope that over the next decade, the mapping of many more hearing-loss genes will permit a better classification of nonsyndromic hearing loss.

Until a better classification emerges, the following classification (modified from Gorlin, Torriello, and Cohen (10) is proposed for NHHL. Given our current knowledge, distinction based on the age at onset of hearing loss appears to be of value only when separated into congenital and noncongenital types. Further categories based on age at onset appear only to confuse the picture further, because the ages are variable even within the extended families of affecteds with similar hearing loss. Congenital malformations of the inner ear, such as Michel aplasia, Schiebe dysplasia, enlarged vestibular aqueduct syndrome, and noncongenital entities such as unilateral vestibular schwannomas, also occur in sporadic and nonsyndromic fashion and only rarely in familial fashion. These disorders have not been included in this classification, although it is possible that they may be included in the future.

Sensorineural Hearing Loss (SNHL)

I. Autosomal Dominant Inheritance
   a. Congenital severe nonprogressive SNHL
   b. Congenital low-frequency progressive SNHL
   c. Noncongenital low-frequency progressive SNHL
   d. Noncongenital mid-frequency progressive SNHL
   e. Noncongenital high-frequency progressive SNHL
   f. Unilateral nonprogressive SNHL
   g. Noncongenital progressive audiovestibular dysfunction or progressive vestibular dysfunction with high-frequency SNHL
   h. Meniere's disease
   i. Mondini's dysplasia
II. Autosomal Recessive Inheritance
   a. Congenital severe-to-profound SNHL
   b. Congenital retrocochlear hearing loss
   c. Congenital moderate nonprogressive SNHL
   d. Congenital progressive SNHL
   e. Noncongenital progressive high-frequency SNHL
III. X-linked Dominant Inheritance
   a. Congenital severe-to-profound SNHL
IV. X-linked Recessive Inheritance
   a. Congenital severe-to-profound SNHL
   b. Noncongenital high-frequency progressive SNHL with moderate impairment
   c. Noncongenital mid-to high-frequency nonprogressive SNHL
V. Mitochondrial Inheritance
   a. Aminoglycoside sensitivity
   b. Type II diabetes and SNHL
VI. Digenomic Inheritance
   a. Maternally derived SNHL

Mixed and Conductive Hearing Loss

1. Autosomal dominant mixed progressive hearing loss.
2. X-linked progressive mixed hearing loss with perilymphatic gusher, recessive.
3. Otosclerosis, possibly autosomal dominant.
4. Familial conductive hearing loss, various types, autosomal dominant and recessive.

As has been shown for autosomal dominant low-frequency progressive SNHL, it is almost certain that one or several genes may be involved in each of these disorders (genetic heterogeneity). It is also likely that a separate category of audiovestibular dysfunction will emerge for some of these subtypes if thorough vestibular examination and testing is performed. It remains to be seen whether molecular genetic technology will corroborate this classification or allow the development of a more practical classification.

GENERAL CONSIDERATIONS IN NONSYNDROMIC HEREDITARY HEARING LOSS

Among NHHLs, most are autosomal recessive. Deaf × deaf matings have produced normal-hearing offspring, indicating tremendous heterogeneity within autosomal recessive SNHL. The estimates of numbers of genes involved in autosomal recessive hearing loss have varied from two to ten or more (15,41–43). Hypothetically, even if three genes were found to be involved in each one of the autosomal recessive subtypes (assuming this classification has molecular genetic validity), a total of 15 genes would be necessary to produce these phenotypes. Additionally, although unlikely, if each subtype has an audiovestibular subtype and assuming that three genes are involved in each, a total of thirty genes emerges. Intralocus heterogeneity within these genes would make large-scale mutation testing a huge endeavor, given current technology.

For dominantly inherited hearing losses, a similar number of genes have been estimated. Here again, if the previous classification is assumed to be valid, many genes appear to be involved. It is also possible that age-related decreases in hearing may be determined in part by autosomal genes in a dominant fashion. In most forms of presbycusis (except the primary strial form), degeneration of neurosensory elements proceeds from the base of the cochlea to the apex, a pattern similar to that of some deaf mice and two important subtypes of *autosomal dominant* nonsyndromic SNHL: progressive high-frequency SNHL and progressive audiovestibular dysfunction (31,32,40).

Generally speaking, most genetic hearing losses are sensorineural, not conductive. Retention of low frequencies is common in recessive hearing losses, which may be more commonly associated with cochleosaccular dysplasia with greater affliction of the basal elements. The hearing losses in dominant disorders appear to be more variable and may be flat, downsloping, or upsloping initially. Another general feature (by no means exclusive) of recessive and dominant hearing losses is that the former usually are present at birth or within the first few years of life, whereas the latter in most cases may have its audiologically tested and often clinical onset in the second or third decade of life. More often than not, the hearing losses are bilateral and mostly symmetric. Further studies should elucidate whether the vestibular decline parallels the audiologic decline in regard to progression and asymmetry. X-linked recessive hearing loss may be associated with retention in all frequencies. Another general characteristic is that in many of the hearing losses, the pathogenetic locus appears to be cochlear.

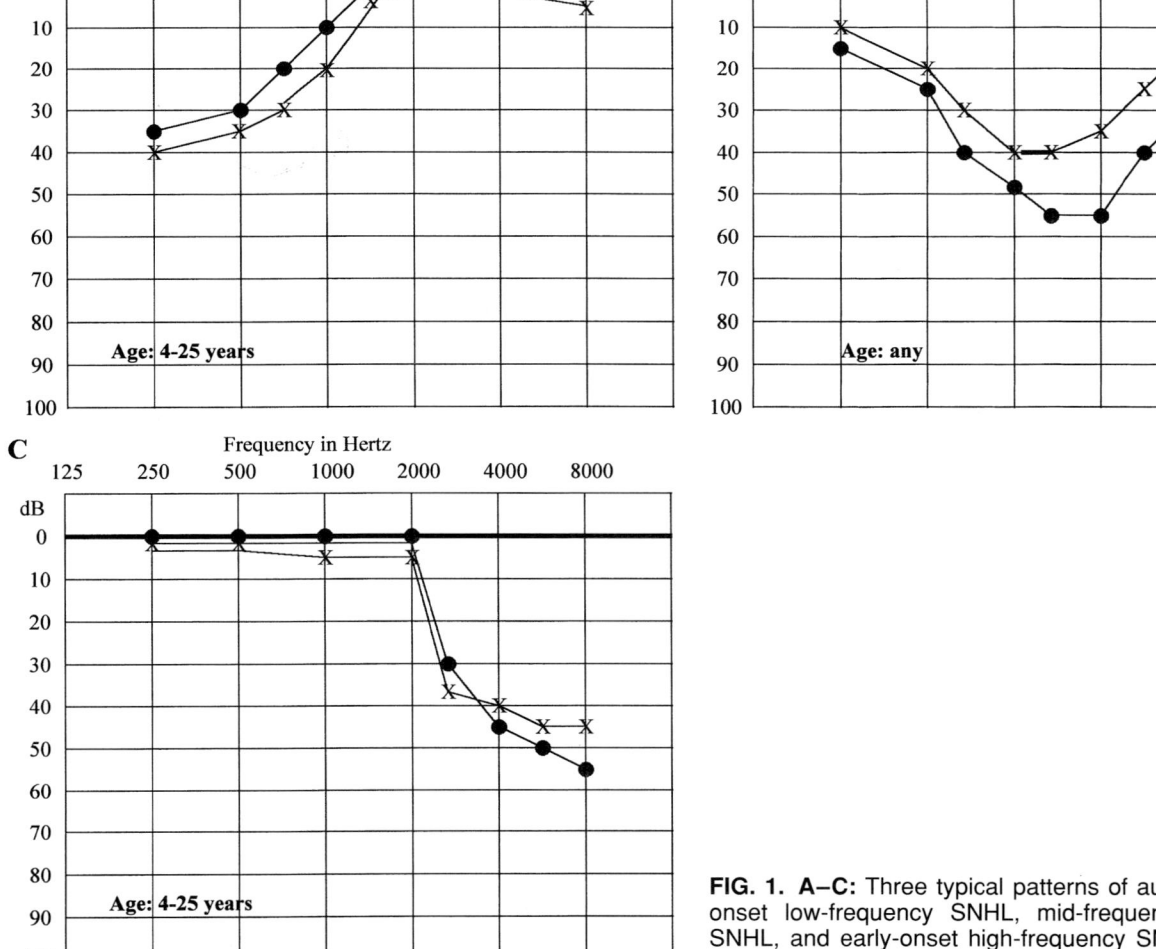

IMPORTANT CONSIDERATIONS IN THE DIAGNOSIS OF NONSYNDROMIC HEREDITARY HEARING LOSS

A hereditary cause should be suspected in *all* cases of hearing loss, even when there appears to be an evident linking, predisposing factor. As the following description of subtypes will show, NHHL does not always manifest at birth or early in life. The suspicion becomes heightened if the hearing loss manifests within the first two or three decades of life and especially if there is a family history of hearing loss. Certain audiometric characteristics should heighten suspicion of NHHL. These are low-frequency (without Meniere accompaniment) or high-frequency SNHL in adolescence or early adulthood, and specifically a mid-frequency or cookie-bite SNHL (Fig. 1). With the exception of rare cases of luetic labyrinthitis, ototoxicity, and prenatal rubella, a U-shaped audiogram should be considered pathognomonic

FIG. 1. A–C: Three typical patterns of audiograms—early-onset low-frequency SNHL, mid-frequency or U-shaped SNHL, and early-onset high-frequency SNHL—that should heighten suspicion of hereditary hearing loss.

TABLE 2. *Medical evaluation of a child with unexplained sensorineural hearing loss*

Pregnancy history
    Material infections (rubella, CMV, toxoplasmosis), potential ototoxic drugs, radiation exposure
    Stress events in the first trimester
    Birth history (hypoxia, kernicterus, trauma, toxemia, prematurity)
Postnatal history
    Head trauma, meningitis, systematic infections (measles, mumps, syphilis, etc.), ototoxic exposure, detailed otologic history
Family history
    Premature hearing loss in blood relations through at least two generations
    Identify consanguinity if present
    All siblings should undergo audiologic evaluation
Physical examination
    Otologic examination to identify malformations, infection, cholesteatoma, or signs of trauma
    General examination by pediatrician to evaluate for systemic disease, pigmentation abnormalities and hypogonadism
    Mental retardation should be assessed for in DFN3 and in Norrie's disease
    Ophthalmologic examination to exclude keratitis (syphilis, Cogan's syndrome, retinitis pigmentosa [Usher's syndrome]), pseudoglioma (Norrie's disease), viral inclusions (CMV, toxoplasma), and to assess visual acuity
Laboratory testing
    Renal function: blood urea nitrogen and creatinine; urinalysis for hematuria and proteinuria (Alport's, polycystic kidney disease, etc.); renal ultrasound in suspected BOR syndrome
    Metabolic function: thyroid function tests (Pendred's syndrome, cretinism); blood and urine glucose (diabetes)
    Complete blood count (anemia, infections)
    Luetic serology
    Immune function: erythrocyte sedimentation rate, antinuclear antibodies, Western blot assay (Cogan's, autoimmune disease)
    Specific immunologic tests if viral disease is suspected (rubella, CMV, etc.)
Electrocardiogram
    Prolonged QT interval of Jervell and Lange-Neilson syndrome or other abnormalities
Computed tomography of temporal bones
    To investigate for malformation (cochlea, semicircular canals, vestibular and cochlear aqueducts, internal auditory canal, middle ear), cholesteatoma, fracture, osteodysplasia (Stickler's disease, osteogenesis imperfecta)

CMV, cytomegalovirus.

of hereditary hearing loss. In an only child or adolescent with unexplained SNHL, history taking, physical examination, and specific laboratory testing may provide important clues toward the diagnosis. A checklist, such as the one shown in Table 2, is invaluable in diagnosing the etiology of an unexplained SNHL. Before designating a hearing loss as nonsyndromic, it is necessary that a thorough physical examination (for disorders such as albinisim-deafness, Waardenburg's, Treacher Collins syndrome, Goldenhar's syndrome, etc.) and appropriate testing be performed to rule out syndromic hearing loss. Some of these tests are urinalysis (Alport's syndrome, BOR), renal ultrasound (BOR), thyroid function tests (Pendred's syndrome), ECG (Jervell and Lange-Nielsen syndrome, Romano-Ward syndrome), fundoscopy or ERG (Norrie's disease, Usher's syndrome), and radiographic examination (osteogenesis imperfecta, Paget's disease, Stickler disease) (Table 2). (The clinical features of many important syndromes associated with hearing loss are described in a separate chapter of this book.) When no evident cause or associated syndromic features are detected, the SNHL is considered to be cryptogenic. The family members should be interviewed and any sibling tested. It is imperative that the parents of an only child be informed that future children should be tested for hearing loss. If the second child is found to have elevated hearing thresholds, the diagnosis of the first child changes from cryptogenic to NHHL (Fig. 2).

In congenital SNHL, many nongenetic etiologies should be considered. These include kernicterus, meningitis, prenatal ototoxic drugs, prenatal rubella, birth trauma, cytomegalovirus (CMV) infection, and otitis media. The development of speech indicates that the hearing loss was most likely postlingual. Low-frequency hearing losses may be secondary to Meniere's disease, inner ear malformations, "viral infections," prenatal rubella, and some retrocochlear disorders. Mid-frequency hearing loss may occur with leutic labyrinthitis, noise trauma, ototoxic drugs, or prenatal rubella. Hereditary high-frequency loss needs to be differentiated from that secondary to CMV, noise trauma, ototoxic drugs, meningitis, previously healed otitis media, presbycusis, and retrocochlear disorders. All frequency hearing loss may be secondary to ototoxins, temporal bone trauma, meningitis, or "viral infections."

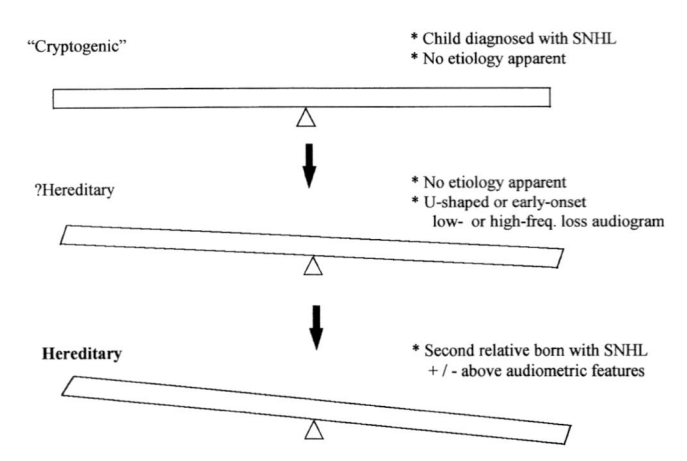

FIG. 2. A hereditary cause should be suspected in any patient with unexplained SNHL especially when the audiogram shows the patterns depicted in Fig. 1. Hereditary hearing loss becomes more likely if the second child is born with SNHL. Modified from Grundfast KG, Lalwani AK. *ENT Journal,* 71: 479–493, 1992, copyright, published with permission.

CHARACTERISTICS OF SUBTYPES OF NONSYNDROMIC HEREDITARY HEARING LOSS

The characteristics and distribution of the many subtypes of NHHL are described here in reference to the audiologic, vestibular, radiologic, temporal bone, and genetic findings. For a further discussion on some of these subtypes, the reader is referred to Gorlin et al.'s catalogue of hereditary hearing loss and its syndromes (10).

Autosomal Dominant Inheritance

Autosomal Dominant Congenital Severe SNHL

This entity was described by Fay (9) and others (44–46). All affected members have nonprogressive hearing losses of greater than 60 dB and delayed speech and language development unless placed in a special rehabilitation facility. Caloric testing generally shows normal responses but may be variable. However, there is a strong need to determine the status of the vestibular system, because there may be subtypes with vestibular abnormalities. There are no published radiologic studies of the temporal bone. Degeneration or dysplasia of the organ of Corti in middle and apical turns and of stria vascularis in basal and middle turns has been found on temporal bone studies (46).

Autosomal Dominant Congenital Low-Frequency Progressive SNHL

This was first described by the Vanderbilt Deafness Study Group (47) and, later, by others (48,49). The hearing loss is congenital and affects the frequency range of 250 to 1,000 Hz maximally. Hearing loss is progressive, and even with progression, the high frequencies may be relatively well preserved. Vestibular findings were variable. Temporal bone tomograms were normal in three patients. Temporal bone findings have not been described.

Autosomal Dominant Noncongenital Low-Frequency Progressive SNHL (DFNA1)

Many families with this hearing loss have been described (44,50,51), the most comprehensive description that of Leon et al. (Fig. 3A) (52–54). The hearing loss typically begins between ages 5 and 20 and is most marked in frequencies of 250 to 1,000 Hz (Fig. 3B). Variable expressivity is seen. Hearing in higher frequencies is normal at younger ages. With advancing age the hearing loss progresses to involve all of the other frequencies until deafness in adult life. Caloric testing appears to be normal, although this has not been performed in all families with this hearing loss. Radiologic or temporal bone findings have not been described. The gene maps to chromosome 5q31 (53,54).

Autosomal Dominant Noncongenital Mid-Frequency Progressive SNHL

Several reports of this phenotype have been documented (Fig. 4A) (55–59). Audiograms show a cookie-bite hearing loss affecting frequencies from 1,000 to 4,000 Hz initially (Fig. 4B). The severity is variable. The age at onset of the hearing loss is usually in the second or third decade of life. The hearing loss progresses to involve the higher frequencies and then the lower frequencies. Vestibular findings were normal in the affected members tested from several different families (56). It is not clear if this subtype can be further

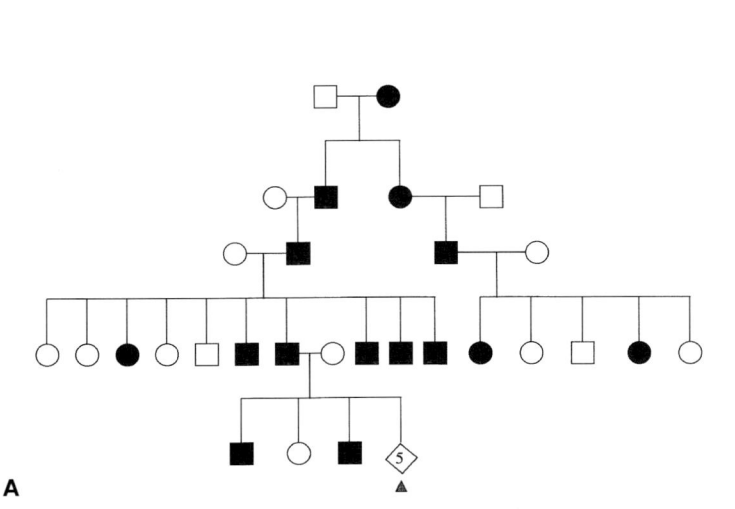

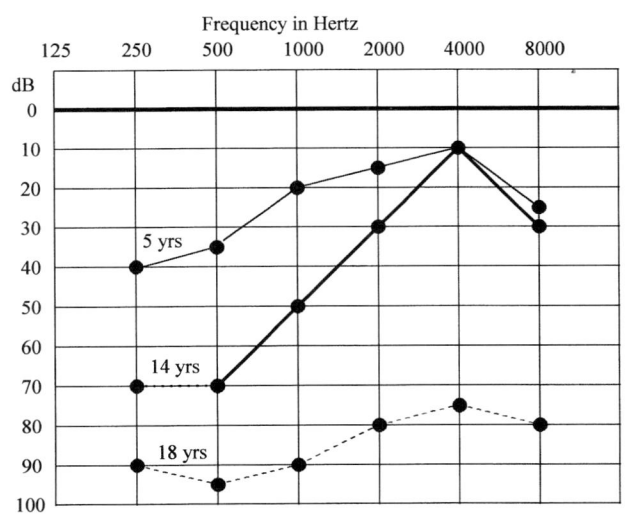

FIG. 3. A, B: Partial pedigree and audiograms of some representative members of noncongenital lowfrequency SNHL. The hearing loss is inherited in an autosomal dominant fashion and is progressive. Modified from Leon et al. *Am J Hum Genet* 33:209–214, 1981, copyright University of Chicago Press, published with permission.

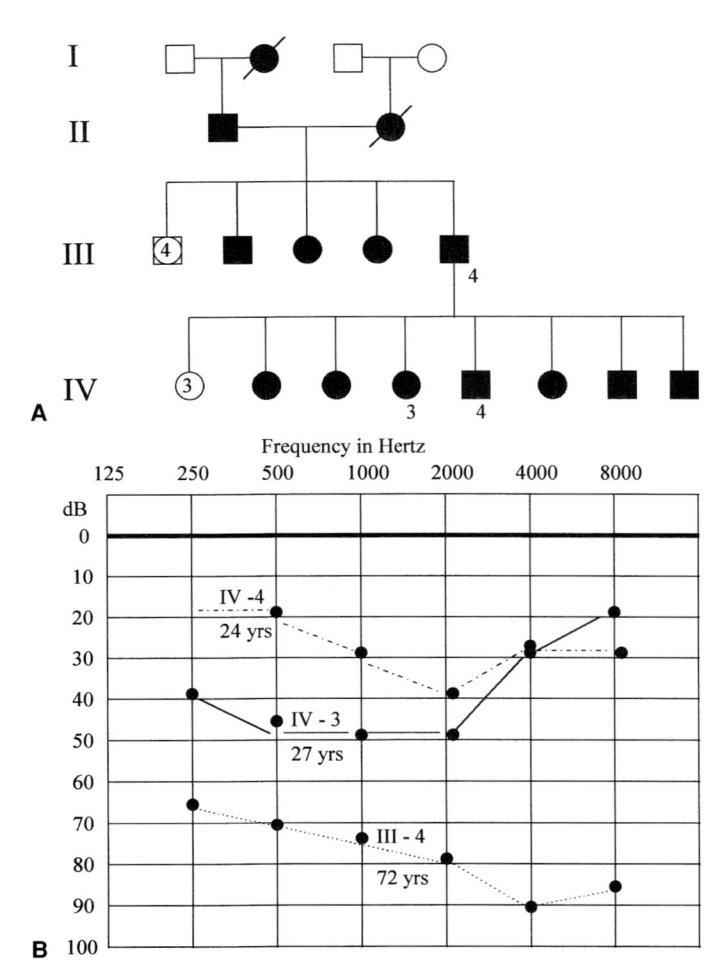

FIG. 4. A, B: Pedigree and audiograms with ages of some representative members with noncongenital mid-frequency SNHL. The hearing loss is inherited in an autosomal dominant fashion and is progressive. Modified from Konigsmark et al. *Ann Otol Rhinol Laryngol* 79:42–53, 1970, family B, copyright Annals Publishing Co., published with permission.

subclassified into different types based on the rate of progression of hearing loss. Radiographic findings have not yet been described.

Temporal bone findings in one individual demonstrated complete loss or clumping of the organ of Corti in all three turns, stria vascularis atrophy, and loss of ganglion cells in the basal turn (58). The vestibular system was intact at the light microscope level. This phenotype may lack a vestibular subtype.

Autosomal Dominant Noncongenital High-Frequency Progressive SNHL

Many such families have been reported (34–36,60–67), the largest being that described by Bu et al. (67). In the latter family, surprisingly, many sibships show generation skipping, and others suggest existence of acquired hearing loss (Fig. 5A). This list is by no means exhaustive. The hearing loss begins in the high frequencies during childhood (usually the second decade or early third decade) and progresses to involve all the remaining frequencies. Children may exhibit a steep loss above 2,000 Hz; adults, losses over 1,000 Hz; and older individuals losses in lower frequencies (Fig. 5B). Some families however, demonstrate gradual progression. Speech discrimination is fairly good until adult life. Vestibular findings are essentially normal (62,68). Using otoacoustic emissions, a pure-tone audiogram, and auditory brainstem audiometry in one affected member of a family with such a hearing loss, Bonfils et al. (66) suggested that the hearing loss in this family was predominantly secondary to inner hair cell loss. This hypothesis assumes an outer hair cell origin of otoacoustic emissions and therefore awaits histologic corroboration. Radiographic findings have not been described. Temporal bone findings include degen-

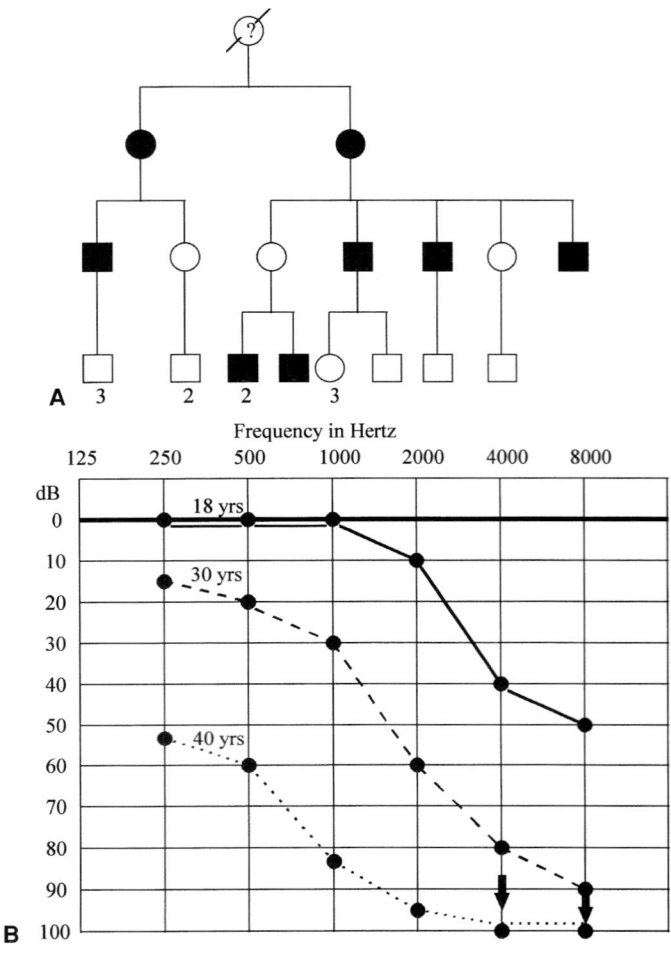

FIG. 5. A: Partial pedigree of autosomal dominant noncongenital high-frequency SNHL. Uncharacteristically, the SNHL appears to skip generations in some sibships in this family. Modified from Bu et al. *Ann NY Acad Sci* 630:310–312, 1991, copyright AAAS, published with permission. **B:** A typical audiogram showing that the hearing loss affects high frequencies at onset and is progressive.

eration of the organ of Corti and cochlear dendrites and neurons in basal and middle turns and a normal vestibular system (61). The findings in one case with "probable" autosomal dominant hearing loss, as described by Paparella, Suguira, and Hoshiro (58), have not been included. Additionally, the findings of Crowe et al. (69) in 79 ears with progressive high-tone loss revealed that the group with steep hearing loss had moderate-to-severe atrophy of the organs of Corti and neurons at the basal end, whereas those with gradual loss have normal organs of Corti with partial atrophy of dendrites. However, genetic information in these ears was not provided and, therefore, these data cannot be strictly admitted under this category.

Dolowitz and Stephens (63) reported a family with gradually progressive high-frequency hearing loss in whom auditory tests indicated a retrocochlear origin. Their clinical findings appear consistent with the histologic findings of Crowe et al. in patients with gradually sloping hearing losses. It may be that heterogeneity exists within this category between abrupt and gradual sloping losses, as suggested by some (34,35), the former cochlear and the latter retrocochlear in locus. An association between HLA B18 and Bw16 and this entity was suggested (70) but has not been studied further or corroborated. Linkage analysis has corroborated the existence of genetic heterogeneity within this subtype. The gene for one type has been mapped to 1p31-32 (71). In an Indonesian family with onset of high-frequency hearing loss in the second decade and in an American family with onset of high-frequency hearing loss from early childhood to adolescence, the gene mapped to 1p31-32. There are notable differences between these two families in the age at onset and severity of hearing loss at identical ages. Vestibular data in these two families were not provided, and, therefore, it is not clear if these two families should be included in this category or in the autosomal dominant noncongenital progressive audiovestibular dysfunction (ADPAVD) category. The Dutch family (36) with the onset of high-frequency hearing loss in affected members between the ages of 5 and 15 does not map to 1p, 5q, or 13q (71). Vestibular data on the Dutch family was reported as normal. These gene mapping data indicate that classification of nonsyndromic hearing loss on the basis of frequency is of value. On the other hand, it appears that the age at onset and severity of hearing loss may be related to intralocus or allelic heterogeneity, stochastic variations or effects of genetic background.

Autosomal Dominant Unilateral SNHL

This entity is somewhat clouded by the fact that some affecteds with unilateral congenital hearing loss have occurred in families with bilateral hearing loss or may be unrecognized Waardenburg's syndrome (72,73). Other familes were reported by Higashi (74) and Everberg (75–77). Unilateral hearing loss appears to be extremely variable in members of the same family, and so are the vestibular results. The hearing loss is congenital and probably nonprogressive. Radiographic or temporal bone findings have not been described. This subtype clearly requires better definition and characterization.

Autosomal Dominant Noncongenital Progressive Audiovestibular Dysfunction

Two groups have defined the nature of this subtype in the recent years: Verhagen and colleagues (Fig. 6) (77–80) and Khetarpal and colleagues (Fig. 7A) (31,32,40). Other possible inclusions in this group are families described by Muller (81), Belal (82), and Gussen (83). The hearing loss in some families begins at about age 20 (31,32,40) and in other families at about age 40 (32,78–81). The onset of hearing loss is in the high frequencies (Fig. 7B), and over time this progresses to involve all of the other frequencies so that patients may be deaf within 10 to 30 years after onset of disease. Most, but not all, patients have dizziness, oscillopsia, and

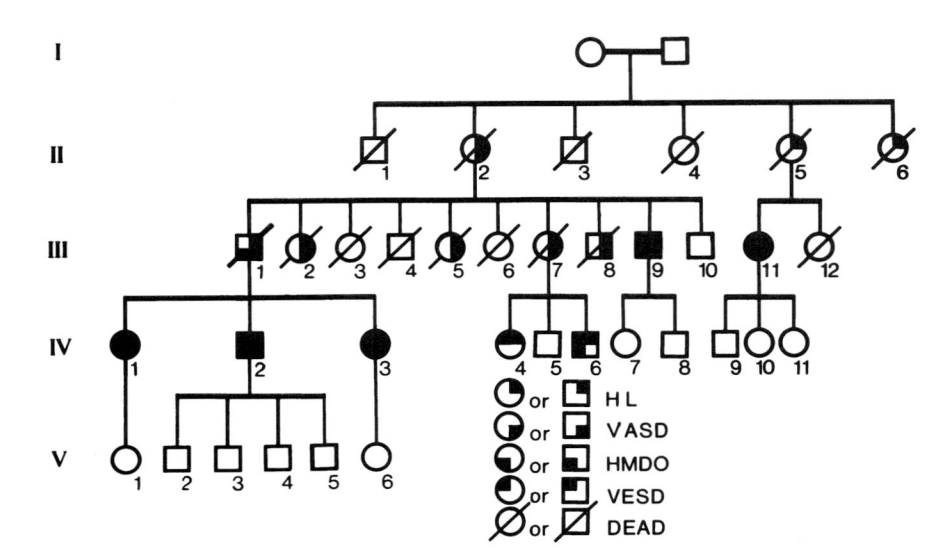

FIG. 6. Pedigree of a family with ADPAVD. *HL,* hearing loss; *HMDO,* head movement dependent oscillopsia; *VASD,* vascular disorders; *VESD,* vestibular dysfunction. From Verhagen WIM, et al. *J Neurol Sci* 92:55–63, 1989, copyright Elsevier Publishers, published with permission.

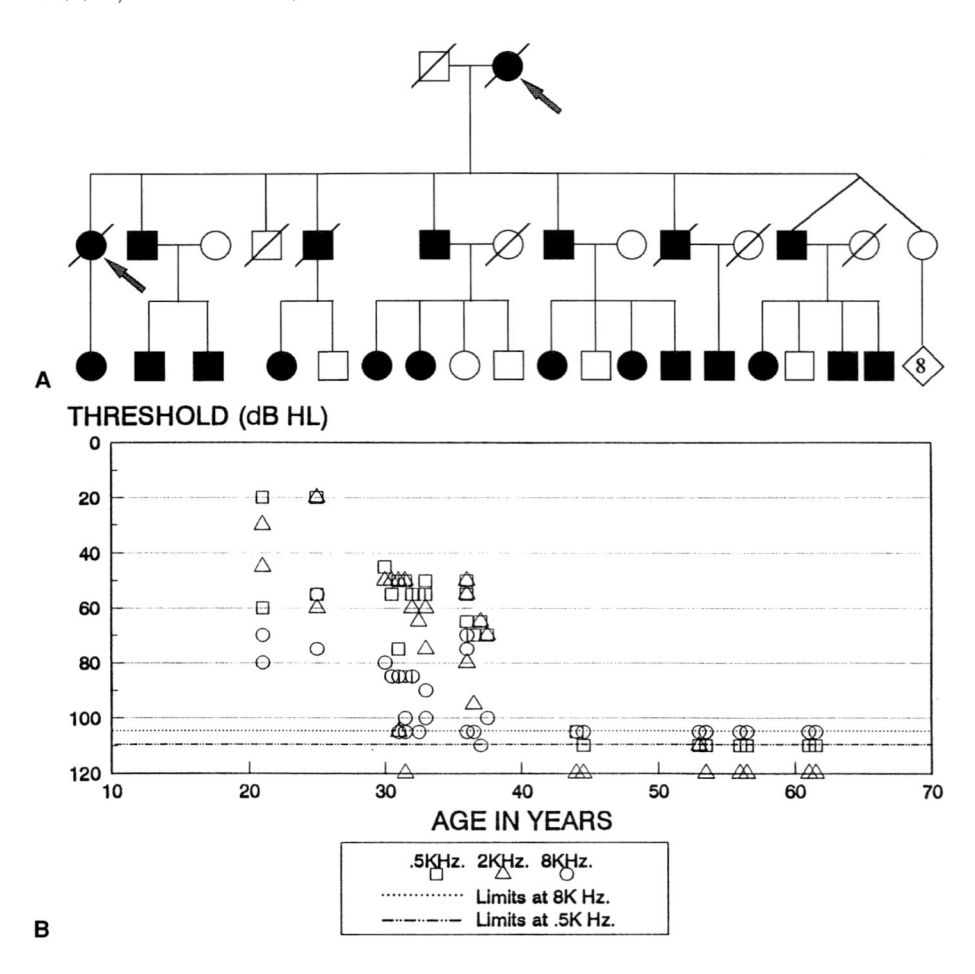

FIG. 7. A, B: Pedigree and audiometric features of a family with ADPAVD. The hearing loss begins at about age 20 in the high frequencies and is progressive and associated with vestibular dysfunction in most affected members. Arrows indicate deceased members whose temporal bones were studied. Modified from Halpin C, Khetarpal U, et al. *Am J Audiol,* in press, copyright ASHA Press, published with permission.

ataxia in the dark or with eyes closed. Vertigo and vomiting were seen in some patients (31,79–81). ABR (Auditory Brainstem Response) was normal in few members tested, with moderate loss indicating that the locus was cochlear. Vestibular testing indicates hypoactive or inactive responses on caloric testing, an absent OKAN (optokinetic after nystagmus), or head movement-dependent oscillopsia (80). One family had a higher incidence of vascular disorders (see Fig. 6). Imaging studies have been negative for inner ear defect. Temporal bone findings were described in two affected members from each of the two kindreds studied (31,32).

In addition to organ of Corti degeneration in all turns (moderate to severe), patchy strial atrophy, degeneration of neurosensory elements in the maculae and cristae, and severe dendritic degeneration of vestibular and cochlear nerves, we found a unique deposit in the spiral ligament, spiral limbus, Rosenthal's canal, osseous and membranous spiral lamina, and the stroma of maculae and cristae (Fig. 8). This deposit was also found to some extent in the stria vascularis and organ of Corti. The deposit is rich in glycosaminoglycans (GAGs). In both temporal bones from one affected, endolymphatic hydrops with obliteration of endolymphatic sac was also reported (32). Importantly, the two kindreds described differed in the age at onset of hearing loss, but all temporal bone had the same GAGs-rich deposit. A similar pathology was described by Linthicum and colleagues (84) in one patient that was implanted. A positive family history in this report indicates that it is inherited as an autosomal dominant trait. Gussen (83) also reported degeration of organ of Corti in middle and basal turns and of macula sacculi, utricle, and cristae. Gussen also noted endolymphatic hydrops but did not detect any deposit in the membranous labyrinth. There appears to be some heterogeneity in this entity in regard to age at onset and histologic findings (presence or absence of deposit). However, the detection of a similar GAGs-rich deposit in members of both pedigrees indicates that the variation in age at onset may be due to intralocus or allelic heterogeneity. Cochlear implantation has been successful in some patients (31). Efforts are ongoing to map the gene(s) for this disorder. Although epidemiologic studies are lacking, this subtype and that of autosomal dominant noncongenital high-frequency progressive SNHL may be the second largest group of NHHL.

Autosomal Dominant Meniere's Disease

The incidence of hereditary Meniere's disease has been reported to vary from 2.5% to 14% (85). Autosomal dominant forms of Meniere's disease were described by several investigators (Fig. 9) (85–90). Penetrance of the gene in

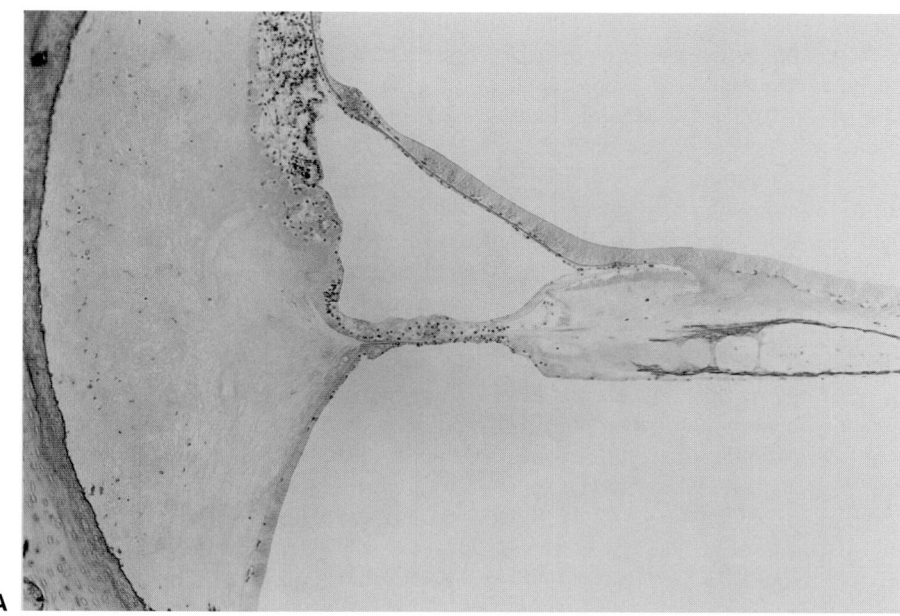

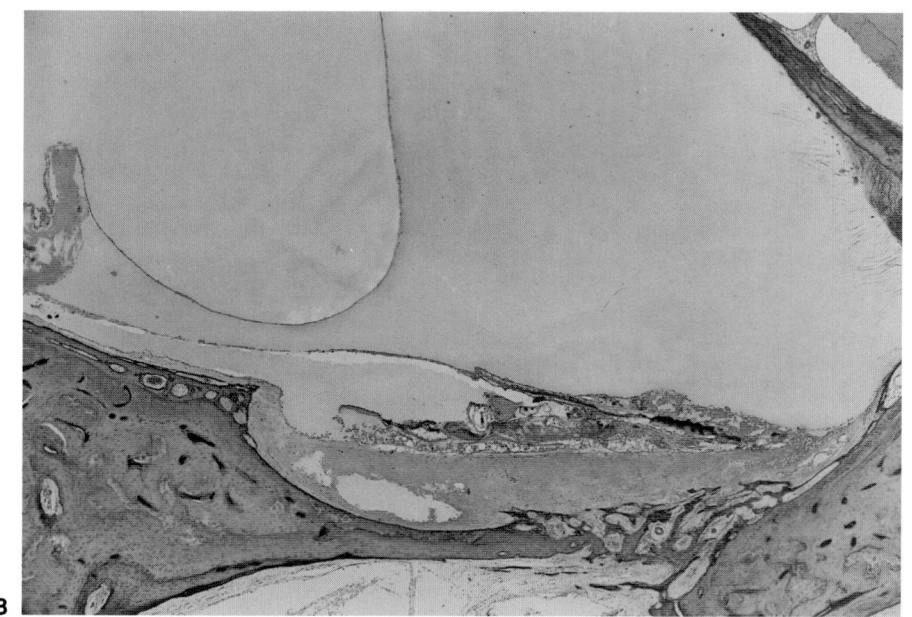

FIG. 8. A, B: Photomicrographs of cochlea and semicircular canal from temporal bone sections from an individual of a family with ADPAVD. These sections show degeneration of the sensory structures with marked loss of dendrites and ganglion cells. A GAGs-rich deposit is detected in the spiral ligament, spiral limbus, membranous spiral lamina, and stroma of saccule and in the cribrose areas. From Khetarpal U, et al. *Arch Otolaryngol Head Neck Surg* 117:1032–1042, 1991, copyright AMA, published with permission.

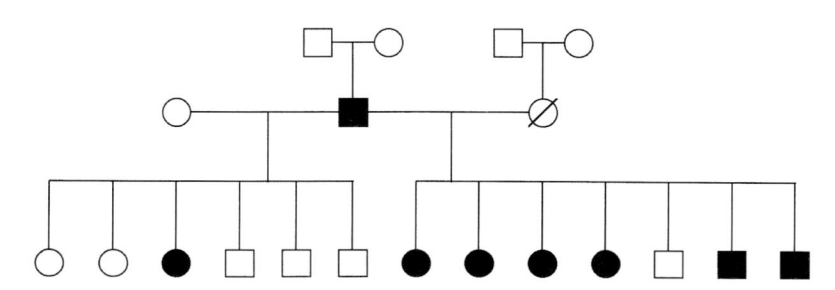

FIG. 9. Pedigree of a family with autosomal dominant Meniere's disease with migraine-like episodes. All affected members had low or flat SNHL. Modified from Oliveira CA, Braga AM. *Ann Otol Rhinol Laryngol* 101;590, 1992, copyright Annals Publishing Co., published with permission.

these families appears to be markedly variable (20–100%). However, most of these families are small. A monogenic-chance-environmental or oligogenic-chance-environmental interaction etiologic model has been proposed and appears to be a plausible one (91). Classical Meniere's disease presents with episodic vertigo, fluctuating hearing loss, tinnitus, sensation of blockage in the affected ear(s), migraine-like episodic headaches in many patients, and low-frequency hearing loss at onset of the disease. The hearing loss progresses until it involves all frequencies. The disease is often unilateral but may be bilateral in up to 50% of the patients on long-term follow-up. Vestibular findings are variable. Lack of demonstration of endolymphatic duct and sac on radiography has been interpreted as evidence for endolymphatic sac dysfunction. Numerous temporal bone findings have shown endolymphatic hydrops with ruptures, hypoplastic endolymphatic sac, and essentially normal organ of Corti at the light microscopic level. Duplication of chromosome 7q was found in a mother and daughter with Meniere's disease (85), but this may be a familial polymorphism. According to one report, HLA-Cw7 has been strongly associated with familial and sporadic Meniere's disease (92). These findings need to be corroborated. There is disagreement regarding the interpretation of Gorlin et al. (10) that a type of familial Meniere's disease has been mapped to chromosome 19 (93,94). The studies of Joutel et al. (93,94) demonstrate mapping of familial hemiplegic migraine to this chromosome and not of Meniere's disease, which may be associated with migraine-like episodic headaches.

Autosomal Dominant Mondini's Dysplasia

Although many cases of nonsyndromic Mondini's dysplasia appear to be sporadic, Chan et al. (95) described a three-generation family with three affected members that had partial to complete SNHL in one ear and normal hearing to partial loss in the opposite ear (Fig. 10). Vestibular system testing revealed abnormalities in all three patients. Radiographically, hypoplasia of the cochlea, flattening of apical turns, scala communis defect (in one patient), dilated vestibules, and a short lateral semicircular canal were reported. The findings varied markedly between the three patients and between the ears of the same patient. Temporal bone findings were not available in this family but have been well described in the literature (Fig. 11). Although the genetics of this condition are unclear except in this report, we propose that nonsyndromic Mondini's dysplasia is a result of a monogenic-chance autosomal dominant model similar to the proposal made by Kurnit, Layton, and Mathysse (96) for endocardial cushion defects (e.g., ventricular septal defects).

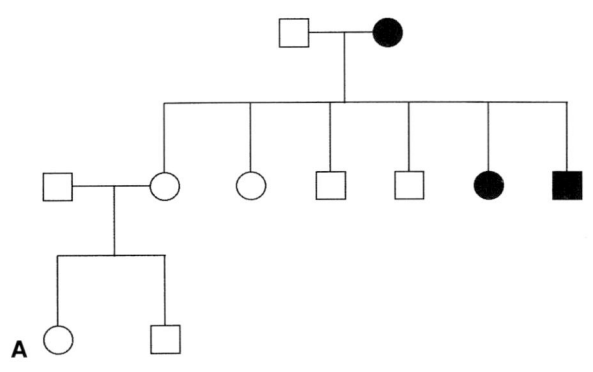

FIG. 10. A–C: Pedigree and audiograms of three individuals with autosomal dominant Mondini's dysplasia. The mother and son had similar audiograms (B), whereas the daughter had a different audiogram (C). Computed tomography findings in all three were consistent with Mondini's dysplasia. Bone and air conduction thresholds were similar therefore only air conduction thresholds are shown. Modified from Chan KH, et al. *Ann Otol Rhinol Laryngol* 100:620–625, 1991, copyright Annals Publishing Co., published with permission.

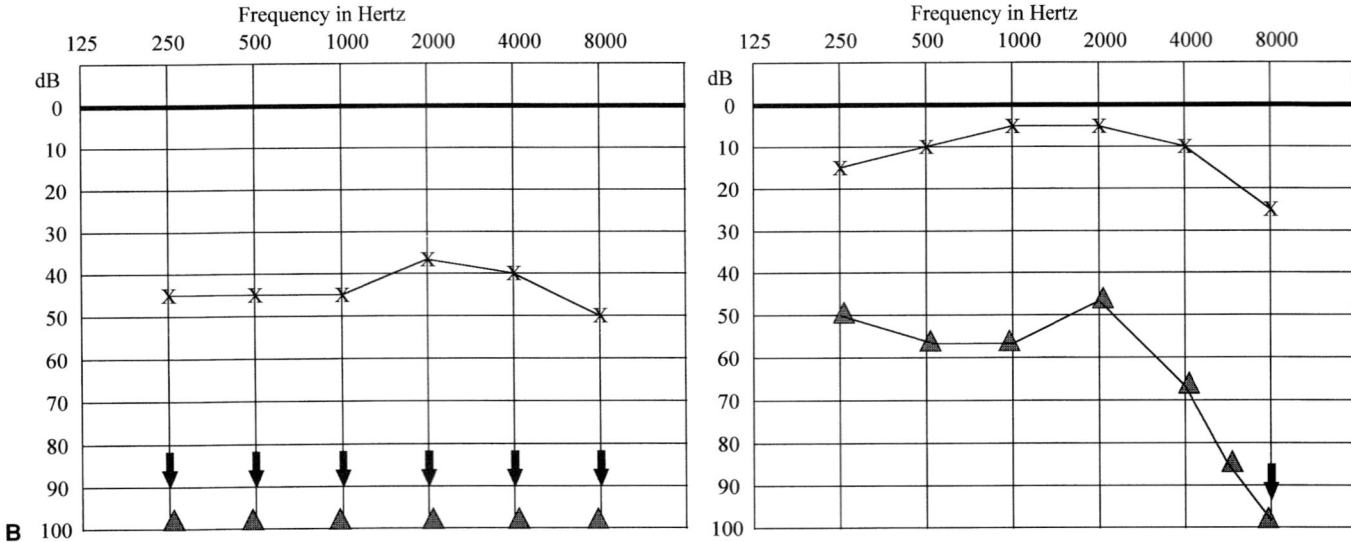

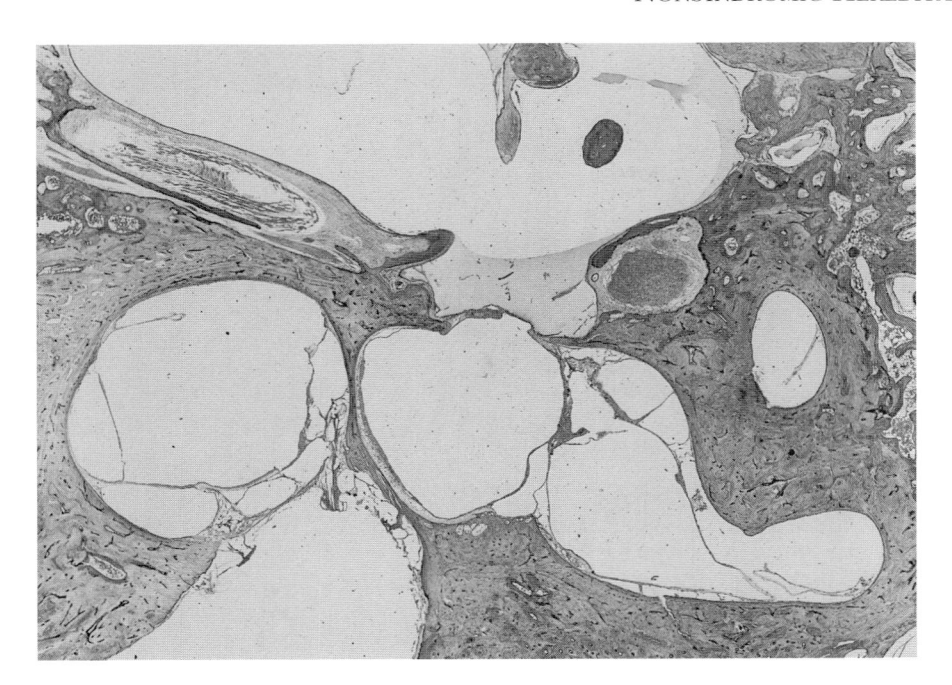

FIG. 11. Photomicrograph of a 20-m temporal bone section from an individual with severe Mondini's dysplasia. A bulbous cochlea without development of any cochlear turns, a rudimentary modiolus, a markedly dilated vestibule, and a defective stapes footplate covered by a thin membrane are seen. Oval window fistulae may result in recurrent meningitis, a dreaded complication of this disorder. Courtesy of Harold F. Schuknecht, Harvard Medical School, Boston.

Stochastic variation within the system may account for the variability in radiographic and audiologic findings or even the lack of penetrance of the gene. The excellent correlation of bony labyrinthine abnormalities between high-resolution CT images and light microscopic morphology of the temporal bone indicates the sensitivity of CT scanning in detecting this entity. The identification of Mondini's dysplasia is extremely important for prognosis. These patients have a high risk of development of perilymphatic fistulaes and recurrent meningitis. To prevent such occurrences in the future, patients with this disease should be forewarned against participating in contact sports, scuba diving, or any activities that may result in implosive or explosive inner ear trauma.

Autosomal Recessive Inheritance

Autosomal Recessive Congenital Severe-to-Profound SNHL

A large number of such families have been described, and it is obvious that there is tremendous heterogeneity within this group (Fig. 12) (12,24,41,43,98–111). They may be separated on the basis of vestibular findings. A few patients in one family complained of vertigo and had a variable age at onset (birth to 16 yr) (111). Because complete audiologic and vestibular data have not been provided in many reports, many of the subtypes of this category appear to be clinically and audiologically indistinguishable. Severe-to-profound SNHL with infrequent preservation in low frequencies is the usual finding (Fig. 12B). Vestibular findings have varied from normal (99,100) to moderate or complete paresis in some members (105,106). Speech development is poor unless some type of rehabilitation has been provided. No radiographic findings are available. Temporal bone findings indicate absence of hair cells, collapse of Reissner's membrane, strial atrophy, and a decreased spiral ganglion cell population (107,108). Although the role of otoacoustic emissions has not been investigated in determining carrier status, it does not appear likely that carriers of these genes can be identified by sophisticated audiologic testing. In isolated inbred communities, the gene frequency may be higher. Three genes have been mapped to 11q13.5, 13q, and 17p-17q12, indicating genetic heterogeneity (109–111). Vestibular test results were not described in any of these three families, although it was reported that some members in one family had vertigo (111). The gene location in this latter family is homologous to the gene location of the mouse shaker 1 (*sh-1*) mutant. *Sh-1* is a fully penetrant, autosomal recessive mutation identified by a characteristic phenotype consisting of neurosensory deafness, hyperactivity, and a vestibular defect causing head shaking and circling behaviour (112). *Sh-1* appears to be due to a defect in the myosin type VII gene (113). It has long been suspected that a type of myosin may function as an adaptive motor associated with hair cell stereocilia tip links. It remains to be seen if this adaptive motor is the type VII molecule. The impact of abnormal myosin on hair cell signal transduction remains to be elucidated. This subtype of hearing loss appears to be the most common of all NHHLs.

Autosomal Recessive Congenital Moderate Nonprogressive SNHL

Such sibships were descibed by Konigsmark and colleagues (114,115). Flat or downsloping, moderate (30–70 dB, low to high frequencies), nonprogressive hearing loss was detected in childhood. Caloric testing was normal. Ra-

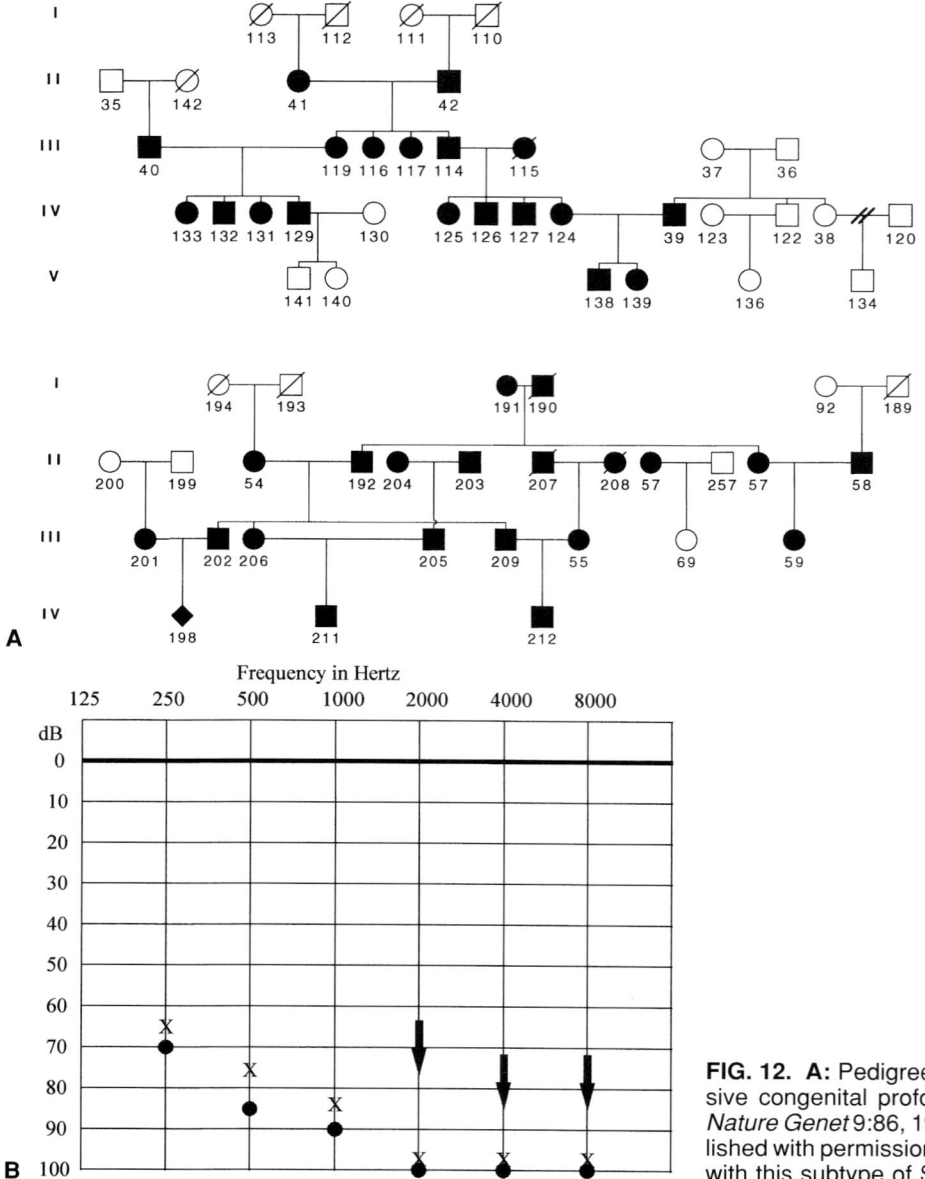

FIG. 12. A: Pedigrees of two families with autosomal recessive congenital profound SNHL. From Friedman TB, et al. *Nature Genet* 9:86, 1995, copyright Nature Publications, published with permission. **B:** A typical audiogram in an individual with this subtype of SNHL.

diographic or temporal bone findings are not available. This appears to be a rare form of disorder.

Autosomal Recessive Congenital Progressive SNHL

This is yet another form of rare disease that was well characterized by Mengel et al. (116) and to a certain extent by Barr and Wedenburg (117). The hearing loss appears to be mild to moderate at birth and then progresses rapidly to deafness by the middle or end of the first decade. Speech pattern is intermediate between that of a congenitally deaf child and a normal-hearing child. Vestibular responses are normal. Radiographic or temporal bone findings have not been described.

Autosomal Recessive Noncongenital Progressive High-Frequency SNHL

These families were described by Cremers et al. (Fig. 13A)(118,119) and Madell and Sculerati (121). Hearing loss was noted at about 5 to 15 years in the high frequencies (Fig. 13B). This progressed rapidly to involve the other frequencies, resulting in poor speech discrimination. Vestibular findings were normal. This must be differentiated from the other recessive and dominant progressive high-frequency losses.

X-linked Inheritance

The majority of X-linked SNHL is congenital, which is easily distinguishable from the rare noncongenital types. It

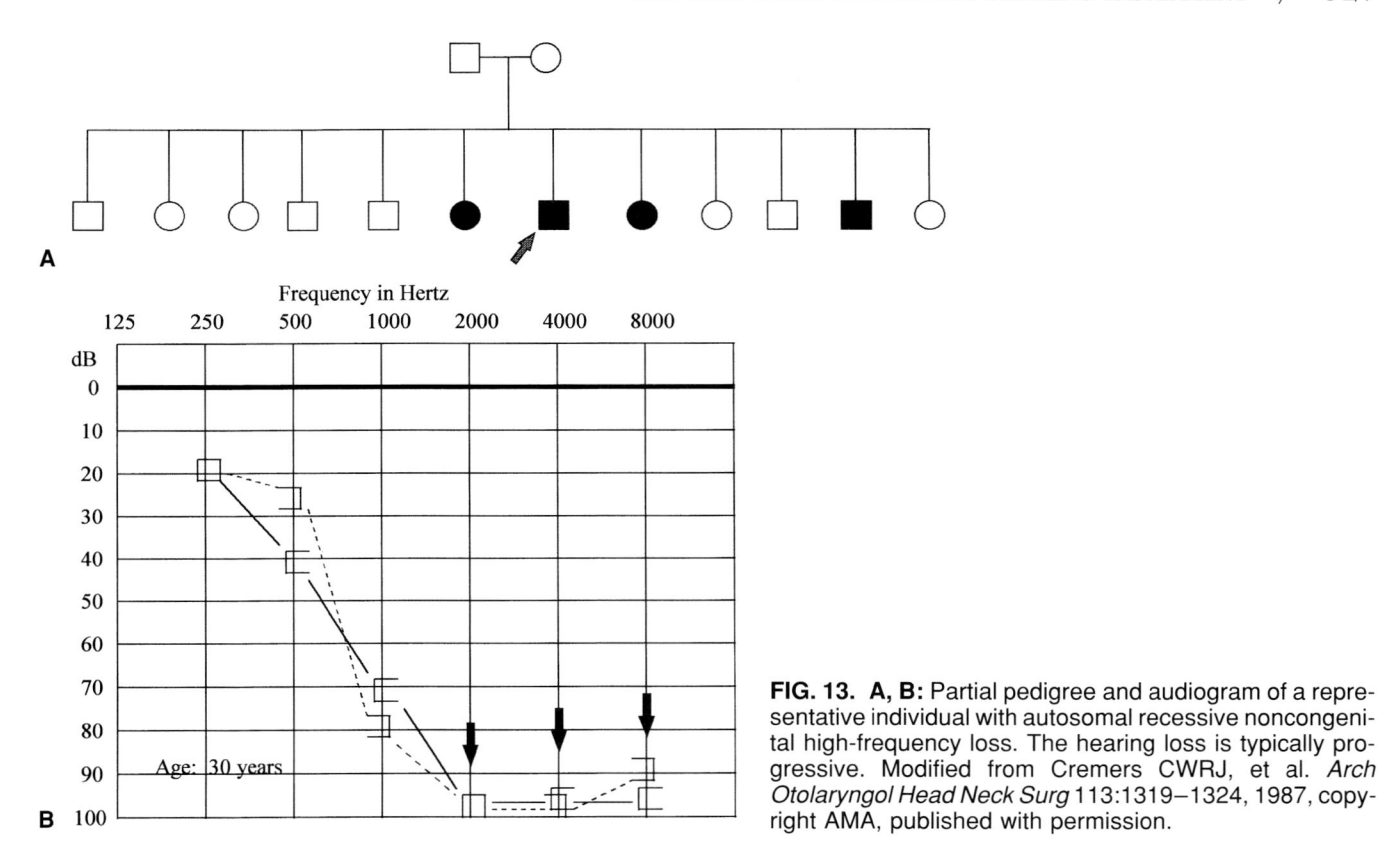

FIG. 13. A, B: Partial pedigree and audiogram of a representative individual with autosomal recessive noncongenital high-frequency loss. The hearing loss is typically progressive. Modified from Cremers CWRJ, et al. *Arch Otolaryngol Head Neck Surg* 113:1319–1324, 1987, copyright AMA, published with permission.

is not clear if the several forms of prelingual nonsyndromic hearing losses are different or identical entities. Reardon et al. (121) have estimated that 50% of all X-linked hearing losses are related to the Xq13-21 region, possibly the X-linked mixed deafness with the perilymphatic gusher (DFN3) gene. An alternate possibility is that there may be more than one gene responsible for hearing loss in the Xq13-21 region. Recent investigation of seven patients with X-linked SNHL has failed to reveal mutations in any of the exons of the POU3F4 gene, the gene for mixed deafness with a perilymphatic gusher (DFN3) (see following discussion) (122). On a clinical basis, there appear to be several different entities. The role of otoacoustic emissions in carrier detection has not been investigated, but it appears unlikely that this testing will detect changes in the presence of normal hearing. Phelps et al. (123) provide compelling evidence for the usage of radiographic criteria in the classification of X-linked recessive hearing loss.

X-linked Dominant Congenital Severe-to-Profound SNHL

This entity was recently described by Lalwani et al. (1994) (Fig. 14). Affected males manifested with congenital bilateral profound SNHL, whereas affected females manifested with bilateral mild-to-moderate (20–50 dB) mid- to high-frequency SNHL, which appears to have its onset after the first decade. The affected females had lesser severity of hearing loss than the affected males, and more variable hearing loss. This suggests that the normal gene on the second X chromosome may play a role in altering the severity and the age at onset of hearing loss. Vestibular findings were not reported. No radiographic abnormalities were found. Temporal bone findings have not been reported. No chromosomal abnormalities were detected in a 850-band karyotype. The gene has been mapped to Xp21.2 (124). Dystrophin appears to be a candidate gene for this hearing loss. However, hearing acuity tested in 51 Duchenne's muscular dystrophy patients (24 ambulatory) by pure-tone audiometry (0.25–6 kHz) was reported as normal (125). Whether this is a dystrophin gene mutation or an alternate novel gene mutation within the dystrophin gene is under investigation. This appears to be a rare X-linked disorder.

X-linked Recessive Congenital Severe-to-Profound SNHL

Several families have been described with this phenotype, although there may be differences (121,126–134). Audiometrically, a 70 to 100-dB loss involving all frequencies is detected on testing. Vestibular abnormalities have been described only in those patients with radiologic cochlear abnormality (123). In some families, high-resolution CT scanning of the temporal bone has revealed a bulbous internal auditory canal incompletely separated from the basal bony coil of the cochlea (121,123). In other families, no radiologic

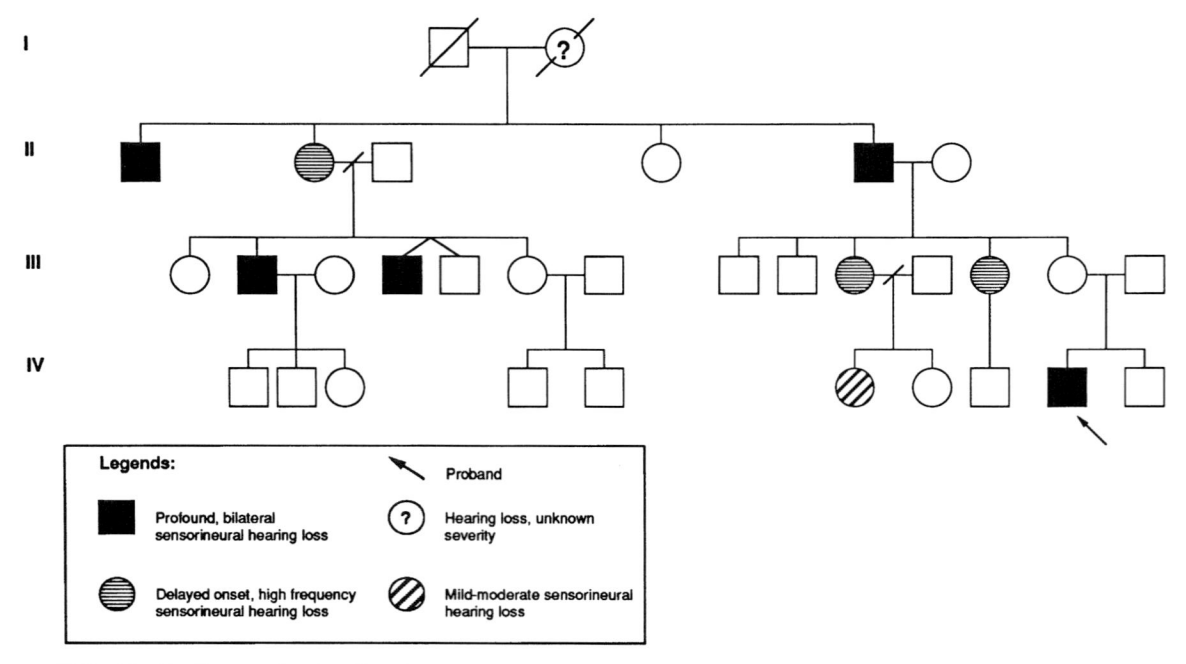

FIG. 14. Pedigree of a family with X-linked dominant congenital severe-to-profound SNHL. Affected male members have profound bilateral SNHL, whereas in affected females, the SNHL is variable. Modified from Lalwani et al. *Am J Hum Genet* 55:685–694, 1994, copyright University of Chicago Press, published with permission.

abnormalities have been found (123,131). Because carriers without hearing loss have been noted to have the radiographic abnormality, the relationship of this temporal bone defect to hearing loss is not clear. Hopefully, temporal bone studies will help clarify their relationship. Mild-to-moderate mental retardation has been observed in some patients (128,129) and choroideremia in some (132). Temporal bone findings have not been described. Fraser (126) estimated that X-linked recessive hearing loss made up about 6.2% of all male patients with profound hearing loss. The results of linkage and candidate gene mutation screening have been varied, suggesting genetic heterogeneity. Deletions have been found in the Xq21 region in patients with isolated SNHL and in patients with SNHL associated with choroideremia (121,132). Robinson et al. (133) found closer linkage to Xq12 than to Xq21 Another report indicated linkage to Xq21 (134). It has been suggested that the gene for SNHL linked to the Xq13-q21 region may be the same as the DFN3 gene (121,135). At the present time, one report has indicated this not to be the case in seven individuals with X-linked SNHL (122) and another report has excluded Xq21 as the defective region in a family with X-linked SNHL (132). Whether these defects are in the exons of POU3F4 gene, its 5' or 3' ends, or its upstream regulator elements, or due to mutations in alternate genes remains to be identified. It is also possible that some families described by Reardon and colleagues (121,123,131), which have been designated X-linked congenital recessive SNHL and show radiologic cochlear abnormality (described earlier), are actually those that may have had mixed deafness if their SNHL was not so severe as to mask the conductive loss.

X-linked Recessive Noncongenital High-Frequency Progressive SNHL with Moderate Impairment

Described by Livan (136) and Pelletier and Tanguay (137), onset occurs around adolescence, with high-frequencies affected to a greater extent than other frequencies. Hearing loss slowly progresses to moderate impairment. Low frequencies appear to be near normal. Caloric testing was normal. No radiographic or temporal bone findings have been reported.

X-linked Recessive Noncongenital Mid- to High-Frequency Nonprogressive SNHL

This is a rare type described by Wellesley and Goldblatt (138) in which the affected males had an abrupt SNHL at about 1.0 to 1.5 kHz, with hearing loss of higher frequencies but not greater than that at about 1.5 kHz. This hearing loss is nonprogressive. Vestibular, radiographic, and temporal findings have not been described.

Mitochondrial Inheritance

In a previous section, the characteristics of mitochondrially inherited disorders were described. Inheritance is maternal. Many families with mitochondrially inherited SNHL have been described (139–143). The hearing loss may be detected in infancy, early childhood, or adulthood; is progressive; and is moderately severe to profound for all frequencies 139–141). Alternatively, the disease may start with elevation of thresholds in the high frequencies, with considerable variability between individuals and no correlation between age and severity of hearing loss (142,143). Vestibular, radiographic, or temporal bone findings have not been described. It has been suggested that the mitochondrial tRNA (Leu(UUR)) (position 3243) mutation is associated exclusively with a subtype of noninsulin-dependant diabetes mellitus associated with SNHL, designated mitochondrially inherited diabetes and deafness (144). However, the same mutation was found in some Japanese diabetic patients, of whom only a few had hearing impairment (145). Additionally, a 10.4-kb mitochondrial DNA deletion was found in one family with type II diabetes and deafness (141). A mutation at site np 7445 in a mitochondrial tRNA gene has been associated with isolated maternally inherited SNHL (143). Additionally, mutations at position 3243 (A–G) have also been detected in a Japanese family with diabetes, SNHL and cardiomyopathy (146). Therefore, testing is recommended for all patients with a family history of maternally inherited diabetes with SNHL for a mutation at position 3243.

Yet another type of mitochondrially inherited deafness is that associated with aminoglycoside toxicity (AGT) (Fig. 15) (28). Polymorphism–mutation at nt 1555 (A–G) in mitochondrial DNA was detected in Japanese pedigrees with AGT, in 4 of 78 cases of sporadic AGT (147) and in 1 of 36 cases of sporadic AGT (148). This suggests that whereas most cases of familial AGT are likely to carry the 1555 mutation, less than 10% of sporadic AGT will bear the same mutation. Whether alternate mutations in mtDNA result in sporadic AGT needs to be investigated. Importantly, therefore, familial association of this hearing loss–vestibulopathy should be sought with extensive history taking. Because mutations in mt tRNA(Leu(UUR)) are also found in patients with myoclonic myopathy, encephalopathy, lactic acidosis, and strokelike episodes, without diabetes or hearing loss, other factors (e.g., a nuclear gene) may also be involved in determining the final phenotype. Even if the yield is poor, routine testing of female patients with AGT will be especially useful in situations in which the mutation is detected. The offspring of the mother carrying the mutation could then be tested for the same mutation and forewarned regarding possible damage from aminoglycosides.

Vestibular, radiographic and temporal bone findings in non-AGT mitochondrial SNHL have not been described. However, temporal bone findings in a patient with Kearns-Sayre syndrome with SNHL (a mitochondrial disease) were described by Lindsay and Hinojosa (150). The membranous labyrinth showed an advanced stage of degeneration of the organ of Corti, with clumping, collapse of Reissner's membrane, and degeneration of stria vascularis and spiral ganglion cells and dendrites.

It is likely that some types of presbycusis and vestibular aging may be related to the accumulation of mitochondrial DNA mutations in the neurosensory or supporting cells, ganglion cells, or secretory cells. This hypothesis should be tested on DNA extracted from temporal bones (membranous cochlea) of patients with known presbycusis. Whether antioxidants have a role in the treatment or prevention of progression in such diseases needs to be defined clearly by well-designed studies.

MIXED AND CONDUCTIVE HEARING LOSS

X-linked Mixed Deafness with Perilymphatic Gusher (DFN3)

Many such families have been described (Fig. 16A) (122,123,150–160), although Nance et al. (158) provided

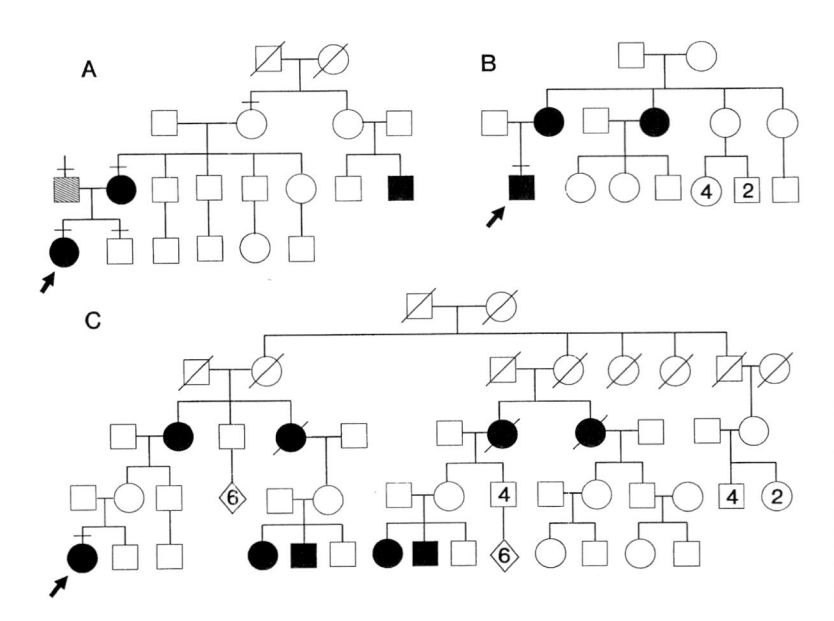

FIG. 15. Pedigree of three families with mitochondrially inherited aminoglycoside-induced toxicity. The mutation was discovered in position 1555 of the mitochondrial DNA. Solid symbols indicate individuals treated with streptomycin before high-frequency SNHL ensued. From Prezant TR, et al. *Nature Genet* 4:289–294, 1993, copyright Nature Publications, published with permission.

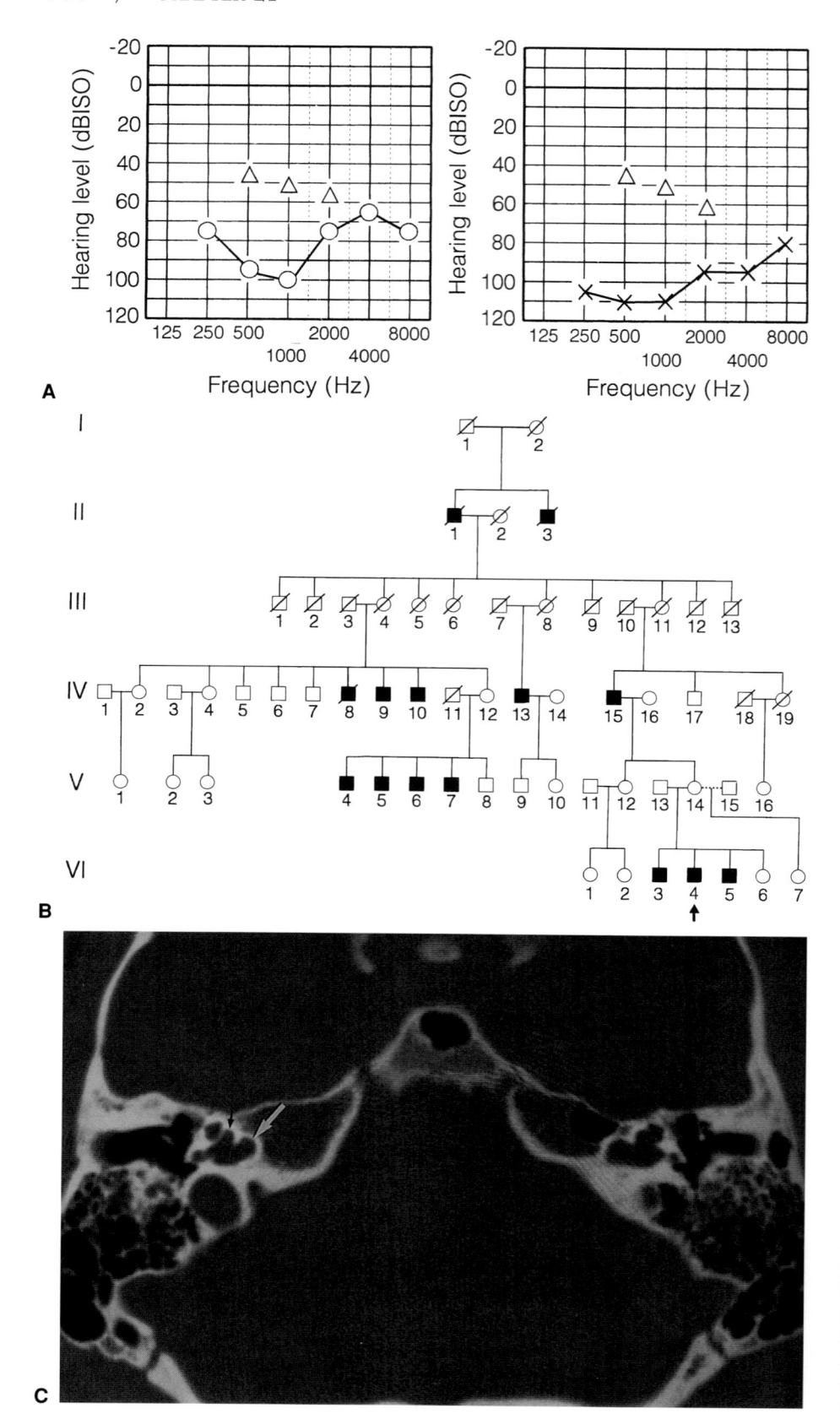

FIG. 16. A: Audiogram of a typical male with X-linked mixed deafness. **B:** A typical pedigree of X-linked mixed deafness with stapes gusher. **C:** Axial CT scan showing incomplete separation of basal turn of cochlea from the fundus of IAC (*arrows*).

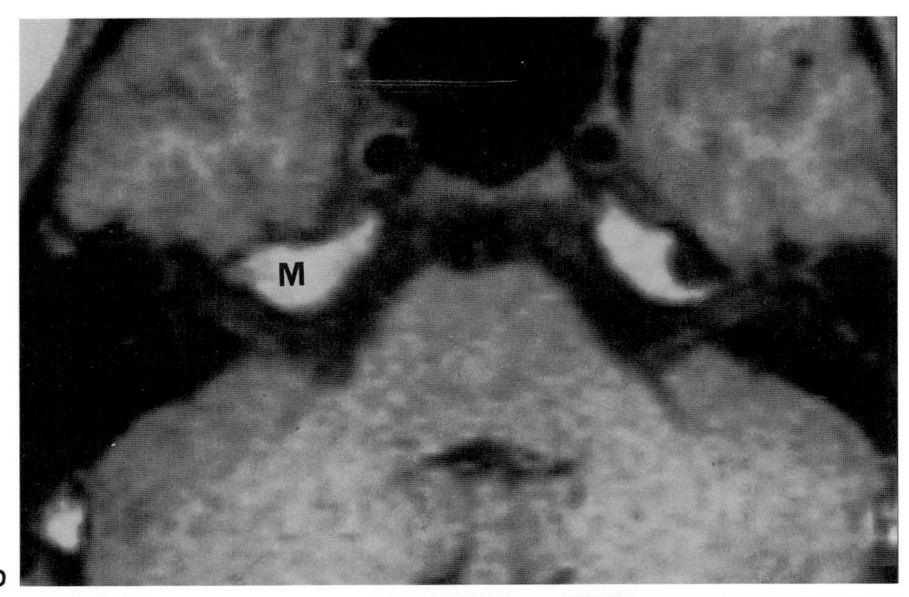

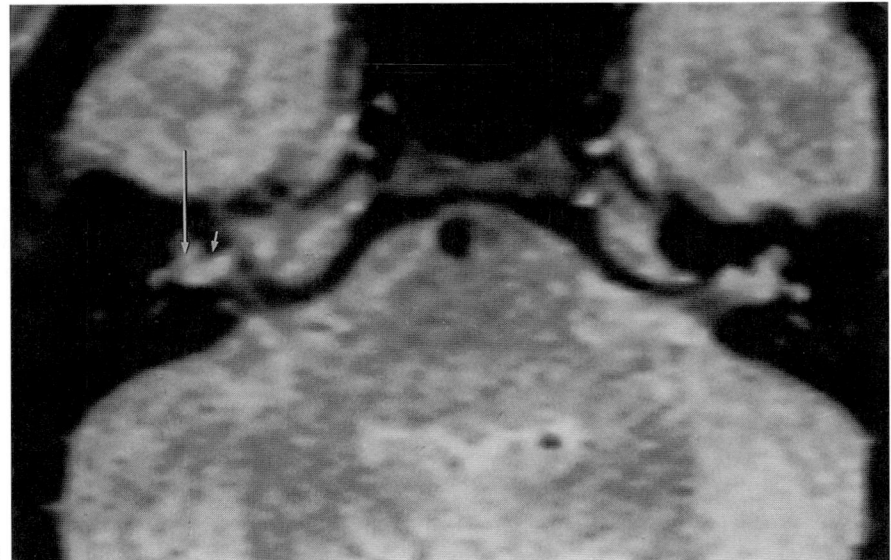

FIG. 16. *Continued.* **D** and **E:** Axial gadolinium-enhanced MRI scans showing marrow in petrous apex (*M*), normal VII and VIII nerves, and bright signal of CSF (on T2-weighted image) in the fundus of IAC and in perilymph of the basal turn of cochlea. From Phelps PD, et al. *Neuroradiol* 33:326–330, 1991, copyright Springer-Verlag, with permission.

the earliest detailed description of this entity. Males have bilateral, mixed loss that may be symmetrical and progressive. Hearing loss begins in the first decade, but there appears to be variability in the severity of hearing loss in different families (153,159,160). The conductive component is usually greater in the lower frequencies (Fig. 16B). Heterozygotic females have a variable mixed loss that is greater in lower frequencies (152). Part of the hearing loss may be due to variable stapes fixation because stapedial reflexes can be elicited in some patients with mild-to-moderate loss (151). However, exploratory tympanotomy reveals fixation of stapes with absence of the annular rim (160). A perilymphatic gusher develops on the performance of a stapedectomy (153,160). Vestibular testing has been found to be abnormal in most males, whereas female heterozygotes have normal findings, indicating an imperfect correlation between vestibular and auditory findings (153). Radiography reveals a widened internal auditory canal with a small cochlea and poor separation of the cochlear turns (Fig. 16C–E) (123). It is suspected that the perilymphatic gusher is a result of abnormal communication between the internal auditory canal and the inner ear (absent cribrose areas) (160), whereas the perilymphatic ooze may be secondary to cochlear aqueduct obstruction or enlargement. The gene has been cloned and mutations found in the POU3F4 gene, a putative transcription factor (122). However, in six individuals with DFN3, point mutations were not found in POU3F4 gene, indicating heterogeneity even in this entity (122). This disorder should be kept in mind with *any* male patient with mixed progressive hearing loss; it can easily be diagnosed by CT scan of the temporal bone. A family history should be sought actively prior to consideration of surgery, because surgical results may be devastating. Most affected individuals function adequately with hearing aids (153).

Otosclerosis

This intriguing disease affects the otic capsule, resulting in stapes fixation with a conductive hearing loss. Often, involvement of the inner ear by secondary mechanisms results in an SNHL giving the pattern of a mixed loss. It is believed to be specific to the temporal bone, although rigorous studies have not been performed indicating this to be the case. Several investigators have proposed that this disease is transmitted in an autosomal dominant fashion with a 25% to 40% penetrance (161–166). Others believe it to be multifactorial in origin (10,167), based on incidence of disease within families with confirmed otosclerosis (168). There is a female predilection, with some worsening of the hearing loss during pregnancy (169). Hearing loss is usually noticed in the second to fourth decades, is progressive, and may be conductive or mixed, with greater sensorineural loss in higher frequencies. Importantly, the stapedial reflex is absent and tympanometry is normal. Vestibular impairment may be found. Polytomography demonstrates a bony bridge covering the oval window and narrowing of the oval window niche (170). Histologically, the otic capsule is replaced by immature, highly vascular woven bone that involves the enchondral layer first at the fissula ante fenestram adjacent to the oval window. The disease may remain quiescent in 90% or spread in 10% to the stapes, annular ligament, or the remaining otic capsule (171). The factors that determine progression of histologic otosclerosis to clinical otosclerosis have not yet been determined. In fact, it is not clear if the histologic otosclerosis group (~10% of all temporal bones studied) is different from the clinical otosclerosis group (~1% of all temporal bones studied). Involvement of the stapes or annular ligament results in stapes fixation. Hyalinization of the spiral ligament is observed whenever the endosteum adjacent to the spiral ligament is involved. Stapedotomy or stapedectomy not only reverses a large part of the conductive loss but also may reverse some of the SNHL at speech frequencies. Although a role for the measles virus in the pathogenicity of the disease has been proposed (172), the evidence requires further corroboration and appropriate controls. In one study, HLA-A11, Bw25, and B15 were found to be associated with familial otosclerosis, (173) but a subsequent study could not confirm this (174). The gene(s) have not been mapped, although efforts in several laboratories are ongoing. If the histologic otosclerosis group does progress to clinical otosclerosis in a minority, this favors the hypothesis of a common gene in the population that predisposes to histologic otosclerosis. Interaction with environmental or other modifying genetic factors may then push it towards clinical otosclerosis. If this assumption is true, the model that otosclerosis would follow is a monogenic-chance-environmental interaction model or a digenic inheritance model.

Familial Conductive Hearing Loss

A number of other hearing disorders, including congenital microtia with external auditory canal stenosis, middle ear abnormalities, and auricular abnormalities, and familial ossicular malformations with conductive hearing loss, have been described. Possible autosomal dominant inheritance has been observed in some families (175–177).

DIAGNOSTIC APPROACH ALGORITHMS

Evaluation of sensorineural/hearing loss begins by obtaining a complete history and a thorough physical examination

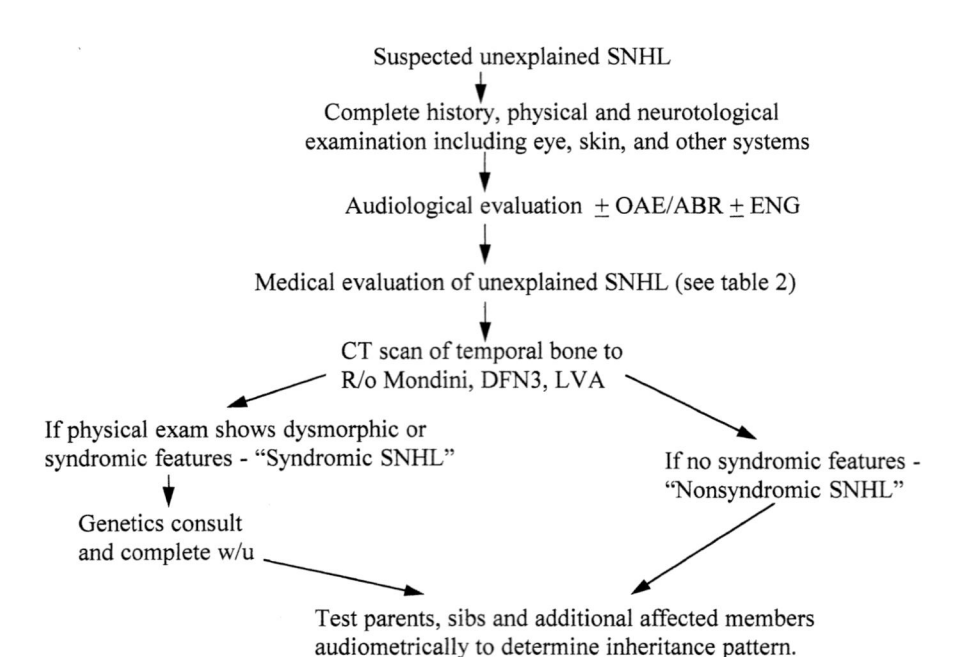

FIG. 17. Diagnostic flow chart for determining the underlying basis of an unexplained SNHL. *LVA*, large vestibular aqueduct; *DFN3*, X-linked mixed deafness with stapes fixation that is typically associated with a bulbous internal auditory canal and a communication of IAC with the cochlea; *ABR*, auditory brainstem response; *ENG*, electronystagmography; *OAE*, otoacoustic emission.

(Fig. 17). In any patient with suspected genetic hearing loss, it is imperative that a family history be assembled and reviewed. This should include information on first-, second- and third-degree relatives. Permission to examine and test the relatives and siblings must be obtained from the consultand. Testing siblings and relatives often allows a more accurate ascertainment of the inheritance pattern of the hearing loss. An accurate pedigree is made and audiometric and vestibular testing is performed. Prior audiograms and vestibular tests, biochemical tests, and radiographic images must be obtained to assess the progression and onset of the disease. The otolaryngologist–geneticist must rule out nongenetic conditions that may have resulted in hearing loss either by history or by specific testing (see Table 2). In the absence of a nongenetic cause, genetic disease must be assumed. If the hearing loss is syndromic, associated systemic features should be diagnosed accurately and supplemented with the help of organ-specific testing and/or radiography. A karyotype should then be performed. A partial listing of situations in which karyotyping may be helpful was compiled by Kimberling and Brookhouser (178). Cost considerations are important in determining the type of karyotype (400- or 800-band karyotypes) to be obtained. Referral should be made to a geneticist if a syndromic hearing loss is suspected. In NHHL the yield from karyotyping is likely to be poor. A high-resolution CT scan of temporal bones should be performed to identify Mondini's dysplasia, and cochleovestibular or ossicular malformations. The benefits of using a CT scan in X-linked deafness cannot be overstated. It should help in gene localization and in understanding the nature of the X-linked hearing loss. Because most nonsyndromic SNHLs occur at the biophysical and histologic level, radiographic analysis will be unremarkable in many. Once a hereditary hearing loss is diagnosed (see Fig. 2), consultation with otolaryngologists and auditory researchers working on the genetics of deafness is highly recommended.

MOLECULAR GENETIC APPROACHES IN GENE MAPPING

Genetic studies in humans have generally been performed in one of three ways: (a) by linkage analysis in well-defined pedigrees to determine if a genetic marker cosegregates with the disease; (b) by affected sib-pair or relative analysis, whereby allele sharing among affected siblings or affected relatives is compared with the alleleic frequency in the general population; and (c) by studying the association between an allele (alternate forms of the same gene or locus) and the disease in a case-controlled study. Although each of these methodologies has advantages and disadvantages, these genetic studies have a limited impact on human diseases that are considered to be etiologically or genetically heterogenous.

In most types of nonsyndromic SNHL, the strategy that has been adopted is that of linkage analysis. Large pedigrees provide the best resource for determination of the disease gene locus. Gene mapping in X-linked diseases is less time consuming and more successful than in autosomes. DNA is obtained from affected and unaffected individuals in the family, and then, by polymerase chain reaction analysis, a genome-wide search using polymorphic markers is performed. These markers have been mapped to specific regions of each chromosome and are available through various sources. Many of these markers are dinucleotide, trinucleotide, or tetranucleotide repeats. Their polymorphicity or heterozygosity and conditions best suited for the reaction are also usually provided along with the products. The cosegregation of the disease with a specific marker or markers provides the first clue toward localizing the suspected gene to a particular chromosome. Various mathematical programs (e.g., LINKAGE, LINKMAP, etc.) are available that determine the tightness of this linkage. In mathematical terms, a value of LOD (logarithm of odds ratio) score of more than 3 indicates linkage to a particular region of chromosome, whereas a value of -2 indicates lack of linkage. An alternative strategy for linkage in autosomal recessive pedigrees in which consanguinity is obvious and higher than in the general population is that of homozygosity mapping. The rationale for this strategy is that genes or markers adjacent to the putative gene will be homozygous at all locations. However, because more than two or three affected siblings in a family is infrequent, multiple families will be required to establish linkage. If genetic heterogeneity is marked, this task may be very difficult. Once linkage is determined by either one of these strategies, effort is then made to identify and isolate the candidate gene either by cosmid or yeast artifical chromosome screening (positional cloning) or by testing candidate genes that have already been mapped to that specific region. After mutations have been detected by molecular methods, the functionality of the mutation is tested by screening other patients or pedigrees with a similar or identical disease, by making mutation-specific constructs and transfecting cells with these constructs and by making transgenic animals. Diagnostic mutation screening can then be performed in the hearing-loss population similar to that performed for cystic fibrosis or Duchenne's muscular dystrophy.

Within the last few years, in addition to mapping and cloning of some genes for syndromic hearing loss, several genes for nonsyndromic SNHL have been mapped (Table 3). These more recent successes foreshadow the cloning of additional genes in the coming years and bring us closer to treating or preventing these diseases.

GENETIC COUNSELING

Clearly, there is an unmet need for genetic counseling in the area of hearing loss. A questionnaire that ascertains the onset of auditory and vestibular symptoms, associated features, progression, family history, environmental factors, ototoxic medication, perinatal causes, and so on, should be completed by the proband and all family members. Genetic counseling is offered only after ascertainment of the inheritance of the hearing loss. Genetic counseling is required not

TABLE 3. *Nonsyndromic hereditary hearing impairment*

Disorder	Pathology	Location	Ref. no.
X-linked recessive			
DFN1	Progressive deafness	Xq21–q22	179
DFN2	Congenital deafness	X	180
DFN3	Stapes fixation with perilymphatic gusher, progressive mixed deafness	Xq21.1	122
DFN4	Congenital deafness	Xp21.2	124
DFN6		Xp22	181
Autosomal dominant			
DFNA1	Early-onset (age 10 yr) low-frequency hearing loss (Monge's deafness), Costa Rican family	5q31	53
DFNA2	Early-onset, high-frequency hearing loss, Indonesian family	1p31–32	71
DFNA3	Early-onset, high-frequency hearing loss, French family	13q12	182
DFNA4	Progressive hearing loss that begins in the second decade, American family	19q13	183
DFNA5	Early-onset hearing loss, Dutch family	7p15	184
DFNA6	Progressive low-frequency hearing loss, American (southeast) family	4p15.3	185
DFNA7	Progressive high-frequency hearing loss, Norwegian family	1q21–q23	179
DFNA8	Moderate-to-severe hearing loss, Austrian family	15q15–q21	186
DFNA9		14q12–q13	187
DFNA10		6q22–q23	188
DFNA11		11q12.3–q21	189
Autosomal recessive			
DFNB1 (NSRD1)	Congenital deafness, Northern Tunisian family	13q12	109
DFNB2	Congenital deafness, Tunisian family	11q13.5	109
DFNB3	Congenital deafness, Indonesian family	17p–17q12	110
DFNB4	Congenital deafness	7q31	190
DFNB5	Consanguineous nuclear families from India with congenital hearing loss	14q12	191
DFNB6	As above	3p21–p14	192
DFNB7	As above	9q13–q21	193
DFNB8	Childhood-onset deafness, Pakistani family	21q22	194
DFNB9	Congenital profound deafness, Lebanese family	2p22–p23	195
DFNB10	Congenital profound deafness	21q22.3	
DFNB11	Congenital profound deafness	9q13–q21	
DFNB12	Congenital profound deafness	10q21–22	
Mitochondrial inheritance			
12S rRNA	Aminoglycoside-induced ototoxicity	A1555G	28
tRNA-Ser(UCN)	Hearing loss of varying severity	T7445C	143
tRNA-Ser(UCN)	Hearing loss, ataxia, and myoclonus	7472insC	196

only for deaf patients, but also for those with partial hearing loss and for those with progressive hearing loss with adult onset. Nance (60,197–199) and, more recently, Arnos et al. (200) and Smith (201) have, in several publications, discussed the needs for counseling in different situations and have stressed the importance of realizing that some in the deaf community do not consider the hearing loss to be a handicap but a microculture. Avoidance of using words such as *deaf, abnormal,* or *affected* and replacement with *nonhearing* has been recommended. In counseling and otherwise, the purpose should be that of providing information and not directing or giving advice. Because a majority of deaf individuals may marry deaf persons, counseling is appropriate, because some of these may have an environmental etiology. Genetic counseling provides estimates of recurrence risks in a family, future offspring and inheritance patterns and of possible diagnostic testing available. It can reassure patients and family members and rule out syndromes and is an opportunity for counselors to correct erroneous perceptions. The availability of a signer is mandatory if the counselor is not adept at Sign Language. Because hearing loss is so heterogenous, addressing these special challenges may require several sessions with the counselor to clarify concepts and provide a better understanding of the genetics of the disease.

Issues regarding consanguinity, deaf × deaf matings in extended pedigrees, childhood or birth trauma, parental questions regarding possible etiologies for the child's hearing loss, and recurrence risks for future offspring should be addressed. Empiric recurrence risks may be calculated by using Bayesian analysis for the family being counseled or by using empiric risk tables devised by Bieber and Nance (202). In general, a fully penetrant gene in a dominantly inherited hearing loss will give a 50-50 chance of an off-

TABLE 4. Recurrent risks for isolated deafness

Parental mating	Number of deaf offspring	Bieber and Nance (202)	Harper (204)	Newton (205)		Fraser (12)
				<80 dB	≥80 dB	
H × H	1	9.8	17	7	11 21	10
	>1	25.0	25		25	—
D × H	0	6.7	5		6	—
	1	40.8	50		—	—
D × D	0	9.7	10		—	10
	1	61.7	>50		—	—

H, hearing; D, deaf.
From Smith SD, *Ann NY Acad Sci* 630:203, 1991, with permission.

spring with hearing loss. In an autosomal recessive disease with heterozygotic hearing parents, there is a 25% risk of inheriting the disease. A male child of a maternal carrier of an X-linked recessive disease has a 50-50 chance of exhibiting the trait, and the daughter has the same likelihood of being a carrier. Predicting recurrence risks in sporadic hearing loss is extremely difficult. The recurrence risk of another offspring with hearing loss in a family with hearing parents and an unexplained nonhearing child has been estimated to be about 9% to 17% (Table 4) (13,201–204). Additional nonhearing offspring emphasize the genetic nature of the hearing loss, thereby increasing the recurrence risk and vice versa. The risk for the offspring of an isolated case to be nonhearing is about 6% (205). However, the differences between 9% and 17% are probably insignificant because couples may not see much practical difference between these risks. The breakdown of recurrence risks into decimal points, although mathematically useful, does not appear to have any clinical significance in terms of counseling.

MULTIDISCIPLINARY REHABILITATION APPROACH

The role of the audiologist is crucial in rehabilitation of hearing impairment. In patients with progressive hearing loss, annual audiologic examination and reassessment of the necessity of hearing aids and the benefit current hearing aids may be providing is mandatory. For children and infants with any level of hearing loss, the goal of early intervention, rehabilitation, and empowering the family to meet the child's needs is to reduce the ultimate cost of providing special education services and to allow the early development of language. These needs can be met only by a multidisciplinary approach that involves otolaryngologists, speech-language pathologists, audiologists, psychologists, family specialists and social workers, special educators, occupational or physical therapists, Sign Language experts, and other consulting members, as deemed necessary. Child educational placement should take into consideration the parents' needs, school personnel, and the rehabilitation required. Parents will need empowerment and possibly counseling in dealing with the feelings of helplessness in the rearing of a nonhearing child that has special needs. Some parents may need to become conversant in Sign Language. Various different communication modalities are available. These include intensive oral and aural education, signing, cued speech, combinations of signing and word–object reading, and total communication (21). Different schools, classrooms, or home-based programs are generally available, and the type of education recommended should be individualized after careful examination of the family and the patient.

ROLE OF COCHLEAR IMPLANTATION

It has been increasingly emphasized that early auditory rehabilitation is critical in enhancing the speech and language development of hearing-impaired individuals and in the establishment of associative networks in the brain. Pediatric cochlear implantation is becoming more commonly available because there is increasing evidence that there may be benefits from early implantation. In the future, many children with genetic hearing loss will receive implantation. Some adults with progressive audiovestibular dysfunction have received cochlear implants with good results postoperatively. Because the pathogenetic locus in most subtypes of nonsyndromic SNHL appears to be cochlear, it is likely that implantation will be of benefit in these disorders on the whole. An unresolved issue under consideration is whether in a given family with progressive hearing loss an implantation should be performed in a patient with moderately severe (not profound) bilateral hearing loss in whom hearing aids have ceased to be of benefit. Further improvements in speech processing and coding should make cochlear implantation in such disorders an even more viable option.

CONCLUSIONS, FUTURE TASKS, AND DIRECTIONS

Genetic hearing loss should be suspected in *all* cases with unexplained SNHL, especially those at an early age. Audiometric characteristics that heighten suspicion of hearing loss include early-onset, low- or high-frequency SNHL or a U-shaped mid-frequency SNHL. Family members should be assessed audiologically, and a CT scan and vestibular tests should performed to aid in classification of the hearing loss in a given family and in preventing devastating complications of meningitis and a perilymphatic gusher.

The current classification of nonsyndromic hearing is simplistic and based largely on inheritance and audiometric patterns. It must be classified and categorized in such a way as to allow gene localization studies. However, this classification is a useful stepping stone for the development of future classifications based on gene localization studies. Comprehensive ascertainment of the nature and type of hearing loss and vestibular manifestations in the family should be an important goal of all otolaryngologists, vestibulologists, and audiologists. This should allow testing of candidate genes or for pooling data for linkage analysis and aid in development of future strategies for treatment, prevention, and genetic counseling of these disorders. Pre- and early postnatal detection of hearing loss should spur preventative intervention strategies.

One of the limitations in most studies is the lack of vestibular data in most types of hearing losses described previously. Vestibular symptoms may be lacking in many, because most of these diseases are either congenital or so slowly progressive that vestibular compensation may occur simultaneously in a fashion somewhat similar to that seen in vestibular schwannomas. Therefore, it is even more important to perform vestibular testing in unaffected and affected members of the family. Future studies should determine if quantifiable vestibular subtypes emerge similar to auditory subtypes and if they will have value in gene localization studies.

As molecular technology continues to improve, gene mapping or testing candidate genes for mutations will be performed much more rapidly. Therefore, it is necessary that we characterize the clinical features and distribution of hearing loss and vestibular manifestations comprehensively to allow such studies to be maximally effective. It is advocated that this be performed in a multidisciplinary fashion including otolaryngologists, ophthalmologists, pediatricians, geneticists, dysmorphologists, neurologists, vestibulologists, and other specialists, as necessary. Clearly, the mapping or identification of genetic mutations has implications in genetic counseling and planning of future progeny. As further genetic data on "multifactorial" audiovestibular diseases are acquired and environmental factors involved are slowly uncovered, our ability to prevent and treat these disorders will increase markedly. Additionally, gene therapies may become a reality for hereditary hearing loss in the not so distant future.

ADDENDUM

Although the classification of genetic diseases into autosomal dominant and recessive types and into syndromic and nonsyndromic diseases (with the underlying assumption that they are caused by different genes) has endured over time, recent molecular genetic evidence for many diseases including hearing losses challenges its validity. For example, nonsyndromic recessive hearing loss (Chinese families), nonsyndromic recessive congenital sensorineural hearing loss (DFNB2) and Usher syndrome type IB are all due to mutations in myosin VIIA gene (206–208). Furthermore, mutations in myosin VIIA in families with nonsyndromic autosomal dominant progressive sensorineural hearing loss (DFNAII) have also been described recently (Kitamura K, personal communication, in press). Additionally, another type of autosomal recessive sensorineural hearing loss (DFNBI) and a type of autosomal dominant sensorineural hearing loss (DFNA3) map to chromosome 13q11-12 (connexin 26, a gap-junction protein) (209). A recessive (DFNB5) and a dominant progressive audiovestibular dysfunction (DFNA9) also map to chromosome 14q12-13 (210,211). These findings suggest that different phenotypes (syndromic vs nonsyndromic, dominant vs recessive) may be determined not by different genes but by different genetic backgrounds or mutations in different regions or alleles of the same gene. As old paradigms are challenged and fall by the wayside, newer ones will emerge until they too are challenged. However, there is no doubt that this new information will provide us a better understanding of the pathophysiology of genetic hearing loss and possibly of nongenetic hearing losses.

REFERENCES

1. Wilson J. Deafness in developing countries. Approaches to a global program of prevention. *Arch Otolaryngol* 1985;111:2–9.
2. Fritsch MH, Sommer A. *Handbook of congenital and early onset hearing loss.* New York: Igaku-Shoin; 1990.
3. Goldstein MA. *Problems of the deaf.* St. Louis: Laryngoscope Press; 1933.
4. Werner H. *Geschichte des Taubstummenproblems bis ins 17 Jahrhundert.* Jena: G. Fischer; 1932.
5. Wilde W. *Practical observations on aural surgery.* Philadelphia: Blanchard and Lea; 1853.
6. Hartmann A. *Taubstummheit und Taubstummenbildung, nach den vorhandenen Quellen, sowie nach eigenen Beobachtungen und Erfahrungen.* Stuttgart: F. Enke; 1880.
7. Politzer A. *Lehrbuch der Ohrenheilkunde fur practische Artze und Studierende.* vol. 2. Stuttgart: F. Enke; 1882.
8. Bell AG. *Memoir upon the formation of a deaf variety of the human race.* Washington DC: National Academy of Sciences; 1884.
9. Fay EA. *Marriages of the deaf in america.* Washington: Volta Bureau; 1898.
10. Gorlin RJ, Torriello HV, Cohen MM. *Hereditary hearing loss and its syndromes.* New York: Oxford University Press; 1995.
11. Proctor C. Diagnosis, prevention and treatment of hereditary sensorineural hearing loss. *Laryngoscope* 1977;87:1–60.
12. Fraser GR. *The causes of profound childhood deafness in childhood.* Baltimore: Johns Hopkins University Press; 1976.
13. Newton VE. Aetiology of bilateral sensorineural hearing loss in young children. *J Laryngol Otol* 1985;10 [Suppl]:1–57.
14. Beighton P. In: *Principles and practice of medical genetics.* Emery AEH, Rimoin DL, eds. New York: Churchill Livingstone; 1990.
15. Majumder PP, Ramesh A, Chinnappan D. On the genetics of prelingual deafness. *Am J Hum Genet* 1989;44:86–99.
16. Nance WE. The genetic analysis of profound prelingual deafness. *Birth Defects* 1980;16:263–9.
17. Parving A. Epidemiology of hearing loss and aetiological diagnosis of hearing impairment in childhood. *Int J Pediatr Otorhinolaryngol* 1983;5:151–65.
18. Taylor IG, Hine WD, Brasier VJ, et al. A study of causes of hearing

loss in a population of deaf children with special reference to genetic factors. *J Laryngol Otol* 1975;89:899–914.
19. Cohen MM, Gorlin RJ. Epidemiology, etiology and genetic patterns. In: *Hereditary hearing loss and its syndromes.* Gorlin RJ, Torriello HV, and Cohen MM ed. New York: Oxford University Press; 1995: 9–21.
20. Arnos KS, Israel J, Cunningham M. Genetic counselling of the deaf. Medical and cultural considerations. *Ann NY Acad Sci* 1991;630: 212–22.
21. Brookhouser PJ: Hereditary hearing loss. In: *Current therapy in otolaryngology—head neck surgery.* 5th ed. Gates GA, ed. St. Louis: Mosby; 1994:44–52.
22. Morton NE. Genetic epidemiology of hearing loss. *Ann NY Acad Sci* 1991;630:16–31.
23. Gorlin RJ, Cohen MM, Levin LS. *Syndromes of the head and neck.* New York: Oxford University Press; 1990.
24. Marres HAM, Cremers CWRJ. Autosomal recessive nonsyndromal profound childhood deafness in a large pedigree: audiometric features of the affected persons and affected carriers. *Arch Otolaryngol Head Neck Surg* 1989;115:591–5.
25. Evans DGR, Harris R. Heterogeneity in genetic conditions. *Q J Med* 1992;84:563–5.
26. Kajiwara K, Berson EL, Dryja TP. Digenic retinitis pigmentosa due to mutations at the unlinked peripherin/RDS and ROM1 loci. *Science* 1994;264:1604–08.
27. Bu X, Shohat M, Jaber L, Rotter JI. A form of sensorineural hearing deafness is determined by a mitochondrial and an autosomal locus: evidence from pedigree segregation analysis. *Genet Epidemiol* 1993; 10:3–15.
28. Prezant TR, Agapian JV, Bohlman MC, et al. Mitochondrial ribosomal RNA mutation associated with both antibiotic-induced and non-syndromic deafness. *Nat Genet* 1993;4:289–94.
29. Soumalainen A, Kaukonen J, Amati P, et al: An autosomal locus predisposing to deletions of mitochondrial DNA. *Nat Genet* 1995;9: 146–51.
30. Konigsmark BW, Gorlin RJ. *Genetic and metabolic deafness.* Philadelphia: WB Saunders; 1976.
31. Khetarpal U, Schuknecht HF, Gacek RR, Holmes LG. Autosomal dominant sensorineural hearing loss: pedigrees, audiologic findings and temporal bone findings in two kindreds. *Arch Otolaryngol Head Neck Surg* 1991;117:1032–42.
32. Khetarpal U. Autosomal dominant sensorineural hearing loss: further temporal bone findings. *Arch Otolaryngol Head Neck Surg* 1993;119: 106–8.
33. Grundfast KM, Lalwani AK. Practical approach to diagnosis and management of hereditary hearing impairment. *Ear Nose Throat J* 1992; 71:479–93.
34. Higashi K. Heterogeneity of dominant high-frequency sensorineural deafness. *Clin Genet* 1988;33:424–8.
35. Niitsu J, Ogasawa M, Tsiuki T, Mukai M. Clinical studies of progression of hereditary deafness. *Audiol Jpn* 1984;27:23–24.
36. (A.) van den Wijngaart WSIM, Verschuure J, Brocaar MP, Huizing EH. Follow up study in a family with dominant progressive hereditary sensorineural hearing impairment, I: analysis of hearing deterioration. *Audiology* 1985;24:336–42; (B.) van den Wijngaart WSIM, Huizing EH, Niermeijer MF, et al. II: Clinical aspects. *Audiology* 1985;24: 336–42.
37. Wilkie AOM, Slaney S, Oldridge M, et al: Apert syndrome results from localized mutations of FGFR2 and is allelic with Crouzon syndrome. *Nat Genet* 1995;9:165–72.
38. Rutland P, Pulleyn LJ, Reardon W, et al. Identical mutations in the FGFR2 gene cause both Pfeiffer and Crouzon syndrome phenotypes. *Nat Genet* 1995;9:173.
39. Jabs EW, et al. Jackson-Weiss syndrome. *Nat Genet* 1994;8:275–79.
40. Halpin C, Khetarpal U, et al. Autosomal dominant progressive sensorineural hearing loss in a large North American family. *Am J Audiol* 1996;5:105.
41. Brownstein Z, Friedlander Y, et al. Estimated number of loci for autosomal recessive severe nerve deafness within the Israeli Jewish population, with implications for genetic counseling. *Am J Med Genet* 1991;41:306–12.
42. Chung CS, Brown KS. Family studies of early childhood deafness, ascertained through the Clarke School for the Deaf. *Am J Hum Genet* 1970;22:630–44.
43. Costeff H, Dar H. Consanguinity analysis of congenital deafness in Northern Israel. *Am J Hum Genet* 1980;32:64–8.
44. Nance WE, Sweeney A. Genetic factors in deafness of early life. *Otolaryngol Clin North Am* 1975;8:19–48.
45. Fraser GR. Profound childhood deafness. *J Med Genet* 1964;1: 118–51.
46. Altmann F. Histologic pictures of inherited nerve deafness in man and animals. *Arch Otolaryngol* 1950;51:852–90.
47. Vanderbilt University Hereditary Deafness Study Group. Dominantly inherited low-frequency hearing loss. *Arch Otolaryngol* 1968;88: 242–50.
48. Parving A, Bak-Pedersen K. Clinical findings and diagnostic problems in sensorineural hearing loss. *Acta Otolaryngol* 1978;85:184–90.
49. Parving A. Inherited low-frequency hearing loss. *Scand Audiol* 1984; 13:47.
50. Parving A, et al. Dominantly inherited low-frequency hearing loss. *Audiology* 1978;17:165–72.
51. Konigsmark BW, Mengel MC, Berlin CI. Familial low-frequency hearing loss. *Laryngoscope* 1971;81:759–71.
52. Leon PE, Bonilla JA, Sanchez JR, et al. Low-frequency hereditary deafness in man with childhood onset. *Am J Hum Genet* 1981;33: 209–14.
53. Leon PE, Raventos H, Lynch E, Morrow J, King MC. The gene for an inherited form of deafness maps to chromosome 5q31. *Proc Natl Acad Sci USA* 1992;89:5181–4.
54. Leon PE, et al. Clinical evaluation of autosomal dominant postlingual deafness and a genetic map of the DFNA1 region of 5q31. *Am J Hum Genet* Suppl 53 1993;(Abst 1031).
55. Cawthorne TE, Hinchcliffe R. Familial perceptive deafness. *Pract Otorhinolaryngol* 1957;19:68–83.
56. Konigsmark BW, Salman S, et al. Dominant mid-frequency hearing loss. *Ann Otol Rhinol Laryngol* 1970;79:42–53.
57. Martensson B. Dominant hereditary nerve deafness. *Acta Otolaryngol* 1960;52:270–4.
58. Paparella M, Suguira S, Hoshino T. Familial progressive sensorineural deafness. *Arch Otolaryngol Head Neck Surg* 1969;90:44–51.
59. Williams F, Roblee LA. Hereditary nerve deafness. *Arch Otolaryngol* 1962;75:69–77. (Same cases as Cawthorne and Hinchcliffe.)
60. Nance WE, McConnell FE. Status and progress of research in hereditary deafness. *Adv Hum Genet* 1974;4:173–250.
61. Rapoport Y, Ruben RJ: Dominant neurosensory hearing loss. *Trans Am Acad Ophthalmol Otolaryngol* 1974;78:423–35.
62. Lenzi P. Sulle sordita ereditaire. *Arch Ital Otol Rhinol Laryngol* 1969; 80:453–85.
63. Dolowitz DA, Stephens FE. Hereditary nerve deafness. *Ann Otol Laryngol* 1961;70:851.
64. Stolbova D, Valvoda M. Detection of normal-hearing carriers of the gene for the autosomal dominant progressive sensorineural hearing loss. *Acta Otolaryngol* 1985;99:509–15.
65. Teig E. Hereditary progressive perceptive deafness in a family of 72 patients. *Acta Otolaryngol* 1968;65:365–72.
66. Bonfils P, Avan P, Londero A, et al. Progressive hereditary deafness with predominant inner hair cell loss. *Am J Otol* 1991;12:203–6.
67. Bu XK, Ying MD, et al. Audiologic investigation of autosomal dominant hereditary sensory hearing loss in a family of 507 members in 6 generations. *Ann NY Acad Sci* 1991;630:310–12.
68. Suga F, Naunton RF, et al. Hereditary progressive sensorineural deafness. *J Laryngol Otol* 1976;90:667–85.
69. Crowe SJ, et al. Observations on the pathology of high-tone deafness. *Bull Johns Hopkins Hosp* 1934;54:315–80.
70. Gross M, Arndt-Hanser A. HLA-Antigene und Schallemfindungsschwerthorigkeit. *Laryngol Rhinol Otol* 1982;61:316–18.
71. Coucke P, Camp GV, Djoyodiharjo B, et al. Linkage of autosomal dominant hearing loss to the short arm of chromosome 1 in two families. *N Engl J Med* 1994;331:425–31.
72. Smith AB. Unilateral hereditary deafness. *Lancet* 1939;2:1172–73.
73. Graf K. Einseitige vererbte Sprachtaubheit als Manifestationsschwankung beidseitiger Sprachtaubheit oder Schwerhörigkeit. *Laryngol Rhinol Otol* 1992;71:242–5.
74. Higashi K: Hereditary unilateral deafness. *Otolaryngology* 1960;58: 133–6.
75. Everberg G. Further studies on hereditary unilateral deafness. *Acta Otolaryngol* 1960;51:615–35.

76. Everberg G. Unilateral anacusis. Clinical, radiological, and genetic investigations. *Acta Otolaryngol* 1960;158 [Suppl]:366–74.
77. Verhagen WIM, Huygen PL, Joosten EM. Familial progressive vestibulo-cochlear dysfunction. *Arch Neurol* 1988;45:766–8.
78. Verhagen WIM, Huygen PL, et al: Hereditary vestibulo-cochlear dysfunction and vascular disorders. *J Neurol Sci* 1989;92:55–63.
79. Verhagen WIM, Huygen PL. Familial progressive vestibulo-cochlear dysfunction. *Arch Neurol* 1991;48:262.
80. Verhagen WIM, Huygen PL, Bles W. A new autosomal dominant syndrome of idiopathic progressive vestibulo-cochlear dysfunction with middle-age onset. *Acta Otolaryngol* 1992;112:899–906.
81. Muller E: Vestibularisstorungen bei erblicher Taubheit. *Arch Ohren Nasen Kehlkopfheilkd* 1936;142:156–63.
82. Belal A. Dandy's syndrome. *Am J Otol* 1980;11:151–6.
83. Gussen R. Delayed hereditary deafness with cochlear aqueduct obstruction. *Arch Otolaryngol Head Neck Surg* 1969;90:429–36.
84. Linthicum FH, Fayad J, Otto SR, Galey FR, House WF. Cochlear implant histopathology. *Am J Otol* 1991;12:256–61.
85. Birgerson L, Gustavson KH, Stahle J. Familial Meniere's disease: a genetic investigation. *Am J Otol* 1987;8:323.
86. Hinchcliffe R. Personal and family medical history in Meniere's disease. *J Laryngol Otol* 1967;81:661.
87. Brown MR. The factor of heredity in labyrinthine deafness and paroxysmal vertigo. *Ann Otol Rhinol Laryngol* 1949;58:665.
88. Martini A. Hereditary Meniere's disease. *Am J Otolaryngol* 1982;3:163.
89. Oliveira CA, Braga AM. Meniere's syndrome inherited as an autosomal dominant trait. *Ann Otol Rhinol Laryngol* 1992;101:590.
90. Bernstein JM. Occurrence of episodic vertigo and hearing loss in families. *Ann Otol Rhinol Laryngol* 1965;74:1011.
91. Khetarpal U. Genes, immunity, environment, chance, endolymphatic hydrops and Meniere's disease. Submitted for publication.
92. Morrison AW, Mowbray JF, Williamson R, et al. On genetic and environmental factors in Meniere's disease. *Am J Otol* 1994;15:35.
93. Joutel A, Bousser MG, Biousse V, et al. A gene for familial hemiplegic migraine maps to chromosome 19. *Nat Genet* 1993;5:40–5.
94. Joutel A, Ducros A, Vahedi K, et al. Genetic heterogeneity of familial hemiplegic migraine. *Am J Hum Genet* 1994;55:1166–72.
95. Chan KH, Eelkema EA, Furman JMR, Kamerer DB. Familial sensorineural hearing loss: a correlative study of audiologic, radiographic and vestibular findings. *Ann Otol Rhinol Laryngol* 1991;100:620–5.
96. Kurnit D, Layton WM, Mathysse S. Genetics, chance and morphogenesis. *Am J Hum Genet* 1987;41:979–95.
97. Lindenov H: *The etiology of deaf-mutism with special references to heredity.* Copenhagen: Munksgaard; 1945.
98. Hopkins LA, Guilder RP. *Clarke school studies concerning the hereditary deafness.* Northampton, MA: Edwards Brothers; 1949.
99. McLeod AC, et al. Autosomal recessive sensorineural deafness: a comparison of two kindreds. *South Med J* 1973;66:141–52.
100. Mengel MC, Konigsmark BW, McKusick VA. Two types of congenital recessive deafness. *EENT Monthly* 1969;48:301–5.
101. Brown KS, Chung CS. Observations on the epidemiology, genetics, and pathogenesis of deafness in children and lower mammals. *Audiology* 1971;10:234–56.
102. Bonaiti C, Demenais F, et al. Studies of an isolated West Indies population. IV. Genetic study of hearing loss. *Genet Epidemiol* 1986;3:113–9.
103. Kabarity S, Hochez J. Autosomal recessive "uncomplicated" profound childhood deafness in an Arabic family with high consanguinity. *Hum Genet* 1981;57:444–6.
104. Stevenson AC, Cheeseman EA. Hereditary deaf-mutism with particular reference to Northern Ireland. *Ann Hum Genet* 1956;20:177–231.
105. Secretan JP. De la surdi-mutite recessive et de ses rapports avec les autres formes de surdi-mutite. *Arch Julius Klaus Stift Vererbungsforsch Socialanthropol Rassenhyg* 1954;29:1–134.
106. Huygen PLM, van Rijn PM, et al. The vestibulo-cochlear reflex in pupils in children at the schools for the hearing-impaired: findings relating to acquired cases. *Int J Pediatr Otorhinolaryngol* 1993;25:39–47.
107. Gray AA, Nelson SH. The pathological conditions found in a case of deaf-mutism. *J Laryngol Otol* 1926;41:7–18.
108. Guli E, Bonetti U. Contributo allo studio dell' anatomia patologica del sordomutismo recessivo. *Folia Hered Pathol (Milano)* 1956;5:102–50.
109. Guilford P, Ben Arab S, Blanchard S, et al. A non-syndromic form of neurosensory, recessive deafness maps to the pericentromeric region of chromosome 13q. *Nat Genet* 1994;6:24–8.
110. Friedman TB, Liang Y, Weber JL, et al. A gene for congenital, recessive deafness DFNB3 maps to the pericentromeric region of chromosome 17. *Nat Genet* 1995;9:86–91.
111. Guilford P, Ayadi H, Blanchard S, et al. A human gene responsible for neurosensory, non-syndromic recessive deafness is a candidate homologue of the mouse sh-1 gene. *Hum Mol Genet* 1994;3:989–93.
112. Lyon MF, Searle AG, eds. In: *Genetic variants and strains of the laboratory mouse.* Oxford: Oxford University Press; 1989.
113. Gibson F, Walsh J, Mburu P, et al. A type VII myosin encoded by mouse deafness gene *shaker-1*. *Nature* 1995;374:62–4.
114. Konigsmark BW: Congenital nonprogressive moderate neural hearing loss. *Birth Defects* 1971;7:140.
115. Konigsmark BW, Mengel MC, Haskins H. Familial congenital moderate neural hearing loss. *J Laryngol Otol* 1970;84:495–505.
116. Mengel MC, Konigsmark BW, et al. Recessive early-onset neural deafness. *Acta Otolaryngol* 1967;64:313–26.
117. Barr B, Wedenberg E. Prognosis of perceptive hearing loss in children with respect to genesis and use of hearing aid. *Acta Otolaryngol* 1964;59:462–74.
118. Cremers CWRJ. Autosomal recessive nonsyndromal progressive sensorineural deafness in childhood: A separate, clinical and genetic entity. *Int J Pediatr Otorhinolaryngol* 1979;1:193–9.
119. Cremers CWRJ, van Rijn PW, ter Haar B. Autosomal recessive progressive high-frequency sensorineural deafness in childhood. *Arch Otolaryngol Head Neck Surg* 1987;113:1319–24.
120. Madell JR, Sculerati N. Noncongenital hereditary hearing loss in children. *Arch Otolaryngol Head Neck Surg* 1991;117:332–8.
121. Reardon W, Roberts S, Phelps PD, et al. Phenotypic evidence for a common pathogenesis in X-linked deafness pedigrees and in Xq13-q21 deletion related deafness. *Am J Med Genet* 1992;44:513–17.
122. de Kok YJM, van der Maarel SM, Bitner-Glindzicz M, et al. Association between X-linked mixed deafness and mutations in the POU domain gene POU3F4. *Science* 1995;267:685–88.
123. Phelps PD, Reardon W, Pembrey M, et al. X-linked deafness, stapes gushers and a distinctive defect of the inner ear. *Neuroradiology* 1991;33:326–30.
124. Lalwani AK, Brister RJ, Fex J, et al: A new nonsyndromic X-linked sensorineural hearing impairment linked to Xp21.2. *Am J Hum Genet* 1994;55:685–94.
125. Allen NR. Hearing acuity in patients with muscular dystrophy. *Dev Med Child Neurol* 1973;15:500–5.
126. Fraser GR. Sex-linked recessive congenital deafness and the excess of males in profound childhood deafness. *Ann Hum Genet* 1965;29:171–96.
127. Deraemaker R. Sex-linked congenital deafness. *Acta Genet (Basel)* 1958;8:228–31.
128. McRae KN, et al. Sex-linked congenital deafness. *Am J Hum Genet* 1969;21:415–22.
129. Parker N. Congenital deafness due to a sex-linked hereditary deafness. *Am J Hum Genet* 1958;10:196–200.
130. Sataloff J, et al. Sex-linked hereditary deafness. *Am J Hum Genet* 1955;7:201–3.
131. Reardon W, Middleton-Price HR, Sandkuijl L, et al. A multipedigree linkage study of X-linked deafness; linkage to Xq13-q21 and evidence for genetic heterogeneity. *Genomics* 1991;11:885–94.
132. Cremers FPM, van de Pol DJR, Diergaarde PJ, et al. Physical fine mapping of the choroideremia locus using Xq21 deletions associated with complex syndromes. *Genomics* 1989;4:41–6.
133. Robinson D, Lamont M, Curtis G, et al. A family with X-linked deafness showing linkage to the proximal Xq region of the X chromosome. *Hum Genet* 1992;90:316–18.
134. Bitner-Glindzicz M, de Kok Y, Summers D, et al. Close linkage of a gene for X-linked deafness to three microsatellite repeats at Xq21 in radiologically normal and abnormal families. *J Med Genet* 1994;31:916–21.
135. Brunner HG, van Bennekom CA, Lambermom EMM, et al. The gene for X-linked progressive mixed deafness with perilymphatic gusher during stapes surgery is linked to PGK. *Hum Genet* 1988;80:337–40.
136. Livan M. Contributo alla conoscenza delle sordita ereditarie. *Arch Ital Otol* 1961;72:331–9.
137. Pelletier LP, Tanguay RB. X-linked recessive inheritance of sensori-

neural hearing loss expressed during adolescence. *Am J Hum Genet* 1975;27:609–13.
138. Wellesley D, Goldblatt J. A new form of X-linked high-frequency sensorineural deafness. *Clin Genet* 1992;41:79–81.
139. Jaber L, Shohat M, Bu X, et al. Sensorineural deafness inherited as a tissue specific mitochondrial disorder. *J Med Genet* 1992;29:86–90.
140. van den Ouweland JM, Lemkes HH, Ruitenbeek W, et al. Mutation in mitochondrial tRNA(Leu) (UUR) gene in a large pedigree with maternally transmitted type II diabetes mellitus and deafness. *Nat Genet* 1992;1:368–71.
141. Ballinger SW, Shoffner JM, Hedaya EV, et al. Maternally transmitted diabetes and deafness associated with a 10.4 kb mitochondrial DNA deletion. *Nat Genet* 1992;1:11–15.
142. Vernham GA, Reid FM, Rundle PA, Jacobs HT. Bilateral sensorineural hearing loss in members of a maternal lineage with mitochondrial point mutation. *Clin Otolaryngol* 1994;19:314–9.
143. Reid FM, Vernham GA, Jacobs HT: A novel point mutation in a maternal pedigree with sensorineural deafness. *Hum Mutation* 1994; 3:243–7.
144. van den Ouweland JM, Lemkes HH, Trembath RC, et al. Maternally inherited diabetes and deafness is a distinct subtype of diabetes and associates with a single point mutation in mitochondrial tRNA(Leu(UUR)) gene. *Diabetes* 1994;43:746–51.
145. Katagiri H, Asano T, Ishihara H, et al. Mitochondrial diabetes mellitus: prevalence and clinical characterization of diabetes due to mitochondrial tRNA(Leu(UUR)) gene mutation in Japanese patients. *Diabetologia* 1994;37:504–10.
146. Kuzuya N, Noda M, Fujii M, Kanazawa Y. [A pedigree with maternally transmitted diabetes mellitus, deafness and cardiomyopathy] [Japanese]. *Nippon Rinsho* 1994;52:2611–15.
147. Hutchin T, Haworth I, Higashi K, et al. A molecular basis for human hypersensitivity to aminoglycoside antibiotics. *Nucleic Acids Res* 1993;21;4174–9.
148. Fischel-Ghodsain N, Prezant TR, et al. Mitochondrial ribosomal RNA gene mutation in a patient with sporadic aminoglycoside ototoxicity. *Am J Otolaryngol* 1993;14;399–403.
149. Lindsay JR, Hinojosa R. Histopathologic features of the inner ear associated with Kearns Sayre syndrome. *Arch Otolaryngol* 1976;102: 747–52.
150. Bento RF, Miniti A. X-linked mixed hearing loss: four case studies. *Laryngoscope* 1985;95:462–68.
151. Clark JL, DeSanto LW, Facer GW. Congenital deafness and spontaneous CSF otorrhea. *Arch Otolaryngol* 1978;104:163–6.
152. Cremers CWRJ, Huygen PLM. Clinical features of female heterozygotes in the X-linked mixed deafness syndrome (with perilymphatic gusher during stapes surgery). *Int J Pediatr Otorhinolaryngol* 1983; 6:179–85.
153. Cremers CWRJ, Homberger GC, Scaf JJ, et al. X-linked progressive mixed deafness with perilymphatic gusher during stapes surgery. *Arch Otolaryngol* 1985;111:249–54.
154. Farrior JB, Endicott JN. Congenital mixed deafness: cerebrospinal fluid otorrhea. Ablation of the aqueducts of the cochlea. *Laryngoscope* 1971;81:684–99.
155. Jensen J, Terkildsen K, Thomsen KA. Inner ear malformation with oto-liquorrhoea: tomographic findings in three cases with a mixed hearing impairment. *Arch Otorhinolaryngol* 1977;214:271–82.
156. Bach I, Brunner HG, Beighton P, et al. Microdeletions in patients with gusher-associated, X-linked mixed deafness (DFN3). *Am J Hum Genet* 1992;51:38–44.
157. Brunner HG, van Bennekom A, Lambermom EM, et al. The gene for X-linked progressive mixed deafness with perilymphatic gusher during stapes surgery (DFN3) is linked to PGK. *Hum Genet* 1988; 80:337–40.
158. Nance WE, Setleff R, McLeod A, et al. X-linked mixed deafness with congenital fixation of the stapedial footplate and perilymphatic gusher. *Birth Defects* 1971;7:64–9.
159. Nance WE, et al. Hereditary deafness: A presentation of some recognized types, modes of inheritance, and aids in counseling. *South Med Bull* 1970;58:41–9.
160. Glasscock ME. The stapes gusher. *Arch Otolaryngol* 1973;98:82–92.
161. Bergman ML. Otosclerosis in identical twins. *Arch Otolaryngol* 1954; 59:316–18.
162. Larsson A. Otosclerosis, a genetic and clinical study. *Acta Otolaryngol* 1960;[Suppl]154:1–86.
163. Morrison AW. Genetic factors in otosclerosis. *Ann R Coll Surg Engl* 1967;41:202–37.
164. Morrison AW, Bundey SE. The inheritance of otosclerosis. *J Laryngol Otol* 1970;84:921–32.
165. Gordon MA. The genetics of otosclerosis. A review. *Am J Otol* 1989; 10:426–38.
166. Fowler EP. Otosclerosis in identical twins. A study of 40 pairs. *Arch Otolaryngol* 1966;83:324–38.
167. Mendlowitz JC, Hirschhorn K. Polygenic inheritance of otosclerosis. *Ann Otol Rhinol Laryngol* 1976;85:281–5.
168. Schroder M, Langenbeck U. Untersuchungen zur Genetik der Otosclerose. *HNO* 1978;26:119–24.
169. Schaap T, Gapany-Gapanavicius B. The genetics of otosclerosis. I. Distorted sex ratio. *Am J Hum Genet* 1978;30:59–64.
170. Brunner S, Rovsing H, Jensen J, et al. Tomographic changes in otosclerosis. *Acta Radiol (Diagn)* 1966;4:632–8.
171. Guild SR. Histologic otosclerosis. *Ann Otol Rhinol Laryngol* 1944; 53:246–67.
172. McKenna MM, Mills BG. Ultrastructural and immunohistochemical evidence of measles virus in active otosclerosis. *Acta Otolaryngol* 1990 [Suppl]470:130–40.
173. Gregoriadis S, Zerves J, Varletzides E: HLA antigens and otosclerosis: a possible new genetic factor. *Arch Otolaryngol* 1982;108:769–71.
174. Dahlqvist A, Diamant H, et al. HLA antigens in patients with otosclerosis. *Arch Otolaryngol* 1985;100:33–5.
175. Higashi K, Yamakawa K, et al. familial ossicular malformations: case report and review of the literature. *Am J Med Genet* 1987;28:655–9.
176. Kumagawa K, et al. A family with hereditary bilateral middle ear malformations. *Otolaryngol (Tokyo)* 1984;59:661–7.
177. Yamada K, et al. Congenital ossicular discontinuity in sibs. *Clin Otol Jpn* 1981;8:92–3.
178. Kimberling WI, Brookhouser PE. Biochemical and cytogenetic techniques of communication disorders. *Laryngoscope* 1981;91:238–49.
179. Tranebjaerg J, Schwartz C, Eriksen H, et al. A new linked recessive deafness syndrome with blindness, dystonia, fractures, and mental deficiency is linked to Xq22. *J Med Genet* 1995;32:257-63.
180. Reardon W. Sex linked deafness: Wilde revisited. *J Med Genet* 1990; 27:376–9.
181. del Castillo I, Villamar M, Sarduy M, et al. A novel locus for nonsyndromic sensorineural deafness (DFN6) maps to chromosome Xp22. *Hum Mol Genet* 1996;5:1283–7.
182. Chaib H, Lina-Granade G, Guilford P, et al. A gene responsible for a dominant form of neurosensory non-syndromic deafness maps to the NSRD1 recessive deafness gene interval. *Hum Mol Genet* 1994; 3:2219–22.
183. Chen AH, Ni L, Fukushima K, et al. Linkage of a gene for dominant non-syndromic deafness to chromosome 19. *Hum Mol Genet* 1995; 4:1073–6.
184. van Camp G, Coucke P, Balemans W, et al. Localization of a gene for non-syndromic hearing loss (DFNA5) to chromosome 7p15. *Hum Mol Genet* 1995;4:2159–63.
185. Lesperance MM, Hall JWR, Bess FH, et al. A hene for autosomal dominant nonsyndromic hereditary hearing impairment maps to 4p16.3. *Hum Mol Genet* 1995;4:1967–72.
186. Kirshhofer K, Hoover D, Kenyon J, et al. Localisation of a gene responsible for an autosomal dominant non-syndromic sensorineural hearing loss to chromosome 15. The Molecular Biology of Hearing and Deafness Meeting, Bethesda, Maryland October 6–8, 1995.
187. Manolis EN, Nadol JB, Eavcy RD, et al. A gene for non-syndromic autosomal dominant progressive postlingual sesorineural deafness maps to chromosome 14q12-13. *Hum Mol Genet* 1996;5:1047–1050.
188. O'Neill ME, Marietta J, Nishimura D, et al. A gene for autosomal dominant late-onset progressive non-syndromic hearing loss maps to chromosome 6-DFNA10. *Hum Mol Genet* 1996;5:853–856.
189. Tamagawa Y, Kitamura K, Ishida T, Tanaka H, Tsuji S, Nishizawa M. A gene for a dominant form of non-syndromic sensorineural deafness (dfna11) maps within the region containing the DFNB2 recessive deafness gene. *Hum Mol Genet* 1996;5:849–52.
190. Baldwin CT, Weiss, S, Farrar LA, Linkage of congenital, recessive deafness (DFNB4) to chromosome 7q31 and evidence for genetic heterogeneity in the Middle Eastern Druze population. *Hum Mol Genet* 1995;4:1637–42.
191. Fukushima K, Ramesh A, Srisailapathy CR, et al. Consanguineous

nuclear families used to identify a new locus for recessive non-syndromic hearing loss on 14q. *Hum Mol Genet* 1995;4:1643–8.
192. Fukushima K, Ramesh A, Srisailapathy CR, et al. An autosomal recessive nonsyndromic form of sensorineural hearing loss maps to 3p-DFNB6. *Genome Res* 1995;5:305–8.
193. Jain P, Fukushima K, Deshmukh D, et al. A human recessive neurosensory nonsyndromic hearing impairment locus is a potential homologue of the murine deafness (dn) locus. *Hum Mol Genet* 1995;4:2391–4.
194. Veske A, Oehlmann R, Younus F, et al. Autosomal recessive nonsyndromic deafness locus (DFNB8) maps on chromosome 21q22 in large consanguineous kindred from Pakistan. *Hum Mol Genet* 1996;5:165–8.
195. Chaib H, Place C, Salem N, et al. A gene responsible for a sensorineural nonsyndromic recessive deafness maps to chromosome 2p22-23. *Hum Mol Genet* 1996;5:155–8.
196. Tiranti V, Chariot P, Carella F, et al. Maternally inherited hearing loss, ataxia and myoclonus associated with a novel point mutation in mitochondrial tRNASer(UCN) gene. *Hum Mol Genet* 1995;4:1421–7.
197. Nance WE. Genetic counseling for the hearing impaired. *Audiology* 1971;10:222–3.
198. Nance WE, et al. Opportunities for genetic counseling through institutional ascertainment of affected probands. In: . Lubs HA, de la Cruz F, eds. *Genetic Counseling* New York: Raven Press; 1977.
199. Nance WE. Genetic counseling of hereditary deafness: an unmet need. In: Bass FH, ed. *Childhood deafness: causation, assessment and management.* New York: Grune & Stratton; 1977:211–6.
200. Arnos KS, Cunningham M, et al. Innovative approach to genetic counseling services for the deaf population. *Am J Med Genet* 1992;44:345–51.
201. Smith SD. Recurrence risks. *Ann NY Acad Sci* 1991;630:203–11.
202. Bieber FR, Nance WE. Hereditary hearing loss. In: Jackson L, Schminke N, eds. *Clinical genetics: a course book for physicians,* New York: John Wiley & Sons; 1979:443–61.
203. Stevenson AC, Davidson BCC. *Genetic counseling,* 1st ed. Philadelphia: JB Lippincott; 1976.
204. Harper PS. *Practical genetic counseling,* 3rd ed, London: Wright; 1988.
205. Newton VE. Genetic counselling for the isolated hearing loss. *J Laryngol Otol* 1989;103:12–5.
206. Liu XY, Walsh J, Mburu P, et al. Mutations in myosin VIIA gene cause non-syndromic recessive deafness. *Nature Genet* 1997;16:188–190.
207. Weil D, Kussel P, Blanchard S, et al: The autosomal recessive isolated deafness, DFNB2, and the Usher 1B syndrome are allelic defects of the myosin VIIA gene. *Nature Genet* 1997;16:191–193.
208. Weil D, Blanchard S, Kaplan J, et al: Defective myosin VIIA gene responsible for Usher syndrome type 1B. *Nature* 1995;374:60–61.
209. Keisell DP, Dunlop J, Stevens HP, et al: Connexin 26 mutations in hereditary non-syndromic sensorineural deafness. *Nature* 1997;387:80–83.
210. Manolis EM, Yandavi N, Nadol JB, et al: A gene for non-syndromic autosomal dominant progressive postlingual sensorineural hearing loss maps to chromosome 14q12-13. *Hum Mol Genet* 1996;5:1047–1050.
211. Fukushima K, Ramesh A, Sarisaliapathy S, et al: Consanguineous nuclear families used to identify a new locus for recessive non-syndromic hearing loss on 14q. *Hum Mol Genet* 1995;4:1643–1648.

CHAPTER 22

Syndromic Hereditary Hearing Impairment

Kenneth M. Grundfast and Helga Toriello

Cherish your exceptions!
Admonition of William Bateson, 1861–1926,
English biologist who coined the term "genetics"

There is a difference between having a syndrome and having a genetic disorder. A syndrome is defined as a set of independent features that occur together and are assumed to have a common cause. There are more than 200 syndromes that include deafness or hearing impairment. Although some syndromes are caused by single gene alterations, others are caused by exogenous or unknown factors. For example, Treacher Collins syndrome (mandibulofacial dysostosis), a relatively common autosomal dominant disorder, is caused by a mutation in the *treacle* gene on chromosome 5; the rubella syndrome and fetal alcohol syndrome result from exogenous teratogenic factors.

A further distinction needs to be appreciated. Individuals with syndromes comprise only about one third of the enitre population of individuals who have inherited hearing impairment. In fact, about two thirds of hereditary hearing impairment (HHI) occurs in individuals with *no associated findings diagnostic of a syndrome,* thus, the term *nonsyndromic.* This means that only one of three patients with HHI has features on physical examination sufficient for diagnosis of a syndrome. Conversely, two of three individuals who have HHI will have a normal phenotype lacking any characteristic anatomic feature that would provide a tell-tale clue that the newborn infant or young child is hearing impaired.

In the evaluation and management of children with otologic disorders, it is important to realize that the otolaryngologist or otologist may be the first physician involved with management of the child to uncover the information that can lead to diagnosis of a syndrome (1). That is, once an abnormality of the eardrum, ossicles, or temporal bone is detected and combined with information about hearing impairment and unusual appearance of the face, an unusual pattern of pigmentation, or, for example, an abnormality of the retina, the constellation of findings may be recognizable as a syndrome. Therefore, an otolaryngologist or otologist working with children has two responsibilites in regard to syndromic hearing impairment. First, the otolaryngologist or otologist should have a working knowledge of the components of commonly occurring syndromes sufficient to detect a syndrome even if it has not yet been apparent to a pediatrician or referring primary care physician. Second, the otolaryngologist or otologist should have a knowledge of the otologic manifestations of commonly occurring syndromes sufficient to provide optimal care based on solid understanding of how the syndrome affects function of the middle ear, the organ of Corti, and the eighth cranial nerve over time.

Understanding that there is a singular importance in recognizing as different and distinctive the physical features diagnostic of a syndrome raises the question of what really makes a physical feature so different from the norm as to be generally accepted as a defining or requisite component of a syndrome. Of course, when an individual is missing a normal anatomic part, such as a child without a pinna or external ear canal (EAC), then the aural atresia quite obviously could be a component of a syndrome such as Goldenhar syndrome. However, if a child with unilateral conductive hearing loss has subtle facial asymmetry, this might be within the realm of normal variation or a finding that can be interpreted along with other findings as diagnostic of a syndrome. The ability to recognize a syndrome depends on knowledge of which physical traits, from the grossly abnormal to the subtle and almost imperceptible, are most often encountered as components of syndromic hearing impairment. A point to remember is this: In evaluating a child for hearing impairment, consider the hearing impairment potentially as one component of a syndrome and proceed through taking the patient's family history, medical history, and doing a physical examination to look for bits of information that might fit with

---

K.M. Grundfast: Department of Otolaryngology and Pediatrics, Georgetown University School of Medicine, Washington, DC 20007.

H. Toriello: Genetic Services, Butterworth Hospital, Grand Rapids, Michigan 49503.

the known hearing impairment to yield the diagnosis of a syndrome. The intent of this chapter is to provide the reader with a method of detecting syndromes in patients who present with hearing impairment. The first portion of the chapter focuses on methods of detecting syndromes and provides examples of common syndromes but does not provide a complete compendium of all syndromes that include hearing impairment. The remaining portion of the chapter provides information on how to manage the otologic aspects of several syndromes that are neither subtle nor difficult to diagnose.

TERMINOLOGY

A syndrome is often named after the individual who first recognized, then described and reported the characteristic findings. When a person's name is used to describe a syndrome, the syndrome name is called an *eponym*. Alternatively, syndromes can be described on the basis of the salient anatomic, morphologic, and pathophysiologic components that comprise the syndrome. Eponomic syndromes that include hearing impairment and that are commonly encountered are: Treacher Collins syndrome (mandibulofacial dysostosis), Goldenhar syndrome (oculoauriculovertebral dysplasia, facioauriculovertebral [FAV] dysplasia, or oculoauriculovertebral spectrum), Alport syndrome (hereditary nephritis), and Waardenburg syndrome, which does not have a specific morphologic descriptive name. Although use of eponyms in describing syndromes has become very much a part of common medical lingo, thinking of syndromes in terms of the morphologic and pathophysiologic components of each disorder helps the clinician to remember the essential features, and in turn, helps to differentiate one syndrome from another.

WHY IDENTIFY A SYNDROME?

Why make an effort to determine whether an individual with hearing impairment has a syndrome? Surely, a child's hearing impairment can be managed by providing amplification with a hearing aid or by operating to correct a congenital ossicular abnormality without even knowing that the child has a syndrome. Nonetheless, there are reasons to look for and identify a syndrome when evaluating a child with hearing impairment.

First, there may be other components, not yet clinically apparent, which may require medical attention. For example, the child with Goldenhar syndrome (oculoauriculovertebral spectrum) may have a renal or vertebral abnormality that will be found when appropriate imaging studies are done.

Second, recognizing a syndrome can affect decision making and management of the otologic aspect of the syndrome. Children with the syndrome known as X-linked mixed hearing loss and perilymphatic gusher are at risk for having decrement rather than improvement in hearing when a surgeon attempts to mobilize or remove the stapes. Not recognizing this syndrome could lead a surgeon to attempt a stapedectomy, encounter a profuse gush of cerebrospinal fluid on removing the stapes, and result in poor outcome for the patient.

Third, identifying a syndrome that has a genetic cause provides potentially useful information for the family about inheritance of hearing impairment. If an autosomal dominant condition such as Treacher Collins syndrome is identified, both parents of the affected child should be carefully examined to look for evidence that one parent might also manifest subtle findings, possibly including hearing impairment previously of unknown cause. If one parent is found to be affected, other children in the family should be evaluated with audiologic testing and careful physical examination to look for subtle clues consistent with diagnosis of a syndrome.

Autosomal dominant syndromes can also arise spontaneously as a new gene mutation. When an autosomal dominant syndrome in a child is found to be the result of a new gene mutation, the likelihood that offspring of the child will have the same syndrome remains at 50%, but the risk of the parents having another child with the same syndrome is low. If a child is found to have an autosomal recessive syndrome such as Usher syndrome and both parents show no sign of having Usher syndrome, then both parents are obligate heterozygote gene carriers because they each must have one of the recessive genes for the syndrome. In this case, when both parents are *unaffected* and they have a child with a syndrome that is known to be autosomal recessive, there is a risk of 25% that each of the next children of the parents will have the syndrome. Therefore, siblings of a child diagnosed with Usher syndrome should be examined carefully for evidence of the syndrome. The examination should include early hearing evaluation, possibly with brainstem auditory evoked response (BAER) tests and even electroretinography (ERG). Syndromes with X-linked recessive inheritance, such as one type of Alport syndrome, generally are more severe in men than in women; affected female heterozygotes may have mild hearing impairment that is not apparent without complete audiolgic testing. For the X-linked recessive syndromes such as X-linked mixed hearing loss with perilymphatic gusher, all of an affected man's daughters will be heterozygous carriers and his sons will be unaffected. A carrier woman has a 50% risk of giving birth to a son that is affected and a 50% risk that each daughter will be a carrier like herself.

Recently, there have been reports about syndromes that include hearing impairment and that are caused by mitochondrial defects. The DNA in mitochondria is not the same as the DNA comprising the genes in the chromosomes within the nucleus of each cell. Mitochondrial DNA is inherited *only* from the mother, *not* from the father. One syndrome caused by mitochondrial DNA mutation defects is the Kearns-Sayre syndrome (ophthalmoplegia plus) characterized by progressive external ophthalmoplegia, atypical pigmentary retinopathy, complete heart block, and, in about 50% of patients, sensorineural hearing loss (see below). Because hearing impairment disorders and syndromes caused by mitochondrial defects can be complicated and difficult to manage, consultation with a medical geneticist is recommended when there is suspicion that a child's hearing impairment might be caused by a mitochondrial defect.

Thus, knowledge of inheritance pattern can be important to parents and families who are concerned about the risk of having another child with hearing impairment. On the other hand, a physician cannot always assume that parents consider deafness as a medical disorder or a risk to be avoided. For example, several large families who have Waardenburg syndrome include many deaf individuals and couples of child-bearing age who are not necessarily concerned about having a deaf child. In general, normal-hearing parents want to have normal hearing children, but when one or more parents are deaf, there may be less concern on the part of the parents about risk for giving birth to a hearing-impaired child. In fact, some individuals with Waardenburg syndrome do not like physicians to refer to them as "patients" or as people having a "disorder" or "medical condition." They simply view themselves and affected family members as different, but not necessarily different in the sense of having a medical condition or disease that needs to be treated or cured.

MAKING A DIAGNOSIS

Relativity in Making the Diagnosis

Just as there is a theory of relativity in physics, there is a concept of relativity that needs to be appreciated in regard to making the diagnosis of syndromic hearing impairment. The ability of a clinician to recognize the presence of a syndrome depends on the following factors:

- Clinician's diagnostic acumen—Ability to discern and comprehend the significance of those aspects of the family and medical history and findings on physical examination that comprise the characteristic components of a syndrome.
- Extent to which the patient's anatomy varies from normal—In genetic disorders with variable expression, the milder the gene expression, the more difficult it is to find abnormalities and make a diagnosis; similarly, in syndromes caused by exogenous factors, there can also be great variability in the teratogenic effect.
- Clinician's fund of knowledge—Familiarity with definitions and descriptions of syndromes. Even though access to a menu-driven, computer database of syndromes can be extremely helpful, a clinician cannot recognize a syndrome that he or she does not know exists.
- Temporal aspects in the evolution of symptoms—All components of a syndrome may not be manifest at the time a patient initially presents for evaluation. For example, a key component of a syndrome can be developmental delay, which becomes apparent only when evidence is uncovered to confirm that a child's development is falling behind the norm or the child fails to meet an expected and predictable milestone. Similarly, loss of function can take time to develop, a child born with normal eyesight and hearing impairment might later become recognized as a child with Usher syndrome when loss of visual acuity becomes apparent.
- Objective test techniques—Electroretinography can help to confirm a suspected diagnosis of retinitis pigmentosa, thereby providing a clue to diagnosis of Usher syndrome. DNA analysis and single-gene tests can be done on blood specimens or buccal smears. However, even though the genes for hearing impairment syndromes such as Usher, Waardenburg, Treacher Collins, and the X-linked mixed hearing loss with stapes gusher syndromes have been located, tests for making the diagnosis for these syndromes are not yet commercially available. Most likely, in the years ahead, confirming the suspected diagnosis of a hearing impairment syndrome will involve use of readily available searches for single-gene defects.

Caution about Cryptogenic versus Cryptogenetic

Cryptogenic, sometimes referred to as cryptogenetic, means "of obscure, doubtful, or unacertainable origin." In about one third to one half the cases of newly diagnosed severe sensorineural hearing impairment presenting during early childhood, there is no clearly apparent cause. Therefore, when a clinician finds no evidence of a syndrome or other apparent cause of a child's hearing impairment, there is the tendency make a notation in the medical record that the child's hearing impairment is "cryptogenic." However, even though no cause for a child's hearing impairment is manifest at the time the child is *initially* evaluated, that does not necessarily mean that the child has no syndrome. In general, the younger the child, the more difficult it can be to recognize that a child has a syndrome. Therefore, when hearing impairment is detected in a child during infancy or under the age of 3 years and no associated findings leading to diagnosis of a syndrome appear to be present, the clinician is advised to remain cautious in labeling the child as having "cryptogenetic" hearing impairment. Not infrequently, as a child grows and develops, additional findings, which then can be recognized as components of a syndrome may become manifested. For this reason, it is important to continually reevaluate all findings each time that a child is seen for follow-up examination—what appeared to be "cryptogenic" hearing loss in the past, might, on reevaluation and uncovering of new findings, turn out to be hearing impairment that is part of a syndrome.

Detecting a Syndrome

To detect that a patient with hearing impairment has a syndrome, specific information is needed from the patient's medical and family history. Then, certain distinguishing physical features must be noticed during the physical examination. Next, the significance of each unusual feature must be analyzed in relationship to the constellation of unusual features that may comprise the requisite components sufficient for diagnosis of a syndrome.

Medical History

The clinical should look for factors that might uncover a specific cause for the hearing impairment by asking the following questions:

1. Did the mother drink alcohol during pregnancy to an extent that might result in the child's being born with fetal alcohol syndrome?
2. Did the mother have rubella during the first trimester of pregnancy, which could have caused the child to be born with rubella syndrome?
3. Were there any problems such as birth weight less than 1,500 grams, asphyxia, hyperbilirubinemia, meningitis, cytomegalovirus, or other postnatal infections all of which could cause hearing impairment that would not ordinarily be part of a syndrome?

Family History

In reviewing the family history, the clinician should keep in mind that individuals with hereditary hearing impairment may falsely attribute hearing impairment in other family members to various causes that are not genetic. For example, it is not uncommon to encounter a child who has congenital deafness and a sibling, father, and aunt who are severely hearing impaired, yet the father of the affected infant says that his hearing loss is from "a high fever" that he had when he was a baby and that the aunt is hearing impaired because she sustained a head injury at a young age. That is, a family member may provide spurious information in response to questions about why other family members are hearing impaired. In general, if two or more family members had significant hearing impairment during childhood, the clinician should suspect a genetic cause and look carefully for findings that could lead to diagnosis of a syndrome.

One should begin taking the family history by asking whether anyone in the patient's immediate family or on either side of the family had hearing impairment or wore a hearing aid at an age younger than 30 years.

If the answer is yes, the following questions should be asked:

1. Are there individuals in prior generations who have eyes that appear to be spaced widely apart (dystopia canthorum), different-color eyes (heterochromia irides), prematurely gray hair (defined as predominance of white hair at an age younger than 30 years), or who have depigmented areas of skin (vitiligo)? These findings can be suggestive of Waardenburg or related syndromes.
2. Are there relatives with renal failure? An affirmative answer might suggest that the patient has one of the many different types of Alport syndrome.
3. Are there siblings or cousins with night blindness, tunnel vision, progressive loss of vision or retinal disorders? An affirmative answer suggests retinitis pigmentosa and Usher syndrome as a possible diagnosis.
4. Are there siblings or cousins with goiter? An affirmative answer suggests that the patient might have Pendred syndrome
5. Are there siblings or cousins who have severe hearing impairment and an abnormal heart rhythm (arrythmia) or history of fainting spells? An affirmative answer suggests that the patient may have Jervell and Lange-Nielsen (JLN) syndrome.

Physical Examination

Detecting a syndrome in a patient with hearing impairment is largely a matter of astute observation during the physical examination, knowing what to look for, and recognizing that a given set of findings fit together as components of a syndrome. During the examination the clinician should systematically examine the following:

- Ears—shape and location of pinnae, size of EACs, appearance of eardrums, shape of the malleus, presence or absence of preauricular pits or tags
- Eyes—eyebrows, distance between the eyes, color of the irides, extraocular movements, fundus, retinal pigmentation
- Face—shape, symmetry
- Skin—texture, pigmentation
- Extremities—shape of fingers and toes, carrying angle of arms

Audiologic Testing

There are certain subtleties involved in regard to audiologic assessment when a diagnosis of hereditary hearing impairment is being considered. A U-shaped ("cookie bite") audiogram classically has been correlated with hereditary hearing impairment (Fig. 1). However, it is important to note that the supposedly characteristic U-shaped audiogram has been described in association with nonsyndromic HHI, not syndromic HHI. Furthermore, a report by Liu and Xu (2) demonstrates that configuration of audiograms associated with nonsyndromic HHI usually are no different from audiograms in individuals with hearing impairment known to be caused by exogenous factors. Similarly, with many of the syndromic types of HHI, there is not necessarily an audiogram configuration that is diagnostic of a particular syndrome.

When evaluating a family for syndromic HHI, testing first-degree relatives of the proband may be worthwhile. If an autosomal dominant syndromic disorder has variable expression, a relative of an individual who has evident stigmata of the syndrome may have clinically inapparent abnormal hearing as the only manifestation of weak gene expression. In X-linked recessive HHI, women who believe they have normal hearing actually may have subtle abnormalities that can be detected with audiologic testing, even though initial analysis of the family pedigree is likely to give the impression that only men are affected with the disorder (3).

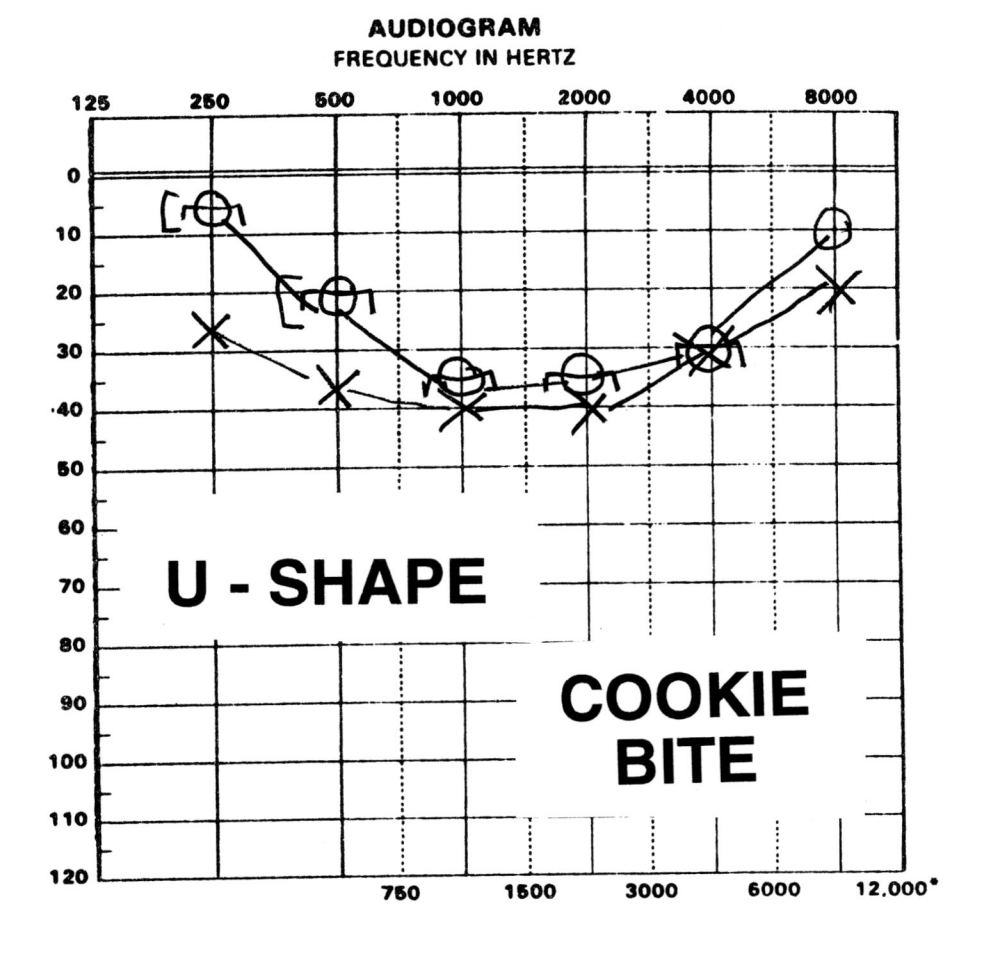

FIG. 1. The U-shape or "cookie-bite" audiogram.

Radiographic Studies

Although the Mondini cochlear abnormality has been described in association with Pendred and other syndromes, in general, findings on computed tomography (CT) of the temporal bones contributes little to the diagnosis of syndromic HHI. On the other hand, before one operates on the middle ear or mastoid in a patient with Goldenhar syndrome (oculoauriculovertebral [OAV] spectrum) or Treacher Collins syndrome, imaging of the temporal bone with CT scan helps to determine the status of a middle ear that may be markedly constricted, a facial nerve that may be in an abnormal location, or ossicles that may be malformed. The one radiographic finding that is helpful in diagnosis of a syndrome is the unusual bulbous shape of the lateral aspect of the internal auditory canal seen in individuals affected with X-linked mixed hearing loss with perilymphatic gusher (Fig. 2).

Cytogenetics and Blood Tests

Although the genes for many of the syndromes that include hearing impairment have already been located (Table 1), simple blood tests are not yet available to be used in confirming or ruling out the diagnosis of a syndrome. Furthermore, even though breaks, deletions, or translocations in chromosomes may be associated with some syndromes, none of the syndromes described here are specifically caused by a discernible chromosomal abnormality (4). Instead, the syndromes that include hearing impairment are the result of point mutations, which are not detectable when using the latest cytogenetic techniques. Therefore, obtaining a karyotype or other cytogenetic evaluation in individuals suspected of having a syndrome is not usually helpful. At present, diagnosis of a syndrome and the conclusion that hearing impairment is part of a syndrome rests almost entirely on synthesis of information obtained from family history and physical examination.

Other Diagnostic Studies

In the evaluation of a patient with newly discovered sensorineural hearing impairment, some otologists routinely order a battery of diagnostic studies including assay of serum glucose, various chemistries, thyroid-function studies, and electrocardiogram. The yield with this approach in terms of uncovering a diagnosis that was previously inapparent is low. That is, without a family history of goiter, it is unlikely that thyroid-function studies alone would lead to a diagnosis of Pendred syndrome. Similarly, because JLN is rarely encoun-

Normal

X-Linked mixed deafness

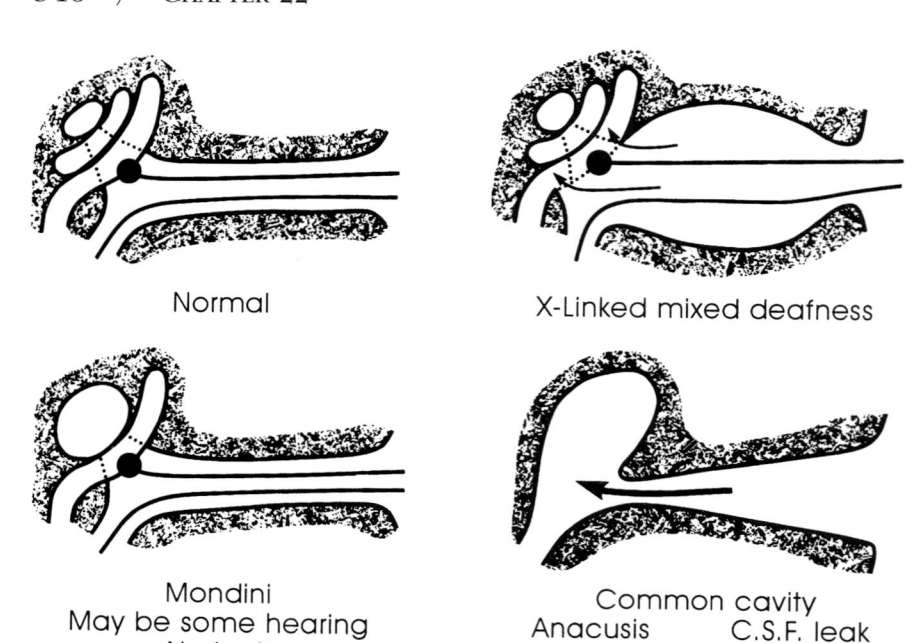

Mondini
May be some hearing
No leak

Common cavity
Anacusis   C.S.F. leak

FIG. 2. Bulbous shape of the internal auditory canal characteristic of X-linked mixed hearing loss with perilymphatic gusher.

tered, sending all patients for an electrocardiogram as a way to find the rare patient with prolonged QT interval may not be judicious. Patients with JLN usually are profoundly deaf at birth and have a history of syncopal episodes beginning during the early childhood years. Urinalysis is a simple, inexpensive, noninvasive test that might uncover asymptomatic hematuria or proteinuria and lead to a diagnosis of Alport syndrome. Although some otologists routinely request serology tests to rule out a diagnosis of syphilis, probably some assessment of the parental sexual activity should be weighed

TABLE 1. Genes located for syndromic hereditary hearing impairment

Disorder	Inheritance	Map	Gene
Albinism-deafness	XLR	Xq	
Alport syndrome	XLR	Xq	COL4A5
Alport syndrome	AD	2q	COL4A3
Alport syndrome	AD	2q	COL4A4
Branchio-otorenal syndrome	AD	8q	EYA1
Crouzon syndrome	AD	10q	FGF
Neurofibromatosis type II	AD	22q	MERLIN
Norries syndrome	XLR	Xp	NDP
Osteogenesis imperfecta	AD	17q	COL1A1
Osteogenesis imperfecta	AD	5p	COL1A2
Pendred syndrome	AR	7q	
Stapes fixation with perilymphatic gusher	XLR	Xq	POU3F4
Stickler syndrome	AD	12q	COL2A1
Stickler syndrome	AD	6p	COL11A2
Tranebjaerg-Mohr (DFN1)	XLR	Xq	DDP
Treacher Collins syndrome	AD	5q	TREACLE
Usher syndrome type Ia	AR	14q	
Usher syndrome type Ib	AR	11q13	MYO7A
Usher syndrome type Ic	AR	11p13	
Usher syndrome type Id	AR	10q	
Usher syndroem type Ie	AR	21q	
Usher syndrome type IIa	AR	1q41	
Usher syndrome type III	AR	3q	
Waardenburg syndrome type I	AD	2q	PAX3
Waardenburg syndrome type II	AD	3p	MITF
Waardenburg-Klein syndrome type III	AD	2q	PAX3
Waardenburg-Shah syndrome type IV	AD	13q	EDNRB

AD, autosomal dominant; AR, autosomal recessive; XLR, X-linked recessive.

instead of requesting a Venereal Disease Research Laboratory (VDRL) test for syphilis in every individual who presents with significant sensorineural hearing loss. Also, the VDRL test is not sufficient for ruling out a diagnosis of congenital syphilis; the fluorescent treponemal antibody (FTA) needs to be done to determine whether a patient has congenital syphilis.

An Aid to Diagnosis

For the otologist not yet familiar with the characteristics of common syndromes, an easy-to-use point-rating system has been developed to assist in recognizing which syndrome a patient may have (Table 2)(4). To use the system, one circles the numbers in *each* column corresponding to findings listed in the rows on the left side that are manifest in the patient being examined. Then total the number of circled points is totaled for each column. A total score of 5 or more points suggests that the patient may have the syndrome that corresponds to the letter at the top of the column (the key to the syndrome is given at the bottom of Table 2). If two or more columns have total points of 5 or higher, the syndrome in the column with the highest total numerical score is the more likely diagnosis.

Consultation with an Ophthalmologist

Approximately 30 syndromes include both hearing impairment and eye abnormalities (Chapter 23). Some eye abnormalities such as coloboma or heterochromia irides are obvious enough to be readily detected. However, abnormalities of the retina might be more difficult for an otologist to detect. Therefore, when there is a family history of sensorineural hearing impairment, it is reasonable to have the patient evaluated by an ophthalmologist, preferably an ophthalmologist with special expertise in diagnosis of genetic disorders. When there is reasonable suspicion that a patient with hearing impairment might have Usher syndrome, the ophthalmologist might proceed with electroretinography (ERG) rather than relying solely on physical examination of the retina (5).

The Clinical Geneticist

Perhaps the most helpful step that can be taken in attempting to figure out whether an individual has a syndromic HHI is to ask for the assistance of a clinical geneticist. A clinical geneticist is trained to look for subtle physical findings that may lead to diagnosis of a syndrome. When there is a family history of hearing impairment and when a child has physical findings that might represent variations from normal, the patient should be referred to a clinical geneticist for further diagnostic evaluation.

Ability to Recognize Salient Features

There has been much discussion about which syndromes that include hearing impairment occur most commonly. Many published reports and textbooks state that Pendred, Usher, and JLN syndromes are the most common syndromes that include congenital deafness, but these syndromes are not commonly encountered. For the clinician involved with diagnosis and managment of ear and hearing disorders in children, knowing how to *recognize* the salient features of certain syndromes is far more important than trying to remember which syndrome is supposedly more common than another syndrome. After all, "new" syndromes are being described at the rate of one or more each week (6) and attempting to keep in mind the rank order of frequency of occurrence of syndromes is not as helpful in clinical practice as is the ability to determine that a child in the office has or does not have hearing impairment associated with a syndrome. Therefore, with emphasis on a practical approach to evaluation of children with syndromic hearing impairment, a description of syndromes grouped in categories with clinical relevance follows.

SYNDROMES WITH FACIAL DYSMORPHISM

In this category are the three syndromes most likely to be encountered in the practice of otolaryngology or otology. Dysmorphism is a term used by geneticists to describe abnormal morphology (unusual appearance). These three syndromes can be diagnosed on the basis of recognizing unusual characteristics of facial appearance. Table 3 provides a summary of the features of these three syndromes. Most important is that each syndrome occurs with great variability. That is, in a given child, the syndrome may be so mild as to be almost imperceptible, possibly going undetected for years, or so severe as to be unmistakable and clearly obvious at birth.

Goldenhar Syndrome

Many terms have been used to describe this syndrome: Goldenhar syndrome, Goldenhar-Gorlin syndrome, hemifacial microsomia, facioauriculovertebral (FAV) dysplasia, OAV spectrum, first arch syndrome, first and second bronchial arch syndrome, and lateral facial dysplasia. The monickers that have become most favored over time seem to be Goldenhar syndrome, FAV syndrome, and hemifacial microsomia. The fact that there are so many different terms to describe the disorder reflects the wide variation that can be seen in individual cases and the different theories on pathogenesis.

Although this syndrome is often thought of as a genetic disorder, in fact, the syndrome usually occurs sporadically; in less than 2% of cases is an a autosomal dominant inheritance pattern seen (7). That the syndrome is frequently encountered in an office practice is supported by epidemiologic

TABLE 2. *Scoring system for syndrome diagnosis*

Findings	A	B	C	D	G	J	P	S	T	U	W	X
Premature gray hair, white forelock											2	
Branchial cleft cyst		2										
Unilateral mandibular hypoplasia					3							
Bilateral mandibular hypoplasia									1		1	
Macrostimia					1				1			
Goiter (large thyroid)							4					
Pigmentary changes, vitiligo, depigmentation											1	
Skeletal abnormalities, enlargement of ankles, knees, wrists								3				
Pain or still joints								1				
Vertebral dysplasia					2							
EKG abnormalities, prolonged QT, interval fainting spells						4						
Stapes surgery, perilymph gusher												4
Chronic nephritis or renal insufficiency	1											
Hematuria	3											
Renal dysplasia or abnormal-shaped kidneys	2	2										
Downward-sloping palpebral fissures									2			
Stapes fixation					1				1			2
Marfanoid habitus								1				
Mental retardation										1		
SNHL without findings listed above			1	1								
Congenital SNHL		1	4			1	1	1		2	1	
Mixed hearing loss		1						1	1			1
Congenital hearing loss		1			1			1	1			1
Progressive hearing loss	1			4								
Vestibular hypofunction										1	1	1
Preauricular pits		2			1							
Deformed external ear/microtia			1		1				3			
Atretic canal					1				1			
Retinitis pigmentosa										3		
Lenticonus, splenophakia, cortical cataracts	1							1				
Widely spaced medial canthorum, dystopia canthorum											1	
Confluent eyebrows (synophrys)											1	
Heterochromia											1	
Congenital/progressive myopia								2				
Retinal detachment								1				
Glaucoma and/or cataracts	1							1				
Coloboma					1				2			
Lateral cilia deficient to coloboma									1			
Flat midface, broad nasal root								1	1		1	
Unilateral facial paralysis					1							
Cleft lip or palate, high arch								1	1		1	
Patient's total score												

A, Alport; B, branchio-otorenal (BOR); C, dominant congenital SNHL; D, autosomal dominant/nonsyndromic; G, Goldenhar; J, Jervell and Lange-Nielson; P, Pendred; S, Stickler; SNHL, sensorineural hearing loss; T, Treacher Collins; U, Usher; W, Waardenburg; X, X-linked mixed hearing loss with stapes gusher.

Source: (ref 4).

TABLE 3. *Four common dysmorphic syndromes*

Syndrome	Inheritance	Face	Eyes	Hearing
Goldenhar, OAV spectrum	Sporadic (not inherited)	Asymmetric; hypoplasia of mandible	Asymmetric position, slant; coloboma; epibulbar dermoids	Usually conductive; ossicular abnormalities, sometimes sensorineural
Treacher Collins, mandibulofacial dystosis	Autosomal dominant	Symmetric, constricted midface	Antimongoloid, down-sloping palpebral fissures	Mixed conductive and sensorineural; may have external auditory canal atresia
Waardenburg	Autosomal dominant	Broad jaw, broad nasal root	Lateral displacement of medial canthi (dystopia canthorum); heterochromia irides	Sensorineural; highly variable audiogram; can have mild or severe hearing loss
Fetal alcohol	Not inherited; teratogenic effect	Long distance, nose to upper lip; faint or absent philtrum	Ptosis of eyelids	Sensorineural, usually mild

data suggesting the frequency of this syndrome in the general population at a range from 1 in 5,600 (8) to 1 in 26,500 (9). Expression varies within families. For example, there are reports of ear and mandibular involvement in two first-degree relatives, and reports of isolated microtia or preauricular tags in one first-degree relative of a patient with ear and mandibular involvement (9). The male-female ratio is at least 3:2, and there is a 3:2 predilection for right-sided ear involvement. Most likely, the cause of Goldenhar syndrome is multifactorial, probably involving some type of intrauterine teratogenic effect and, in some cases, combined with a genetic predilection. Some reports suggest that the intrauterine problem involves a vascular mechanism (10).

Although there is no universally accepted set of diagnostic criteria, the appearance (phenotype) of the patient's face is characteristic when enough manifestations are present. There is extreme variability of expression. About 50% of affected individuals have other anomalies besides the main features described below (9).

Face

Marked facial asymmetry is present in 20% of patients, some degree of asymmetry is present in 65% of patients, and the disorder is almost always more severe on one side. However, the asymmetry may be subtle and inapparent in the infant but become more noticeable when the child reaches age 3 or 4 years. The maxillary, temporal, and malar bones on the more severely involved side are somewhat reduced is size and flattened. There may be hypoplasia or aplasia of the mandibular ramus and condyle (Fig. 3).

Eye

Narrowing of the palpebral fissure (blepharoptosis) occurs on the affected side in about 10% of patients (11). Epibulbar dermoids, either unilateral or bilateral, are found in about 35% of patients (12). The dermoids usually are located in the inferotemporal quadrant of the limbus and appear as solid yellowish or pinkish white ovoid masses varying in size from a tiny spot to 8 to 10 mm in diameter. Unilateral colobomas of the upper lid are noted in about 20% of patients.

Ear

Abnormality of the ear may be as slight as a flattened helical rim of the pinna or as severe as complete anotia. Preauricular skin tags and protuberant small mounds of cartilage underneath skin are extremely common. Supernumerary skin appendages (ear tags) may occur anywhere along a line from the tragus to the lateral commisure of the mouth. The EAC may be slightly narrow or completely atretic. Conductive hearing impairment is the most common finding, but sensorineural hearing impairment is found in 15% of pa-

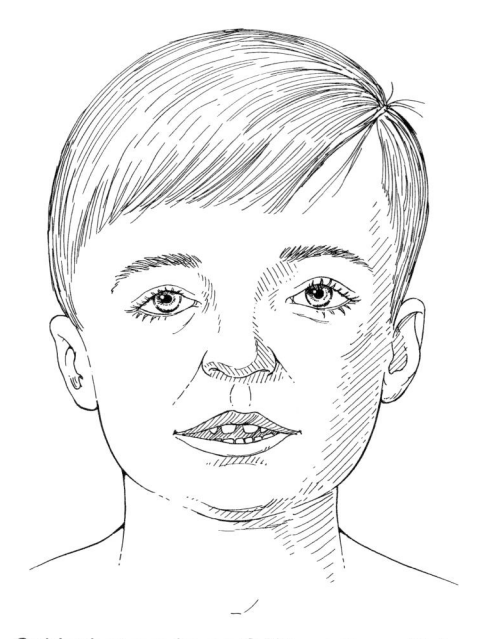

FIG. 3. Goldenhar syndrome OAV spectrum. Note asymmetry of the face and hypoplasia of the mandible.

tients. Aberrant location of the facial nerve and associated skull-base anomalies have also been reported (13).

Central Nervous System

Although mental retardation is not a part of the syndrome, an association between Goldenhar syndrome and mental retardation can be seen in 5% to 15% of patients (14). There may be involvement of cranial nerves, and facial weakness is seen in 10% to 20% of patients (15).

Renal System

The variety of renal abnormalities reported includes absent kidney, double ureter, crossed renal ectopia, anomalous blood supply to the kidney, hydronephrosis, and hydroureter.

Skeletal System

Facial anteroposterior and vertical dimensions are usually reduced on the affected side, and the temporomandibular joint may be anteroinferiorly displaced. The orbit is often reduced in size and vertically dislocated. Cervical spine and cranial base anomalies are common, 20% to 35% of patients have cervical vertebral fusion and 30% have platybasia (16).

Oral Manifestations

Macrostomia and pseudomacrostomia can be seen. There may be agenesis of the ipsilateral parotid gland, displaced salivary gland tissue, or salivary fistulas. The palatal and tongue muscles may be unilaterally hypoplastic, paralyzed, or both. Unilateral or bilateral cleft lip, cleft palate, or both occurs in 7% to 15% of patients (17). Tooth development can be delayed and third molars or other teeth can be missing on the affected side. Velopharyngeal insufficiency is reported in 35% of patients (18).

Other

In addition to the abnormalities described above, various associated abnormalities involving the heart, lung, and the gastrointestinal system have been reported.

Clues to Detection in Subtle Cases

An important clue that should raise suspicion of Goldenhar syndrome is the detection that an individual with conductive or mixed conductive and sensorineural hearing impairment has asymmetry of the face. Sometimes, the asymmetry can be extremely subtle. Two aspects of the physical examination can be used to detect Goldenhar Syndrome when the individual is minimally affected. First, if slight facial asymmetry is suspected, one should first look at the individual in full-face view, then put the patient in the sitting position, go behind the patient, and look down over the top of the patient's head at both malar eminences. If the patient has Goldenhar syndrome, the malar eminence on the involved side is slightly flatter and less prominent than the malar eminence on the opposite side. The second aspect to pay attention to during the physical examination is the size and shape of the patient's EAC. If the EAC is slightly smaller or more tortuous on the side with unilateral hearing loss, Goldenhar syndrome should be suspected. In fact, if a patient with unilateral conductive or mixed conductive and sensorineural hearing loss has an EAC that admits an ear

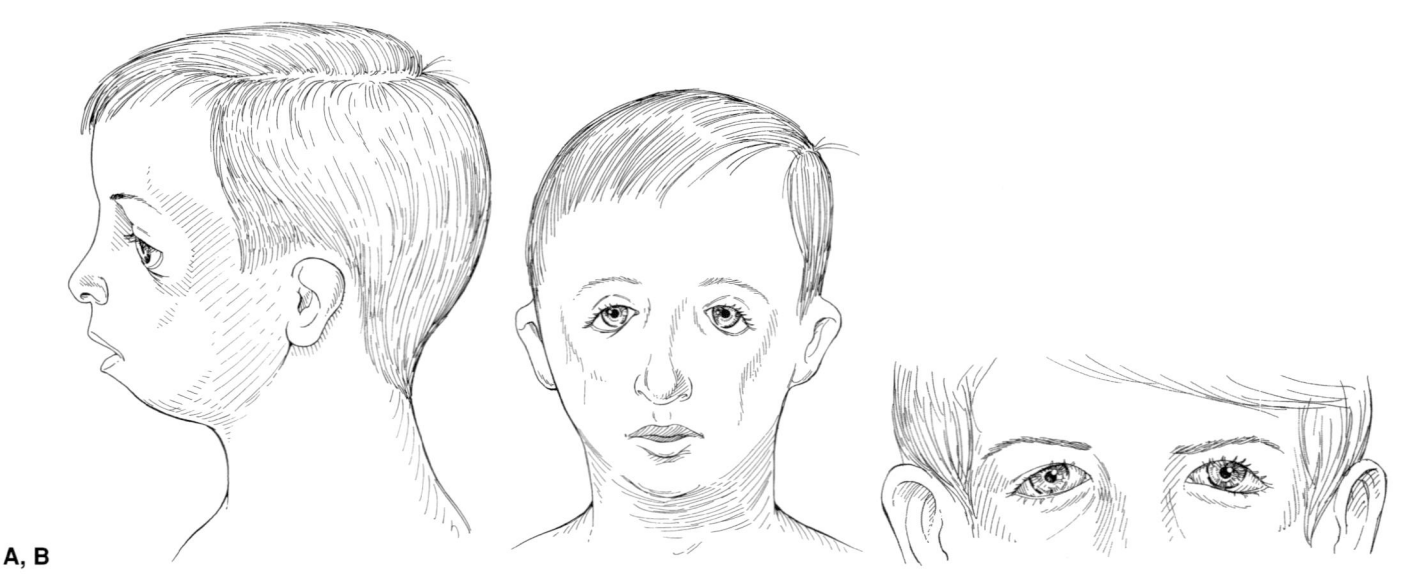

FIG. 4. Treacher Collins syndrome (mandibulo-facial dysostosis). Note the antimongoloid down-sloping palpebral fissures, constricted midface, cup-shaped pinnae. **A:** lateral view, **B:** front face view, **C:** subtle antimongoloid slant of eyes seen in child with mild Treacher Collins syndrome.

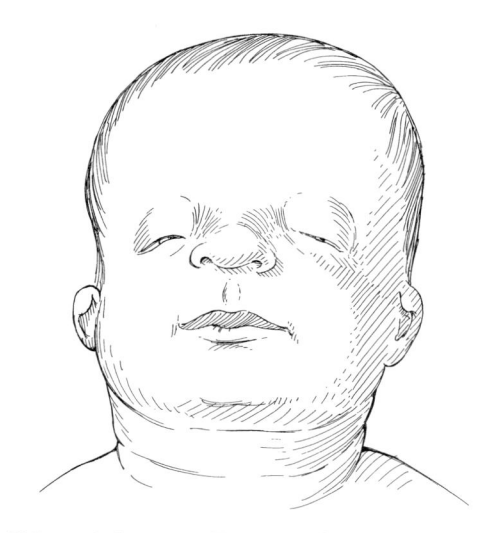

FIG. 5. Infant with Treacher Collins syndrome.

speculum no larger than a size No. 3 but the EAC on the opposite side can accept a larger size speculum, the patient has Goldenhar syndrome until proven otherwise.

Treacher Collins Syndrome

Treacher Collins syndrome, sometimes referred to as Franceschetti-Zwahlen-Klein syndrome, or mandibulofacial dysostosis, involves structures derived from the first and second pharyngeal arch, groove, and pouch. Inheritance is autosomal dominant with variable expressivity. Approximately 60% of cases apparently are caused by new mutations and therefore might appear to be sporadic (19). The gene that causes the syndrome has been located and mapped to 5q31–34 (20). Typical findings are described below.

Face

Abnormalities are bilateral and usually symmetric. The palpebral fissures are down-sloping, the face is narrow, the cheek bones are depressed. The midface is small and constricted. The nose looks large because the zygoma and orbital rims are hypoplastic. The pinnae are malformed, the chin recedes, and the mouth has a down-turned appearance (Figs. 4, 5, and 6).

Skull

Supraorbital ridges are poorly developed. The body of the malar bones are usually symmetrically underdeveloped but may be totally absent. The zygomatic process of the frontal bone and the lateral pterygoid plates and pterygoid muscles are hypoplastic. The mastoids are not well pneumatized and are likely to be markedly sclerotic. The paranasal sinuses are small and may be completely undeveloped. The orbits are hyperteloric. The mandibular condyle is severely hypoplastic.

Eyes

The palpebral fissures are short, slope laterally downward, and there is usually a coloboma in the outer third of the lower lid. About half of affected individuals have deficiency

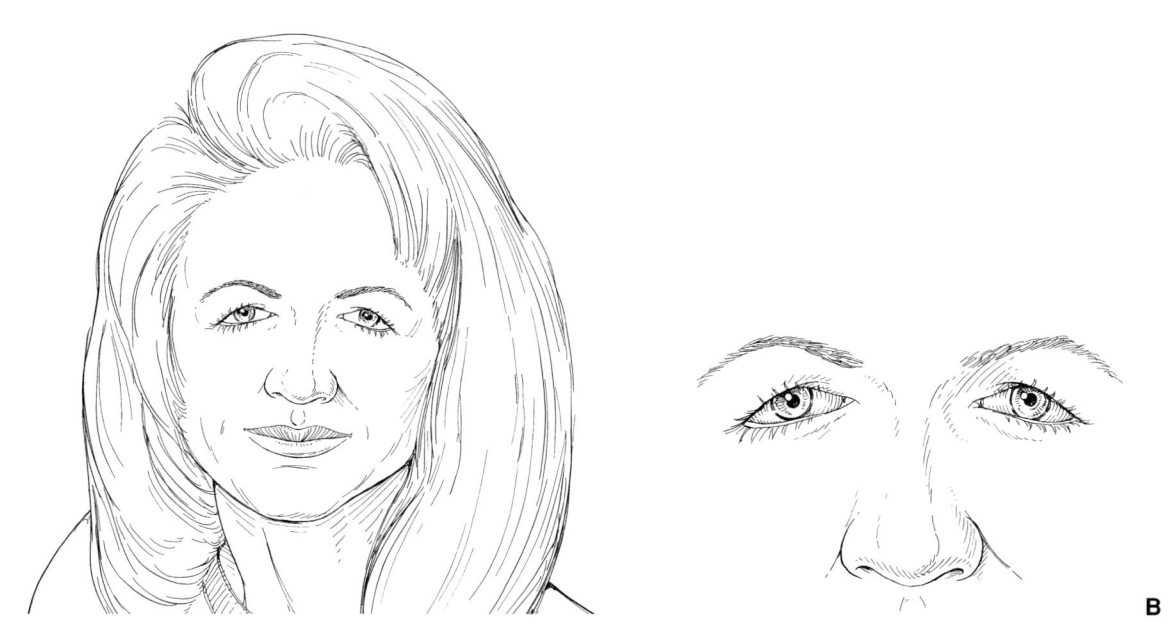

FIG. 6. A: Mother of a child severely affected with Treacher Collins syndrome. Note subtle findings of the autosomal dominant syndrome. Gene expression in this woman consists only of mild sensorineural hearing loss and antimongoloid down-sloping palpebral fissures. **B:** Close-up view of subtle, down-sloping palpebral fissures.

of cilia medial to the coloboma (21). The lower lacrimal points, the meibomian glands, and the intermarginal strip may be absent.

Ears

The pinnae are usually malformed, rather cup-shaped and tilted forward or misplaced toward the angle of the mandible. Most affected individuals have narrow or tortuous ear canals, and in more than one third of patients the EAC is absent (22). In most cases, the middle-ear cleft is markedly constricted, the ossicles are abnormal, and the cochlea and labyrinths may be malformed or partially absent. The mastoid antrum is markedly underdeveloped and the mastoid air cells may be absent so that the mastoid appears completely sclerotic on x-ray. Ossicular abnormalities that have been observed include agenesis or malformation of the malleus, incus, or both, monopodal stapes, absence of the stapes and oval window, ankylosis of the stapes in the oval window, deformed superstructure of the stapes, complete absence of the middle ear and epitympanic space, and a small middle-ear space filled only with connective tissue (23). Extra ear tags and blind fistulas may occur anywhere along a line between the tragus and the angle of the mouth.

Nose

The nasofrontal angle usually is obliterated by the bridge of the nose, which is more prominent than usual. The nares are narrow and the alar cartilages hypoplastic. The nose appears large because of lack of development of the malar bones and hypoplastic supraorbital ridges. Choanal atresia has been reported (24).

Oral Manifestations

Cleft palate is found in 35% of patients and congenital palatopharyngeal incompetence has been reported in an additional 30% to 40% of patients (25). Macrostomia may be unilateral or bilateral. the levator muscles of the upper lip are deficient (26). Radiographic studies demonstrate that the mandibular condyle is malformed and the inferior surface of the body of the mandible can be concave. The angle of the mandible is more obtuse than normal, and the ramus may be deficient. The coronoid and condyloid processes are flat or aplastic.

Mental Status

Intelligence is usually normal although there have been reports of mental retardation in a few patients (27).

In managing Treacher Collins syndrome, one should not be quick to attempt tympanoplasty with ossiculoplasty to improve a conductive hearing loss or attempt repair of EAC atresia in patients with anotia or severe microtia (R. Jahrsdoerfer, *personal communication*; see also Chapter 35).

Waardenburg Syndrome

The syndrome described in detail by an ophthalmologist, Petrus Johannes Waardenburg, in 1951 (28) has characteristic findings including pigmentary abnormalities such as heterochromia irides, hypopigmented areas of skin, or white forelock and hearing impairment. Inheritance is autosomal dominant with almost complete penetrance and variable expressivity. The variation in gene expression can be so marked that one affected individual in a family may manifest findings that are immediately obvious, but another individual in the same family who also has the gene for Waardenburg syndrome may have physical findings so subtle as to give the impression that the gene was nonpenetrant even though pedigree analysis suggests that the seemingly unaffected family member is likely to have the gene for Waardenburg syndrome.

Waardenburg syndrome has been subdivided into two different types on the basis of whether the affected individual has lateral displacement of the medial canthi, dystopia canthorum. Affected individuals *with* dystopia canthorum have Waardenburg syndrome type I; individuals who manifest characteristic traits but who do *not* have dystopia canthorum are diagnosed with Waardenburg syndrome type II. Estimates of prevalence suggest that Waardenburg syndromes may be found in 2% to 5% of all congenitally deaf persons (29). An analysis of audiologic findings in children with Waardenburg syndrome revealed no auditory system changes that were specifically characteristic of either Waardenburg syndrome type I or type II (30). The gene for Waardenburg syndrome type I has been located and mapped to chromosome 2q and the gene for Waardenburg syndrome type IIA has been located at 3p (31).

Characteristic features are described below.

Face

Individuals with Waardenburg syndrome type I have a striking facial appearance because of the lateral displacement of the medial canthi (dystopia canthorum), synophrys (confluent eyebrow across bridge of the nose), heterochromia irides (different-color eyes), broad nasal root, hypoplastic alar cartilages, and mild mandibular prognathism (Fig. 7).

Eyes

Individuals with Waardenburg syndrome type I have dystopia canthorum, an abnormally wide distance between the medial canthi of the eyes. The dystopia canthorum is a result of lateral displacement of the medial canthi. Dystopia canthorum differs from hypertelorism. In contrast to individuals with hypertelorism, individuals with dystopia canthorum have normal interpupillary distances and the measurable distance between outer (lateral) canthi is normal (Fig. 8). True ocular hypertelorism has been found in about 10% of indi-

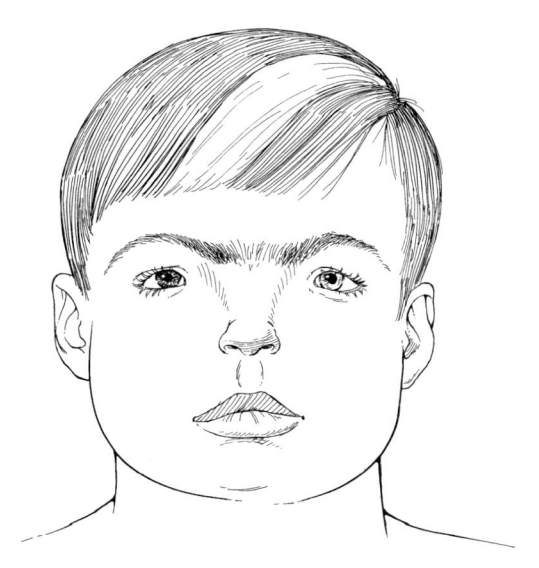

FIG. 7. Waardenburg syndrome type I. Note white forelock, laterally displaced medial canthi (dystopia canthorum), confluent eyebrow (synophrys), broad nasal root, hypoplastic nasal alae.

viduals with Waardenburg syndromes (32). The inferior lacrimal points are displaced laterally, sometimes as far as the cornea, and there is an increased susceptibility to dacryocystitis. Hyperplasia of the medial portions of the eyebrows or synophrys (confluence) of the eyebrows is present in 85% of individuals with type I and in 25% of individuals affected with type II (33). There may be two eyes of different color, for example, one blue eye and one brown eye, or one eye with a pie shaped segment of different color. Both eyes may have an unusually brilliant (sapphire) blue color, sometimes referred to as "Waardenburg eyes."

Hair and Skin

Although a white forelock is the most distinctive characteristic feature, it is seen in only 30% to 40% of affected individuals (33). Premature gray hair beginning around age 20 years is seen in 20% to 35% of cases of type I and in 5% of type II cases (33). Hypopigmented areas of skin (vitiligo) is seen in 15% to 20% of persons affected with either type (34).

Ears

Bilateral congenital sensorineural hearing loss has been observed in 20% of individuals with type I and in 55% of individuals with type II (33). An analysis of audiologic findings in children with Waardenburg syndrome revealed no auditory system changes that were characteristic specifically of either Waardenburg syndrome type I or type II (33). At least half the individuals with Waardenburg syndrome have normal hearing, and only 20% have hearing impairment severe enough to require amplification (Hereditary Hearing Impairment Resource Registry and National Institute on Deafness and Other Communication Disorders, *personal communication,* 1995). In most cases, vestibular function is normal.

Skeletal System

Various skeletal abnormalities including the Sprengel deformity have been reported in association with Waardenburg syndrome.

Gastrointestinal System

An association between both types of Waardenburg syndrome and Hirschsprung's disease has been reported (35). Hirschsprung's disease, sometimes called congenital megacolon, is a disorder of intestinal motility characterized by absence of parasympathetic ganglion cells in the submucosal and myenteric plexuses of the gut.

Oral Manifestations

The lower lip may be full and protruding. The mandible usually is prognathic. Cleft lip, palate, or both is about eight times more frequent in persons with Waardenburg syndromes as compared with frequency in the general population (36).

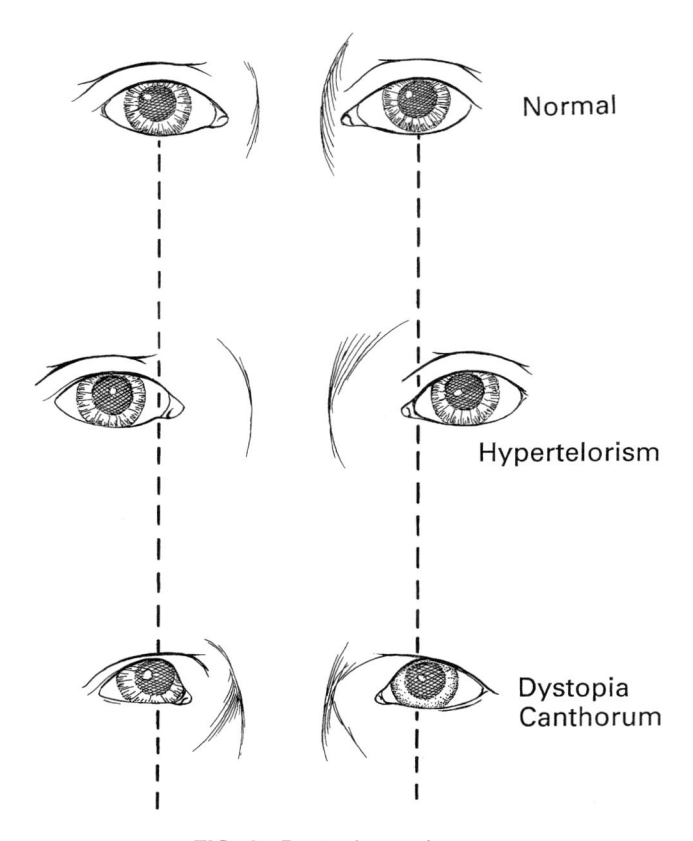

FIG. 8. Dystopia canthorum.

Clinical Clues

- When encountering a child with congenital unilateral or bilateral hearing impairment, the clinician should ask about family history of pigmentary abnormalites such as premature gray hair or areas of depigmented skin.
- In examining children with sensorineural hearing impairment, the clinician should look at pigmentation of the iris, not only in the child but also in the parents and siblings.
- Waardenburg syndrome type I can be differentiated from Waardenburg syndrome type II by measuring a patient's intercanthal distance and referring to a table of norms. If the distance between the medial canthi is more than two standard deviations greater than the norm, the patient has dystopia canthorum; if other requisite findings are present, the patient has Waardenburg syndrome type I rather than Waardenburg syndrome type II (37).
- A simpler but not definitive way for an otolaryngologist or otologist to determine that a patient is likely to have dystopia canthorum is to compare the amount of white sclera that is seen medial and lateral to the iris. In patients without dystopia canthorum, the amount of white sclera seen medial and lateral to the iris is approximately the same; patients with dystopia canthorum generally have less white sclera visible medial to the iris than lateral to the iris.

Fetal Alcohol Syndrome

Fetal alcohol syndrome is not an inherited disorder. The syndrome, characterized by an unusual facial appearance and sometimes sensorineural hearing loss, is caused by the teratogenic effect of alcohol ingestion by the mother during pregnancy (Fig. 9). depicts the appearance of the face with

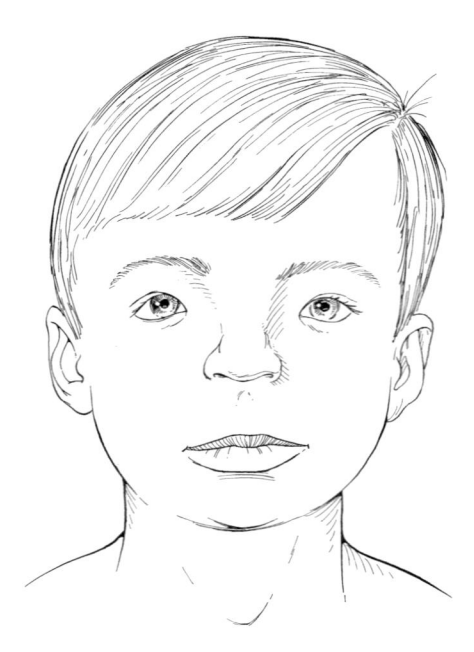

FIG. 9. Fetal alcohol syndrome. Note long distance between the nose and the upper lip, and faint, almost absent, philtrum.

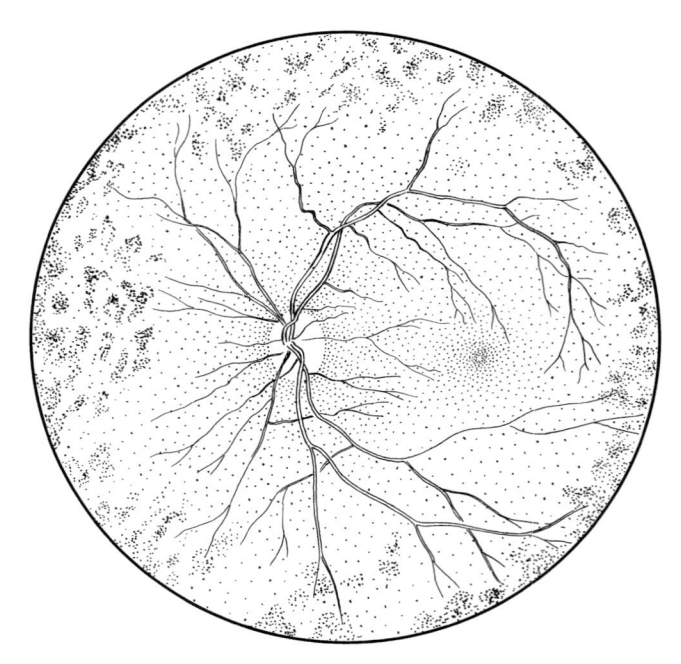

FIG. 10. Usher syndrome.

long distance between the nose and the upper lip and faint or absent philtrum, and ptosis of the eyelids. Affected individuals may also have hypoplasia of the nail on the fifth finger, learning disabilities, and behavior problems.

SYNDROMES FREQUENTLY DISCUSSED, INFREQUENTLY ENCOUNTERED

This section discusses three autosomal recessive syndromes. Much attention has been focused on these syndromes, but children with these disorders are not commonly seen by otolaryngologists and otologists. Because the syndromes are autosomal recessive, parent's of an affected child are not likely to manifest hearing impairment or other aspects of the syndrome.

Usher Syndrome

Usher syndrome is an autosomal recessive disorder that includes retinitis pigmentosa and hearing impairment (Fig. 10). Usher syndrome has been subdivided into three types. Table 4 provides a summary of the characteristic features of the different types of Usher syndrome. An ophthalmologist may help in making the diagnosis of retinitis pigmentosa and ERG may provide objective evidence of retinitis when findings on examination are equivocal or in infants in whom examination is difficult to accomplish.

Pendred Syndrome

Described by Pendred in 1896, this autosomal recessive syndrome includes nontoxic goiter and profound congenital sensorineural hearing loss. The goiter is usually evident before puberty (Fig. 11). About 50% of affected individuals

TABLE 4. *Different types of Usher syndrome*

	Type I	Type II	Type III
Hearing impairment	Profound hearing impairment usually corner audiogram	Congenital sloping sensorineural loss from mild loss in low frequencies to severe profound loss in high frequencies	Possible normal hearing at birth or mild hearing loss that gets worse over a decade or more; sloping sensorineural pattern on audiogram
Balance	Absent vestibular response	Normal vestibular function	Progressive vestibular dysfunction
Vision loss from retinitis pigmentosa	Night blindness in early childhood; blind spots by late childhood or teens; legally blind by early adulthood	Night blindness in teens; blind spots by late teens or early adulthood; legally blind in early to mid-adulthood	Timing of progression may vary, but night blindness precedes daytime loss
Gene location	1a: 14q 1b: 11q (most common) 1c: 11q (Acadians) 1d: 10q 1e: 21q	2a: 1q 2b: not yet localized	3q

are euthyroid and 50% are hypothyroid (38). The defect in the organic binding of iodine is demonstrable with the perchlorate discharge test. There is an association between the Mondini deformity of the cochlea and Pendred syndrome, but the frequency of this association is not known precisely.

Jervell and Lange-Nielsen Syndrome

Jervell and Lange-Nielsen described this autosomal recessive syndrome that includes congenital bilateral profound sensorineural hearing impairment, the electrocardiographic abnormality of prolonged QT interval repeated syncopal episodes, and, in the past, sudden unexplained death in childhood. Affected children have syncopal attacks and sudden lapses of consciousness beginning around 3 to 5 years of age. In the past, most affected individuals died by age 15 years, but prognosis may be better now that affected patients can be treated with beta-adrenergic blocking agents to reduce the chance of developing a fatal arrythmia. The gene for hereditary prolonged QT interval has been mapped to chromosome 11 (39).

SYNDROMES SEEN FREQUENTLY

Although this chapter is not intended to provide a complete compendium of syndromes that include hearing loss, ten syndromes occur relatively frequently, and the otologic surgeon should be familiar with them and know how to manage the otologic aspects of these syndromes.

Syndromes with Problematic Otitis Media

In this category are syndromes and disorders that include otitis media worse than the common type of otitis media that affects children who have normal anatomy. Children affected with these syndromes and disorders need special attention for management of the otitis media and otologic sequelae.

Stickler Syndrome

Individuals with Stickler syndrome usually are tall and thin, almost Marfanoid, have a flat midface, and severe myopia requiring thick glasses (corrective lenses) (Fig. 12). However, about 25% of affected individuals are not tall (40). Sometimes there is an associated cleft palate or Pierre Robin sequence. Joint hypermobility is common during childhood and arthritis can develop later in life. Inheritance is autosomal dominant and affected individuals often develop retinal detachments, cataracts, or both. Progressive sensorineural hearing loss has been reported in as much as 80% of affected

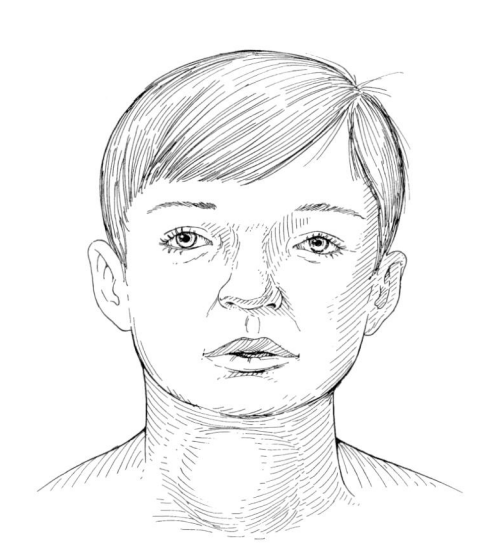

FIG. 11. Pendred syndrome.

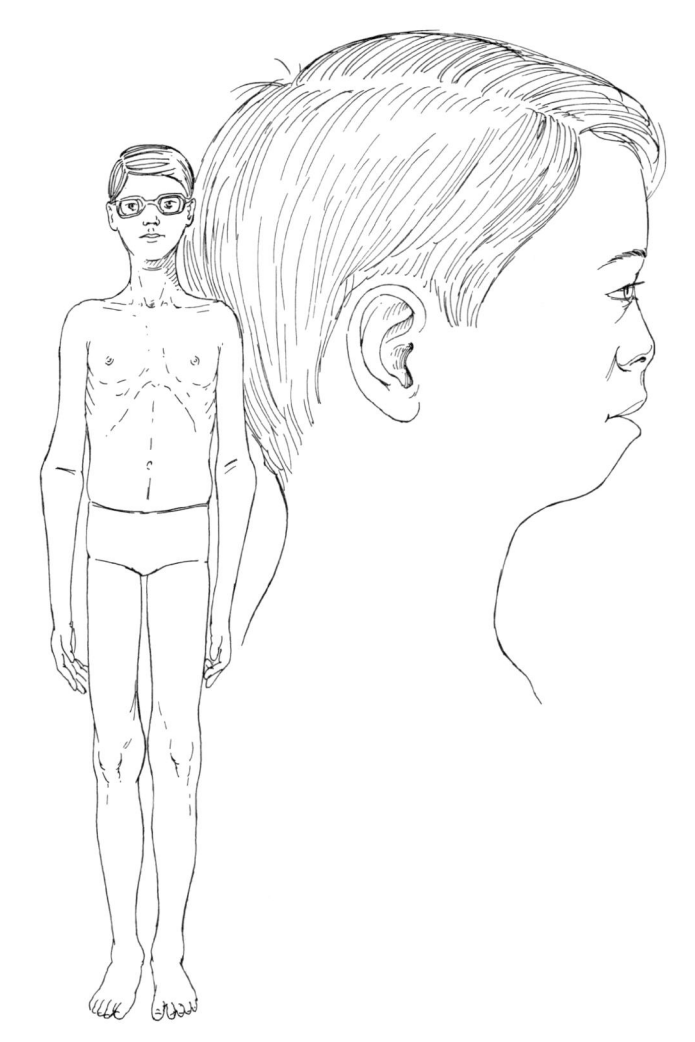

FIG. 12. Stickler syndrome. Note flat face profile, thick glasses to correct severe myopia.

individuals (41) conductive hearing loss has also been reported (42).

Velocardiofacial Syndrome

Children with velocardiofacial (VCF) (Shprintzen) syndrome have cardiovascular anomalies, cleft palate or submucous cleft palate, learning disabilities, and a characteristic facial appearance. The face is long and myopathic with a laterally full nose having a prominent bridge and hypoplastic alae (Fig. 13.). The eyes sometimes appear almond-shaped. Hypotonia in infancy and childhood is common. Cardiac anomalies include right-sided aortic arch, venriculoseptal defect, tetralogy of Fallot, and aberrant left subclavian artery. The hands and fingers are slender and tapered. About 50% of affected children have short stature (43). Otologic findings include small pinnae, thickening of the helical rims, frequently persistent otitis media that is attributed to eustachian tube dysfunction related to the cleft palate, and (less commonly) sensorineural hearing loss. Inheritance is autosomal dominant and the syndrome is caused by a deletion found at location 22q11.2 (44). Some research laboratories already have available molecular probes that can help to confirm a tentative diagnosis of VCF syndrome. The test used to help confirm a clinical impression of VCF is the fluorescent in situ hybridization (FISH) test, which is a cytogenetic evaluation that is based on having cloned the gene for VCF.

Turner Syndrome

Turner syndrome (Ullrich-Turner syndrome) is characterized by short stature and gonadal dysgenesis with streak ovaries, primary amenorrhea, sexual infantalism, and a karyotype that is either 45,X or a structural abnormality of the X or Y chromosome. The face is often hypotonic and expressionless with ptosis of the upper eyelids and downslanting palpebral fissures and corners of the mouth. The neck is broad and short, sometimes with pterygium colli (also known as "web neck"). Coarctation of the aorta is frequent, as are renal abnormalities. External ears are relatively long and narrow, often protruding more in the lower portions of the auricle especially if the patient has pterygium colli. The EAC may be displaced anteriorly and inferiorly. Hearing loss definitely can be a part of the syndrome, but the type of hearing loss seen is highly variable. The hearing loss is usually mild or moderate and can be conductive, sensorineural, or mixed. Otitis media and chronic middle-ear effusions occur in most affected individuals. Some evidence suggests that children with Turner syndrome are more likely than other children to develop cholesteatoma.

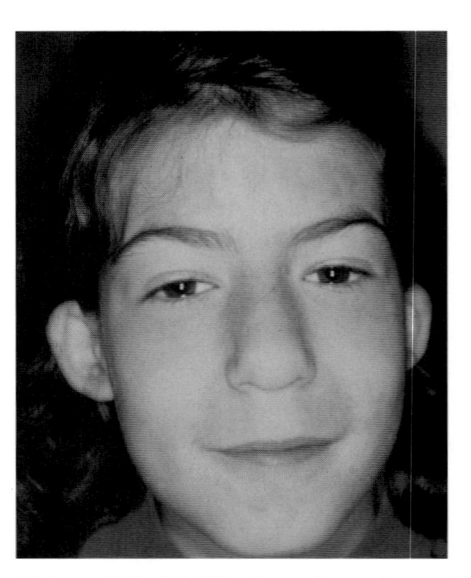

FIG. 13. Velocardiofacial (Shprintzen) syndrome. The face is long with vertical maxillary excess, malar flatness, and mandibular retrusion. The nose is prominent with a squared nasal root and hypoplastic nasal alae. There is a long philtrum and thin upper lip. (Courtesy of Robert Shprintzen, State University of New York, Upstate Medical Center, Syracuse, New York.)

Achondroplasia

Achondroplasia is a form of short-limbed dwarfism associated with enlarged head, depressed nasal bridge, short, stubby, trident hands with inability to approximate terminal digits, lordotic lumbar spine, prominent buttocks, and protuberant abdomen. Inheritance is autosomal dominat, but more than 80% of cases are sporadic, most likely representing new mutations (42). A smaller than normal foramen magnum and narrow spinal canal predisposes affected children to neurologic complications with advancing age. Mild ventricular dilation or significant hydrocephalus can occur (45). Perhaps related to this propensity for neurologic abnormalities, there is a relatively higher incidence of sudden infant death during infancy and early childhood (46).

Stura et al. found in a study on hearing in 18 children with achondroplasia that 10 had hearing loss, of which 7 was conductive loss and 3 sensorineural loss (47). However, the main concept to keep in mind in managing the child with achondroplasia is that bilateral otitis media with effusion and signficant conductive hearing loss is virtually pervasive among in children with achondroplasia and often persists beyond the early years of childhood (48). Most children with achondroplasia benefit from insertion of ventilation tubes; use of longterm tubes is often advisable. When inserting tympanostomy tubes in the ears of a young child with achondroplasia, one must keep in mind that the child may have a smaller than normal foramen magnum and spinal canal. Thus, one must take special caution in the administration of anesthesia; it is preferable to select an anesthesiologist familiar with the special needs of children with achondroplasia. One must also take care not to overly rotate the patient's head in an attempt to view the entire surface area of the eardrum.

Down Syndrome

Down syndrome is probably the genetic disorder most commonly encountered by otolaryngologists and otologists. This genetic disorder is caused by having three copies (trisomy) of chromosome 21 and is characterized by upslanting palpebral fissures; lax joints; mental retardation; congenital heart anomalies, including ventricular septal and subendocardial cushion defects; and stenotic EACs. The pinnae are often abnormal (relatively broad), the lobule is hypoplastic or absent, and the helix folded. Numerous reports document a correlation between severity of the pinna abnormality and severity of the child's hearing loss (49). Certainly children with Down syndrome have more problems with persistent otitis media than do other children. There have also been reports suggesting that some children with Down syndrome also have ossicular abnormalities and sensorineural hearing loss (50). Management of the otologic aspects of Down syndrome requires keeping in mind several points:

- Ear canals can be so stenotic early in life that visualization of the eardrums, even with an otomicroscope, is difficult or not possible.
- Because the stenotic ear canals can make testing of otoacoustic emissions problematic and because mental retardation is a component of the syndrome, behavioral audiologic testing can be difficult; BAER testing may be needed to assess hearing. When BAER tests show bilateral mild or moderate hearing loss after the child has had insertion of tubes in the ears, use of hearing aid(s) should be considered.
- Because delay in acquisition of speech and language skills commonly occurs, an attempt should be made to maximize a child's ability to hear, which usually means early insertion of tympanostomy tubes. If the child has markedly stenotic ear canals, tympanostomy tubes may have to be inserted several times.
- Even after insertion of tubes in the ears and despite the fact that the child has normal or nearly normal hearing, there still may be a significant delay in speech development as a result of the mental retardation. Some children with Down syndrome are learning American Sign Language as a means of communicating during the early childhood years.

Kabuki Syndrome

Kabuki syndrome was initially described independently by Niikawa et al. and Kuoki et al. in 1981. Although they used the term ''Kabuki make-up syndrome,'' the genetic disorder is referred now simply as Kabuki syndrome. The characteristic distinctive facial appearance consists of long palpebral fissures, eversion of the lower eyelid, and short nasal septum (Fig. 14). Ears are often large, poorly folded, or both. Visceral abnormalities are not common but may include cardiac defects, renal anomalies, and genital defects. Most affected individuals have growth retardation and mild

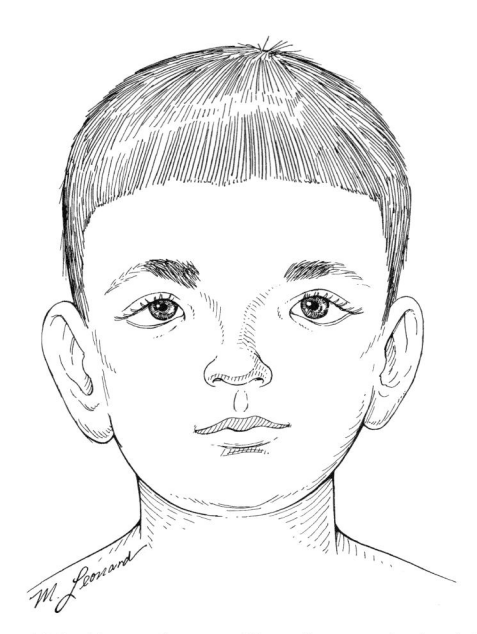

FIG. 14. Kabuki syndrome. Note long palpebral fissures, eversion of lower eyelid, short nose, large ears.

to moderate mental retardation. Conductive hearing loss, usually from otitis media, is present in 25% of patients (51).

SYNDROMES DIFFICULT TO DETECT

In this category are syndromes characterized by components that may not be readily apparent at the time a child is initially evaluated and found to have hearing impairment. That is, children with these syndromes do not necessarily have dysmorphic features that provide tell-tale clues to diagnose the syndrome.

Alport Syndrome

Alport syndrome, which includes hereditary progressive glomerulonephritis and sensorineural hearing impairment, can have an autosomal dominant or an X-linked recessive inheritance pattern. The six different types of Alport syndrome are summarized in Table 5. An account diagnosis of Alport syndrome can be made if an individual has three of the four criteria listed below:

- Positive family history of hematuria, with or without renal failure
- Electron microscopic evidence of glomerulonephritis on renal biopsy
- Characteristic ophthalmologic signs
- High-frequency sensorineural hearing loss, which usually begins during childhood and is progressive

Immunohistochemical methods can be used to identify the X-linked dominant form of Alport syndrome.

X-Linked Mixed Hearing Loss with Perilymph Gusher

Characteristically, this type of hearing loss is a mixed hearing loss present at birth and then becomes progressively worse as the thresholds for bone conduction become higher. About half the carrier women who have been studied have a mild mixed or purely sensorineural hearing loss. Women with hearing loss have normal vestibular responses, but men have an absent or strongly reduced vestibular response (Hereditary Hearing Impairment Resource Registry and National Institute on Deafness and Other Communication Disorders, *personal communication,* 1995). The conductive component of the mixed hearing loss is greater at the lower frequencies (52) and may be a result of dampened movement of the stapes footplate secondary to higher than normal pressure of the perilymph against the inner surface of the footplate. The leak of perilymph that can occur with stapedotomy or stapedectomy apparently is a result of abnormal communication between the internal auditory canal and the vestibule of the inner ear (53). A patient does not have to have stapes surgery and develop a perilymph gusher to be diagnosed with this disorder. The otologist should think of this inherited disorder whenever two men in a family have mixed hearing loss. A CT scan can help in diagnosis. Phelps described an abnormality that is highly correlated with this disorder seen on x-ray (54). The lateral aspect of the internal auditory canal is bulbous and there may be incomplete bony separation from the base of the modiolus and the coils in the cochlea (Fig. 15). Other forms of X-linked mixed hearing loss differ in age of onset, severity, and have more normal vestibular function. If perilymph gusher is thought to be a likely possibility, Cremers et al. (55) recommend carefully touching or slightly moving the stapes footplate to look for a transient small gush of perilymph fluid before attempting stapedotomy or stapedectomy.

Kearns-Sayre Syndrome

Kearns-Sayre syndrome (KSS) (ophthalmoplegia plus) is known to be caused by a defect in mitochondria. Genetic defects in mitochondria are inherited in a way that is unique and different from the common types of mendellian inheritance. Mitochondria replicate independently from their host cell and contain their own DNA, which differs from the genomic DNA in the nucleus of each cell. At the time of fertilization of an oocyte, mitochondria is contributed to the zygote only from the mother because male mitochondria, located in the neck of the sperm, do not enter the zygote. Only the head of the sperm enters the zygote. Therefore, mitochondrial inheritance is characterized by transmission of the disorder only from a mother to her sons and daughters, never to the offspring of a man who may manifest the disorder.

In 1951, Kearns and Sayre described a syndrome of progressive external opthalmoplegia, retinitis pigmentosa, and complete heart block. Subsequently, Kearns and Sayre found other abnormalities associated with those originally reported. In recent years, criteria have been established (56) for diagnosis of KSS:

- Onset before 20 years
- Progressive external ophthalmoplegia

TABLE 5. *Types of Alport syndrome*

Type	Hereditary	End-stage renal disease	Hearing loss	Other
I	AD	Juvenile	Yes	Ocular
II	XL	Juvenile	Yes	Ocular
III	XL	Adult	Yes	None
IV	XL	Adult	No	None
V	AD	Adult	Yes	Macrothrombocytopenia
VI	AD	Juvenile	Yes	Ocular

AD, autosomal dominant; XL, X-linked.

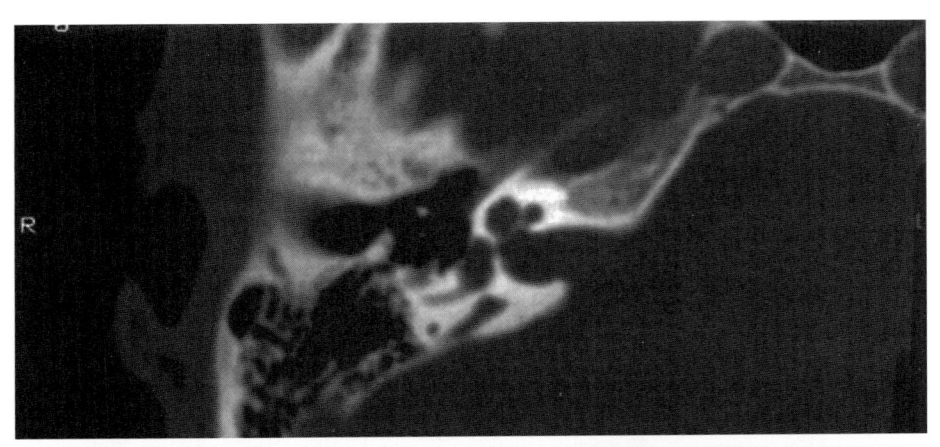

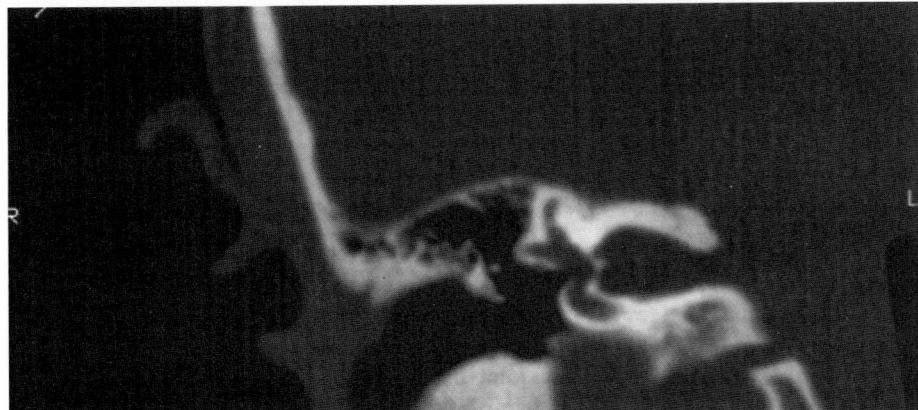

FIG. 15. Radiographic findings in a patient with X-linked mixed hearing loss with perilymphatic gusher. Note bulbous lateral aspect of internal auditory canals.

- Atypical pigmentary retinopathy
- One or more of ataxia, complete heart block, and elevated cerebrospinal fluid (CSF) protein

Though sensorineural hearing loss is not listed as one of the criteria requisite for diagnosis, about 50% of individuals with KSS have sensorineural hearing loss; occasionally, the hearing loss is a presenting symptom of the disorder. The hearing loss is worse in the higher frequencies and is slowly progressive. Vestibular testing has revealed markedly diminished or absent responses to caloric stimulation in about 85% of patients tested (57). Histopathologic changes in the inner ear include severe cochleosaccular degeneration with almost complete absence of the Organ of Corti in all turns and reduction in the number of spiral ganglion cells (58).

Children with KSS are usually short in stature and slightly built. Ptosis of the eyelids followed by progressive symmetric external ophthalmoplegia is usually the first sign of the disorder. Retinal pigmentary degeneration and optic atrophy often appear soon after the ophthalmoplegia becomes manifest. Cerebrospinal fluid protein is often elevated to greater than 100 mg/dl, and lactic acidosis is often present. Currently, the best way to confirm a suspected diagnosis is with muscle biopsy that demonstrates "ragged red fibers" (RRF) when stained by the modified Gomori trichrome method (59). Detection of mitochondrial deletions using polymerase chain reaction (PCR) technique may help in making the diagnosis.

OTHER SYNDROMES AND GENETIC DISORDERS

The syndromes and disorders in this section may not be encountered frequently by the practicing otolaryngologist or otologist, but they should be recognizable when encountered.

Branchio-Otorenal Syndrome

The term branchio-otorenal syndrome (BOR), was first used in 1975 by Melnick to describe the disorder, which includes *b*ranchial cleft fistulas or cysts, *o*tologic anomalies including malformed pinna, preauricular pits or sinuses, hearing impairment, and *r*enal anomalies of various types (Fig. 16). Inheritance is autosomal dominant with variable expressivity.

CHARGE Association

The mneumonic CHARGE describes a set of abnormalities first described by Hall in 1979, and later named the CHARGE association by Pagon in 1981. The abnormalities are: *c*oloboma, *h*eart defects, *a*tresia of the choanae, *r*etarded growth and development, *g*enital hypoplasia, and *e*ar anomalies (60). The fact that this disorder is described as an "association" instead of a syndrome means that components of the disorder are believed to be a nonrandom association of

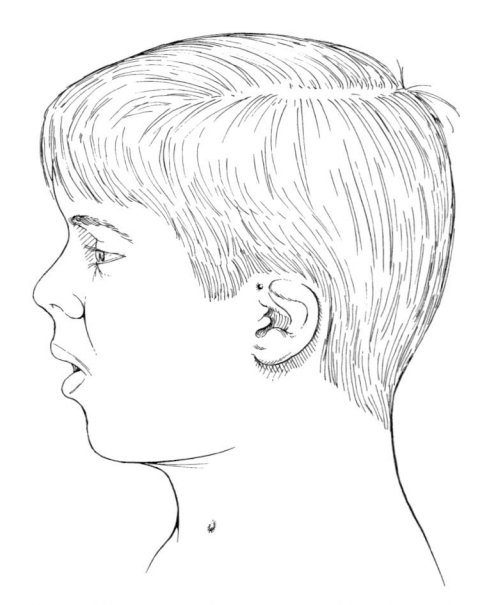

FIG. 16. Branchio-otorenal syndrome. Note long face, preauricular pit, and branchial cleft sinus with orifice in the neck.

defects for which an etiology cannot be defined. Children with CHARGE association have small or absent ear lobes, unusual shaped pinnae (Fig. 17), and preauricular tags. In rare cases, an affected child has microtia with atresia of the EAC. About one third of patients have facial paralyisis (60) and approximately 85% have hearing loss (61). The hearing loss is usually mixed conductive and sensorineural and varies in severity from mild unilateral to bilateral profound hearing loss. The majority of patients have a down-sloping audiogram configuration with worst hearing at the higher frequencies. Although some hearing loss is usually present at birth, the sensorineural component of a mixed hearing loss can progress. Thelin et al. described a "wedge" audiogram believed to be a unique part of the CHARGE association,

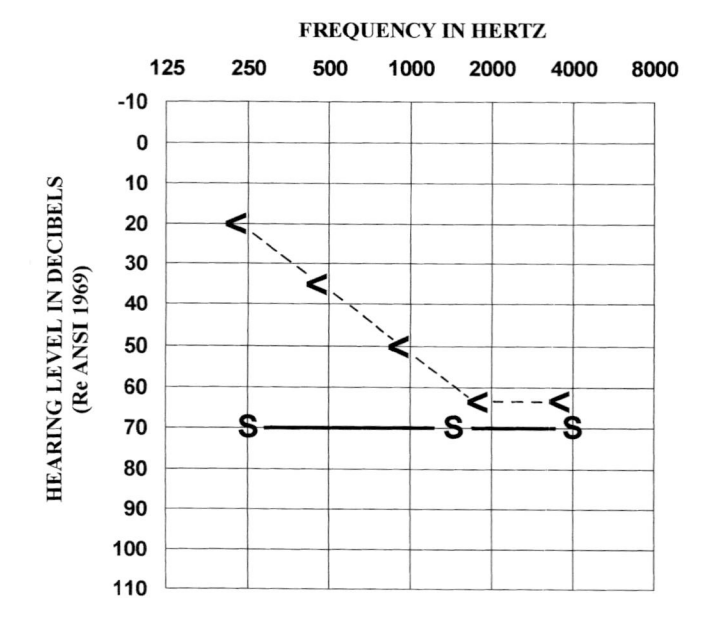

S SOUND FIELD RESPONSE
< RIGHT UNMASKED BONE CONDUCTION RESPONSE

FIG. 18. The "wedge" audiogram believed to be characteristic of CHARGE association.

apparently the result of conductive hearing loss from otitis media combined with congenital sensorineural hearing loss (Fig. 18) (61).

Osteogenesis Imperfecta

Osteogenesis imperfecta (OI) is not simply the classic disorder characterized by brittle bones, blue sclera, and conductive hearing loss. Rather, OI occurs in many different forms

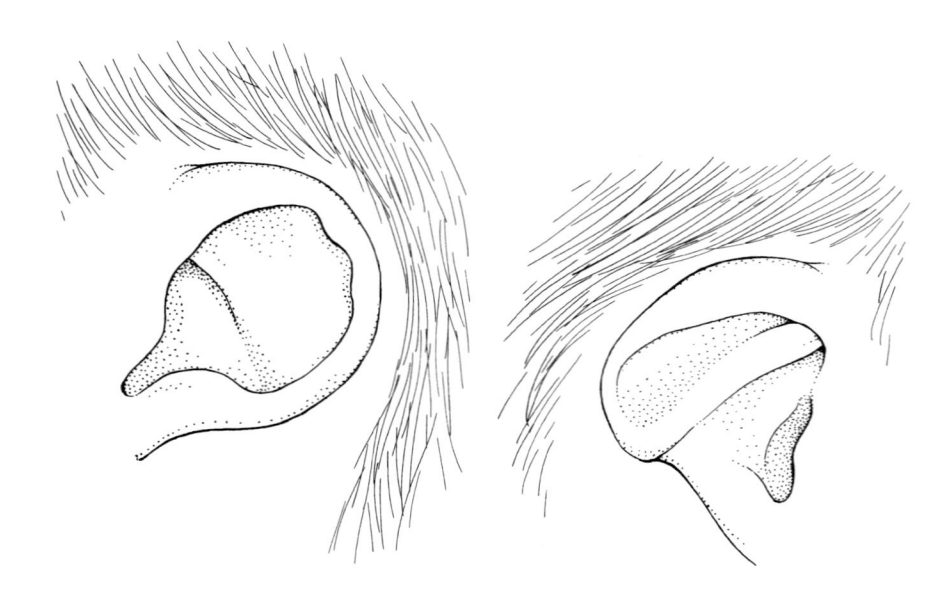

FIG. 17. Shape of the pinnae are characteristic of CHARGE association.

TABLE 6. *Major types of osteogenesis imperfecta*

Type	Salient features
IA	Mild to moderately severe bone fragility Blue sclerae Hearing loss Normal teeth
IB	Mild to moderately severe bone fragility Blue sclerae Hearing loss Opalescent teeth
IC	Mild to moderately severe bone fragility Blue sclerae Hearing loss Dentition resembles dentin dysplasia, type II
IIA, B, C	Very severe bone fragility Blue sclerae Stillborn or death shortly after birth
III	Moderately severe to severe bone fragility Blue sclerae in infancy that fades with age Generally not lethal in infancy, but death in first decades of life not uncommon
IVA	Mild to moderately severe bone fragility Normal sclerae, but may be pale blue in early childhood Hearing loss Normal teeth
IVB	Mild to moderately severe bone fragility Normal sclerae, but may be pale blue in early childhood Hearing loss Opalescent teeth

as an autosomal dominant inherited group of abnormalities of connective tissue associated with bone fragility. The four major types of OI are summarized in Table 6. Hearing loss usually begins after age 10 years and is initially a conductive hearing loss. Later, as the child becomes older, a sensorineural component to the hearing loss develops so that the adolescent or young adult manifests a mixed hearing loss.

Sometimes, stapedectomy or stapedotomy is considered in management of the child with OI and bilateral conductive or mixed hearing loss. Since there have not been reported results of large series of patients with OI who have had stapes surgery, there is no definitive information available to contraindicate or advise stapes surgery in patients with OI. Although a new method of gaining practical information about otologic surgery, an Internet discussion group, has revealed that several otologic surgeons have achieved good improvement in hearing when operating on patients with OI, reporting successful results on the Internet is anecdotal, and the surgeons usually do not specify the type of OI for the patients who have had stapedectomy surgery. Further, since data suggest that many patients with OI have progressive sensorineural hearing loss, the otologic surgeon must be careful in recommending stapes surgery for patients with OI.

DIDMOAD Syndrome

The DIDMOAD syndrome Wolfram Syndrome derives its name from the the components of the syndrome: *d*iabetes *i*nsipidus, *d*iabetes *m*ellitus, *o*ptic *a*trophy, and "*d*eafness." Children with this autosomal recessive syndrome are small, underweight, and have delayed sexual maturation, gonadal dysgenesis, or both. Unfortunately, they have bilateral progressive loss of visual acuity leading to blindness caused by the optic atrophy which is a constant feature of the syndrome. The hearing loss is bilateral sensorineural and typically progresses slowly from moderate to severe during the second decade of life (62). Vestibular hypofunction and nystagmus have also been reported (63). Children with this syndrome become deaf and blind. Cochlear implantation may be helpful, but there is some evidence that the hearing loss can have a retrocochlear component (64). Thus, caution is recommended in selecting a child with DIDMOAD for cochlear implantation.

Lacrimoauriculodentodigital Syndrome

Lacrimoauriculodentodigital (LADD) syndrome is an autosomal dominant syndrome characterized by cup-shaped ears, nasolacrimal duct abnormalities, dental anomalies, and mixed hearing loss. The nasolacrimal duct abnormalities include duct hypoplasia or aplasia, duct obstruction, absent lacrimal puncta usually associated with chronic epiphora, dacryocystitis, recurrent conjuctivitis, and keratoconjunctivitis. Nasolacrimal duct fistulae have also been reported (65). There can be associated abnormalities of the fingers, such as duplicated phalanx of the thumb, digitalized thumb, exaggerated interdigital cleft between the second and third fingers, syndactyly of the second and third digits, or fifth finger clynodactyly. Dental abnormalities include hypodontia, pegshaped incisors, and enamel dysplasia of deciduous and permanent teeth. The cup-shaped ears with short helix and underdeveloped antihelix are an almost constant feature of the syndrome although this abnormality is sometimes unilateral. The mixed conductive and sensorineural hearing impairment ranges in severity from mild to severe, and, in some patients, is predominantly sensorineural. Patients with LADD syndrome may need to be differentiated from patients who have BOR syndrome or Townes-Brock sydrome.

ADDITIONAL RESOURCES

Compendium of Syndromes that Include Hearing Loss

A compendium of the syndromes that include hearing impairment is available. *Hereditary Hearing Loss and Its Syndromes* (42) is a comprehensive textbook that describes almost all hereditary syndromes that include hearing impairment. The text is well written, illustrated, and indexed so that it is valuable for a clinician seeking to identify syndromes on the basis of information gleaned from evaluation of patients in the office setting.

CD-ROM Assistance in Diagnosis of Syndromes

The ability of an otolaryngologist or otologist to make a diagnosis of a syndrome depends, in part, on his or her knowledge base. That is, if one has never heard of or learned about the existence of a certain syndrome, one cannot recognize that a patient with hearing loss has the syndrome. However, in this era of electronic data storage and retrieval, every clinician has access to a vitually limitless database that can help in making the diagnosis of a syndrome. Two relevant databases available on CD-ROM are the London Dysmorphology Database (66) and Pictures of Standard Syndromes and Undiagnosed Malformations (POSSUM) (67) from the Royal Victoria Children's Hospital in Melbourne, Australia. One can key in the findings identified in a patient and the software tells whether the findings constitute a syndrome. Conversely, one can use the databases to provide the components of syndromes as a self-teaching tool for the syndromes likely to be encountered.

Hereditary Hearing Impairment Resource Registry

To facilitate collection and dissemination of information on HHI, the National Institute on Deafness and Other Communication Disorders (NIDCD) has established the Hereditary Hearing Impairment Resource Registry (HHIRR). The HHIRR is a national resource for the biomedical research community in the study of genetic hearing impairment and deafness. Located at the Boys Town National Research Hospital in Omaha, Nebraska, the HHIRR collects and maintains genetic, medical, audiologic, epidemiologic, and demographic data on individuals and families with HHI. Investigators who wish to have access to the information can submit an application for collaboration describing their research project and what information is being requested. The HHIRR matches investigators attempting to locate a gene that causes a specific type of HHI with individuals and families who have the type of HHI known to be the result of expression of the gene being sought. In addition, the HHIRR disseminates information about HHI to professionals and families. (For more information, contact the HHIRR directly at: NIDCD HHIRR, 555 N. 30th Street, Omaha, Nebraska 68131; 1-800-320-1171 (Voice or TDD), 402-498-6331, e-mail: NIDCD HHIRR@boystown.org; WWW URL: http://www.boystown.org/hhirr/.)

Genetic Counseling

The question often arises of possible need for genetic counseling when a child is diagnosed with an inherited syndrome. Genetic counseling helps family members to understand how the syndrome is transmitted through the generations to learn the risk of having additional offspring that will be affected. For further information on genetic counseling, see Chapter 23.

SUMMARY

More than 200 syndromes include deafness or hearing impairment. This chapter provides information to assist in detecting a syndrome in a child with hearing impairment and offers some advice on how to manage hearing impairment in children diagnosed with a syndrome. To provide optimal care for children with hearing impairment, the otolaryngologist and otologist should be vigilant in looking for associations between hearing impairment or other findings that are manifest and the yet-to-be-discovered findings that could lead to diagnosis of a syndrome. Advances in computer database technology and ever expanding clinical applications of molecular biology, markedly enhance clinicians' ability to recognize syndromes.

REFERENCES

1. Lalwani AK, Grundfast KM. A role for the otolaryngologist in identification and discovery of genetic disorders and chromosomal abnormalities. *Arch Otolaryngol Head Neck Surg* 1993;119:1074.
2. Liu X, Xu L. Nonsyndromic hearing loss—an analysis of audiograms. *Ann Otol Rhinol Laryngol* 1994;103:428.
3. Lalwani AK, Brister JR, Fex J et al. A new nonsyndromic X-linked sensorineural hearing impairment linked to Xp21.2. *Am J Human Genet* 1994;55:685.
4. Grundfast KM, Josephson GD. Hereditary hearing loss. In: Hughes GB, Pensak ML, eds. *Clinical otology.* New York: Thieme; 1997:269–287.
5. Young NM, Johnson JC, Mets MB, Hain YC. Cochlear implants in young children with Usher's syndrome. *Ann Otol Rhinol Laryngol Suppl* 1995;24:342.
6. Toriello HV. New syndromes from old: the role of heterogeneity and variability in syndrome delineation. *Am J Med Genet Suppl* 1988;1:50.
7. Allanson J. Genetic hearing loss associated with external ear abnormalities. In: Gorlin RJ, Toriello HV, Cohen MM, eds. *Hereditary hearing loss and its syndromes.* New York: Oxford University Press, 1995:72.
8. Grabb WC. The first and second branchial arch syndrome. *Plast Reconstr Surg* 1965;36:485.
9. Melnick M. The etiology of external ear malformation and its relation to abnormalities of the middle ear, inner ear and other organ systems. *Birth Defects* 1980;16:4:303.
10. Gorlin RJ, Cohen MM, Levin LS. *Syndromes of the head and neck.* New York: Oxford University Press; 1990:641.
11. Mansour AM, et al. Ocular findings in the facio-auriculovertebral sequence (Goldenhar-Gorlin syndrome). *Am J Ophthalmol* 1985;100:555.
12. Baum JL, Feingold M. Ocular aspects of Goldenhar's syndrome. *Am J Ophthalmol* 1973;75:250.
13. Bassila MK, Goldenberg R. The association of facial palsy and/or sensorineural haring loss in patients with hemifacial microsia. *Am J Med Genet* 1989;36:287.
14. Shokier MHK. The Goldenhar syndrome: a natural history. *Birth Defects* 1977;13:67.
15. Yovich J, et al. Goldenhar syndrome and overlapping dysplasias in vitro fertilization and ovopathy. *J Med Genet* 1997;24:616–620.
16. Avon SW, Shirley JL. Orthopedic manifestations of Goldenhar syndrome. *J Pediatr Orthop* 1988;8:683.
17. Figueroa AA, Friede H. Craniovertebral malformations in hemifacial microsomia. *J Craniofac Genet Dev Biol Suppl* 1985;1:167.
18. Luke, et al. Velopharyngeal insufficiency in hemifacial microsomia. *Plast Reconstr Surg* 1977;60:602.
19. Jones KL, et al. Older paternal age and fresh gene mutation: data on additional disorders. *J Pediatr* 1976;86:84.
20. Dixon J, Edwards SJ, Anderson I, et al. Identification of the complete coding sequence and genomic organization of the Treacher Collins syndrome gene. *Genome Res* 1997;7(3):223–34.
21. Mann I, Kilner TP. Deficiency of the malar bones with defect of the lower lids. *Br J Opthalmol* 1943;27:13.
22. Stovin JJ, et al. Mandibulofacial dysostosis. *Radiology* 1960;74:225.
23. Hutchinson JC, et al. The otologic manifestations of mandibulofacial synostosis. *Trans Am Acad Ophthalmol Otolaryngol* 1977;84:520.
24. McNeil KA, Wynter-Wedder DL. Choanal atresia—a manifestation of the Treacher-Collins syndrome. *J Laryngol Otol* 1953;67:365.

25. Peterson-Falzone S, Pruzansky S. Cleft palate and congenital palatopharyngeal incompetency in mandibulofacial dysostosis. *Cleft Palate J* 1976;13:354.
26. Herring SE, et al. Anatomical abnormalities in mandibulofacial dysostosis. *Am J Genet* 1979;3:225.
27. Stovin JJ, et al. Mandibulofacial dysostosis. *Radiology* 1960;74:225.
28. Waardenburg PJ. A new syndrome combining developmental anomalies of the eyelids, eyebrows and nose root with congenital deafness. *Am J Hum Genet* 1951;3:195.
29. DeSave M, et al. Waardenburg syndrome in South Africa. *S Afr Med J* 1984;66:256.
30. Pilcus A, Grundfast KM, Newton V. Collaborative analysis of unpublished data.
31. Hughes AE, Newton VE, Liu XZ, Read AP. A gene for Waardenburg syndrome type 2 maps close to the human homologue of the microphthalmia gene at chromosome 3p12–14.1. *Nat Genet* 1994;7:509–512.
32. Olivelli A, Silenz M. Hypertelorism and Waardenburg's syndrome. *Helv Paediatr Acta* 1969;24:123.
33. Hageman MJ, Delleman JW. Heterogeneity in Waardenburg syndrome. *Am J Hum Genet* 1977;29:468.
34. Pantke OA, Cohen MM. The Waardenburg syndrome. *Birth Defects* 1971;7(7):147.
35. Branski D, et al. Hirschsprung's disease and Waardenburg syndrome. *Pediatrics* 1979;63:803.
36. Giacola JP, Klein SW. Waardenburg's syndrome with cleft lip. *Am J Dis Child* 1969;117:344.
37. Hall JG, Froster-Oskenius U, Allanson J. *Handbook of normal physical measurements.* New York: Oxford Medical Publications; 1989.
38. Johnson T, et al. Pendred's syndrome—acoustic, vestibular and radiological findings in 17 unrelated patients. *J Laryngol Otol* 1987;101:1187.
39. Neyroud N, Tesson F, Denjoy I, Leibovici M, et al. A novel mutation in the potassium channel gene KVLQT1 causes the Jervell and Lange-Nielsen cardioauditory syndrome. *Nat Genet* 1997;15:186–189.
40. Hermann J, et al. The Stickler syndrome (hereditary ophthalmopathy). *Birth Defects* 1975;11:76.
41. Temple IK. Stickler's syndrome. *J Med Genet* 1989;26:119.
42. Gorlin RJ, Toriello HV, Cohen MM. *Hereditary hearing loss and its syndromes.* New York: Oxford University Press; 1995:236.
43. Lipson AH, et al. Velocardiofacial (Shprintzen) syndrome—an important syndrome for the dysmorphologist to recognize. *J Med Genet* 1991;28:596.
44. Ravnan JB, Chen E, Golabi M, Lebo RV. Chromosome 22q11.2 microdeletions in velocardiofacial syndrome patients with widely variable manifestations. *Am J Med Genet* 1996;66(3):250–6.
45. Mueller SM, et al. Achondroplasia and hydrocephalus. *Neurology* 1977;27:430.
46. Bland JD, Emery JL. Unexpected death of children with achondroplasia after the perinatal period. *Dev Med Child Neurol* 1982;24:489.
47. Stura M, et al. Problemi audiologici negli acondroplasici. *Minerva Pediatr* 1987;39:499.
48. Berkowitz RG, Grundfast KM, Scott G, Rosenbaum KA. Middle ear disease in childhood achondroplasia. *Ear Nose Throat J* 1991;70:305.
49. Maniglia JM, et al Congenital deafness in 13-5 syndromes. *Arch Otolaryngol* 1970;92:181.
50. Sando I, et al. Temporal bone histopathological findings in trisomy 13 syndrome. *Ann Otol Rhinol Laryngol* 1975;84(Suppl 21):1.
51. Philip N, Meinecke P, David A, Dean J, Ayme S, Clark R, et al. Kabuki make-up (Niikawa-Kurodi) syndrome—a study of 16 nonJapanese cases. *Clin Dysmorphol* 1992;1:63–78.
52. Cremers CWRJ. Audiologic features of the X-linked progressive mixed hearing deafness syndrome with perilymphatic gusher during stapes surgery. *Am J Otolaryngol* 1985;6:243.
53. Glasscock ME. The stapes gusher. *Arch Otolaryngol Head Neck Surg* 1973;98:82.
54. Phelps PD, et al. X-linked deafness, stapes gushers and a distinctive defect of the inner ear. *Neuroradiology* 1991;33:326.
55. Cremers CWRJ, et al. X-linked progressive mixed deafness with perilymphatic gusher during stapes surgery. *Arch Otolaryngol Head Neck Surg* 1985;111:249.
56. Moraes CT, et al. Mitochondrial DNA deletions in progressive external ophthalmoplegia and Kearns-Sayre syndrome. *N Eng J Med* 1989;320:1293.
57. Berenberg RA, et al. Lumping or splitting Ophthalmoplegia-plus or Kearns-Sayre syndrome? *Ann Neurol* 1977;1:37.
58. Lindsay JR, Hinojosa R. Histopathologic features of the inner ear associated with Kearns-Sayre syndrome. *Arch Otolaryngol* 1976;102:747.
59. Dobyns WB. Genetic hearing loss associated with nervous system disorders. In: Gorlin RJ, Toriello HV, Cohen MM, eds. *Hereditary hearing loss and its syndromes.* New York: Oxford University Press; 1995:308.
60. Pagon RA, et al. Coloboma, congenital heart disease, and choanal atresia with multiple anomalies—CHARGE Association. *J Pediatr* 1981;99:223.
61. Thelin JW, et al. CHARGE syndrome—Part II, hearing loss. *Int J Pediatr Otorhinolaryngol* 1986;12:145.
62. Cremers CWRJ, et al. Juvenile diabetes mellitus, optic atrophy, hearing loss, diabetes insipidus, atonia of the urinary tract and bladder, and other abnormalities (Wolfram syndrome)—a review of 88 cases from the literature and personal observation on 3 patients. *Acta Paediatr Scand Suppl* 1977;264:3.
63. Rose RC, et al. The association of juvenile diabetes mellitus and optic atrophy—clinical and genetic aspects. *Q J Med* 1986;35:385.
64. Grosse Aldenhovel HB, et al. Juvenile onset diabetes mellitus, central diabetes insipidus and optic atrophy (Wolfram syndrome)—neurological findings and prognostic implications. *Neuropediatrics* 1991;22:103.
65. Kreutz JM, Hoyme HE. Levy-Hollister syndrome. *Pediatrics* 1988;82:96.
66. Baraitser M, Winter RM. *London Dysmorphology Database and London Neurogenetics Database.* New York: Oxford University Press; 1992.
67. Bankier A. *Pictures of Standard Syndromes and Undiagnosed Malformations.* (POSSUM). Melbourne, Australia: Royal Victoria Children's Hospital; 1995.

CHAPTER 23

Oculoauditory Syndromes

Scott R. Schoem and Kenneth M. Grundfast

Hereditary hearing impairment (HHI) can be associated with eye abnormalities, including irregularities of the palpebral fissures, synophrys, myopia, glaucoma, heterochromia irides, lens opacities, pigmentary retinopathy (retinitis pigmentosa), and optic atrophy. Because the optic and otic placodes are both derived simultaneously from neuroectoderm, any perturbation in embryogenesis can result in concomitant eye and ear abnormalities (1).

The ability of an otolaryngologist to recognize syndromic types of HHI depends on the detection of distinctive and unusual physical features, some of which may be unfamiliar or subtle. To recognize many of the syndromes that include hereditary hearing loss, the otolaryngologist needs to be familiar with those eye abnormalities that represent components of the common types of syndromic HHI.

This chapter presents an organized approach toward recognizing altered eye and other facial characteristics associated with HHI and provides illustrative examples of commonly encountered disorders, including Waardenburg's syndrome, Usher's syndrome, oculo-auriculo-vertebral (Goldenhar's) syndrome and the Duane's retraction syndrome. A guide of eye findings found in these common disorders is offered as a quick reference for the clinician.

ANATOMY AND EMBRYOLOGY

Anatomically, the eye consists of three primary layers. The outer layer, composed primarily of collagen-elastic tissue, provides a protective outer wall. The cornea comprises the anterior one sixth, and the sclera forms the posterior five sixths of this layer. The middle layer, the uvea, consists of three portions: the iris, the ciliary body, and the choroid. When separated from the outer layer, the middle layer has a purple color and rounded contour, resembling a grape. Hence the name *uvea,* derived from the Latin word *uva,* for grape. The uvea provides vascular supply to the eye. The inner layer and the optic nerve are anterior projections from the brain, derived from the bilayered, neuroectodermal optic cup. This inner layer consists of the sensory retina, the retinal pigment epithelium, and the epithelium of the iris and ciliary body.

The first evidence of primitive eye formation occurs as the anterior portion of the neural tube closes during the third week of gestation. The optic pit is a small depression that forms on either side of the midline in the ventrolateral region of the primitive forebrain (prosencephalon). Each optic pit rapidly enlarges to form a globular projection, the primary optic vesicle. During the fourth week of gestation, the optic vesicle invaginates to form a more cup-shaped structure. By the sixth week, most of the basic elements of the eye are present. Thereafter, most ocular development is by differentiation and modification of existing structures (1).

Figure 1 parallels development of the primitive eye with that of the inner ear during embryogenesis. A familiarity with normal sequential development helps in understanding alterations in embryogenesis that involve both the eye and ear in development.

RECOGNIZING ALTERED EYE AND FACIAL CHARACTERISTICS

Certain congenital abnormalities occur with increased frequency in association with some chromosomal aberrations. For instance, many autosomal defects are associated with microcephaly, short stature, and mental retardation. Ocular abnormalities, including microphthalmos, colobomas, and hypertelorism are features of many autosomal

---

S.R. Schoem: Department of Otolaryngology, Head and Neck Surgery, National Naval Medical Center, Bethesda, Maryland 20889-5000.
K.M. Grundfast: Department of Otolaryngology and Pediatrics, Georgetown University Medical Center, Washington, DC 20007.
*This work was performed while employed by the Department of the Navy. The views expressed in this report are those of the author and do not reflect the official policy or position of the Department of the Navy, Department of Defense, or the United States Government.

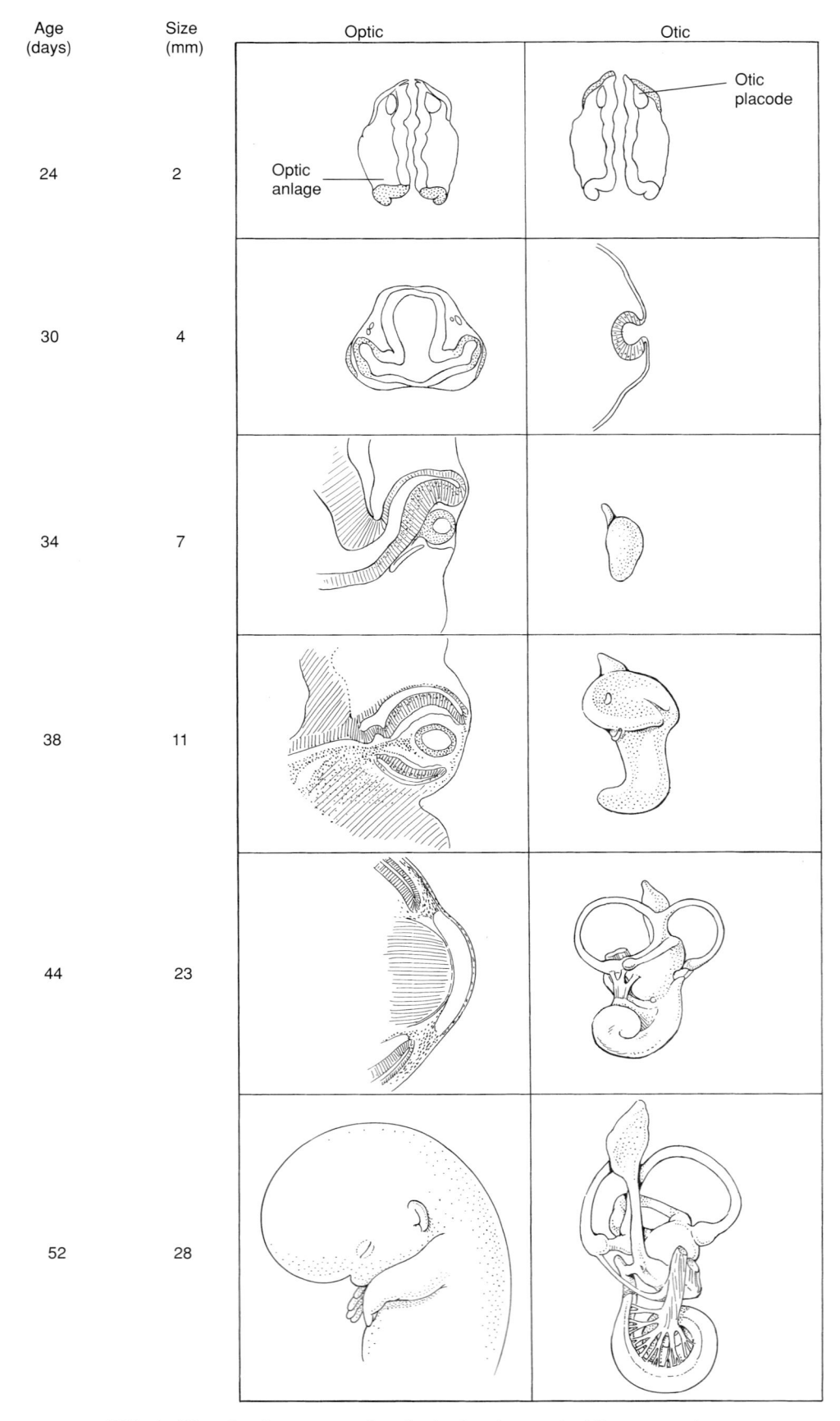

Age (days)	Size (mm)	Optic	Otic
24	2	Optic anlage	Otic placode
30	4		
34	7		
38	11		
44	23		
52	28		

FIG. 1. The simultaneous embryologic development of the eye and ear.

chromosomal alterations. If the clinician reviews an extensive listing of known entities and their respective associated physical abnormalities, lines of distinction quickly blur without use of a system of categorization. (See Appendix A.)

Chromosomal defects alter the facial features in a consistent manner so that individuals with specific syndromes tend to resemble each other more than members of their own family or ethnic group. However, phenotypic analysis is a skill that is best learned through pattern recognition. Analysis of facial features begins by describing each specific facial and ocular feature, and continues by comparison of these altered components with family members and individuals who have the same disorder.

Terminology should be precise. For example, the concept of "widely spaced eyes" has caused considerable confusion in the literature. *Widely spaced eyes* may connote (a) true ocular hypertelorism (increased interpupillary distance), as seen in Crouzon's and Apert's syndromes, (b) dystopia canthorum or primary telecanthus (lateral displacement of the medial canthi), as seen in type I Waardenburg's syndrome, or (c) merely the appearance of downward sloping of the palpebral fissures, as seen in mandibulofacial dysostosis (Treacher Collins syndrome). See Fig. 2 for details.

The developmental embryologic pathways that lead to specific ocular abnormalities are complex and diverse. They may result from multiple chromosomal abnormalities with overlapping phenotypic features (2). Yet, an otolaryngologist can learn to detect obvious and even some subtle alterations in ocular features by close examination. Figure 3 presents the authors' preferred method of evaluating a child newly diagnosed with sensorineural hearing loss (SNHL). Additionally, several basic handbooks easily provide a framework of quick examination for the clinician (3,4).

The following is a modification of the quick, yet comprehensive eye examination recommended by the American Academy of Ophthalmology. Using easily obtained equipment, the clinician can perform a detailed and sophisticated screening examination. There are seven components to the examination. The first six are done with only a penlight and simple laminated vision cards. Because most HHI disorders with eye findings are nonretinal in nature, without even removing the ophthalmoscope from your office wall rack, you would have screened for the vast majority of inherited hearing loss syndromes with associated eye findings. The seven basic steps are

1. Facial features gestalt
2. External eye examination
3. Visual acuity
4. Confrontation visual fields
5. Pupillary examination
6. Motility and alignment examination
7. Ophthalmoscopic examination

1. *Facial features gestalt:* Note any features of head shape or facial disharmony. Specifically search for cranial bone abnormality, hemifacial asymmetry, maxillary or mandibular hypoplasia, low ear position or external ear shape irregularity, and hair texture changes or early graying.

2. *External eye examination:* Inspect the eyebrows and eyelids for synophrys (eyebrow hair confluency), coloboma (notch or defect that may occur in the eyelid or iris), epibulbar dermoid, ptosis of eyelid, symmetry, contour and slant of the palpebral fissures, and both symmetry and color homogeneity of the iris. Figure 4 depicts an iris coloboma.

3. *Visual acuity:* Common hereditary causes of visual acuity problems include cataracts, amblyopia, optic neuropathy, and macular degenerative disorders. The following represents age-appropriate visual acuity levels:

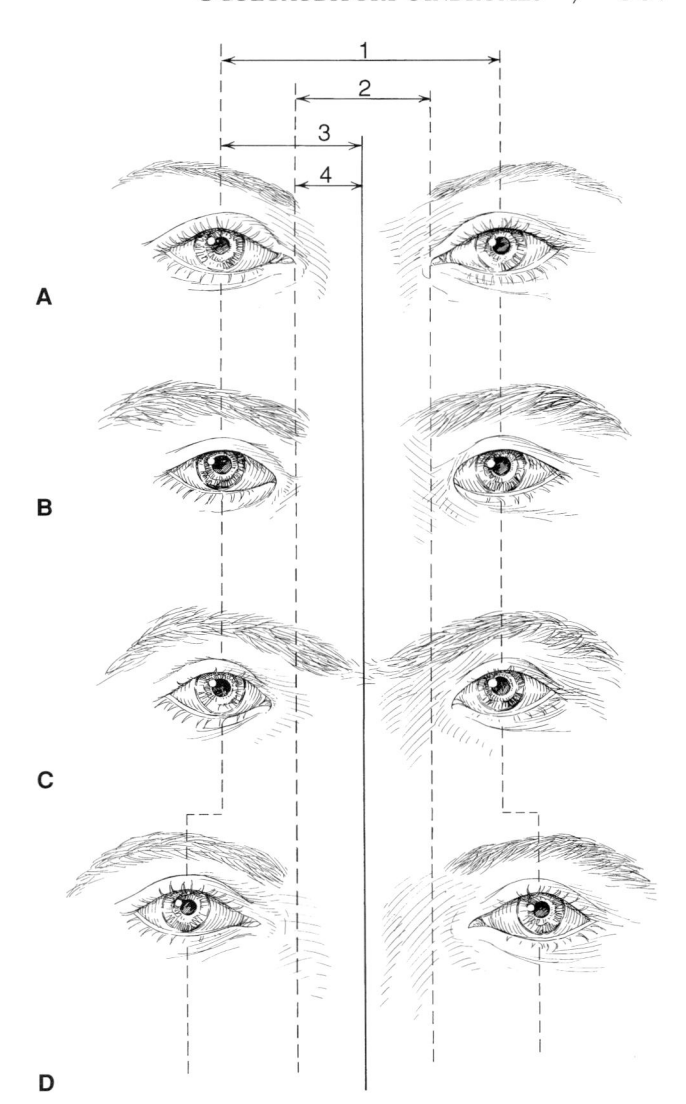

FIG. 2. Precise measurement of the medial intercanthal distance and the interpupillary distance distinguishes primary telecanthus from true ocular hypertelorism. A, normal; B, epicanthal folds; C; dystopia canthorum (primary telecanthus); D, ocular hypertelorism; 1, interpupillary distance; 2, intercanthal distance; 3, distance of pupil to midline; 4, medial canthus to midline.

```
                        Newly diagnosed SNHL *
                                  |
                        CT scan, Urinalysis ^
              ┌───────────────────┴───────────────────┐
    Family history of SNHL?                  Altered Facial or Eye #
        ┌────┴────┐                             Characteristics?
        No       Yes                          ┌────┴────┐
        |         |                          Yes        No
   No further     └──────────────┬────────────┘          |
   initial evaluation            |                   No further
                                 |                   initial evaluation
                         (1) Genetic counseling
                         (2) Ophthalmology consultation
                          ( ERG at discretion of consultant )
```

Eye Characteristics: **Eyebrows** - hair color, texture, confluence (synophrys)
Palpebral fissures - upslant(Down s.) v. downslant (Treacher Collins)
Distance between eyes Intercanthal (Dystopia canthorum)
Sclera - color: blue (Osteogenesis imperfecta)
Cornea - lens opacities (Alport)
Iris pigmentary changes - heterochromia, segmental
Extraocular muscle dysfunction - CN VI paralysis (Duane)
Irregularities - colobomas of iris (OPD II), eyelid (FAV)
  - epibulbar dermoids (FAV)
Retinal changes - pigment (Usher)
  - detachment (Stickler)

* SNHL - sensorineural hearing loss: audiologic reevaluation and treatment depends on degree of loss, developmental progress and family dynamics

^ CT scan - to assess any bony structural abnormality
Urinalysis - to assess proteinuria, hematuria

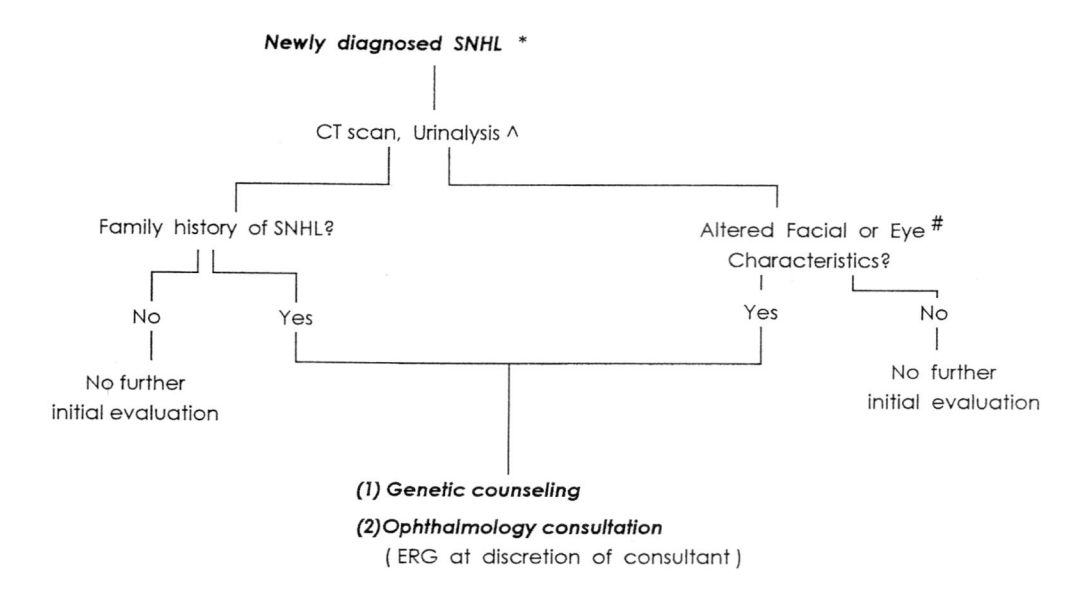

FIG. 3. Algorithm for childhood, nonmeningitic SNHL. ERG-electroretinogram.

Age Group	Normal Visual Acuity
6 mo–3 yr	Fix and follow face, toy, or light
2–5 yr	≥20/40
>5 yr	≥20/30

a. Fixation and following: For the 6-month- to 2-year-old child, use finger counting or light perception acuity. Observe the patient first with both eyes open, then with one eye closed at a time to determine if the child stares (fixates) at a stationary object (toy or light) and follows a moving target.
b. Picture chart: Between 2 and 4 years old and in mentally delayed children, patients can identify pictures of diminishing size by pointing to the identical one in a series.
c. Tumbling "E" chart: This test is more accurate than the picture chart for children 3 to 5 years old or mentally delayed patients. The child identifies orientations of the letter "E" by pointing the hand in the direction of the open E spokes. Figure 5 demonstrates the picture chart and the tumbling E chart.
4. *Confrontation visual fields:* This portion can be performed reliably only on older children to detect gross visual pathway disturbances. The patient identifies the number of stationary fingers within the normal boundary of each field quadrant.
5. *Pupillary examination:* There are three components to this examination. First, measure each pupil size in dim

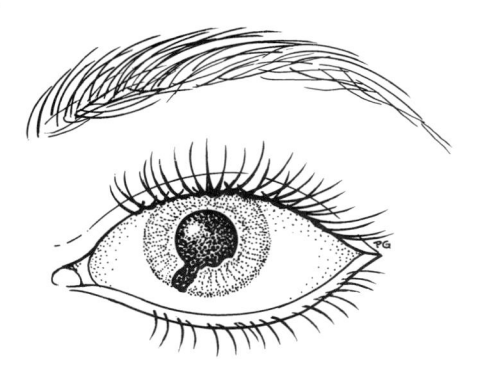

FIG. 4. An iris coloboma.

light. *Anisocoria* is defined as a difference in pupillary size of greater than 1 mm. Second, assess the pupillary response to direct light stimulation. This measures both the sensory and motor reflex arcs. And third, assess the sensory limb of the reflex arc by performing the swinging light test, checking for abnormal dilation rather than the expected pupillary constriction.

Few hereditary problems cause pupillary abnormalities. A pupillary examination may uncover benign idiopathic aniscoria, cranial nerve III paralysis and optic nerve atrophy.

6. *Motility and alignment examination:* The two parts of this examination are the motility (ocular movement) and the alignment.
   a. Ocular movement can easily be checked in most school age children by following a penlight or finger. This quick, but important step may reveal a previously missed Duane's retraction syndrome.
   b. Alignment: The corneal light reflex test compares the location of the light reflex in each eye. If the eyes are not aligned, one image will be displaced. For example, if the eye points inward (esotropia), the corneal reflex will appear outwardly displaced due to greater show of the outer sclera. Likewise, if the corneal show is abnormally greater inside, the ocular alignment is outwardly displaced (exotropia). If the corneal light reflex is either upwardly or downwardly displaced, there is vertical misalignment (hypertropia).
7. *Ophthalmoscopic examination:* A good retinal examination will be difficult to perform on most small children. However, even noting the presence or absence of the normal red reflex provides valuable information. If a red reflex is present, the eye can be safely deemed to be free of opacities, there is no large refractive error, and the eyes are grossly aligned. In reality, most non-ophthalmologists will not be capable of adequately screening for hereditary pigment retinopathies. This requires expertise even beyond the scope of most general ophthalmologists.

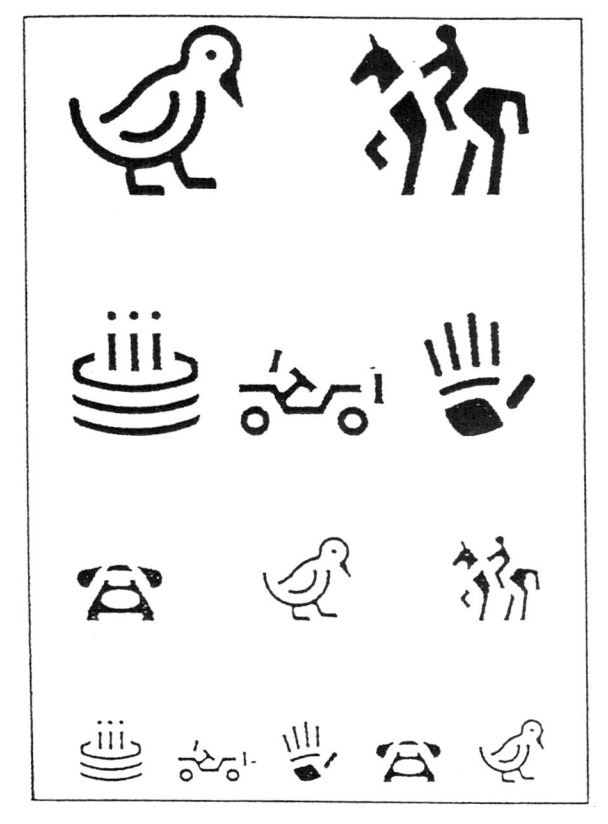

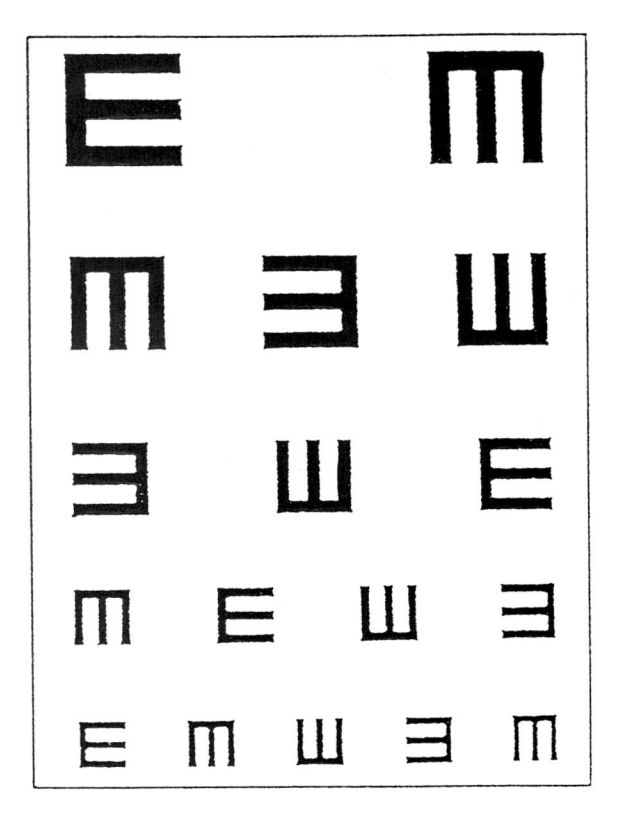

FIG. 5. Use of the picture chart and the tumbling "E" chart.

Colobomas, epibulbar dermoids, and iris pigmentary changes are easy to recognize. Unfortunately, some important ocular abnormalities are not as easy to detect. Early cataract formation or the early peripheral changes seen in retinal pigmentary disease requires a high level of examiner sophistication. For this reason, any child with newly diagnosed, severe unilateral or bilateral neurosensory hearing loss, with or without a family history of an oculoauditory syndrome, should have a baseline ophthalmologic evaluation. This should be performed, preferably, by an ophthalmologist trained in ophthalmogenetics.

COMMON DISORDERS

The following are four relatively common entities that otolaryngologists may encounter in their clinical practices. They are presented as models to further understand the associated oculoauditory embryologic defects within specific disorders.

Waardenburg Syndromes

In 1951, the Dutch ophthalmologist, Johann Waardenburg, described an autosomal dominant condition marked by dystopia canthorum (lateral displacement of the medial canthi), synophrys (confluent eyebrows), broad prominent nasal root, heterochromia of the iris, white forelock (hair hypopigmentation), poliosis (early graying of hair), vitiligo, eye fundal pigmentation abnormalities, and congenital deafness (5).

Waardenburg's syndrome recently has been determined to be of two heterogeneous types. Type I, linked to chromosome 2q35-37, has complete expression of dystopia canthorum, whereas Type II has absence of dystopia canthorum (6–12). Within Type II alone, there exists genetic heterogeneity (13). Type III is associated with unilateral ptosis and multiple skeletal abnormalities, including camptodactyly (permanent flexion of finger interphalangeal joints), syndactyly, scoliosis, and severe growth retardation (Klein-Waardenburg) (14).

Hearing loss occurs in 20% of individuals with Waardenburg's syndrome. Hearing impairment is more common in Type II than Type I. Whereas the hearing loss is usually moderate in Type II patients, mostly involving the lower to middle frequencies, affected type I patients have severe-to-profound hearing loss. Inner ear findings include an abnormal or absent organ of Corti, strial atrophy, a decreased number of cochlear neurons, and spiral ganglia atrophy (14).

Figure 2 demonstrates the difference between interpupillary and intercanthal disorders. This helps to highlight that Waardenburg's syndrome is not marked by ocular hypertelorism, but rather by a widening of the intercanthal distance due to the lateral displacement of the medial canthi. Figure 6 shows the features of synophrys, broad prominent nasal root, and iris heterochromia.

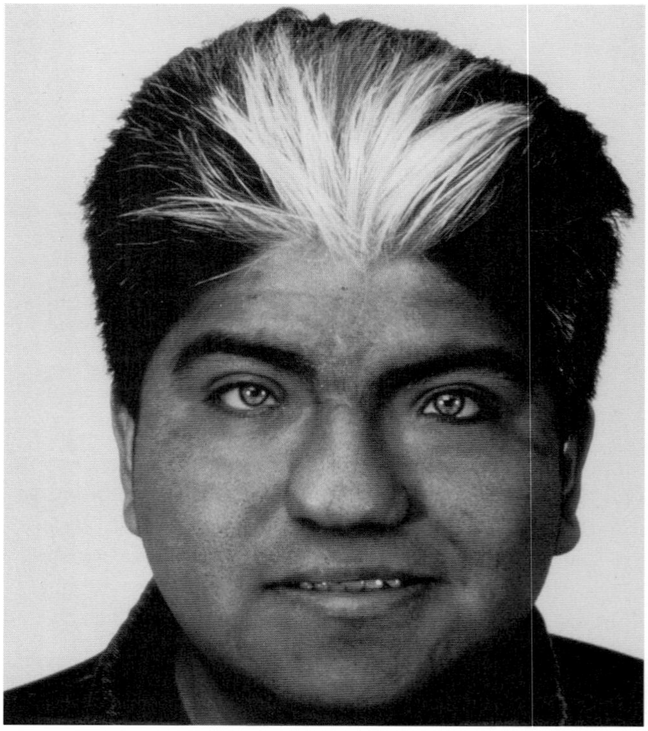

FIG. 6. Waardenburg syndrome type I: Note the findings of dystopia canthorum, prominent broad nasal root, and synophrys. Courtesy of Theresa San Agustin, MD, National Institutes of Health.

Goldenhar's Syndrome (Oculo-Auriculo-Vertebral Spectrum, Hemifacial Microsomia)

Goldenhar's syndrome usually occurs sporadically; however, autosomal dominant transmission may occur. The incidence is approximately 1 per 5,600 live births. There is a male preponderance. Physical abnormalities range from mild to severe. Typical eye findings include epibulbar dermoids and colobomas (notches or defects) of the upper eyelids. Facial asymmetry is marked by unilateral hypoplasia of the mandibular ramus and condyle. Lateral cleftlike extensions from the corner of the mouth give the appearance of macrosomia. There may be either fusion or absence of cervical vertebrae. Cleft lip, cleft palate, congenital cardiac disease, and renal disease may occur. Ear findings include multiple preauricular skin tags from the tragus to the corner of the mouth, microtia, stenosis or atresia of the external auditory canal, tympanic membrane abnormalities, and ossicular malformations. The hearing impairment is conductive (14).

Formation of an eyelid coloboma follows classic embryologic growth arrest. At 5 to 6 weeks' gestation, the optic vesicle invaginates the distal and inferior margin, leading to the optic cup and the ventral embryonic ocular fissure (1). Formation of a coloboma usually results from an arrest in the normal process of invagination of optic neuroectoderm just prior to the point of embryonic fissure closure. Figure

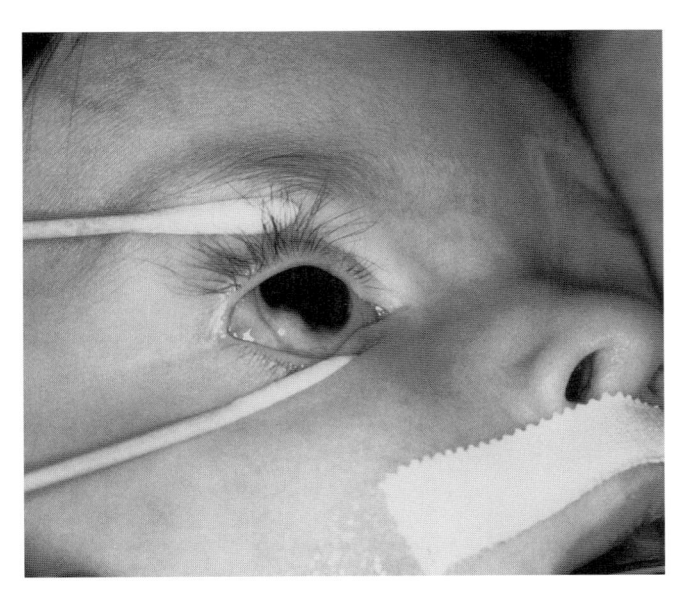

FIG. 7. An epibulbar dermoid in a child with the oculo-auriculo-vertebral spectrum.

7 depicts an epibulbar dermoid in a child with the oculo-auriculo-vertebral spectrum.

Usher Syndromes

The constellation of Usher syndromes are inheritable, progressive pigmentary retinopathies (retinitis pigmentosa) with initial nyctalopia (night blindness) and later development of visual field constriction and ultimate loss of central vision. Von Graefe (15) and Liebreich (16) noted the high frequency of combined deafness and blindness in Berlin Jews. The British ophthalmologist, Charles Usher, noted that 11 of his 69 retinitis pigmentosa patients were deaf, and he emphasized the hereditary nature of the disease (17). Usher syndromes are a heterogeneous set of diseases with autosomal recessive inheritance (18,19). In the United States, the general incidence is 4.4 per 100,000 population. Three percent to 6% of the deaf population and 66% of all deaf and blind people have a form of the Usher syndromes (20).

Usher's syndrome Type I is the most common form. Recent genetic studies link Type I to chromosome 14q (long arm) in French families, 11p (short arm) in isolated Louisiana Acadians, and 11q in other families from Sweden, Iceland, South Africa and the United States (21–23). Type II has been localized to chromosome 1q (24,25). The term *retinitis pigmentosa,* itself, is a misnomer because there is little or no evidence of histopathologic inflammation. Rather, *pigmentary degeneration* or *dystrophy of retinal pigment* are more accurate descriptive terms. Most patients develop pigment deposition in the walls of sclerosed retinal vessels. This gives the characteristic "bone spicule" pattern. However, the retinal pigment deposition is a secondary effect of the disease process and may not be the actual cause of the retinal deterioration (26). Figure 8 demonstrates the predominantly lateral pigmentary deposits seen on the retina.

Early diagnosis by an ophthalmologist is essential. Most useful tests include the electroretinogram, electrooculogram, dark adaptation recordings, visual field testing, and best corrected visual acuity (27,28). The ERG measures the health of the total retinal pigmentary epithelium. Because this is severely affected early in the disease process, it remains the gold standard for early diagnosis. Once the disease process affects 30% to 40% of the retinal pigmentary epithelium, the test becomes abnormal.

Hearing impairment is neurosensory and bilateral (28,29). Temporal bone histopathology demonstrates degeneration of the striae vascularis, organ of Corti and spiral ganglion atrophy, and central nerve degeneration (30). Cochlear implantation in four type I patients has recently been reported with promising results (31). The Merin classification (Table 1) outlines typical findings of the various Usher types (32).

A screening ERG for the infant or child with a family history of any retinal pigmentary disease may detect early peripheral abnormalities. The ERG is strongly recommended by the Usher Syndrome Consortium for any suspected individual (33). However, because only 3% to 6% of the profoundly hearing impaired population have a form of Usher syndromes, routine comprehensive ERG screening may not be cost effective in the evaluation of a child suspected of having an oculoauditory disorder. Therefore, the use of ERG as a screening test should be at the discretion of the examining ophthalmogeneticist.

Duane's Retraction Syndrome

Of all congenital oculomotor abnormalities, Duane's retraction syndrome is the most common. One percent of all patients with congenital strabismus have the disorder, which consists of limitation of lateral rectus abduction, slight limitation of adduction, either elevation or depression on adduction (upshoot or downshoot), and retraction of the globe on attempted adduction (34,35). Visual acuity is usually normal. The palpebral fissure typically narrows on attempted adduction. Most patients with Duane's retraction syndrome and strabismus in the primary position adopt a head turn to achieve single binocular vision. This maneuver avoids the development of amblyopia (36). The left eye is usually affected, though the reason for this is unclear. The mode of inheritance is unknown. Some degree of sex linkage may exist, with most series demonstrating about a 60:40 female to male ratio (37,38). However, sporadic onset appears to be more common than hereditary origin (35). Though numerous theories abound, the etiology for this condition is still uncertain.

Duane's retraction syndrome represents one component of the cervico-oculo-acoustic (Wildervanck) syndrome. The triad also includes fused cervical vertebrae (Klippel-Feil) and moderate to severe congenital hearing loss (39–41). Approximately 5% of patients with solely the Duane's retraction syndrome component have severe neurosensory hearing impairment. Another 5% have high-frequency hearing loss (35,42). Those patients who also have the cervical vertebral

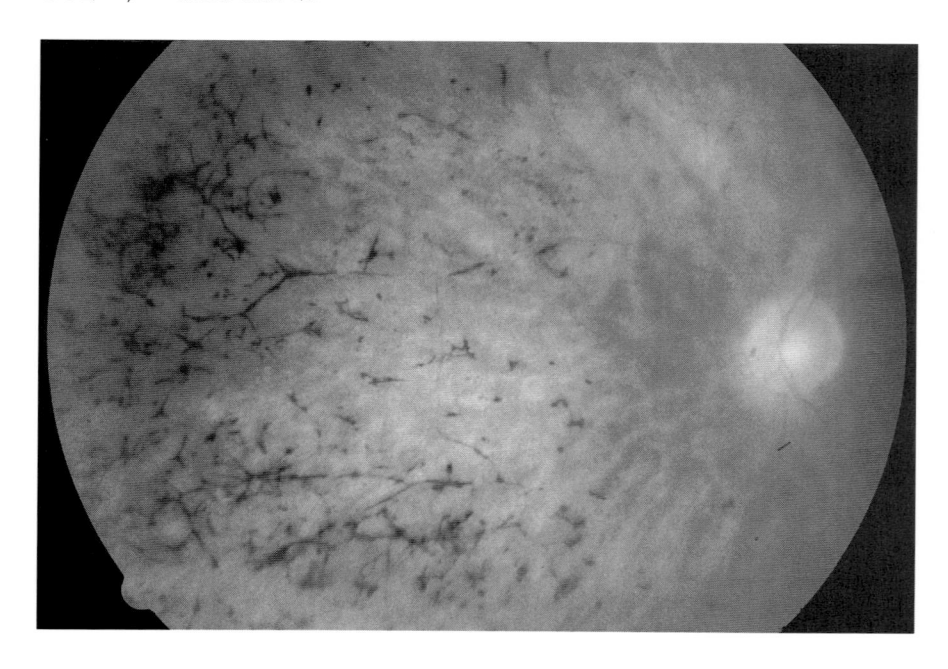

FIG. 8. This retinal photograph depicts the "bone spicules" of pigmentary deposits seen in Usher syndromes. Courtesy of Muriel Kaiser-Kupfer, MD, National Eye Institute, National Institutes of Health.

element of the Wildervanck triad should be suspected of having possible conductive hearing loss secondary to ossicular abnormalities, including stapes footplate fixation (41). Neurosensory hearing loss has been shown to be associated with several cochlear, vestibular and internal auditory canal anomalies (43–45). Figures 9 and 10 demonstrate the computed tomographic (CT) features of common cochleovestibular cavity and narrowed internal acoustic canal seen in a patient with Duane's retraction syndrome associated with severe neurosensory hearing loss.

SUMMARY

Because the optic and otic placodes simultaneously develop in utero and are often adversely affected together, an abnormality in one merits a full examination in the other. Otolaryngologists can learn to discern the physical features of certain ocular abnormalities seen in common oculoacoustic syndromes. Systematic examination starts with an overall facial gestalt and recollection of previously examined children with any similar facial or ocular abnormalities. The clinician then notes any specific eye findings, beginning with the soft tissues around the eyes, followed by focusing on the ocular structures.

Even though the otolaryngologist may pick up important clues on the history and physical examination, consultation with an ophthalmologist trained in genetic disorders is necessary to provide the appropriate, complete evaluation of the child with newly diagnosed, severe unilateral or bilateral

TABLE 1. *Typical findings of various Usher's syndrome types*

	Eye Findings	Hearing	Vestibular	Other
Type I	Retinitis pigmentosa Nyctalopia-onset 1st or early 2nd decade Visual field loss: 1st decade ERG: nondetectable	Congenital, total	No function	
Type II	Retinitis pigmentosa	Congenital, partial	Normal	
	Nyctalopia-onset 2nd or early 3rd decade Visual field loss-variable ERG-variable, from nondetectable to subnormal	Congenital, partial almost straight line drop-off from low to high frequencies	Normal	
Type III (Hallgren)	Retinitis pigmentosa	Congenital, total	Vestibulo-cerebellar ataxia	Possible psychoses (schizophrenia) (retardation)
Type IV (Infantile phytanic acid storage)	Retinitis pigmentosa	Congenital, total		Hypotonia Mental retardation Serum levels less than in Refsum

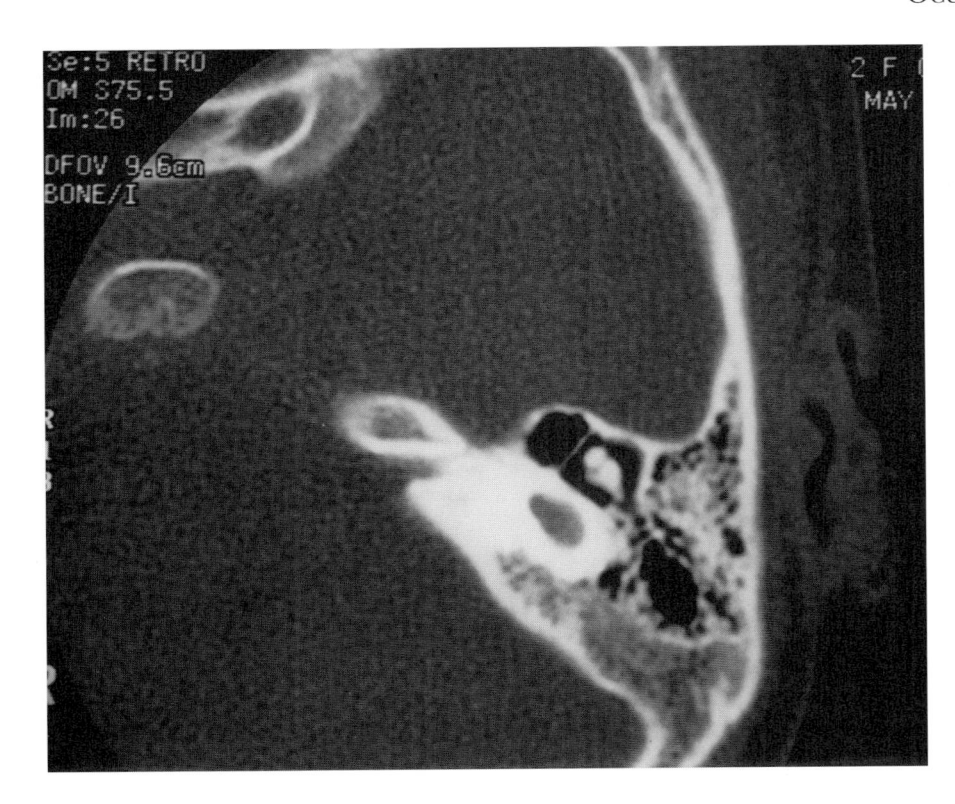

FIG. 9. A CT scan of the left common cochleovestibular cavity in a patient with Duane's retraction syndrome and severe left neurosensory hearing loss.

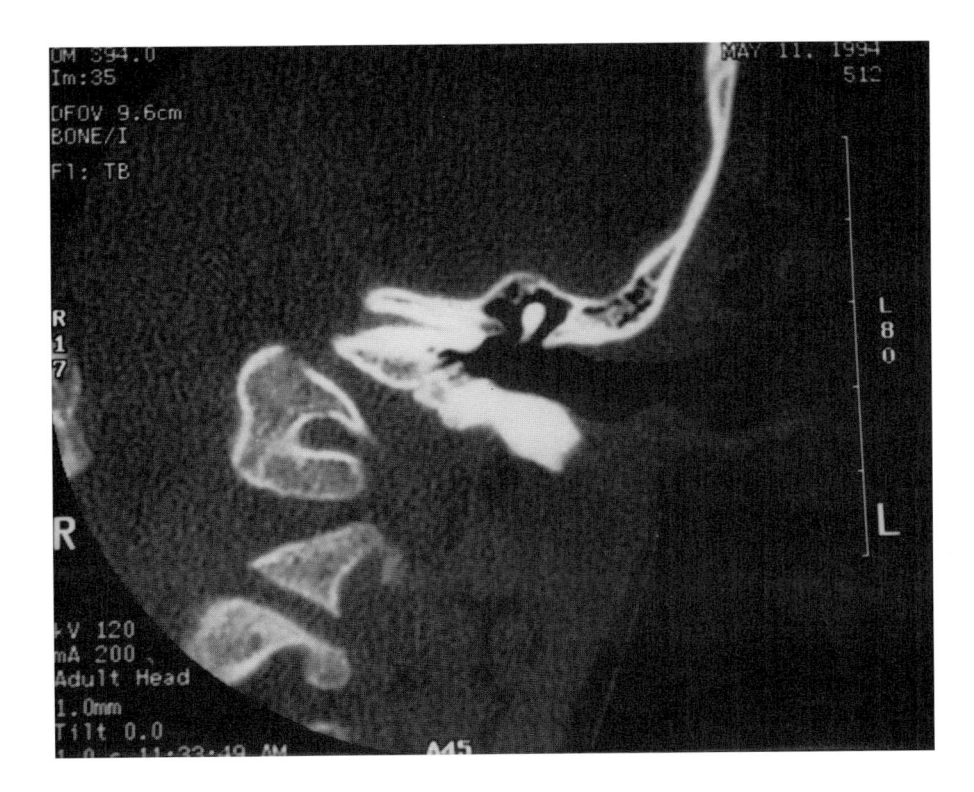

FIG. 10. A CT scan showing a narrowed left internal acoustic canal in the same patient as in Fig. 9.

neurosensory hearing loss. An ERG is strongly recommended in any individual suspected of having a retinal pigmentary disturbance. In addition, consultation with a geneticist may prove valuable in diagnosis, treatment, and counseling for the patient and family.

REFERENCES

1. Hamming NA, Apple D. Anatomy and embryology of the eye. In: Peyman GA, Sanders DR, Goldberg MF, eds. *Principles and practice of ophthalmology.* vol 1. Philadelphia: WB Saunders, 1980.
2. Gieser SC, Carey JC, Apple DJ. Human chromosomal disorders and the eye. In: Renie WA, Goldberg MF, eds. *Goldberg's genetic and metabolic eye disease.* 2nd ed. Boston: Little, Brown, 1986.
3. Vaughan D, Asbury T. *General ophthalmology.* 10th ed. Los Altos, CA: Lange Medical, 1983.
4. Trobe JD. *The physician's guide to eye care.* American Academy of Ophthalmology, 1993.
5. Waardenburg PJ. A new syndrome combining developmental anomalies of the eyelids, eyebrows, and nose root, with pigmentary defects of the iris and head hair and with congenital deafness. *Am J Hum Genet* 1951;3:195–253.
6. Fisch L. Deafness as part of an hereditary syndrome. *J Laryngol Otol* 1959;73:355–383.
7. Arias S. Genetic heterogeneity in the Waardenburg syndrome. *Birth Defects* 1971;7:87–101.
8. Arias S, Mota M. Apparent non-penetrance for dystopia in Waardenburg syndrome type I with some hints on the diagnosis of dystopia canthorum. *J Genet Hum* 1978;26:101–131.
9. Arias S. Waardenburg syndrome. Two distinct types. [Letter to the Editor] *Am J Med Genet* 1980;6:99–100.
10. Dellman JW, Hageman MJ. Ophthalmological findings in 34 patients with Waardenburg syndrome. *J Pediatr Ophthalmol Strabismus* 1978;15:341–345.
11. Hageman MJ, Dellman JW. Heterogeneity in Waardenburg syndrome. *Am J Hum Genet* 1977;29:468–485.
12. Hageman MJ. Audiometric findings in 34 patients with Waardenburg's syndrome. *J Laryngol Otol* 1977;91:575–584.
13. Farrer LA, Grundfast KM, Amos J, et al. Waardenburg syndrome (WS) type I is caused by defects at multiple loci, one of which is near ALPP on chromosome 2: first report of the WS consortium. *Am J Hum Genet* 1992;50:902–913.
14. Grundfast KM, Lalwani AK. Practical approach to diagnosis and management of hereditary hearing impairment (HHI). *Ear Nose Throat J* 1992;71:479–493.
15. von Graefe A. Exceptionelles Verhalten des Gesichtsfeldes bei Pigmententartung der Netzhaut. *Graefes Arch Clin Ophthalmol* 1858;4:250–253.
16. Liebreich R. Abkunft aus Ehen unter blutsverwandten als grund van retinitis pigmentosa. *Dtsch Klin* 1861;13:53.
17. Usher CH. On the inheritance of retinitis pigmentosa with notes of cases. *R Lond Ophthal Hosp Rep* 1914;19:1930–2036.
18. Dahl SP, Weston MD, Kimberling WJ, Gorin MB, Shugart YY, Kenyon JB. Possible genetic heterogeneity of Usher syndrome type II: a family unlinked to chromosome 1q markers. Washington, DC: 8th International Congress of Human Genetics, 1991.
19. Fishman GA, Kumar A, Joseph ME, Torok N, Anderson RJ. Usher's Syndrome: Ophthalmic and neuro-otologic findings suggesting genetic heterogeneity. *Arch Ophthalmol* 1983;101:1367–1374.
20. Merin S, Auerbach E. Retinitis pigmentosa. *Surv Ophthalmol* 1976;20:303–345.
21. Kaplan J, Gerber S, Bonneau D, et al. A gene for Usher syndrome type I (USHIA) maps to chromosome 14q. *Genomics* 1992;14:979–987.
22. Evans KL, Fantes J, Simpson C, et al. Human olfactory marker protein maps close to tyrosinase and is a candidate gene for Usher syndrome type I. *Hum Mol Genet* 1993;2(2):115–118.
23. Smith RJH, Lee EC, Kimberling WJ, et al. Localization of two genes for Usher syndrome type I to chromosome 11. *Genomics* 1992;14:995–1002.
24. Kimberling WJ, Weston MD, Moller, et al. Localization of Usher syndrome type II to chromosome 1q. *Genomics* 1990;7:245–249.
25. Lewis RA, Otterud B, Stauffer D, et al. Mapping recessive ophthalmic diseases: Linkage of the locus for Usher syndrome type II to a DNA marker on chromosome 1q. *Genomics* 1990;7:250–256.
26. Marshall J, Heckinlively JR. Pathologic findings and putative mechanisms in retinitis pigmentosa. In: *Retinitis pigmentosa.* Heckinlively JR, ed. Philadelphia: JB Lippincott, 1988.
27. Heckinlively JR. The diagnosis and classification of retinitis pigmentosa. *Retinitis pigmentosa.* Philadelphia: JB Lippincott, 1988.
28. Samuelson S, Zahn J. Usher's syndrome. *Ophthal Paediatr Genet* 1990;11(1):71–76.
29. Vernon M. Usher's syndrome—deafness and progressive blindness. *J Chron Dis* 1969;22:133–151.
30. Schuknecht HF. *Pathology of the ear.* Cambridge, MA: Harvard University Press, 1974.
31. Hinderlink JB, Mens LH, Brokx JP, van den Broek P. Results from four cochlear implant patients with Usher's syndrome. *Ann Otol Rhinol Laryngol* 1994;103:285–293.
32. Merin S, Abraham FA, Auerbach E. Usher's and Hallgren's syndromes. *Acta Genet Med Gemellol (Roma)* 1974;23:49–55.
33. Smith RJH, Berlin CI, Hejtmancik JF, et al. Clinical diagnosis of the Usher syndromes. *Am J Med Genet* 1994;50:32–38.
34. Duane A. Congenital deficiency of abduction, associated with impairment of adduction, retraction movements, contraction of the palpebral fissure and oblique movements of the eye. *Arch Ophthalmol* 1905;34:133–159.
35. Shauly Y, Weissman A, Meyer E. Ocular and systemic characteristics of Duane's syndrome. *J Pediatr Ophthalmol Strabismus* 1993;30:178–183.
36. Kowal VO, McKeown CA. Duane's syndrome. *Int Ophthalmol Clin* 1992.
37. Pfaffenbach DD, Cross HE, Kearns TP. Congenital anomalies in Duane's retraction syndrome. *Arch Ophthalmol* 1972;88:635–639.
38. Kirkham TH. Inheritance of Duane's syndrome. *Br J Ophthalmol* 1970;54:323–329.
39. Wildervanck LS. Een geval van aandoening van Klippel-Feil, gecombineerd met abducensparalyse, retractio bulbi en doofstomheid. *Ned Tijdschr Geneeskd* 1952;96:2752–2756.
40. Wildervanck LS. Een cervico-oculo-acusticussyndroom. *Ned Tijdschr Geneeskd* 1960;104:2600–2605.
41. Cremers WRJ, Hoohland GA, Kuypers W. Hearing loss in the cervico-oculo-acoustic (Wildervanck) syndrome. *Arch Otolaryngol* 1984;110:54–57.
42. Ro A, Chernoff G, MacRae, Orton RB, Cadera W. Auditory function in Duane's retraction syndrome. *Am J Ophthalmol* 1990;109:75–78.
43. Schuknecht H. Mondini dysplasia–a clinical and pathological study. *Ann Otol* 1980;89[Suppl 65]:3–23.
44. Schild JA, Mafee MF, Miller MF. Wildervanck syndrome—the external appearance and radiologic findings. *Int J Pediatr Otorhinolaryngol* 1984;7:305–310.
45. West PDB, Gholkar A, Ransden RT. Wildervanck's syndrome—unilateral Mondini dysplasia identified by computed tomography. *J Laryngol Otol* 1989;103:408–411.

CHAPTER 24

The Acquired Hearing Losses of Childhood

Richard M. Irving and Robert J. Ruben

Hearing loss in childhood is important because of its profound effects on child development. Initially, hearing loss may result in impaired language and communication skills, which in turn can lead to poor social and educational progress. Early diagnosis and treatment is essential so that the effects of the hearing loss on the child can be minimized.

Hearing loss has been defined by the International Association of Physician Audiologists as loss greater than 20 dB, average of 0.5, 1, 2, and 4 kHz in the better ear (1). This is called the better ear hearing level (BEHL). The reported prevalence of hearing loss in childhood using this definition is 5.9% (at age 8 yr) and 12% (at age 18 yr) (2). The incidence of severe to profound hearing loss (> 80 dB at 0.5, 1, 2, and 4 kHz) is reported as 1 in 1,000 children at birth, doubling in the first few years of life, and doubling again to 4 in 1,000 children by the end of their adolescence (3).

Measuring hearing loss in this way, as a pure-tone average, is far from ideal, because hearing loss implies a hearing level that has a deleterious effect on the child's development. Children of different abilities respond variably to hearing loss; the age of onset and fluctuation of the hearing loss are also important (4). It is recognized that hearing loss tends to have a lesser effect in older children (1). At present, no true definition of hearing loss takes these additional factors into account.

The presentation of hearing loss is protean. Some children present with an obvious otologic history, either recurrent ear infections or a suspicion of deafness. In 70% of patients, the parents suspect that their child may have a hearing loss. Others are detected by infant or child screening programs, or are picked up by the child's teacher. Developmental delay, particularly for speech and language, and behavioral disturbance are less frequent modes of presentation.

R.M. Irving: Department of Otolaryngology, University Hospital, Birmingham NHS Trust, Birmingham, United Kingdom.
R.J. Ruben: Departments of Otolaryngology and Paediatrics, Albert Einstein College of Medicine and Montefiore Medical Center, Bronx, New York 10467.

The variability of presentation makes the diagnosis difficult—an alarming number of children with hearing loss are diagnosed in late childhood. In a European study of children born in 1969, only 55% of children with losses of 50 dB (BEHL) or greater were found to be identified by 3 years of age (4). In a study from the United States, looking exclusively at sensorineural impairment, 40 to 80 dB (BEHL) losses were not diagnosed until an average age of 8.8 years (5), and 20 to 40 dB (BEHL) losses were first detected at an even later age.

Hearing loss is hereditary in approximately one third of patients, acquired in one third of patients, and of unknown etiology in the remaining third (6). The acquired losses have been classified according to the time at which the auditory damage occurred (Table 1).

GENETIC HEARING LOSS

Genetic diseases can present in childhood with a progressive hearing loss that can be difficult to distinguish from acquired deafness. Some of these disorders may occur congenitally and progress throughout life; others only become apparent later in childhood or adolescence.

It is a reflection on the complexity of ear development that in some 30% of cases of genetic deafness there are associated clinical features comprising a syndrome. The diagnosis of genetic deafness in such cases is relatively straightforward. In contrast, nonsyndromic deafness, in which hearing loss is the sole presenting feature, is frequently inseparable from an acquired hearing loss. An attempt should be made to distinguish these types, although in a large proportion of patients a specific diagnosis can not be made.

The syndromic and the nonsyndromic progressive losses may be inherited as autosomal recessive, autosomal dominant, sex-linked or mitochondrial loss. The most frequently diagnosed autosomal recessive progressive losses are Usher's type III and Pendred syndrome (7). Hearing loss associated with mitochondrial diseases is observed in about half the

TABLE 1. *Acquired hearing losses of childhood*

Prenatal
    Rubella
    Cytomegalovirus
    Toxoplasmosis
    Congenital syphilis
    Inner-ear teratogenesis
Perinatal
    Severe perinatal disease
    Persistent fetal circulation
    Kernicterus
Postnatal
    Otitis media with effusion
    Meningitis
    Viral infections
    Chronic otitis media
    Autoimmune
    Ototoxic drugs
    Head trauma
    Acoustic trauma
    Perilymph fistula
    CPA and petrous apex lesions
    Ménière's disease

CPA, cerebellopontine angle.

patients with the main associated syndromes: Kearns-Sayre syndrome (8); myoclonic epilepsy associated with ragged red fibers (MERRF) (9), mitochondrial encephalopathy, lactic acidosis and stroke-like episodes (MELAS) (10) and mitochondrial diabetes (11). Mitochondrial mutations of ribosomal RNA (1555 A–G) are associated with increased susceptibility to aminoglycoside induced ototoxic deafness (12). This RNA mutation can explain why an occasional patient has sensorneural hearing loss (SNHL) following standard dosage of an aminoglycoside. There is no readily available screen for this condition. In a group of hearing-impaired children with a presumed 40% genetic etiology, studies have shown that two thirds of the children have a progressive loss in a 5-year period (13). Children with presumed genetic losses therefore need to be followed into early adult life with continued audiometric monitoring.

ACQUIRED PRENATAL HEARING LOSS

Rubella

Congenital rubella syndrome describes a triad of eye defects, cardiac abnormalities and deafness. The hearing loss usually has a flat configuration, is severe or profound, and may be asymmetric. In the past, Rubella accounted for approximately 10% of childhood SNHL (14). Characteristically, SNHL follows a maternal infection in the second or third months of pregnancy; more than 50% of the children born from these pregnancies are deaf (15). Infection after the second month of pregnancy can also result in hearing loss for the child, but usually the other features of the congenital rubella syndrome are absent (14). Hearing loss can also follow a subclinical maternal infection. In patients who have isolated deafness, the diagnosis is suspected if the patient's mother had a rash during the first trimester of pregnancy, but a clear diagnosis can be made only if an increase in the maternal rubella antibody titer is also demonstrated. Alternatively, an ophthalmologic examination of the infant may reveal evidence of pigment abnormalities diagnostic of rubella embryopathy.

Cytomegalovirus

Infection with the cytomegalovirus (CMV), a herpes virus, is recognized as the most common fetal viral illness, with an incidence of 1% of all live births (16). Infection is usually acquired in utero, although some cases follow exposure to infected maternal genital secretions during delivery or occur as a result of ingesting breast milk containing CMV. Transmission following CMV-infected blood transfusion has also been described. The majority of women with infection remain asymptomatic, but in 5% of CMV infections the illness is clinically recognizable in the neonate as a more virulent form of the disease. Known as cytomegalic inclusion disease (CID) (16) this condition is characterized by low birth weight, prematurity, microcephaly, chorioretinitis, purpura, icterus, and hepatosplenomegaly. A further 5% have atypical clinical involvement, but 90% have no clinical manifestations at birth (16).

Maternal CMV infection during pregnancy differs from other viral infections, such as rubella or toxoplasmosis, because it can arise as a primary infection or as a result of reinfection or reactivation of latent virus. Maternal immunity in recurrent cases may be present but inadequate to prevent reinfection. It can however, influence the fetal illness, and a congenital infection is more likely to be serious in the neonate if it results from a primary rather than a recurrent infection (16). Hearing loss occurs in 30% to 60% of cases of CID but can also follow atypical or subclinical CMV infection (16). The true incidence of hearing loss following subclinical infection is unknown but estimated to be about 10% of patients (16–18). The hearing loss varies in severity from mild to profound and is often unilateral.

Cytomegaloviral infections, like other herpes virus infections, are characterized by dormancy and reactivation, and the clinical course of the disease is characteristically chronic with periodic exacerbations. The resulting hearing loss may be progressive in nature, and in some cases can develop after the first year of life (19). Regular audiometric evaluation, at least until the age of six (16) is advised for these children.

The most sensitive and specific method of diagnosis is viral isolation, either from the urine or saliva, and detection of CMV DNA by polymerase chain reaction. Antibody detection can also confirm CMV infection, but this serologic analysis should be carried out in the first few weeks of life. Because exposure to the virus is very common in young infants, seropositivity later in childhood can not be regarded as confirmation that CMV was the agent responsible for the hearing loss (18).

Toxoplasmosis

Toxoplasmosis is an infection caused by the obligate intracellular parasite *Toxoplasma gondii*. It is most often acquired following the ingestion of material contaminated with feces from infected cats. If a woman is infected for the first time during pregnancy, the fetus may be affected. The majority of maternal infections are subclinical; what proportion of the infections result in fetal infection is not known. About 5% to 10% of infected neonates show evidence of severe involvement at birth, the central nervous system, retina and choroid are the common sites of involvement. Neonates with subclinical infection at birth go on to develop signs of the infection, notably retinal abnormalities, in the majority of cases by the age of 16 years.

Unilateral, bilateral, and frequently progressive SNHL has been reported in 14% to 26% of infected patients (20,21). Calcium deposits have been identified in the spiral ligament of the cochlea, similar to the areas of cerebral calcification seen in congenital toxoplasmosis (22). The progressive nature of the hearing loss is thought to be due to the continued inflammatory response to the parasite within the cochlea and also to its replication. The diagnosis is made by a combination of characteristic clinical findings, including chorioretinitis, cerebral calcifications, and serologic testing.

Congenital Syphilis

In 1917 Sir William Osler observed that 20% of stillbirths and 22% of infant deaths in the United States resulted from syphilis (23). Now, in the postantibiotic era, syphilis has become a rarity in most areas, but it does remain endemic in certain populations. Syphilis in neonates and children closely parallels the disease in adults, and there are large differences between racial and socioeconomic groups. Infants with syphilis are more likely to be born of mothers who are black or Hispanic and have multiple pregnancies. There is also an association with lower socioeconomic status and drug abuse (23).

In primary or secondary maternal syphilis, there is nearly a 100% chance of transplacental infection of the fetus. This follows exposure to the pathogen during the second half of pregnancy. The severe form of the disease manifests before the age of 2 years with a fulminant course. The majority of cases of congenital syphilis, however, manifest in the second or third decades of life.

Syphilitic labyrinthitis can result either from prenatal or acquired exposure to the spirocete *Treponema pallidum*. Because of the effectiveness of antibiotc therapy in the control of disease, the vast majority of cases are believed to be prenatal in origin (24).

The hearing loss is sensorineural and usually, but not always, symmetric and fluctuating. This may be associated with vertigo, and endolymphatic hydrops may occur, with a similar clinical presentation to Ménière's disease. The hearing loss can be rapidly progressive over weeks or months, rarely presenting as sudden deafness. It is an important diagnosis to make because treatment can prevent hearing loss and, in some patients, improve the hearing.

Inner Ear Teratogenesis

Malformations of the inner ear occur when the development of the inner ear is arrested. In many patients, the cause is inborn genetic error, but some cases result from external influences during the first trimester of pregnancy. Teratogenic influences known to affect inner-ear organogenesis include viral infections such as rubella, chemicals such as thalidomide, (25) and exposure of the fetus to radiation. Inner-ear anomalies can be considered as limited to the membranous labyrinth or involving both the osseous and membranous labyrinth. The latter can be classified according to radiographic appearance (26).

ACQUIRED PERINATAL HEARING LOSS

Severe Perinatal Disease

There is little doubt about the association between a traumatic perinatal period and hearing loss. In such infants there may be a history of hypoxia, sometimes even severe asphyxia, complicated often by kernicterus and treatment with aminoglycosides and diuretics. All are likely to have a synergistic effect on the cochlea. Hearing loss is also demonstrated to occur more frequently with low birth weight (less than 1500 grams) (27) and in children who have had neonatal convulsions (28). The relative contribution of these factors to hearing loss has proved difficult to entangle and is likely to be multifactorial in most of these infants. Hypoxia is associated with neurodevelopmental deficits in childhood, usually manifested by mental retardation and neuromuscular disorders. In severe hypoxia, hearing loss has been reported in 4% of surviving neonates (29).

The characteristics of a hearing loss following a traumatic perinatal period have not been well defined, but the hearing loss may be progressive and present months after discharge from the newborn intensive care unit (NICU) (23). It has been recommended that infants who had severe respiratory distress at birth be screened for hearing loss throughout their first year of life (30).

Persistent Fetal Circulation

Persistent fetal circulation is characterized by continued severe hypoxemia despite ventilatory support and is usually seen in full-term infants. It is associated with a variety of diagnoses. A rate of SNHL of 20% to 50% has been demonstrated in infants who survive this condition; in many patients, the loss is profound (31,32). These children are treated with aggressive hyperventilation, pulmonary vasodilators, and diuretics; they appear to be a subgroup of sick neonates who are at particularly high risk for perinatal acquired hearing loss. In most cases, hearing loss is delayed and progressive; thus, early, serial audiometric evaluation is advised for these infants.

Kernicterus

Hearing loss can occur following exposure to high levels of circulating unconjugated bilirubin in the newborn. This is usually a result of rhesus incompatibility in rhesus-negative mothers but occurs occasionally after blood group incompatibility and is more common in premature babies. Unconjugated bilirubin can cross the immature blood-brain barrier and becomes deposited primarily in the basal ganglia. In kernicterus, the hair cells are characteristically normal and the auditory pathway is thought to be damaged at the level of the auditory nuclei; in some patients, the auditory nerve appears to be involved (33).

The full syndrome is characterized by choreoathetosis, asymmetrical spasticity, disturbed eye movements, and hearing loss. Hearing loss, however, can also be an isolated finding in mild cases (34). The pattern of loss observed is usually mild to severe and is greater for the high frequencies. Carhart described the characteristic audiometric features: a plateau of good hearing in the low frequencies, a sharp decline between 500 and 2,000 Hz, and a plateau of more severe hearing loss in the high frequencies (35).

ACQUIRED POSTNATAL HEARING LOSS

Otitis Media with Effusion

Hearing loss as a result of otitis media with effusion (OME) is the most common cause of acquired hearing loss in childhood and has a prevalence of 10% in children ages 3 to 5 years. There are numerous predisposing factors, such as Down syndrome, cleft palate, adenoid hypertrophy, and passive smoking.

With observation alone, 60% to 80% clear in 3 months, but there is currently a lack of consensus as to the appropriate management of cases that persist. No medical treatment has been shown to significantly influence the outcome of OME other than in the short term (36–38). Ventilation tubes improve hearing while they are in situ, but there is no good evidence to suggest that they influence the course of the disease process. Adenoidectomy has been shown to promote resolution of OME, and evidence suggests that children between the ages of 4 and 8 years are most likely to benefit (39).

A poor outcome is associated with parental smoking, onset of OME before the age of 30 months and a long duration of preoperative hearing loss. In children who present at ages 4 to 8 years and do not undergo adenoidectomy, there is also a significantly poorer outcome. These children are also at increased risk of developing atelectasis and cholesteatoma, with resultant lifelong hearing impairment.

Meningitis

Meningitis and its associated labyrinthitis is the cause of 25% of all severe and profound acquired SNHL in children. Meningitis is mainly bacterial or viral in origin. Bacterial cases tend to have a more serious course and patients are left with more residual symptoms. Despite current medical therapy, there is still considerable morbidity and mortality associated with this disease.

Bacterial meningitis is a disease of young children; 90% of patients are between the age of birth and 5 years. The common causative organisms are *Haemophilus influenzae, Escherichia coli, Neisseria meningitides,* and *Streptococcus pneumoniae.* Neonatal meningitis is most commonly caused by *E. coli,* but after 1 month of age, *H. influenzae* is the predominant organism.

Deafness can result from direct involvement of the cochlear nerve or more commonly, by bacterial invasion of the labyrinth through the cochlear aqueduct, the internal auditory canal (IAC) or the bloodstream. The mechanism of the hearing loss appears to be also partly an immune reaction to invading bacteria (40).

Following bacterial meningitis, hearing loss is noted in 5% to 13% of children; children who have low cerebrospinal (CSF) glucose or a delay in the commencement of antibiotic therapy of 48 hours from the onset of first symptoms are at an increased risk (41).

The use of dexamethasone in the management of acute meningitis has received a great deal of attention in the literature recently. Most studies suggest that the incidence of SNHL is reduced in children treated with dexamethasone (42–49) but some studies indicate no obvious benefit (45). Current evidence is strongly suggestive of benefit when the causative organism is *H. influenzae,* however, there is at present too little evidence to confirm benefit in children with pneumococcal or viral meningitis (46). Published series indicate that the earlier a patient with meningitis is diagnosed and treated, the lesser the probability of SNHL. A 2-day regimen of dexamethasone, 0.15 mg/kg every 6 hours for 4 days, has been proposed as adequate (47) and maximal benefit has been demonstrated if steroids are started before the administration of antibiotics (48). There is, however, individual variability. Some children who have been diagnosed and treated early have had SNHL, but others who were diagnosed late had no SNHL.

Meningitic labyrinthitis is a progressive disorder. The continuing process of ossification of the scalae of the cochlea is one expression (Fig. 1). The hearing loss may continue in an episodic and fluctuating fashion years after the initial infection (49) and serial audiometric evaluations are required for these children.

Treatment of progressive hearing losses with corticosteroids is appropriate on the basis of its effectiveness in the

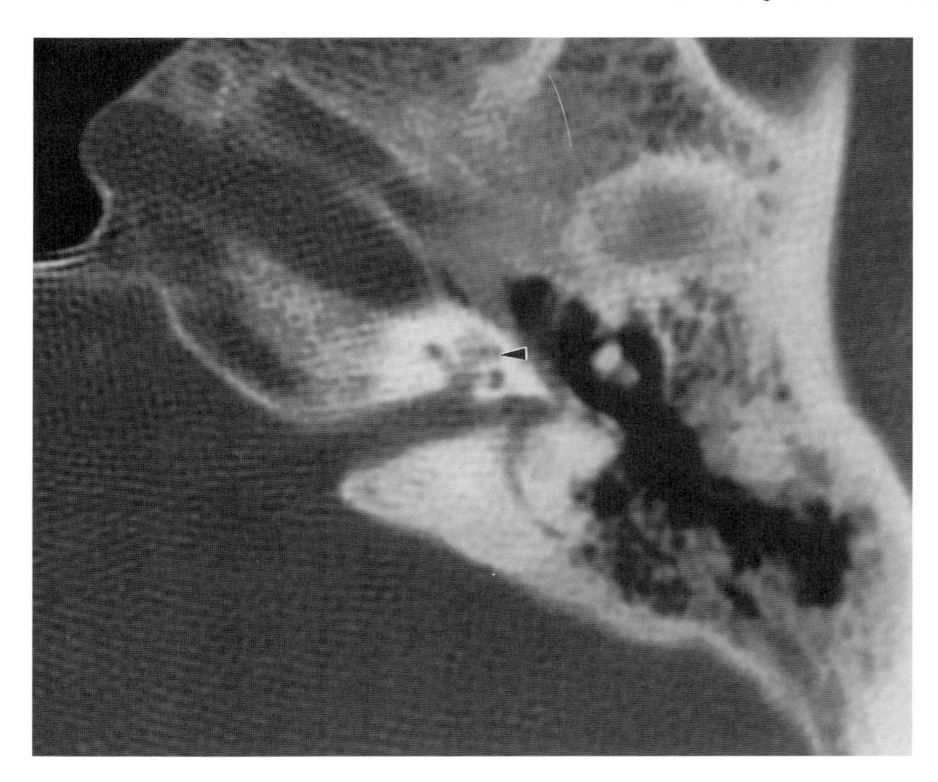

FIG. 1. Transaxial CT scan demonstrating labyrinthitis ossificans involving the basal and apical turns of the cochlea.

acute stage and evidence that the losses may in part result from an immune reaction. The possibility of late hearing improvement has also been reported, although this is a rare occurrence (50).

Viral Infections

The most common cause of viral-acquired SNHL is mumps. Studies from Japan (51) show that 3% of all sudden deafness reported is attributable to mumps; most of the cases were unilateral. Sensorineural hearing loss associated with measles infection has been reported from nonindustrialised countries (52). There are also reported cases of SNHL following immunization with measles, mumps, and rubella vaccine (53).

Chronic Otitis Media

The majority of cases of acute otitis media resolve with no sequelae. A small number of patients are left with conductive hearing loss caused either by a persistent tympanic-membrane perforation or damage to the ossicular chain. Children with repeated episodes of bacterial otitis media are also found to have an increased incidence of SNHL (54,55) predominantly for the high tones, but in most patients this loss is not clinically significant (56). Hearing loss is thought to be caused by bacterial endotoxins (57), but there may be an ototoxic component in some patients (58). Irreversible atelectasis resulting from persistent tubal dysfunction also causes conductive loss, which is bilateral in many patients.

Atelectasis may follow OME despite prompt treatment with adenoidectomy and ventilation tubes.

Cholesteatoma in very young children is usually congenital. Acquired cholesteatoma may also occur following OME with chronic middle-ear dysfunction or, in some patients, with no otologic history. If the disease is detected early, prompt removal can be achieved with little or no loss of hearing. However, if the disease has spread to involve the ossicles and mastoid, a significant hearing loss may result.

There is some evidence to suggest that the prompt and continued use of a tympanostomy tube may help to prevent cholesteatoma. Dominguez and Harker (59) showed that the prevalence of cholesteatoma in children with cleft palate in Iowa was 9.2% from 1947 to 1968. During the period 1969 to 1977, the prevalence was 2.6%. This threefold difference has been attributed to the early use of tympanostomy tubes; however, there is also evidence to suggest that the incidence of acquired cholesteatoma in the general population has not declined since the introduction and widespread use of the ventilation tube (60,61).

Autoimmune Disease

There are numerous reports in the literature of children with nonsyndromic hearing loss and serum abnormalities compatible with an autoimmune process (62–64). Systemic vasculitis can also involve the inner ear, and SNHL in children has been documented in Cogan syndrome (65) and Takayasu's disease (66).

Autoimmune mechanisms have also been found to be a

factor in several syndromic forms of hearing loss, such as parvo virus infection (67), scleroderma (68) and Kawasaki disease (69). In the latter, there is the possibility that salicylate may have contributed to the SNHL and that its withdrawal may have accounted for the improvement. Nevertheless, collective reports suggest that children with autoimmune diseases and systemic vasculitis should be evaluated for the possibility of hearing loss, which can present early in childhood; the youngest reported case of suspected autoimmune hearing loss is at age 19 months (64). Reports also indicate that the prognosis for these diseases can be improved by treating the SNHL with corticosteroids, although whether therapy will be effective is difficult to predict; and what constitutes an effective regimen is also unknown.

Ototoxicity

The most commonly reported agents causing ototoxicity in children are aminoglycosides, diuretics, salicylates, and cytotoxic agents. In the majority of cases, the cochlea is more susceptible to damage than is the vestibular apparatus (Table 2). Many of these agents have a synergistic effect, and toxicity is also potentiated by coexistent renal disease. Some patients have a hereditary susceptibility to aminoglycosides and an associated mitochondrial small ribosomal RNA gene mutation (12). Toxicity directly relates to drug levels; therefore, careful blood monitoring, especially for susceptible patients, is mandatory to reduce the risk of ototoxicity from systemic agents.

The hearing loss from ototoxicity is sensorineural, is usually symmetric, and manifests initially in the high frequencies. Ototoxicity may also be associated with tinnitus and vestibular symptoms. The use of ototoxic antibiotics in the middle-ear cleft has been associated with SNHL (55,58,70,71). Whether the reported hearing loss is related to repeated applications of ototoxic drugs or to middle-ear sepsis is unknown. However, it seems prudent to use an antibiotic that does not contain an ototoxic agent for a patient who has a tympanostomy tube or tympanic-membrane perforation.

TABLE 2. *Ototoxic drug characteristics*

Drug	Cochleotoxic	Vestibulotoxic
Streptomycin	+	+ +
Gentamycin	+	+ + +
Dihydrostreptomycin	+ +	+
Neomycin	+ + + +	+
Kanamycin	+ + +	+
Erythromycin	+	−
Vancomycin	+ +	+
Furosemide	+	±
Quinine	+	−
Cisplatin	+	−
Salicylates	+	+

Trauma

Conductive losses occurring as a result of injury to the middle ear are another cause of acquired losses in children. A commonly seen cause is perforations of the tympanic membrane or damage to ossicles from foreign bodies in the ear canal (from the foreign body itself or as a result of an attempt to remove the object). Temporal bone fractures can result in mixed hearing losses and are seen as a result of motor vehicle accidents, most commonly in young children age under 2 years of age and in adolescent boys (72) (Fig. 2). Hearing loss can also result from irradiation of pediatric intracranial tumours, particularly for lesions involving the brainstem.

Acoustic Trauma

Sound trauma (73,74) causes a significant amount of acquired SNHL in childhood. Sound-induced SNHL has been reported in a child of 14 months from a firecracker, and 26% of a series of patients with SNHL from noise were less than 10 years of age. The most commonly reported cases of hearing loss, both bilateral and unilateral, are fireworks, firearms, music at discotheques and rock concerts, recreational vehicles (primarily snowmobiles), power tools, and other power equipment (75). Other sources of potential sound trauma from music are the portable tape cassette and compact disc players and boom boxes; the output of the latter may exceed 120 dB.

Perilymphatic Fistula

Perilymphatic fistula (PLF) has been reported as a cause of acquired, genetic, and idiopathic progressive SNHL in childhood. Hereditary PLF has been reported in one set of identical twins (76). Most commonly, however, PLF is associated with no known etiology. Trauma is believed to be the major cause of acquired PLF. Several cases (unpublished observations) of acquired PLF have been surgically diagnosed in infants and young children who have sustained minor head injury. The injuries resulted in a progressive SNHL in the first year of life. At surgery, the children were found to have displaced stapes with an active loss of perilymph fluid from the oval window.

The diagnosis of PLF depends on a history of progressive SNHL. The progression of the hearing loss may be episodic and can be associated with true rotatory vertigo. An audiogram usually shows severe to profound SNHL with markedly poor speech discrimination. Vestibular function may also be abnormal (76,77). The use of imaging techniques to detect a PLF has not proved useful (78–80).

Controversy surrounds the diagnosis and management of PLF in children. The candidate group for exploratory tympanotomy are children with rapidly or intermittently progressive SNHL and abnormality of vestibular function. The outcome following surgical repair of a congenital or acquired PLF is variable, but usually the vestibular symptoms are relieved. In some patients, restoration of hearing or the halt-

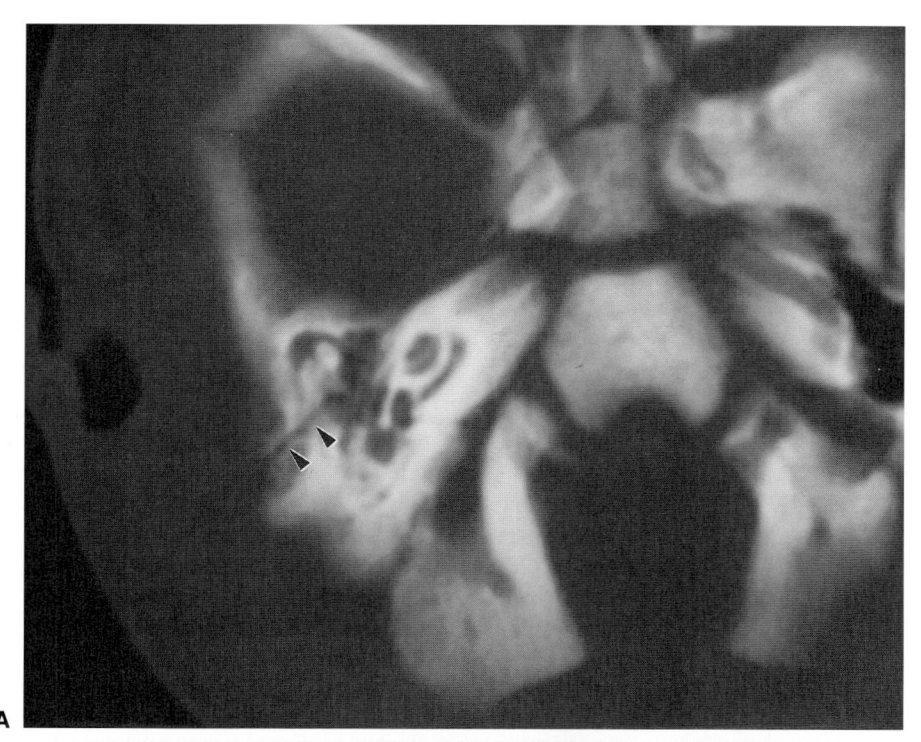

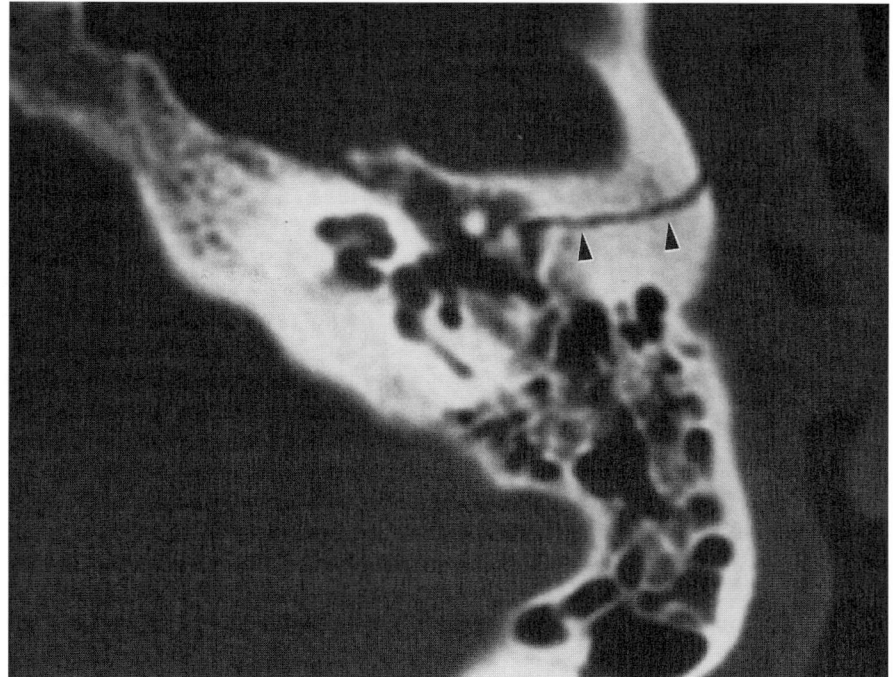

FIG. 2. High-resolution transaxial CT scans demonstrating classic longitudinal temporal bone fractures; **A:** in a neonate; **B:** in a teenage boy. In the neonate, the fracture was the result of forceps trauma. In both patients, the fracture extended through the roof of the external auditory meatus. The incudomalleal joint in B is disrupted and the incus is laterally and posteriorly rotated.

ing of progression of SNHL can be achieved (76) but the hearing results are generally disappointing.

Temporal Bone, Petrous Apex, and CPA Lesions

Progressive unilateral SNHL in childhood should alert the clinician to the rare possibility of a retrocochlear lesion. The most common cerebellopontine angle (CPA) lesions reported in childhood are medulloblastoma and vestibular schwannoma. These are rare tumors. If a vestibular schwannoma is seen in childhood, a diagnosis of neurofibromatosis type II should be strongly suspected. Petrous apex lesions and temporal bone diseases are also rare occurrences in childhood. The most common reported etiologies are fibrous dysplasia (81), and Langerhans' cell histiocytosis (82).

Ménière's Disease

Pediatric Ménière's disease has been estimated to comprise 3% of all cases. The majority present in adolescence; the condition is extremely rare in children under the age of 5 years (83). The evaluation of children presenting with fluctuating hearing loss and vertigo should include a routine work-up including a glucose tolerance test, thyroid function test, and syphilis serology.

MANAGEMENT OF ACQUIRED HEARING LOSS

Investigation

The diagnosis of a conductive hearing loss in a child is usually evident following a thorough history and examination. The difficulty arises when the child has a SNHL. As mentioned earlier, SNHL can be genetically acquired or unknown in etiology; these occur in roughly equal proportions. The investigation pertinent to acquired causes should include toxoplamosis, rubella, cytomegalovirus, and herpes simplex (TORCH) serology, blood and urine glucose, and tests of immune function such as erythrocyte sedimentation rate (ESR) and antinuclear antibodies. Computed tomography (CT) is useful to demonstrate inner-ear malformations or the extent of a cholesteatoma. Other imaging may be required to delineate rare temporal bone or CPA lesions. An examination by an ophthalmologist should be requested to exclude keratitis or retinal anomalies, and a review by a pediatrician to look for evidence of systemic disease may be helpful. In the clinical setting, investigations to look for detectable genetic diseases should also be carried out.

Preventative

The emphasis in prenatal infectious disease control has been appropriate screening and prevention by immunization. It is hoped that immunization against measles, mumps, and rubella will reduce the number of cases of acquired hearing loss, there is already evidence of a dramatic fall in the incidence of congenital rubella as a result (84). It is hoped that congenital rubella will cease to be a major cause of hearing loss.

CMV however presents a problem for immunization. The ability of the latent virus to reactivate means that attempted prevention of maternal and intrauterine infection with a live vaccine would probably be of little value. The morbidity attributable to CMV at present far exceeds that produced by congenital rubella, thus, CMV is likely to continue as a major cause of early childhood hearing loss.

A dramatic reduction in the number of cases of *Haemophilus* meningitis has occurred following the introduction of the *Haemophilus influenzae* type B (HIB) vaccine (85). The development of safe vaccines against *S. pneumoniae* and *N. meningitidis* would be an important next stage in the reduction of hearing loss from meningitis.

Screening for syphilis in all women in the first trimester of pregnancy has been recommended, and it is also suggested that women at high risk be screened again in their third trimester and at delivery (86). It is unfortunate, however, that the women at highest risk are also the women least likely to attend prenatal care regularly.

Perinatal problems have proved more difficult to control. However, the routine administration of antirhesus immunoglobulin to all rhesus-negative mothers who give birth to a rhesus-positive child should reduce the incidence of icterus neonatorum and associated hearing loss in subsequent births.

Medical Treatment

Many of the acquired hearing losses of childhood respond to medical treatment; the importance of an accurate and early diagnosis can not be overemphasised. Treatment for CMV remains a problem. Antiviral agents have been tried and there is some preliminary data to suggest that gancyclovir may prove effective (87). For congenital toxoplasmosis, there is some evidence to suggest that antimicrobial therapy, sulfonamide, and pyrimethamine, continued for one year can substantially improve the outcome for affected neonates (88).

Treatment of congenital syphilis is with penicillin or ampicillin, and high doses have been suggested as necessary to cross the blood perilymph barrier and sterilize the inner ear (83). This treatment should be combined with steroids and continued for 4 weeks. If the patient's hearing continues to deteriorate or fluctuate in spite of antibiotic and oral steroid, long-term corticotropin (ACTH) may be useful (89). There is presently evidence to suggest that corticosteroids also have a role in the prevention of hearing loss from meningitis and in the management of autoimmune SNHL, particularly for *H. influenzae* type B meningitis and possibly for other pathogens.

Approximately two thirds of children with SNHL of genetic, acquired, and unknown causes, have a progressive loss in a 5-year period (90,91). Children with SNHL should therefore have continued audiometric monitoring throughout early childhood.

Hearing Aids

The mainstay of nonsurgical management remains aggressive rehabilitation with hearing aids. In patients with unilateral hearing loss, evidence suggests that there is an associated linguistic morbidity (92). This occurs equally regardless of whether the loss is conductive, sensorineural, or mixed and comes from the difficulty that the unilaterally hearing-impaired child has in hearing speech in noise. The younger the child with unilateral hearing loss, the greater the effect.

For bilateral hearing losses, bilateral amplification hearing aids should be provided and fitted. They need to be regularly checked; in young children, the molds may have to be changed every 6 months. It is now accepted that rehabilitation of the hearing impairment, including fitting hearing aids, should be started as early as possible, ideally within the first 6 months of life. There is already evidence to suggest that this practice improves the prognosis for the intelligibility of a child's speech (93). The goal, therefore, is to detect and treat all causes of hearing loss as early as possible.

For bilateral profound hearing losses that are beyond the limits of conventional amplification, cochlear implantation has an important role. There are, however, some important considerations in cochlear implantation in acquired hearing loss. In some children deafened by meningitis, there is progressive ossification within the cochlea, which may prevent full electrode insertion. Evidence of progressive ossification by CT or magnetic resonance imaging (MRI) is therefore an indication for early implantation. The acquired hearing losses in many instances, such as tomoplasmosis, CMV, and kernicterus, have the potential to cause multilevel damage to the auditory system, which may influence the results of cochlear nerve electrical stimulation. Inner-ear malformations also require careful consideration. In cochlear abnormalities there is an increased risk of CSF leakage and a poor result from electrical stimulation. A narrow IAC has been considered a relative contraindication to cochlear implantation (94).

Education

It is essential to develop a close working relationship with the educational services involved in the care of the hearing-impaired child. Even for unilateral and mild bilateral hearing loss, having the child sit at the front of the class often does not suffice. If the hearing can not be restored medically or surgically, the use of a frequency modulated (FM) hearing aid system in the school setting is desirable so that the child may have the least restrictive environment for learning (95). The microphone is attached to the teacher, the speaker to the pupil, thus, the child can always optimally hear the teacher regardless of what is going on in the room.

Surgical Treatment

Surgery has a demonstrable role in the management of OME, chronic suppurative otitis media (CSOM), including cholesteatoma, and in conductive hearing loss secondary to trauma. In the management of PLF, surgery has been shown to be reasonably effective in controlling the vertigo, but the hearing results have been generally poor.

FUTURE PROSPECTS

During the past decade there have been major advances in our understanding of the molecular mechanisms that underlie disease processes. These basic science studies have laid the foundations for molecular interventions that may effect protection from damage, may repair, and may even replace of sensory and neural cells. Any strategy requires delivery of the substance in an active and safe form to the diseased cell and tissue and may require repeated applications. The experimental techniques include the use of osmotic pumps connected to the scala tympani, infusion into the middle-ear cleft, and transfection using retroviruses.

Protection is conceived as placing a substance in the inner ear before a pathologic event occurs to prevent or minimize further loss, and may be applicable to both genetic and acquired diseases characterized by a progressive SNHL. Currently under investigation is the use of antioxidants to prevent ototoxicity and the use of toughening to prevent sound trauma.

Animal and human studies indicate that in a number of types of SNHL the sensory cells are present but not functioning. This finding was clearly shown in the Sh-1 mouse (96). Evidence from humans is largely inferred from the ability of some patients to regain their hearing following an insult, for example, after sudden hearing loss (97) and after treatment for autoimmune disorders. It is assumed that recovery is based on a population of nonfunctioning or marginally functioning sensory and neural cells. Molecular therapies that could be devised to assist in repair and recovery may improve the prognosis in conditions following a recent hearing loss. The ultimate goal in SNHL is cell replenishment. The sensory cells of hearing can be replenished in a number of species (98) and recent reports of in vitro studies suggest cell replenishment may also be possible in mammals (99,100).

REFERENCES

1. Parving A, Christensen B. On criteria for hearing impairment in children. *Int J Pediatr Otorhinolaryngol* 1992;24:1–9.
2. Montgomery JK, Fujikawa S. Hearing thresholds in the second, eight, and twelth grades. *Lang Speech Hear Serv Schools* 1992;23:61–63.
3. Haggard M, Hughes E. Screening children's hearing: a review of the literature and implications of otitis media. Medical Research Council. HMSO, London, 1991;10170:252–268.
4. Martin JAM, Bentsen O, Colley JRT, et al. Childhood deafness in the European Community. *Scand Audiol* 1991;10:165–174.
5. Ruben RJ, Levine R, Baldinger E, et al. Moderate to severe sensorineural hearing impaired child: analysis of aetiology, intervention, and outcome. *Laryngoscope* 1982;92:38–46.
6. Fraser GR. Profound childhood deafness. *J Med Genet* 1964;1:118–151.
7. Brookhouser PE, Worthington DW, Kelly WJ. Fluctuating and/or progressive sensorineural hearing loss in children. *Laryngoscope* 1994;104:958–964.
8. Zeviani M, Moraes CT, DiMauro S, et al. Deletions of mitochondrial DNA in Kearn-Sayre syndrome. *Neurology* 1988;38:1339–1346.
9. Tiranti V, Chariot P, Carella F, et al. Maternally inherited hearing loss, ataxia, and myoclonus associated with a novel point mutation in mitochondrial tRNA$_{ser(ucn)}$ gene. *Hum Mol Genet* 1995;4:1421–1427.
10. Gold M, Rapin I, Shanske S. Mitochondrial inheritance of acquired deafness. *Ann N Y Acad Sci* 1991;630:301–302.
11. Yamaasoba T, Yoshitomo O, Katsounri T, Masaichi N, Kaga K. Auditory findings in patients with maternally inherited diabetes and deafness harboring a point mutation in the mitochondrial transfer RNA$_{LEU(UUR)}$ gene. *Laryngoscope* 1996;106:49–53.
12. Bacino C, Prezant TR, Bu X, Fournier P, Fischel-Ghodsian N. Susceptibility mutations in the mitochondrial small ribosomal RNA gene in aminoglycoside induced deafness. *Pharmacokinetics* 1995;5:165–172.
13. Schaefer GB. Ten syndromes most commonly associated with hearing impairment. *Advances in the genetics of deafness.* National Institute

on Deafness and Other Communication Disorders and Hereditary Hearing Impairment Resource Registry; 1995:1–4.
14. Newton VE. Aetiology of bilateral sensorineural hearing loss in young children. *J Laryngol Otol* 1985;Suppl 10:1–57.
15. Sheppard S, Smithells RW, Peckham CS, Dudgeon JA, Marshall WC. National congenital rubella surveilance 1971–1975. *Health Trends* 9: 38–41.
16. Stagno S, Pass RF, Dworsky ME, Alford CA. Congenital and perinatal cytomegalovirus infections. *Semin Perinatol* 1983;7:31–42.
17. Hicks T, Fowler K, Richardson M, Dahle A, Adams L, Pass R. Congenital cytomegalovirus infection and neonatal auditory screening. *J Pediatr* 1993:779–782.
18. Stern H, Elek SD. The incidence of infection with cytomegalovirus in a normal population: a serological study in Greater London. *J Hyg (Lond)* 1965;63:79–87.
19. Williamson WD, Demmler GJ, Percy AK, Catlin FI. Progressive hearing loss in infants with asymptomatic congenital cytomegalovirus infection. *Pediatrics* 1992;90:862–866.
20. Eichenwald HF. A study of congenital toxoplasmosis, with particular emphasis on clinical manifestations, sequelae, and therapy. In: Sim JC, ed. *Human toxoplasmosis* Copenhagen: Munksgaard; 1964:41.
21. Wilson CB, Remington JS, Stagno S, et al. Development of adverse sequelae in children born with subclinical toxoplasma infection. *Pediatrics* 1980;66:767.
22. Keleman G. Toxoplasmosis and congenital deafness. *Arch Otolaryngol* 1958;68:547–561.
23. Starling SP. Syphilis in infants and young children. *Pediatr Ann* 1994; 23:334–340.
24. Schuknecht HF. *Pathology of the ear.* Cambridge: Harvard University Press; 1993:2–266.
25. Jorgensen MB, Kristensen HK. Thalidomide induced aplasia of the inner ear. *J Laryngol Otol* 1964;78:1095–1101.
26. Jackler RK, Luxford WM, House WF. Congenital malformations of the inner ear: a classification based on embryogenesis. *Laryngoscope* 1987;97(suppl 40):2–14.
27. Abramovich SJ, Gregory S, Slemick M, Stewart A. Hearing loss in very low birth weight infants treated with neonatal intensive care. *Arch Dis Child* 1979;54:421–426.
28. Bergman I, Hirsch RP, Fria TJ, Shapiro SM, Holzmann I, Painter MJ. Cause of hearing loss in the high risk premature infant. *J Pediatr* 1985;106:95–101.
29. Nelson KB, Ellenberg JH. Apgar scores as predictors of chronic neurologic disability. *Pediatrics* 1981;68:36–44.
30. Kawashiro N, Tsuchihashi N, Koga K, Ito Y, Kawano H. Idiopathic deafness or hearing loss of unknown aetiology following discharge from the NICU. *Acta Otolaryngol Suppl* 1994;541:81–84.
31. Naulty CM, Weiss IP, Herer GR. Progressive sensorineural hearing loss in survivors of perstent fetal circulation. *Ear Hear* 1986;7:74–77.
32. Hendricks-Munoz KD, Walton JP. Hearing loss in infants with persistent fetal circulation. *Pediatrics* 1988;81:650–656.
33. Ahdab-Barmada M, Moossy J. The neuropathology of kernicterus in the premature neonate: diagnostic problems. *J Neuropathol Exp Neurol* 1984;43:45–56.
34. Hyman CB, Keaster J, Hanson V, et al. CNS abnormalities after neonatal haemolytic disease or hyperbilirubinaemia. *Am J Dis Child* 1969; 117:395–405.
35. Carhart R. Probable mechanisms underlying kernicteric hearing loss. *Acta Otolaryngol Suppl* 1967;221.
36. Healey GB. Antimicrobial therapy for chronic otitis media with effusion. *Int J Pediatr Otorhinolaryngol* 1984;8:13–17.
37. Persico M, Podoshin L, Fradis M. Otitis media with effusion: a steroid and antibiotic trial before surgery. *Ann Otol Rhinol Laryngol* 1978; 87:191–196.
38. Stangerup SE, Sederberg-Olsen J, Balle V. Autoinflation as a treatment of secretory otitis media: a randomized controlled study. *Arch Otolaryngol Head Neck Surg* 1992;118:149–152.
39. Maw A, Parker AJ. A model to refine the selection of children with otitis media with effusion for adenoidectomy. *Clin Otol* 1993;18: 164–170.
40. Harris JP, Woolf NK, Ryan AF. Elaboration of systemic immunity following inner ear immunization. *Am J Otolaryngol* 1985;6: 148–152.
41. Nadol JB. Hearing loss as a sequela of meningitis. *Laryngoscope* 1978;88:739–755.
42. Lebel MH, Freij BJ, Syrogiannopoulous GA, et al. Dexamethasone therapy for bacterial meningitis. Results of two double blind placebo controlled trials. *N Engl J Med* 1988;319:964–971.
43. Kanra GY, Ozen H, Secmeer G, Ceyhan M, Ecevit Z, Belgin E. Beneficial effects of dexamethasone in children with pneumococcal meningitis. *Pediatr Infect Dis J* 1995;14:490–494.
44. Yurkowski PJ, Plaisance KI. Prevention of auditory sequelae in pediatric bacterial meningitis: a meta analysis. *Pharmacotherapy* 1993; 13:494-499.
45. Wald ER, Kaplan SL, Mason EO, et al. Dexamethasone therapy for children with bacterial meningitis. *Pediatrics* 1995:9521–9528.
46. Schaad UB, Kaplan SL, McCracken GH. Steroid therapy for bacterial meningitis. *Clin Infect Dis* 1995;20:685–690.
47. Syrogiannopolous GA, Lourida AN, Theodoridou MC, et al. Dexamethasone therapy for bacterial meningitis in children: 2 versus 4 day regimen. *J Infect Dis* 1994;169:853–858.
48. Odio CM, Faingezicht I, Paris M, et al. The beneficial effects of early dexamethasone administration in infants and children with bacterial meningitis. *N Engl J Med* 1991;324:1525–1531.
49. Silkes ED, Chabot J. Progressive hearing loss following *Haemophilus infleunza* meningitis. *Int J Pediatr Otorhinolaryngol* 1985;9:249–256.
50. McCormick B, Gibbin KP, Lutman ME, O'Donohue GM. Late partial recovery from meningitic deafness after cochlear implantation: a case study. *Am J Otol* 1993;14:610–612.
51. Yanagita N, Nakashima T, Ohno Y, Kanazaki J, Shitara T. Estimated annual number of patients treated for sensorineural hearing loss in Japan. *Acta Otolaryngol Suppl* 1994;514:9–13.
52. Elango S, Chand RP, Purohit GN. Childhood deafness in Malaysia. *Int J Pediatr Otorhinolaryngol* 1992;24:11–17.
53. Stewart BJ, Prabhu PU. Reports of sensorineural deafness after measles, mumps and rubella immunization. *Arch Dis Child* 1993;69: 153–154.
54. English MG, Northern JL, Fria T. Chronic otitis media as a cause of sensorineural hearing loss. *Arch Otolaryngol Head Neck Surg* 1973; 97:18–22.
55. Harada T, Yamasoba T, Yagi M. Sensorineural hearing loss associated with otitis media with effusion. *ORL* 1992;54:61–65.
56. Noordzij JP, Dodson EE, Ruth RA, Arts HA, Lambert PR. Chronic otitis media and sensorineural hearing loss: is there a clinically significant relation. *Am J Otol* 1995;16:420–423.
57. Darrow DH, Keithley EM, Harris JP. Effects of bacterial endotoxin applied to the guinea pig cochlea. *Laryngoscope* 1992;102:683–688.
58. Podoshin L, Fradis M, Ben David. J Ototoxicity of ear drops in patients suffering from chronic otitis media. *J Laryngol Otol* 1989;103:46–50.
59. Dominguez S, Harker LA. Incidence of cholesteatoma with cleft palate. *Ann Otol Rhinol Laryngol* 1988;97:659–660.
60. Padgham N, Mills RP, Christmas HE. Has the increasing use of grommets influenced the frequency of surgery for cholesteatoma? *J Laryngol Otol* 1989;103:1034–1035.
61. Roland NJ, Philips DE, Rogers JH, Singh SD. The use of ventilation tubes and the incidence of cholesteatoma surgery in the paediatric population of Liverpool. *Clin Otol* 1992;17:437–439.
62. Kanzaki J, Inoue Y, O-Uchi T. Immunological findings of serological tests in steroid-responsive sensorineural hearing loss. *Acta Otolaryngol Suppl* 1994;514:66–69.
63. Ruben RJ, Balogun AO. Autoimmune inner ear disease: Results of testing and therapy. *The 23rd meeting of the society of ear nose and throat advances in children,* 1995 (abst 80).
64. Hughes GB, Barna BP, Kinney SE, Calabrese LH, Nelepa NL. Predictive value of laboratory tests in "Autoimmune" inner ear disease. Preliminary report. *Laryngoscope* 1986;96:502–505.
65. Podder S, Shepherd RC. Cogan's syndrome: a rare systemic vasculitis. *Arch Dis Child* 1994;71:163–164.
66. Siglock TJ, Brooker KH. Sensorineural hearing loss associated with Takayasu s disease. *Laryngoscope* 1987;97:797–800.
67. Cotter CS, Singleton GT, Corman LC. Immune mediated inner ear disease and parvo virus B19. *Laryngoscope* 1994;104:1235–1239.
68. Beetham WP, Osmet LS, Wisner WH. Progressive systemic scleroderma in a child: a case report. *South Med J* 1967;60:236–240.
69. Sundel RP, Cleveland SS, Beiser AS, Newberger JW, et al. Audiologic profiles of children with Kawasaki disease. *Am J Otol* 1992;13: 512–515.
70. Tommerup B, Moller K. A case of profound hearing impairment fol-

70. lowing the prolonged use of framycetin ear drops. *J Laryngol Otol* 1984;98:1135–1137.
71. Lind O, Kristiansen B. Deafness after treatment with ear drops containing neomycin, gramicidin and dexamethasone. A case report. *ORL* 1986;48:52–54.
72. Williams WT, Ghorayeb BY, Yeakley JW. Pediatric temporal bone fractures. *Laryngoscope* 102:600–603.
73. Davis AC, Fortnum HM, Coles RRA, et al., eds. *Damage to hearing from leisure noise: a review of the literature.* Nottingham: University of Nottingham; 1985.
74. Anon. Consensus conference, noise and hearing loss. *JAMA* 1990; 263:3185–3190.
75. Brookehouser PE, Worthington DW, Kelly WJ. Noise induced hearing loss in children. *Laryngoscope* 1992;102:645–655.
76. Ruben RJ, Yankelowitz SM. Spontaneous perilymphatic fistula in children. *Am J Otol* 1989;10:198–207.
77. Wall C, Casselbrant M. System identification of perilymphatic fistulae in an animal model. *Am J Otol* 1992;13:443–448.
78. Reilly JS. Congenital perilymphatic fistula: a prospective study in infants and children. *Laryngoscope* 1989;99:393–397.
79. Pappas DG, Simpson LC, Godwin GH. Perilymphatic fistula in children with pre-existing sensorineural hearing loss. *Laryngoscope* 1988; 98:507–510.
80. Weissman JL, Weber PC, Bluestone CD. Congenital perilymphatic fistula: computed tomography appearance of middle ear and iner ear anomalies. *Otolaryngol Head Neck Surg* 1994;111:243–249.
81. Megerian CA, Sofferman RA, McKenna MJ, Eavy RD, Nadol JB. Fibrous dysplasia of the temporal bone: ten new cases demonstrating the spectrum of otologic sequelae. *Am J Otol* 1995;16:408–419.
82. Irving RM, Broadbent V, Jones NS. Langerhan's cell histiocytosis in childhood: management of head and neck manifestations. *Laryngoscope* 104;64–70.
83. Meyerhoff WL, Paparella MM. Ménière's disease in children. *Laryngoscope* 1978;88:1504–1511.
84. Kvaerner KJ, Arnesen AR. Hearing impairment in Oslo born children 1989–1991. *Scand Audiol* 1994;23:233–239.
85. Bent JP, Beck RA. Bacterial meningitis in the paediatric population: paradigm shifts and ramifications for otolaryngology head and neck surgery. *Int J Pediatr Otorhinolaryngol* 1994;30:41–49.
86. Centers for Disease Control and Prevention. 1993 sexually transmitted diseases treatment guidelines. *MMWR* 1993;42:21–46.
87. Nigro G, Scholz H, Bartmann U. Gancyclovir therapy for symptomatic congenital cytomegalovirus infection in infants: a two-regimen experience. *J Paediatr* 1994;318–322.
88. McGee T, Wolters C, Stein L, et al. Absence of sensorineural hearing loss in treated infants and children with congenital toxoplasmosis. *Otolaryngol Head Neck Surg* 1991;III:75–80.
89. Chan YM, Adams DA, Kerr AG. Syphilitic Labyrinthitis—an update. *J Laryngol Otol* 1995;109:719–725.
90. Ruben RJ, Fishman G. Otological care of the hearing impaired child. *Proceedings of third Elk's international conference on early management of hearing loss.* New York: Grune & Stratton, 1980:105–119.
91. Levi H, Tell L, Feinmesser M. Progressive hearing loss in hard of hearing children. *Audiology* 1993;32:132–136.
92. Bess FH, Tharpe AM. Unilateral hearing impairment in children. *Pediatrics* 1984;74:206–216.
93. Markides, A. Age at fitting of hearing aids and speech intelligibility. *Br J Audiol* 1986;20:165–168.
94. Jackler RK, Luxford WM, House WF. Congenital malformations of the inner ear: sound detection with cochlear implant in five ears of four children with congenital malformations of the cochlea. *Laryngoscope* 1987;97(Suppl 40):15–17.
95. Updike CD. Comparison of FM auditory trainers, CROS aids and personal amplification in unilaterally hearing impaired children. *J Am Acad Audiol* 1994;5:204–209.
96. Mikaelian DO, Ruben RJ. Hearing degeneration in the shaker-1 mouse. *Arch Otolaryngol* 1964;80:418–430.
97. Mattox DE, Simmons FB. Natural history of sudden sensorineural hearing loss. *Ann Otol Rhinol Laryngol* 1977;86:463–480.
98. Cotanche DA. regeneration of hair cell sterociliary bundles in the chick cochlea following severe acoustic trauma. *Hear Res* 1987;30: 181–195.
99. Lefebvre PP, Malgrange B, Straecker H, Moonen G, Van Der Watter TR. Retinoic acid stimulates regeneration of mammalian auditory hair cells. *Science* 1993;260:692–695.
100. Lefebvre PP, Van Der Watter TR, Straecker H, et al. Nerve growth factor stimulates neurite regeneration but not survival of adult auditory neurons in vitro. *Acta Otolaryngol* 1992;112:288–293.

CHAPTER 25

Central Auditory Disorders

Brad A. Stach

Childhood central auditory disorders can be classified into two groups: those associated with identifiable neuropathology and those of idiopathic origin that present as communication disorders. Central auditory disorders related to neuropathologic conditions are rare. Chapter 33 of this textbook provides a summary of neuropathologies that occur in children. When neoplasms affect the auditory nervous system, they are usually diagnosed with radiographic techniques and on the basis of associated medical problems. Treatment strategies for such disorders are often similar to those that would be appropriate in adults with similar pathology.

There are relatively few reports of central auditory disorder in children with CNS lesions due, in part, to the rarity of the lesions and, presumably, because hearing disorders tend to be a relatively minor aspect of the generally deteriorated health of such children. Jerger (1) summarized results of an audiometric battery in 21 children with documented CNS lesions. Result showed patterns of abnormality consistent with those found in adults with similar lesions. Specifically, those children with extra- and intra-axial gliomas had abnormal, degraded monotic speech perception, and those with temporal lobe lesions had abnormal dichotic speech perception. Most other reports corroborate these findings that children and adults tend to exhibit similar patterns of abnormality (2,3), although some have suggested that auditory deficits in children with CNS lesions may be more generalized and less severe than in adults with similar lesions (4). Regardless, the probability of encountering such children in a clinical setting is low, and auditory disorders are likely to be a minor component of care, except in such extreme cases as bilateral acoustic tumors.

The vast majority of childhood central auditory disorders do not result from documented neuropathologic conditions. Rather, they present as a communication disorder that resembles hearing impairment. The specific hearing impairment is related to an idiopathic dysfunction of the central auditory nervous system and is commonly referred to as central auditory processing disorder (CAPD). Although the auditory symptoms and clinical findings in children with CAPD may mimic those of children with auditory disorders due to discrete pathology in the central auditory nervous system, they result from no obvious pathologic condition that requires medical intervention. Nevertheless, physicians with a practice in otology will evaluate a number of these children who present with the symptomatology of hearing loss, yet have normal pure-tone audiograms.

OVERVIEW OF CENTRAL AUDITORY PROCESSING DISORDER

Central auditory processing disorder can be thought of as a hearing disorder that occurs as a result of dysfunction of the central auditory nervous system. Although some children may be genetically predisposed to CAPD, it is more likely to be a developmental delay or disorder, resulting from inconsistent or degraded auditory input during the critical period for auditory perceptual development. This disorder is symptomatic in nature and is often confused with an impairment of hearing sensitivity. It can be an isolated disorder, or it can coexist with attention-deficit disorders, learning disabilities, and language disorders. Clinically, CAPD is operationally defined most often on the basis of speech audiometric results. Recent advances in speech audiometry and recent studies of auditory evoked potentials hold promise for refinement in the diagnosis. Functionally, children with CAPD act as if they have hearing-sensitivity deficits, although they are usually capable of hearing faint sounds. In particular, they exhibit difficulty in perceiving spoken language or other sounds in hostile acoustic environments. Thus, a common age of identification is early in the children's academic lives, when they enter a conventional classroom situation and are unable to understand instructions from the teacher. Once properly diagnosed as a hearing disorder, treatment takes one of at least three forms. For milder

---

B.A. Stach: Nova Scotia Hearing and Speech Clinic, Halifax, Nova Scotia B34 1L1 Canada.

cases, environmental manipulation aimed at overcoming hostile acoustic conditions may be all that is necessary to assure effective audition. In more severe cases, special amplification systems that enhance the acoustic environment may be necessary. In all cases, children may benefit from treatment related to the development of compensatory skills. Although children may develop such compensatory strategies naturally as they get older, intervention should be pursued promptly, because the child with CAPD is at risk for academic achievement problems.

DEFINING CENTRAL AUDITORY PROCESSING DISORDER

Problems

The concept of CAPD emerged from several different perspectives, including those of the audiologist, speech pathologist, educational diagnostician, and neuropsychologist, which naturally led to diverse developments in assessment tools and rehabilitative strategies. Historically, the term *central auditory processing disorder* has been used to describe many different types of communication problems in children. The controversy over its definition stemmed from at least two factors. First, for an acoustic signal to be understood as a spoken word by an individual, a significant amount of processing must occur. There are many models that attempt to define how an acoustic signal is detected by the auditory sensory system, processed through the central auditory nervous system, and perceived as language. Processing of the acoustic signal begins at the outer ear, where sounds reach the two ears at different intensities and arrival times. Processing continues at the sensitive cochlea and beyond, through complex auditory brainstem and cortical pathways. Brought to bear on these neural impulses are linguistic constructs, developed through experience and potentiated by intelligence and attention. The identification of an acoustic signal as a word that has meaning is the result of a complex set of factors acting on the auditory reception of this signal.

It is easy to imagine that a breakdown in any one of these processes could result in the signal not being identified correctly. For example, if the child were not attending to the signal, if the child did not have the word in his or her vocabulary, or if the child could not remember the word that was heard, the result would be a lack of identification of the acoustic information. Thus, theories of audition attempt to account for the complexity of receiving spoken language. This has led some to suggest that any factors that are involved in the reception of auditory signals must be considered as components of auditory processing and that a disorder at any level must be considered a disorder of auditory processing. That is, they suggest that, in a general sense, any disorder that prevents the acoustic signal from being understood as a spoken word falls into a complex of disorders known as auditory processing disorders. By such thinking, an attention deficit, a language deficit, or a cognitive deficit could all be considered auditory disorders if they interfered with this process. While this idea is of interest from a theoretical perspective, it is intractable from a clinical perspective.

A second factor that confounded the definition of CAPD was the perspective of those doing the evaluation. Individuals who were evaluating and treating children with attentional deficit disorders, learning disabilities, and speech and language impairments noted that some of these children appeared to have difficulty hearing speech and perceiving it accurately. As a result, disordered auditory processing was classified as a subset of these more global disorders. Simultaneously, those who evaluated hearing were identifying increasing numbers of children, with or without concomitant problems, who, despite normal hearing sensitivity, had difficulty in the processing of auditory stimuli. Patterns of auditory abnormality emerged that were quite similar to those found in children and adults with known neurologic disorders of the central auditory nervous system. Thus, the definition of CAPD became entangled in a theoretical tug-of-war. Is it a language deficit? A cognitive impairment? An attentional disorder? A hearing impairment?

Jerger, Martin, and Jerger (5) provided an interesting perspective when they described CAPD in the context of two theoretical models of learning disability. One theoretical approach is termed the *linguistic model*. Individuals who ascribe to the linguistic model believe that CAPD is a conceptual problem, that the deficit is in representational or symbolic behavior, and that linguistic–cognitive factors are the primary problem involved in CAPD. Another theoretical approach is the auditory model. Individuals who ascribe to the auditory model contend that CAPD is an auditory problem, that the deficit is in behaviors that are precursory to language, and that linguistic–cognitive factors are secondary. The remainder of this chapter will treat CAPD from the auditory-model perspective.

Definition

As our understanding of CAPD has progressed, we have begun to better define its true nature and to agree on clinical, operational definitions of the disorder. Although controversy remains, consensus is beginning to emerge on a definition of CAPD that distinguishes it from language-processing disorders and other neuropsychological disorders. One classification scheme that I have found useful for categorizing disorder types is shown in Table 1. Under this scheme, CAPD is defined as an auditory disorder that results from deficits in central auditory nervous system function. *Receptive language processing disorder* is defined as a deficit in linguistic-processing skills and may affect language comprehension and vocabulary development. *Neuropsychological disorders,* such as auditory attention and auditory memory, are defined as deficits in cognitive ability. Clearly, overlap exists among these disorders; they may coexist, and they are often difficult to separate. For example, the change from percep-

TABLE 1. *Categories of disorders related to turning sound into meaning*

Disorder	Nature of disorder	Types of deficits
Central auditory processing disorder	Auditory	Reduced understanding in noise Difficulty with low redundancy signals Difficulty in localizing/lateralizing sound Dichotic deficits Reduced temporal process
Receptive language processing disorder	Linguistic	Auditory comprehension deficits Auditory integration deficits
Neuropsychologic disorder	Cognitive	Attention-deficit hyperactivity disorder Auditory memory deficits

tion to comprehension must occur on a continuum, and deciding where one ends and the other begins can only be defined operationally. Similarly, the relation of memory and attention to either perception or comprehension is difficult to parse. Nevertheless, distinguishing among these classes of disorders is important clinically, because they tend to have different sequelae and to be treated differently (6–10).

Central auditory processing disorder, then, can be thought of as an auditory disorder that occurs as a result of dysfunction in the manipulation and utilization of acoustic signals by the central auditory nervous system. It is broadly defined as an impaired ability to process acoustic information that cannot be attributed to impaired hearing sensitivity, impaired language, or impaired intellectual function.

Central auditory processing disorders have been characterized based on models of deficits in children and adults with acquired lesions of the central auditory nervous system (11). Such deficits include reduced ability to understand in background noise, to understand speech of reduced redundancy, to localize and lateralize sound, to separate dichotic stimuli, and to process normal or altered temporal cues. Children with CAPD exhibit deficits similar to those with acquired lesions, although they may be less pronounced in severity and are more likely to be generalized than ear-specific.

The etiology of CAPD is not known. There have been anecdotal reports of families with CAPD, including parents and siblings. In addition, in larger series of children with CAPD, there is an indication of a high prevalence of chronic otitis media. Until further evidence can be gathered, it remains only a conjecture that children who have aperiodic disruption in auditory input during the critical period for auditory development may be at risk for developing CAPD. However, several reports have shown convincing delays in auditory processing ability in children with a history of chronic otitis media (12–15).

In general, children with CAPD will act as if they have a hearing-sensitivity loss, even though most will have normal audiograms. They will ask for repetition, fail to follow instructions, and so on, particularly in the presence of background noise or other factors that reduce the redundancy of the acoustic signal. To the extent that such difficulties result in frustration, secondary problems may develop related to their behavior and motivation in the classroom. Some children with CAPD will have concomitant speech and language deficits, learning disabilities, and attention-deficit disorders (10). Thus, CAPD may be accompanied by distractibility, attention problems, memory deficits, language comprehension deficits, restricted vocabulary, and reading and spelling problems.

DIAGNOSIS OF CENTRAL AUDITORY PROCESSING DISORDER

Problems

Diagnosis of CAPD is challenging because there is no biologic marker. Its diagnosis relies on operational definitions, which are based primarily on behavioral speech audiometric measures. The interpretation of such measures, when administered in an uncontrolled manner, can be confounded by nonauditory influences such as language delays, attentional deficits, and impaired cognitive functioning. Administered properly, however, measures of CAPD can, in most instances, validly and reliably separate CAPD from these other disorders.

Much of the controversy that surrounds diagnosis of CAPD results from the lack of a universally accepted clinical approach to controlling nonauditory influences on CAPD test interpretation. This lack of control has reduced the predictive value of a positive test. That is, too many children who do not have CAPD fail the tests. This results in a large number of false-positive test results, which not only burdens the health-care system with children who do not need further testing, but also muddles the issue of CAPD and its contribution to a child's problems.

The main reason for less than optimal predictive values is that results on CAPD measures can be influenced by the nonauditory factors of attention, cognition, and language skills. An excellent illustration of the problem was provided in an article by Gascon, Johnson, and Burd (16). They evaluated a group of nine children who were considered to be hyperactive and have attentional deficit disorders. The children were evaluated with several speech audiometric tests of auditory processing ability. In addition, they were evaluated with several measures of attention, including motor impersistence, finger localization, face and/or hand extinction, visual tracking, and pointing span of objects in sequence. Both the CAPD test battery and the attention test battery were administered before and after the children were medicated with stimulants to control hyperactivity. Results showed that 79% of the children improved on the CAPD test battery following stimulants. In contrast, 50% of the children improved on the attentional battery, and 53% showed improvement in their communication and attention behavior. What these results indicate, of course, is that the CAPD tests are very sensitive to the effects of attention. Stated another way, children who have attentional disorders often perform poorly on these CAPD measures even if they do not have CAPD, because they cannot attend to the task thoroughly enough for the auditory system to be evaluated. As a result, the effects of auditory processing disorder cannot be separated from the effects that attentional deficits have on a child's ability to complete these particular test measures.

Similar influences of nonauditory factors on auditory test results have been reported on other CAPD tests as well. For example, results from clinical trials with the SCAN test (17), which was designed as a screening test for auditory processing disorders, showed that scores on the test were significantly correlated with scores on the Peabody Picture Vocabulary Test. These results can be interpreted in one of at least three ways: (a) children with CAPD are likely to have vocabulary deficits; (b) children with vocabulary deficits are likely to have CAPD; or (c) children who do not have the vocabulary necessary to perform this test score poorly on it. In the case of the latter interpretation, abnormal test results would be uninterpretable with regard to CAPD in children who have vocabulary deficits. A second finding from the same study showed that subjects with attentional deficit disorders scored significantly worse on the test than those who did not have attentional disorders. Once again, this may mean that the two are correlated, so that children who are more likely to have one are more likely to have the other. Or it may mean that test results cannot be interpreted for CAPD because they are confounded by attentional deficit disorders. Finally, another study of the SCAN (18) showed significant improvement in scores in hyperactive children when they were on stimulants, similar to the data from Gascon, Johnson, and Burd (16), indicating that the test is sensitive to the effects of attention. What these studies suggest is that if a child has a language deficit or an attentional deficit, that child is likely to fail this screening test for CAPD, regardless of his or her auditory processing ability. If the goal of assessment is to identify children with language deficits, attentional deficits, and CAPD, such a test might be appropriate. If the goal is to test exclusively for CAPD, however, the influences of attention, cognition, and language skills must be controlled during the evaluation process.

It seems important to emphasize that the actual tests that are used may not be the main problem, assuming that the vocabulary level is appropriate for the child being tested. Rather, it is often the clinical approach that dictates whether a particular test will be effective.

Fortunately, evidence is emerging that well-controlled speech audiometric testing, in conjunction with auditory evoked potential measures, may be a powerful diagnostic tool for assessing CAPD. Nevertheless, the problem that remains in the diagnosis of CAPD is that there is no single gold standard against which to judge the effectiveness of any particular test. Although CAPD can be operationally defined on the basis of behavioral and electrophysiologic test results, and although nonauditory factors can be controlled to a certain extent, without a standard against which to compare the operational definition, agreement about the accuracy of CAPD diagnosis remains elusive.

Successful Diagnostic Strategies

There are a number of speech audiometric measures of CAPDs (19–21). Most of them evolved from adult measures that were designed to aid in the diagnosis of neurologic disease in the pre–magnetic resonance imaging era. The application of many of these adult measures to the pediatric population has not been altogether successful, largely because of a lack of control over linguistic and cognitive complexity in applying them to young children.

In recent years, however, speech audiometric approaches have been developed that have proven to be valid and reliable. When they are administered under properly controlled acoustic conditions, with materials of appropriate language age, and with testing strategies that control for the influences of attention and cognition, these measures permit an accuracy in diagnosis that was not attainable previously. Diagnostic strategies have advanced to a point that some researchers are beginning to identify distinguishable types of CAPD (22) and assign them estimates of severity.

When appropriate tests are administered correctly, a diagnosis of CAPD can be made quite effectively in those with auditory disorders. Conversely, in those who do not have auditory processing problems, CAPD can be ruled out. In a small percentage of children, however, cognitive problems, language delays, or attentional deficits may preclude testing or may render test results uninterpretable.

Speech Audiometry

One test battery is described briefly here in an effort to illustrate an approach to the diagnosis of CAPD that has proven successful clinically. While it is by no means the only strategy that exists, it is successful because it controls the influences of cognition, attention, and language ability, thereby isolating auditory disorder from nonauditory influences on test interpretation. Such a strategy could readily be applied to any of a number of existing tests of CAPD.

The test battery is summarized in Table 2. The concept behind this test-battery approach is one of varying several parameters across a continuum to sensitize the speech mate-

TABLE 2. *A speech audiometric battery for evaluating children for central auditory processing disorders*

Test measure	Auditory parameter
Speech audiometric measures: Younger children	
PSI-ICM words at +10 and +4 dB MCR	Signal-to-noise ratio
PSI-ICM words performance-intensity function	Intensity
PSI-ICM sentences at +10 and 0 dB MCR	Signal-to-noise ratio
PSI-ICM words versus sentences	Extrinsic redundancy
PSI-CCM sentences	Dichotic listening
Speech audiometric measures: Older children	
PB words performance-intensity function	Intensity
SSI sentences at +10 and 0 dB MCR	Signal-to-noise ratio
PB words versus SSI sentences	Extrinsic redundancy
DSI	Dichotic listening

rials. The goal of this approach is to provide a test battery that is both sensitive to auditory processing disorders and that provides tester control over nonauditory influences. The parameters include intensity, signal-to-noise ratio, redundancy of informational content, and monotic versus dichotic performance.

For younger children, the Pediatric Speech Intelligibility (PSI) test (23) is used. Words are presented with an ipsilateral competing message (ICM) at message-to-competition ratios (MCRs) of +10 and +4 dB. Testing at +10 dB MCR provides an easier listening condition to assure that the child knows the vocabulary, is cognitively capable of performing the task, and can attend adequately enough to complete the procedure. Then the MCR is reduced to +4 dB to challenge the integrity of the auditory nervous system. At the more difficult MCR, a performance-versus-intensity function is obtained to evaluate for "rollover" of the function, or poorer performance at higher intensity levels. This assessment in the intensity domain is also designed to assess auditory nervous system integrity.

Sentences are also presented with both ipsilateral (ICM) and contralateral competing messages (CCM). The word-versus-sentence comparison assesses the child's ability to process speech signals of different redundancy. The ipsilateral-versus-contralateral competition comparison assesses the difference between monotic and dichotic auditory processing ability.

For older children, adult speech audiometric materials are used. These include single-syllable words from phonetically balanced (PB) lists presented in quiet, the Synthetic Sentence Identification (SSI) test (24) with ipsilateral competing message, and the Dichotic Sentence Identification (DSI) test (25). Performance-versus-intensity functions of the PB word lists and SSI test are completed to assess high-intensity-level processing and word-versus-sentence processing. The SSI is carried out at two MCRs, +10 and 0 dB, to assess processing along the signal-to-noise ratio continuum. Finally, SSI and DSI comparisons are made to assess monotic versus dichotic performance.

The manner in which these speech audiometric measures can be designed to assess auditory processing ability while controlling the nonauditory effects of language, cognition, and attention is probably best illustrated in an individual patient. Audiometric data from a 4-year, 1-month-old child who was diagnosed with CAPD are shown in Fig. 1. Although hearing sensitivity was within normal limits in both ears, speech audiometric results were strikingly abnormal. In the right ear, the performance-intensity functions for both

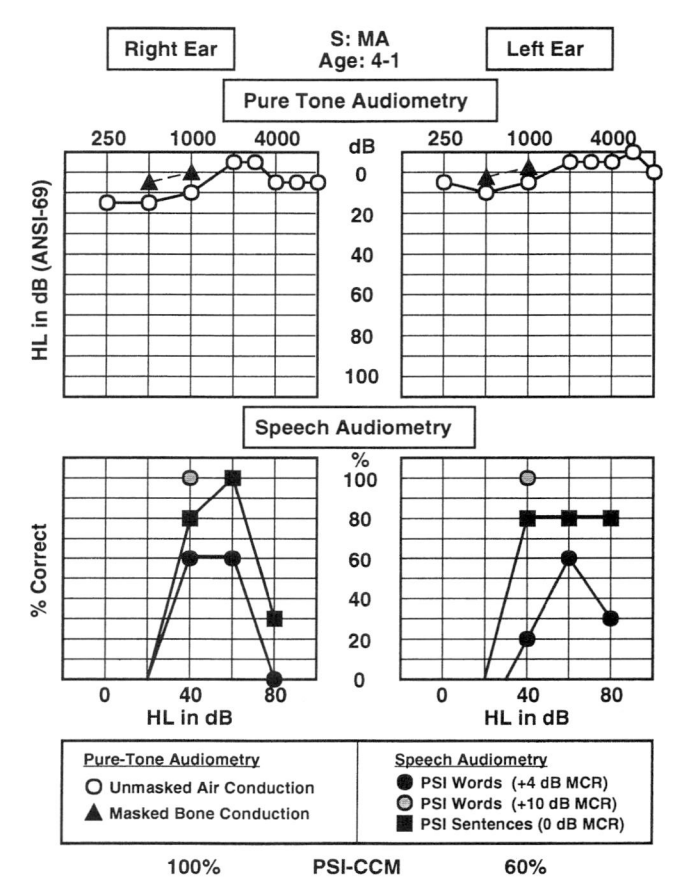

FIG. 1. Pure-tone and speech audiometric results in a 4-year, 1-month-old child with a diagnosis of central auditory processing disorder (CAPD). The Pediatric Speech Intelligibility (PSI) test was carried out at several message-to-competition ratios (MCR)s, designated in decibels. The Pediatric Speech Intelligibility (PSI) sentence test was also carried out with a centralateral competing message (CCM).

words and sentences showed rollover. Rollover of these functions cannot be explained as attention, linguistic, or cognitive disorders without invoking some theory of intensity-level dependence of one of these types of disorders. In other words, it is difficult to reconcile that a language, cognition, or attention deficit could be present at one intensity level and not at another. In addition, in the left ear, there was a substantial discrepancy between understanding of sentences and understanding of words. This was obviously not a language problem, because at 60 dB HL, the child understood all of the sentences correctly and, at an easier listening condition of +10 dB MCR, the child identified all of the words correctly. The child was clearly capable of doing the task linguistically and cognitively. Thus, use of performance-intensity functions, various MCRs, and word-versus-sentence comparisons permitted the assessment of auditory processing ability in a manner that reduced the likelihood of nonauditory factors influencing the interpretation of test results.

Auditory Evoked Potentials

Some studies have suggested the possibility that auditory evoked potentials might be used to corroborate speech audiometric testing. Specifically, the auditory middle latency response (MLR), late vertex response (LVR), and auditory P3 response (26,27) have been found to be abnormal in children who have CAPD. As an example, some of my colleagues and I reported results from 44 children who were diagnosed as having CAPD based on patterns of speech audiometric results (28). The auditory brainstem response (ABR) was normal in all children. However, the later auditory evoked potentials were abnormal in 84% of the children tested. Of these 37 children, both the MLR and LVR were abnormal in 73%, the MLR was abnormal in isolation in 13.5%, and the LVR was abnormal in isolation in 13.5%.

Although encouraging, a lack of sufficient normative data on young children reduces the ease of interpretation of auditory evoked potentials on an individual basis at this point in time. Advances in recording strategies, such as topographic brain mapping, are likely to enhance CAPD diagnosis.

Our clinical experience with this diagnostic strategy has been encouraging. In conjunction with thorough speech, language, and neuropsychological evaluations, the use of well-controlled speech audiometric measures and auditory evoked potentials has proven to be quite powerful in defining the presence or absence of an auditory processing disorder.

Other Assessment Approaches

When consensus is reached on methods for diagnosing CAPD, the next challenge will be that of identifying those who are at risk for the disorder, so that diagnostic testing can be implemented. Because CAPD is, by its very nature, symptomatic, some would argue that it need not be screened, but rather that the presence of its symptomatology be systematically investigated. Thus, one alternative to the use of a screening test is simply to assess the symptoms. Several efforts have been made to use checklists or performance scales, designed to be completed by teachers or parents, to evaluate the symptomatology of CAPD. For example, Smoski and colleagues (29) developed the Children's Auditory Processing Performance Scale for such a purpose. In this approach, the presence or absence of the symptoms is evaluated, and the child is referred for diagnostic testing if symptoms are present. Although this alternative has been largely untested, it appears to have merit as a method for identifying those children who are at risk for CAPD.

FUNCTIONAL CONSEQUENCES OF CENTRAL AUDITORY PROCESSING DISORDER

Consequences of CAPD can range from mild difficulty understanding a teacher in a noisy classroom to substantial difficulty understanding speech in everyday listening situations at home and school. One of the most important deficits in children with CAPD is difficulty understanding in background noise. In an acoustic environment that would be adequate for other children, a child with CAPD may have substantial difficulty understanding what is being said. Thus, parents will often complain that the child cannot understand them while the television is on, while riding in the car, or while the parents are speaking from another room. The teacher will complain of the child's inability to follow directions, distractibility, and general unruliness. In effect, the complaints will be similar to those expressed by parents or teachers of children with impairments of hearing sensitivity. In a quiet environment, with one-on-one instruction, a child with CAPD may thrive in a manner consistent with academic potential. In a more adverse acoustical environment, a child with CAPD will struggle.

It seems likely that the presence of CAPD in a child will have an adverse impact on speech and language development. Some even argue that it is unlikely that a child could have CAPD and not have some consequent language disorder. Evidence suggests that CAPD is prevalent in groups of children with speech and language disorders. A causal relationship, while implied, has not been confirmed. Evidence also suggests that CAPD can occur in isolation, suggesting that CAPD and language disorder are not necessarily consequential (5).

TREATMENT OF CENTRAL AUDITORY PROCESSING DISORDER

Central auditory processing disorder can be thought of as an auditory disorder that has as one of its main components the difficulty in understanding speech in background noise. Treatment strategies that focus on this component are often effective in forestalling or changing the expected outcome related to the presence of CAPD.

Intervention strategies directed toward enhancement of signal-to-noise ratio (SNR) have proven successful in the treatment of children with CAPD (30,31). There are at least two approaches to this type of intervention. The first approach is to alter the acoustic environment in order to enhance the SNR. Environmental alterations include such practical approaches as preferential seating in the classroom and manipulation of the home environment so that the child is placed in more favorable listening situations. Alterations also may include equipping the classroom with sound field speakers to provide amplification of the teacher's speech.

It is not uncommon in children with CAPD for the diagnosis itself to serve as the treatment. That is, once parents and teachers become aware of the nature of the child's problem and that the solution is one of enhancement of SNR, they manipulate the environment in such a manner that the problem situations are eliminated, and the child's auditory processing difficulties become inconsequential.

In other cases, however, when severity of the auditory processing disorder is greater, the use of remote microphone technology may be indicated. Personal FM systems, which use remote microphones for SNR enhancement, have been used to assist these children in overcoming their deficit in understanding speech in background noise.

In 1987, some of my colleagues and I summarized our experience at the Neurosensory Center of Houston with intervention in children with CAPD (32). Of those children who were considered to have CAPD, 30 were successfully treated by enhancing the awareness of parents and teachers to the need for environmental alteration to reduce background noise. In 11 others, however, the more aggressive approach of personal FM-system use was taken. These were relatively young children whose average age was 7 years. Although some of the children had slight, low-frequency hearing loss, all had pure-tone averages that were within normal limits. The majority (72%) also had a history of chronic otitis media. Evidence of improvement in nine of the children using FM systems was gathered from interviews with parents and teachers. In eight of the nine children, improved grades and improved behavior were reported anecdotally by the teacher and parents. In addition, two of the children were reported to have improved speech and language abilities, two had improved attention, and, in two, there was a school placement change from a special-education classroom to a regular classroom.

Children with CAPD may also benefit from auditory-training therapy, directed toward enhancement of the ability to process auditory information (33) and to development of compensatory skills (9). While it may seem counterintuitive to try to train away a sensory deficit, there is convincing evidence of functional plasticity of the maturing central auditory nervous system (34). It seems likely that stimulation of the auditory system through therapy could exploit such neural plasticity.

Because children with CAPD often have concomitant deficits in speech, language, attention, learning, and cognition, comprehensive approaches to treatment are recommended. Treatment for memory, vocabulary, comprehension, listening, reading, and spelling are often necessary in children with multiple involvement.

SEQUELAE OF CENTRAL AUDITORY PROCESSING DISORDER

One of the most often asked questions regarding CAPD is whether the child will *grow out of it*. It is an emerging clinical impression that children do not grow out of the disorder, although they appear to develop compensatory skills as they get older. In many cases, the course of action with a child who has been diagnosed as having CAPD is based on both the lack of an answer to this question and the sense of urgency to solve the immediate problems of difficulty in the classroom. In general, it appears that it is better to try to forestall achievement problems than to wait to see if the child will grow out of it.

Sequelae of CAPD in younger children are related to appropriate speech and language development. Although data on outcomes are limited, anecdotal evidence suggests that early detection results in early referral for speech and language evaluation and monitoring. Sequelae of CAPD in older children are related mostly to the extent to which the auditory problem affects hearing in the classroom. Successful intervention is expected to reduce achievement problems, while undetected or unmanaged problems are likely to result in academic underachievement.

CASE HISTORY

The following case illustrates an approach to diagnosis and treatment of CAPD that we have found to be efficacious in the clinic. In addition, it serves to illustrate some of the questions that remain in our search for an understanding of this elusive disorder. Results are from a 5-year-old girl with a speech and language disorder who also had symptoms of hearing impairment (35). Diagnostic testing was completed in a manner that limited the influence of speech and language deficits on test interpretation. Results revealed a deficit in speech understanding in the presence of background competition and abnormal late-latency auditory evoked potentials. In both speech treatment sessions and in the classroom, the child used a personal FM amplification system as a means of enhancing the SNR. Anecdotal reports suggested that the device was of benefit in her learning environments.

Description of Subject

JC was 5 years, 2 months old when her hearing was first evaluated. Her mother had been concerned about her speech for over 2 years. JC's perinatal history was unremarkable. During early childhood, she had numerous bouts of rhinitis. Her medical history was otherwise unremarkable. Although her mother reported normal language milestones, she also reported that she was the only one who could understand JC because of JC's poor articulation.

A speech–language evaluation indicated that JC had moderate dysarthria and possible apraxia that resulted in a moderate-to-severe articulation disorder, with limited speech intelligibility related to deficiencies in oral-motor timing and range of motion. She may also have had a mild expressive language disorder with deficits noted in morphologic (plurals) and syntactic (grammatical) structures, although such deficits are difficult to separate from the influence of an articulation disorder. In addition, receptive language skills were within normal limits for her age.

Audiologic Results

The overall pattern of results from the audiologic test battery was consistent with CAPD. In addition, the child had middle ear disorder on the left, accompanied by a mild, low-frequency conductive hearing loss. The CAPD was characterized by depressed speech understanding of single-syllable words presented in competition, and by a dichotic deficit. Depressed speech understanding was accompanied by abnormality in the late-latency auditory evoked potentials.

Acoustic immittance measures consisted of tympanometry, static immittance, and acoustic reflex thresholds. Results indicated normal middle ear function in the right ear. Left ear results indicated middle ear disorder, consistent with fixation of the ossicular chain, characterized by a type A tympanogram, low static immittance, and absent acoustic reflexes.

Results of pure-tone and speech audiometry are shown in Fig. 2. Pure-tone sensitivity was within normal limits in the right ear. The left ear showed a mild, low-frequency conductive hearing loss.

The PSI test was used to assess auditory processing ability. Performance-intensity functions were obtained for both words and sentences in the presence of ipsilateral competition at 4dB and 0 dB MCR, respectively. Initial practice was carried out at a 10 dB more favorable MCR to assure that JC was capable of performing the task. Performance on the PSI sentence task was also measured with a CCM over a range of 0 to −20 dB MCR. Results were abnormal in both ears. Although JC's ability to identify sentences in the presence of competition was within normal limits, her ability to identify words in competition was abnormal for both ears. The right ear performance-intensity function showed rollover. For the left ear, the absolute score at the point of maximum performance was abnormally depressed. In addition, for the dichotic listening task, wherein sentences are presented with a CCM, performance was markedly abnormal, with a score of 0% in the left ear and 100% in the right ear.

Auditory evoked potentials were measured using conventional signal and recording parameters. Click stimuli were used to elicit ABRs, and tone-burst stimuli were used to elicit MLRs and LVRs. Results of the auditory evoked potential assessment (Fig. 3) showed that both the MLRs and ABRs were well formed and had peaks at appropriate and symmetric latencies. However, late vertex responses were not identifiable for either ear.

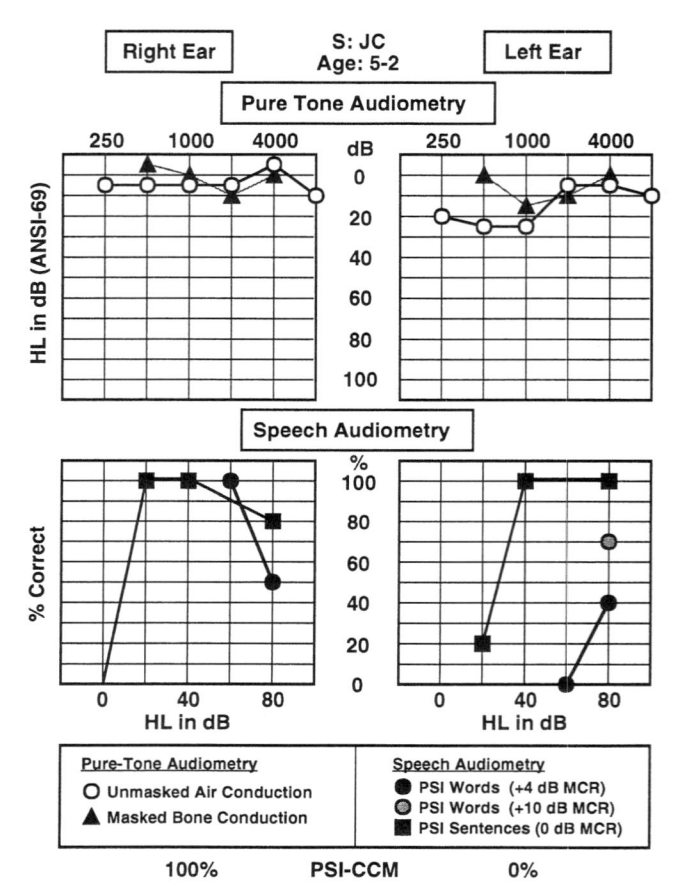

FIG. 2. Pure-tone and speech audiometric results in a 5-year, 2-month-old child with a diagnosis of CAPD. See Fig. 1 for explanation.

Rehabilitative Assessment and Course

Because JC demonstrated difficulty in understanding speech in the presence of background competition, our next clinical goal was to determine the extent to which she could benefit from an enhancement in SNR.

JC reported that she had difficulty understanding the teacher when she wrote on the board and that she could not listen to her teacher and write at the same time. Coupled with parental and teacher concerns over progress in the classroom, the decision was made to implement trial use of an FM system in the classroom. JC appeared enthusiastic about the trial and began using the device at school on a regular basis.

After wearing the device for a month, reports from the teacher and parents suggested that its use was having a noticeable impact. Evidence of FM system benefit included (a) a reduction in the number of emotional outbursts in the classroom; (b) an improvement in the care in which her assignments were carried out; and (c) improvement in the quality of her overall classroom performance.

For the next 2 years, JC continued FM-system use and

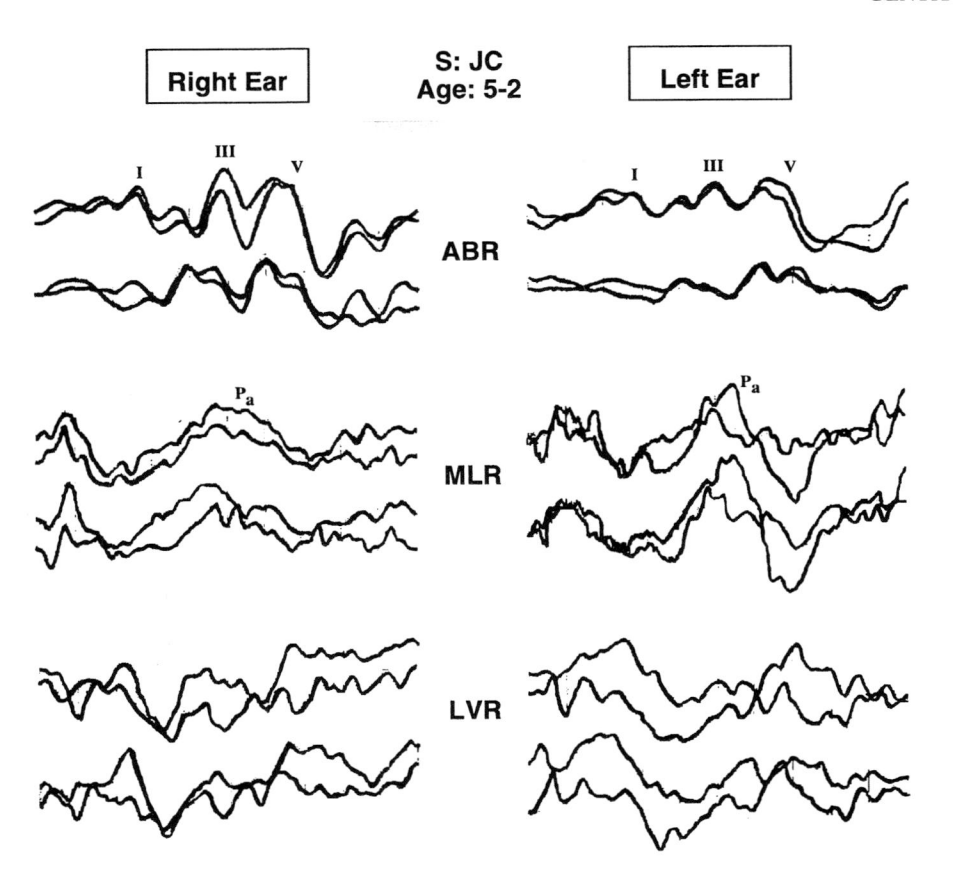

FIG. 3. Auditory evoked potentials in a 5-year, 2-month-old child with a diagnosis of central auditory processing disorder (CAPD) including the auditory brainstem response (ABR) with its component peaks I, III, and V; the middle latency response (MLR) with its component peak Pa; and the late vertex response (LVR).

speech treatment. Continual progress was noted in her motor speech ability, and her academic achievement flourished. Hearing sensitivity was monitored and showed no significant change.

Audiologic Reevaluation

A complete audiologic evaluation was carried out at age 8 years, 2 months (3 years after the initial diagnosis of CAPD). Pure-tone audiometry showed normal sensitivity in the right ear and a mild conductive loss in the left ear. Immittance measures continued to be normal on the right and consistent with middle ear disorder on the left, characterized by an increase in the stiffness of the middle ear mechanism. Results on the SSI test were within normal limits and were considered somewhat exceptional for a child of this young age. Because the abnormal results from the initial evaluation were obtained with the PSI-ICM for word identification and with the PSI-CCM for dichotic ability, both tests were administered again. As expected in an 8 year old, PSI-ICM maximum scores were 100% for both ears, as were PSI-CCM scores at −20 dB MCR. Auditory evoked potential testing was also carried out, but with an expanded protocol. Results of ABR testing remained normal. Both the MLR and LVR were recorded with multiple electrodes and topographic mapping of brain activity. Responses were similar to those obtained when JC was first diagnosed with CAPD.

Although middle latency responses were normal, LVRs continued to show no response in the left ear and a very delayed negative response, at 267 ms, in the right ear.

Comment

JC was not unlike many children who are referred for audiologic assessment to rule out CAPD. While some have no apparent speech and language deficits, others have language deficits that are considerably more severe. Her audiologic profile and the course of her treatment and progress over a 3-year period serve to illustrate several critical concepts in the clinical diagnosis and treatment of children with CAPD. They also serve to illustrate some of the questions that remain unanswered regarding this disorder.

One concept illustrated by JC's results is that speech audiometric strategies can be used that permit the assessment of auditory processing ability in a manner that reduces the likelihood of nonauditory factors influencing the interpretation of test results. Results showed rollover of the PSI word function in the right ear and a substantial discrepancy between word and sentence understanding in the left ear. This is obviously not a language problem, because, at 60 dB HL in the right ear, the child identifies all of the words correctly. The child is clearly capable of doing the task linguistically and cognitively and has the attentional ability to complete the task. Thus, the deficit appears to be in her auditory processing ability. In this case, the nature of the disorder was an increased difficulty in identifying words in competition, presumably due to more limited redundancy in words than in sentences.

Another concept that is illustrated by this case study is that intervention strategies directed toward enhancement of SNR ratio can be effective in the treatment of children with CAPD. In the case of JC, due to the severity of the auditory processing disorder, the use of remote-microphone technology was indicated and proved to be effective in overcoming her deficit in understanding speech in background noise in the classroom.

The case of patient JC also illustrates one of the most pressing and elusive questions related to the diagnosis and treatment of CAPD: Will the child grow out of it? It is our clinical impression that children do not grow out of the disorder, although they appear to develop compensatory skills as they get older. Our course of action with JC was based on both our lack of knowledge of the answer to this question and our sense of urgency at solving the immediate problem of difficulty in the classroom. That is, we took the approach that it was better to try to forestall achievement problems than to wait to see if she would grow out of it. Our clinical evidence was actually conflicting. Speech audiometric results improved over the 3-year period. This improvement could be interpreted to suggest (a) that she no longer has the disorder, (b) that the speech audiometric measures lost sensitivity for the disorder as she became older, or (c) that her compensatory skills developed to an extent that she could then perform well on these measures. On the other hand, auditory evoked potentials remained abnormal over the 3-year period, suggesting that, in fact, the disorder remained.

REFERENCES

1. Jerger S. Validation of the pediatric speech intelligibility test in children with central nervous system lesions. *Audiology* 1987;26:298–311.
2. Goodglass H. Binaural digit presentation and early lateral brain damage. *Cortex* 1967;3:295–306.
3. Bergman M, Costeff H, Koren V, Koifman N, Reshef A. Auditory perception in early lateralized brain damage. *Cortex* 1984;20:233–42.
4. Woods B. Dichotic listening ear preference after childhood cerebral lesions. *Neuropsychologia* 1984;22:303–10.
5. Jerger S, Martin RC, Jerger J. Specific auditory perceptual dysfunction in a learning disabled child. *Ear Hear* 1987;8:78–86.
6. Young ML, Protti-Patterson E. Management perspectives of central auditory problems in children: top-down and bottom-up considerations. *Semin Hear* 1984;5:251–61.
7. Dalebout SD, Nelson NW, Hletko PJ, Frentheway B. Selective auditory attention and children with attention-deficit hyperactivity disorder: effects of repeated measurement with and without methylphenidate. *Lang Speech Hear Services Schools* 1991;22:219–27.
8. Grundfast KM, Berkowitz RG, Conners CK, Belman P. Complete evaluation of the child identified as a poor listener. *Int J Pediatr Otorhinolaryngol* 1991;21:65–78.
9. Chermak GD, Musiek FE. Managing central auditory processing disorders in children and youth. *Am J Audiol* 31992;1(3):61–5.
10. Keller WD. Auditory processing disorder or attention-deficit disorder?, In: Katz J. Stecker N, Henderson D, eds. *Central auditory processing: a transdisciplinary view.* St Louis: Mosby Year Book 1992:107–14.
11. Jerger J, Johnson K, Loiselle L. Pediatric central auditory dysfunction: comparison of children with confirmed lesions versus suspected processing disorders. *Am J Otol* 1988 [Suppl] 9:63–71.
12. Jerger S, Jerger J, Alford BR, Abrams S. Development of speech intelligibility in children with recurrent otitis media. *Ear Hear* 1983;4:138–45.
13. Hall JW, Grose JH, Pillsbury HC. Long-term effects of chronic otitis media on binaural hearing in children. *Arch Otolaryngol* 1995;121:847–52.
14. Schilder AGM, Snik AFM, Straatman H, van den Broek P. The effect of otitis media with effusion at preschool age on some aspects of auditory perception at school age. *Ear Hear* 1994;15:224–31.
15. Brown DP. Speech recognition in recurrent otitis media: results in a set of identical twins. *J Am Acad Audiol* 1994;5:1–6.
16. Gascon GG, Johnson R, Burd L. Central auditory processing and attention deficit disorder. *J Child Neurol* 1986;1:27–33.
17. Keith RW, Rudy J, Donahue PA, Katbamna B. Comparison of SCAN results with other auditory and language measures in a clinical population. *Ear Hear* 1989;10:382–86.
18. Engineer P, Keith RW. Effects of methylphenidate on auditory processing abilities of children with attention deficit—hyperactivity disorder. *Audiology Today* 1991;3:44 (abst).
19. Willeford J. Assessing central auditory behavior in children: a test battery approach, In: Keith R ed. *Central auditory dysfunction.* New York: Grune and Stratton; 1977:43–72.
20. Musiek F, Geurkink N, Keitel S. Test battery assessment of auditory perceptual dysfunction in children. *Laryngoscope* 1982;92:251–7.
21. Stecker NA. Central auditory processing: implications in audiology. In: Katz J, Stecker N, Henderson D, eds. *Central auditory processing: A transdisciplinary view.* St Louis: Mosby Year Book 1992:117–27.
22. Katz J. Classification of auditory processing disorders. In Katz J, Stecker N, Henderson D, eds. *Central auditory processing: A transdisciplinary view.* St Louis: Mosby Year Book 1992:81–91.
23. Jerger S, Lewis S, Hawkins J, Jerger J. Pediatric speech intelligibility test. I. Generation of test materials. *Int J Pediatr Otorhinolaryngol* 1980;2:217–30.
24. Jerger J, Speaks C, Trammel J. A new approach to speech audiometry. *J Speech Hear Disord* 1968;33:318–27.
25. Fifer RC, Jerger JF, Berlin CI, Tobey EA, Campbell JC. Development of a dichotic sentence identification test for hearing-impaired adults. *Ear Hear* 1983;4:300–5.
26. Jirsa RE, Clontz KB. Long latency auditory event-related potentials from children with auditory processing disorders. *Ear Hear* 1990;11:222–32.
27. Musiek F, Bornstein S. Auditory event-related potentials in central auditory disorders. In: Katz J, Stecker N, Henderson D, eds. *Central auditory processing: a transdisciplinary view.* St Louis: Mosby Year Book 1992:151–60.
28. Stach BA, Loiselle LH, Jerger JF. Auditory evoked potential abnormalities in children with central auditory disorder. *ASHA* 1988;30:133 (abst).
29. Smoski WJ, Brunt MA, Tannahill JC. Listening characteristics of children with central auditory processing disorders. *Lang Speech Hear Services Schools* 1992;23:145–152.
30. Stach BA, Loiselle LH, Jerger JF, Mintz SL, Taylor CD. Clinical experience with personal FM assistive listening devices. *Hear J* 1987;40:24–30.
31. Stach BA. Hearing aid amplification and central processing disorders. In: Sandlin RE, ed. *Handbook of Hearing Aid Amplification.* Vol. II: *Clinical considerations and fitting practices.* Boston: College-Hill Press; 1990:87–111.
32. Stach BA, Loiselle LH, Jerger JF. FM system use by children with central auditory processing disorder. *ASHA* 1987;29:69 (abst).
33. Schneider D. Audiologic management of central auditory processing disorders. In: Katz J, Stecker N, Henderson D, eds. *Central auditory processing: a transdisciplinary view.* St Louis: Mosby Year Book 1992:161–8.
34. Aoki C, Siekevitz P. Plasticity in brain development. *Sci Am* 1988;259:56–64.
35. Stach BA, Loiselle LH. Central auditory processing disorder: Diagnosis and management in a young child. *Semin Hear* 1993;14:288–95.

CHAPTER 26

Diagnosis and Management of Sensorineural Hearing Disorders

Thomas J. Balkany and Michal Luntz

Without sound, part of the continuity and logic of life is lost. Hearing is essential to children for language acquisition, socialization, and cognitive development, as well as material to safety and enjoyment of many of life s greatest pleasures. Loss of this critical sense in infants is among the most handicapping and prevalent of disabilities (1). In the United States each year, 4,000 children are born deaf and 37,000 more are born with milder degrees of hearing loss (HL); enough to impair normal development of language and speech. In all, 6 children in 1,000 are born with significant hearing impairment (2,3).

CLASSIFICATION

The most important features to consider in classifying childhood hearing loss are degree, age of onset, and etiology. These factors are highly correlated with the impact sensorineural hearing loss (SNHL) has on the child and family. In general, the greater the degree of bilateral hearing loss and the earlier its onset, the more severe the consequences. Thus, prelingual, profoundly deaf children experience the greatest impact on language development, education, and lifestyle. However, even mild conductive hearing loss associated with otitis media with effusion can result in delayed language acquisition (see Chapter 41). Classification by etiology is also useful in treating, predicting progression, and establishing the risk of SNHL in family members. It is estimated that 50% of childhood SNHL is genetic, 20% to 25% acquired, and 25% to 30% of unknown cause (4).

GENETIC HEARING LOSS

Since genetic SNHL was first established 150 years ago, a progressively greater proportion of SNHL has been found

T.J. Balkany: Department of Otolaryngology, University of Miami Ear Institute, and Neurological Surgery and Pediatrics, University of Miami, Miami, Florida 33101.
M. Luntz: Department of Otolaryngology—Bnai Zion Medical Center, Faculty of Medicine Technion, Haifa, Israel 31048.

to be of genetic etiology (5). Genetic SNHL may be congenital (for the purposes of this chapter, congenital refers to HL present at birth) or delayed in onset; syndromic (associated with other anomalies) or nonsyndromic (6). About 75% to 80% of genetic HL is transmitted in an autosomal recessive mode, 18% to 20% is autosomal dominant. The rest are X-linked or are the result of chromosomal disorders (4). The main difficulty in the diagnosis of genetic hearing loss is its variability in expression, including both recessive transmission and erratic penetrance of dominant transmission (7).

Syndromic Sensorineural Hearing Loss

Syndromic SNHL accounts for 7% to 12% of children with SNHL (8,9), and is classified on the basis of the other organ systems involved (e.g., craniofacial, cervical, skeletal, ocular, neurologic, renal, metabolic, etc.) and on the mode of inheritance. Although approximately 1% of newborns have multiple anomalies, only 40% of the anomalies are recognized as syndromes. It is estimated that new syndromes are being described at a rate of more than one per week (10), and many include SNHL. Due to recessive transmission and variation in expression, not all symptoms are present in affected individuals.

Autosomal Dominant Syndromes

Waarendenburg syndrome consists of hearing impairment, heterochromasia (two different colors of the eyes), white forelock (poliosis) and telecanthus. Two types of Waarendenburg syndrome are recognized. Type I, without hypertelorism, is responsible for 2% of congenital deafness; type II, with true hypertelurism, is less common. In type I, SNHL occurs in 20% of patients, and type II in 50% of patients. Hearing loss can be unilateral or bilateral, vary from mild to profound, and can also be progressive. The gene for type I has been located to chromosome 2 (4,11–13).

Branchio-otorenal syndrome is hearing impairment with earpits, structural defects of the outer ear or middle ear (fixed stapes and fused ossicles) or with inner-ear anomalies (cochlear dysplasia) and renal anomalies (mild hypoplasia to complete agenesis). The gene for this abnormality is found on chromosome 8. The frequency of the syndrome is approximately 1 in 40,000. Hearing loss can be conductive, sensorineural or mixed (4,11,12,14).

Stickler syndrome is a connective tissue disorder that includes progressive sensorineural or mixed hearing loss in 15% of the patients, and retinal detachment, cataract, myopia, cleft palate, micrognathia, hypermobility, enlargement of the joints, and early adult onset of arthritis. Genes responsible for this syndrome were identified on chromosomes 12 and 6 (4,12,15).

Osteogenesis imperfecta is a disorder of bone fragility, blue eclera, hyperelasticity of joints and ligaments, and a progressive, usually bilateral mixed hearing loss. There are four clinical types of osteogenesis imperfecta. The incidence of HL varies by type. In osteogenesis imperfecta type I, HL is 43%. The severe congenital type may be present with intrauterine fractures. Van der Hoeve syndrome is a subtype in which hearing loss begins in early childhood and progresses. The most significant otologic finding in osteogenesis imperfecta is the fixation of the stapes. Stapes surgery is often less satisfactory in patients with osteogenesis imperfecta as compared to surgery in patients with otosclerosis (4,11,12,16).

Treacher Collins syndrome is the result of bilateral defects of first and the second branchial arch derivatives. The clinical features are malar hypoplasia, mandibular hypoplasia, projection of scalp hair onto cheek, defect in the lower lid (coloboma), downward obliquity of palpebral fissures, microtia, aural atresia, hearing loss, cleft palate, ear tags, and first branchial arch fistulas. Hearing loss is usually conductive but SNHL and vestibular dysfunction may also be present. The frequency of Treacher Collins syndrome among profoundly deaf children is 0.7% (17). Its gene is located on chromosome 5 (4,12,18).

Autosomal Recessive Syndromes

Usher syndrome (USH) consists of hearing impairment with retinitis pigmentosa. Its frequency is 4.4 in 100,000 in the United States. About half of the deaf-blind population in the US have Usher syndrome. It is the causal factor in 3% to 6% of deaf children. Seven different genes have been identified for this impairment. Clinically, three subtypes exist: type I presents with congenital profound hearing loss and absent vestibular function, type II with moderate hearing loss and normal vestibular function, and type III (which is extremely rare) with progressive hearing loss (4,11,12,19).

Pendred syndrome is SNHL-associated with abnormal iodine metabolism resulting in euthyroid goiter (4). The gene for this syndrome is probably on chromosome 8 (18) and it is found in 0.5% of profoundly deaf children (17).

Jervell and Lange-Nielsen syndrome is severe congenital SNHL with cardiac conduction defect, which may produce syncopal episodes and even sudden death in infancy. The electrocardiogram (ECG) demonstrates large T waves and prolongation of QT interval.

Hurler syndrome (mucopolysaccharidosis type I) is a storage disease in which the child is born normal. However, the lack of lysosomal enzyme for degradation of a glycosaminoglycan molecule causes mental retardation, coarse face, corneal clouding, and progressive hearing loss. It becomes clinically evident by the second year of life (11).

X-Linked Syndromes

Alport syndrome is hearing impairment with nephritis and may also include ocular (lenticonus and macular flecks) and hematologic abnormalities (macrothrombocytopenia) or leiomyomatosis of the esophagus. Through a separate method of inheritance it is also occasionally seen in women. Both hearing loss and kidney disease are progressive; however, their severities are not correlated. The hearing loss is usually diagnosed in the second decade as high-tone loss that becomes rapidly progressive. The renal disease may cause hematuria in infancy but generally remains asymptomatic until several years before onset of renal insufficiency (4,11,12,20).

Hunter syndrome (mucopolysaccharidosis type II) is a storage disease, similar but less severe than *Hurler syndrome*. Hearing loss is progressive, mixed or sensorineural (21).

Nonsyndromic Sensorineural Hearing Loss

Nonsyndromic SNHL is thought to be the cause in 20% to 36% of children with SNHL (8,9). Diagnosis of nonsyndromic hearing loss may be difficult and is based on comparing audiometric configuration (21), age at onset, and progression, preferably over three generations (7).

The pattern of audiometric configuration may be helpful in establishing the diagnosis of genetic nonsyndromic SNHL. The pattern can be sloping, flat, residual (residual hearing in the low or high frequencies) or "cookie-bite pattern" (U-shaped audiograms) (6). The latter configurations, when seen, are relatively specific but not sensitive indications of genetic SNHL, which is present in only a minority of cases (6). Dominant progressive hearing loss (DPHL) is one of the most common forms of nonsyndromic genetic deafness. Like presbyacousia, but with earlier onset, DPHL is actually a group of disorders, which vary among different families in rate of progression, initial frequencies involved, and ultimate severity of the loss. However, the characteristics are relatively consistent with a given family.

Cochlear Dysplasia

Cochlear dysplasia (inner-ear structural malformation) causes SNHL, which may be diagnosed by high-resolution computed tomography (HRCT), and is sometimes treatable. Michel dysplasia is aplasia of the cochlea. Various bony anomalies of the inner ear have been lumped under the term *Mondini dysplasia*. The classification suggested by Jackler, Luxford, and House (22), which uses the terms common cavity, incomplete parition, and "hypoplasia," is based on the theory that these malformations result from an arrest of development during varying stages of inner-ear organogenesis. *Scheibe dysplasia* is a malformation limited to the membranous labyrinth; therefore, the CT scan is normal. Schiebe dysplasis has been reported in several syndromes including Usher and Waardenburg, and it is the predominant anomaly in rubella deafness (23). Some inner-ear malformations isolated to the membranaceous labyrinth, and which are not demonstrated on HRCT, scan have also been described. *Bing-Seibenman malformation* is characterized by normal abnormal membranous labyrinth of both the pars inferior (cochlear duct) and superior (semicircular ducts). The bony labyrinth is normal (24). Alexander dysplasia is characterized by a defect in the development of the organ of Corti and the ganglion cells limited to the basal coil. Therefore, the CT scan is normal and hearing loss is limited to the high frequencies (4,25).

NONGENETIC HEARING LOSS

Nongenetic hearing loss in children may be associated with infection, ototoxic drugs, noise trauma, metabolic disorders, autoimmune inner-ear disease, perilymphatic fistula, or the cause may be unknown.

Infections

Infections that cause SNHL can be congenital (toxoplasmosis, cytomegalovirus, rubella, herpes simplex encephalitis, and syphilis) or may occur later in life (bacterial meningitis, mumps, measles).

Congenital cytomegalovirus is currently the most common infectious cause of congenital SNHL, occurring in about 1% to 2% of live births (26), 90% of which have no overt signs of disease in the neonatal period. The incidence of hearing loss in this group of infants is 5% to 15% (23). In 1% to 5% of the infected patients, cytomegalic inclusion disease develops; SNHL occurs in as much as 50% of this group. In patients with congenital cytomegalovirus, SNHL tends to be more pronounced in the high frequencies and is usually bilateral (23). Hearing may continue to deteriorate for years (26). Diagnosis is made by isolation of cytomegalovirus from cord blood or fresh urine during the first 1 to 2 weeks of life, therefore making the diagnosis unlikely in the majority of cases.

Congenital rubella is highly associated with severe to profound SNHL that is often progressive (11). It is usually associated with first-trimester maternal rubella, but second-trimester maternal rubella may also cause SNHL. About 50% of mothers in whom virus is isolated are asymptomatic. Hearing loss is the only defect found in 22% of the rubella population. When the virus is clinically isolated, 57% of the infants have hearing loss. Hearing loss is sensorineural and varies in degree. Most typical is the cookie-bite audiometric configuration with greatest loss in the middle frequencies. The mandatory administration of rubella vaccine has reduced significantly the incidence of rubella (4). The diagnosis is achieved by isolation of rubella virus from urine or throat cultures during the first weeks of life, identification of IgM antibodies against rubella in serum from the neonate, or increased antibody titer to rubella virus in the infant during the first few months of life (23).

Although *congenital toxoplasmosis* is subclinical in 90% of patients, when symptoms are present they can be severe and often include SNHL (4). Maternal toxoplasmosis is diagnosed by maternal seroconversion and is treated by pyrimethamine and sulfonamide. Fetal infection is diagnosed by amniotic fluid and fetal blood inoculation into mice and maternal and fetal IgG studies. The treatment of congenitally infected infants is administration of alternative courses of pyrimethamine and sulfonamide.

Neonatal herpes simplex encephalitis is known to have a predilection for the temporal and frontal areas of the brain. Only 50% of neonatal herpes simplex virus infections are related to a recognized maternal infection. Diagnosis is made clinically in the presence of fever, altered mental state, abnormal cerebrospinal fluid (CSF) findings, and focal meningoencephalitis as shown by electroencephalogram (EEG), CT scan and magnetic resonance imaging (MRI). Treatment consists of high-dose intravenous acyclovir (4).

Congenital syphilis causes hearing loss in 38% of infected patients. In 37%, hearing loss develops before the age of 10 years. The hearing loss is often sudden, bilateral and profound (27). The fluorescent treponemal antibody-absorption (FTA-ABS) test, which detects antibodies that react with treponemal antigens, has a 98% specificity and nearly 100% sensitivity in cases of otologic syphilis (28).

Post-natal bacterial meningitis has been estimated to be responsible for 90% of acquired hearing impairment diagnosed by the age of 3 years (29). Approximately 6% to 8% of all childhood hearing impairment is due to bacterial meningitis (30,31,32). The incidence of hearing impairment in children surviving bacterial meningitis has been reported to be from 3.5% to 37.2% (33,34–38). Hearing loss following meningitis is usually bilateral, but can be asymmetric or unilateral (33,36,37). Progressive and fluctuating cases have also been noted (33,36). For bilateral profound losses, the incidence is 1% to 4% (39). Patients who have initial low concentration of glucose in their CSF during the disease carry a much higher risk of hearing impairment (36,39). It is commonly accepted that the incidence of hearing loss after pneumococcal meningitis is higher (31%) than after *Neisseria* meningitis (10.5%) or *Haemophilus influenzae* meningitis (6%) (23). Bacterial meningitis has been reduced by immunization for *H. influenzae* (39,40).

In severe cases of hearing loss, damage is most likely

to occur as a result of direct spread of infection from the subarachnoid space to the inner ear, thus causing suppurative labyrinthitis. Occasionally, reversible SNHL occurs. In such cases, it is postulated that toxic or serous labyrinthitis is responsible (39). Recent studies on experimental animals have shown that lysis of bacterial cells by antimicrobial agents produces endotoxin that initiates an inflammatory reaction which may be responsible for the hair-cell damage (41,42). The notion that the concomitant use of steroids with antibiotics decreases inner ear inflammation and thereby lessens damage to the inner ear (39,41) has been challenged by studies that failed to show a beneficial effect of steroids for audiologic, neurologic, or developmental outcomes in children with bacterial meningitis (43).

Deafness from mumps is estimated to be associated with hearing loss in 5 of every 10,000 patients with mumps (44). Hearing loss is unilateral in 80% of cases, very often profound and permanent. The vestibular system is occasionally involved but this condition is clinically resolved after several weeks.

Rubeola virus (measles) has been reduced since the introduction of vaccine. Measles presents with abrupt, usually bilateral, hearing loss at the time of the rash. The degree of hearing loss varies, but 45% of patients have profound loss. Diagnosis is made by isolation of rubeola virus from the throat, identification of rubeola viral antigen by immunofluorescent staining of exfoliated perithelial cells obtained by swabbing the pharynx, conjunctiva, or buccal cavity, and by demonstration of a fourfold or greater serologic rise in measles antibody titer taken between acute and convalescent serum samples (23).

Noise-Induced Sensorineural Hearing Loss

Noise-induced SNHL occurs in older children as a result of exposure to personal music players, noisy toys, fireworks, and recreational devices. Thus, noise-induced SNHL in children is preventable. Only 26% of children diagnosed as having noise-induced hearing loss were found to be under 10 years of age (45).

Ototoxic Drugs

Although the list of potentially ototoxic drugs is long (4), those that are relevant in infants and children are aminoglycosides, diuretics, and (occasionally) antimetabolites. When given together, potentiation occurs. Children receiving these drugs are often in the intensive care unit.

Metabolic Disorders

Hyperbilirubinemia in the neonatal period has long been associated with progressive SNHL (11). Fluctuating SNHL is associated with lipid levels in children and is reversible with dietary control of the cholesterol levels (46). Other metabolic disturbances responsible for SNHL in infants and children are congenital hypothyroidism, rare enzymatic disorders (e.g., galactosemia) (9) and glycogen-storage disorders.

Perilymph Fistula

Perilymph fistula (PLF) is an abnormal passage of perilymph from the inner to the middle ear. Perilymph fistula is suspected in children with SNHL when HRCT demonstrates cochlear dysplasia. When such dysplasia is found, exploration of the middle ear is indicated. Obliteration of PLF is indicated for prevention of bacterial meningitis, for control of vestibular symptoms that may accompany hearing loss, and for prevention of further deterioration of hearing. Middle-ear exploration may also be indicated for progressive SNHL in the absence of inner-ear dysplasia, especially when SNHL is accompanied by vestibular symptoms. This finding, however, is less clear, and explanation regarding the controversy should be offered to the parents.

CHARGE Association, a term first introduced by Pagon in 1981 (47) consists of four of the following anomalies: ocular *c*oloboma, *h*eart defect, choanal *a*tresia, *r*etarded growth or development (or both), *g*enital hypoplasia and *e*ar anomalies, possibly with hearing loss. The etiology of this disease entity is unknown and has been reported as both teratogenic and genetic (48). Hearing loss appears in 21% to 95% of individuals (48,49). Various malformations of the inner ear and middle ear, including ossicular anomalies absence of oval window and Mondini malformation, have been described in histological studies (50).

EARLY INDENTIFICATION OF HEARING LOSS

The 10% to 15% reduction in income for the 350,000 deaf and the 21,000,000 hard of hearing in the United States costs an estimated $76.5 billion annually. Because deaf people with normal hearing until 3 years of age earn 5% more than persons born deaf, early identification and intervention is estimated to reduce this burden by $3.9 billion (51,52).

Perinatal risk factors are present in 33% to 57% of children educated in residential schools for the deaf (53,54). Low birth weight, hyperbilirubinemia, low Apgar score, requirement for mechanical ventilation, and fetal respiratory distress syndrome are most commonly defined as such risk factors. However, most reasons for admitting a newborn into the neonatal intensive care unit (NICU) can be considered as risk factors for SNHL. As much as 7% of NICU graduates have SNHL (55–57).

It is also estimated that universal newborn screening would detect 41,000 children born deaf or hard of hearing and would cost $381 million. This is still ten orders of magnitude less than the $3.9 billion that would be saved annually with early identification and treatment of hearing loss achieved through universal screening.

The Joint Committee on Infant Hearing of the American Academy of Otolaryngology—Head and Neck Surgery endorsed in December 1994 (58) the goal of universal detection

TABLE 1. *Indicators associated with sensorineural and conductive hearing loss (58)*

Neonates (birth through age 28 days) with no universal screening
  Family history of hereditary congenital childhood SNHL
  Mother's in utero infection (cytomegalovirus, rubella, syphilis, herpes, toxoplasmosis)
  Craniofacial anomalies, including morphologic abnormalities of the pinna and ear canal
  Birth weight less than 1,500 gm (3.3 lb)
  Hyperbilirubinemia at a serum level requiring exchange transfusion
  Ototoxic medication including aminoglycosides in multiple courses or in combination with loop diuretics
  Bacterial meningitis
  Apgar score of 0–4 at 1 minute or 0–6 at 5 minutes
  Mechanical ventilation for 5 days or longer
  Stigmata/other findings associated with syndrome including SNHL and/or conductive hearing loss
Infants (age 29 days through 2 years) with health conditions requiring rescreening
  Parent/caregiver's concern regarding hearing, speech, language and/or developmental delay
  Bacterial meningitis
  Head trauma associated with loss of consciousness or skull fracture
  Stigmata/other findings associated with syndrome including SNHL and/or conductive hearing loss
  Ototoxic medication including aminoglycosides in multiple courses or in combination with loop diuretics
  Recurrent/persistent otitis media with effusion for at least 3 months
Infants (age 29 days through 3 years) requiring periodic hearing monitoring[a]
  Family history of hereditary childhood hearing loss
  Mother's in utero infection (cytomegalovirus, rubella, syphilis, herpes, and toxoplasmosis)
  Neurofibromatosis type II and neurodegenerative disorders

[a] Infants with these indicators require hearing evaluation at least every 6 months until age 3 years, and at appropriate intervals thereafter.

of infants with hearing loss as early as possible. The committee determined that all infants with hearing loss should be identified before 3 months of age and should receive intervention by 6 months of age. Universal audiometric screening of all newborns with otoacoustic emissions or auditory brainstem response was also recommended as a goal by the National Institutes of Health (NIH) consensus conference statement on early identification of hearing impairment in infants and young children (59). When universal screening is not available, high-risk registers can be used to identify infants who should be tested (Table 1). Of children with educationally significant SNHL only 50% to 60% have one of these risk factors (53,60). Unfortunately, 40% to 50% of hearing-impaired children do not exhibit any risk factor (53).

MANAGEMENT OF CHILDREN WITH SENSORINEURAL HEARING LOSS

Management of SNHL is in large part individualized and based on the age of the patient and degree of hearing loss. Most children with mild to severe losses should have normal language development and educational achievement with early identification and intervention. In children under the age of 6 months, this may require that amplification be based on preliminary audiometric findings, often prior to obtaining definitive auditory thresholds.

The goals of management of SNHL are to (a) determine the type and degree; (b) identify the etiology (focusing on treatable causes); (c) institute early medical treatment when possible; (d) provide early amplification and (re)habilitation; (e) involve the parents in all aspects, including the diagnostic and therapeutic plans, appropriate expectations for their child's future, and provide access to appropriate resources, support, and educational organizations.

Determining the Type and Degree

Audiometric testing may be instituted within days of birth (Chapter 39). Once auditory threshold levels are estimated, amplification is begun and a plan for management can be developed for the child. This process should not be delayed pending definitive audiometric results.

Audiometry is repeated monthly until definitive thresholds are obtained. Because progression has been reported in 25% to 50% of children with SNHL (61–63), and in 78% of ears of children with hereditary SNHL (61), testing (aided and unaided) is repeated every 3 months until thresholds are shown to be stable. Once stable, testing should be repeated every 6 months until the child is 36 months of age (the heart of the critical period for language development), and then yearly. If fluctuation or progression occurs, the child should be tested every 3 months until stable.

Identifying the Etiology

Primary efforts are to identify treatable causes of hearing loss. Next, attention is paid to congenital causes, which may effect family planning. Finally, identifying other causes of SNHL is helpful to the family in accepting their child's condition and in predicting long-term hearing levels.

The usual admonitions regarding a complete history including genetic pedigree, consanguinity, perinatal maternal fever, rash or other illness, and complete physical examination with attention to craniofacial anomalies, digits, and skin are well established. In question are which of the dozens of available tests should be performed when the child is referred to the otolaryngologist, usually between 6 and 18 months of age.

I routinely perform serologic testing for syphilis (although the yield is low); HRCT for inner-ear malformation, which may be associated with PLF; electrocardiography for the slight chance of sudden chance death due to Jervell and Lange-Neilson syndrome; and urinalysis, ultrasound, or both for renal abnormalities. Thyroid functions are performed when other signs of cretinism accompany SNHL. Pediatric ophthalmologic consultation is obtained due to the high incidence of visual problems in children with SNHL and because it may aid in the diagnosis (e.g., rubella, retinitis pigmentosa). Lipid profiles are not currently obtained and await further reports to verify utility.

When a treatable etiology is not identified, the child is evaluated by a geneticist. Viral screening is usually not helpful at the time the patient is seen by the otolaryngologist. However, if the child is seen early, the toxoplasmosis, rubella, cytomegalovirus, herpes (TORCH) screen is ordered. In spite of every effort, the etiology is identified in less than 50% of children.

Medical Treatment

Syphilis is treated with penicillin or a substitute antimicrobial following lumbar puncture and complete evaluation. Imaging evidence of inner-ear malformation associated with progressive SNHL is an indication for middle-ear exploration. The progress of SNHL can be slowed or halted by repair of PLF. In addition, repair is necessary to obviate otitic meningitis. Children with abnormal ECG are managed by a pediatric cardiologist and may require permanent pacing. Likewise, abnormalities of the eyes and kidneys are managed by the appropriate specialist. It is important to carefully control otitis media because its additional conductive hearing problem may cause the aggregate hearing loss to exceed the range of the hearing aids.

Early Amplification

Too often critical time is lost between identification of SNHL and the pinpointing of definitive auditory thresholds. Once thresholds are estimated, amplification should be initiated. If it is not possible to estimate threshold, I use moderate gain aids binaurally as a clinical trial. Parents, audiologists, therapists, and educators then work together to determine whether the child is responding. If the child does not respond, more powerful aids are tried.

Family Consultation

For a child with SNHL, the parents may have just begun to accept the fact of their perfect child s serious flaw. It is important to establish that the problem is not rare and that expertise and help are available.

The otolaryngologist should anticipate and discuss the family's four basic questions: How severe is the hearing loss? What is the cause of the hearing loss? Will the hearing get worse? What are we going to do? To the extent that the otolaryngologist can anticipate these issues, articulate them, and propose a rational plan of action, an excellent relationship can be established, relieving anxiety and leading to appropriate management. Unfortunately, the divorce rate among parents of deaf children is approximately 80% in my practice; and thus, parents need to avoid both recrimination and placing their total focus on the child.

Parents should understand the value of establishing an etiologic diagnosis, although this is possible in fewer than half the of children in my practice. It is impossible to predict the progression of hearing loss; however, most SNHL tends to get worse over time. Serial audiograms give an indication of the rate of progression. The plan is to establish the etiology, determine the precise degree of hearing loss (and language developmental level in older infants and children), and begin rehabilitation simultaneously. Purely unilateral SNHL acquired after the first year of life tends to remain unilateral.

An initial language evaluation is undertaken followed by appropriate habilitation. This should always include home language stimulation under the direction of a rehabilitative audiologist or speech-language therapist. Otologic follow-up is important to treat otitis media with effusion aggressively because it may add enough additional hearing loss to impede development. In my opinion, all hearing-impaired children should have an opportunity for oral education. Those who are unable to progress should be considered for cochlear implantation. Nonetheless, parents of deaf children should be introduced to the deaf community. Typically, a representative of the deaf culture proposes using American Sign Language rather than concentrating on oral education.

REFERENCES

1. Mandell JR. Identification and treatment of very young children with hearing loss. *Infants Young Child* 1988;1:20–30.
2. Grundfast KM, Epstein S. Comment on the Joint Committee Statement. *AAO-HNS J* December 1994.
3. Northern JL, Hayes D. Universal screening for infant hearing impairment: necessary, beneficial and justifiable. *Bull Am Acad Audiol* 1994;6:10–13.
4. Brookhouser PE. Sensorineural hearing loss in children. In: Cummings CW. ed. *Otolaryngology—head and neck surgery*. 2nd ed. Vol 4. St. Louis: Mosby–Year Book; 1993:3080–3102.
5. Ruben RJ. The history of the genetics of hearing. In: Ruben RJ, Van De Water TR, Steel KP, eds. *Genetics of hearing impairment.* New York: New York Academy of Sciences; 1991:6–15.
6. Liu X, Xu L. Nonsyndromic hearing loss: an analysis of audiograms. *Ann Otol Rhinol Laryngol* 1994;103:428–433.
7. Cremers CWRJ, Marres HAM, van Rijn PM. Nonsyndromal profound genetic deafness in childhood. In: Ruben RJ, Van De Water TR, Steel KP, eds. *Genetics of hearing impairment.* New York: New York Academy of Sciences; 1991:191–196.
8. Parving A. Longitudinal study of hearing-disabled children. A follow-up investigation. *Int J Pediatr Otolaryngol* 1988;15:233–244.
9. Das VK. Aetiology of bilateral sensorineural deafness in children. *J Laryngol Otol* 1988;102:975–980.
10. Cohen MM. The process of syndrome delineation and the heterogeneity of hearing loss. In: Ruben RJ, Van De Water TR, Steel KP, eds. *Genetics of hearing impairment.* New York: New York Academy of Sciences 1991:133–142.
11. Meyerhoff WL, Cass S, Schwaber MK, Sculerati N, Slattert WH. Progressive sensorineural hearing loss in children. *Otolaryngol Head Neck Surg* 1994;110:569–579.
12. Kimberling JK. Current progress in finding gene involved in hearing impairment. *Adv Genet Deaf* 1995;1:1–7.
13. Asher JH, Morell R, Friedman TB. Confirmation of the location of a Waardenburg syndrome type I Mutation on human chromosome 2q. In: Ruben RJ, Van De Water TR, Steel KP, eds. *Genetics of hearing impairment.* New York: New York Academy of Sciences; 1991: 295–297.
14. Comeau K, Kimberling WJ, Cremers CWRJ, Shugart Y. The search

for branchiootorenal syndrome on chromosomes 1 and 8. In: Ruben RJ, Van De Water TR, Steel KP, eds. *Genetics of hearing impairment.* New York: New York Academy of Sciences; 1991:288–289.
15. Shaver Arnos K, Israel J, Cunningham M. Genetic counseling of the deaf.In: Ruben RJ, Van De Water TR, Steel KP, eds. *Genetics of hearing impairment.* New York: New York Academy of Sciences 1991: 212–222.
16. Garretesen TJTM, Cremers CWRJ. Clinical and genetic aspect in autosomal dominant inherited osteogenesis imperfecta. In: Ruben RJ, Van De Water TR, Steel KP, eds. *Genetics of hearing impairment.* New York: New York Academy of Sciences; 1991:240–248.
17. Beighton P, Viljoen I, Winship I, Beighton G, Sellars S. Profound childhood deafness in Southern Africa. In: Ruben RJ, Van De Water TR, Steel KP, eds. *Genetics of hearing impairment.* New York: New York Academy of Sciences; 1991:290–291.
18. Marion RW. The genetic anatomy of hearing. In: Ruben RJ, Van De Water TR, Steel KP, eds. *Genetics of hearing impairment.* New York: New York Academy of Sciences; 1991:32–37.
19. Weston MD, Kimberling WJ, Moller CG, Pieke Dahl S, Smith RJ, Martini A, et al. A progress report on the localization of Usher syndrome type II to chromosome $1q_a$. In: Ruben RJ, Van De Water TR, Steel KP, eds. *Genetics of hearing impairment.* New York: New York Academy of Sciences; 1991:284–287.
20. Brunner HG, Smeets B, Smeets D, Nelen M, Cremers CWRJ, Popers HH. Molecular genetics of X-linked hearing impairment. In: Ruben RJ, Van De Water TR, Steel KP, eds. *Genetics of hearing impairment.* New York: New York Academy of Sciences; 1991:176–190.
21. Konigsmark BW, Gorlin RJ. *Genetic and metabolic deafness.* Philadelphia: WB Sauders, 1976:7–48.
22. Jackler RK, Luxford WM, House WF. Congenital malformation of the inner ear: a classification based on embryogenesis. *Laryngoscope* 1987; 97 (suppl 40):2–14.
23. Davis LE. Infections of the labyrinth. In: Cummings CW, ed. *Otolaryngology—head and neck surgery.* St. Louis: Mosby Year–Book; 1993: 2795–2807.
24. Beal DD, Davey PR, Lindsay JR. Inner ear pathology of congenital deafness. *Arch Otolaryngol* 1967;85:134–142.
25. Valvassori GE, Mafee MF. Imaging of the neck. In: Ballenger JJ ed. *Diseases of the nose, throat, ear, head and neck.* Philadelphia: Lea & Febiger; 1991:899.
26. Hickson LMH, Alcock D. Progressive hearing loss in children with congenital cytomegalovirus. *J Paediatr Child Health* 1991;27:105–107
27. Karmody CS, Schuknecht HF. Deafness in congenital syphilis. *Arch Otolaryngol* 1966;83:44–53.
28. Hughes and Rutherford I. Predictive value of serologic tests for syphilis in Otologt. *Ann Otol Rhinol Laryngol* 1986;95:250–259.
29. Davis A, Wood S. The epidemiology of childhood hearing impairment: factors relevant to planing od services. *Br J Audiol* 1992;26:77–90.
30. Vernon M. Meningitis and deafness: the problem, its physical and audiological, psychological and educational manifestations in deaf children. *Laryngoscope* 1967;77:1856–1874.
31. Das VK. Aetiology of bilateral sensori-neural deafness in children. *Scand Audiol Suppl* 1988; 30:43–52.
32. Martin JAM, Bentzen O, Colley JRT, et al. Childhood deafness in the European community. *Scand Audiol* 1981;10:165–167.3
33. Brookhouser PE, Auslander MC, Meskan ME. The pattern and stability of postmeningitis hearing loss in children. *Laryngoscope* 1988;98: 940–948.
34. Spanjaard L, Bol P, De Jong MCJY, Zanen HC. Bacterial meningitis in 366 children in the Netherlands, 1982–1983. Epidemiology and antibiotic therapy. *Tijdschr Kindergeneeskd* 1986;54:108.
35. Finitzo-Hieber Y, Simhadri R, Hieber JP. Abnormality of the auditory brainstem response in post-meningitis infants and children. *Int J Pediatr Otorhinolaryngol* 1981;3:275–86.
36. Berlow SJ, Caldarelli DD, Matz GJ, Meyer DH. Bacterial meningitis and sensorineural hearing loss: a prospective investigation. *Laryngoscope* 1980;90:1445–1452.
37. Fortnum H, Davis A. Hearing impairment in children after bacterial meningitis: incidence and resource complications. *Br J Audiol* 1993; 27:43–52.
38. Naess A, Halstensen A, Nyland H, Pedersen SHJ, Moller P, Borgmann R, et al. Sequelae one year after meningococcal disease. *Acta Neurol Scand* 1994;89:139–142.
39. Fortum HM. Hearing impai rment after bacterial meningitis: a review. *Arch Dis Child* 1992;67:1128–1133.
40. Bent JP III, Beck RA. Bacterial meningitis in the pediatric population: paradigm shift and ramification for otolaryngology-head and neck surgery. *Int J Pediat Oto Laryngol* 1994;30:41–49.
41. Tarlow MJ, Comis SD, Osborne MP. Endotoxin induced damage to the cochlea in guinea pigs. *Arch Dis Child* 1991;66:181–184.
42. Roos KL. Dexamethasone and non-steroidal anti-inflammatory agents in the treatment of bacterial meningitis. *Clin Ther* 1990;12:290–296.
43. Wald ER, Kaplan SL, Mason EO, Sabo D, Ross L, Arditi M, et al. Dexamethasone therapy for children with bacterial meningitis. *Pediatrics* 1995;95:21–31.
44. Everberg G. Deafness following mumps. *Acta Otolaryngol* 1957;48: 397.
45. Brookhouser PE, Worthington DW, Kelly WJ. Noise induced hearing loss in children. *Laryngoscope* 1992,102:645–655.
46. Strome M, Topf P, Vernick DM. Hyperlipidemia in association with childhood sensorineural hearing loss. *Laryngoscope* 1988;98:165–169.
47. Pagon RA, Graham JM, Zonana J, Yong LS. Cloboma, congenital heart disease and choanal atresia with multiple anomalies: CHARGE association. *J Pediatr* 1981;99:223–227.
48. Brown DP, Israel SM. Audiologic findings in a set of fraternal twins with CHARGE association. *J Am Acad Audiol* 1991;2:183–188.
49. Thelin JW, Mitchell JA, Hefner MA, Davenport SLH. CHARGE syndrome. Part II. Hearing loss. *Int J Pediatr Otorhinolaryngol* 1986;12: 145–163.
50. Wright CG, Brown OE, Meyerhoff WL, Rutledge JC. Auditory and temporal bone abnormalities in CHARGE association. *Ann Otol Rhinol Laryngol* 1986;95:480–486.
51. Downs MP. Benefits of screening at birth: economic, educational and functional factors. *NIH Consensus Development Conference on Early Identification of Hearing Impairment in Infants and Young Children.* National Institute of Health; 1993.
52. Schein JD, Delk MT. *The deaf population of the United States.* Silver Spring, MD: National Association of the Deaf; 1974.
53. Mauk GW, White KR, Mortensen LB, Behrens TR. The effectiveness of screening programs based on high-risk characteristics in early identification of hearing impairment. *Ear Hear* 1991;12:312–319.
54. U.S. Department of Health and Human Services. *Healthy People 2000: National Health Promotion and Disease Prevention Objectives.* Washington, DC: Public Health Service, 1990.
55. Stein L, Ozdamar O, Kraus N, Paton J. Follow-up of infants screened by auditory brainstem response in the neonatal intensive care unit. *J Pediatr* 1983;103:447–453.
56. Galambos R, Hicks G, Wilson MJ. Hearing loss in graduates of a tertiary intensive care nursery. *Ear Hear* 1982;87–90.
57. Shulman-Galambos C, Galambos R. Brain stem evoked response audiometry in newborn hearing screening. *Arch Otolaryngol* 1979;105: 86–90.
58. Joint Committee on Infant Hearing. The 1994 Position Statement. *AAO-HN J* December 1994.
59. Early identification of hearing impairment in infants and young children. *NIH Consensus Statement.* National Institute of Health; 1993:11.
60. Frasier GR. The genetics of congenital deafness. *Otolaryngol Clin North Am* 1971;4:227–247.
61. Brookhouser PE, Worthington DW, Kelly WJ. Fluctuating and/or progressive sensorineural hearing loss in children. *Laryngoscope* 1994; 104:958–964.
62. Barr B, Wedenberg E. Perceptive hearing loss in children with respect to genesis and use of hearing aid. *Acta Otolaryngol Rhinol* 1965;59: 462–467.
63. Levi H, Tell L, Feinmesser M. Progressive hearing loss in hard of hearing children. *Audiology* 1993;32:132–136.

CHAPTER 27

Autoimmune Inner Ear Diseases

Jeffrey P. Harris

Rapidly progressive bilateral deafness in a child creates enormous anxiety and distress for an involved family. Despite the consultation of many specialists, the search for a cause of this affliction often turns up empty. While hearing aids provide considerable benefit initially, the instability of these ears may lead to their continual decline in function. The future well-being of a child from an educational, psychological, and socioeconomic standpoint often becomes a central issue and one that may result in considerable parental guilt, because there will always be lingering questions about whether every avenue has been investigated to the fullest extent possible. The single most important aspect of autoimmune inner ear disease (AIED) as a potential cause of rapidly progressive bilateral sensorineural hearing loss (SNHL) from a physician's standpoint is to consider it in the differential diagnosis. This is of utmost importance because we have now come to the realization that once recognized, this condition is potentially treatable.

Of paramount importance then is the ability for a clinician to be aware of this condition, know how to diagnose it, and institute prompt and effective treatment. In doing so, the opportunity to reverse, or at least stabilize, hearing is maximized. Because the inner ear subserves a balance function as well as hearing, it is not surprising that many individuals afflicted with immune-mediated inner ear disease also suffer from vestibular symptoms. Oftentimes untreated children complain of vertigo or unexplained spells of dizziness or disequilibrium, and as most practitioners realize, this is uncommon in the pediatric population.

There is no doubt, from results of experimental studies, that immunologic responses within the inner ear are deleterious to the functioning of the delicate sensory structures responsible for hearing and balance, and it is our goal as clinicians to minimize the risks of this occurring through early intervention.

J.P. Harris: Division of Otolaryngology—Head and Neck Surgery, University of California—San Diego Medical Center, La Jolla, California 92037-1300.

CLINICAL AUTOIMMUNE DISEASE OF THE INNER EAR

Over the years, there have been sporadic reports of sudden or rapidly progressive hearing losses that have been found to be immune-mediated or in the setting of other systemic autoimmune disease. Reports exist that link illnesses such as polyarteritis nodosa, Cogan's syndrome, relapsing polychondritis, systemic lupus erythematosis, and rheumatoid arthritis with SNHL and dizziness, but these cases have all been in adults. Several studies also reported that immunosuppressive drugs could reverse cases of deafness, which suggested an immune basis for their hearing loss.

Autoimmune disease that affects the ear may be either the result of organ-specific disease or the result of a systemic disorder. When examining patients for this disorder, one must attempt to classify such patients into either of these categories.

Veldman et al. (1) reported autoimmune SNHL that resulted from immune complex-induced vasculitis, a defect in polymorphonuclear neutrophil (PMN) leukocytes, and postvaccination serum sickness. Each of these three etiologies are systemic disorders that cause inner ear dysfunction as a manifestation of their illness. Other reports of immune-complex disorders associated with SNHL have surfaced and suggest that steroids may be beneficial in their treatment (2).

The following cases represent the spectrum of immune-mediated disease that has been seen in the pediatric age group and underscore the relative *lack* of specific clinical features, which would suggest that these children are exhibiting anything other than progressive sensorineural deafness often seen in the pediatric population.

Case History 1

RB, an 11-year-old boy with a history of serous otitis media for which pressure equalization tubes were placed at an early age, developed vertigo following an upper respiratory infection. Within several weeks, he began to experience fluctuating hearing in his right ear, which rapidly deteriorated despite diuretics. Several months later, he began to lose the hearing in his left ear (Fig. 1). Prednisone 40 mg/day was instituted, and the hearing in his left ear improved dramatically. He was gradually tapered down to 20 mg every other day, but attempts to reduce this drug further were associated with tinnitus and declining hearing (Fig. 2). A Western blot assay was obtained, which was positive, as was his ANA (1/160). All other laboratory tests were normal. His hearing remained relatively stable over several years (Fig. 3).

Comment

In case history 1, an 11-year-old has a new onset of autoimmune deafness following an upper respiratory infection (URI). There are no outward manifestations of other rheumatologic diseases, and the only evidence for this etiology is his positive Western blot and the markedly elevated ANA in so young a child. The relationship of the URI to the development of this disorder is unknown; however, there appears to be some association of such an antecedent event with a number of these cases.

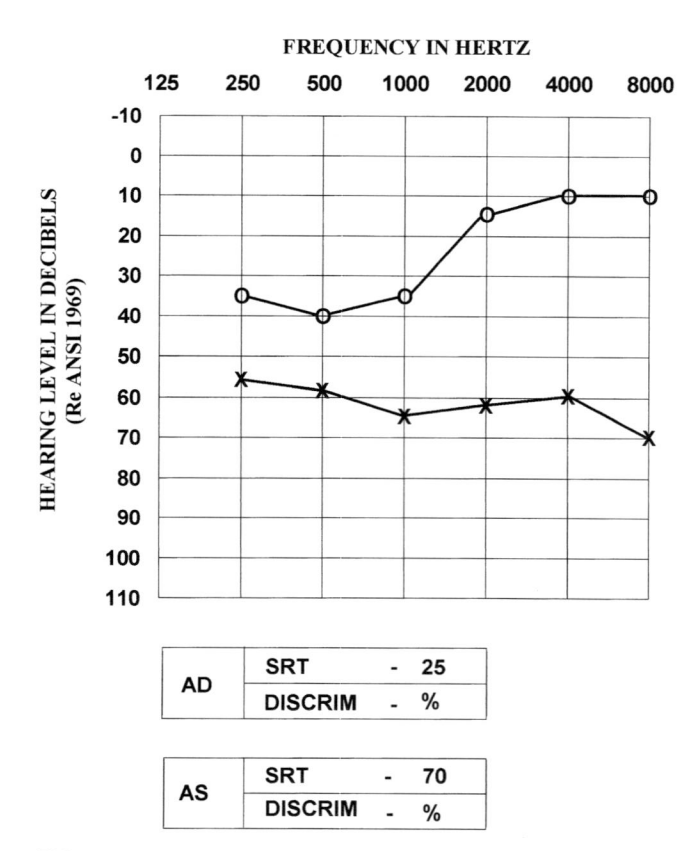

FIG. 1. Baseline audiogram of patient RB. Patient reports to have excellent discrimination.

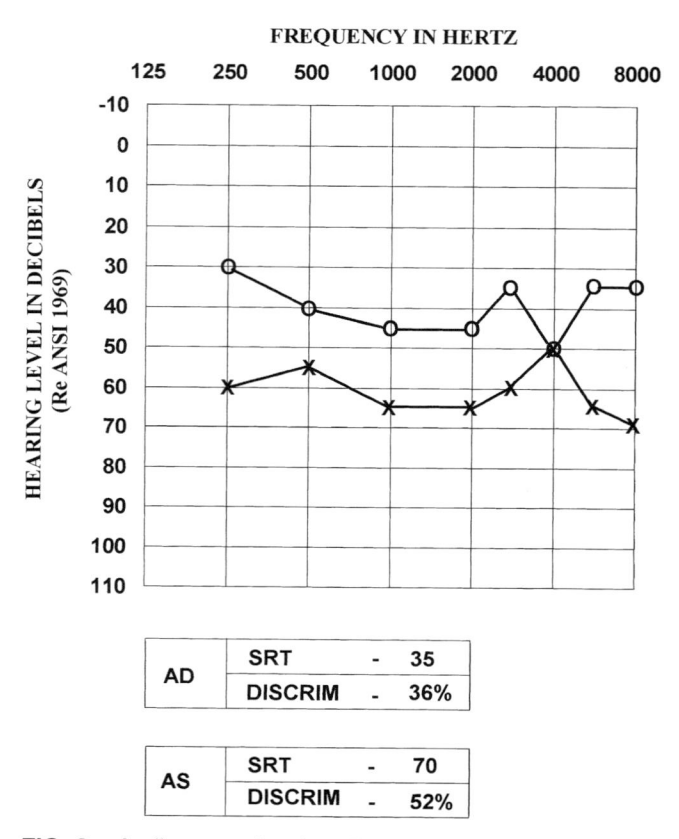

FIG. 2. Audiogram of patient RB obtained following significant drops in speech discrimination.

Case History 2

NH, an 8-year-old boy who was diagnosed as having bilateral SNHL since the age of 2, began to develop a marked decline in the low-frequency hearing thresholds bilaterally (Fig. 4). The etiology for his underlying moderate SNHL was unknown and required hearing aid usage. The recent drop in hearing was unexplained, and he was sent for new, stronger hearing aids. Because of this sudden and continued progression of the hearing loss, laboratory tests were obtained, which were all normal except for the Western blot, which was positive. Prednisone 20 mg/day was instituted, and after 3 weeks his hearing began to improve gradually. After 2 months, his hearing was back at the level it had been before the sudden decline, and his medication was stopped. He has been relatively stable since that time (Fig. 5).

Comment

In case history 2, a child with early-onset, bilateral SNHL became unstable for unknown reasons. The drop in hearing

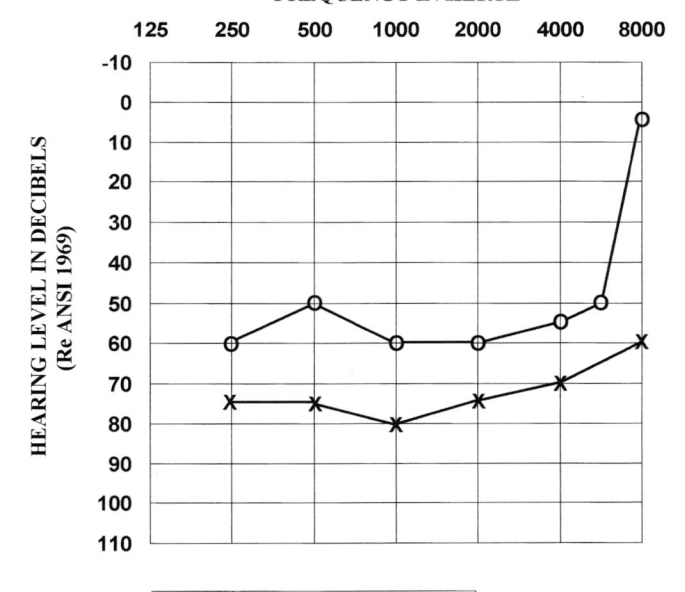

FIG. 3. Audiogram of patient RB obtained approximately 2.5 years following treatment.

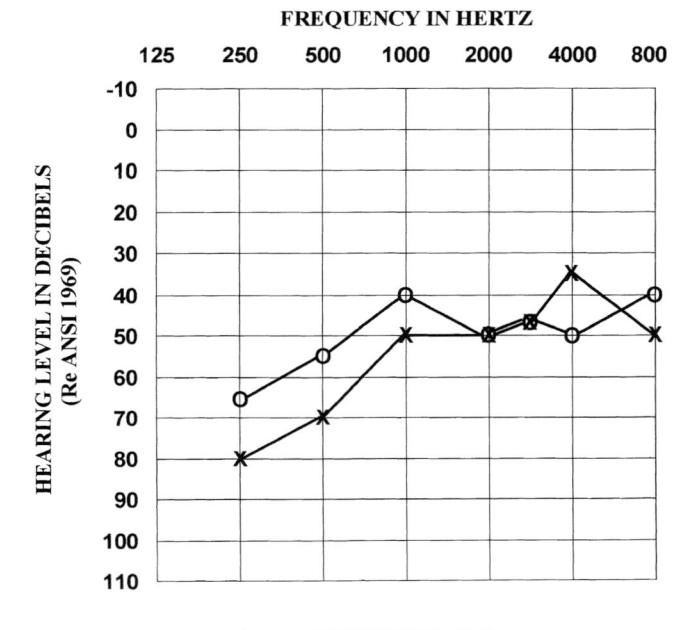

FIG. 4. Audiogram of patient NH, obtained after sudden drop in low-frequency hearing bilaterally.

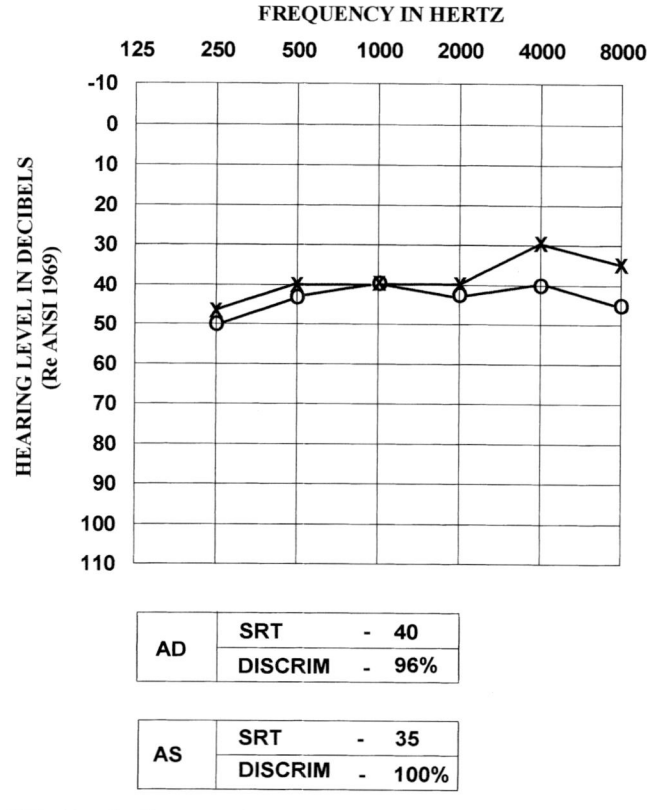

FIG. 5. Audiogram of patient NH, obtained several months following prednisone therapy. The patient is now back to his baseline levels.

suggested the development of a hydropic condition, and the positive Western blot suggested that it had an immune basis. The underlying pathogenesis of the hearing loss is unknown, but one could speculate that earlier or ongoing trauma (viral?) initiated the immune response, which was now causing progressive hearing loss.

Case History 3

AF, a 12-year-old girl, experienced acute onset of vertigo with nausea and vomiting. One week later, she developed SNHL in her left ear. Subsequently, she developed acute otitis in her right ear associated with aural polyps. This was treated and cleared by antibiotic therapy; however, SNHL developed in her right ear as well (Fig. 6). Routine laboratory testing was normal, including tests for syphilis, ANA, and rheumatoid factor, except for an elevated IgE. Radiologic imaging was also normal. Lymphocyte transformation test (LTT) was reported to be 1.7 (slightly positive), and Western blot against 68-kD antigen was also positive. She was started on high-dose steroids, and her hearing markedly improved. However, when this was tapered, her hearing regressed (Fig. 7). She has had a relentless downhill course despite repeated short courses of prednisone, although she uses hearing aids bilaterally (Fig. 8).

Comment

This case history demonstrates the importance of long-term aggressive therapy once the diagnosis is made and the possible association of prior inflammatory processes in the middle ear. The elevated IgE has not been seen in other cases, but raises a possible allergic association as well.

Case History 4

RM, an 11-year-old boy, was in excellent health, except for a history of adenoidectomy with pressure equalization tubes and tonsillectomy. He had normal hearing until 6 months earlier, when he developed episodic vertigo. Four months later, he began to experience bilateral fluctuating SNHL (Fig. 9). Laboratory and radiologic testing was normal, except for a sedimentation rate of 30, a weakly positive ANA (1/16), elevated circulating immunoglobulins, and a positive Western blot against 68-kD inner ear antigen. He was started on prednisone 40 mg, and his hearing improved (Fig. 10). He was slowly tapered over 1 year and did well until the prednisone was discontinued, when he again developed dizziness and hearing loss. Steroids were resumed, and his hearing improved in one ear but not in the other to any appreciable degree. He has since been fitted with bilateral

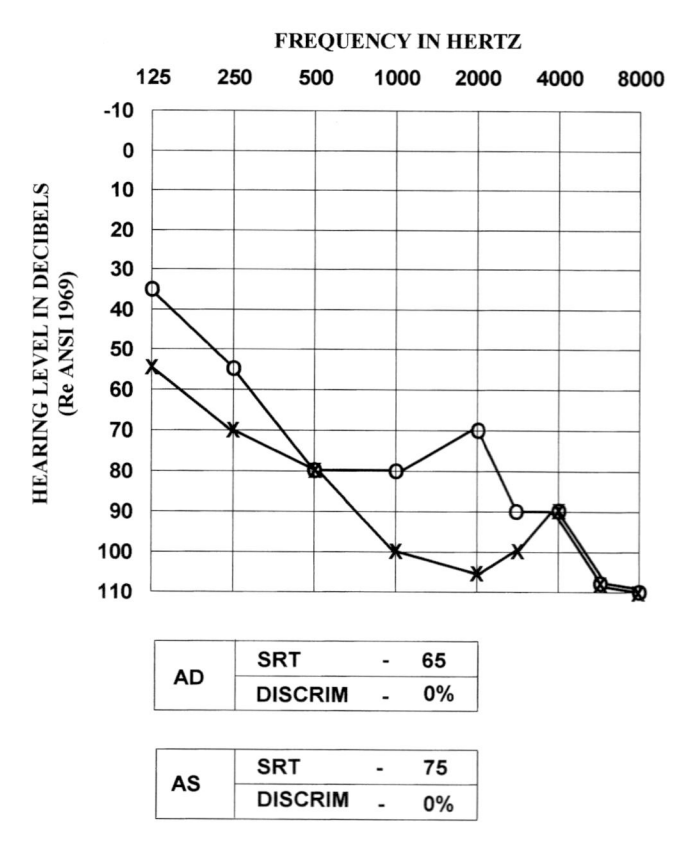

FIG. 6. Audiogram of patient AF, obtained at onset of hearing instability, showing extremely poor speech discrimination.

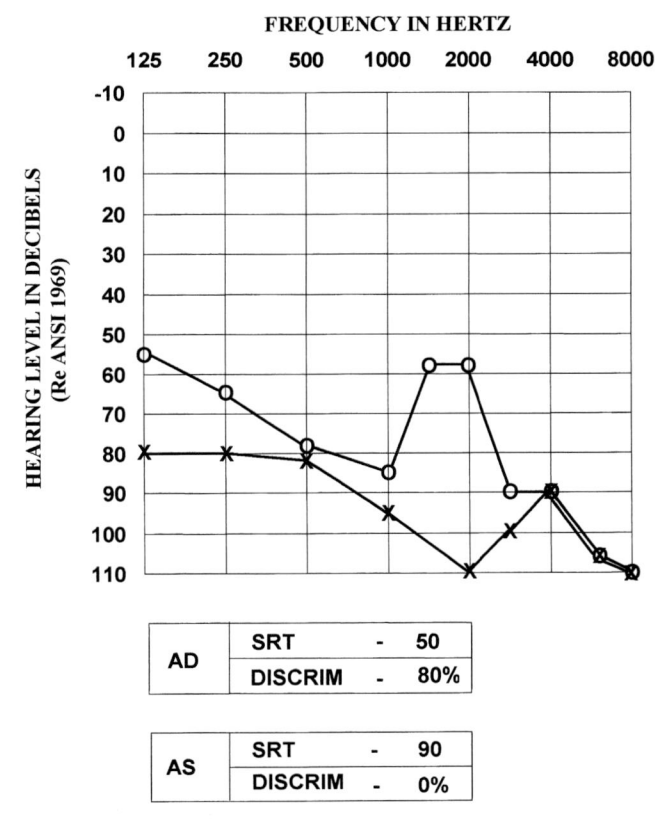

FIG. 7. Audiogram of patient AF, showing improved speech discrimination *(AD)* following immunosuppression therapy.

hearing aids and has been stable except for occasional drops in hearing following URIs. He has not required any further steroid therapy in 6 years, has functional hearing with amplification, and has just graduated from college.

Comment

This boy had evidence of circulating immunoglobulins and an elevated sedimentation rate, as well as a positive Western blot. He may have developed a vasculitis that damaged his inner ear vasculature. With aggressive long-term therapy, he eventually outgrew the disorder and has gone into long-term remission. This case provides sufficient long-term results, which support the presumption that the benefits of careful aggressive treatment outweigh the risks.

Case History 5

This 6-year-old boy was diagnosed with a medulloblastoma. He underwent surgery and full-course radiotherapy and had a partial tumor response. He lost his hearing in one ear from the radiation therapy, and several years later he began to complain of progressive hearing loss in his only hearing ear. Prednisone was instituted and his hearing recovered. When it was clear that he was steroid-sensitive, a work-up for AIED was initiated. All laboratory tests were normal except for a positive Western blot against 68-kD inner ear antigen. He has received repeated courses of prednisone, and his hearing has remained relatively stable. Two similar, additional cases have been seen with positive Western blots following radiation therapy for CNS malignancies.

Comment

This case points out the possibility that radiation-induced damage to the inner ear can expose inner ear tissue to the immune system, resulting in an immunologic response to the contralateral inner ear, so-called contralateral delayed endolymphatic hydrops. Alternatively, the positive Western blot may have no etiologic significance except as reflective of inner ear damage and that the cause of the contralateral deafness is in fact radiation-induced labyrinthitis.

Organ-Specific Autoimmune Inner Ear Disease

To establish organ-specific autoimmunity, cell-mediated or humoral immunity must be evident against the body's own tissue antigen(s). In the case of vestibuloauditory autoimmunity, there should be autoantibodies or evidence of cell-mediated immune responses (lymphocyte transforma-

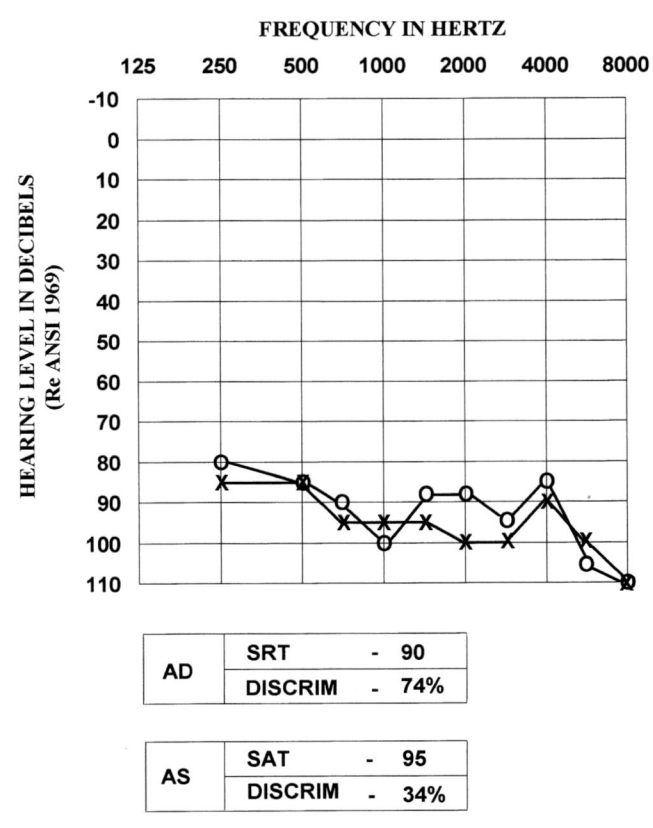

FIG. 8. Audiogram of patient AF, showing further decline in hearing thresholds.

PATIENT – **R.M.**
DATE – **7-1-85**

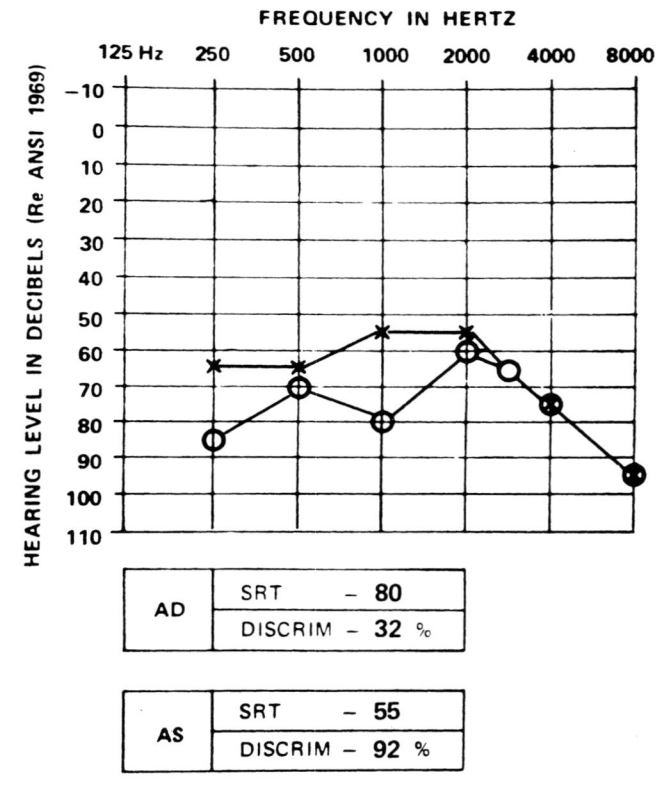

FIG. 9. Audiogram of patient RM, showing drop in hearing. Reprinted with permission from *Laryngoscope* 100, May 1990.

tion, lymphokine production, or delayed hypersensitivity) directed against inner ear antigens (cochlea, vestibular, or both).

The report by McCabe (3) brought attention to the possibility that a new, previously unrecognized form of specific autoimmune SNHL represented a treatable form of deafness. It is of interest to note that his original patient with this disorder had undergone a mastoidectomy, which had not healed despite revisions of the wound. After review of the pathology from the nonhealing wound, which revealed evidence of vasculitis, systemic steroids were instituted. Not only did the wound heal, but the associated SNHL improved. This serendipitous observation led to McCabe's speculation that a distinct entity existed in which the inner ear was the target of an autoimmune disease. However, as early as 1958, Lehnhardt (4) speculated that cases of bilateral deafness were due to anticochlear antibodies; yet, no evidence emerged to support this hypothesis. Attempts at creating animal models of autoimmune allergic labyrinthitis failed, as previously discussed (5,6). In 1974, Schiff and Brown (7) speculated that amelioration of sudden deafness by ACTH and heparin treatments was evidence of an autoimmune vasculitis etiology (7). Again, no specific testing was done to confirm this hypothesis or its organ specificity. In McCabe's original series, the bilateral SNHL was asymmetric and progressive over weeks to months and was associated with electronystagmographic evidence of vestibulopathy. In addition, a small percentage showed a coexistent facial paralysis (3). None of these cases involved children.

Diagnosis

While there was initial enthusiasm for lymphocyte migration inhibition assay as a means of demonstrating organ-specific autoimmunity toward inner ear antigens, more recently its specificity and sensitivity have been questioned, and Hughes et al. (8) have promoted lymphocyte transformation as a more sensitive assay. The LTT assumes that circulating lymphocytes, which have been sensitized to inner ear proteins, will respond to the putative antigen(s) in vitro. When a previously sensitized lymphocyte receives a second similar antigen exposure, a proliferative response and release of lymphokines are identified as a positive test. Unfortunately, this test was available only at the Cleveland Clinic and is no longer being performed by these investigators,

PATIENT – **R.M.**
DATE – **8–2–85**

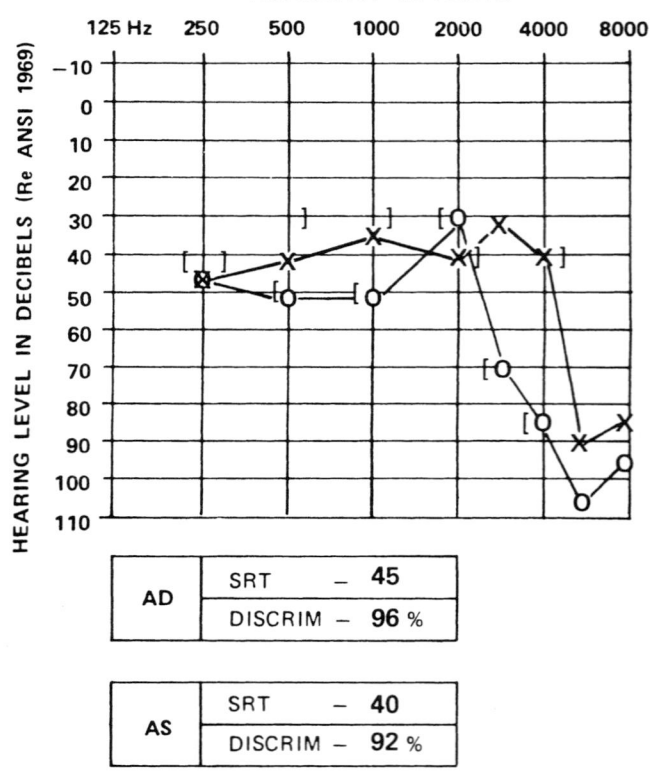

FIG. 10. Audiogram of patient RM, showing improved hearing following a 1-month trial of prednisone. Reprinted with permission from *Laryngoscope* 100, May 1990.

who have opted instead to use Western blotting (discussion follows). Despite this, the specificity of the LTT has been reported to be 93%, with a sensitivity estimated to be between 50% to 80% during the active phase of the disease. The predictive value of a positive LTT in a high-risk patient is estimated to be 56% to 73% (9). Berger et al. (10) reported the usefulness of LTT against type II collagen as a sensitive means of diagnosing autoimmune SNHL. In this study, 34 of 68 tested patients with progressive SNHL showed stimulation indices of greater than 2.5, with a mean of 4.7. This reflects an apparent "sensitization" of the host to this antigen and possibly will prove to be an important adjunct in its diagnosis. Additionally, Helfgott et al. (11) reported the presence of antibodies to type II collagen as predictive of steroid responsiveness in this disorder. However, Sujita et al. (12) were unable to confirm this finding because only one of eight patients with steroid-responsive inner ear disease had anti-type II collagen antibodies. Arnold, Pfaltz, and Altermatt (13) incubated serum from patients with suspected "autoimmune" SNHL onto sections of nonrelated, healthy human temporal bones and demonstrated positive immunofluorescence labeling in 15 of 21 patients. The five patients who were tested by lymphocyte transformation against inner ear antigen were found to be negative.

In a subsequent study, 119 serum samples from patients with hearing loss were similarly investigated by immunofluorescence microscopy, and 54% showed labeling against sections of healthy temporal bones. Despite these findings, only 27% of patients treated with prednisolone showed some improvement in hearing (14). Other authors have also utilized decalcified temporal bones for immunohistochemistry to demonstrate specific targets of autoimmunity within the inner ear (15–18). There remains a problem in interpreting these results because antigen degradation occurs with prolonged decalcification, and human leukocyte antigen (HLA) differences between the patients and the cadavers could account for the observed labeling. If the specificity of staining is confirmed, humoral autoantibodies are implicated in the pathogenesis of this disease. In contrast, cell-mediated immunity is implicated by the studies of Hughes et al. (8) and Berger et al. (10). A number of other studies have looked for the presence of autoantibodies (ANA, anticardiolipin, antismooth muscle, antiendoplasmic reticulum) in a variety of inner ear disorders and the incidence of one or more of these being positive is surprisingly high (19–22). Because many of these tests are nonspecific and are increasingly positive with age in the normal population (e.g., ANA), the results of these studies are difficult to interpret. However, the presence of a significantly abnormal autoantibody or multiple autoantibodies in the sera of a suspected patient is helpful in identifying patients who may be at risk for an immune-mediated disorder.

The Western blot immunoassay has also been used to identify serum antibodies that may be reacting against inner ear antigen(s). In this assay, inner ear antigen(s) are electrophoresed onto a gel and then incubated over several hours with a dilute concentration of patient's serum. If a specific antibody is present in the serum to an antigen derived from the inner ear, then antibody will tightly bind to its target antigen. This in vitro antigen–antibody complex can then be developed and stained, revealing one of several bands on a gel. Originally, Harris and Sharp (23) reported the use of this technique in 54 patients with progressive SNHL and found that 19 (35%) showed evidence of a specific anticochlear antibody in their serum (Fig. 11). Of note, the inner ear antigenic epitope, against which their serum reacted, was the same by molecular weight determination (62–68,000), as was found in the experimental autoimmune SNHL produced in animals. Furthermore, by two-dimensional gel electrophoresis they were able to show that a pediatric patient with steroid-responsive autoimmune deafness had autoantibodies that reacted against an inner ear antigen not only with the same molecular weight, but also with the identical isoelectric point as the hearing-loss animals (Fig. 12).

This is compelling evidence that some patients with rapidly progressive SNHL have autoantibodies to a particular antigenic epitope within the inner ear and that this is a true organ-specific autoimmune event. This observation was confirmed by Moscicki et al. (24) in 11 patients who demonstrated this antibody on Western blot analysis and whose hearing improved on immunosuppressive therapy. Since then, Harris' laboratory has extended the original observation to include 279 patients with rapidly progressive SNHL, in whom 90 (32%) were positive by Western blot, and of the positive patients, there was a distinct female predominance (63%) (25). This is again in keeping with the female prevalence seen in other autoimmune conditions of the body. Analysis of these positive patients reveals that a spectrum exists from patients with deafness and florid clinical and laboratory evidence of systemic autoimmune disease to those who exhibit hearing loss as their only detectable manifestation of autoimmunity. Controls consisted of several groups of patients: individuals with no evidence of hearing loss (10/200, 5%); patients with rheumatologic disease (rheumatoid arthritis, systemic lupus erythematosis) (5/71, 7%); and female controls (8/100, 8%) (26). Statistical comparison of the experimental patient group with the control population reveals a significant difference ($p < 0.001$). Based on this, it can be concluded that this assay appears to be highly specific (95%) but rather insensitive when used in the general population. In a group of patients who have unexplained progressive deafness, however, there is about a one-third chance of there being an immune etiology for their hearing loss. Further work from this laboratory has shown several other antigens against which these patients' sera react, but recent analysis of these antigens, (33–35 kD, 50 kD, 55kD, 62 kD, and 220 kD) has failed to demonstrate a statistically significant difference compared with controls.

Moscicki et al. (27) reported that 89% of patients with active progressive bilateral SNHL had antibodies to 68-kD antigen, while those patients with inactive disease were uniformly negative. Of the Western blot–positive patients, 75%

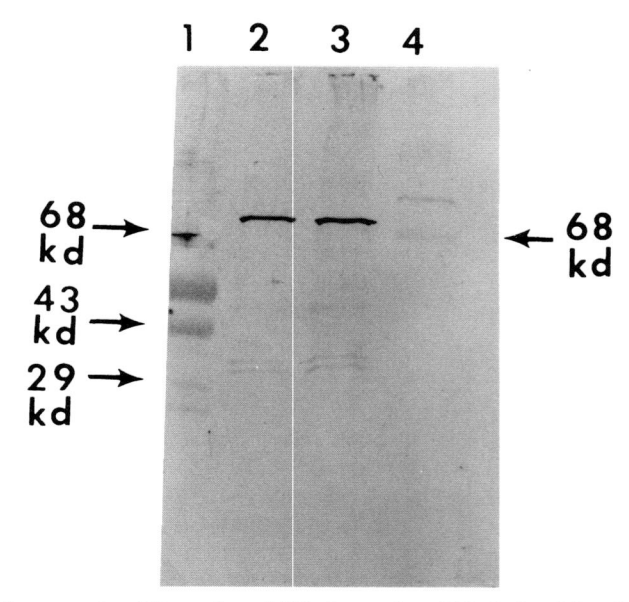

Lane 1: Standard Molecular Weight Markers
Lane 2: 9.5ug of Inner Ear Antigen
Lane 3: 19ug of Inner Ear Antigen
Lane 4: 10.3ug of Bovine Serum Albumin

FIG. 11. Positive Western blot immunoassay of a patient with rapidly progressive SNHL.

responded to steroids compared with 18% that were 68-kD antibody negative (27). Billings et al. (28) reported that the 68-kD antigen, which has also been associated with renal tissue, is either heat shock protein-70 (HSP-70) or an antigen that is bound to it. Quite independently, Bloch and coworkers (28a) found that HSP-70 was the protein identified when the 68-kD antigen was sequenced. Thus, preliminary work now suggests that HSP-70 is either the target of the autoimmune response or that it represents an epiphenomenon that develops as a result of inner ear damage. Regardless, the presence of this autoantibody in the sera of patients with progressive deafness is diagnostic of an immune-mediated cause of deafness and predicts steroid sensitivity. As previously stated, this is a disease usually found in middle-aged women, but there have been several patients in their sixth and seventh decades, as well as eight children in the author's personal experience, with steroid-sensitive progressive deafness.

Pathology

The pathology of autoimmune SNHL awaits description of a temporal bone from a patient with deafness and no signs of systemic disease. However, Schuknecht (29) reported a patient who died with bilateral progressive SNHL and systemic eosinophilia. These temporal bones showed hydrops, mononuclear and plasma cell infiltrates in the scalae, osteoneogenesis in the scala tympani adjacent to the round window membrane, and perivascular infiltrates surrounding the spiral modiolar veins. Of interest was a dense bone formation surrounding the spiral modiolar vein and modiolus, which we have also seen experimentally in ears that have undergone chronic antigen stimulation (23). Of particular interest has been the recent finding that in a review of the National Temporal Bone Registry, the only diagnosis in which 100% of the temporal bones show evidence of osteoneogenesis within the inner ear was autoimmunity (personal communication, E. Keithley, Ph.D.)

Manifestations of Disease

The typical afflicted patient with this disease is a middle-aged woman. In the series by Hughes et al. (30), 65% were women and 35% were men. This is in keeping with the Western blot results in our series of patients, in whom 63% were women (23). However, we suspect that with increased awareness, the incidence of this disorder in the pediatric population will grow. As of now, the author has experience with approximately ten pediatric patients who have been Western blot–positive. In the usual presentation, the patient may develop rapidly progressive SNHL over a several-week period. Occasionally, there is a concomitant serous otitis media, which may confuse the picture, because a complication of otitis media becomes a consideration and occasionally these patients are started on antibiotics empirically. De-

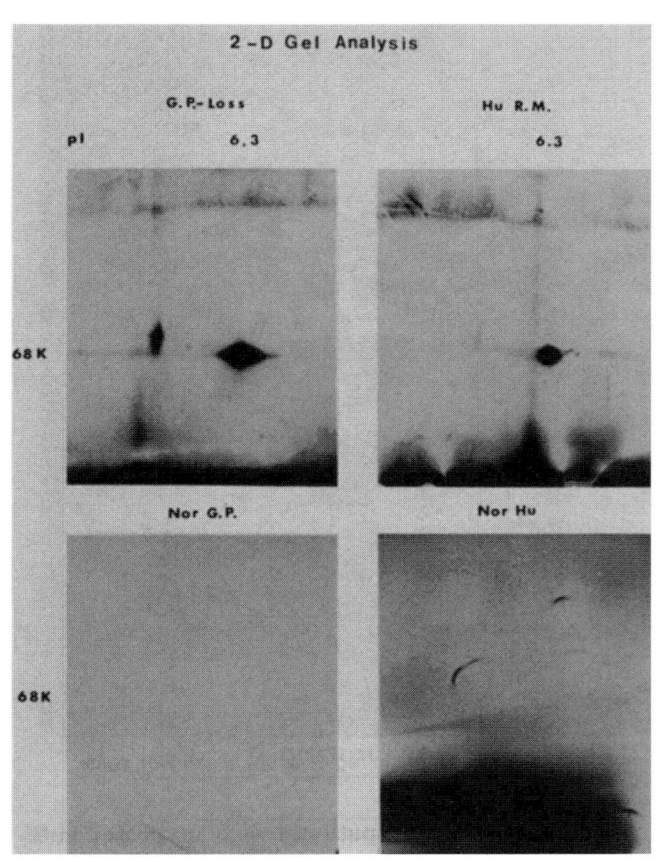

FIG. 12. Two-dimensional gel analysis. *GP loss*, sera from guinea pigs with hearing loss following immunization with bovine inner ear antigens; *Hu RM*, serum from patient RM (see Figs. 9, 10); *Nor GP*, serum from normal guinea pigs; *Nor Hu*, serum from normal human control. All reacted against bovine inner ear antigen. Reprinted with permission from Laryngoscope 100, May 1990.

spite this therapy, and even in the absence of serous otitis media, the hearing may continue to drop, with obvious fluctuations apparent. These fluctuations and the presence of dizziness and aural fullness in approximately one fourth to one half of the patients often lead to the diagnosis of Ménière's disease. In the typical patient, this may become a poorly functioning ear over time and is given up for lost, when suddenly the hearing in the good ear drops precipitously. It is usually at this point that the practitioner considers an immune-mediated inner ear disease and institutes prednisone or like therapy. Bilateral hearing loss occurs in the majority of patients (79%), and in approximately one third of patients, there are no associated vestibular symptoms (30). Due to the gradual loss of vestibular function bilaterally, rare patients may develop ataxia typical of Dandy's syndrome. However, the majority of patients have some initial symptoms typical of Ménière's disease, which dissipate over time. In one series, the coexistence of other systemic autoimmune disease occurs in upwards of 29% of patients (30).

Ménière's Disease

Ménière's disease is a capricious disorder with a high incidence of bilaterality and a waxing and waning course. These characteristics have led many to wonder if it might also have an autoimmune etiology (31). It is clear that a number of non–organ-specific autoimmune causes of deafness may have a Ménière's disease–like presentation (i.e., Cogan's syndrome, polyarteritis nodosa), and only with the passage of time will the other stigmata of a systemic autoimmune disorder become evident. Hughes et al. (32) reported two of ten patients with Ménière's disease with a slightly increased stimulation index on lymphocyte transformation assay. In a subsequent study, Hughes et al. (33) reported that approximately half of the patients with autoimmune SNHL presented as Ménière's disease. There have also been reports of elevated circulating immune complexes and other immunologic abnormalities in patients with this disorder. Brookes (34) reported 54% of patients with Ménière's disease with elevated immune complexes, as compared with 2.9% in controls. More recently, Derebery et al. (35) found that 96% of patients with Ménière's disease showed elevated circulating immune complexes. If immune complexes are involved in the etiology of this disease, it should be relatively easy to document this through immunohystochemical demonstration of immune complexes in the sacs of Ménière's patients. Evidence of this relationship is still lacking.

Xenellis et al. (36) reviewed 671 patients with Ménière's disease and compared them with 689 age- and sex-matched controls. In this study, there was a slightly higher incidence of other associated autoimmune disorders (10.3% vs. 4%) among the patients with Ménière's disease. Furthermore, there was a highly significant association of the major histocompatibility complex class I HLA allele CW7 and Ménière's disease. The association of this HLA allele has also been reported for autoimmune inner ear disease in general (37). Gottschlich et al. (26) has also examined patients with Ménière's disease by Western blot and have found an inordinately high incidence of a positive anti-68-kD autoantibody (32%). This would suggest that a subgroup of patients with Ménière's disease has an immune etiology. Additionally, Harris and Aframian (38) found positive Western blots in six of seven patients with delayed endolymphatic hydrops, in which the only hearing ear has become unstable. This variant of Ménière's disease is, therefore, most probably an autoimmune disorder and should be treated aggressively to save the only hearing ear from further deterioration.

Yoo et al. (39) reported an elevated type II collagen autoantibody level in patients with Ménière's disease and otosclerosis. Autoimmunity to type II collagen experimentally produced in animals has resulted in widespread inner ear dysfunction (i.e., hearing loss, vestibular dysfunction, and endolymphatic hydrops). This form of autoimmunity needs to be considered as an additional feature of AIED, but it is unclear at this time if this represents a primary or secondary autoimmune event.

Clearly, while typical Ménière's disease is not a common disorder of childhood, children do give histories of experiencing dizziness and vertigo. Several reports in the literature substantiate the development of this condition, but more often in children over the age of 10, and it can occur bilaterally, although rarely (40).

NON–ORGAN-SPECIFIC AUTOIMMUNE INNER EAR DISEASE

Polyarteritis Nodosa

Polyarteritis nodosa (PAN), a systemic disorder affecting the small- and medium-sized arteries throughout the body, rarely affects children. Its cause is unknown, although it has been associated with prior drug exposure, hepatitis B antigen, streptococcal infections, and serous otitis media. It has only rarely been associated with cochlear injury. For example, Malamud and Foster (41) reviewed 300 cases of PAN and found only two patients with SNHL. Although this is a systemic disorder, hearing loss may be the sole presenting symptom (42–44). Temporal bone histopathologic studies have been reported in PAN. Gussen (45) found arteritis in the internal auditory artery with widespread cochleovestibular ischemic changes, and osteoneogenesis and fibrous tissue in the basilar turns. Jenkins, Pollak, and Fisch (46) reported similar pathologic findings, but these findings were restricted to the cochlea.

In a temporal bone study, Yanagita et al. (47) reported a case of bilateral deafness associated with nephritis and a B-cell lymphoma. In this patient, necrotizing vasculitis was seen in small- and medium-sized arteries throughout the body in association with PAN, and there was complete disappearance of the organ of Corti, atrophy or absence of the stria vascularis, collapse of Reissner's membrane, distortion of the tectorial membrane, and bone formation and fibrosis of the apical turn. Many of these findings have been experimentally produced by the aforementioned immunologic challenges of the cochlea, as well as by sudden interruption of cochlear blood flow (48,49). Thus, from these temporal bone findings, one can conclude that vasculitis is one clearly definable cause of profound hearing loss, and a search for such an etiology should be made in patients with profound unexplained deafness.

Cogan's Syndrome

Cogan's syndrome is a disorder of young adults and is characterized by nonsyphilitic interstitial keratitis (IK) and vestibuloauditory dysfunction (50–52). This disorder has not been seen in the pediatric population per se. Interstitial keratitis develops suddenly with photophobia, lacrimation, and eye pain, and gradually resolves with occasional flairs. The vestibuloauditory symptoms are characterized by acute episodes of vertigo, tinnitus, and hearing loss, with the hearing loss progressing to deafness over a 1- to 3-month period. Patients may develop the vestibuloauditory symptoms 1 to 6 months before or after the onset of IK. It should be noted, however, that these symptoms may precede or follow the eye symptoms by as much as 2 years, in which case, the disorder is classified as atypical Cogan's syndrome. Vestibuloauditory symptoms occurring in association with eye disease other than IK (e.g., episcleritis, uveitis, conjunctivitis, etc.) are also considered atypical Cogan's syndrome. Cogan's syndrome occasionally may be associated with systemic symptoms, which include arthritis, PAN, glomerulonephritis, inflammatory bowel disease, and splenomegaly (52).

The temporal bone findings in this disorder consist of endolymphatic hydrops, plasma cell and lymphocytic infiltration of the spiral ligament (53), saccular rupture, osteoneogenesis of the round window, spiral ganglion cell degeneration, and cystic degeneration of the stria vascularis (54). In addition, Zechner (55) found degeneration of the organ of Corti, as well as fibrosis and osteoneogenesis within the perilymphatic space. In another temporal bone study, bilateral cochlear osteoneogenesis and ectopic bone tissue within the vestibular semicircular canals were found in a patient with Cogan's syndrome (56). This disorder may not be confined to the peripheral auditory system but may have CNS manifestations, as evidenced by a report of electrophysiologic changes localized to bilateral pontocerebellar regions (normal wave I on brainstem-evoked audiometry) (57).

The etiology of Cogan's syndrome is thought to be a hypersensitivity response to one or more infectious agents and is associated with vasculitis (58). The finding of lymphocyte transformation on exposure of a patient's lymphocytes to corneal antigen, scleroprotein (59,60), and inner ear antigen has been reported (61). This may be evidence that this disorder is organ-specific, with autoimmunity directed against the eye and ear. It must be remembered, however, that the presence of autoantibodies or sensitized lymphocytes may not be the primary event involved in injury to that tissue. Rather, one may have a non-organ-specific event (i.e., immune complex–induced vasculitis) that injures the tissue, releasing antigens to which the immune system then responds. Western blotting against inner ear tissue has been uniformly negative against 68-kD antigen in Cogan's syndrome.

The responsiveness of this disorder to treatment probably relates to how long the disease has been active prior to diagnosis. Obviously, if the aforementioned histopathologic features of these "late" cases develop, one should not expect significant improvement with steroid treatment. If, on the other hand, a limited vasculitis results in labyrinthine ischemia, one can predict a beneficial response to treatment.

A condition that has similarities to Cogan's syndrome is the Vogt-Koyanagi-Harada syndrome. It is characterized by SNHL, dizziness, granulomatous uveitis, depigmentation of the hair and skin around the eyes, loss of eyelashes, and aseptic meningitis. In distinction, CSF abnormalities are uncommonly present in Cogan's syndrome (54). The etiopathogenesis of this condition is thought to involve autoimmunity to the melanocytes, involving tissues containing these cells, such as uvea, skin, meninges, and inner ear (62).

Wegener's Granulomatosis

The classic triad of Wegener's granulomatosis consists of (a) necrotizing granulomas with vasculitis of the upper and lower respiratory tracts, (b) systemic vasculitis, and (c) focal necrotizing glomerulitis (63,64). McDonald and DeRemee (88) pointed out that ear manifestations occurred in one fifth of their series of 108 patients and were most often serous otitis media associated with infection or obstruction of the nasopharynx. Although the resultant conductive hearing loss was common, nine patients had sensorineural losses and five improved with prednisone therapy.

The otologic symptoms of Wegener's granulomatosis have been reported by others, with serous otitis and middle ear involvement being the most common manifestations (65,66). Kempf (67) reported a higher incidence of low-to-moderate SNHL in 21 of 26 ears examined audiologically. Karmody (68) suggested that in children, otitis media appears to be the heralding condition, which after being refractory to treatment will lead to a mastoidectomy and the submission of tissue that is diagnostic of Wegener's.

The etiology of the inner ear disease is unknown. However, if the endolymphatic sac is a mucosal-type immune site, as is found in the upper and lower respiratory tracts and the kidney, perhaps the necrotizing vasculitis would also have a predilection for involving the vasculature of the endolymphatic sac as well (69).

Because the otologic manifestations may be the sole presenting symptom of these patients, a thorough and repeated search for evidence of the aforementioned classic triad of Wegener's granulomatosis should be performed on patients with unexplained, sudden otologic disease. A test has been described that recognizes antibodies to azurophilic granules in neutrophils. This antineutrophil cytoplasmic antibody (ANCA) test is positive in 95% of patients with Wegener's granulomatosis (70).

Behçet's Syndrome

Behçet's syndrome is a chronic disorder, the hallmark of which is the development of oral and genital mucosal ulcerations and eye lesions. This condition is rare in children. The systemic manifestations may include the skin, joints, vasculature, and CNS (66,71). One report described inner ear involvement in this disorder, but because of the small patient sample size, no definitive conclusion could be reached about the association of this disorder with progressive SNHL and disequilibrium, or whether the patients had coexistent presbycusis or idiopathic SNHL (one patient) (72).

Relapsing Polychondritis

Relapsing polychondritis is a rare disease characterized by recurrent episodes of inflammatory necrosis affecting cartilaginous structures of the ears, nose, upper respiratory tract, and peripheral joints (73). This illness, while rare, has been reported in a few pediatric cases. This disease destroys supporting cartilage, resulting commonly in saddle nose and tracheal collapse. The auricular inflammation must be distinguished from bacterially caused perichondritis; however, the association of vestibuloauditory symptoms helps point toward an immune-mediated rather than an infectious cause. The most life-threatening manifestation is the airway obstruction resulting from loss of cartilaginous support of the trachea. Laboratory abnormalities include increased erythrocyte sedimentation rate (ESR), mildly increased serum immunoglobulins, and biologically false-positive VDRL (Veneral Disease Research Laboratory) test. The finding of antibodies to cartilage and to types II and IX collagen, as well as the induction of lymphocyte activation on exposure to cartilage, is the basis for this being considered an autoimmune disorder (74,75). The finding of type II collagen in the tectorial membrane and in the otic capsule provides a rationale for occurrence of an inner ear disorder in the presence of specific autoimmunity directed against collagen (39,76–78). Antiinflammatory agents have been used with success in reversing the inflammation and SNHL in this disorder.

There are a variety of other rare types of systemic vasculitis, including giant-cell arteritis, Takayasu's arteritis, postvaccination vasculitis, and serum sickness in which an occasional incidence of vestibuloauditory dysfunction has been seen (79,80). The basic underlying pathologic condition is vasculitis, with the ultimate consequence being ischemic injury to the inner ear.

Systemic Lupus Erythematosus

Systemic lupus erythematosus (SLE) is a multisystem disease that has protean manifestations. This disorder of altered immune regulation is thought to be genetically determined, but also with a possible underlying viral pathogenesis. It occurs in childhood in 20% of patients and usually occurs over the age of 8 years. It may have an insidious onset or may be fulminant and rapidly progressive. In children, the most common presenting symptoms are fever, malaise, arthritis, and rash. The malar "butterfly rash" is pathognomonic but presents in relatively few patients. Polyarthralgia, arthritis, pleuritis, pericarditis, pneumonitis, myocarditis, endocarditis, nephritis, cranial nerve palsies, meningitis, cerebrovascular accidents, neuritis, scleritis, retinal degeneration secondary to vasculitis, and inflammatory bowel disease are all part of the clinical spectrum of this disease (81,82). The otologic manifestations include chronic otitis media with necrotizing vasculitis and progressive SNHL and/or disequilibrium (3). The laboratory abnormalities include increased ESR, evidence of circulating immune complexes, and multiple autoantibodies (see immunoassays). The association of a decreased level of suppressor T cells in patients with SLE is intriguing in light of autoantibody formation, although this does not prove causality, because it may be caused by anti-T cell antibodies also present during the course of their disease.

Rheumatoid Arthritis

Rheumatoid arthritis (RA) is a chronic systemic inflammatory disease that mainly affects the joints. In the pediatric population, it is referred to as juvenile rheumatoid arthritis (JRA). The disease is thought to be due to an infection with an as yet unidentified microorganism or a hypersensitivity or autoimmune reaction to unknown stimuli. Juvenile rheumatoid arthritis affects a quarter million children. This disorder characteristically affects the small joints of the hands and feet and then progressively involves other joints in a symmetric fashion. Extra-articular manifestations include vasculitis, muscle atrophy, subcutaneous nodules, lymphadenopathy, splenomegaly, and leukopenia and are present in 20% of children with JRA. Rheumatoid factors (RF), 19S and 7S IgM and 7S IgG, react against abnormal IgG produced by lymphocytes usually found in the synovia. Rheumatoid factor serum titers are present in 75% of patients. The presence of RF-IgG complexes within the joint space activate the complement system, resulting in inflammation and tissue injury. This, together with mononuclear cell infiltrates and PMN leukocytes, perpetuates the cycle. The titer of RF may also be of diagnostic value because the very high titers (1:640) are highly diagnostic of RF, while lower titers (1:20 to 1:160) may be present in chronic inflammatory states such as liver disease. In children with RF-positive disease, ANA is also positive in approximately 75% of cases.

Otologic manifestations of RA have been sporadically reported and include loosening of the transducer mechanism (83) and vestibuloauditory dysfunction (61,84). No temporal bone studies have been reported, and the relationship of RA with inner ear dysfunction is not confirmed, because there is no proof that patients with RA have any greater likelihood of developing an isolated ear disorder than does the general population. This holds true for a number of other autoimmune disorders that have been associated with vestibuloauditory dysfunction, including ulcerative colitis, idiopathic thrombocytic purpura, polymyositis, and dermatomyositis.

As an initial step in the evaluation of a suspected patient with AIED, a battery of serologic tests are employed as a screen for the presence of systemic immunologic disorders. The following tests have been found to be most often helpful in this regard:

ANA
Sedimentation rate
C1Q binding
Raji cell assay
Rheumatoid factor
Cryoglobulins
Urinalysis
FTA-ABS
Western blot against 68-kD inner ear antigen

TREATMENT

Patients in whom there is clear-cut evidence of autoimmunity and whose deafness and disequilibrium is disabling should be started on an immunosuppressive regimen. The suggested treatment protocols have not been determined by clinical trials but by individual preferences. High-dose steroids are generally agreed on, although the recommended dose and duration of treatment varies. Generally, 1 to 2 mg/kg/day of prednisone for 4 weeks will provide an initial therapeutic trial. Patients with a beneficial response should be maintained on a high dose for an additional 1 to 2 months and then tapered down slowly at 2.5-mg increments. The risks of chronic steroid therapy are not trivial and can represent significant morbidity to the patient; therefore, they should be thoroughly discussed.

In nonresponsive but desperate cases, consideration should be given for the use of cytotoxic drugs. Unlike in adults, for whom cytoxan has been recommended as a first-line drug after prednisone, the potential for neoplasia and the likelihood of permanent sterility prohibits its use in children. Therefore, methotrexate (MTX), a folic acid antagonist, has been the drug of choice for treating AIED in children when steroids either have become ineffective or have resulted in significant toxicity. Several reports have demonstrated that MTX is efficacious in the treatment of other autoimmune diseases of childhood, such as JRA (85). Methatrexate inhibits peripheral blood mononuclear cell proliferation and T- and B-cell response to mitogens, causing significant immunosuppression. Many of its known immunosuppressive actions result in the reduction of several important mediators of inflammation. Oral MTX has been recommended at a dosage schedule of either 5 mg/m^2/wk or 10 mg/m^2/wk for "resistant" cases of JRA with 1 mg/day of folate supplement to help prevent bone marrow suppression.

Clinical monitoring should include: complete blood cell (CBC) count, liver enzyme determinations, renal function tests, and urinalysis at baseline. Thereafter, weekly for 2 weeks, then biweekly for 1 month, then monthly determinations of CBC, AST, and ALT are recommended. Complications include liver and pulmonary interstitial fibrosis. Some initial rise in a liver function test can occur, but stabilization should quickly ensue. If not, the drug should be withheld until they again normalize. On rare occasions liver biopsy will be required if enzyme levels continue to rise. In some situations, oral dosage ceases to be effective, and this will need to be changed to either an intramuscular or subcutaneous route. It often takes as long as 30 days before the MTX effect will be seen; therefore, oral steroid usage should continue until the beneficial effect is seen, and then a slow steroid taper can be initiated. The use of MTX in AIED in adults was reported by Sismanis et al. in 1994 (86).

There has been wider experience with cytoxan than MTX for the treatment of adult AIED. For instance, McCabe (87) reported on 66 patients with progressive bilateral deafness who responded to immunosuppression. In his experience, patients more readily improved with cyclophosphamide than with prednisolone. In McCabe's treatment regimen, patients are given an initial trial of high-dose steroids for 3 weeks. Those who respond are then escalated to a cyclophosphamide–prednisolone combination for a 3-month period. The cyclophosphamide is then discontinued, and the prednisolone is slowly tapered. Any drop in hearing is followed by the reinstitution of the full combination of drugs at their original dosages. Administration of cyclophosphamide has been associated with the development of hemorrhagic cystitis and malignancies of the urinary tract; therefore, careful monitoring of the patient is indicated during therapy. The effects of chronic administration of alkylating agents has been shown to be leukemogenic, although, of this class of agents, cyclophosphamide has been found to be one of the weakest leukemogens (88). However, regardless of which of these agents is selected, the patient should be appropriately informed of their risks and managed in concert with a rheumatologist or hematologist–oncologist.

In recalcitrant cases, in which humoral immune mechanisms appear to be at play (i.e., autoantibodies and circulating immune complexes), plasmopheresis can be considered (30,89). The frequency and duration of treatment depends on the class of immunoglobulin and its equilibrium characteristics. For example, IgG is widely distributed both intravascularly and extravascularly. Therefore, repeated plasmapheresis treatments over a period of time are necessary to reduce the total-body IgG. One can approach reduction to approximately 20% of total-body IgG after eight treatments. A typical protocol would prescribe daily pheresis for 5 days, then every other day for 2 weeks, followed by twice a week for a total of ten runs in 1 month. One can usually assess the benefits of treatment by 1 month. If a beneficial response is seen, maintenance treatment can be done every 10 days or less. During plasmapheresis, immunosuppressive drugs should be continued in order to maximize the immunosuppressive effect and to prevent the continued production of antibody.

The experience at The National Institutes of Health in treating a variety of autoimmune types of vasculitis, including Wegener's granulomatosis and Cogan's syndrome, with systemic necrotizing vasculitis has been that aggressive immunosuppressive therapy be maintained for 1 year after the disappearance of active disease (63,90). In general, this proven method for managing potentially life-threatening autoimmune conditions should serve us well in the management of disabling vestibuloauditory dysfunction.

In the management of hearing loss associated with Cogan's syndrome, it has been recommended that if hearing acuity is poor, a trial of prednisone 2 mg/kg/day in divided doses be instituted for 5 to 7 days and, regardless of the response, tapered to 1 mg/kg/day over the next week, and, if after 2 weeks there has been no response, the prednisone should be rapidly tapered and stopped (52). However, a consensus has developed among otolaryngologists treating autoimmune SNHL that some patients will not respond to this short a course of immunosuppression and that cessation of the drug so quickly may result in a serious and perhaps permanent relapse.

SUMMARY

Autoimmune inner ear disease appears to be recognized as one important cause of progressive vestibuloauditory dysfunction in childhood. These patients may initially masquerade as progressive SNHL attributed to a childhood infection or inherited genetic deafness. The rapid progression, the asymmetrical nature of the hearing loss, and often the presence of previously normal hearing before instability developed should alert one to the possibility of AIED. In this setting, the clinician should have a high index of suspicion, obtain laboratory confirmation, and begin immunosuppressive therapy as soon as possible in order to preserve function. Due to the uncertainties of diagnosis, some patients may receive these drugs empirically, which then in itself serves to confirm the diagnosis if an ameliorative affect is achieved. The development of specific and sensitive laboratory tests to further identify these patients and to monitor their response to treatment appears to hold great promise. Increased experience with these patients will hopefully provide, in the near future, a precise and highly efficacious treatment regimen.

ACKNOWLEDGMENTS

I wish to thank my colleagues for their contributions to this research. Funding was provided by NIH-NIDCD grants DC00193 and DC00139, and by the Research Service of the Veterans Administration.

REFERENCES

1. Veldman JE, Roord JJ, O'Connor AF, et al. Autoimmunity and inner ear disorders: an immune-complex mediated sensorineural hearing loss. *Laryngoscope* 1984;94:501–7.
2. Kanzaki J, Ouchi T. Steroid-responsive bilateral sensorineural hearing loss and immune complexes. *Arch Otorhinolaryngol* 1981;230:5–9.
3. McCabe BF. Autoimmune sensorineural hearing loss. *Ann Otol Rhinol Laryngol* 1979;88:585–9.
4. Lehnhardt E. Plotzliche Horstorungen, auf beiden Seiten gleichzeitig oder nacheinander aufgetreten. *Z Laryngol Rhinol Otol* 1958;37:1–16.
5. Beickert P. Zur Frage der Empfindungsschwerhorigkeit und Autoallergie. *Z Laryngol Rhinol Otol* 1961;40:837–42.
6. Terayama Y, Saski Y. Studies on experimental allergic (isoimmune) labyrinthitis in guinea pigs. *Acta Otolaryngol* 1963;58:49–64.
7. Schiff M, Brown M. Hormones and sudden deafness. *Laryngoscope* 1974;84:1959–81.
8. Hughes GB, Barna BP, Calabrese LH, et al. Predictive value of laboratory tests in autoimmune inner ear disease: preliminary report. *Laryngoscope* 1986;96:502–5.
9. Hughes GB, Moscicki R, Barna BP, et al. Laboratory diagnosis of immune inner ear disease. *Am J Otol* 1994;15:198–202.
10. Berger P, Koja S, Rogowski M, et al. The lymphocyte transformation test for detecting immunologic inner ear deafness. *HNO* 1989;37:153–7.
11. Helfgott SM, Moscicki RA, San Martin J, et al. Correlation between antibodies to type II collagen and treatment outcome in bilateral progressive sensorineural hearing loss. *Lancet* 1991;337:387–9.

12. Sutjita M, Peter JB, Baloh RW, et al. Type II collagen antibodies in patients with sensorineural hearing loss. *Lancet* 1992;339:559–60.
13. Arnold W, Pfaltz R, Altermatt HJ. Evidence of serum antibodies against inner ear tissues in the blood of patients with 42. certain sensorineural hearing disorders. *Acta Otolaryngol* 1985;99:437–44.
14. Arnold W, Pfaltz R. Critical evaluation of the immunofluorescence microscopic test for identification of serum antibodies against human inner ear tissue. *Acta Otolaryngol* 1987;103:373–8.
15. Soliman AM. An improved technique for the study of immunofluorescence using non-decalcified frozen guinea pig cochlea. *J Laryngol Otol* 1988;102:215–8.
16. Soliman AM. A comparative immunofluorescent study of fixed decalcified tissue from the guinea pig cochlea. *Arch Oto Rhino Laryngology* 1988;244(6):337–41.
17. Gebbers JO, Altermatt HJ, Arnold WW, et al. Binding of serum immunoglobulins to human inner ear tissue in inner ear hearing loss: methodologic limits. *HNO* 1987;35:487–91.
18. Soliman AM, Zanetti F. Improvements of a method for testing autoantibodies in sensorineural hearing loss. *Adv Otol Rhinol Laryngol* 1988;39:13–7.
19. Elies W, Plester D. Sensorineural hearing loss and immunity. In: Veldman JE, et al., eds. *Immunobiology, autoimmunity, transplantation in otorhinolaryngology*. Berkeley, California: Kugler; 1985:111–7.
20. Zanetti F, Klein R, Berg PA. Progressive inner ear diseases sequelae of a secondary autoimmune process? Significance of antibodies to endoplasmic reticulum. *HNO* 1987;35:34–7.
21. Kempf HG, Hornig T. Immunologic findings and therapeutic results in chronic progressive inner ear hearing loss. *HNO* 1987;35:38–42.
22. Plester D, Soliman AM. Autoimmune hearing loss. *Am J Otol* 1989;10:188–92.
23. Harris JP, Sharp P. Inner ear autoantibodies in patients with rapidly progressive sensorineural hearing loss. *Laryngoscope* 1990;97:63–76.
24. Moscicki R. Western blot analysis of serum antibody to inner ear antigens in patients with idiopathic progressive bilateral sensorineural hearing loss (IPBSNHL). American Neurotology Society Meeting, Palm Beach, Florida, April 27–29, 1990.
25. Harris JP, Ryan AF. Fundamental immune mechanisms of the brain and inner ear. *Otolaryngol Head Neck Surg* 1995;112:639–53.
26. Gottschlich S, Billings PB, Keithley EM, et al. Assessment of serum antibodies in patients with idiopathic progressive sensorineural hearing loss and Ménière's disease. *Laryngoscope* 1995;105:1347–52.
27. Moscicki RA, San Martin JE, Quintero CH, et al. Serum antibody to inner ear proteins in patients with progressive hearing loss. *JAMA* 1994;272:611–6.
28. Billings PB, Keithley EM, Harris JP. Evidence linking the 68kD antigen associated with progressive sensorineural hearing loss with the highly inducible hsp70. *Ann Otol Rhinol Laryngol* 1995;104:181–8.
28a. Bloch DB, San Martin JE, Rauch SD, Moscicki RA, Bloch KJ: Serum antibodies to heat shock protein 70 in sensorineural hearing loss. *Archives of Oto Laryngology-Head & Neck Surgery*, 1995;121(10):1167–71.
29. Schuknecht H. Ear pathology in autoimmune disease. In: Pfaltz CR, Arnold W, Kleinsasser O, eds. *Bearing of basic research on clinical otolaryngology*. Basel; Karger, New York; 1991:50–70.
30. Hughes GB, Barba BP, Calabrese LH, et al. Clinical Diagnosis of Immune Inner Ear Disease. *Laryngoscope* 1988;98:251–3.
31. Ryan AF. Immunological factors in Ménière's disease. In: Bernstein J, Ogra P, eds. *Immunology of the ear*. New York: Raven Press; 1987:453–61.
32. Hughes GB, Kinney SE, Barna BP, et al. Autoimmune reactivity in Ménière's disease: a preliminary report. *Laryngoscope* 1983;3:410–7.
33. Hughes GB, Kinney SE, Barna, BP, et al. Autoimmune vestibular dysfunction: preliminary report. *Laryngoscope* 1985;95:893–7.
34. Brookes GB. Circulating immune complexes in Ménière's disease. *Arch Otolaryngol* 1986;112:536–540.
35. Derebery MJ, Rao VS, Siglock TJ, et al. Ménière's disease: An immune complex-mediated illness? *Laryngoscope* 1991;101:225–9.
36. Xenellis J, Morrison AW, McClowskey D, et al.: HLA antigens in the pathogenesis of Ménière's disease. *J Laryngol Otol* 1986;100:21–4.
37. Bowman C, Nelson R: HLA antigens in autoimmune sensorineural hearing loss. *Laryngoscope* 1987;97:7–9.
38. Harris JP, Aframian D. Role of autoimmunity in contralateral delayed endolymphatic hydrops. *Am J Otol* 1995;15:710–6.
39. Yoo TJ, Stuart JM, King AH, et al. Type II collagen autoimmunity in otosclerosis and Ménière's disease. *Science* 1982;17:1153–5.
40. Kitahara M, Matsubara T, Takeda T, et al. Bilateral Ménière s disease. Abstracts, Barany Society Ordinary Meeting in Uppsala, Sweden, June 1–2, 1978:39–40.
41. Malamud N, Foster DB. Periarteritis nodosa: a clinic-pathological report with special reference to the central nervous system. Preliminary Report-University Hospital Bulletin, Ann Arbor, 1941;7:102–4.
42. Lake-Bazaar G. Polyarteritis nodosa presenting with bilateral nerve deafness. *J R Soc Med* 1978;71:144–7.
43. Paterson E, Carlson BH. Hearing impairment as the initial sign of polyarteritis nodosa. *Acta Otolaryngol* 1966;61:189–95
44. Wolf M, Kronenburg J, Engelberg S, et al. Rapidly progressive hearing loss as a symptom of polyarteritis nodosa. *Am J Otolaryngol* 1987;8:105–8.
45. Gussen P. Polyarteritis nodosa and deafness: a human temporal bone study. *Arch Otorhinolaryngol* 1977;217:263–71.
46. Jenkins HA, Pollak AM, Fisch U. Polyarteritis nodosa as a cause of sudden deafness: a human temporal bone study. *Am J Otolaryngol* 1981;2:99–107.
47. Yanagita N, Yokoi H, Koide J, et al. Acute bilateral deafness with nephritis: a human temporal bone study. *Laryngoscope* 1987;97:345–52.
48. Alford BR, Shaver EF, Rosenburg JJ, et al. Physiologic and histopathologic effects of microembolism of the internal auditory artery. *Ann Otol Rhinol Laryngol* 1965;74:728–48.
49. Kimura R, Perlman HB. Arterial obstruction of the labyrinth. I. Cochlear changes. II. Vestibular changes. *Ann Otol Rhinol Laryngol* 1958;67:5–40.
50. Cody DT, Sones DA. Relapsing polychondritis: audiovestibular manifestations. *Laryngoscope* 1971;81:1208–2.
51. Cogan DG. Syndrome of nonsyphilitic interstitial keratitis and vestibuloauditory symptoms. *Arch Ophthalmol* 1945;33:144–9.
52. Haynes BF, Kaiser-Kupfer MI, Mason P, et al. Cogan's syndrome: studies in thirteen patients, long-term follow-up, and a review of the literature. *Medicine* 1980;56:426–41.
53. Fisher ER, Hellstrom HR. Cogan's syndrome and systemic vascular disease: Analysis of pathologic features with reference to its relationship to thromboangitis obliterans. *Arch Pathol* 1961;72:572–92.
54. Wolff D, Bernhard WG, Tsutsumi S, et al. The pathology of Cogan's syndrome causing profound deafness. *Ann Otol Rhinol Laryngol* 1965;74:507–20.
55. Zechner G. Zum Cogan-syndrome. *Acta Otolaryngol* 1980;89:310–6.
56. Rarey KE, Bicknell JM, Davis LE. Labyrinthine osteogenesis in Cogan's syndrome. *Am J Otolaryngol* 1986;4:387–90.
57. Benitez JT, Arsenault MD, Licht JM, et al. Evidence of Central vestibulo-auditory dysfunction in atypical Cogan's syndrome: a case report. *Am J Otology* 1990;11:131–4.
58. Cheson BD, Bluming AZ, Alroy J. Cogan's syndrome: a systemic vasculitis. *Am J Med* 1976;60:549–55.
59. Brinkman CJ, Broekhuyse RM. Cell-mediated immunity after retinal detachment as determined by lymphocyte stimulation. *Am J Ophthalmol* 1978;86:260–5.
60. Cogan DG, Sullivan WR Jr.: Immunologic study of nonsyphilitic interstitial keratitis with vestibuloauditory symptoms. *Am J Ophthalmol* 1975;80:491–4.
61. Hughes GB, Kinney SE, Barna BP, et al. Autoimmune reactivity in Cogan's syndrome: a preliminary report. *Otolaryngol Head Neck Surg* 1983;91:24–32.
62. Hiraki Y, Kuwasaki N, Shoji H, et al. Each one case of Vogt Koyanagi-Harada disease with vestibular and cerebellar ataxia, and multiple cranial nerve palsies. *Rinsho Shinkeigaku* 1989;29:54–8.
63. Fauci AS, Wolff SM. Wegener's granulomatosis studies in eighteen patients and a review of the literature. *Medicine* 1973;52:535–61.
64. McDonald TJ, DeRemee RA. Wegener's granulomatosis. *Laryngoscope* 1983;93:220–31.
65. Campbell SM, Montanaro A, Bardana EJ. Head and neck manifestations of autoimmune disease. *Am J Otolaryngol* 1983;4:187–216.
66. Kornblut AD, Wolff SM, Fauci AS. Ear disease in patients with Wegener's granulomatosis. *Laryngoscope* 1982;92:713–7.
67. Kempf HG. Ear involvement in Wegener's granulomatosis. *Clin Otolaryngol* 1989;14:451–6.
68. Karmody, CS. Wegener's granulomatosis: presentation as an otological problem. *Trans AAOO* July-August, 1978.

69. Leone CA, Feghali JG, Linthicum F. Endolymphatic sac: possible role in autoimmune sensorineural hearing loss. *Ann Otolaryngol* 1984;93: 208–9.
70. Schur P. Serologic tests in the evaluation of rheumatic diseases. *Immunol Allergy Prac* 1991;13:9–16.
71. O'Duffy J, Lehner T, Barnes CG. Summary of the Third International Conference on Behçet's Disease. *J Rheumatol* 1983;10:154–8.
72. Brama I, Fainaru M. Inner ear involvement in Behçet's disease. *Arch Otolaryngol* 1980;106:215–7.
73. McAdam LP, O'Hanlan MA, Bluestone R, et al. Relapsing polychondritis: prospective study of 23 patients and a review of the literature. *Medicine* 1976;55:193–215.
74. Ebringer R, Rook G, Swana GT, et al. Autoantibodies to cartilage and type II collagen in relapsing polychondritis and other rheumatic diseases. *Ann Rheum Dis* 1981;40:473–9.
75. Rogers PH, Boden G, Tourtellotte CD. Relapsing polychondritis with insulin resistance and antibodies to cartilage. *Am J Med* 1973;55:243–8.
76. Thalmann I, Thallinger G, Comegys TH, et al. Collagen: the predominant protein of the tectorial membrane, ORL. *J Otorhinolaryngol Relat Spec* 1986;48:107–15.
77. Yoo TJ, Tomoda K, Stuart JM, et al. Type II collagen-induced autoimmune otospongiosis: a preliminary report. *Ann Otol Rhinol Laryngol* 1983;92:103–8.
78. Yoo TJ, Tomoda K, Stuart JM, et al. Type II collagen-induced autoimmune sensorineural hearing loss and vestibular dysfunction in rats. *Ann Otol Rhinol Laryngol* 1983;92:267–71.
79. Mair IWS, Elverland HH. Sudden deafness and vaccination. *J Laryngol Otol* 1977;91:323–9.
80. Rosen E. Interstitial keratitis and vestibuloauditory symptoms following vaccination. *Arch Ophthalmol* 1949;41:24–31.
81. Steinberg A (moderator), Raveche ES, Laskin CA, Smith HR, et al. (discussants). NIH conference: systemic lupus erythematosus; insights from animal models. *Ann Intern Med* 1984;100:714–27.
82. Tan EM, Cohen AS, Fries JF, et al. The 1982 revised criteria for the classification of systemic lupus erythematosus. *Arthritis Rheum* 1982; 25:1271–7.
83. Moffat DA, Ramsden RT, Rosenberg JN, et al. Oto-admittance measurements in patients with rheumatoid arthritis. *J Laryngol Otol* 1977; 91:917–27.
84. McCabe BF. Autoimmune inner ear disease. In: Bernstein J, Ogra P. eds. *Immunology of the ear*. New York: Raven Press; 1987:427–35.
85. Weisman MH, Weinblatt ME, eds. *Treatment of rheumatic disease: companion to the textbook of rheumatology*. Philadelphia: W.B. Saunders, 1995.
86. Sismanis A, Thompson T, Willis HE. Methotrexate therapy for autoimmune hearing loss: a preliminary report. *Laryngoscope* 1994;104: 932–4.
87. McCabe BF. Autoimmune inner ear disease: therapy. *Am J Otol* 1989; 10:196–7.
88. Kaldor, Day NE, Pettersson F, et al. Leukemia following chemotherapy for ovarian cancer. *N Engl J Med* 1990;322:1–6.
89. Luetje CM. Theoretical and practical implications for plasmapheresis in autoimmune inner ear disease. *Laryngoscope* 1989;99(11):1137–46.
90. Fauci AS, Haynes B, Katz P. NIH conference: the spectrum of vasculitis; clinical, pathologic, immunologic, and therapeutic considerations. *Ann Intern Med* 1978;89:660–76.

PART VII

Vestibular Dysfunction

CHAPTER 28

Vertigo, Dizziness, and Disequilibrium

Phillip A. Wackym and David G. Cyr

Dizziness and vertigo are relatively uncommon in children. This chapter presents various causes and mechanisms of types of dizziness and vertigo. The chapter also discusses ways to distinguish the peripheral causes of dizziness and vertigo from their central etiologies.

In attempting to establish the diagnosis of vertigo, it is essential to obtain an accurate and detailed history. In most instances, this is the most revealing aspect of the work up and should give a good indication of the diagnosis. In obtaining the patient's history, it is very important that the child be encouraged to describe symptoms as well as having the parents describe the episodes, their duration, and the progression of the child's balance dysfunction and associated signs and symptoms (Table 1 and Table 2). Vertigo is most broadly defined as a hallucination of motion of any kind and in any direction. The definition of vertigo does *not* include lightheadedness, nausea, a feeling of faintness, or a feeling that the subject may fall; thus, the word ''dizzy'' should not be accepted without a detailed description.

Vertigo is an extremely frightening symptom to the child, and the fear is shared by the parents. Regardless of its cause, the physician therefore needs to provide support and reassurance to both the child and the parents. If the patient's fear and anxiety can be alleviated, the symptom is less distressing. Although children with vertigo have no intuitive insight into its etiology, the parents often suspect that their child has a brain tumor or another life-threatening neurologic disorder. In most patients, these possibilities can be ruled out after the history and physical examination have been completed. The physician can then inform the child and the parents that the condition is not life threatening and that it can be treated.

The child with acute vertigo should be told to lie still in bed in a darkened, quiet room. In fact, many children lie rigid in bed, frightened, on experiencing vertigo. Explaining to the older child how head movements and position changes exacerbate the vertigo during th acute stage is often helpful. However, in younger children and any child who experiences panic with the episodes of vertigo, general vestibular suppression and sedation may be necessary. Fortunately, the central nervous system (CNS) has a remarkable ability to compensate for most types of vestibular imbalance, and therefore, regardless of its cause, acute vertigo usually resolves within a few days. Experimental studies have demonstrated that vestibular suppression does not impair the process of compensation (1).

As the acute vertiginous episode subsides, rehabilitation should begin promptly. Since vertigo is aggravated by head movements, patients typically hold themselves stiffly when turning and moving about. They also tire easily with physical activity. At this point the child and the parents must be made aware that a gradual return to normal physical activity is vital to recovery. For the CNS to recalibrate the relationship between visual, auditory, proprioceptive, and vestibular signals, repeated head, eye, and body movements are essential. Children may suffer developmental delay or drift into a state of chronic invalidism if they are unaware of this requirement.

DIFFERENTIATING BETWEEN PERIPHERAL AND CENTRAL LESIONS

When a child presents with vertigo as a major complaint, one of the earliest differentiations that must be made is whether there is an abnormality of the peripheral component or the and central component of the vestibular system. In a peripheral lesion, vertigo of any significance is accompanied by nystagmus, and the two are usually directly proportional. Furthermore, spontaneous vertigo and nystagmus of peripheral origin rarely last longer than 3 weeks. Also, because of the close anatomic relationship of the peripheral vestibular and cochlear systems, the presence of concomitant auditory symptoms suggests a peripheral lesion. The reader is referred

---

P.A. Wackym: Ear Service (Otology and Neuro-otology), Department of Otolaryngology, Mount Sinai School of Medicine, New York, New York 10029-6574.

D.G. Cyr: Vestibular Laboratory, Boys Town National Research Hospital, Omaha, Nebraska 68131.

TABLE 1. *Causes of dizziness and vertigo in children*

Symptom	Cause
Vertigo	Benign positional vertigo, labyrinthitis, vestibular neuronitis, Ménière's disease, otosyphilis, Ramsay Hunt syndrome, migraine, brainstem or cerebellar infarction
Presyncopal light-headedness	Hyperventilation associated with panic disorders or chronic anxiety, postural hypotension, congestive heart failure, diffuse cerebrovascular disease
Disequilibrium	Ototoxic drugs, peripheral neuropathy cerebellar atrophy, cerebellar infarction, posterior fossa tumors, meningitides
Visual distortion	New refractive prescription, congenital cataract, ototoxic drugs, extraocular muscle dysfunction, corneal disease
Multisensory dizziness	Psychophysiologic dizziness, diabetes mellitus, systemic vasculitis, adverse drug reaction

Adapted with permission, Wackym PA, Blackwell KE, Nyerges AM. Pharmacotherapy of vestibular dysfunction. In: Jackler RK, Brackmann DE (Eds.), Neurotology. Mosby-Year Book, Inc., St. Louis, MO, 1994:544.

to several topical reviews of subsets of children with vestibular dysfunction (2–7).

VERTIGO OF PERIPHERAL ORIGIN

The following entities should be considered in the differential diagnosis of dizziness and vertigo of peripheral origin (Table 3).

TABLE 2. *Mechanisms of various types of dizziness and vertigo in children*

Symptom	Mechanism
Vertigo	Imbalance of tonic vestibular signals
Presyncopal light-headedness	Diffuse ischemia of the brain
Disequilibrium	Symmetric vestibular loss, proprioceptive loss, cerebellar damage
Visual distortion	Visual and vestibular input mismatch
Multisensory dizziness	Integrative dysfunction involving visual, proprioceptive and/or vestibular systems

Adapted with permission, Wackym PA, Blackwell KE, Nyerges AM. Pharmacotherapy of vestibular dysfunction. In: Jackler RK, Brackmann DE (Eds.), Neurotology. Mosby-Year Book, Inc., St. Louis, MO, 1994:544.

TABLE 3. *Peripheral causes of dizziness and vertigo in children*

Benign positional vertigo
Ménière's disease
Vestibular neuronitis
Ramsay Hunt syndrome (herpes zoster oticus)
Otitis media
    Serous otitis media
    Serous labyrinthitis
    Circumscribed labyrinthitis
    Acute suppurative labyrinthitis
Other infections
    Mumps
    Meningitis
Posttraumatic conditions
Drug or heavy metal-induced toxicity
    Gentamicin
    Lead
    Streptomycin
    Phenytoin
    Vancomycin
Genetic peripheral vestibular disorders
    Syndromic and nonsyndromic hearing loss
    Congenital malformations
        Spectrum of labyrinthine malformations
        Enlarged vestibular aqueduct syndrome
        Mondini dysplasia
    Degenerative
        Scheibe dysplasia
        Usher syndrome type I
Perilymph fistula

Benign Paroxysmal Positional Vertigo

Benign paroxysmal positional vertigo, also called benign positional vertigo (BPV) is the single most common cause of vertigo of peripheral origin in adults; however, BPV is rare in children. The condition results from several different insults to the inner ear (e.g., after a virus or after a head injury). In our experience, true BPV in children is limited to individuals who have had head injury prior to the onset of the disorder. Clinical response to the canalith repositioning maneuver or to vestibular exercises is equivalent to the response of adults with BPV (described later). A clear distinction should be made between BPV and that termed benign paroxysmal vertigo of childhood. The latter disorder is one of central dysfunction and its etiology is associated with migraine; this disorder is discussed in detail later in the chapter.

In BPV, the vertigo is brought on by turning the head to a particular position, but the symptoms last only several seconds. In most cases, this is the only symptom, and it is inconsistent. An observant patient may volunteer that repeated movements of the head to the critical position either bring on vertigo of progressively lesser severity or lead to a symptom-free period lasting several hours. In many instances, careful questioning may elicit a history of a recent mild head injury. Routine clinical and audiometric examinations are usually normal.

The only component of the electronystagmography (ENG) test battery that may be abnormal, and which is characteristic of this entity, is the positional test—provided both horizontal and vertical electroculography leads are employed. A typical positive response, on suddenly placing the patient's head in the critical position using the Hallpike manuever (see Chapter 11), is a latent period of 5 to 10 seconds, followed by gross vertigo and nystagmus that attenuates rapidly and ceases after about 20 seconds. The nystagmus persists in the same direction when the test is repeated or if the head position is changed. The nystagmus is highly characteristic with rotatory (torsional) in the ipsilateral eye (side turned toward the examiner) and vertical in the contralateral eye (side opposite the examiner). Repeating the test may produce a similar response but of lesser severity and of shorter duration until, after the second or third time, the response may not be occur; however, it may again be induced after 1 or 2 hours. This fatiguability is characteristic of the disease.

In addition, abnormalities in sensory interaction measured by posturography have been described in children with BPV (8). The condition is believed to be due to a displacement of otoconia and debris, originating from the utricle, into the ipsilateral posterior semicircular canal, the cupula of the posterior canal crista ampullaris (9–11). The symptoms usually subside spontaneously without treatment after about 1 year; within 2 months with use of Cawthorne's exercises; or immediately after canalith repositioning maneuvers (10).

Ménière's Disease

Ménière's disease (Ménière syndrome, endolymphatic hydrops) is an idiopathic condition of the membranous labyrinth and is characterized by spontaneous bouts of prolonged vertigo, fluctuating hearing loss, and tinnitus. Histologically, there is excessive endolymph within the scala media (Fig. 1) (9,12–14). In 1938, Hallpike and Cairns (15) and Yamakawa (16) independently observed histologic endolymphatic hydrops in the temporal bones of patients with Ménière's disease. In the same year, Samuel Crowe at the Johns Hopkins Hospital was the first to report a case of Ménière's disease affecting a 6-year-old child (17). Although Ménière's disease primarily affects adults between the ages of 30 and 60, children are also affected. In fact, 3% to 5% of patients with Ménière's disease experience the onset of signs and symptoms during childhood (18,19). The disease rarely affects children under the age of 10, but in our experience, high dietary sodium or renal dialysis are risk factors for the clinical expression of Ménière's disease in the pediatric population. More commonly, however, we encounter post-traumatic endolymphatic hydrops in children (see below).

Ménière's disease is unilateral in approximately 80% of patients; when it is bilateral, the second ear usually becomes affected within 3 years of the first episode. Bilateral involvement has been reported in 16% to 50% of patients (20). By far the most common pattern is involvement of both the vestibular and the cochlear labyrinths; however, in very rare instances, the disease may produce vestibular symptoms alone or be manifested by episodes of fluctuating hearing loss alone. In these uncommon presentations, the other portion of the labyrinth eventually becomes symptomatic as the disease progresses. The vertiginous episodes last anywhere from 15 minutes to several hours. In an extraordinarily rare subset of pediatric Ménière's disease, patients experience vestibular otolith dysfunction, termed an otolithic crisis of Tumarkin. Most of these patients develop a sudden disorientation relative to the earth; some patients have the illusion of being violently pushed to the ground.

The pattern of occurrence of the spells varies. Some children exhibit long remissions between attacks, but others

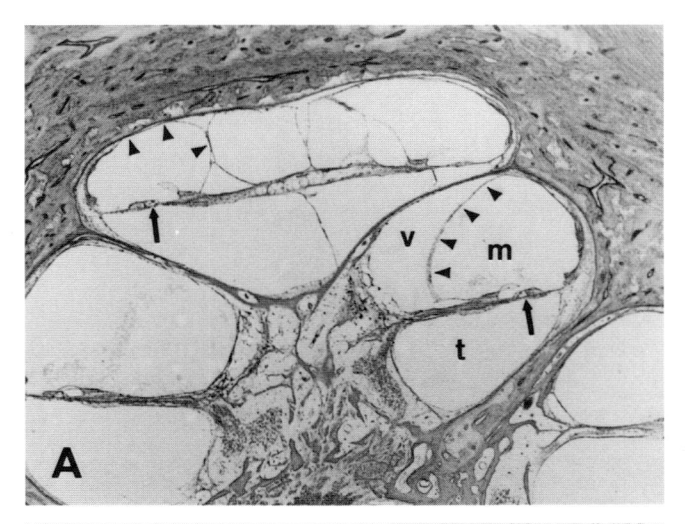

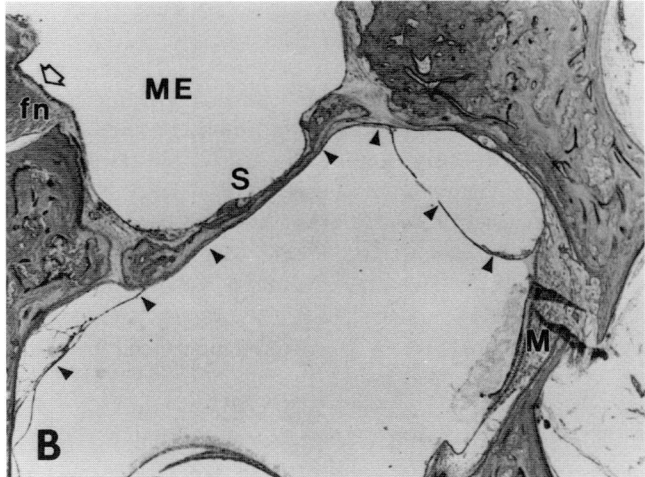

FIG. 1. Photomicrographs from a patient with Ménière's disease affecting the left ear. **A:** the midmodiolar level, endolymphatic hydrops has resulted in the characteristic distension of the scala media *(m)* with displacement of Reissner's membrane *(arrowheads)* into the scala vestibuli *(v)*. The organ of Corti *(arrow)* rests on the basilar membrane which separates the scala media from the scala tympani *(t)*. **B:** Within the vestibule, center, the displaced saccular membrane *(arrowheads)* has become adherent to the oval window membrane beneath the stapes footplate *(S)*. The macula of the saccule *(M)* with its overlying otoconia are seen lower right. Within the middle ear *(ME)* of this patient, the bony wall of the Fallopian canal containing the facial nerve *(fn)* is dehiscent at the level of the oval window *(open arrow)*. H & E, ×20. Published with permission, copyright © 1994 P.A. Wackym.

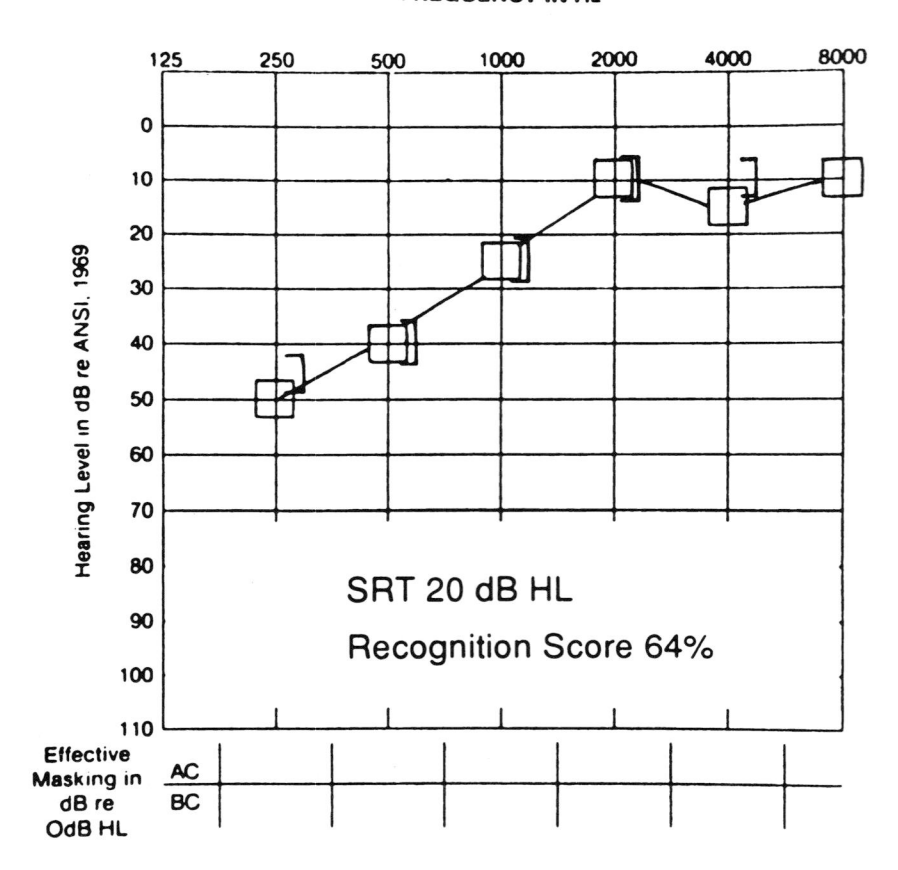

FIG. 2. Air □—□ and bone ( ]—]) conduction pure-tone threshold sensitivity as a function of frequency, showing the relationship between pure-tone air conduction average hearing loss (500–2,000 Hz) and speech recognition measures in a sensorineural hearing loss due to Ménière's disease. Published with permission, copyright © 1994 P.A. Wackym.

show a clustering of attacks with long symptom-free periods between attacks. A classic spell is usually preceded by an aura consisting of pressure on the side of the head on the affected side, tinnitus, and hearing loss. The spell comes on suddenly, with severe whirling vertigo accompanied by diaphoresis and nausea. In the early stages of the disease, the nausea may progress to vomiting. Head motion usually accentuates the symptoms. The hearing loss is characterized by a distortion of sound, which is results in poor speech perception. This distortion may also be present between spells, especially when the volume of sound is raised. Loud sounds may be so intolerable that they are painful. In the intervals between spells, the hearing loss may fluctuate considerably, especially in the early stages of the disease before much destruction of the cochlear labyrinth occurs. Most patients are controlled medically. with a low-sodium diet (1,000–1,500 mg/day), with or without a diuretic. Less than 10% of patients fail medical therapy and become candidates for a vestibular denervation procedure (e.g., labyrinthectomy or vestibular neurectomy). The cause of Ménière's disease remains unknown (9,12–14,20,21).

The general physical examination is usually normal, thus, the diagnosis has to depend on an accurate history and on the results of audiometric and vestibular tests. Pure-tone audiometry usually shows a sensorineural loss in the affected ear and has a flat or rising curve (Fig. 2). Fluctuation in hearing level is elicited on repeated testing at varying intervals of time. Speech audiometry invariably demonstrates a drop in discrimination, out of proportion to the level of the sensorineural loss. Audiograms performed before and after the child ingests 1.2 ml of glycerol/kilogram of body weight often show an improvement in speech reception threshold and word discrimination. In older children, tuning fork and whisper tests can corroborate the sensorineural nature of the loss and can also demonstrate the discrimination problem and recruitment.

Tests for vestibular function during quiescence may, on caloric stimulation, demonstrate hypofunction on the affected side. Subjectively, the caloric test duplicates the spontaneous episode, although it may be less severe. The most difficult lesions to differentiate from Ménière's disease, in its early stages at least, are an acoustic neuroma, sporadic or early neurofibromatosis type 2, or other cerebellopontine angle tumor. These tumors cause vertiginous episodes in less than 20% patients, but may produce auditory abnormalities similar to those found in Ménière's disease.

Secondary Endolymphatic Hydrops

Endolymphatic hydrops with associated vertiginous symptoms may also be seen in children after head injury or with congenital syphilis. Typical symptoms of endolymphatic hydrops develop after trauma in a small percentage of patients. These children usually respond well to medical treatment, and glycerol dehydration testing may provide further diagnostic data. In our experience, this is the most common clinical history associated with hydropic signs and symptoms in children. Late congenital syphilis may closely mimic Ménière's disease. In contradistinction to the 16% to 50% incidence of bilaterality in Ménière's disease, syphilis usually affects both ears. Syphilitic hearing loss also has an earlier age of onset and may give a positive fistula test in the presence of an intact tympanic membrane. Large doses of systemic steroids can evoke a good but transient improvement in hearing (22,23).

Vestibular Neuronitis

This condition is characterized by a sudden onset of sustained and severe vertigo, made worse with head movements. Vestibular neuronitis usually affects subjects in early middle age or slightly later and is usually unilateral; however, 3% to 7% of all cases occur in children, with the youngest reported case affecting a 3-year-old (24–26). It presents with varying degrees of severity. Thought to be caused by a viral infection of Scarpa's ganglion, the condition often is preceded or accompanied by an obvious viral infection and may affect several individuals in a community at the same time—hence the term endemic vertigo or endemic labyrinthitis. The most severe period of the attack usually lasts from 1 to 3 weeks and is characterized by an improvement of the symptoms from day to day, although they may be made worse by sudden movements of the head. There is no accompanying deafness or tinnitus, and the CNS is normal. The spontaneous nystagmus has its fast component to the opposite side (destructive nystagmus), and the caloric response in the affected ear is either reduced or absent.

Vestibular neuronitis is frequently called acute viral labyrinthitis or labyrinthine apoplexy, particularly by emergency department physicians, but both viral and bacterial labyrinthitis are quite rare. In addition to acute vestibular dysfunction, patients with labyrinthitis experience sudden, profound hearing loss in the affected ear. Although the vertigo subsides after 3 weeks, in certain instances it may still be provoked by sudden movements of the head. As a general rule, however, compensation occurs after 3 weeks, with complete recovery from symptoms, especially in younger age groups. During the active period of disease, patients should be treated with symptomatic pharmacotherapy (23). Although some patients have complete resolution, others maybe left with permanent hypofunction detectable by the caloric test in the affected ear, although the deficit is invariably asymptomatic after central vestibular compensation. There is some evidence that children recover caloric function, compensate better (or both) than do their adult counterparts (27–29).

Histopathologically, degenerative changes in the vestibular nerve, Scarpa's ganglion, vestibular neuroepithelium, and decreased synaptic density within the ipsilateral vestibular nuclei are consistent findings (30,31). Epidemiologic and serologic data suggest a viral etiology (26,32). The latent virus (e.g., herpes simplex virus) is thought to remain dormant within the vestibular primary afferent neuron ganglion of Scarpa. Although all the evidence has been circumstantial, recent demonstration of varicella-zoster viral DNA in the spiral and geniculate gangia of patients with Ramsay Hunt syndrome (herpes zoster oticus) by using archival temporal bone sections suggests that similar studies from Scarpa's ganglia neurons from patients with vestibular neuronitis can be completed (33,34).

Ramsay Hunt Syndrome

James Ramsay Hunt (35) first postulated that the etiology of herpes zoster oticus was recrudescence of herpes zoster in the geniculate ganglion. In our experience, Ramsay Hunt syndrome is very rare in young children (Fig. 3), but may be encountered in teenagers. Clinically, Ramsay Hunt syndrome may have a variety of manifestations. However, the original four classifications of the disease were (a) disease affecting the sensory portion of cranial nerve VII; (b) disease affecting the sensory and motor divisions of the cranial nerve VII; (c) disease affecting the sensory and motor parts of the cranial nerve VII with auditory symptoms (hearing loss); and (d) disease affecting the sensory and motor divisions of the cranial nerve VII with both auditory (hearing loss) and vestibular (vertigo) symptoms. Hunt's classification assumed that the pathologic process of the disease occurred in the geniculate ganglion. Involvement of the vestibular nerve has been documented clinically and histopathologically (36,37). Recent molecular temporal bone pathology studies have demonstrated varicella-zoster viral DNA in archival temporal bone sections through Scarpa's and the spiral ganglia and in sections through the geniculate gangia of patients with Ramsay Hunt syndrome (herpes zoster oticus) (34).

Experience with the use of intravenous acyclovir during the acute presentation of Ramsay Hunt syndrome suggests that antiviral medications in combination with oral steroids may facilitate recovery and minimize the morbidity associated with the facial paralysis (38–41). The intravenous route has more inherent expenses than does an oral route of administration. However, tissue levels of acyclovir delivered via an oral route are not high enough to treat varicella-zoster infections. Alternate antiviral agents, such as famciclovir, that achieve adequate levels via an oral route are now available as an alternative to intravenous acyclovir for the treatment of patients with Ramsay Hunt syndrome. Since the oral route is much more cost effective, this route is preferred.

Otitis Media

Otitis media affects two thirds of American children by 2 years of age, making it the most common diagnosis in children and the second most common diagnosis in medicine

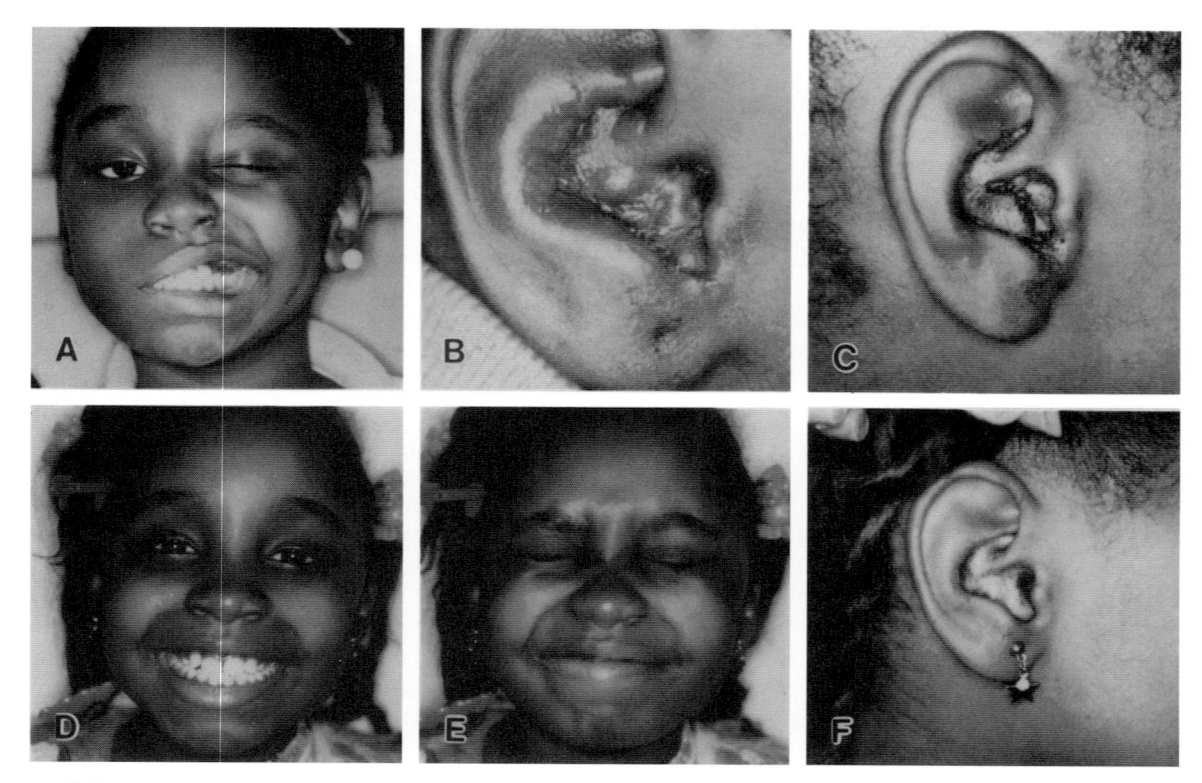

FIG. 3. An 11-year-old girl with Ramsay Hunt syndrome. **A:** Initial presentation with complete right facial paralysis. **B:** Early rescrudescence of varicella-zoster virus, visible as vesicles within the concha of the affected side. **C:** By 1 week, the vesicles were well demarcated and beginning to superficially crust. **D** and **E:** At 3 months after presentation and treatment with oral prednisone, she had fully recovered her facial nerve function. **F:** Her conchal skin had returned to normal. Courtesy of Dr. Kenneth Grundfast, Georgetown University School of Medicine, Washington, DC. Published with permission, copyright © 1995 P.A. Wackym.

(42). A spectrum of vestibular dysfunction is associated with otitis media in children; these disorders are discussed below in order of decreasing frequency of occurrence.

Serous Otitis Media

Serous otitis media (otitis media with effusion) is a common cause of vestibular dysfunction in children. It does not result in true vertigo; rather, these children experience disequilibrium or clumsiness. The signs and symptoms have been shown to resolve after removal of the effusions and placement of tympanostomy tubes (43). In our experience, this is a fairly common phenomenon, especially in toddlers. The balance disorder is mild, and typically there is a delay in recognizing the dysfunction in young children (43,44). As expected, objective, quantitative changes measured with rotatory testing were not statistically different for children with effusions and those without effusions (45). Although the mechanism responsible for the balance dysfunction is not known, one possibility is that changes in middle-ear pressure are transmitted to the inner ear. Casselbrant et al. studied postural control, with use of platform posturography, in 41 children with otitis media before and after insertion of tympanostomy tubes (46). The 41 children with otitis media were compared to 50 children without ear disease. The researchers found that the sway velocity was statistically increased in children with otitis media. However, much work remains to be completed to understand the relationship between otitis media and balance disorders, motor development, and accident proneness.

Serous Labyrinthitis

Serous labyrinthitis represents an irritation of the inner ear without bacterial or viral invasion and is usually secondary to direct trauma or to adjacent infection. A classic example is vestibular irritation following an operation on the labyrinth, such as stapedectomy, or accompanying acute suppurative otitis media, in which diffusion of toxic products of the infection is thought to occur across the round window membrane. In either instance, recovery is the rule, although hypofunction may persist in response to caloric stimulation. In serous labyrinthitis, vertiginous symptoms may be constant and may last for hours or for several days. The hearing may be decreased, but usually not severely. The accompanying nystagmus is irritative and may last for days. The response to caloric testing may be diminished but is not lost.

Circumscribed Labyrinthitis

Circumscribed labyrinthitis is considered present whenever a fistula test is positive in the presence of chronic suppurative otitis media. In the fistula test, compressing the air in the patient's external auditory canal leads to transient conjugate deviation of the eyes to the opposite side; negative pressure causes deviation toward the affected ear. In this condition, a cholesteatoma or an inflammatory process has eroded bone of the otic capsule down to, but not through, the endosteum of the labyrinth. Invariably, this takes place over the lateral semicircular canal (Fig. 4). Consequently, compression of the air of the external auditory canal leads to compression of the membranous semicircular duct, thus causing the nearby cupula to be deflected toward the utricle. Ampullopetal deflection causes the eyes to deviate to the opposite side. A labyrinthine fistula may be symptom-free, but when vertigo is present, the older child may describe it as periodic waves of mild dizziness. Occasionally, the patient may complain of a bizarre gait, in which he feels displaced in the direction opposite to the involved ear; alternatively, the child's parents may observe a change in gait, which may signify the erosive process of the cholesteatoma. These cases require prompt operative removal of the cholesteatoma, the source of the infection, or both, before the condition progresses to acute suppurative labyrinthitis.

Acute Suppurative Labyrinthitis

Bacterial invasion of the labyrinth always results in total loss of both auditory and vestibular functions. In modern times, loss of function is more likely to follow chronic otitis media rather than acute suppurative otitis media. Acute suppurative labyrinthitis is characterized by sudden prostration with violent vertigo, nausea, vomiting, and nystagmus. The crisis is usually ushered in with a fever. Initially, the hearing may still be present because the quick component of the nystagmus is toward the affected ear (irritative nystagmus). Hearing is gradually lost over a period of hours when the direction of the nystagmus changes to the opposite side (destructive nystagmus).

Treatment consists of large intravenous doses of appropriate bactericidal antibiotics and must be followed by a complete mastoidectomy and insertion of a tympanostomy tube, possibly with labyrinthotomy to prevent intracranial spread of the infection (47–49). Postoperatively, the destructive nystagmus continues toward the opposite side until compensation occurs within about 3 weeks. Interestingly, although the spiral ganglion cell survival is only 28% to 40% following viral or bacterial labyrinthitis, the Scarpa's ganglion cell survival is approximately 80% (50).

Other Infections and Ototoxicity

Bacterial, fungal, or viral infections as well as various ototoxic medications can result in unilateral or bilateral vestibular paresis or paralysis. Acute unilateral loss results in true vertigo, but bilateral losses rarely cause vertigo because the brain does not perceive an asymmetric firing rate between the two sides. However, children with bilateral lesions have difficulty with imbalance and clumsiness. The most serious problem that children with bilateral vestibular paralysis experience is disorientation while swimming, because

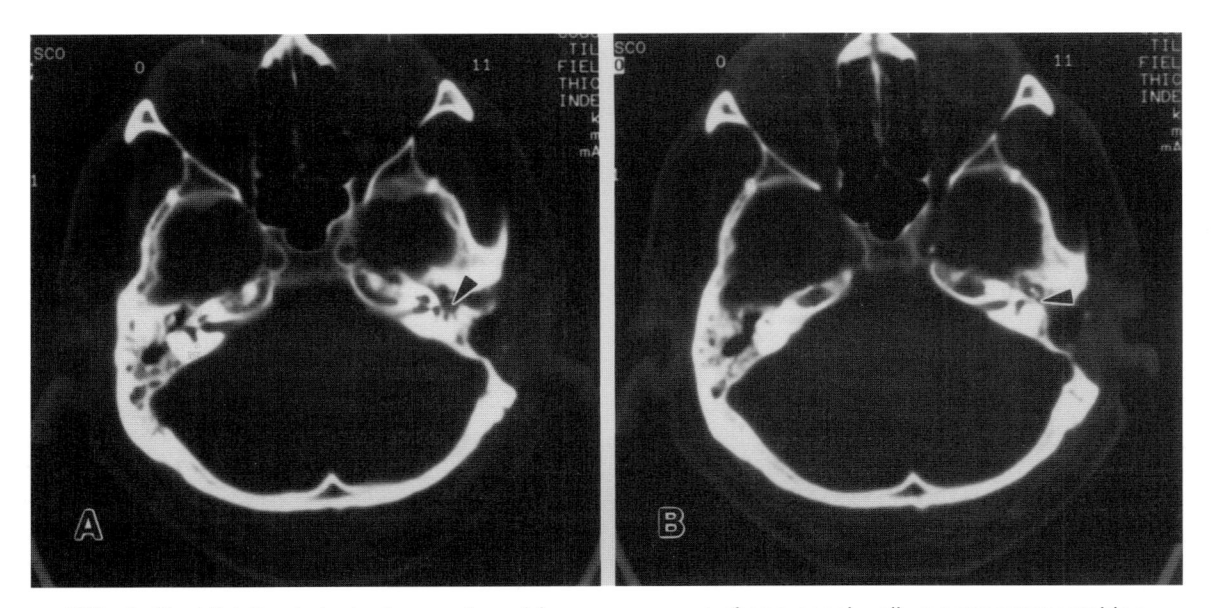

FIG. 4. Recidivistic cholesteatoma referred for management after a canal wall up tympanomastoidectomy. Exertional vertigo and progressive sensorineural hearing loss. **A:** Axial temporal bone CT without contrast shows loss of stapes and erosion of the lateral (horizontal) semicircular canal *(arrowhead)*. **B:** Lateral semicirzcular canal erosion and cholesteatoma evident *(arrowhead)*. Published with permission, copyright © 1996 P.A. Wackym.

they depend solely on vision and proprioception to remain oriented relative to the surface.

Mumps

Mumps is an acute, contagious, systemic paramyxovirus infection, usually causing painful swelling of the parotid glands. Mumps is rare under the age of 2 years due to maternal immunologic protection. Infected children can have later complications (e.g., orchitis in postpubertal boys) and pancreatitis, prostatitis, nephritis, myocarditis, and meningoencephalitis. An unexplained feature of mumps labyrinthine involvement is the typical unilateral infection (51). The degree of impairment varies from mild high-frequency hearing loss to profound deafness. Because of the asymmetry of mumps labyrinthitis, the children are acutely vertiginous; however, compensation is usually complete.

Meningitis

Meningitis secondary to ear disease is primarily a disease of infants and young children with acute otitis media (49,52,53). Although all the bacteria associated with acute and chronic otitis media can cause meningitis, pneumococcal meningitis *(Streptococcus pneumoniae)* is the most serious of the common forms of bacterial meningitis, with a mortality rate of 7% to 10% in children (52). In addition, 20% to 30% of survivors have otologic sequelae (49,52,53). Of the 23 children with auditory or vestibular dysfunction after pneumococcal meningitis reported in one series, 9 had vertigo and 13 had complete bilateral loss of peripheral vestibular function, but only 17 had hearing loss (52). Although bilateral vestibular loss may result in delay in reaching the developmental landmarks of standing and walking, no evident postural difficulties are noted by the teenage years. However, studies have compared postural control in these children to that of normal controls, and increased body sway has been reported (54,55).

Drug-Induced Ototoxicity

Peripheral vestibular dysfunction of the inner ear is produced by a group of ototoxic drugs, primarily antibiotic, chemotherapeutic, and diuretic agents. Damage from heavy metals or from quinine is now seldom seen, but lead exposure should always be considered in children with postural balance abnormalities (56,57). Children with ototoxic injury rarely experience vertigo because both labyrinths are involved equally, although disequilibrium and ataxia are common, especially with impairments of proprioception or vision (5).

The best clinical, pathologic, and experimental information has come from studies of the aminoglycoside group of antibiotics—streptomycin, dihydrostreptomycin, neomycin, kanamycin, and gentamicin—because of the magnitude and frequency of the end-organ damage that these agents produce in the labyrinth. Ototoxicity is usually dose related, and because aminoglycosides are excreted by the kidneys, the plasma level of the drugs reflects renal function. These drugs are concentrated in the labyrinthine fluids and persist there at a much higher concentration and for a longer duration than they do in plasma. Therefore, special consideration should be given to the child receiving long-term peritoneal dialysis (58).

The aminoglycosides cause striking pathological changes in the sensory elements of the inner ear. Gentamicin, the most frequently used aminoglycoside is far more vestibulotoxic than cochleotoxic (23,59). In the vestibular labyrinth, there is a dramatic loss of hair cells in the ampullary cristae and the utricular and saccular maculae. There is also a change in the number and size of otoconia. Neural degeneration occurs and is presumed to be secondary to hair-cell loss. In the organ of Corti, outer hair cells are destroyed in all turns, especially in the first and second rows of the basal turn. Inner hair cells may also be destroyed at the apex. Other changes in the cochlea similar to those seen in renal tubular cells after administration of similar toxic drugs have been observed and may reflect a disturbance of the ionic equilibrium. In our experience, an increased frequency of bilateral vestibulopathy in children is being encountered due to the increased use of gentamicin as a cost-saving measure in treating chronic infections, such as osteomyelitis, that require prolonged administration of intravenous antibiotics. Other antibiotics known to cause severe end-organ damage are vancomycin and the tuberculostatic agent viomycin. Use of these agents should be avoided, but if there is no alternative, the physician is obligated to be vigilant in monitoring the cochleotoxicity during administration (60). In addition, there is evidence of genetic susceptibility to aminoglycoside ototoxicity in some patients due to a specific mitochondrial DNA defect (34,61,62).

Nonantibiotic ototoxic agents are nitrogen mustard, which produces cochlear damage and injures the vestibular organ to a lesser extent, and ethacrynic acid, which has caused both transient and permanent sensorineural hearing loss. Transient losses have been noted with use of furosemide.

Tinnitus usually precedes noticeable hearing loss or decrease in discrimination and should be viewed with alarm, although in young children this information is rarely volunteered. Because tinnitus heralds significant cochlear damage, the drug should be discontinued if possible. Audiometrically, losses are first noted in the upper frequencies, but they soon involve the lower ones. Discrimination ability is impaired, and progression may be very rapid. There may be no warning of impending or early damage in the vestibular system because of symmetrical damage to bilateral end organs. When the patient has the eyes closed, however, marked disequilibrium is noticed because normal equilibrium depends on proprioception and visual cues in addition to vestibular information. As a result, a subject can easily ambulate with two of the three senses intact, but not with only one. Consequently, periodic gait and posture tests should be performed during therapy with ototoxic drugs.

Electronystagmographic recordings with caloric stimulation can also demonstrate bilateral decrease in function; however, in young children, rotational chair testing is better tolerated than caloric stimulation. If possible, the drug should be stopped at the first evidence of decreased response. The following guidelines may be helpful in the use of ototoxic drugs:

1. Use the drug only for lifesaving measures; prophylactic use is not justified;
2. Inform the parents and the child at the outset of the ototoxic potential of the drug and warn them of the early symptoms of toxicity;
3. Administer the drug by milligrams per kilogram of body weight;
4. Reduce the dosage in the presence of impaired renal function;
5. Keep the child well hydrated;
6. Avoid using more than one ototoxic drug at a time;
7. Avoid using ototoxic drugs in children with existing end-organ disease;
8. Have the patient evaluated before therapy to establish baselines for hearing (clinical and audiometric tests), vestibular and statokinetic systems (gait, stance, and caloric tests), and renal function (blood urea nitrogen and creatinine clearance tests);
9. Evaluate the child during therapy with the same tests: daily clinical hearing evaluation and inquiry about tinnitus, weekly audiometry, weekly renal studies (more often if abnormal) and biweekly vestibular (especially rotatory chair) and posturography tests;
10. Discontinue the drug at the onset of toxicity.

Posttraumatic Vestibular Dysfunction

Trauma to the temporal bone, common even in minor head injury (63), can result in a variety of peripheral vestibular dysfunctions such as temporal bone fractures, labyrinthine concussion, posttraumatic positional vertigo, perilymph fistulae, and delayed endolymphatic hydrops. In addition, central vestibular dysfunction such as dizziness due to brainstem trauma, postconcussion syndrome, or cervical vertigo are common (64).

GENETIC PERIPHERAL VESTIBULAR DISORDERS

Chapters 5, 21, and 22 focus on the molecular genetics and clinical features of syndromic and nonsyndromic hearing losses. In addition to auditory impairment, many of these genetic disorders, with or without inner ear anomalies, are associated with vestibular dysfunction. Children with bilateral vestibular deficits are known to stand and walk later than do other children, yet by teenage years, they have no evident postural difficulties (54,55). Motor development, visual cues, and proprioceptive and CNS development appear to be important for the acquisition of compensatory strategies (65–68).

Congenital Malformations

Spectrum of Labyrinthine Malformations

Developmental abnormalities of the temporal bone may involve the external auditory canal, middle ear, cochlear or the labyrinthine portions of the inner ear (or both), and the internal auditory canal (69). Because Chapter 13 focuses on the classification of these malformations, and together with Chapters 21, 22, and 23, the auditory aspects of these congenital abnormalities are detailed, only the vestibular aspects of several bony or membranous malformations and degenerative disorders of the inner ear disorders are discussed in this chapter. Malformations such as bilateral aural atresia present additional diagnostic challenges for the assessment of vestibular function (70).

Occasionally, while attempting surgical correction of conductive hearing loss, the otologist may encounter a flow of cerebrospinal fluid (CSF), ranging from an ooze to a jet-like stream, from the oval window. This is commonly referred to as a perilymph gusher. On the basis of morphometric and qualitative data from temporal bone pathology studies, it is unlikely that CSF enters the perilymphatic space via the cochlear aqueduct; rather, the origin is most likely via a defect in the fundus of the internal auditory canal (71).

Enlarged Vestibular Aqueduct Syndrome

Although enlarged vestibular aqueducts that are radiographically obvious are commonly associated with Mondini dysplasia, they may occur in isolation. This anomaly is usually bilateral and the clinical course of children with this condition includes bilateral progressive hearing loss and mild to severe true vertigo (72–76). Although the temporal bone pathology remains to be identified, it is believed on the basis of radiographic findings and clinical features, that endolymphatic hydrops characterizes this syndrome. Clinical failure of endolymphatic sac shunt surgery in children with this condition led to the abandonment of this management option (72).

Mondini Dysplasia

An inner ear deformity first described by Mondini in 1791, Mondini dysplasia is characterized by bony and membranous anomalies of the inner ear. The diversity of the anomalies ranges from cochlear hypoplasia to aplasia, incomplete cochlear partition, or a common cochlear cavity; incompletely developed vestibular end organs; and deformed or absent semicircular canals. Clinically, children with Mondini dysplasia exhibit a wide range of auditory and vestibular dysfunction. Mondini deformities may be unilateral or bilateral and are easily diagnosed with computed tomography (CT). In the more severe forms, progressive sensorineural hearing loss accompanied by vertigo may be observed. Instead of the five ultrastructurally distinct epithelial cell types normally present within the endolymphatic sac (ES) (77), the ES in Mondini dysplasia is distended, and there is a single flattened epithelial cell type (78). On the basis of histopathologic observation of ES distension in Mondini dysplasia, this disorder was initially thought to be amenable to ES shunt surgery; however, an outcomes analysis of a series of patients with this disorder suggested that ES shunt surgery should not be undertaken (79). A recent study associated Mondini dysplasia with cytomegalovirus infection, although much study remains to demonstrate causality (80).

Degenerative Malformations

Scheibe Dysplasia

Scheibe dysplasia is the most common malformation of the inner ear; it is also known as cochleosaccular dysplasia. In this disorder, only the cochlea and the saccule are affected; radiographically, the temporal bone appears normal (81). The utricle and all the semicircular canal cristae are normal in histologic appearance and function. The primary afferent neuron populations usually remain normal, but cochlear and saccular hair cell loss has been reported (82). The severity of the hearing loss varies, and the vestibular component is limited to symptoms of otolith dysfunction, such as an illusion of tilt or linear motion. Phenotypically, children with Scheibe dysplasia also exhibit pigmentary anomalies.

Usher Syndrome Type I

Usher syndrome represents the association of hearing loss and visual loss due to retinitis pigmentosa. The retinitis pigmentosa is usually diagnosed by the age of 10 years because of visual field defects or night blindness. It is an autosomal recessive disorder and has several distinct clinical subsets. Children with Usher syndrome type 1 have bilateral sensorineural hearing loss, retinitis pigmentosa, and bilateral vestibular paresis or paralysis (83). Early in the course, postural instability dominates; later ataxia increases in frequency due to the combination of bilateral vestibular loss and blindness. Vestibular therapy targeted at maximizing proprioceptive function is the most effective strategy in rehabilitating these children.

Perilymph Fistula

Traumatic or spontaneous perilymphatic fistulae represent an abnormal communication between the perilymphatic space and the middle ear. However, few areas in otology are surrounded with more controversy than spontaneous perilymph fistula (PLF) (with or without an associated minimal trauma). Because Chapter 44 is devoted to PLF, we mention here some diagnostic dilemmas related to vestibular dysfunction and potential tools to aid in the diagnosis of PLF. A child with PLF may have a variety of clinical presentations including fluctuant or sudden sensorineural hearing loss with or without vertigo or imbalance (84–88). A clinical presentation that is frequently reported in pediatric PLF is sensorineural hearing loss and transient or intermittent spatial disorientation (84,89,90).

A fundamental difficulty in establishing a diagnosis of PLF is in the absence of a reliable objective test; moreover, many children with PLF have subjective symptoms that may be considered to be similar or the same as those experienced by patients with Ménière's disease (91,92). An additional clinical difficulty is in differentiating true PLF from dependent accumulation of subcutaneously injected epinephrine solution. If middle ear exploration for PLF is undertaken, the future holds promise for objective perilymph specific protein markers that will facilitate the establishment of a diagnosis (87,93,94).

VERTIGO OF CENTRAL ORIGIN

When an otologist is confronted by a patient suffering from vertigo, one of the most important things is to exclude the possibility of a CNS disorder. Although only a few of the peripheral causes of vertigo may be dangerous to health, most factors responsible for central vertigo are not only associated with serious disease, but may also be life threatening. In addition to the common central causes of vertigo (Table 4), many other conditions, such as systemic metabolic disorders (5), craniovertebral junction disorders (7), and focal seizure disorders (5) may cause dizziness or vertigo. Even though vertigo may be a prominent symptom in these patients, other features often indicate a lesion within the central nervous system. Therefore, the complaint of vertigo may be overlooked. Spontaneous nystagmus due to involvement of the central vestibular pathways in the brainstem may persist indefinitely, even though the vertigo may not be in proportion to the nystagmus; or vertigo may not even be a symptom at the time of examination. Additional balance disorders may result from CNS pathology or dysfunction and may present with symptoms such as ataxia, imbalance, or motion intolerance.

Brainstem and Posterior Fossa Lesions

Tumor

In children, 60% to 70% of intrinsic brain tumors are found in the posterior fossa; in adults, most tumors are supratentorial (95). The clinical presentations of the tumors commonly reflect either CSF obstruction with hydrocephalus and accompanying headaches, nausea, and vomiting or features of direct involvement of the cerebellum or brainstem, such as ataxia, limb clumsiness, diplopia, facial numbness or weakness, dysphagia, hearing loss, or vertigo.

Primary brainstem tumors, such as gliomas, usually grow slowly and infiltrate the brain stem nuclei and fiber tracts

TABLE 4. *Central causes of dizziness and vertigo in children*

Brainstem and posterior fossa lesions
  Tumor
  Chiari malformations
  Vascular disorders
    Vascular anomalies
    Vasculitis
    Cerebrovascular disease without structural lesions
    Migraine
  Trauma
Demyelinating disease
  Acquired immunodeficiency syndrome
  Multiple sclerosis
Hereditary disorders
  Dyslexia/learning disabilities
  Cerebellar vermal agenesis (Joubert syndrome)
  Cerebellar vermal atrophy or hypoplasia
  Familial periodic cerebellar ataxia and vertigo
  Spinocerebellar disease
Tumors of the cerebellopontine angle
  Acoustic neuroma (vestibular schwannoma)
    Sporadic
    Neurofibromatosis type 2
  Meningioma
  Other cerebellopontine angle tumor
Other disorders
  Hydrocephalus
  Motion intolerance
  Seizures

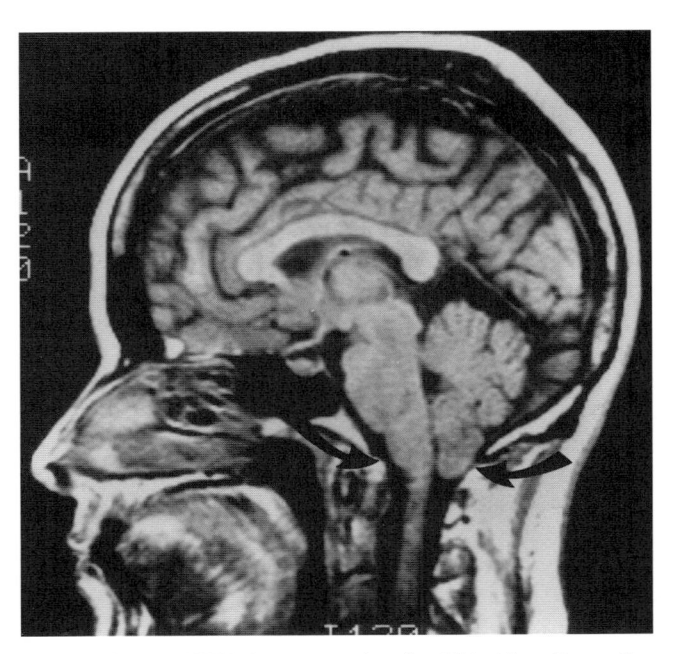

FIG. 6. Sagittal MRI demonstrating the Chiari I malformation with tonsillar herniation. The arrows represent the level of the foramen magnum. Published with permission (Wackym PA, Blackwell KE. Abnormalities of the craniovertebral junction. In: Jackler RK, Brackmann DE, (Eds.), Neurotology, Mosby–Year Book, Inc., St. Louis, MO, 1994:1213).

producing multiple signs and symptoms (Fig. 5). In adults gliomas comprise approximately 1% of intracranial tumors; however, in children, they are 5 to 10 times more common. Vestibular and cochlear signs and symptoms are common, occurring in approximately 50% of patients. The brainstem site of origin can usually be determined on the basis of associated neurologic findings, and the tumors may be classified as focal or diffuse. The focal tumors may be further divided into mesencephalic, medullary, dorsally exophytic, and pontine. Mesencephalic brainstem gliomas usually present with hydrocephalus; medullary tumors usually present with anorexia, upper respiratory infections, swallowing dysfunction, vomiting, vocal fold paresis or paralysis, hemi- or quadriparesis, and ataxia; dorsally exophytic tumors usually present with vomiting and multiple cranial neuropathies; and pontine tumors (rarest) may present with isolated pure motor hemiparesis, facial nerve paresis or paralysis, unilateral hearing loss, or true vertigo. Diffuse brainstem gliomas may present in a fulminant manner with ataxia, and multiple bilateral cranial nerve palsies and hemiparesis are commonly seen (see Fig. 5). The prognosis of diffuse tumors is much worse than the prognosis for focal tumors.

Tumors adjacent to the fourth ventricle can produce vestibular signs and symptoms by compressing the vestibular nuclei. These tumors include: medulloblastomas, cerebellar astrocytomas, ependymomas, papillomas, teratomas, epidermoid cysts, and cysticercosis. Most present with ataxia, head tilt, nausea, and vomiting rather than vertigo.

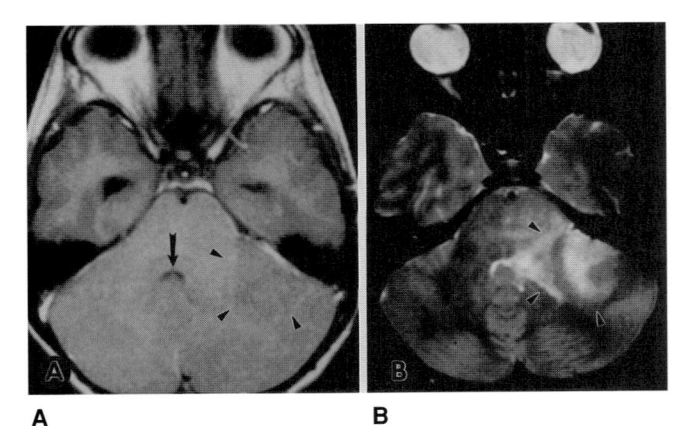

FIG. 5. Axial MRI of diffuse brainstem glioma. **A:** Short-relaxation-time, contrast-enhanced image of left diffuse brainstem glioma. The tumor has extended posterolaterally *(arrowheads)* and shifted the fourth ventricle to the right *(heavy arrow)*. **B:** Long-relaxation-time, contrast-enhanced image shows differentiation between tumor, cerebellum, and brainstem *(arrowheads)*. Original MRI courtesy of Dr. Scott Atlas, Mount Sinai School of Medicine, New York. Published with permission, copyright © 1996 P.A. Wackym.

Chiari Malformations

The Chiari malformations constitute a group of posterior fossa congenital herniation syndromes. They are classified into four types of malformations of the hind brain. In type I, there is downward herniation of long, thin cerebellar tonsils through the foramen magnum (Fig. 6). In type II, also referred to as Arnold-Chiari malformation, the cerebellar vermis extends through the foramen magnum, and there is caudal displacement of the lower pons and medulla, often overlapping the upper portion of the upper cervical spinal cord. A portion of the fourth ventricle extends into the spinal canal and the upper cervical rami course cephalad before leaving the spinal canal. In type III, the cerebellum herniates through a bony defect in the occipital bone; type IV shows cerebellar hypoplasia (96,97).

The type II, III, and IV malformations cause florid symptoms and signs and are likely to be recognized in infancy or early childhood. The type II malformation is the most common. Most cases are associated with myelomeningocele, spina bifida, and hydrocephalus. Type III is equivalent to an occipital meningoencephalocele; type IV is sometimes classified as a variant of the Dandy-Walker syndrome (98). Type I is the least severe manifestation and may present during late childhood or early adult life, although type I cases have been seen in children as young as 10 years old. The Chiari malformations are frequently associated with other abnormalities of the craniovertebral junction, such as syringomyelia, basilar impression, atlanto-occipital fusion, and the Klippel-Feil deformity (99). In a series of 60 patients, Chiari malformations had the following presenting symptoms (100): headache (42%); neck pain (23%); suboccipital pain (17%); limb pain 23%), arm or leg pain (5%); limb weakness (32%); limb numbness (47%); unsteadiness, vertigo, or ataxia (42%); leg stiffness (7%); blurred vision or diplopia (23%); dysphagia (27%); tinnitus (8%); and dysarthria (3%).

Most cases of Chiari malformation are amenable to posterior decompression by suboccipital craniectomy and C-1–C-2 laminectomy. In cases of anterior impingement, transoral anterior decompression may be beneficial (99). In cases accompanied by syringomyelia, patients may additionally benefit from a shunting procedure to redirect the flow of CSF away from the syrinx cavity. In their extensive review of the literature, Levy, Mason, and Hahn (101) found that 46% of cases improved, 32% remained clinically stable, and 20% worsened after surgical intervention.

Vascular Disorders

Pediatric neurovascular disorders may result in vertigo, dizziness, or disequilibrium. This broad group of diseases can be divided into three groups: vascular anomalies, vasculitis, and cerebrovascular disease without structural lesions. The vestibular or balance dysfunction reflects the nature of the underlying disorder: vertigo with unilateral processes, dizziness with CNS hypoperfusion or metabolic disorders, or disequilibrium with brainstem or cerebellar compression.

Vascular anomalies that involve the posterior fossa and that may result in vestibular dysfunction include saccular, traumatic, mycotic, and giant aneurysms; arteriovenous malformations (AVM); moyamoya disease; fibromuscular dysplasia; carotid dissections; and vertebral dissections. The etiologies of vasculitis that involve the posterior fossa and that may result in vestibular dysfunction include idiopathic; acquired immunodeficiency syndrome (AIDS); drug abuse; Wegener's granulomatosis; immune-related diseases (e.g., polyarteritis nodosa, systemic lupus erythematosus, juvenile-onset rheumatoid arthritis); conditions related to Crohn's disease; and granulomatous angiitis.

Cerebrovascular disease without structural lesions that involve the posterior fossa and that may result in vestibular dysfunction can be divided into five categories: heart disease, metabolic disorders, hematologic disorders, infections, and other disorders. Dizziness may result from primary cardiac defects such as cyanotic heart defects, valvular diseases, endocarditis patent ductus arteriosis, septal defects, patent foramen ovale, or cardiac tumors. Metabolic disorders such as homocystinuria or diabetes mellitus can also result in the symptom of dizziness. Ischemic or hemorrhagic strokes involving the cerebellum or brainstem can result from hematologic disorders such as sickle-cell disease, leukemia, hemophilia, pregnancy-related conditions, or conditions related to contraceptive use. Migraine is the most significant clinical entity in the "other disorders" category and can cause episodic vestibular-related symptoms, migraine is therefore considered separately later.

In children, cerebral infarction, both ischemic and hemorrhagic, is usually manifested by an acute event that causes a focal deficit. The overall incidence of childhood stroke has been estimated to be 2.7 cases in 100,000 each year (102). Vascular occlusion of the ipsilateral vertebral artery results in a lateral medullary infarction (Wallenberg syndrome). Major symptoms include vertigo, nausea, vomiting, intractable hiccuping, ipsilateral facial pain, diplopia, dysphagia, and dysphonia. One or all of the following physical findings may be present: ipsilateral Horner syndrome; ipsilateral loss of pain and temperature sensation of the face; ipsilateral paralysis of the palate, pharynx, and larynx; ipsilateral facial and lateral rectus weakness; ipsilateral dysmetria, dysrhythmia, and dysdiadochokinesia; and contralateral loss of pain and temperature sensation on the body. The lesion occurs caudal to the cochlear nuclei and cochlear nerve root entry zone, and therefore hearing loss does not occur. Patients with Wallenberg syndrome experience a prominent motor disturbance characterized by their body and extremities to strongly deviate toward the side of the lesion.

Vascular occlusion of the anterior inferior cerebellar artery usually results in an infarction of the dorsolateral pontomedullary region and the inferior lateral cerebellum. Because the labyrinthine artery supplying the cochlea arises from the anterior inferior cerebellar artery in 80% to 90% of patients, infarction of the membranous labyrinth is common. Major symptoms include severe vertigo, nausea, and vomiting. Other symptoms may include unilateral hearing loss, tinnitus, and facial paralysis. The physical examination reveals: ipsilateral hearing loss, facial weakness, cerebellar dysfunction, ipsilateral loss of pain and temperature sensation of the face, and decreased pain and temperature sensation on the body.

Vascular occlusion of the vertebral artery, the posterior inferior cerebellar artery, or the anterior inferior cerebellar artery results in cerebellar infarction without brainstem involvement. The initial symptoms are severe vertigo, vomiting, and ataxia. Brainstem signs and symptoms are absent; therefore, an erroneous diagnosis of a peripheral vestibular disorder may be made. The unique differentiating feature is the presence of cerebellar signs.

Transient ischemic attacks initially presenting in childhood are most frequently associated with an identifiable underlying disorder. Moyamoya disease, fibromuscular dysplasia, and migraines can present with recurrent, transient ischemic events. Other than these disorders, recurrent vestibular symptoms are unusual in pediatric cerebrovascular disease. When the transient ischemic attacks involve the territories of the vertebrobasilar system, recurrent vertigo may result. Children with these attacks often manifest short-lived symptoms such as vertigo, diplopia, dysarthria, bilateral limb weakness, gait ataxia, variable (and often bilateral) sensory disturbance, and memory loss (103).

Migraine

Migraine is a common cause of episodic vertigo and disequilibrium in children. However, the nomenclature that evolved in identifying this disorder is confusing. Pediatric neurologists and pediatricians often refer to this entity as benign paroxysmal vertigo of childhood (104,105), which should not be confused with benign paroxysmal positional vertigo.

Migraine has long been considered a vascular disorder, with vasoconstriction responsible for the neurologic symptoms, and vasodilation responsible for the headache. Basilar artery migraine produces symptoms related to areas of the CNS supplied by the posterior circulation. The vertigo usually lasts for minutes, but the disequilibrium may last for several hours. Headache is not a major clinical feature in these patients; however, they may experience visual disturbances (photophobia or visual field cuts), flushing, nausea, and vomiting. Most important, there is often a family history of classic migraine headaches (104,107–109). Diagnosis of migraine remains a diagnosis of exclusion.

Demyelinating Diseases

Multiple Sclerosis

For patients with multiple sclerosis, vertigo is the initial symptom in approximately 5% and is reported sometime during the course of the disease in as much as 50% of patients (110,111). Although multiple sclerosis is uncommon in children, as much as 10% of all cases manifest during childhood. In a series of pediatric patients with multiple sclerosis, 20% initially presented with vertigo (112). The duration of the vertigo is usually several hours to several days. Hearing loss occurs in approximately 10% of patients, and it can be acute (hours to days), subacute (over months), or slowly progressive in nature. Partial or complete remission after the onset of hearing loss is common. Plaques involving the vestibular and cochlear nerve root entry zones are commonly seen on magnetic resonance imaging (MRI), and can explain the frequent findings of unilateral caloric hypoexcitability and hearing loss. In addition, diplopia, weakness, numbness, and ataxia are also frequently seen early in the disease process.

Hereditary Disorders

Dyslexia/Learning Disabilities

Because developmental dyslexia represents a serious problem for approximately 2% of the school population, investigators have studied the oculomotor and vestibular function in this clinical group (113). Jerabek and Krejcová found both visual pursuit impairment and abnormal otokinetic nystagmus in subpopulations of these patients (113). Nonspecific vestibular suppression using antimotion-sickness medications such as meclizine, cyclizine, and dimenhydrate has been reported to improve the symptoms associated with the dyslexia (114).

Cerebellar Vermal Agenesis

Cerebellar vermal agenesis (Joubert syndrome) is a nonprogressive, autosomal recessive disorder. Because of the cerebellar agenesis, these patients experience ataxia, disequilibrium, and mental retardation (115,116). In addition, episodic tachypnea, hypotonia, and nystagmus may be observed shortly after birth.

Cerebellar Vermal Atrophy

Cerebellar vermal atrophy (Hypoplasia) is a nonprogressive, autosomal dominant disorder. In contrast to Joubert syndrome, the ataxia is mild and is accompanied by upbeat nystagmus (117,118). In these patients, during rotational chair testing, the vestibulo-ocular reflex is normal or increased; however, the smooth pursuit and optokinetic nystagmus is decreased.

Familial Periodic Cerebellar Ataxia and Vertigo

Familial periodic cerebellar atxia and vertigo is an autosomal dominant disorder. Patients with this disorder experience episodic dysarthria, limb ataxia, and disequilibrium that lasts several hours. Interestingly, the disorder is remarkably responsive to acetazolamide and it is thought that there is a specific defect in cerebellar pH homeostasis (119–122). The vestibulo-ocular reflex can be at the upper limit of normal or increased. A single positron emission tomography (PET) scan has been reported after resolution of the ataxic spell. One study demonstrated a decrease in glucose metabolism in the whole cerebellum, the inferior portion of the temporal lobes, and the thalami (122).

Tumors of the Cerebellopontine Angle

These tumors can give rise to marked and persistent disequilibrium, ataxia, or vertigo. It should be noted, however, that acoustic neuromas (vestibular schwannomas), which are by far the most common neoplasms of the posterior fossa, result in vertigo in less than 20% of patients although up to 50% of patients experience imbalance; however, these tumors are unusual in children. Other cerebellopontine angle tumors are seen, including: meningiomas, epidermoid cysts, cholesterol granulomas, and neurofibromas.

Acoustic Neuroma

Although acoustic neuromas (AN) (vestibular schwannomas) comprise an estimated 6% to 8% of all intracranial tumors, they are infrequently found in children who do not have neurofibromatosis type 2 (NF2). The terms acoustic neuroma and vestibular schwannoma are used interchangeably to identify the tumor that develops from the superior or inferior division of the vestibular nerve; however, vestibular schwannoma is more precise. Both sporadic and familial NF2 AN share the same genetic defect in the schwannomin gene on chromosome 22 (123–125).

Sporadic

Acoustic neuromas are usually detected during adulthood, with unilateral hearing loss and poor speech discrimination the most frequent presentations. Approximately 20 cases of sporadic AN have been reported in children; however, careful family histories should be completed because unilateral AN in NF2 can occur (126,127). As is the case with any unilateral AN, the vestibular deafferentation that occurs as a result of the tumor and the surgical resection is of limited long-term consequence because vestibular compensation is the rule. However, patients with AN experience some unsteadiness with rapid angular acceleration tasks, and the unsteadiness is minimized best with visual cues.

Neurofibromatosis Type 2

An autosomal dominant disease, NF2 predisposes the formation of multiple tumors in both the central and the peripheral nervous system. The presence of bilateral ANs is considered to be the hallmark of the disease (Fig. 7), although NF2 is also associated with other neural tumors such as meningiomas and neurofibromas, as well as with juvenile posterior subcapsular cataracts and retinal hamartomas. von Recklinghausen's disease (NF1) and NF2 are clinically and genetically distinct diseases. The genetic defect in NF1 is located on chromosome 17; the genetic defect in NF2 is located on chromosome 22 (123–125). The incidence of NF1 is 1 in 4,000 individuals; the incidence for NF2 is 1 in 40,000 individuals. Clinical heterogeneity of NF2 has been reported on the basis of age at onset, presence or absence of CNS tumors other than AN, and presence or absence of retinal hamartomas (128,129). Preliminary evidence suggests that a 163-bp deletion of the schwannomin gene is associated with the variable phenotypes observed in NF2 (125).

Aside from the auditory management issues related to hearing preservation surgery, use of cochlear implants to stimulate viable cochlear afferent dendrites, and the use of the auditory brain stem implant for the rehabilitation of patients with NF2, there are clinically significant issues related to balance. Because patients with NF2 develop bilateral vestibular paralysis, visual and proprioceptive function become increasingly important. Because patients with NF2 fre-

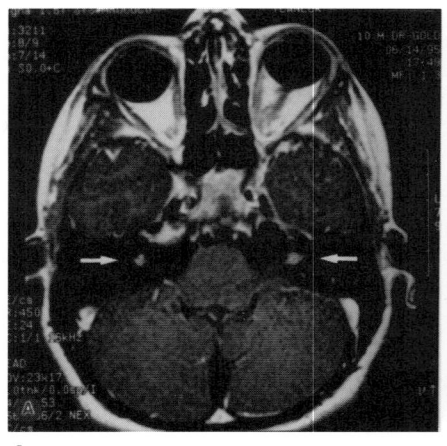

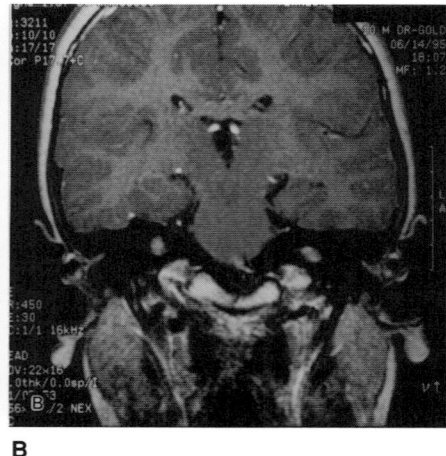

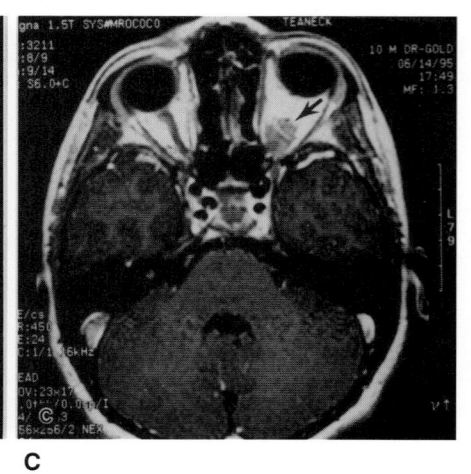

FIG. 7. Bilateral acoustic neuromas in a 10-year-old child with neurofibromatosis type 2 (NF2). **A:** Short-relaxation-time, contrast-enhanced axial MRI image shows bilateral tumors *(white arrows).* **B:** Short-relaxation-time, contrast-enhanced coronal image shows bilateral tumors. **C:** Short-relaxation-time, contrast-enhanced axial image shows left optic glioma *(black arrow).* Published with permission, copyright © 1996 P.A. Wackym.

quently develop ocular manifestations, especially cataracts and optic nerve gliomas, most patients become solely dependent on proprioceptive cues to maintain balance, which is further confounded by motor dysfunction resulting from spinal tumors (130,131). Although spinal tumors, café-au-lait (coffee with milk) macules in the skin, or both are less frequently encountered than than they are in patients with NF1, patients affected with NF2 can also have these conditions (130,131).

Meningioma

Meningiomas in children are especially rare, with an incidence of 0.3 in 100,000, and of these, posterior fossa meningiomas represent only 10% of all intracranial meningiomas (132). Cerebellar compression with ataxia is the most common etiology of balance dysfunction in this subset of patients.

Other Cerebellopontine Angle Tumors

Posterior fossa arachnoid cysts are rare lesions, representing 1% of all intracranial masses. As these CSF-filled cysts expand, they may produce ataxia, unsteadiness, headache, nausea, and/or vomiting. Posterior fossa arachnoid cysts may be classified by location. Supracerebellar cysts are located in the tentorial notch; retrocerebellar cysts are located in the superior or inferior midline and posterior to the cerebellar hemispheres; laterocerebellar cysts are located within the cerebellopontine angle; and clival cysts are located anterior to the brainstem. Symptomatic cysts can be treated surgically; several options are available. Needle aspiration, resection of the cyst wall, and shunting are all currently performed at various centers (133).

Other Disorders

Hydrocephalus

Vestibular function in hydrocephalic children has been studied after long-term shunt placement (134). A complete ENG test battery including recording of spontaneous and positional nystagmus, pendular eye tracking tasks, saccadic eye movements, and optokinetic and bithermal caloric responses were measured. Thirty-one children (82%) had ENG pathology suggesting central dysfunction; 12 (44%) of the 27 successfully studied had pathologic caloric function. Ten (26%) children had a combination of both central and peripheral pathology. These findings are particularly relevant because hydrocephalic children often have impaired motor development.

Motion Intolerance

Motion sickness or motion intolerance is believed to result from sensory mismatch between vision and vestibular cues (135). Motion intolerance is often induced when one experiences passive motion, particularly in the back seat of an automobile or while fixed in position with the visual surrounding moving, as in the vestibular laboratory when one is presented with a rotating optokinetic stimulus. Clinically children with motion intolerance experience autonomic dysfunction with nausea, diaphoresis, pallor and occasionally vomiting. During the episodes, the children may experience dizziness or imbalance. Interestingly, there is a much higher incidence of motion intolerance in patients with migraine (107,108). General vestibular suppression with diazepam or meclizine may be necessary.

REFERENCES

1. McCabe BF, Ryu JH, Sekitani T. Further experiments on vestibular compensation. *Adv Otorhinolaryngol* 1973;19:195.
2. Eviatar L, Eviatar A. Vertigo in children: differential diagnosis and treatment. *Pediatrics* 1977;59:833.
3. Fried MP. The evaluation of dizziness in children. *Laryngoscope* 1980;90:1548.
4. Cyr D. The vestibular system: pediatric considerations. *Semin Hear* 1983;4:33.
5. Baloh RW, Honrubia V. *Clinical neurophysiology of the vestibular system*. Philadelphia: FA Davis; 1990.
6. Tusa RJ, Saada AA, Niparko JK. Dizziness in childhood. *J Child Neurol* 1994;9:261.
7. Wackym PA, Blackwell KE. Abnormalities of the craniovertebral junction. In: Jackler RK, Brackmann DE, eds. *Neurotology*. St. Louis: Mosby-Year Book; 1994:1203.
8. Norré ME. Sensory interaction posturography in patients with benign paroxysmal positional vertigo. *Clin Otolaryngol* 1993;18:226.
9. Schuknecht HF. *Pathology of the ear*. 2nd ed. Philadelphia: Lea & Febiger; 1993.
10. Parnes LS, Price-Jones RG. Particle repositioning maneuver for benign paroxysmal positional vertigo. *Ann Otol Rhinol Laryngol* 1993;102:325.
11. Wackym PA, Morgan DE, King WA. Neuro-otology. In: Youmans JR, Becker DP, Dunsker SB, Friedman WA, Hoffman HJ, Smith RR, et al. eds. *Neurological Surgery*. 4th ed. Philadelphia: W.B. Saunders; 1995:374.
12. Wackym PA, Linthicum FH, Ward PH, House WF, Micevych PE, Bagger-Sjöbäck D. Re-evaluation of the role of the human endolymphatic sac in Ménière's disease. *Otolaryngol Head Neck Surg* 1990;102:732.
13. Wackym PA, Schuknecht HF, Ward PH, et al. Blinded, controlled study of endolymphatic duct and sac fibrosis in Ménière's disease. In: Filipo R, Barbara M, eds. *Ménière's Disease: Perspectives in the 90's*. Amsterdam: Kugler; 1994:209.
14. Wackym PA. Histopathologic findings in Meniere's disease. *Otolaryngol Head Neck Surg* 1995;112:90.
15. Hallpike CS, Cairns H. Observations on the pathology of Meniere's syndrome. *J Laryngol Otol* 1938;53:625.
16. Yamakawa K. Über die pathologische Veränderung bei einem Meniere-Kranken. *J Otorhinolaryngol Soc Jpn* 1938;44:2310.
17. Crowe SJ. Meniere's disease: study based on examinations made before and after intracranial division of the vestibular nerve. *Medicine (Baltimore)* 1938;17:1.
18. Meyerhoff WL, Paparella MM, Shea D. Ménière's disease in children. *Laryngoscope* 1978;88:1504.
19. Matsuoka I, Kurata K, Kaxama N, Nakamura T, Sugimaru T, Satah M: The beginning of Meniere's disease. *Acta Otolaryngol Suppl (Stockh)* 1991;481:505.
20. Wackym PA. Ménière's disease. *ASHA* 1992;21:19.
21. Wackym PA, Storper IS, Fu Y-S, House WF, Ward PH. Differential diagnosis of virus-like particles in the human inner ear. *Am J Otol* 1992;13:431.
22. Smith ME, Canalis RF. Otologic manifestations of AIDS: the otosyphilis connection. *Laryngoscope* 1989;99:365.
23. Wackym PA, Blackwell KE, Nyerges AM. Pharmacotherapy of vestibular dysfunction. In: Jackler RK, Brackmann DE, eds. *Neurotology*. St. Louis: Mosby-Year Book; 1994:543.
24. Coats AC. Vestibular neuronitis. *Acta Otolaryngol Suppl (Stockh)* 1969;251:5.

25. Harrison M. Vestibular neuronitis. *Acta Otolaryngol (Stockh)* 1969;67:379.
26. Sekitani T, Imate U, Noguchi T, Inokuma T. Vestibular neuronitis: epidemiological survey by questionnaire in Japan. *Acta Otolaryngol Suppl (Stockh)* 1993;503:9.
27. Okinaka Y, Sekitani T, Okazaki H, Miura M, Tahara T. Progress of caloric response of vestibular neuronitis. *Acta Otolaryngol Suppl (Stockh)* 1993;503:18.
28. Tahara T, Sekitani T, Imate Y, Kanesada K, Okami M. Vestibular neuronitis in children. *Acta Otolaryngol Suppl (Stockh)* 1993;503:49.
29. Imate Y, Sekitani T. Vestibular compensation in vestibular neuronitis. Long-term follow-up evaluation. *Acta Otolaryngol (Stockh)* 1993;113:463.
30. Nadol JB Jr. Vestibular neuritis. *Otolaryngol Head Neck Surg* 1995;112:162.
31. Baloh RW, Lopez I, Ishiyama A, Wackym PA, Honrubia H. Vestibular neuritis: clinical-pathologic correlation. *Otolaryngol Head Neck Surg* 1996;114:586.
32. Shimizu T, Sekitani T, Hirata T, Hara H. Serum viral antibody titer in vestibular neuronitis. *Acta Otolaryngol Suppl (Stockh)* 1993;503:74.
33. Wackym PA, Popper P, Kerner MM, Grody WW. Varicella-zoster DNA in temporal bones of patients with Ramsay Hunt syndrome. *Lancet* 1993;342:1555.
34. Wackym PA. Molecular temporal bone pathology. *Laryngoscope* 1996;Suppl: 1997;107:1156.
35. Hunt JR. On herpetic inflammations of the geniculate ganglion. A new syndrome and its complications. *J Nerv Ment Dis* 1907;34:73.
36. Zajtchuk J, Matz G, Lindsay J. Temporal bone pathology in herpes oticus. *Ann Otol Rhinol Laryngol* 1972;81:331.
37. Proctor L, Perlman H, Lindsay J, Matz G. Acute vestibular paralysis in herpes zoster oticus. *Ann Otol Rhinol Laryngol* 1979;88:303.
38. Stafford FW, Welch AR. The use of acyclovir in Ramsay Hunt syndrome. *J Laryngol Otol* 1986;100:337.
39. Dickins JRE, Smith JT, Graham SS. Herpes zoster oticus: treatment with intravenous acyclovir. *Laryngoscope* 1988;98:776.
40. Inamura H, Aoyagi M, Tojima H, Koike Y. Effects of aciclovir in Ramsay Hunt syndrome. *Acta Otolaryngol Suppl (Stockh)* 1988;446:111.
41. Uri N, Greenberg E, Meyer W, et al. Herpes zoster oticus: treatment with acyclovir. *Ann Otol Rhinol Laryngol* 1992;101:161.
42. Schappert SM. Office Visits for Otitis Media: United States, 1975–1990. Washington, DC: US Dept of Health and Human Services, Public Health Service, Centers for Disease Control, National Center for Health Statistics, 1992.
43. Golz A, Westerman ST, Gilbert LM, Joachims HZ, Netzer A. Effect of middle ear effusion on the vestibular labyrinth. *J Laryngol Otol* 1991;105:987.
44. Nield LS. Diagnosis: balance disturbance secondary to middle ear effusion. *Pediatr Rev* 1994;15:369.
45. Ben-David J, Podoshin L, Fradis M, Faraggi D. Is the vestibular system affected by middle ear effusion? *Otolaryngol Head Neck Surg* 1993;109:421.
46. Casselbrant ML, Furman JM, Rubenstein E, Mandel EM. Effect of otitis media on the vestibular system in children. *Ann Otol Rhinol Laryngol* 1995;104:620.
47. Feuerman T, Wackym PA, Gade GF, Dubrow TJ. Craniotomy improves outcome in subdural empyema. *Surg Neurol* 1989;32:105.
48. Wackym PA, Canalis RF, Feuerman T. Subdural empyema of otorhinologic origin. *J Laryngol Otol* 1990;104:118.
49. Kangsanarak J, Fooanant S, Ruckphaopunt K, Navacharoen N, Teotrakul S. Extracranial and intracranial complications of suppurative otitis media. report of 102 cases. *J Laryngol Otol* 1993;107:999.
50. Chiong CM, Xu W-Z, Glynn RJ, Nadol JB Jr. Survival of Scarpa's ganglion in the profoundly deaf human. *Ann Otol Rhinol Laryngol* 1993;102:425.
51. Lindsay JR, Davey PR, Ward PH. Inner ear pathology in deafness due to mumps. *Ann Otol Rhinol Laryngol* 1960;69:918.
52. Rasmussen N, Johnsen NJ, Bohr VA. Otologic sequelae after pneumococcal meningitis: a survey of 164 consecutive cases with a follow-up of 94 survivors. *Laryngoscope* 1991;101:876.
53. Naess A, Halstensen A, Nyland H, et al. Sequelae one year after meningococcal disease. *Acta Neurol Scand* 1994;89:139.
54. Magnusson M, Enbom H, Pyykkö I. Postural compensation of congenital or early acquired vestibular loss in hearing disabled children. *Acta Otolaryngol Suppl (Stockh)* 1991;481:433.
55. Enbom H, Magnusson M, Pyykkö I. Postural compensation in children with congenital or early acquired bilateral vestibular loss. *Ann Otol Rhinol Laryngol* 1991;100:472.
56. Bhattacharya A, Linz DH. Postural sway analysis of a teenager with childhood lead intoxication—a case study. *Clin Pediatr* 1991;30:543.
57. Bhattacharya A, Shukla R, Dietrich KN. Functional implications of postural disequilibrium due to lead exposure. *NeuroToxicol* 1993;142:179.
58. Warady BA, Reed L, Murphy G, et al. Aminoglycoside ototoxicity in pediatric patients receiving long-term peritoneal dialysis. *Pediatr Nephrol* 1993;7:178.
59. Thomas RJ. Neurotoxicity of antibacterial therapy. *South Med J* 1994;87:869.
60. Shrimpton SB, Milmoe M, Wilson APR, et al. Antimicrobial practice. Audit of prescription and assay of aminoglycosides in a UK teaching hospital. *J Antimicrob Chemother* 1993;31:599.
61. Hu D-N, Qiu W-Q, Wu B-T, et al. Genetic Aspects of Antibiotic Induced Deafness: Mitochondrial Inheritance. *J Med Genet* 1991;28:79.
62. Wackym PA, Chen CT, Kerner MM, Bell TS. Characterization of DNA extracted from archival celloidin-embedded human temporal bone sections. *Am J Otol* 1995;16:14.
63. Feuerman T, Wackym PA, Gade GF, Becker DP. Value of skull radiography, head computed tomographic scanning, and admission for observation in cases of minor head injury. *Neurosurgery* 1988;22:449.
64. Oosterveld WJ, Kortschot HW, Kingma GG, deJong HAA, Saatci MR. Electronystagmographic findings following cervical whiplash injuries. *Acta Otolaryngol (Stockh)* 1991;111:201.
65. Tsuzuku T, Kaga K. The relation between motor function development and vestibular function tests in four children with inner ear anomaly. *Acta Otolaryngol Suppl (Stockh)* 1991;481:443.
66. Berger W, Discher M, Trippel M, Ibrahim IK, Dietz V. Developmental aspects of stance regulation, compensation and adaptation. *Exp Brain Res* 1992;90:610.
67. Assaiante C, Amblard B. Ontogenesis of head stabilization in space during locomotion in children: influence of visual cues. *Exp Brain Res* 1993;93:499.
68. Woods LA, Haller RJ, Hansen PD, Fukumoto DE, Herman RM. Decreased incidence of scoliosis in hearing-impaired children. Implications for a neurologic basis for idiopathic scoliosis. *Spine* 1995;20:776.
69. Jackler RK, Luxford WM, House WF. Congenital malformations of the inner ear: a classification based on embryogenesis. *Laryngoscope* 1987;97:2.
70. Kaga K, Suzuki JI. Bilateral congenital atresia. Auditory and vestibular testing and surgical approach. *Acta Otorhinolaryngol Belg* 1991;45:51.
71. Schuknecht HF, Reisser C. The morphologic basis for perilymphatic gushers and oozers. *Adv Otorhinolaryngol* 1988;39:1.
72. Jackler RK, De la Cruz A. The large vestibular aqueduct syndrome. *Laryngoscope* 1989;99:1238.
73. Levenson MJ, Parisier SC, Jacobs M, Edelstein DR. The large vestibular aqueduct syndrome in children. *Arch Otolaryngol Head Neck Surg* 1989;115:54.
74. Arcand P, Desrosiers M, Dube J, Abela A. The large vestibular aqueduct syndrome and sensorineural hearing loss in the pediatric population. *J Otolaryngol* 1991;20(4):247.
75. Okumura T, Takahashi H, Honjo I, Takagi A, Mitamura K. Sensorineural hearing loss in patients with large vestibular aqueduct. *Laryngoscope* 1995;105:289.
76. Zalzal GH. Tomaski SM, Vezina LG, Bjornsti P, Grundfast KM. Enlarged vestibular aqueduct and sensorineural hearing loss in childhood. *Arch Otolaryngol Head Neck Surg* 1995;121:23.
77. Wackym PA, Friberg U, Bagger-Sjöbäck D, Linthicum FH Jr, Friedmann I, Rask-Andersen H. Human endolymphatic sac: possible mechanisms of pressure regulation. *J Laryngol Otol* 1987;101:768.
78. Gussen R. The endolymphatic sac in the Mondini disorder. *Arch Otorhinolaryngol* 1985;242:71.
79. Jackler RK, Luxford WM, Brackmann DE, Monsell EM. Endolymphatic sac surgery in congenital malformations of the inner ear. *Laryngoscope* 1988;98:698.

80. Bauman NM, Kirby-Keyser LJ, Dolan KD, et al. Mondini dysplasia and congenital cytomegalovirus infection. *J Pediatr* 1994;124:71.
81. Nomura Y, Kawabata I. Schiebe dysgenesis of the inner ear. *J Laryngol Otol* 1980;94:1345.
82. Schuknecht HF. Dysmorphogenesis of the inner ear. In: Gorlin RJ, ed. *Morphogenesis and malformation of the ear.* New York: Alan R. Liss; 1980:47.
83. Well D, Blanchard S, Kaplan J, et al. Defective myosin VIIA gene responsible for Usher syndrome type 1B. *Nature* 1995;374:60.
84. Grundfast KM, Bluestone CD. Sudden or fluctuating hearing loss and vertigo in children due to perilymph fistula. *Ann Otol Rhinol Laryngol* 1978;87:761.
85. Brookhouser PE, Worthington DW, Kelly WJ. Unilateral hearing loss in children. *Laryngoscope* 1991;101:1264.
86. Brookhouser PE, Worthington DW, Kelly WJ. Fluctuating and/or progressive sensorineural hearing loss in children. *Laryngoscope* 1994;104:958.
87. Weber PC, Perez BA, Bluestone CD. Congenital perilymphatic fistula and associated middle ear abnormalities. *Laryngoscope* 1993;103:160.
88. Weissman JL, Weber PC, bluestone CD. Congenital perilymphatic fistula: computed tomography appearance of middle ear and inner ear anomalies. *Otolaryngol Head Neck Surg* 1994;111:243.
89. Knight NJ. Severe sensorineural deafness in children due to perforation of the round-window membrane. *Lancet* 1977;2(8046):1003.
90. Pashley NRT, Shapiro R. Spontaneous perilymphatic fistula. *J Otolaryngol* 1978;7:110.
91. Black FO, Pesznecker S, Norton T, et al. Surgical management of perilymph fistulas. A new technique. *Arch Otolaryngol Head Neck Surg* 1991;117:641.
92. Kohut RI. Perilymph fistulas. *Arch Otolaryngol Head Neck Surg* 1992;118:687.
93. Skedros DG, Cass SP, Hirsch BE, Kelly RH. Sources of error in use of beta-2 transferrin analysis for diagnosing perilymphatic and cerebral spinal fluid leaks. *Otolaryngol Head Neck Surg* 1993;109:861.
94. Thalmann I, Kohut RI, Ryu J, Comegys TH, Senarita M, Thalmann R. Protein profile of human perilymph: in search of markers for the diagnosis of perilymph fistula and other inner ear disease. *Otolaryngol Head Neck Surg* 1994;111:273.
95. Childhood Brain Tumor Consortium. A study of childhood brain tumors based on surgical biopsies from ten North American institutions: sample description. *J Neurooncol* 1988;6:9.
96. Rydell RE, Pulec JL. Arnold-Chiari malformation: neurotologic symptoms. *Arch Otolaryngol* 1971;94:8.
97. Sclafani AP, Dedio RM, Hendrix RA. The Chiari I malformation. *Ear Nose Throat J* 1992;70:208.
98. Longridge NS, Mallinson AI. Arnold-Chiari malformation and the otolaryngologist: place of magnetic resonance imaging and electronystagmography. *Laryngoscope* 1985;95:335.
99. Kohno K, Sakaki S, Shirashi T. Successful treatment of adult Arnold-Chiari malformation associated with basilar impression and syringomyelia by the transoral approach. *Surg Neurol* 1990;33:284.
100. Saez RJ, Onofrio BM, Yanagihara T. Experience with Arnold-Chiari malformation, 1960 to 1970. *J Neurosurg* 1976;45:416.
101. Levy WJ, Mason L, Hahn JF. Chiari malformation presenting in adults: a surgical experience with 127 cases. *Neurosurgery* 1983;12:377.
102. Schoenberg BS, Mellinger JF, Schoenberg DG. Cerebrovascular disease in infants and children: a study of incidence, clinical features, and survival. *Neurology* 1978;28:763.
103. Oas JG, Baloh RW. Vertigo and the anterior inferior cerebellar artery syndrome. *Neurology* 1992;42:2274.
104. Basser LS. Benign paroxysmal vertigo of childhood (a variety of vestibular neuronitis). *Brain* 1964;87:141.
105. Fenichel GM. Migraine as a cause of benign paroxysmal vertigo of childhood. *J Pediatr* 1967;71:114.
106. Koenigsberger MR, Chutorian AM, Gold AP, Schvey MS. Benign paroxysmal vertigo of childhood. *Neurology* 1970;20:1108.
107. Harker LA, Rassekh CH. Migraine equivalent as a cause of episodic vertigo. *Laryngoscope* 1988;98:160.
108. Olsson JE. Neurotologic findings in basilar migraine. *Laryngoscope* 1991;101(suppl. 52):1.
109. Parker W. Migraine and the vestibular system in adults. *Am J Otol* 1991;12:25.
110. Ward PH, Cannon D, Lindsay JR. The vestibular system in multiple sclerosis. A clinical-histopathological study. *Laryngoscope* 1965;75:1031.
111. Shepard NT, Telian SA, Smith-Wheelock M. Balance disorders in multiple sclerosis: assessment and rehabilitation. *Semin Hearing* 1990;11:292.
112. Molteni RA. Vertigo as a presenting symptom of multiple sclerosis in childhood. *Am J Dis Child* 1977;131:553.
113. Jerabek J, Krejcov H. Oculomotor and vestibular findings in developmental dyslexia. *Acta Otolaryngol Suppl (Stockh)* 1991;481:513.
114. Levinson HN. Dramatic favorable responses of children with learning disabilities or dyslexia and attention deficit disorder to antimotion sickness medications: four case reports. *Percept Mot Skills* 1991;73:723.
115. Joubert M, Eisenring J, Robb JP, et al. Familial agenesis of the cerebellar vermis. *Neurology* 1969;19:813.
116. Lambert SR, Kriss A, Gresty M, et al. Joubert syndrome. *Arch Ophthalmol* 1989;107:709.
117. Furman JM, Baloh RW, Yee RD. Eye movement abnormalities in a family with cerebellar vermian atrophy. *Acta Otolaryngol (Stockh)* 1986;101:371.
118. Rivier F, Echenne B. Dominantly inherited hypoplasia of the vermis. *Neuropediatrics* 1992;23:206.
119. Farmer TW, Mustian VM. Vestibulocerebellar ataxia. *Arch Neurol* 1963;8:471.
120. Baloh RW, Winder A. Acetazolamide-responsive vestibulocerebellar syndrome: clinical and oculographic features. *Neurology* 1991;41:429.
121. Bain PG, O'Brien MD, Keevil SF, Porter DA. Familial periodic cerebellar ataxia: a problem of cerebellar intracellular pH homeostasis. *Ann Neurol* 1992;31:147.
122. Van Bogaert P, Van Nechel C, Goldman S, Szliwowski HB. Acetazolamide-responsive hereditary paroxysmal ataxia: report of a new family. *Acta Neurol Belg* 1993;93:268.
123. Trofatter JA, MacCollin MM, Rutter JL, et al. A novel moesin-, ezrin-, radixin-like gene is a candidate for the neurofibromatosis 2 tumor suppressor. *Cell* 1993;72:791.
124. Rouleau GA, Merel P, Lutchman M, et al. Alteration in a new gene encoding a putative membrane-organizing protein causes neurofibromatosis type 2. *Nature* 1993;363:515.
125. Kluwe L, Pulst SM, Koppen J, Mautner VF. A 163-bp deletion at the C-terminus of the schwannomin gene associated with variable phenotypes of neurofibromatosis type 2. *Hum Genet* 1995;95:443.
126. Neurofibromatosis Conference Statement. National Institutes of Health Consensus Development Conference. *Arch Neurol* 1987;45:575.
127. Kim DK, Born DE, Berger MS, Mayberg MR. Unilateral vestibular schwannoma in a child with prior orbital rhabdomyosarcoma. *Surg Neurol* 1994;42:125.
128. Evans DGR, Huson SM, Donnai D. A genetic study of type 2 neurofibromatosis in the United Kingdom. I. Prevalence, mutation rate, fitness, and confirmation of maternal transmission effect on severity. *J Med Genet* 1992;29:841.
129. Parry DM, Eldridge R, Kaiser-Kupfer MI, Bouzas EA, Pikus A, Patronas N. Neurofibromatosis 2 (NF2): clinical characteristics of 63 affected individuals and clinical evidence for heterogeneity. *Am J Med Genet* 1994;52:450.
130. Mautner VF, Tatagiba M, Guthoff R, Samii M, Pulst SM. Neurofibromatosis 2 in the pediatric age group. *Neurosurgery* 1993;33(1):92.
131. Roos KL, Muckway M Neurofibromatosis. *Dermatol Clin* 1995;13(1):105.
132. Longstreth WT Jr, Dennis LK, McGuire VM, et al. Epidemiology of intracranial meningioma. *Cancer* 1993;72:639.
133. Harsh GR IV, Edwards MSB, Wilson CB. Intracranial arachnoid cysts in children. *J Neurosurg* 1986;64:835.
134. Löppöen H, Sorri M, Serlo W, von Wendt L. ENG findings of shunt-treated hydrocephalus in children. *Int J Pediatr Otorhinolaryngol* 1992;23:35.
135. Brandt T, Daroff RB. The multisensory physiological and pathological vertigo syndromes. *Ann Neurol* 1980;7:19.

PART VIII

Trauma

CHAPTER 29

Injuries of the Auricle, Middle Ear, and Temporal Bone

Rick A. Friedman and William M. Luxford

Accidental injuries have become a significant problem in the pediatric population as society has become increasingly mechanistic. Vehicular accidents and falls are responsible for a great deal of morbidity and mortality in children. The ear and temporal bone are uniquely vulnerable to injury during childhood. The prominent pinna is subject to injury during athletic events, the middle ear can be injured during playful experimentation, and the temporal bone is especially vulnerable during early childhood due to the relatively large size of the cranium and skull base. This chapter reviews the diagnosis and management of a variety of injuries to the ear and temporal bone in children.

AURICULAR HEMATOMA

The prominence of the pinna renders it vulnerable to injury. Blunt trauma, lacerations, avulsions, and burns can result in significant auricular deformity. Auricular hematoma typically results from direct blunt trauma to the external ear. Although physical contact in a variety of sports may lead to auricular hematoma, high school and collegiate wrestling are the most common sources of this injury.

Auricular hematoma was described in ancient Greek lore, with the thickened pinna of the wrestler being his "earmark." With the worldwide popularity of wrestling has come the dilemma over management of the hematoma. It was common for wrestlers to have theirre ears drained repeatedly with needles after each match. The discomfort of this practice led many to avoid treatment and accept the permanent disfigurement.

Patients with auricular hematoma typically present with a soft, fluctuant mass on the outer surface of the pinna. The hematoma most often accumulates in the scaphoid fossa, the triangular fossa, or the concha. In addition to the pain of the blow, the patients often express a feeling of warmth in the involved pinna from the accumulated blood.

The pathophysiology of the acute injury can be explained by the local anatomy. The skin overlying the anterior surface of the pinna is adherent to the underlying perichondrium. Unlike the posterior surface, which can withstand a shearing force due to the layer of subcutaneous loose connective tissue, the full impact of the blow to the anterior surface is transmitted directly to the adherent perichondrium and cartilage.

Left untreated the so-called "cauliflower ear" will develop. Many theories on the pathogenesis of this entity have been put forth. In a convincing set of experiments, Ohlsen, Skoog, and Sohn (1) demonstrated that blood placed in the subcutaneous tissue of a rabbit s ear, between the skin and perichondrium, resolved without deformity. A similar deposit of blood placed between the auricular cartilage and its overlying perichondrium resulted in the accumulation of chondrocytes, chondroneogenesis, and the "cauliflower ear." It is, therefore, imperative to efficiently and expeditiously treat these injuries.

The treatment of auricular hematoma is aimed at evacuation of the blood and the prevention of its reaccumulation. Many forms of therapy have been described, including simple aspiration, incision and drainage, aspiration or incision followed by bolster placement, suction drainage, or posterior transcartilaginous incision. It is clear that aspiration alone results in a high rate of treatment failure. Giffin (2) describeds incision of the auricle anteriorly in a cosmetic location, followed by evacuation of the hematoma, excision of the newly formed fibrocartilage and overlying perichondrium, and placement of cotton bolsters. Schuller, Dankle, and Strauss (3) described a technique of evacuation by incision and drainage, followed by the immediate placement of a pressure dressing consisting of molded dental rolls secured

---

R.A. Friedman: Department of Otolaryngology, University of Cincinnati College of Medicine, Cincinnati, Ohio 45267.

W.M. Luxford: House Ear Clinic, Los Angeles, California 90057.

with through-and-through sutures. This technique allows the athleteathelete to return to activity immediately. In those patients treated in this fashion for a 14-day period, no recurrences of hematoma or subsequent auricular deformity were encountered.

AURICULAR FROSTBITE

Frostbite is a term used to describe a cold injury to tissue resulting in ice crystal formation. The injury results from exposure to temperatures below freezing. The helical rim is the area of the ear most commonly involved. A detailed classification scheme of frostbite injuries has been proposed. However, most authors feel characterizationlassification of injuries as superficial orand deep is most useful.

There are two major theories regarding the pathogenesis of frostbite injuries. One theory suggests that the tissue damage is secondary to blood vessel endolthelial injury. The other theory states that the cold acts directly on the tissue, resulting in a thermal injury.

The treatment of frostbite injuries has undergone significant revolution. Previously, these injuriesMany people were treated by slow thawing with cold water or ice baths. More recently, Sessions et al. (4) described a method of rapid thawing of the frozen pinna by soaking with warm, wet, sterile cotton pledgets between 38°C and 42°C. This rapid warming is quite painful and may require a general anesthetic in young children. After thawing, no attempt should be made to debride the area and no dressing should be applied. Antibiotics are reserved for evidence of infection.

AURICULAR AVULSION

The majority of auricular avulsions in children result from animal bites. Partial auricular loss due to avulsion, left unrepaired, results in an unsightly defect for the patient and a reconstructive problem for the surgeon. Every attempt should be made to salvage auricular avulsion injuries. Small avulsion injuries, particularly of the helix, can be managed by wedge excision and closure, helical advancement, or conchal chondrocutaneous advancement flaps (5). A pinna that has been partially avulsed should be reattached. The extensive blood supply to the pinna will likely support the injured segment, even through a small retained pedicle.

There are many reports in the literature of successful replantation of the severed pinna. The revascularization of the grafted pinna, like other free grafts, is supported by plasmatic imbibition for the first 24 to 48 hours, followed by inosculation and permanent vessel-to-vessel anastomoses. In a series of nine patients, Bernstein and Nelson (6) reported excellent results with primary replantation of severed pinnae. Their protocol included minimal debridement of exposed cartilage, cleansing in povidone–iodine solution, surface cooling with iced gauze pads, and anticoagulation with subcutaneous heparin and dextran 40. Venous congestion, a major cause of graft failure, was relieved by multiple stab incisions or medicinal leeches.

Delayed reconstruction of auricular defects utilizing the pocket principle has proven efficacious in several small series. Mladick and Carraway (7) reported the successful repair of a 3-year-old suffering an auricular avulsion from a dog bite. After dermabrasion of the avulsed segment, the amputated portion was reattached and then buried in a postauricular subcutaneous pocket. After 7 to 14 days, the repaired pinna was bluntly dissected from the pocket, dressed with antibiotic gauze, and allowed to re-epitheilialize.

Recent advances in microvascular anastamosis have led to the successful repair of auricular avulsion by microsurgical replantation. The auricle has a generous blood supply which is derived from anterior and posterior branches of the superficial temporal artery. These vessels are suitable for microvascular anastamoses. Turpin (8) suggests identification of arteries in the superior one third of the auricle and veins in the lower one third. Additionally, as with all microvascular anastamoses, careful handling of the vessels and postoperative anticoagulation with intravenous heparin for 4 to 10 days is essential.

Venous congestion is the primary cause of failure of microvascular replantation and must be treated early. Frequent drainage incisions or medicinal leeches (Leeches, USA, New York) are useful for relief of venous congestion. Medicinal leeches, *Hirudo medicinalis,* inject a local anesthetic and anticoagulant called hirudin. The leeches are applied for 45 minutes every 8 hours. They relieve venous congestion both by consumption of blood and by injection of hirudin, which provides lasting local anticoagulation. Leeches are colonized by *Aeromonas hydrophila,* and patients should, therefore, receive antibiotic prophylaxis with either trimethoprim-sulfamethoxazole or ciprofloxacin.

AURICULAR BITE WOUNDS

Approximately 1 million animal bite victims seek medical attention each year, and the majority are in the pediatric population. Dogs account for the large majority of these injuries. Although far less common, human auricular bite wounds occur with some frequency secondary either to rough play or assault. In a review of bite wounds in children, Brook (9) described the microbiology of 21 animal bites and 18 human bites. Six of the 39 wounds occurred on the head and neck. Mixed aerobic and anaerobic flora were most commonly cultured from the wounds of both animal and human bites. The most frequent isolates from animal bites were, in descending order, *Staphylococcus aureus, Pasteurella multocida,* and anaerobic cocci. The most frequent isolates from human bites were *S. aureus,* gamma-hemolytic streptococci, anaerobic cocci, *Fusobacterium* spp., and *Bacteroides* spp. *P. multocida* and *Pseudomonas fluorescens* group were notably absent in human wounds in contrast to animal wounds.

The bacteria isolated from infected bite wounds are those that colonize the skin of the victim and the oral cavity of the assailant. Polymicrobial aerobic and anaerobic flora infect synergistically, making the infection more difficult to treat. Furthermore, 41% of the 39 wounds in Brook's study contained beta-lactamase–producing organisms.

No single antimicrobial eradicates all of the pathogens responsible for bite wound infections. Treatment should be directed at specific isolates through appropriate bacterial cultures. Penicillin and ampicillin are the best agents for the treatment of *P. multocida* and other oral flora. *S. aureuas* and a large percentage of *Bacteroides* spp. are resistant to penicillins. The combination of amoxicillin and clavulanic acid is very effective against most uncomplicated animal and human bite wounds.

Early treatment of all bite wounds is essential for the prevention of infection and the optimal cosmetic result. Stucker et al. (10) described their comprehensive management of bite wounds. Their treatment begins with immediate jet lavage, debridement of all devitalized tissue, and intravenous antibiotics (Timentin). The decision regarding method and timing of repair depends on the site and severity of the wound, the source of the wound, and the time elapsed between the injury and the implementation of treatment. Stucker et al. advocate primary repair of clean nonhuman bites if performed within 5 hours of injury. All human bite wounds and avulsion injuries are managed in a delayed fashion.

Rabies prevention, including hyperimmune serum and immunization, should be instituted for animal bites. For all wounds, a tetanus toxoid booster is given if the child has been immunized within the past 10 years. In unimmunized patients, tetanus immune globulin should be administered.

TRAUMATIC INJURIES TO THE TYMPANIC MEMBRANE AND OSSICLES

Vehicular trauma is the leading cause of death of people less than 20 years of age. Falls are a frequent cause of injury in children less than 5 years of age. The head injuries associated with these accidents are frequently accompanied by damage to the ear and temporal bone (11,12).

Children are especially prone to injuries of the tympanic membrane. Toddlers and preschool-age children are well known for their experimentation with placing various objects into their ear canals. Older children are not immune to tympanic membrane injuries. In a review of 57 cases of traumatic tympanic membrane rupture, Armstrong (13) found the cotton-tipped applicator to be the leading offender. Tympanic membrane rupture can occur from indirect trauma as well. A shock wave in the external auditory canal from an explosion, such as a firecracker, or a blow to the ear that occludes the meatus, compressing the air column, can subsequently stretch the tympanic membrane beyond its elastic limit, leading to rupture. Regardless of the mechanism, these injuries require immediate attention.

Microscopic examination of the ear after a suspected injury is recommended within the first 24 hours (14). When examining a child, all aspects of the procedure should be explained and demonstrated priorproir to commencement. The ear speculum, microscope light, cerumen currette, and suction aspirator can all be demonstrated to the child in an effort to avoid suprises and familiarize the child with the planned examination. Most painful procedures, depending on the age of the patient, will require a general anesthetic.

Fortunately, traumatic tears of the tympanic membrane tend to heal spontaneously. Even large perforations can heal without surgical repair (14). Despite the resilience of the injured drum, certain injuries require closer attention. Armstrong (13), in a review of 57 traumatic tympanic membrane ruptures, recommended the immediate repair of all large perforations, and perforations, of the posterior-superior quadrant. Furthermore, the use of steroid-containing otic drops were felt to inhibit healing and were, therefore, contraindicated.

Examination, under either local or general anesthesia, involves aspiration of blood clots, sterile irrigation, inspection of the drum and middle ear, and palpation of the ossicular chain. Medially displaced flaps can be replaced to their original position (14). These flaps can be held in place with a cigarette paper patch or gelfoam.

A tympanic membrane that has healed incompletely, depending on the size, can be treated with chemical cauterization with 50% trichloroacetic acid or 10% silver nitrate. When using silver nitrate, it is recommended that the acid be neutralized with a cotton-tipped applicator soaked in saline solution to prevent further injury. Slightly larger perforations can be repaired by utilizing the technique of fat myringolplasty.

Larger perforations or those unresponsive to the aforementioned techniques can be treated by utilizing with standard myringoplasty techniques. For small posterior perforations, an underlay technique may suffice. For most other perforations of the tympanic membrane, we utilize the lateral surface grafting technique (15).

Following a traumatic rupture of the tympanic membrane, a mild conductive hearing loss (10–30 dB), will be observed on audiometric testing. Small perforations are associated with very slight degrees of conductive loss. The presence of a perforation in the posterior-superior quadrant or conductive losses exceeding 35 dB should alert the physician to the possibility of ossicular injury. Armstrong (13) found 13 cases of ossicular injury associated with tympanic membrane rupture.

Blunt nonpenetrating trauma to the ear or temporal bone is frequently associated with ossicular injury. Longitudinal temporal bone fractures are often accompanied by ossicular subluxation or fracture. Cremin (16) found the most common cause of conductive hearing loss after head injury to bewas hemotympanum and external canal laceration. In patients with persistent conductive loss after head injury ossicular injury should be suspected. Ossicular injury after head trauma is well described in children. Hough et al. (17) found 50% of their study patients with ossicular injury to be under the age of 13 years. Furthermore, 70% were under the age of 21 years.

The mechanism of ossicular injury with penetrating trauma is self-evident. However, the mechanism of injury withat for blunt trauma is speculative. Hough et al. (17) hypothesized several mechanisms acting individually or in concert: (a) the explosive effects of concussion, producing temporary tissue weakening and separation; (b) the effects of inertia on the patient's head during reaction to acceleration and deceleration; (c) the tetanic contraction of the intratympanic muscles; and (d) the torsion effect of skull fracture, causing shifting of the middle ear structures.

Regardless of the mechanisms leading to injury, posttraumatic ossicular injury and subsequent conductive hearing loss is well described. The most common site of injury, in most series, is the incudostapedial joint (16,18–20). Hough et al. (17) identified incudostapedial joint separation to be etiologic in 82.3% of cases of conductive hearing loss after skull fracture. The point of disarticulation or fracture is determined by the strength of each ossicle and its soft tissue support. The malleus is supported by its five ligaments and its attachments to the tympanic membrane at the umbo and short process. The stapes is supported by its annular ligament and the stapedius tendon. The incus is left spanning the distance between the malleus and stapes, supported only by its articulation with the malleus and its supporting ligaments in the attic and fossa incudis. The incus, therefore, is the ossicle most commonly disrupted in temporal bone trauma.

The stapes is the second most frequently injured ossicle (16). Because the footplate is secured in the oval window by the annular ligament, the site of stapedial injury is most often the crura. Crural fracture is most often associated with incudostapedial joint injury or incus dislocation. Several series describing traumatic ossicular injury have identified stapedial fracture to be somewhat more frequent in children. Elbrond and Aastrup (21) noted that seven of 11 patients with stapes crural fracture were under 15 years old. Does and Bottema (20) found fracture of the stapes crura in four of 13 patients, three of which were 15 years old or younger. They hypothesized the malleability of the pediatric skull to result in greater excursion of the incus during trauma, predisposing the stapes suprastructure to fracture.

Subluxation of the stapes footplate, although uncommon, is an otologic emergency (22) (see Fig. 1). Footplate subluxation is often associated with sensorineural hearing loss, tinnitus, and vertigo with nystagmus (23). The exposed vestibule should be covered as soon as the patient is suitable for surgery. Early intervention may prevent deafness, resolve vertigo, and provide a barrier to infection for the inner ear and adjacent CSF.

The recognition and repair of traumatic middle ear injuries were realized with the advent of the operating microscope and tympanoplastic techniques. The first desciptions traumatic ossicular injuries due to head trauma were made independently in 1956, first by Thornburn (24), and shortly thereafter by Hough (17). A variety of techniques for repair have been described, including ossicular repositioning, type III tympanoplasty, and incus replacement prostheses. At the House Ear Clinic, we believe that children with unilateral conductive hearing loss and normal contralateral hearing can be managed conservatively until they are old enough to participate in the decision and postoperative care of ossicular

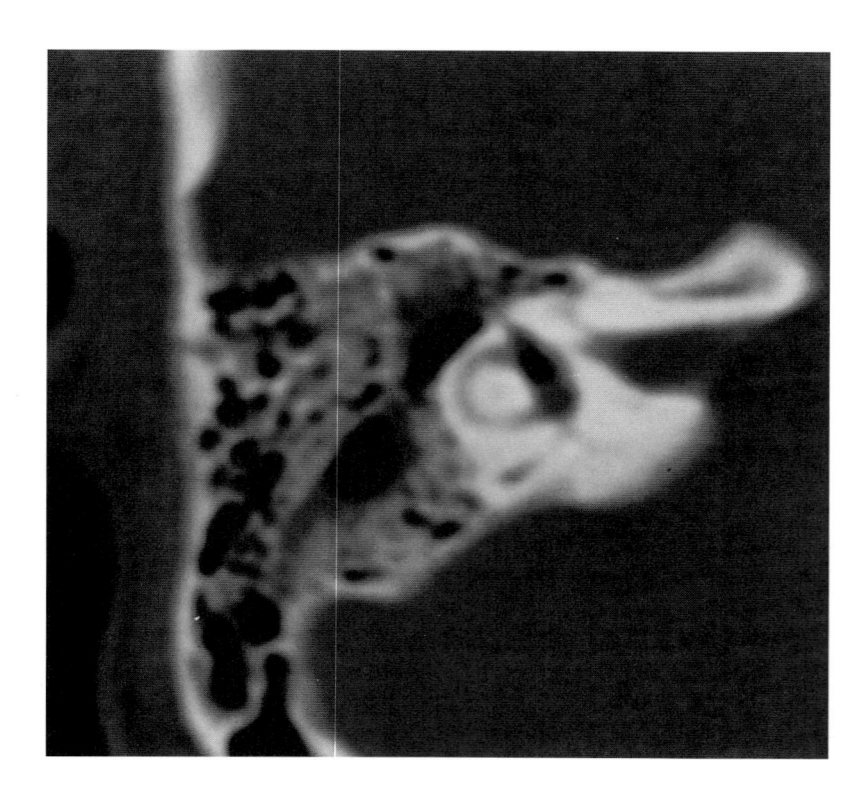

FIG. 1. Temporal bone computed tomography scan (axial image) in a patient with a longitudinal temporal bone fracture and stapes subluxation demonstrating air in the vestibule.

reconstruction. Additionally, surgery for conductive hearing loss should not be performed on an only-hearing ear.

In general, we prefer a postauricular approach for tympanoplasty. The type of reconstruction will depend on the surgical findings. For the most common injury, incudostapedial joint dislocation, we have utilized the Applebaum hydroxylapatite I-S joint prosthesis. If the incus is more severely subluxed, it is removed and continuity restored by either reshaping the incus and placing it between the malleus and stapes, placement of a hydroxylapatite incus replacement prosthesis, or placement of a prosthesis from the undersurface of the drum to the stapes (POP or TOP). The latter technique is favored in cases with an anteriorly positioned malleus. Injuries to the incus and stapes suprastructure are reconstructed with a TOP. Autologous cartilage is placed on the platform of all partial and total ossicular reconstruction prostheses to prevent extrusion and to reinforce the tympanic membrane in this group of patients prone to eustachian tube dysfunction.

TEMPORAL BONE FRACTURES AND THEIR COMPLICATIONS

Craniofacial trauma in the pediatric population is not a frequent occurrence. The use of car seats and safety belts is the likely explanation for the low incidence of trauma in young children. Despite the low incidence, intracranial injuries and base of skull fractures are frequent consequences of craniofacial trauma in children. In a review of 72 children under the age of 16, who were treated for maxillofacial injuries, McGraw and Cole (25) found intracranial injuries and temporal bone fractures to be most common in young children. Forty-one percent of the children under 6 years of age had temporal bone fractures. Older children in their series were more likely to have mid- and lower facial injuries.

Craniofacial development is the likely reason for the pattern of injury in pediatric craniofacial trauma. The craniofacial ratio decreases from 8:1 in infants to 2.5:1 in adults, rendering the cranial contents and base of skull vulnerable to injury (25). Fractures of the skull base occur in approximately 10% of children with head trauma (26). Several series report the most common etiology of these injuries to be pedestrian versus vehicle or vehicle accidents (25,27,28).

Studies of the mechanisms and anatomic distributions of temporal bone fractures reveal that they tend to occur in specific locations and result in characteristic signs and symptoms (29). The petrous portion of the temporal bone forms approximately two thirds of the floor of the middle cranial fossa and one third of the floor of the posterior cranial fossa. The foramina at the base of the skull are areas of stress concentration; consequently, fractures tend to occur in their vicinity.

Temporal bone fractures have classically been described as longitudinal, transverse, and mixed. Approximately 90% of fractures are of the longitudinal type (30–32). Longitudinal fractures are associated with a temporal or parietal blow

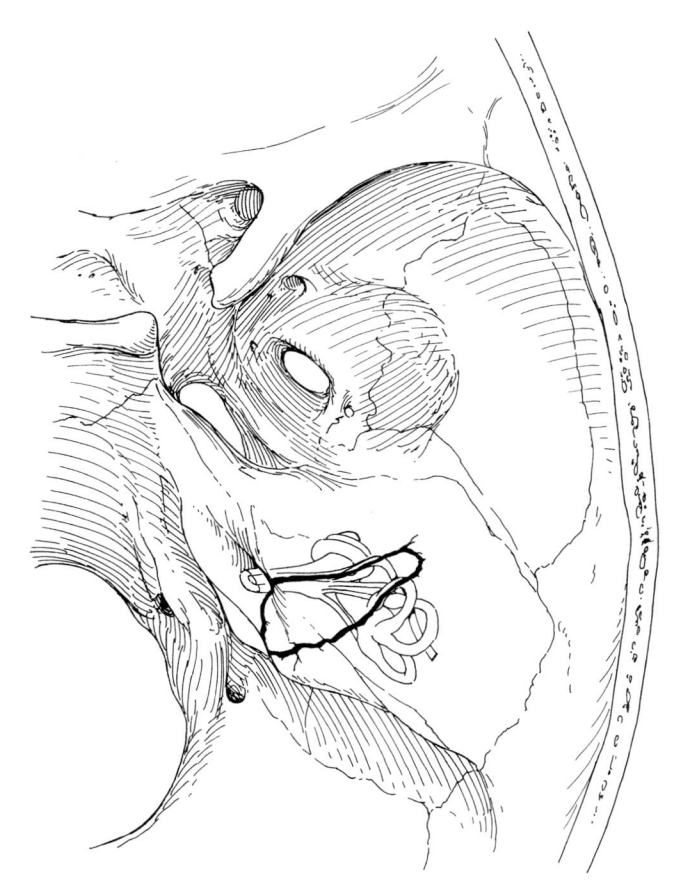

FIG. 2. Schematic diagram of a longitudinal temporal bone fracture. Note the fracture line anterior and lateral to the otic capsule.

and result in a fracture of the petrous bone extending anteromedially along the petrous ridge to the foramen lacerum and foramen ovale (Fig. 2). The fracture line often begins in the squamous portion, extends through the posterior and superior walls of the external canal, traverses the tegmen tympani, and extends anterior to the otic capsule on its way to the petrous apex (29). The facial nerve is injured in approximately 15% of cases, usually in the perigeniculate region (30,31). Longitudinal fractures are often associated with the "Traumatic Conductive Triad" described by Hough et al. (17) as follows: (a) loss of hearing, (b) bleeding from the ear through a lacerated tympanic membrane, and (c) unconsciousness.

Transverse fractures are less frequent, comprising 10% to 15% of temporal bone fractures (30,31). Frontal or occipital blows result in a fracture that extends from the posterior cranial fossa to the middle cranial fossa at a right angle to the petrous bone (29) (Figs. 3, 4). The fracture may run from the foramen magnum or jugular foramen across the internal auditory canal to the foramen lacerum or foramen spinosum. Other fractures begin at the internal acoustic meatus and cross the vestibule to the region of the oval or round windows (33). Regardless of the path, most series reveal anacusis in

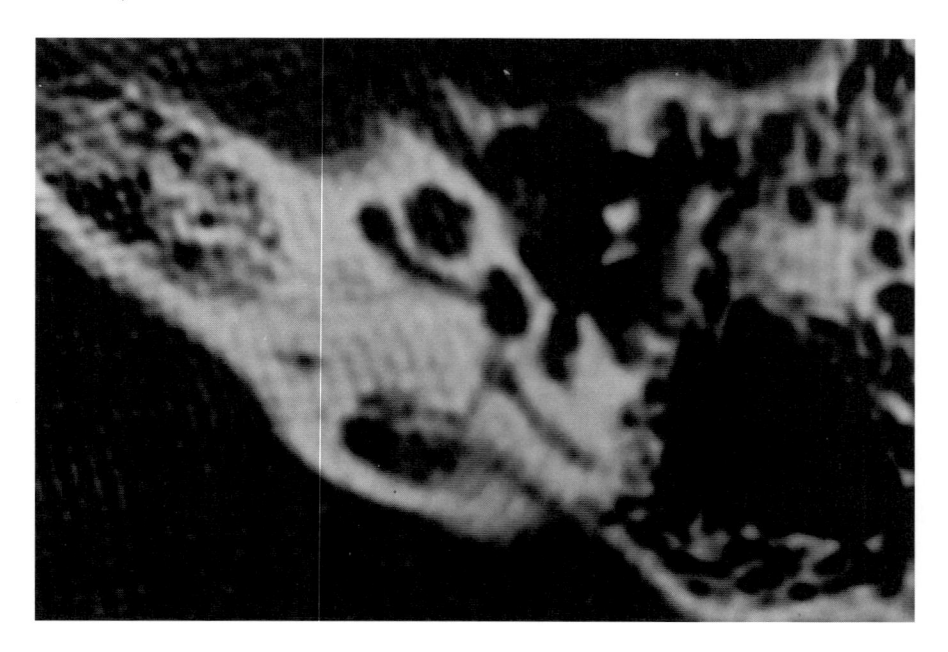

FIG. 3. Temporal bone computed tomography scan (axial image) demonstrating a transverse fracture extending through the ampulla of the posterior semicircular canal and ending in the vestibule.

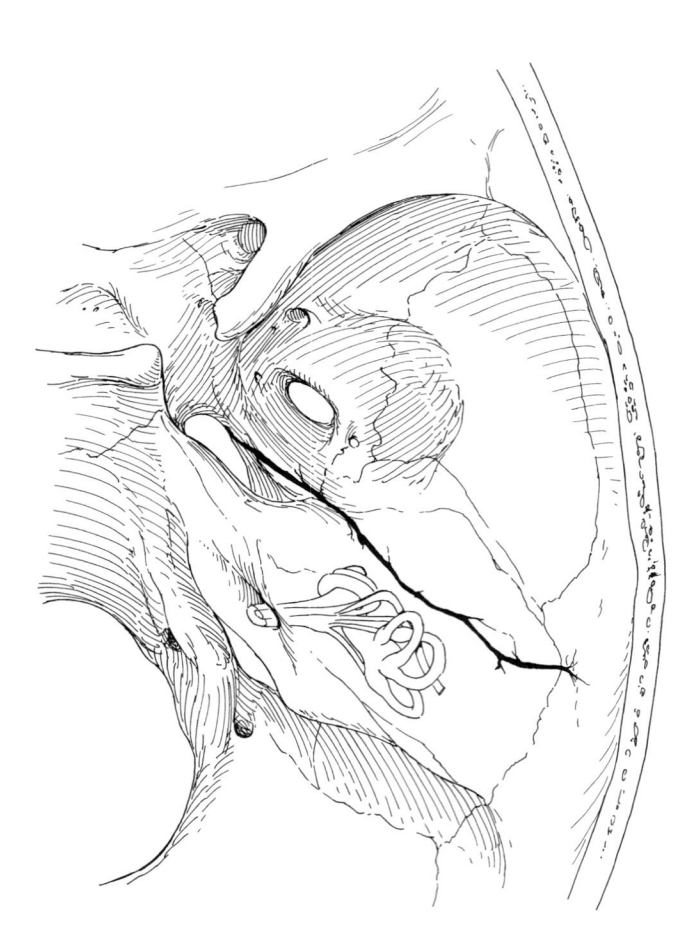

FIG. 4. Schematic diagram of a transverse temporal bone fracture. Note the potential for the fracture line to cross the vestibule and enter the middle ear cleft.

all affected ears. These fractures are often associated with hemotympanum but not otorrhea, because the tympanic membrane is intact (29). The facial nerve is injured in approximately 50% of cases, usually proximal to the geniculate ganglion (29–32,34,35).

Many fractures of the temporal bone are not uniform. Tos (31) found that approximately 50% of transverse fractures were actually mixed. In a review of 25 pediatric temporal bone fractures using three-dimensional computed tomography (CT) reconstruction, Williams, Ghorayeb, and Yeakley (28) identified oblique fractures as the most common type. These fractures are oriented in a vertical direction to the temporal bone, extending antero-inferior across the external auditory canal to the glenoid fossa. Regardless of the anatomic classification of the fracture, management depends on the injury to the contents of the temporal bone, which overlaps considerably in each of the fracture types.

Initial management of children with head injury involves the establishment of a safe airway and adequate ventilation. Following airway, hemodynamic, and neurologic stabilization, the work-up of a suspected temporal bone fracture may commence.

High-resolution CT scans of the temporal bone, axial and coronal, provide excellent anatomic detail (36). When stable, all children suffering head injury should undergoundergoe pure-tone air, bone, and speech audiometry with appropriate masking. Finally, as discussed in subsequent sections, facial nerve testing may be indicated if decompression is contemplated.

Hearing Loss

According to Barber (37), damage to the inner ear is the most common sequel of head injury (Table 1). Several early

TABLE 1. *Complications of temporal bone fracture*

Hearing loss
   Conductive loss
   Sensorineural loss
Vestibular injury
Facial nerve injury
CSF fistula and meningitis

studies revealed hearing loss in 33% to 50% of patients after head injury (29,30,38). Studies with more sophisticated audiologic data indicate that between 20% and 40% of head-injured patients will suffer from hearing loss (11,39). In a review of 199 children with head injury, Vartiainen, Karjalainen, and Karja (40) found a similar incidence of posttraumatic hearing loss.

The incidence of hearing loss with head trauma is related to the force of the injury and the location of the fracture. Podoshin and Fradis (11) found hearing loss in 71% of patients with temporal bone fractures compared with 45% of those patients with skull fractures not involving the temporal bone. Proctor, Gurdjian, and Webster (29) and Grove (30) demonstrated an approximately 40% incidence of hearing loss in patients sustaining skull fractures not involving the temporal bone. Barber (37) demonstrated a higher incidence of hearing loss in patients with skull fractures. However, he found that approximately 40% of the patients without fractures sustained a hearing loss. Griffiths (38), in a study of hearing loss in minor head trauma, found a 56% incidence. Finally, in a review of 304 patients with brain concussion without skull fracture, Podoshin and Fradis (11) found 14.7% suffered from hearing loss.

Tos (31), in a review of 248 temporal bone fractures, 92% of which were longitudinal, found a 67% incidence of hearing loss. Eighty-five percent of the losses were conductive, 7% sensorineural, and 7% mixed. Williams, Ghorayeb, and Yeakley (28) reviewed 27 pediatric temporal bone fractures, the majority of which were oblique, and found that 70% of the children displayed a purely conductive loss, 15% sensorineural, and 15% mixed. In their review of 120 children with temporal bone fractures, McGuirt and Stool (41) noted a 43% incidence of conductive hearing loss, a 54% incidence of sensorineural loss, and a 5% incidence of mixed loss.

When longitudinal fractures are considered alone, conductive hearing loss seems to be most common. The mechanisms most frequently csited are hemotympanum, ruptured tympanic membrane, and ossicular disruption. Hemotympanum, the most frequent cause of conductive loss, usually presents with a 30- to 45-dB loss, with complete recovery within 6 weeks (31).

The prognosis for conductive hearing loss is good. Mc Guirt and Stool (41) found complete resolution of hemotympanum by 3 weeks in 19 children and a 63% spontaneous rate of improvement in all cases with conductive hearing loss. Tos (31) revealed an 80% rate of spontaneous resolution of conductive hearing loss in his series. He emphasized that one should be suspicious of an ossicular injury if the air–bone gap exceeds 50 dB at presentation or 30 dB at 6 weeks follow-up. The patterns of ossicular injury and techiques of repair were described in a previous section.

High-frequency sensorineural hearing loss after head injury has been documented in 10% to 24% of adult patients (11,37). This type of hearing loss was reported in 7% of children with head injuries reported by Vartiainen, Kajarlainen, and Karja (40). Transverse temporal bone fractures are almost universally followed by anacusis in the involved ear (31,38,41,42).

The pathophysiology of sensorineural hearing loss in transverse fractures is self-evident. However, the pathophysiology in longitudinal fractures and head injuries without fracture has been the subject of much debate. Several authors describe sensorineural loss resulting from "commotio labyrinth," or labyrinthine concussion (29,30,43). In 1950, Schuknecht (44) found histopathologic changes in the organ of Corti and spiral ganglion cells in cats after head trauma. The injury occurred in the mid-basal portion of the cochlea and was similar to that resulting from acoustic trauma (4–8 kHz). Although he did find blood in the scalae, its location did not coincide with the areas of injury, and he concluded that the hearing loss in these cats was due to excessive stimulation of the inner ear.

Several studies have implicated a retrocochholear origin for posttraumatic hearing loss. Kirikae et al. (45) found extensive hemorrhage in the inferior colliculae, lateral lemnisci, and superior olivary nuclei of five patients suffering fatal head injuries. In clinical and laboratory reviews of head injury and hearing loss, Makishima and Snow (46) cited hemorrhage in and laceration of the eighth nerve at the brainstem as the most likely source of the loss.

Although fluctuating sensorineural hearing loss after head trauma has been reported, these losses are not progressive (47). Griffiths (38) grouped posttraumatic sensorineural losses according to type: type As were low tone only, type Bs were high tone only, and type Cs had both low- and high-tone losses with higher thresholds for the higher tones. In type A, the hearing fully recovered in 86%;, in type B, 25% had partial recovery; and no improvement was noted in type C. Reviewing the prognosis for recovery of sensorineural loss in children, Vartiainen, Karjalainen, and Karja (40) documented improvement in one third of their patients, and McGuirt and Stool (41) noted improvement in 53%.

Vestibular System Injury

Although dizziness is a frequent complication of head injury, virtually all of the literature is devoted to adults. Tuohimaa (48) found dizziness in 78% of 82 patients with head injury. Griffiths (38) noted a lower incidence of 24%. Barber (37) studied 110 patients with electronystagmography (ENG) and divided them into mild head injury, amnesia less than 1 hour, and severe head injury. He demonstrated that 59% of the patients had spontaneous or positional nystagmus. Spontaneous nystagmus, occurring in 23%, was felt to be an important sign because it was found only in patients with severe trauma. He also found benign positional nystagmus in 20% of the patients. The symptom of dizziness did not depend on the severity of the injury. Transverse fractures werare most often accompanied by an absent response on ENG.

The pathogenesis of the vestibular injury is not completely understood. Most authors feel that, like injury to the auditory system, there are both peripheral and central components to the vestibular injury. Unlike the prognosis in auditory injury, however, that for posttraumatic vestibular injury is good. Barber (37) found the majority of patients to be free of symptoms with resolution of ENG abnormalities by 6 to 12 months. Nonsurgical management with physical therapy will, in most cases, lead to resolution.

Facial Nerve Injury

The facial nerve is more often paralyzed than any other motor nerve. This is likely due to its long course in the bony confines of the fallopian canal. In a review of facial palsy after head injury, Potter (49) found a 1% incidence of facial nerve injury in 2,712 cases. Virtually all of the cases of facial nerve palsy were associated with skull base fractures. The incidence of facial nerve injury in children, like the incidence of temporal bone fracture in general, is highest in the younger age group (50) (Kornblut). Facial nerve paralysis in adults is seen in 10% to 18% of longitudinal fractures and 30% to 50% of transverse fractures (30,51). The incidence of facial nerve injury in pediatric temporal bone trauma is lower than that in adults, occurring in 6% to 32% of temporal bone fractures. The lower incidence is felt to be due to decreased ossification, hence, greater resistance to deformation.

The mechanisms of injury to the facial nerve are different for longitudinal and transverse fractures. Fisch (52) found transection of the nerve in 100% of the transverse fractures. In contrast, the pathology in the group of longitudinal fractures revealed intraneural hematoma in 50%, bony impingement in 17%, and complete transection in 26%. He concluded that lesions of the facial nerve in temporal bone fractures, particularly longitudinal, were the result of traction on the greater superficial petrosal nerve. In support of this, Grobman et al., in a postmortempostmortum pathologic study of a longitudinal fracture, identified demyelinization and swelling of the facial nerve beginning at the meatal foramen, the narrowest portion of the fallopian canal. They concluded that the delayed paralysis in this case was not due to injury at the fracture site but to traction of the greater superficial petrosal nerve leading to edema and entrapment of the nerve at the meatal foramen. This proposed mechanism helps to explain the overwhelming incidence of perigeniculate lesions of the facial nerve in several large series examining temporal bone fractures (36,52–54).

The treatment of facial nerve injuries in pediatric temporal bone fractures is similar to that in adults and is is equally controversial. The decision to proceed with surgical decompression is based on the neurologic status of the patient, the onset and severity of the paralysis, the radiographic findings, and the results of electrical testing. Coker et al. (36) describe an algorithm for the management of temporal bone fractures complicated by facial paralysis that includes high-resolution CT, axial and coronal views, of the temporal bone, audiometric evaluation, and electrical testing with either nerve excitability or electroneuronography (ENoG) (Fig. 5). Facial nerve testing may not always be obtainable in infants and children. Eavey et al. (55) have shown, however, that ENoG was obtainable and reliable in 95% of tested children aged 3 months through 16 years.

In general, the prognosis for spontaneous recovery of posttraumatic facial paralysis in children is quite favorable (41,50). In 1944, Turner (56) reviewed 70 cases of traumatic facial paralysis, 34 of which were delayed, and found that 32 of the 34 (94%) delayed-onset palsies recovered spontaneously. Similarly, McKennan and Choale (57) found 94% of their patients with delayed-onset facial paralysis recovered (House grade I) without surgical intervention. May (58) advocates surgical exploration in cases of immediate-onset paralysis without response on maximal stimulation within 5 days of injury and evidence of fracture or bony impingement on high-resolution CT. Lambert and Brackmann (54) and Coker et al. (36) recommend surgery based on the results of electrical testing. Early exploration is indicated, if after a fracture, more than 90% degeneration of facial nerve fibers is demonstrated on electroneuronography within 6 days of the onset of the palsy (52). Lambert and Brackmann (54), like Fisch (52), recommend decompression in cases of delayed paralysis within 6 months if no evidence of regeneration is present on electromyography.

The timing of surgery is also a controversial issue. McCabe (53) recommended delaying repair of facial nerve paralysis in temporal bone fracture for 21 days, the amount of time necessary for the nerve cell body to push axoplasmic filaments across the nerve gap. More recent work suggests that the optimum time for repair is dictated by the overall condition of the patient.

The approach to repair is dictated primarily by the status of the hearing. Patients with nonserviceable sensorineural loss undergoe decompression via the transmastoid–translabyrinthine approach. Those patients with normal hearing or conductive loss undergoe the middle cranial fossa-transmastoid approach. In cases of edema or hematoma, decompression is facilitated by removing the bone of the fallopian canal and slitting the epineural sheath at the injured site (52). Partial transections greater than one third the diameter and complete transections should be repaired either by rerouting and direct anastamosis or by interposition grafting. Moderate-

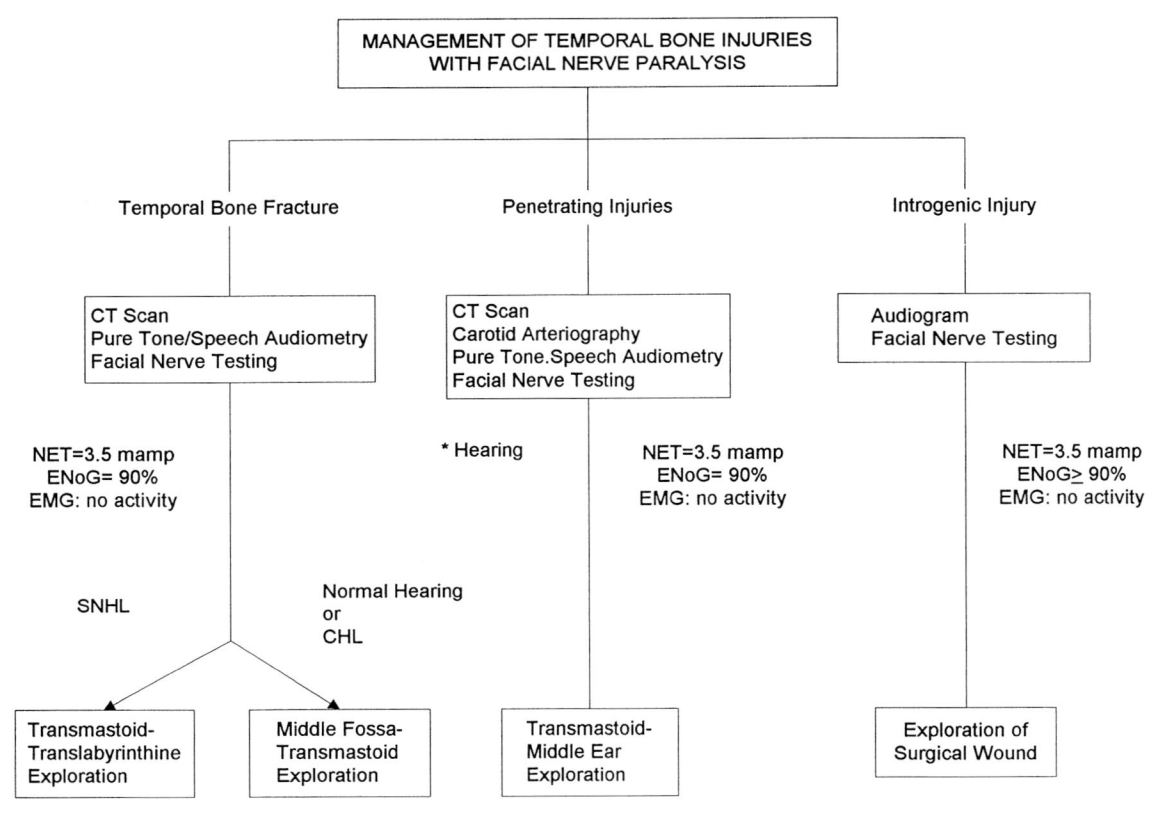

FIG. 5. Recommended mamagement scheme for temporal bone trauma with facial nerve paralysis. SNHL, sensorineural hearing loss; CHL, conductive hearing loss; EMG, electromyelogram; NET, nerve excitability test. Reproduced with permission from Coker NJ, Kendall KA, Jenkins HA et al. Traumatic intratemporal facial nerve injury: Management rationale for preservation of function. Otolaryngol Head Neck Surg 1987;97:262, Figure 3.

to-severe dysfunction (House grade IV) is the likely outcome in cases requiring grafting (36).

The role of steroids in the management of traumatic facial nerve injury is undefined. There are no randomized prospective trials available that demonstrate efficacy. Therefore, at the present time, no specific recommendations can be made for the use of steroids in traumatic facial nerve injury.

Cerebrospinal Fluid Fistula and Meningitis

Cerebrospinal fluid otorhinorrhea with resultant meningitis is a potentially lethal complication of temporal bone fracture. In a 1992 review, Jones, McGill, and Healy (59) identified CSF leaks in only 0.26% of 10,561 children admitted for head trauma. The low incidence of CSF leak in the pediatric population has been attributed to the greater pliability of the child's skull, lessening the risk of fracturefracturea and dural tear.

The diagnosis can be made by the observation of clear otorrhea or rhinorrhea, the presence of a double-ring sign, or laboratory evaluation for total protein, glucose, and β-2-transferrin. High-resolution CT scans with with intrathecal metrizamide are sensitive for identifying subtle leaks.

The incidence of meningitis associated with CSF leaks in children ranges from 15% to 24% in reported series (59,60). The most common etiologic organism is *Streptococcus pneumoniae* (59,61,62). There is much controversy in the literature regarding the use of prophylactic antibiotic therapy. Tos (63) reported on 113 patients treated prophylactically with penicillin and 80 patients who were not. Meningitis occurred in 8% and 5% of the patients, respectively. In a placebo-controlled double-blind study evaluating the efficacy of prophylactic penicillin in 52 patients with CSF leak after head injury, Klastersky, Sadeghi, and Brihaye (64) found no cases of meningitis in the treated group and one case in the placebo group. Jones, McGill, and Healy (59) found four cases of meningitis in 27 pediatric patients with posttraumatic CSF fistulae. Fifteen of the 27 patients were placed on antibiotics at the time of admission and all four cases of meningitis occurred in that group. The opinion of the associates at the House Ear Clinic is that prophylaxis is not indicated in posttraumatic CSF fistula without signs or symptoms of meningitis.

The treatment of CSF leaks complicating temporal bone trauma is nonsurgical in the vast majority of cases. The treatment consists of bed rest, elevation of the head, stool softeners, and avoidance of straining. Many advocate placement of a lumbar drain for leaks persisting beyond 1 week. However, Jones, McGill, and Healy (59) found that those leaks not resolving within 7 days did not resolve with the placement of a lumbar drain. Nonsurgical therapy resulted in spontaneous resolution of the CSF leaks in 70% and 93% of children in two large series (41,59). Surgical therapy is recommended for leaks persisting beyond 2 to 3 weeks, large bony defects, recurrent meningitis, late-onset leaks, and brain herniation. Surgical repair can be accomplished through a transmastoid or middle cranial fossa approach. The dura can be repaired primarily or patched with fascia and reinforcedreinforced with muscle or fat. If hearing has been lost, the middle ear and eustachian tube can be obliterated with muscle (65). This procedure can be combined with blind sac closure of the external canal for cases of persistent otorrhea.

REFERENCES

1. Ohlsen L, Skoog T, Sohn SA. The pathogenesis of cauliflower ear. *Scand J Plast Reconstr Surg* 1975;9:34.
2. Giffin CS. The wrestler s ear (acute auricular hematoma). *Arch Otolaryngol* 1985;11:161.
3. Schuller DE, Dankle SD, Strauss RH. A technique to treat wrestlers auricular hematoma without interrupting training or competition. *Arch Otolaryngol Head Neck Surg* 1989;115:202.
4. Sessions DG, Stallings JO, Mills WJ, Beal DD. Frostbite of the ear. *Laryngoscope* 1971;81:1223.
5. Pless J. Laminate-plasty reconstruction of partial auricular defects. *Scand J Plast Reconstr Surg* 1975;9:40.
6. Bernstein L, Nelson RH. Replanting the severed auricle. *Arch Otolaryngol* 1982;108:587.
7. Mladick RA, Carraway JH. Ear reattachment by the modified pocket principle. *Plast Reconstr Surg* 1973;51:584.
8. Turpin IM. Microsurgical replantation of the external ear. *Clin Plast Surg* 1990;17:397.
9. Brook I. Microbiology of human and animal bite wounds in children. *Pediatr Infect Dis J* 1987;6:29.
10. Stucker FJ, Shaw GY, Boyd S, Shockley WW. Management of animal and human bites in the head and neck. *Arch Otolaryngol Head Neck Surg* 1990;116:789.
11. Podoshin L, Fradis M. Hearing loss after head injury. *Arch Otolaryngol* 1975;101:15.
12. Hough JVD, Stuart WD. Middle ear injuries in skull trauma. *Laryngoscope* 1968;78:899.
13. Armstrong BW. Traumatic perforations of the tympanic membrane: observe or repair? *Laryngoscope* 1970;82:1822
14. Bellucci RJ. Traumatic injuries of the middle ear. *Otolaryngol Clin North Am* 1983;16:633.
15. Sheehy JL. Surgery of chronic otitis media. In: English GM, ed. *Otolaryngology.* New York: Harper and Row; 1984:1:(chap.20).
16. Cremin MD. Injuries of the ossicular chain. *J Laryngol Otol* 1969;83:845.
17. Hough JVD. Restoration of the hearing loss after head trauma. *Ann Otol* 1969;78:210.
18. Bauer F. Dislocation of the incus due to head injury. *J Laryngol* 1958;72:676.
19. Flisberg K, Floberg LE. Traumatic luxation of the incus in children. *Acta Otolaryngol* 1963;182[Suppl]:43.
20. Does IES, Bottema T. Posttraumatic conductive hearing loss. *Arch Otolaryngol* 1965;82:331.
21. Elbrond E, Aastrup JE. Isolated fractures of the stapedial arch. *Acta Otolaryngol* 1973;75:357.
22. Silverstein H. Trauma of the tympanic membrane and ossicles. In: Nadol JD, Schuknecht HF, eds. *Surgery of the ear and temporal bone.* New York: Raven Press, 1993;325.
23. Sade J. Traumatic fractures of the stapes. *Arch Otolaryngol* 1964;80:258.
24. Thornburn IB. Post-traumatic conduction deafness. *J Laryngol* 1957;71:542.
25. McGraw BL, Cole RR. Pediatric maxillofacial trauma. *Arch Otolaryngol Head Neck Surg* 1990;116:41.
26. Liu-Shindo M, Hawkins DB. Basilar skull fractures in children. *Int J Pediatr Otorhinolaryngol* 1989;17:109.
27. Shapiro RS. Temporal bone fractures in children. *Otolaryngol Head Neck Surg* 1979;87:323.
28. Williams WT, Ghorayeb BY, Yeakley JW. Pediatric temporal bone fractures. *Laryngoscope* 1992;102:600.
29. Proctor B, Gurdjian ES, Webster JE. The ear in head trauma. *Laryngoscope* 1956;66:16.
30. Grove WE. Skull fractures involving the ear. A clincial study of 211 cases. *Laryngoscope* 1939;49:833.
31. Tos M. Prognosis of hearing loss in temporal bone fractures. *J Laryngol Otol* 1971;85:1147.
32. Cannon CR, Jahrsdoerfer RA. Temporal bone fractures. Review of 90 cases. *Arch Otolaryngol* 1983:109:285.
33. Olson JE, Shagets FW. Blunt trauma of the temporal bone. *Am Acad Otolaryngol* 1980;14.
34. Fredrickson JM, Griffith AW, Lindsay JR. Transverse fracture of the temporal bone. *Arch Otolaryngol* 1963;78:54.
35. Kelemen G. Fractures of the temporal bone. *Arch Otolaryngol* 1944;40:333.
36. Coker NJ, Kendall KA, Jenkins HA, et al. Traumatic intratemporal facial nerve injury: Management rationale for preservation of function. *Otolaryngol Head Neck Surg* 1987;97:262.
37. Barber HO. Head injury audiological and vestibular findings. *Ann Otol Rhinol Laryngol* 1969;78:239.
38. Griffiths MV. The incidence of auditory and vestibular concussion following minor head injury. *J Laryngol Otol* 1979;93:253.
39. Kochhar LK, Deka RC, Kacker SK, Raman EV. Hearing loss after head injury. *Ear Nose Throat J* 1990;69:537.
40. Vartiainen E, Karjalainen S, Karja J. Auditory disorders following head injury in children. *Acta Otolaryngol (Stockh)* 1985;99:529.
41. McGuirt WF, Stool SE. Temporal bone fractures in children: a review with emphasis on long-term sequelae. *Clin Pediatr* 1992;1:12.
42. Wiet RJ, Valvassori GE, Kotsanis CA, Parahy C. Temporal bone fractures. State of the art review. *Am J Otol* 1985;6:207.
43. Ward PH. The histopathology of auditory and vestibular disorders in head trauma. *Ann Otol Rhinol Laryngol* 1969;78:227.
44. Schuknecht HF. Mechanism of inner ear injury from blows to the head. *Ann Otol Rhinol Laryngol* 1969;78:253.
45. Kirikae I, Eguchi K, Okamoto M, Nakamura K. Histopathological changes in the auditory pathway in cases of fatal head injury. *Acta Otolaryngol* 1969;67:341.
46. Makishima K, Snow JB. Pathogenesis of hearing loss in head injury. Studies in man and experimental animals. *Arch Otolaryngol* 1975;101:426.
47. Clark SK, Rees TS. Pottraumatic endolymphatic hydrops. *Arch Otolaryngol* 1977;103:725.
48. Tuohimaa P. Vestibular disturbances after acute mild head injury. *Acta Otolaryngol* 1978;359[Suppl]:1.
49. Potter JM. Facial palsy following head injury. *J Laryngol Otol* 1964;78:654.
50. Kornblut AD. Facial nerve injuries in children. *J Laryngol Otol* 1974;88:717.
51. McHugh HE. The surgical treatment of facial paralysis and traumatic conductive deafness in fractures of the temporal bone. *Ann Otol Rhinol Laryngol* 1959;68:855.
52. Fisch U. Facial paralysis infractures of the petrous bone. *Laryngoscope* 1974;84:2141.
53. McCabe BF. Injuries to the facial nerve. *Laryngoscope* 1972;82:1972.
54. Lambert PR, Brackmann DE. Facial paralysis in longitudinal temporal bone fractures: a review of 26 cases. *Laryngoscope* 1984;94:1022.
55. Eavey RD, Herrmann BS, Joseph JM, Thornton AR. Clinical experience with electroneurography in the pediatric patient. *Arch Otolaryngol Head Neck Surg* 1989;115:600.

56. Turner JWA. Facial palsy in closed head injuries. *Lancet* 1944;1:156.
57. McKennan KX, Chole RA. Facial paralysis in temporal bone trauma. *Am J Otol* 1992;13:167.
58. May M. Total facial nerve exploration: transmastoid, extralabyrinthine, and subtemporal. Results. *Laryngoscope* 1979;89:906.
59. Jones DT, McGill TJ, Healy GB. Cerebrospinal fistulas in children. *Laryngoscope* 1992;102:443.
60. MacGee EE, Cauthen JC, Brackett CE. Meningitis following acute traumatic cerebrospinalfluid fistula. *J Neurosurg* 1970;33:312.
61. Brawley BW, Kelly WA. Treatment of basal skull fractures with and without cerebrospinal fluid fistulae. *J Neurosurg* 1967;26:57.
62. Leech PJ, Paterson A. Conservative and operative management for cerebrospinal-fluid leakage after closed head injury. *Lancet* 1973;1:1013.
63. Tos M. Course of and sequelae to 248 petrosal fractures. *Acta Otolaryngol* 1973;75:353.
64. Klastersky J, Sadeghi M, Brihaye J. Antimicrobial prophylaxis in patients with rhinorrhea or otorrhea: a double-blind study. *Surg Neurol* 1976;6:111.
65. Brackmann DE, Rodgers GK. Management of postoperative cerebrospinal fluid leaks. In: Brackmann DE, Shelton C, Arriaga MA, eds. *Otologic Surgery*. Philadelphia: WB Saunders; 1994:709.

PART IX
Facial Paralysis

CHAPTER 30

Disorders of the Facial Nerve

Barry M. Schaitkin, Andrew Shapiro, and Mark May

On first examination of a child with facial paralysis, the otolaryngologist may be tempted to follow the same diagnostic protocol used for evaluation of facial paralysis in adults, in whom this condition is more familiar. Nevertheless, although Bell's palsy is the most frequent diagnosis in both adults and children with facial palsy, differential diagnosis of this condition in a child requires an increased awareness of infections and of congenital and developmental factors that may be contributing to the problem.

This chapter presents an approach to facial paralysis developed during the past 30 years of evaluating and managing the condition in 2,350 patients, including 537 younger than 18 years of age. With few exceptions, all of these patients underwent complete medical and otoneurologic evaluations and were followed for 6 months or longer.

DEVELOPMENTAL AND PATHOPHYSIOLOGIC CONSIDERATIONS

An understanding of facial nerve embryology and a grasp of nerve pathophysiology are important to evaluating and treating facial nerve dysfunction in children.

Embryology of the Facial Nerve

Normal and abnormal presentations of the facial nerve can best be understood through an awareness of its embryonic development (1,2). The main features of the nerve's complex course, branching pattern, and relationships are established in the first 3 months of prenatal life. During this period, the muscles of facial expression differentiate, become functional, and actively contract. Important steps in facial nerve development occur throughout gestation, but the nerve is not fully developed until approximately 4 years after birth.

Congenital anomalies can be understood by relating them to embryologic development. The facial nerve develops within the second pharyngeal arch during the time that closely adjacent derivatives of the first arch and first external groove and internal pouch are forming external and middle ear structures. Anomalies of the facial nerve within the temporal bone should therefore be anticipated whenever there is an associated malformation of the external or middle ear. For example, if the stapes or incus is deformed, the surgeon should be on guard for a possibly misplaced and exposed facial nerve; a soft-tissue mound over the footplate of the stapes or the promontory may actually be the facial nerve (3).

A variety of facial nerve presentations have been encountered within the temporal bone (4). The nerve may course with the chorda tympani nerve, bifurcate, trifurcate, or take innumerable other aberrant pathways within the temporal bone. For example, when the chorda tympani nerve is larger than normal, it may be because the nerve is carrying motor fibers to the face. In such instances, the vertical segment of the facial nerve just distal to the point where the chorda tympani nerve branches off may be narrowed to a fibrous strand and lie in a narrowed fallopian canal. This condition has been encountered in children born with facial paralysis. Alternatively, the facial nerve may be dehiscent and may herniate into the middle-ear cavity (5). This presentation of the facial nerve, when encountered during otologic surgery, must not be mistaken for a facial nerve schwannoma. Excision or biopsy of such a structure would cause an iatrogenic facial paralysis.

Neuropathophysiology

Injuries to the facial nerve, which carries some 10,000 fibers including 7,000 myelinated motor axons (6), can present across a broad spectrum. Despite the variety of symptoms, however, types of injury to a nerve can be categorized. Seddon (7) classified nerve injuries into three types: neuropraxia, axonotmesis, and neurotmesis. Sunderland's (8) clas-

---

B.M. Schaitkin: Department of Otolaryngology, University of Pittsburgh, Pittsburgh, Pennsylvania 15232.
A. Shapiro: Department of Surgery, Milton S. Hershey Medical Center, Hershey, Pennsylvania 17033.
M. May: Pittsburgh, Pennsylvania 15232.

TABLE 1. *Five degrees of nerve injury and facial nerve function test results*

Degree of injury	Pathology of injury[a]	Test response[b]	Mechanisms of recovery	Time	Results[c]
1	Compression, axoplasm damming, no morphologic changes (neuropraxia)	Normal	No morphologic changes noted	1–4 wk	Grade I; complete, no evidence of faulty regeneration
2	Compression persists, increased intraneural pressure, axons lost but tubules intact (axonotmesis)	0%–10% normal	Axons grow 1 mm/day into intact tubules	1–2 mo	Grade II; fair, volitional or spontaneous movement evidences minimal faulty regeneration
3	Increased pressure in nerve destroys myelin tubes (neurotmesis)	No response	Loss of tubes leads to growth of some axons into other tubes	2–4 mo	Grades III–IV; moderate to poor, facial movement is noticeably abnormal (degree varies) with moderate to marked synkinesis (mouth movement with eye closure)
4	Compression, loss of tubes, disruption of perineurium (partial transection)	No response	Some axons grow into other tubes, plus scarring impairs axon growth in some cases	4–18 mo	Grade V; little facial movement perceptible
5	Loss of tubes, disruption of perineurium and epineurium (complete transection)	No response	Scarring at transection site prevents regrowth of axons	Never	Grade VI; no spontaneous recovery of facial function

[a] Classification according to Seddon (7).
[b] Results of evoked electromyography and maximal stimulation.
[c] Grades of recovery modified from House and Brackmann (72).

sification is more exact, however, because it describes five possible degrees of peripheral nerve injury.

As Table 1 shows, changes in responses to electrical testing can be associated with the degree of injury to the nerve and are predictive of the type of recovery that can be expected. Sunderland (8), for example, suggested that inflammatory conditions result from external pressure on the nerve. This pressure causes impaired flow of axoplasm, in turn leading to compression of venous drainage and further pressure on the nerve. Eventually, endoneurial tubules can be lost and lead to third-degree injury.

Nerves with fourth or fifth degree injury show significant disruption of endoneurial tubules and disturbance of the perineurium; with fifth-degree injuries, the changes are also accompanied by significant disruption in the epineurium. No matter how well such severe injuries are managed, the recovery of facial function after fourth- or fifth-degree injury is never as good as after a first-, second-, or third-degree injury.

Objective Tests to Evaluate Facial Nerve Injury

Early tests developed to evaluate facial nerve injury sought to determine the status of the nerve by testing various functions, such as tearing (9), taste (10), and salivary flow (11) as popularized by Tschiassny (12). However, unless these tests are used to evaluate function soon after the onset of nerve paralysis, the results indicate little about the status of the facial nerve. In addition, contrary to a previous report (14), results of such functional tests have limited prognostic value, for several reasons: (a) due to individual variations in anatomy, axons may regrow in a number of ways; (b) the lesion in the facial nerve may be diffuse rather than focal; (c) different parts of the nerve may recover at different times; and (d) the tests may not give reliable results.

Unlike the results of facial nerve function tests, the results of serial electrical testing allow quite accurate estimation of the status of the facial nerve. The results of serial electrical testing therefore help determine the time and quality of spontaneous facial nerve regeneration and whether surgical repair of the nerve should be considered. Electrical tests that may be used include the maximal stimulation test (MST), evoked electromyography (EEMG), and electromyography (EMG). More recently, magnetic stimulation of the facial nerve has been evaluated.

Maximal Stimulation Testing

Serial evaluations using the MST provides quite accurate information about the degree of facial nerve degeneration when testing is begun soon after the onset of facial paralysis.

For this test, the examiner applies a stimulus of increasing intensity and notes the intensity (usually 1–5 mA) at which facial muscles twitch in response to the stimulus or the patient complains of discomfort. The stimulus is applied first to an area on the normal side of the face and then to the corresponding area on the affected side; results are stated for the affected side as a percentage of normal.

In the authors' series, when responses to MST remained equal during the first 10 days after onset of Bell's palsy, 92% of patients had complete spontaneous return of facial nerve function, but when the response was lost within the first 10 days after onset of palsy, all patients had incomplete return of facial nerve function. A marked decrease in the response during the first 10 days resulted in incomplete return of facial nerve function in 73% of patients (14).

Others, who reported the results of serial MST evaluations using a five-point scale, found the test to be 94% accurate in predicting the outcome of Bell's palsy (15).

Evoked Electromyography

Evoked electromyography, which Fisch and Esslen (16,17) popularized as "electroneurography," is similar to MST in that it involves evaluation of muscle compound action potentials (muscle CAPs). With MST the examiner evaluates the response visually, but with EEMG the response is recorded electrically. If the amplitude of the muscle CAPs decreases on serial testing, increasing slope of the decrease parallels worsening prognosis for spontaneous recovery of facial nerve function. May, Klein, and Taylor (18) showed that patients with Bell's palsy have a 98% chance of satisfactory return of facial nerve function if they maintain 25% or more of normal CAP amplitude on the affected side for up to 10 days after the onset of facial nerve paralysis. Chances of satisfactory recovery drop to 84% if the response decreases to between 11% and 24% of normal during the first 10 days; if response drops below 10% of normal during this time, the patient has only a 21% chance of satisfactory recovery.

These results were confirmed for 387 patients in the authors' series: 97% of patients with EEMG responses 25% or more of normal for the first 14 days had satisfactory return of facial function; 63% of those with responses between 11% and 24% of normal had satisfactory return, and only 30% of those with 10% or less of normal EEMG responses had satisfactory return.

Electromyography

When voluntary action potentials appear on EMG recordings from facial muscles in the first few days after injury to the facial nerve, the nerve lesion is incomplete. However, if fibrillation potentials appear, usually 10 to 21 days after nerve injury, significant nerve degeneration has occurred. These characteristics of EMG responses make the test the most reliable for following the course of facial muscle denervation after severe injury to the facial nerve.

Electromyography also provides the first evidence of recovery of facial nerve function, in the form of decreased fibrillation potentials followed by the appearance of prolonged polyphasic voluntary motor unit action potentials (19). As reported by May, Blumenthal, and Klein, Silliman, and Fisch (14,20,21), when voluntary motor unit action potentials appeared early on the EMG, even though EEMG results showed loss of 90% of function, patients had a good prognosis for spontaneous return of facial nerve function.

Magnetic Nerve Stimulation

Stimulating the facial nerve magnetically rather than electrically has been investigated by several clinicians, including Metson et al. (22), Kartush et al. (23), and Rimpilainen et al. (24). The advantages of magnetic stimulation over electrical stimulation include (a) stimulation of the proximal portion of the facial nerve rather than the peripheral nerve, which theoretically allows (b) obtaining evidence of nerve degeneration earlier in its course, and (c) less patient discomfort than with EEMG if a small magnetic coil is used and positioned properly over the root exit zone of the nerve. Magnetic stimulation has not become widely used, however, so it is not currently useful in predicting when surgical decompression of the nerve might be indicated.

Imaging Techniques to Evaluate the Facial Nerve

A number of imaging techniques may be used to evaluate the paralyzed facial nerve. Computed tomography (CT) provides excellent definition within the temporal bone. The most helpful technique for extratemporal lesions, however, is magnetic resonance imaging (MRI) with gadolinium enhancement. Using this technique, Murphy and Teller (25) found increased signal intensity in the facial nerve, usually localized to the labyrinthine geniculate ganglion and proximal tympanic segment, in 18 of 25 patients with Bell's palsy. Patients who did not have evidence of enhancement tended to have a better outcome. Weber and McKenna (26) also noted enhancement of the facial nerve on MRI in patients with Ramsey Hunt syndrome.

Weber and McKenna (26) also pointed out the value of MRI in helping to distinguish among neoplastic lesions affecting the facial nerve. They found, for example, that a neuroma, the most common neoplasm affecting the facial nerve, appeared brightly enhanced by gadolinium and showed expansion in the labyrinthine segment and geniculate ganglion region. A neuroma in the parotid gland could be similarly differentiated from a pleomorphic adenoma on MRI.

DIAGNOSTIC CONSIDERATIONS IN CHILDREN

In addition to the diagnostic considerations that must be entertained in adults, a variety of congenital and developmental anomalies may be associated with facial nerve disorders in the pediatric population. A systematic approach to diagnosis is essential, beginning with a careful history and physical examination.

History and Physical Examination

In infants and young children, evaluation may be complicated by the difficulty in obtaining accurate information. The elasticity of newborn skin combined with generous buccal fat may delay recognition of facial weakness for weeks to months, thus making it difficult to assess whether the dysfunction was congenital or more recent in onset. A further difficulty is that young children are unable to describe symptoms of facial nerve injury such as pain and disturbances in sensation, gustatory ability, or auditory and vestibular function.

Nonetheless, a history of the onset of facial paralysis can provide much of the information needed to arrive at a diagnosis. Determining the age of onset, time course (e.g., rapid vs. slow) of onset, and the duration of paralysis allows distinction between congenital or acquired etiology and may significantly shorten the list of differential diagnoses. In addition, the child's history should be reviewed carefully for any previous episodes of facial paralysis, cervicofacial trauma, central nervous system disorder, or otologic disease.

Physical examination of even the youngest child may reveal much about the status of the facial nerve. Careful attention to facial movement during crying, particularly while the child is sitting or held upright, can reveal asymmetries in facial movement and tear production. In cooperative children, facial movements can often be elicited by asking the child to mimic the expressions of the examiner. Spontaneous facial movement can be observed during play or by tickling the child. The tongue should be examined for atrophy of taste papillae on the ipsilateral surface to provide evidence of chorda tympani nerve dysfunction.

Tests to Evaluate Facial Nerve Function

The presence of a hearing loss and the type of loss may provide useful information about the site of pathology in the facial nerve. Facial nerve dysfunction in association with sensorineural hearing loss may indicate a lesion involving the internal auditory canal or central nervous system. Conductive hearing loss implicates the middle ear as a potential location.

Advances in auditory assessment allow evaluation of hearing in almost all children. If behavioral audiometry is unable to be performed, auditory brainstem testing or otoacoustic emission testing can be utilized. When indicated, vestibular testing, including electronystagmography, posturography, and rotatory testing may be performed in selected children as young as 3 years of age.

Electrical testing, as discussed in the previous section, provides an objective means by which the degree of facial nerve dysfunction can be monitored, even in cases of complete paralysis. Furthermore, electrophysiologic tests can be helpful in differentiating the causes of complete facial paralysis during the perinatal period. Facial nerve conduction studies demonstrate immediate abnormalities in patients with developmental anomalies of the facial nerve, whereas patients who have suffered traumatic injuries usually manifest normal excitability within the first few days after birth. Electrophysiologic testing can be performed without sedation in cooperative children, particularly if the stimulus intensities are kept below a level that causes discomfort. If testing is necessary in an uncooperative child, a short-duration anesthetic may be administered.

DIAGNOSIS AND MANAGEMENT OF CONGENITAL FACIAL PARALYSIS

Between 0.8 and 1.8 in 1,000 infants are estimated to have facial paralysis at birth (27–29). Congenital paralysis can be classified broadly as *traumatic* or *developmental* in origin, a distinction that carries important prognostic, therapeutic, and medicolegal implications.

Diagnosis of Traumatic Facial Paralysis

In the majority of patients with congenital facial paralysis, the condition is attributed to trauma to the facial nerve during the mother's pregnancy or delivery (27, 29). Traumatic facial paralysis typically involves the entire distribution of the facial nerve. Congenital traumatic facial nerve injuries are often associated with a prolonged and difficult labor; the classic case is delivery of a large infant from a primiparous mother. A significant proportion of the injuries have been associated with forceps deliveries, but it remains unclear whether forceps are truly the cause, or simply reflect the difficult nature of these deliveries (27,29,30).

A less common cause of congenital traumatic facial nerve injury may be compression of the nerve due to intrauterine positioning. Parmalee (31) suggested that the pressure of the maternal sacrum on the facial nerve of the infant could lead to paralysis.

Physical examination of a newborn who has suffered traumatic facial nerve injury may reveal stigmata of injury to the temporal bone or face, such as hematomas or lacerations, hemotympanum, or ecchymosis overlying the mastoid. Any portion of the facial nerve may be injured during birth, but the most common site is probably the intratemporal portion, where the thin bone of the fallopian canal is prone to collapse and compress the underlying nerve. Transection of the facial nerve during birth has never been recorded, accounting for the high (90% or greater) rate of spontaneous recovery of nerve function after birth trauma (32).

In the rare cases in which the facial nerve does not recover spontaneously from birth trauma, surgical intervention may be considered. However, complete decompression is indicated only (a) when complete paralysis is present at birth,

(b) EEMG demonstrates a complete loss of facial nerve function by 3 to 5 days after birth, (c) paralysis and absence of electrical activity persist at 5 weeks of age, (d) physical examination reveals evidence of temporal bone trauma, and radiologic imaging demonstrates a fracture. This conservative course of action maximizes the opportunity for spontaneous recovery while allowing adequate return of function should decompression be required.

Inherited or Developmental Disorders of Facial Nerve Function

Facial nerve dysfunction in the newborn can be the result of an inherited disorder or disturbances in fetal development. Whether the paralysis is unilateral or bilateral, the presence of accompanying anomalies helps to determine the diagnosis.

When facial paralysis is due to an inherited or developmental anomaly, abnormalities are usually present in associated craniofacial structures, such as the external or middle ear, palate or other maxillary structures, and other cranial nerves (33). The lesion may have occurred at the cortical, brainstem, or peripheral level. Hypoplasia of the facial musculature may occur, either primarily or as a result of lack of neural stimulation during development.

The diagnosis of inherited or developmental facial palsy can often be established by clinical evaluation alone. Consultation with a dysmorphologist may be helpful in identifying specific syndromes in addition to assisting in comprehensive evaluation of other organ systems. Electrophysiologic testing may be performed to confirm a developmental etiology in questionable cases; when palsy is due to inherited or developmental abnormalities, the electromyogram (EMG) (EEG) evidences electrical silence with no fibrillation potentials. Results of EEMG are also abnormal at birth, and serial testing shows no change in contrast electrical testing following birth trauma produces a progressive decrease in the amplitudes of compound action potentials over time.

Auditory brainstem response testing should be performed to evaluate sensorineural and conductive hearing loss in any child with congenital facial palsy. Abnormalities in the interwave latencies and the amplitudes of waves I and V are typical findings when such a loss is present (34). A poorly developed or nonexistent fallopian canal, with or without other temporal bone anomalies, may show on CT.

Inherited Disorders

Two types of facial paresis are inherited, myotonic dystrophy and Albers-Schönberg Disease.

Myotonic Dystrophy

Myotonic dystrophy is an autosomal dominant disorder characterized by progressive muscle weakness, wasting, and variable degrees of mental impairment. Facial muscle weakness is usually one of the first symptoms noted, and facial diplegia is often present at birth.

Albers-Schönberg Disease

Albers-Schönberg disease is a sporadic or autosomal recessive disease (osteopetrosis) affecting bone metabolism. Increased bone density and lack of primary bone resorption lead to bony compression of nerves and often result in blindness, deafness, and facial paralysis when cranial nerves are affected.

Developmental Abnormalities

Poor facial muscle function is also a feature of several congenital syndromes, including Mobius syndrome, CHARGE syndrome, oculoauriculovertebral (OAV) syndrome, and asymmetric crying facies.

Mobius Syndrome

Mobius syndrome is characterized by the presence of unilateral or bilateral facial paralysis in conjunction with sixth cranial nerve palsy. Often the inferior aspect of the face is relatively spared. A number of other anomalies are associated with the Mobius syndrome, including other neuropathies of other cranial nerves (specifically, cranial nerves III, IV, V, IX, X, and XII), and malformed extremities or absence of the pectoralis muscles in 50% of patients. The diagnosis is usually established in infancy, although the absence of asymmetry in bilateral facial palsy may delay recognition of the disorder.

The cause of Mobius syndrome is unknown, although agenesis of the facial nucleus, nerve, or musculature has been implicated as the primary aberration (35). A number of teratogens, particularly thalidomide, can produce anomalies identical to the findings in this disorder.

CHARGE Association

The association of *c*olobomata, *h*eart defects, *a*tresia choanae, *r*etarded growth, *g*enital hypoplasia, and *e*ar anomalies has been widely reported. Approximately 43% of patients with CHARGE association manifest facial nerve dysfunction. In some cases, the associated anomalies also meet criteria for Mobius syndrome (36).

Oculoquriculovertebral Syndrome (OAV)

Oculoauriculovertebral syndrome consists of a spectrum of disorders characterized by unilateral malformation of first and second branchial arch derivatives. Physical findings include hypoplasia of the bone and soft tissues of the maxilla and mandible, microtia, and microstomia. This syndrome may not be clinically apparent until facial growth has progressed enough that asymmetry becomes apparent. Facial weakness is only one of a number of central nervous system abnormalities associated with these disorders.

Goldenhar syndrome, consisting of epibulbar dermoids and vertebral anomalies in addition to the unilateral malformations described, accounts for approximately 10% of cases of OAV. Facial weakness is nearly universal in the subset of children with Goldenhar syndrome.

Asymmetric Crying Facies

One of the more common conditions associated with facial nerve dysfunction, asymmetric crying facies is also known as congenital unilateral lower lip palsy (CULLP) or hypoplasia of the depressor anguli oris. Clinically, the diagnosis becomes apparent when the patient's lower lip fails to depress with crying.

No particular functional deficit results from asymmetric crying facies, but the condition should be noted because it is frequently associated with other defects. Deformities of the external ear most often accompany asymmetric crying facies. Cardiac anomalies are present in about 10% of affected children and may be severe.

Treatment of Developmental Facial Palsy

The treatment of patients with developmental palsy of the facial nerve is controversial. Often, patients with mild palsies and segmental deficits do not need surgery, although they may benefit from working with a therapist trained in facial muscle motor-sensory reeducation. For patients with more severe deficits, a variety of surgical interventions may be considered.

Surgical exploration of a facial nerve that has developed abnormally generally reveals a tapered, fibrous filament unsuitable for grafting or decompression (35,37). Furthermore, patients with this type of nerve abnormality usually have associated abnormalities of the facial musculature, which preclude attempts to restore facial function by nerve grafting.

On the other hand, a recent study of temporal bones from children with developmental facial palsy demonstrated necrotic lesions involving the facial nerve, and evidence of aberrant axonal regeneration (38). These findings suggest that an insult late in development may be responsible for some cases of developmental palsy. If this is the case, early nerve exploration and grafting might be of benefit in selected patients. Techniques for reconstruction are described later in the chapter.

FACIAL PARALYSIS OCCURRING BEYOND THE NEWBORN PERIOD

Facial paralysis occurring after the newborn period usually is idiopathic (Bells's palsy) or results from infection or trauma.

Bell's Palsy

In approximately 40% of 300 patients younger than 18 years of age in the series, the cause of facial paralysis was determined to be Bell's palsy (idiopathic) (39). Although Bell's palsy is a diagnosis of exclusion, it is considered to be caused by inflammatory edema of the facial nerve compressed within the confines of the fallopian canal. Certain features are often associated with the disorder: (a) a family history or previous episode of facial paralysis (present in 10% of patients), (b) a preceding viral prodrome, and (c) identification of a red chorda tympani nerve on otoscopy (40).

The facial weakness of Bell's palsy usually progresses over 3 weeks or less. The palsy is often accompanied by pain or paresthesias involving the ipsilateral cervicofacial region, tongue, shoulder, or a combination of these areas in 50% of patients; hyperacusis and decreased tearing are not uncommon. When the history and physical examination rule out other causes for facial paralysis, the diagnosis of Bell's palsy can usually be made without laboratory testing or imaging studies.

The majority of patients with Bell's palsy can expect a satisfactory recovery; in the series by Peiterson, 84% recovered House grade I or II function (41). Patients in whom paralysis remains incomplete can expect an excellent recovery. When paralysis is complete and EEMG levels are less than 10%, an unsatisfactory outcome is much more likely; 50% to 75% of these patients have House grade III or IV results.

Another characteristic of Bell's palsy that helps predict outcome is the time at which facial function starts to return. If recovery begins within 3 weeks, it is usually complete. Final results are usually satisfactory when facial function begins to return between 3 weeks and 2 months after onset of palsy, but if onset of recovery is delayed until 2 to 4 months after paralysis occurs, some permanent residual effects are likely. If the return of facial function is delayed beyond 6 months after onset of Bell's palsy, other causes for the paralysis should be sought.

About 10% of individuals who have an episode of Bell's palsy experience recurrent facial paralysis, typically on the contralateral side. Because ipsilateral recurrence of Bell's palsy is less common, it should be evaluated thoroughly to be sure it does not represent Melkersson-Rosenthal syndrome or a neoplasm involving the facial nerve.

The treatment of Bell's palsy remains controversial. A glucocorticoid drug is often prescribed, although the results of drug efficacy studies are generally equivocal (42,43). Serial electrophysiologic testing may be used to follow the progress of recovery in patients with complete paralysis. There is evidence that patients with poor prognostic signs may benefit from early steroid administration, which in some studies has been shown to reduce the number of patients experiencing denervation and poor outcomes (House grade IV or V) (44). Fisch (45) recommended middle fossa and transmastoid decompression of the facial nerve in patients with complete paralysis and EEMG results demonstrating greater than 90% denervation within 3 weeks of the onset of paralysis.

Infection

Infections are responsible for a larger proportion of cases of facial paralysis in children than in adults. A number of specific conditions account for this difference.

Acute Otitis Media

Facial paralysis as a complication of acute otitis media is most often seen in young children. The facial nerve may become inflamed through erosion of the thin bone of the fallopian canal, through congenital dehiscences, or by spread along another structure such as the stapedius nerve, chorda tympani nerve, or posterior tympanic artery (46). Inflammation of the nerve leads to edema, which results in compression of the facial nerve within the canal.

Facial nerve palsy due to acute otitis media is managed by immediate performance of a wide myringotomy to drain the middle-ear effusion and obtain a culture of the exudate, followed by administration of antibiotic drugs. The initial antibiotic drug should be effective against *Streptococcus pneumoniae* and *Haemophilus influenza*; when the results of exudate culture are known, an alternative antibiotic agent may be substituted or added to the regimen. Placement of a tympanostomy tube is recommended for patients with a history of recurrent otitis media.

Only rarely is more extensive surgery indicated to treat acute otitis media. Criteria for mastoidectomy are independent of the facial paralysis and include continued otorrhea and coalescent mastoiditis. The authors have performed mastoidectomy in rare cases of facial paralysis when responses to electrical testing were lost precipitously (EEMG < 10% normal) and CT scans suggested formation of an abscess.

The prognosis for recovery of facial function after facial paralysis secondary to acute otitis media is less favorable than the prognosis for idiopathic facial paralysis: approximately 40% of patients with acute otitis media and facial palsy have incomplete return of facial nerve function. The usefulness of therapy with steroids for this condition has not been established.

Chronic Otitis Media

In older children, cholesteatoma or, less commonly, granulation tissue may compress the facial nerve and cause facial palsy. Surgical removal of the offending tissue followed by decompression of the facial nerve proximal and distal to the site of lesion usually results in good recovery of facial nerve function.

Herpes Zoster Oticus

Rapidly progressive facial paralysis, vesicular eruptions in the ear canal and pinna, and severe pain are characteristic of herpes zoster infection of the facial nerve. Infection of the eighth cranial nerve, resulting in hearing loss and vertigo, often occurs concurrently. Herpes zoster oticus (Ramsay Hunt Syndrome) accounts for at least 3% to 12% of cases of facial paralysis (47).

The diagnosis of herpes zoster oticus can usually be established on the basis of clinical presentation, although antibody titers or complement fixation studies are increasingly being used to confirm the diagnosis. Steroid drugs and the antiviral medication acyclovir have been used to treat this condition, but their efficacy has not been tested in controlled studies 48,49). Of patients with this condition, 30% to 50% have persistent weakness of facial muscles.

Lyme Disease

Acute facial palsy is the most frequent focal neurologic manifestation of Lyme disease, a tick-borne illness caused by infection with the spirochete *Borellia burgdorferi*. Lyme disease is found worldwide; and in some study populations, it was the leading cause of facial paralysis in children (50).

In 60% to 80% of patients with Lyme disease, a characteristic expanding erythematous skin lesion appears at the site of inoculation. Within several weeks, a variety of symptoms may appear, such as rashes, headache, stiff neck, migratory arthralgias, and fatigue. Facial paralysis usually occurs during this stage, particularly when the site of inoculation was in the cervicofacial area (51,50). Facial paralysis occurs more often in children than in adults with Lyme disease, perhaps because children are more likely to be inoculated in the head and neck region.

Confirmation of a diagnosis of Lyme disease is usually sought by enzyme-linked immunoadsorbent assay (ELISA) for IgG and IgM antibodies to the spirochete. Although in some cases serum analysis results are sufficient (50). This infection is usually treated effectively by tetracycline or macrolide antibiotics.

Autoimmune Deficiency Syndrome

Facial paralysis occurs in individuals affected with the human immunodeficiency virus (HIV) or acquired immunodeficiency syndrome (AIDS). It has been reported as complications of herpes zoster oticus (52), progressive multifocal leukoencephalopathy (53), or neoplasm (54).

Tumors

Tumors were the cause of facial paralysis in 6% of the pediatric patients in the May's series (54a). In children, tumors causing facial paralysis were more often benign than malignant and were usually derived from the nerve sheath.

Facial paralysis usually has a more rapid onset when caused by a malignant tumor than a benign lesion.

The most common malignancies affecting the facial nerve are leukemia involving the temporal bone (which causes direct compression or infiltration of the facial nerve) (55) and rhabdomyosarcoma of the head and neck (56). In addition, brain tumors, particularly those arising infratentorially, may produce weakness of the facial muscles.

Patients in our series whose facial paralysis was caused by a tumor consistently had signs and symptoms of the neoplasm for some time before the diagnosis was made. Clearly, careful monitoring of the progress of facial paralysis and evaluation for neoplastic or other causes are crucial to providing effective treatment in a timely manner. A tumor involving the facial nerve should be suspected as the cause of facial paralysis that (a) progresses slowly for more than 3 weeks, (b) does not resolve after 6 months, (c) recurs on the same side, (d) is associated with facial twitching, or (e) is associated with other neurologic signs.

Idiopathic Diseases

Facial paralysis is characteristic of two diseases of unknown origin: Melkersson-Rosenthal syndrome and Kawasaki disease.

Melkersson-Rosenthal Syndrome

Melkersson-Rosenthal syndrome is characterized by a triad of relapsing, alternating facial paralysis; recurrent facial edema; and fissured tongue. The disease is rare, with facial paralysis usually appearing first, during the teenage years (57). A familial tendency to Melkersson-Rosenthal syndrome has been recorded, although the specific pattern of inheritance has not been identified (58).

The facial paralysis of Melkersson-Rosenthal syndrome may be partial or complete, unilateral or bilateral, and may precede the other features by months to years. Histologic examination of edematous tissue has revealed noncaseating granulomas (57). Although spontaneous resolution of the facial paralysis is expected, complete decompression of the nerve has been recommended for patients with multiple recurrences (59).

Kawasaki Disease

Symptoms of Kawasaki disease include persistent high fever, cervical adenitis, erythema of the oral mucosa, injection of the conjunctiva, and upper and lower extremity edema and desquamation. Peripheral neuropathy, particularly facial paralysis, has been noted in some cases. The facial paralysis typically resolves completely with resolution of the underlying illness (60).

Traumatic Facial Nerve Injuries

Facial paralysis may result from traumatic injury to the nerve. Common mechanisms of injury in children include temporal bone fracture and facial wounds that involve the nerve.

Temporal Bone Fracture

Fracture of the temporal bone has been reported in 6% to 14% of children with head trauma (61), and head injuries have been reported to be the leading cause of acquired facial paralysis in children in a recent series from Switzerland (62). In this series, unilateral peripheral palsy occurred in 8.3% of 132 children with temporal bone fracture (62).

Although temporal bone fractures may be longitudinal or transverse, in 90% of facial nerve injuries, the fracture was longitudinal. Typically, this fracture parallels the long axis of the petrous bone, involving the tegmen and external auditory canal and passing lateral to the otic capsule.

The site of facial nerve injury may be at the geniculate ganglion, tympanic portion, or, less frequently, at the second genu in the mastoid segment. Paralysis may be immediate or delayed in onset. Hemotympanum, ossicular discontinuity, or tympanic membrane perforation may also occur and cause conductive hearing loss. In rare cases, sensorineural hearing loss and vertigo due to labyrinthine concussion or subluxation of the stapes footplate may occur.

Transverse fractures, which cause more severe injury and are often fatal, disrupt the otic capsule. This results in sensorineural hearing loss and vertigo; approximately 50% of patients also have facial paralysis.

Patients who have suffered a temporal bone fracture should be evaluated for facial nerve injury as soon as possible. Physical examination for facial muscle tone and eye closure should be supplemented by electrical testing and evaluation of CT and MRI results for evidence of decreased function. Facial movement of any type is an excellent indication that the facial nerve has not been transected (63), but because children may retain good facial muscle movement even when the facial nerve has been transected, assessment for signs of facial nerve injury should be ongoing.

When complete loss of facial nerve function is evident, EEMG should be repeated daily. If function remains greater than 10% of normal for 5 days, the nerve probably has not been completely transected, and spontaneous recovery of satisfactory function is likely. If EEMG responses deteriorate during this time, however, surgical intervention is indicated. The facial nerve should be explored and decompressed from the meatus to the stylomastoid foramen. A translabyrinthine approach is appropriate if the patient has a profound sensorineural hearing loss, but when hearing is intact, a transmastoid-middle fossa approach is most often used. The authors have found a transtemporal–sub-middle fossa approach can be used for decompression with preservation of hearing.

If the facial nerve is found to be injured, it should be repaired by direct anastomosis or grafting, depending on the extent of injury. Repair of tears in the tympanic membrane, ossicular disruptions, cerebrospinal fluid leaks, and other injuries may also be necessary.

Facial Wounds

When the extracranial facial nerve is injured, the wound should be explored as soon as possible (but within the first 3 days after injury). If the wound is clean, the nerve should be repaired at this time by primary anastomosis or interposition grafting. In a contaminated wound, the nerve ends should be tagged with clips or nonabsorbable sutures and the wound allowed to heal by secondary intention. The nerve can then be repaired as long as 3 weeks after injury with better results than if repair is attempted in a contaminated wound immediately after injury.

Iatrogenic Injury

Even by experienced surgeons, the facial nerve can be injured during surgery on the ear or in the parotid region.

Otologic Surgery

During surgical procedures on the ear, the facial nerve is most often injured at the second genu in the mastoid, followed by the portion that passes through the anterior epitympanum. Injury is more likely when the course of the nerve is aberrant or altered by the presence of pathology. However, even the use of landmarks (64,65) or neurophysiological monitoring techniques does not ensure protection of the facial nerve.

When facial paralysis occurs unexpectedly in a patient who has undergone otologic surgery, dressings should be checked to be sure they are not compressing the nerve extracranially; if the first evaluation is less than 2 hours after the end of the procedure, the patient should be evaluated again after 2 hours, when anesthetic effects have more fully dissipated.

Whether the patient is returned to surgery for exploration of the nerve depends on the degree of certainty with which the nerve was identified during the initial operation. If the nerve was positively identified and preserved, as documented by response to stimulation at the end of the procedure, exploration is unnecessary. However, if the nerve was not positively identified, exploration is indicated. This may be undertaken the next day to allow the patient to recover somewhat from the initial operation, to discuss the situation with the patient and family, and possibly to request consultation with another physician.

Decompression should begin several millimeters proximal to the injury and proceed distally to the stylomastoid foramen. Simple decompression should be adequate to treat contusions and other injuries that have left the endoneurial contents intact. A transected nerve is treated by freshening the injured edges and epineurial repair or nerve grafting to achieve tension-free reapproximation of nerve ends.

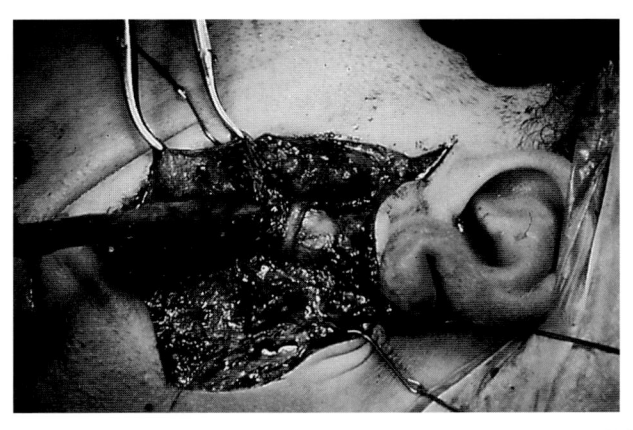

FIG. 1. First branchial sinus tract with facial nerve at risk travelling between the soft tissue and cartilogenous portion.

Parotid Surgery

The facial nerve is at high risk during any surgery on the parotid gland of a young child because the nerve fibers are microscopic in size, the mastoid tip is not well developed, and the lower division of the nerve lies more superficially over the angle of the mandible, thus making it especially vulnerable to injury.

As during otologic surgery, the facial nerve should be protected during surgery on a child's parotid gland by identifying and monitoring the location of the nerve at each step of the procedure. In addition, the main trunk of the nerve should be stimulated at the conclusion of the procedure. If the whole side of the child's face moves, the nerve is intact, thus, even if movement is lost postoperatively, it should return without further treatment.

If the face does not move, however, the nerve branch(es) to paralyzed parts of the face should be explored at the initial surgery and injuries repaired by primary anastomosis or interposition grafting. Results of such repair are usually excellent (66).

The most common tumors of the parotid gland are hemangiomas and lymphangiomas. These tumors tend to send multiple projections into the gland, thus making dissection of the facial nerve difficult, especially in a child. Whenever possible, management of the lesion by a therapy such as administration of steroid agents or interferon should be tried before surgery is undertaken.

The patient who presents with a pit at the angle of the jaw in a first branchial cleft anomaly provides a unique challenge. The child's facial nerve is more superficial to begin with and further involvement with the first branchial cleft sinus tract can be disorienting for the surgeon. Figure 1A shows the external canal reduplication with the facial nerve draped over it. The nerve is seen traveling just beneath the adipose tissue and across the sinus tract. For this reason, our clinic sees more patients with first branchial clefts for treatment of the facial paralysis than for treatment of the branchial lesion itself. The first branchial cleft anomaly is much less common than the second branchial cleft anomaly, and surgeons are generally less familiar with it. An extreme sense of care and meticulous dissection is required to avoid a devastating injury in a young child.

MANAGEMENT OF FACIAL PARALYSIS

Because most patients with facial paralysis recover spontaneously, clinicians frequently approach this facial paralysis with no particular urgency. However, occasionally a patient with facial paralysis has an underlying life-threatening disorder. In other cases, such as facial paralysis secondary to cholesteatoma, delay of treatment until the facial nerve is electrophysiologically dead—which can occur as soon as the second or third day after onset of paralysis—condemns the patient to permanent disability. For this reason, a diagnosis should be established as quickly as possible so that if definitive treatment is available, it can be instituted rapidly.

In addition, the patient and family should be given a prognosis for return of facial function. If the permanent deficit is expected to be mild, the patient and family usually suffer minimal psychological distress. However, more marked deficits can cause significant interpersonal problems, even when function is minimally affected. In these cases, it is essential to provide the family with a realistic assessment of the expected degree of recovery and the options available for treatment and rehabilitation. Regardless of the degree of disability expected, many families benefit from referrals to a support group or psychological counseling.

Eye Care

Patients with congenital facial paralysis are unlikely to develop ophthalmologic problems as a result of the paralysis, even though lacrimation may be decreased. On the other hand, children with acquired paralysis need to practice the same procedures for eye care that are required in adults. Meticulous eye care is particularly important when the patient lacks *B*ell's phenomenon, corneal *a*nesthesia is present, and the eye is *d*ry because of inadequate tear production (BAD syndrome) (67).

The purpose of the eye-care regimen is to protect the eye from exposure and drying. Artificial tears should be instilled frequently during the day, and a lubricating ophthalmic ointment should be applied before sleep. A moisture chamber (Pro-Optics, Palatine, IL) is also effective in protecting the eye from exposure and drying.

Another way to prevent the eye from drying is to hold it closed. The classic way to achieve this has been tarsorrhaphy, and a temporary tarsorrhaphy may be indicated for some patients. Patients may try to obtain the same effects without surgery by taping the eye shut or patching, but these techniques are less effective and may be irritating. For other patients, a small semicircle of tape on the upper eyelid may provide enough weight to overcome the pull of the superior levator muscle and allow the eyelid to protect the cornea.

If these conservative measures fail, and the patient develops keratitis, or if the prospects for spontaneous return of function are poor, surgery is usually indicated. As an alternative to tarsorrhaphy, the upper eyelid may be reanimated by placement of a gold weight or spring. Children generally maintain excellent tone in the lower eyelid, and ectropion is rare, so children with facial paralysis usually do not need a lower eyelid procedure. If the lower eyelid does become lax, a lid tightening procedure or placement of an auricular cartilage graft may be performed (68,69).

Medications

Without question, antimicrobial agents play an important role in the management of facial paralysis secondary to acute suppurative otitis media. In conjunction with wide myringotomy, antibiotics may provide rapid resolution of facial paralysis in these patients.

Corticosteroid drugs have been used extensively in the management of facial paralysis, in particular Bell's palsy and herpes zoster oticus. They have been reported to be beneficial in providing pain relief and improving both the duration and outcome of the paralysis. Nonetheless, several studies in large numbers of patients have failed to show any definite improvement in the rate or extent of recovery of facial function when steroid drugs were administered. Thus, the use of steroids will continue to be debated until a well-controlled, randomized study is conducted to determine the benefits provided by these drugs (42).

Acyclovir has been proposed to treat both Ramsey Hunt syndrome and Bell's palsy, on the theory that both these disease processes are caused by the herpes zoster virus. Several published reports indicate that acyclovir is beneficial in these cases, but the studies reported were conducted in a small number of patients and without controls, so the results cannot be considered definitive (48,49). Controlled studies must be conducted in large series of patients to determine the possible benefits and harms of acyclovir for either disorder.

Surgery

A variety of surgical procedures have been developed to treat facial paralysis.

Facial Nerve Decompression

Fisch (45) has suggested that the facial nerve be decompressed when facial paralysis is 90% complete, to prevent total degeneration. However, no randomized, controlled clinical trial with a sufficient number of patients has been performed to show whether surgical decompression of the facial nerve is effective in relieving facial paralysis due to any pathologic condition that does not interrupt the nerve. Thus, the benefit of surgery has not been established for idiopathic (Bell's) palsy, herpes zoster cephalicus, acute sup-

```
                        FACIAL REANIMATION DECISION TREE
                                  facial weakness
                                        ↓
                                        ↓
                                        ↓
                     status of proximal + distal neuromuscular system
                                        ↓
                                        ↓
systems intact proximal + distal to area of injury              systems not intact
―――――――――――――――――――――――――――――――――――――――――――――――――――――――――――――――――――――――――――――――――
            ↓                                                           ↓
            ↓                                                           ↓
         deficit                                                        ↓_____
   ―――――――――――――――――――――――――――――――――――――――――              
    short          long          only proximal          neither proximal      only distal
    segment        segment       intact                 or                    intact
       ↓             ↓              ↓                   distal available         ↓
       ↓             ↓              ↓                         ↓                  ↓
    reanastomosis  interposition  free flap             temporalis            XII-VII
                   nerve          innervated            muscle                interpositional
                   graft          by ipsilateral        transposition         jump graft*
                                  cranial               free flap                ↓
                                  nerve VII*            or                       ↓
                                                        static                   ↓
                                                        suspension*              ↓
                                                            ↑                    ↓
                                              ← ← ←if xii not available ← ←
```

*Reanimate eye separately.

FIG. 2. Decision tree for facial reanimation surgery.

purative otitis media, necrotizing external otitis, or facial paralysis following iatrogenic or external temporal bone trauma.

Nevertheless, when facial paralysis is the result of an ongoing process such as chronic suppurative otitis media, paralysis cannot resolve unless the primary process is eradicated. Thus, surgery should be performed in such patients before nerve function has deteriorated to the point that recovery of facial function is jeopardized. Specifically, surgery must not be delayed if the palsy has progressed from incomplete to complete and if the response to EEMG is less than 25% of normal or is dropping precipitously after the third day following onset. In addition, surgery is absolutely indicated in two situations: (a) to rule out or treat facial nerve transection or (b) when a tumor is suspected to involve the facial nerve.

Rehabilitation of the Paralyzed Face

Figure 2 diagrams the surgeon's decision-making process in evaluating options for rehabilitating the paralyzed face. Patients with facial paralysis require an individualized approach to rehabilitation; one must take into consideration the etiology and duration of the paralysis as well as the functional and emotional needs of the patient. If the paralysis is likely to be long-standing, a variety of surgical techniques are available to improve cosmesis and function. Unfortunately, even the most successful procedures cannot restore "normal" facial function; it is essential before surgery is undertaken, that patients and families be educated to have realistic expectations of the surgical outcome.

The timing for facial reanimation procedures varies according to the cause and duration of facial paralysis. Patients with a recent injury benefit from rapid reinnervation. On the other hand, children with congenital paralysis or absence of suitable muscle may be best served by waiting until facial growth is completed. In general, when discussing options for rehabilitation of the paralyzed face, the procedures described below should be considered. The procedures are presented in order of preference from most successful to least likely to provide "normal" facial function.

Direct Facial Nerve Anastomosis

If the facial nerve has been sharply transected secondary to surgery or trauma, debridement and direct anastomosis without tension should be performed as early as possible. Within 72 hours the distal nerve stumps may be electrically stimulated, thereby aiding localization. We have found that repair can be performed with satisfactory results for at least several months after injury. However, results have generally been poor if repair is delayed for more than 1 year following injury, due to fibrosis of the distal nerve and atrophy of the facial muscles.

Interposition Grafting

Blunt trauma or removal of a tumor involving the facial nerve may cause damage to or require resection of a significant length of the facial nerve. We prefer to close the resulting gap by placement of a nerve graft, typically from the cervical cutaneous or sural nerve, rather than perform extensive surgery to mobilize the facial nerve in an attempt to achieve tension-free primary anastomosis. In these cases, two suture lines are no disadvantage over a single anastomosis.

Nerve Transposition

Although best results are achieved by restoring the continuity of the facial nerve, other cranial nerves may be "hooked" to the distal facial nerve if the proximal portion of the facial nerve is unavailable. The success of this technique depends on the patient's facial musculature being intact; thus, this procedure is inappropriate for most cases of developmental paralysis or paralysis of greater than 2 years' duration.

Nerve transposition is especially useful to manage injury to the facial nerve at the brainstem. The phrenic, spinal accessory, contralateral facial, and hypoglossal nerves have been transposed to animate the distal facial nerve. Theoretically, the best results would be obtained with a cross-facial nerve graft, which could provide for segmental input to the facial musculature and allow involuntary facial movement. Unfortunately, the outcome of such procedures has been inconsistent in our experience, probably because the procedures were performed so late after the onset of paralysis that facial muscles had atrophied.

We have obtained the best results of nerve transposition surgery to reanimate the paralyzed face by using the hypoglossal nerve. Of patients who underwent such a procedure, 90% regained facial symmetry and tone, and 77% had satisfactory motor function (69). Despite these positive results, loss of motor innervation to the ipsilateral tongue has frequently been a source of significant morbidity. To overcome this problem, we use a hypoglossal-facial "jump graft" technique that avoids tongue paralysis and allows the performance of bilateral hypoglossal-facial anastomoses if necessary (Fig. 2).

Microneurovascular Free Muscle Transfer

The most satisfactory procedure currently in use to reanimate the faces of patients whose facial musculature has atrophied or who have a developmental facial paresis is a free muscle transfer with neurovascular anastomosis. The most experience has been reported with a two-stage procedure in which crossed facial nerve grafting is performed first; muscle transfer is performed when axons have reached the ipsilateral face. The gracilis muscle is most often used for this procedure, although the flexor digitorum and serratus muscles may be used. The results of this procedure have been rated excellent in 50% to 60% of patients (70,71).

A more attractive option may be a one-stage procedure to place a hypoglossal-facial jump graft. Our preliminary results with this procedure have been very satisfactory. However, these procedures are technically challenging and require specialized training in microvascular surgery, and long-term results, particularly in children, have not yet been assessed.

Pedicled Temporalis or Masseter Transpositions

The indications for a pedicled temporalis or masseter muscle transposition procedure are the same as indications for microneurovascular free muscle transfer. These transpositions have been successful in providing excellent tone in facial muscles, and when the patient spends time training muscles to create a smile and other facial expressions, voluntary movement is satisfactory. Transposition procedures are most appropriate for rehabilitating the lower half of the face, but the procedures described above to reanimate the eye have provided excellent functional and cosmetic results for the upper face.

Case Histories

The following case reports offer vignettes of treatment choices and outcomes for managing facial paralysis due to a variety of causes.

Case History 1

A child who was involved in a motor vehicle accident suffered lacerations by glass in the preauricular area and presented with a facial weakness. The wound was explored, the ends of the lacerated upper division of the facial nerve were debrided, and the nerve was repaired primarily (Fig. 4). Evaluation 1 year after surgery showed some persistent weakness with eye closure (Fig. 5) and smiling (Fig. 6).

Case History 2

A young man underwent resection of a facial nerve schwannoma through a combined transmastoid-middle fossa approach (Fig. 7). A section of the sural cutaneous nerve was harvested for grafting by using the lateral malleolus (Fig. 8) and the lesser saphenous vein (Fig. 9) as landmarks. The sural nerve graft was sutured into the facial nerve in the middle fossa (Fig. 10). The patient had symmetry on eye closure (Fig. 11) and was able to produce a spontaneous

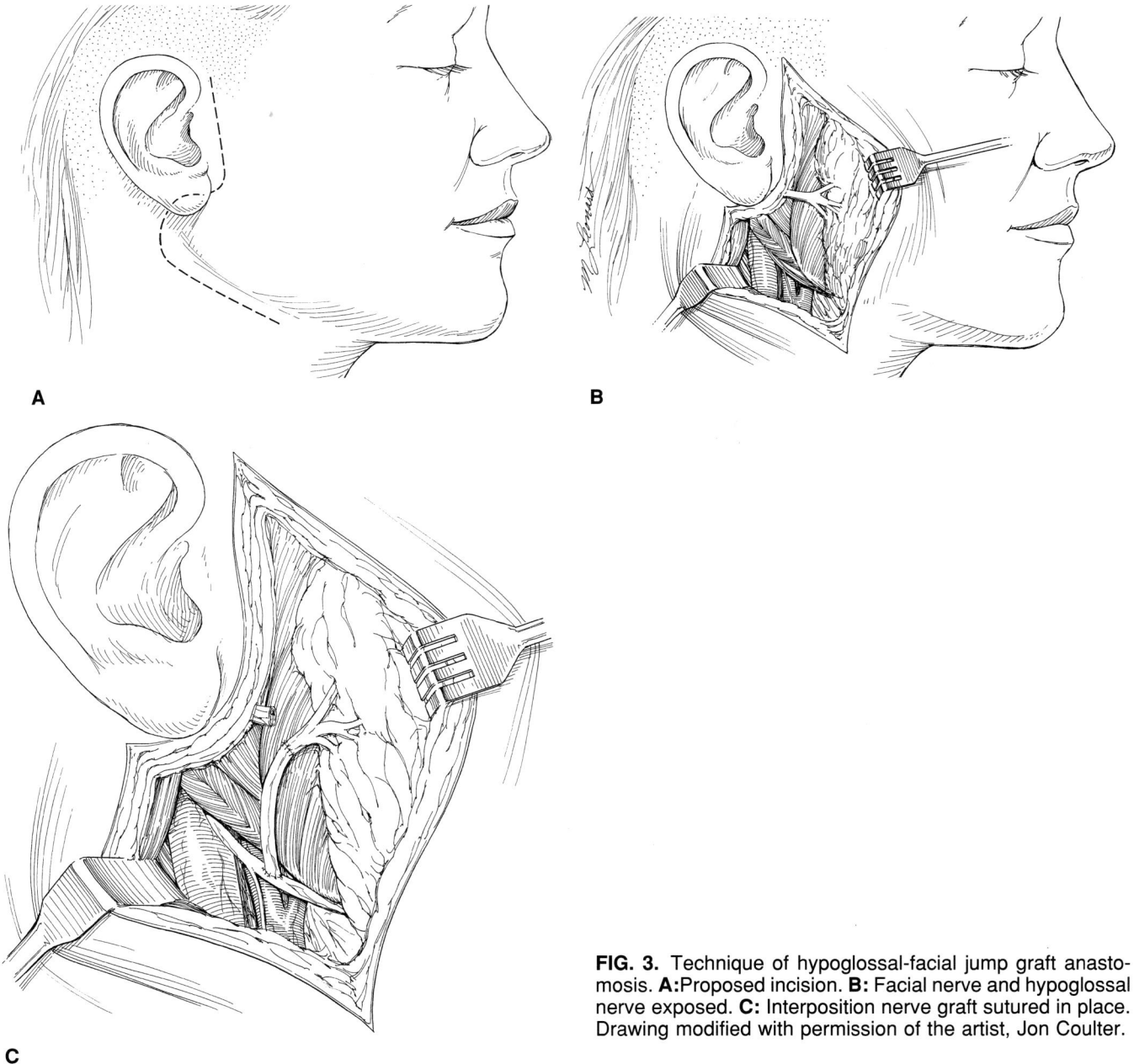

FIG. 3. Technique of hypoglossal-facial jump graft anastomosis. **A:** Proposed incision. **B:** Facial nerve and hypoglossal nerve exposed. **C:** Interposition nerve graft sutured in place. Drawing modified with permission of the artist, Jon Coulter.

smile (Fig. 12). Best results are achieved by reestablishing the continuity of the facial nerve, regardless of the length of graft or number of anastomoses required.

Case History 3

A 15-year-old underwent resection of a large acoustic neuroma (Fig. 13). The facial nerve was resected as part of the tumor (Fig. 14) and the patient was referred for early reanimation. There was no proximal seventh nerve to which to attach a graft, so a hypoglossal-facial jump graft was placed within the first month of injury. One year after reanimation surgery, this adolescent had excellent facial function (Fig. 15–18). These results demonstrate the importance of early reinervation of the transected facial nerve, especially when the facial nerve cannot be repaired.

Case History 4

A 20-year-old woman presented with right-sided facial weakness (Fig. 19). Synkinesis of her platysma and periorbicular area suggested that the incomplete paralysis was traumatic in origin, but it was in fact developmental. Surgery was performed. It is necessary to overcorrect the tension on the temporalis muscle (Fig. 20), and 9 months postoperatively she had a more balanced smile (Fig. 21). Recently, we have used an innervated free gracilis muscle flap for such procedures.

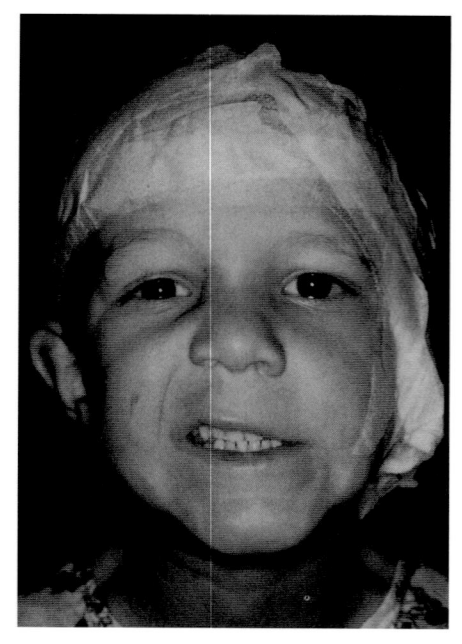

FIG. 4. Immediate postoperative view of child with traumatic facial nerve injury.

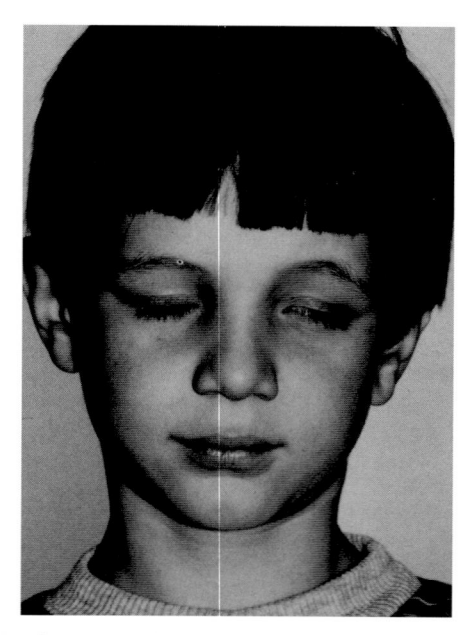

FIG. 5. One year after neurorrhaphy, with eyes closed.

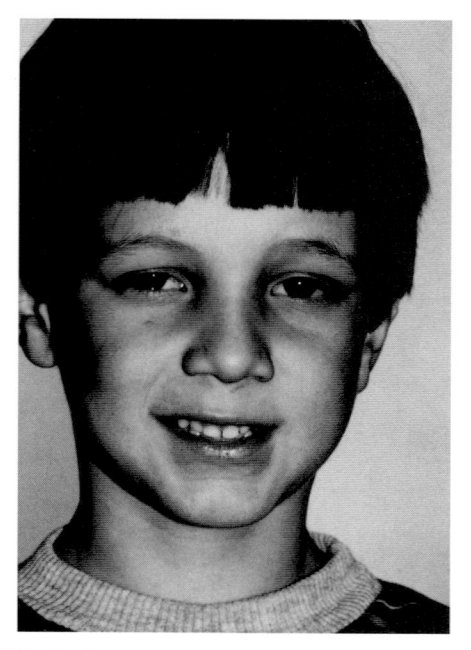

FIG. 6. One year after neurorrhaphy, smiling.

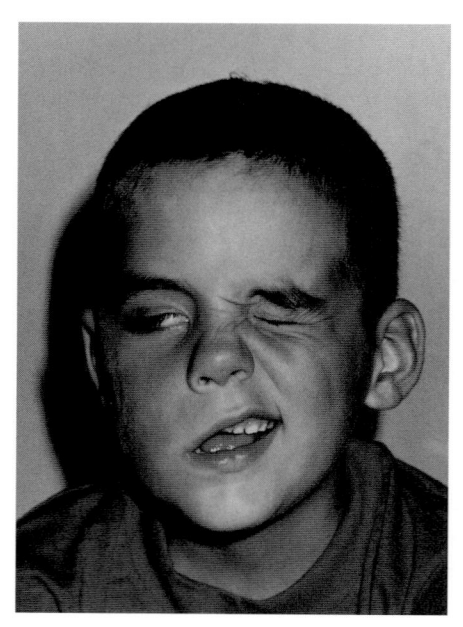

FIG. 7. Right-sided facial paralysis after resection of a facial nerve schwannoma.

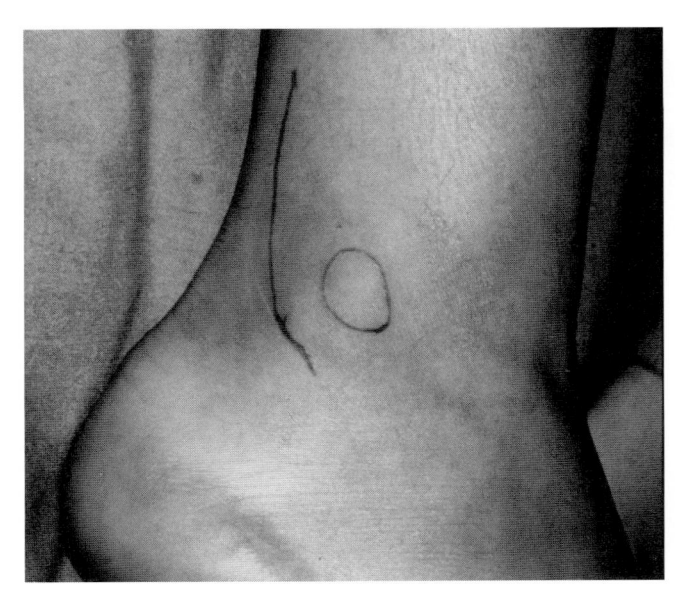

FIG. 8. Lateral malleus was used as a landmark to locate the sural cutaneous nerve.

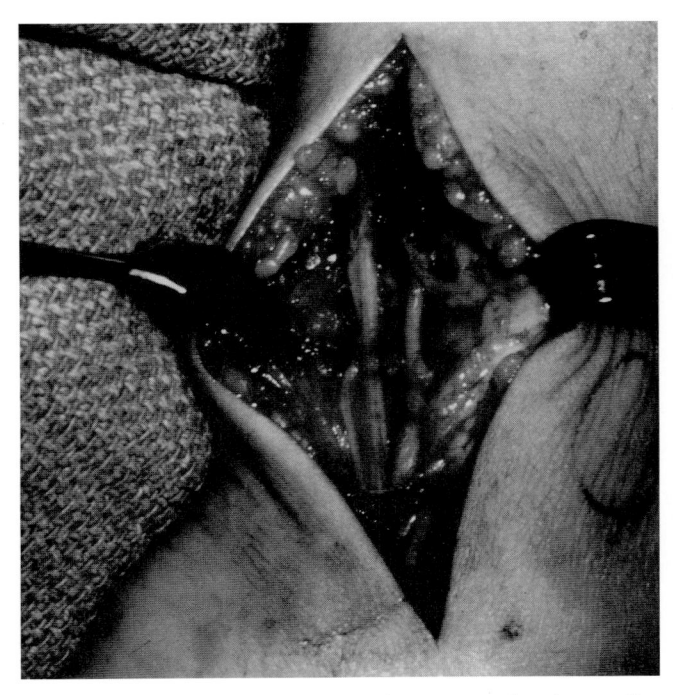

FIG. 9. The lesser saphenous vein was used to locate the section of sural cutaneous nerve to be harvested as a graft for the facial nerve.

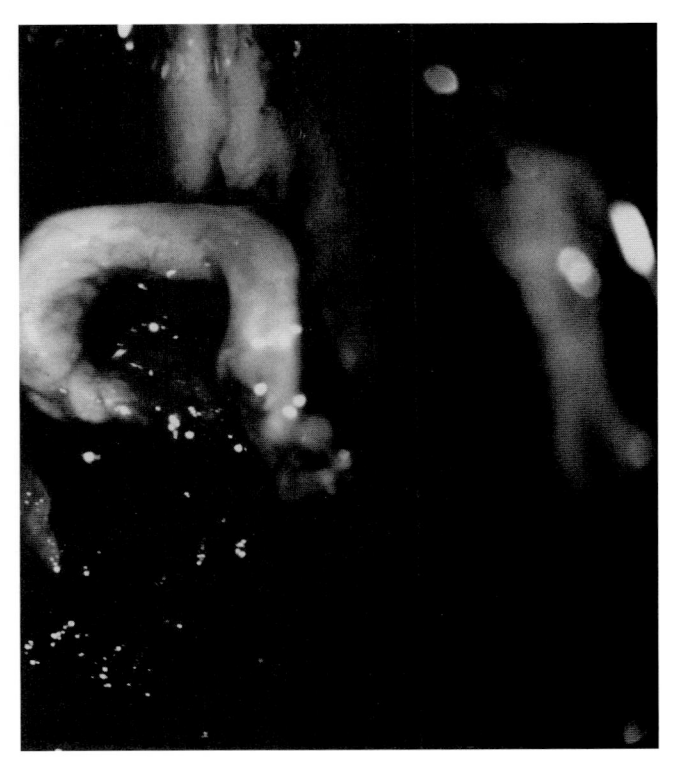

FIG. 10. The sural nerve graft is sutured in place to restore continuity of the facial nerve in the middle fossa.

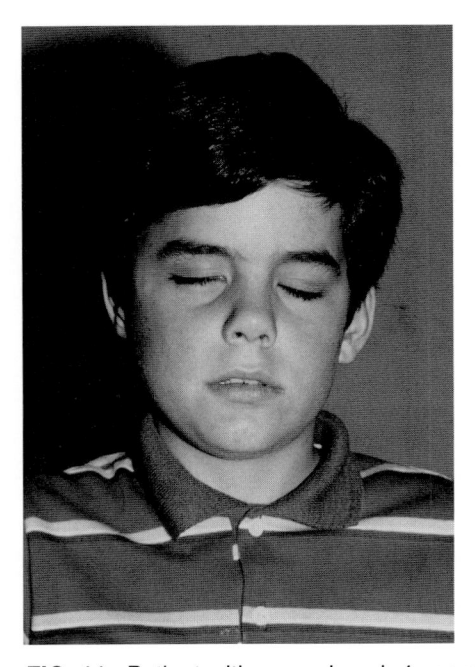

FIG. 11. Patient with eyes closed, 4 years after surgery.

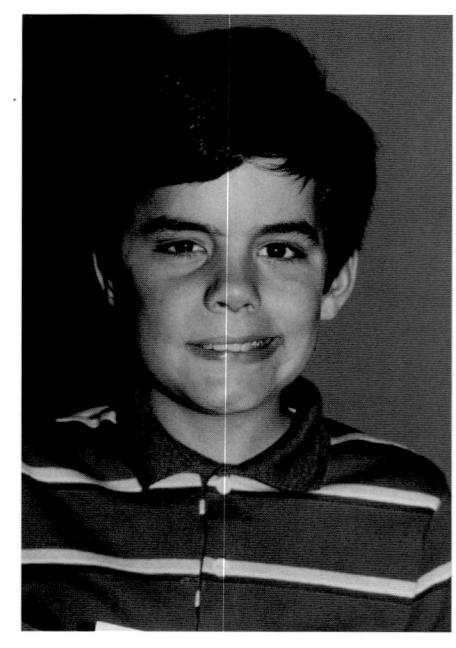

FIG. 12. Patient smiling 4 years after surgery.

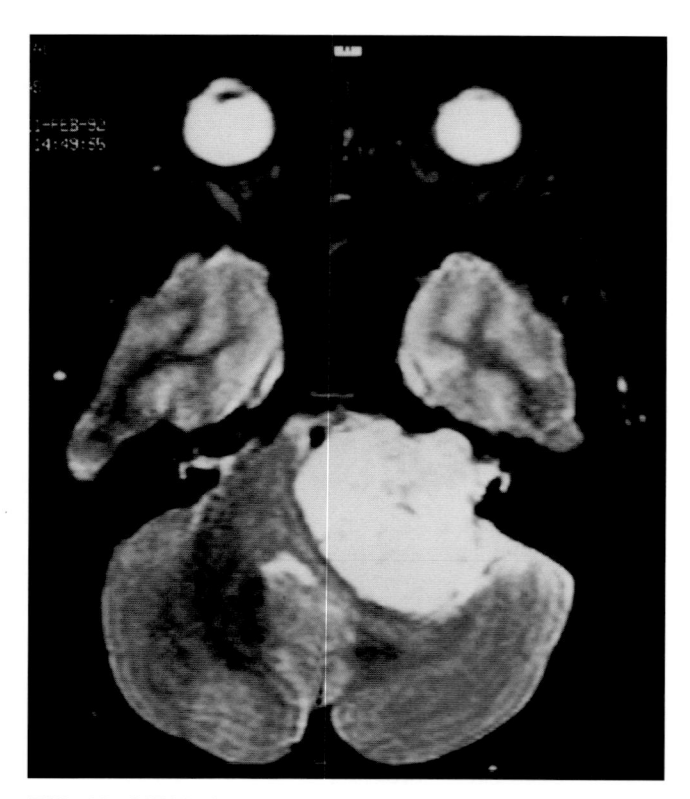

FIG. 13. MRI before tumor resection shows large lesion in the cerebellopontine angle.

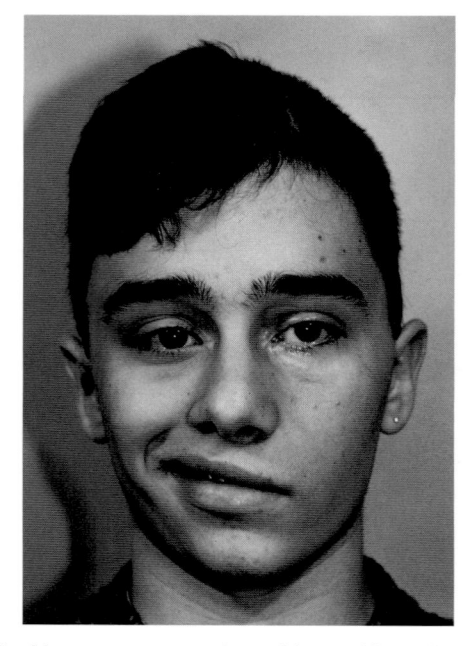

FIG. 14. After tumor resection with sacrifice of a segment of the facial nerve on the left, patient had left-sided facial paralysis.

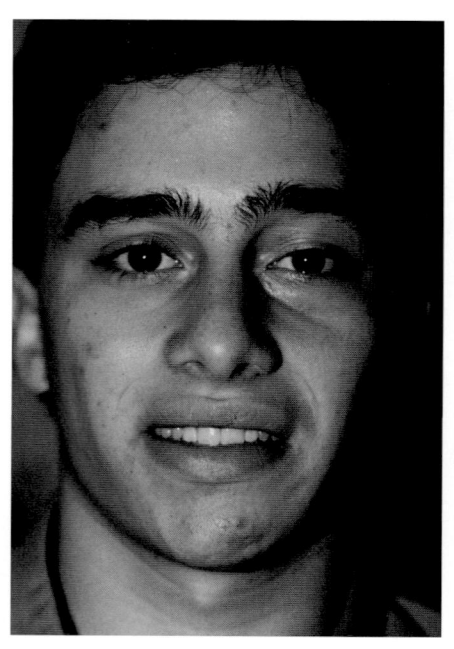

FIG. 15. One year after reanimation of the left face by a hypoglossal-facial jump graft procedure, patient has excellent facial function.

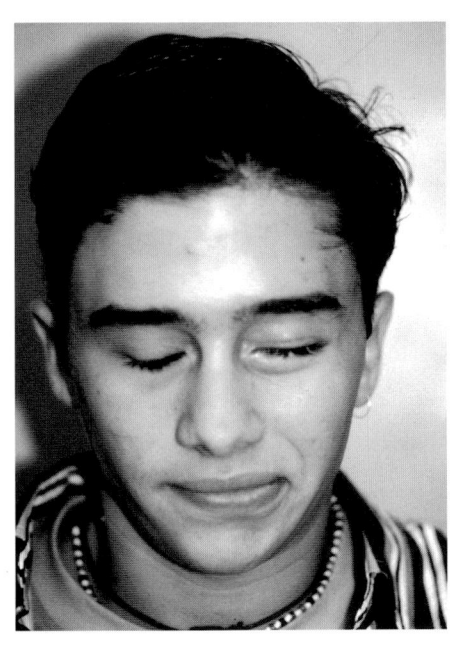

FIG. 16. One year after reanimation of the left face by a hypoglossal-facial jump graft procedure, patient has excellent facial function.

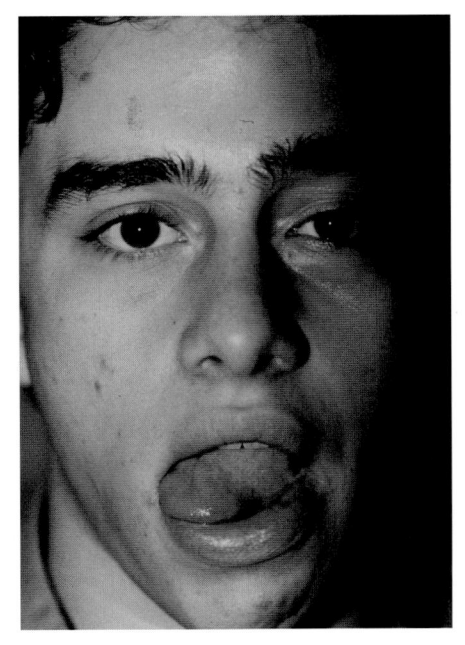

FIG. 17. One year after reanimation of the left face by a hypoglossal-facial jump graft procedure, patient shows excellent tongue movement.

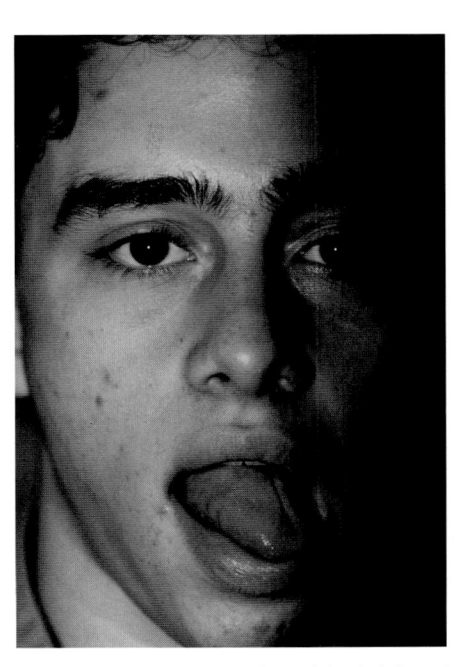

FIG. 18. One year after reanimation of the left face by a hypoglossal-facial jump graft procedure, patient shows excellent tongue movement.

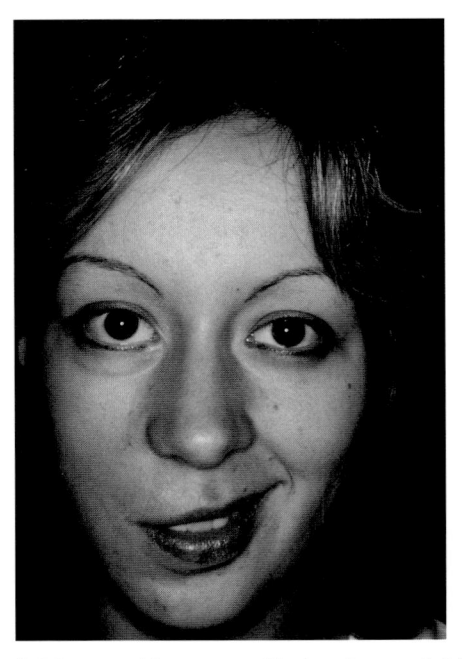

FIG. 19. A 20-year-old woman with developmental facial paralysis.

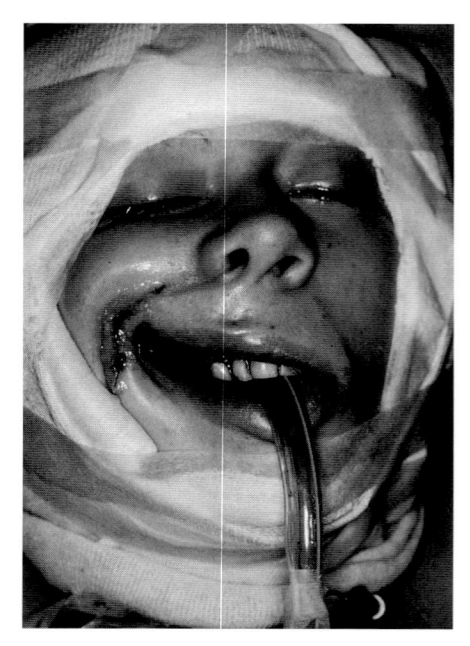

FIG. 20. A right temporalis muscle flap was used to animate the face. The flap was sutured to overcorrect the smile at the time of surgery.

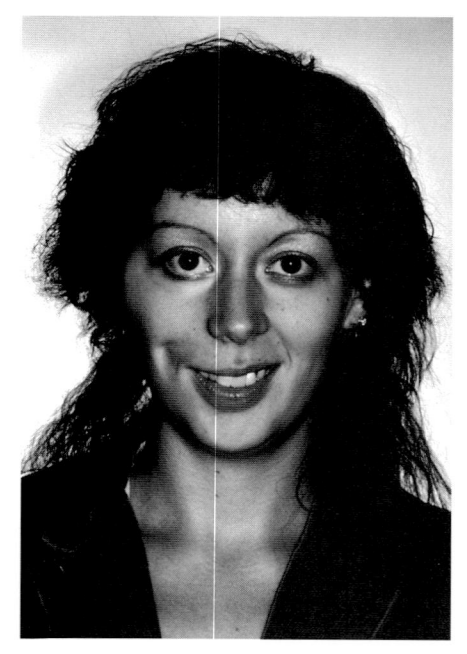

FIG. 21. Nine months after surgery to place a right temporalis muscle flap, the patient has a more balanced smile.

REFERENCES

1. Gasser RF. The development of the facial nerve in man. *Ann Otol Rhinol Laryngol* 1967;76:37–56.
2. Gasser RF. The development of the facial muscles in man. *Am J Anat* 1967;120:357–376.
3. Jahrsdoerfer RA. The facial nerve in congenital middle ear malformations. *Laryngoscope* 1981;91:1217–1224.
4. Proctor B, Nager GT. The facial canal: normal anatomy, variations and anomalies. *Ann Otol Rhinol Laryngol Suppl* 1982;93:33–61.
5. Johnson LG, Kingsley RC. Herniation of the facial nerve in the middle ear. *Arch Otolaryngol* 1970;91:598–602.
6. Van Buskirk C. The seventh nerve complex. *J Comp Neurol* 1945;82:303–333.
7. Seddon HJ. Three types of nerve injury. *Brain* 1943;66:237–288.
8. Sunderland S. *Nerve and nerve injuries,* 2nd ed. London: Churchill Livingstone; 1978:88–89, 96–97, 133.
9. Zilstorff-Pedersen K. Quantitative measurements of the nasolacrimal reflex in normal and in peripheral facial paralysis. *Arch Otolaryngol* 1965;81:457–462.
10. Kvarup V. Electro-gustometry: a method for clinical taste examinations. *Acta Otolaryngol (Stockh)* 1958;49:294–305.
11. Blatt IM. Bell's palsy. I. Diagnosis and prognosis of idiopathic peripheral facial paralysis by submaxillary salivary flow—chorda tympani nerve testing. A study of 102 patients. *Laryngoscope* 1965;75:1081–1091.
12. Tschiassny K. Eight syndromes of facial paralysis and their significance in locating lesions. *Ann Otol Rhinol Laryngol* 1953;62:677–691.
13. May M, Blumenthal F, Taylor RH. Bell's palsy: surgery based upon prognostic indicators and results. *Laryngoscope* 1981;91:2092–2103.
14. May M, Blumenthal F, Klein SR. Acute Bell's palsy: prognostic value of evoked electromyography, maximal stimulation, and other electrical tests. *Am J Otol* 1983;1:1–7.
15. Ruboyianes JM, Adour KK, Santos DQ, von Doersten PG. The maximal stimulation and facial nerve conduction latency tests: predicting the outcome of Bell's palsy. *Laryngoscope* 1994;104:1–6.
16. Fisch U, Esslen E. The surgical treatment of facial hyperkinesia. *Arch Otolaryngol* 1972;95:400–404.
17. Fisch U, Esslen E. Total intratemporal exposure of the facial nerve: pathologic findings in Bell's palsy. *Arch Otolaryngol* 1972;95:335–341.
18. May M, Klein SR, Taylor FH. Idiopathic (Bell's) facial palsy: natural history defies steroid or surgical treatment. *Laryngoscope* 1985;95:406–409.
19. Blumenthal F, May M. Electrodiagnosis. In: May M, ed. *The facial nerve.* New York: Thieme; 1986.
20. Fisch U. Prognostic value of electrical tests in acute facial paralysis. *Am J Otol* 1984;5:494–498.
21. Sillman JS, Niparko JK, Lee SS, Kileny PR. Prognostic value of evoked and standard electromyography in acute facial paralysis. *Otolaryngol Head Neck Surg* 1992;107:377–381.
22. Metson R, Rebeiz E, West C, Thornton A. Magnetic stimulation of the facial nerve. *Laryngoscope* 1991;101:25–30.
23. Kartush JM, Bouchard KR, Graham MD, Linstrom CL. Magnetic stimulation of the facial nerve. *Am J Otol* 1989;10:14–19.
24. Rimpilainen I, Karma P, Laranne J. Eskola H, Hakkinen V. Magnetic facial nerve stimulation in Bell's palsy. *Acta Otolaryngol (Stockh)* 1992;112:311–316.
25. Murphy TP, Teller DC. Magnetic resonance imaging of the facial nerve during Bell's palsy. *Otolaryngol Head Neck Surg* 1991;105:667–674.
26. Weber AL, McKenna MJ. Radiological evaluation of the facial nerve. *Isr J Med Sci* 1992;28:186–192.
27. Falko NA, Erickson E. Facial nerve palsy in the newborn: incidence and outcome. *Plast Reconstr Surg* 1990;85:1–4.
28. Harris LE, Stayura LA, Ramirez-Talavera PF, et al. Congenital and acquired abnormalities observed in live born and stillborn neonates. *Mayo Clin Proc* 1975;50:85–90.
29. Smith JD, Crumley R, Harker L. Facial paralysis in the newborn. *Otolaryngol Head Neck Surg* 1981;89:1021–1024.
30. Hepner WR Jr. Some observations on facial paresis in the newborn infant: etiology and incidence. *Pediatrics* 1951;8:494–497.
31. Parmalee AH. Molding due to intra-uterine posture: facial paralysis probably due to such molding. *Am J Dis Child* 1931;42:443–445.

32. Bergman I, May M, Wessel HB, Stool SE. Management of facial palsy caused by birth trauma. *Laryngoscope* 1986;96:381.
33. Bergstrom L, Baker BB. Syndromes associated with congenital facial paralysis. *Otolaryngol Head Neck Surg* 1981;89:336–342.
34. Harris JP, Davidson TM, May M, Tria T. Evaluation and treatment of congenital facial paralysis. *Arch Otolaryngol* 1983;109:145–151.
35. May M. Facial nerve disorders in the newborn and children. In: May M ed. *The facial nerve.* New York: Thieme; 1986.
36. Byerly KA, Pauli RM. Cranial nerve abnormalities in CHARGE association. *Am J Med Genet* 1993;45:751–757.
37. Narcy P, Tran-Ba-Huy E, Margoloff B, et al. Indications therapeutiques dans les paralysies faciales du nouveau-ne. *Ann Otolaryngol Chir Cervicofac (Paris)* 1982;99:377–382.
38. Saito H, Takeda T, Kishimoto S. Neonatal facial nerve defect. *Acta Otolaryngol Suppl (Stockh)* 1994;510:77–81.
39. May M, Fria T, et al. Facial paralysis in children. *Otolaryngol Head Neck Surg* 1981;89:841–848.
40. May M. Red chorda tympani nerve and Bell's palsy. *Laryngoscope* 1974;84:1507.
41. Peitersen E. The natural history of Bell's palsy. *Am J Otol* 1982;4:107.
42. Adour K. Medical management of idiopathic (Bell's) palsy. *Otolaryngol Clin North Am* 1991;24:663–674.
43. Stankiewicz JA. A review of the published data on steroids and idiopathic facial paralysis. *Otolaryngol Head Neck Surg* 1987;97:481–485.
44. Austin JR, Peskind SP, Austin SG, Rice DH. Idiopathic facial nerve paralysis: a randomized double blind controlled study of placebo versus prednisone. *Laryngoscope* 1993;103:1326–1333.
45. Fisch U. Surgery for Bell's palsy. *Arch Otolaryngol Head Neck Surg* 1981;107:1–11.
46. Tschiassny K. Facial palsy, when complicating a case of acute otitis media, indicative for immediate mastoid operation? *Cincinnati J Med* 1944;25:262.
47. Robillard RB, Hilsinger RL Jr, Adour KK. Ramsay Hunt facial paralysis: clinical analysis of 185 patients. *Otolaryngol Head Neck Surg* 1986; 95:292–297.
48. Dickins J, Smith J, Graham S. Herpes zoster oticus: treatment with intravenous acyclovir. *Laryngoscope* 1988;98:776–779.
49. Uri N, Greenberg E, Meyer W, Kitzes-Cohen R. Herpes zoster oticus: treatment with acyclovir. *Ann Otol Rhinol Laryngol* 1992;101:161.
50. Christen HJ, Bartlau N, Hanefield F, et al. Peripheral facial palsy in childhood; Lyme borreliosis to be suspected until proven otherwise. *Acta Paediatr Scand* 1990;79:1219–1224.
51. Steele AC. Lyme disease. *N Engl J Med* 1989;321:586–596.
52. Mishell JH, Applebaum EL. Ramsay Hunt syndrome in a patient with HIV infection. *Otolaryngol Head Neck Surg* 1990;102:177–179.
53. Langford-Kuntz A, Reichert P, Pohle HD. Impairment of cranio-facial nerve due to AIDS. *Int J Oral Maxillofac Surg* 1988;17:227–229.
54. Linstrom CJ, Pincus RL, Leavitt EB, Urbina MC. Otologic neurotologic manifestations of HIV-related disease. *Otolaryngol Head Neck Surg* 1993;108:680–687.
54a. Shapiro A, Schaitkin B, and May M. Facial paralysis in children. In: Bluestone, Stool, Kema. Pediatric Otolaryngology, 3e Saunders, Philadelphia, 1996.
55. Lilleyman JS, Antoniou AG, Sugden PJ. Facial nerve palsy in acute leukemia. *Scand J Hematol* 1979;22:87–90.
56. Feldman BA. Rhabdomyosarcoma of the head and neck. *Laryngoscope* 1982;92:424–440.
57. Woorsae N, Christensen KC, Schiodt M, Reibel J. Melkersson-Rosenthal syndrome and cheilitis granulomatosa. *Oral Surg* 1982;54:404.
58. Carr RD. Is the Melkersson-Rosenthal syndrome hereditary? *Arch Dermatol* 1966;93:426.
59. Graham MD, Kartush JM. Total facial nerve decompression for recurrent facial paralysis: an update. *Otolaryngol Head Neck Surg* 1989; 101:442.
60. Kleinman MB, Passo MH. Incomplete Kawasaki disease with facial nerve paralysis and coronary artery involvement. *Pediatr Infect Dis J* 1988;7:301–302.
61. Hendrick EB, Harwood-Hash MR. Head injuries in children. *Clin Neurosurg* 1964;11:1964.
62. Glarner H, Meuli M, Hof E, et al. Management of petrous bone fractures in children: analysis of 127 cases. *J Trauma* 1994;36:198–201.
63. McKennan, KX, Chole RA. Facial paralysis in temporal bone trauma. *Am J Otol* 1992;13:167–172.
64. Rulon JT, Hallberg OE. Operative injuries to the facial nerve. Explanation for its occurrence during operations on the temporal bone and suggestions for its prevention. *Arch Otolaryngol Head Neck Surg* 1962; 76:131.
65. Glasscock ME. Unusual facial nerve problems. Some thoughts on identifying the nerve in the temporal bone. *Laryngoscope* 1971;81:8669.
66. May M, Sobol S, Mester SJ. Managing segmental facial nerve injuries by surgical repair. *Laryngoscope* 1990;100:1062–1067.
67. Levine RE, May M. Ophthalmologic Medical Management. In: May M, ed. The Facial Nerve, Thieme, 1986, 399.
68. May M. Gold weight and wire spring implants as alternatives to tarsorrhaphy. *Arch Otolaryngol Head Neck Surg* 1987;113:656–660.
69. May M, Sobol SM, and Mester SJ. Hypoglosal facial nerve interposition-jump graft for facial reanimation without tongue atrophy. *Otolaryngol Head neck surg* 1991;104:818.
70. Aviv J, Urken M. Management of the paralyzed face with microneurovascular free muscle transfer. *Arch Otolaryngol Head Neck Surg* 1992; 118:909–912.
71. O'Brien B, Pederson W, et al. Results of management of facial palsy with microvascular free muscle transfer. *Plast Reconstr Surg* 1990;86: 12–22.
72. House JW, Brackmann DE. Facial nerve grading system. *Otolaryngol Head Neck Surg* 1985;93:146–147.

PART X
HIV Infection

CHAPTER 31

Otologic Disorders in the HIV-Positive Child

J. Christopher Post and Garth D. Ehrlich

Acquired immunodeficiency syndrome (AIDS) is characterized by a decrease in the patient's ability to fight infections and by infections with opportunistic organisms and organisms not normally found in an immunocompetent host. Otologic findings in the human immunodeficiency virus (HIV)-positive child include recurrent otitis media (OM), unsusual infections of the temporal bone, and sensorineural hearing loss. Because the number of children with AIDS is increasing, it is of great interest to health-care providers to know the incidence of OM in the pediatric AIDS population and the severity of disease in an immunoincompetent host. It is also important to know whether the causal organisms are the same or different from the usual organisms that cause otologic infections in children. The answers to these questions have important implications for treatment.

OTITIS MEDIA

Otitis media is one of the most common infections in children and results from a complex interplay of infectious agents, host immune and anatomic factors, and environmental influences. It is the most common primary diagnosis made by pediatric practitioners in the United States for children under the age of 15 years (1). Speech and language development can be affected adversely by the hearing loss resulting from OM (2). Otitis media is the most common reason children receive antimicrobial therapy and surgery, and the economic impact of OM is substantial, with over $3.5 billion spent annually in the United States. for the medical and surgical treatment of this disease (3).

Acute OM is characterized by otalgia, fever, and other constitutional signs and symptoms. Physical examination reveals a red or opaque tympanic membrane with decreased mobility. Acute OM is extremely common in normal children, with 83% of children followed to age 3 years experiencing at least one episode and 46% of 698 children documented as having at least three episodes (4). Otitis media with effusion (OME) is a more chronic condition characterized by the presence of fluid in the middle ear cavity for a prolonged period with minimal constitutional symptoms except for hearing loss (2). Physical examination will show a dull, semiopacified tympanic membrane with fluid behind it, and occasionally air bubbles will be seen. Tympanometry performed on children with either acute AOM or OME will demonstrate decreased tympanic membrane mobility. The pathogenesis of OME appears to be multifactorial, involving immature anatomy, initiating viral infections that induce eustachian tube dysfunction, retrograde movement of bacteria from the oropharynx into the middle-ear cavity, and host physiologic factors.

HUMAN IMMUNODEFICIENCY VIRUS

Acquired immunodeficiency syndrome first came to medical attention with the hospitalization of five homosexual men in Los Angeles with *Pneumocystis carinii* pneumonia (5). Other reports of followed opportunistic infections and unusual cancers, such as Kaposi's sarcoma, in homosexual men (6). Cases were then reported among intravenous drug users and hemophiliacs, suggesting that the cause of AIDS could be a blood-borne pathogen. Acquired immunodeficiency syndrome then began to appear in the pediatric population (7,8). The predominant route of pediatric infection is

---

J.C. Post and G.D. Ehrlich: Center for Genomic Sciences, Department of Otolaryngology, Allegheny University of the Health Sciences, Pittsburgh, Pennsylvania 15212-4772.

by vertical transmission from the mother, with contaminated blood products another mode of transmission. Almost all children born to HIV-infected mothers are HIV antibody–positive at birth, but only 15% to 30% of these children are actually infected with HIV (9). Because maternally derived IgG antibody can persist for as long as 18 months of age in the child, antibody testing cannot reliably indicate the child's infectious status before 18 months of age. Conversely, virus culture and the polymerase chain reaction (PCR) can identify nearly 100% of infected infants by the age of 3 to 6 months (10).

The primary etiologic agent of AIDS is a retrovirus, HIV type 1 (HIV-1). Earlier names for HIV include human T-cell lymphotrophic virus III (HTLV-III) or lymphadenopathy-associated virus. This virus is characterized by an extremely high mutation rate, which results in its very rapid evolution and ability to evade the hosts' immune system. A second human retrovirus with a slightly different genomic structure, termed *HIV-2,* is responsible for a small percentage of AIDS cases worldwide. This pathogen is primarily confined to certain West African populations and immigrants from those locales in Western Europe. Fewer than 50 cases of HIV-2 infection have been detected in the United States, whereas the number of HIV-1 cases has been estimated at greater than 2 million.

Both HIV-1 and HIV-2 are in the retroviral subfamily Lentivirinae. The lentiviruses are distinguished from the oncoviruses, the second major pathogenic subfamily of retroviruses, in that they are associated with chronic cytopathic infections of the immune and central nervous systems. In contrast, the Oncovirinae are transforming viruses, which result in immortalization and transformation of the cells that they infect. Examples of human oncoviruses include human T-cell lymphoma/leukemia viruses types I and II (HTLV-I and -II). The former is associated with adult T-cell lymphoma/leukemia and the latter with large granular lymphomas.

The sine qua non of retroviruses is their unique life cycle. The infectious viral particle contains a diploid single-stranded RNA genome and a unique DNA polymerase, termed *reverse transcriptase* (RT). The RT is an RNA-dependent DNA polymerase that utilizes the ssRNA within the viral particle as a template for the synthesis of a double-stranded DNA provirus with long terminal repeats, which facilitate control of the various viral genes. The provirus is then inserted into the host's genome where it can direct production of viral particles (horizontal transmission) and can also be passed on to daughter cells when the infected cell replicates its DNA and divides (vertical transmission).

Human immunodeficiency virus 1, as with all of the human retroviruses, is transmitted by an exchange of body fluids and tissues via sexual intercourse, intravenous drug abuse, organ donation, blood, and blood product donation. Almost the entire population of factor VIII–requiring hemophiliacs in the United States during the first half of the 1980s became infected with HIV-1. This occurred because most of the individuals who donated blood for factor VIII were paid donors and a very high percentage of these individuals were intravenous drug abusers (IVDAs) who sold their blood to buy illicit drugs. These IVDA populations were ravaged very early in the HIV-1 epidemic because of their sharing infected needles.

All health-care workers are at risk for contracting HIV-1 infection through body fluid contact, and these considerations led to the promulgation and adoption in 1984 of universal biohazard precautions. Universal biohazard precautions state that all body fluids from all individuals, whether known to be infected or not, are considered infectious and treated accordingly. Surgeons and surgical teams are at elevated risk of acquiring HIV-1 infections because of the extent of and length of contact with body fluids. In a prospective study of middle ear pathogens in adults, four HIV-positive patients developed OM and underwent tympanocentesis (11). All four middle ear effusions were positive for both HIV DNA and RNA, by PCR-based and RT PCR–based assays, respectively. These results demonstrate the importance of using universal precautions when dealing with any fluid from HIV-positive patients. However, causality of OM cannot be inferred from these data.

Human immunodeficiency virus 1 infection is characterized by a brief incubation period followed by seroconversion illness during which the patient may present with flulike syndromes and CD4+ lymphocytopenia. During this seroconversion illness, HIV titers can reach titers of greater than 1012 particles/ml. During this seroconversion illness, infected persons are extremely infectious but are not detectable as HIV-1 infected when using standard antigen-based ELISA screening assays, which detect anti-HIV-1 antibody. In one famous case, an individual who died of other causes prior to the development of anti-HIV-1 antibodies, and was, therefore, not detected as being HIV-1–positive, transmitted HIV-1 to 17 other individuals who received his organs and tissues through transplant procedures. This case has led to a joint program between the National Heart Lung and Blood Institute and the Food and Drug Administration to support the development and licensure of direct nucleic acid–based screening tests for HIV-1 infection to augment current serologic detection modalities. It is felt that such direct testing, which does not rely on the body's ability to direct an immune response, will substantially reduce the period between infection and detection of infection.

The primary target of infection by HIV-1 is the CD4− helper lymphocyte; however, HIV-1 can infect numerous other cell types, including macrophages, microglial cells, endothelial cells, and follicular dendritic cells. It is currently felt that HIV-1 is through its infection of dendritic cells early in the disease that it is rapidly spread through the body, because dendritic cells are professional antigen-presenting cells and may contact hundreds of CD4+ lymphocytes as part of the antigen presentation process. The dendritic cells pass throughout all of the tissues of the body, carrying their deadly cargo with them.

Convincing evidence has accumulated that the best predictor of how long an HIV-1 infected individual will remain AIDS-free, following the seroconversion illness, is the extent to which the primary immune response can reduce the viral titer. Employing very accurate quantitative measures of viral RNA it is possible to predict the disease-free survival time of individuals. Earlier attempts at quantitative measures of viral levels focused on the provirus; these analyses did not prove to be predictive.

During the asymptomatic stage of infection, the virus does not enter a latent period; rather, the infectious pathogenic process is largely confined to the lymphatic tissues, primarily the lymph nodes. During this time, a very reactive process rages wherein huge numbers of CD4+ cells are produced and killed by HIV-1 infection. Gradually, over time, the virus gains the upper hand in this battle through two processes: mutation and escape from immune detection. As previously stated HIV-1 has a phenomenally high mutation rate; the error rate for the HIV-1 RT is the highest ever described for a DNA polymerase. Due to this high mutation rate, strains eventually will arise that are more cytopathic and have higher replication rates (the two phenomena are probably linked). These strains then reduce the number of immune cells that can fight the infection, setting up a vicious cycle in which fewer CD4+ cells are available to combat ever more viral particles. In individuals who can control the primary infection to a greater extent, it takes much longer to develop a more cytopathic strain, because there a fewer replicating viruses to begin with, thereby minimizing the pool for mutation.

It is likely that the phenotype of the infecting strain plays a major role in how effective the immune system is in controlling postseroconversion viral titers. Evidence suggest that if a person is infected by an individual with frank AIDS, or by an individual who will progress rapidly to AIDS, they are more likely to experience rapid disease progression themselves than somebody who is infected by an individual who is starting a long asymptomatic period. These observations would explain the epidemiology of the infection observed in the major coastal cities of the United States in the early 1980s, where huge numbers of individuals perished in very short periods. These individuals would have been spreading highly pathogenic strains of HIV-1 that resulted in rapid disease progression thereby limiting time for spread. As often happens with highly virulent parasites, it burned itself out because it did not keep the host alive long enough to ensure spread once the high-risk populations were saturated. Less pathogenic strains ensure a healthy host for an extended period, which increases their chance of transmission.

CLASSIFICATION OF HUMAN IMMUNODEFICIENCY VIRUS INFECTION IN CHILDREN

As understanding of the disease has progressed, the classification systems for HIV infection in children have been refined and expanded. Recognizing differences between adult and pediatric AIDS, in 1987 the Center for Disease Control (CDC) adopted a separate classification system for HIV infection for children under 13 years of age in (12). This system classified children into three classes: class P-0 (indeterminate infection); class P-1 (asymptomatic infection); and class P-2 (symptomatic infection). Class P-1 was divided into three subclasses based on immune function, and class P-2 was divided into multiple subclasses and categories, based largely upon the presence of specified infections or cancers.

In 1994, the CDC (9) revised the classification for children, based on additional knowledge of the progression of pediatric AIDS, and progress made in diagnosis, to better reflect the disease process. This new system classifies HIV-infected children into categories based on three parameters: (a) infection status, (b) clinical status, and (c) immunologic status. Under this new system, a child's placement into a specific classification has prognostic significance and attempts to balance medical accuracy with a simple-to-use system. Determination of the child's infectious status is accomplished by the use of HIV culture, HIV PCR, or HIV antigen determination for children less than 18 months old; HIV-antibody positivity is considered proof in children older than 18 months of age. The classification system also takes into account perinatally exposed children (<18 mo of age and HIV antibody–positive) and seroreverters (asymptomatic children born to HIV-positive mothers who become HIV antibody–negative after 6 mo of age). Clinical status is divided into four mutually exclusive groups: category N (not symptomatic), category A (mildly symptomatic), category B (moderately symptomatic), and category C (severely symptomatic). Immunologic status classification reflects the normal decline in CD4− counts as the child matures and the observation that children can develop opportunistic infections at higher CD4− levels than can adults. Age-specific CD4− T-lymphocyte counts and percentage of total lymphocytes are used to divide children into three immunologic categories: (a) no evidence of suppression, (b) evidence of moderate suppression, and (c) severe suppression. Thus, infected children can be divided into groups ranging from N1 (no signs or symptoms with no evidence of immunologic suppression) to C3 (severe signs and symptoms with severe immunologic suppression).

IMMUNOLOGIC DEFECTS OF ACQUIRED IMMUNODEFICIENCY SYNDROME

Patients with AIDS suffer from infections with opportunistic and unusual organisms from several reasons. Lymphopenia, reversed T-cell helper–suppressor-cell ratios, decreased cell-mediated immunity, and hyperimmunoglobinemia are noted in affected individuals. The lymphopenia is due to a decrease in the absolute number of CD4+ lymphocytes. This reduction leads to an inversion of the CD4+/CD8+ (helper/suppressor) ratio and can serve as a marker of disease progression. Qualitative defects in helper cells are also noted. B-cell lymphocyte function is abnormal, with an increase in spontaneous secretion of immunoglobulins noted, but with a decrease responsiveness to in vivo and in vitro stimulation. These defects in B-cell function can predispose to infection with encapsulated bacteria, such as *Streptococcus pneumoniae* and *Haemophilus influenzae*. This is one of the reasons that recurrent bacterial infections are common early manifestations of HIV infection in children (13). In addition, monocyte and macrophage chemotaxis and intracellular killing capacity are impaired, and granulocytopenia is not uncommon.

PREVALENCE, CLINICAL MANIFESTATIONS, TREATMENT, AND MICROBIOLOGY OF OTITIS MEDIA IN THE HUMAN IMMUNODEFICIENCY VIRUS–POSITIVE CHILD

Barnett and coworkers (14) compared the number of episodes of acute OM in a population of 28 HIV-infected children with that of 33 children who seroreverted to HIV antibody–negative status. There were no differences between the groups in terms of age or risk factors for the mother's HIV status. In the HIV-positive children, the mean number of acute OM episodes per year increased from 1.89 to 2.40, whereas in the control group, the mean number of episodes decreased from 1.33 to 0.13. By age 3 years, 80% of the HIV-positive children had experienced six or more episodes of OM, whereas none of control children had experienced that many episodes. CD4+ lymphocyte counts were predictive of number of infectious episodes, in that children with low counts had a nearly threefold increased risk of recurrent OM, compared with HIV-infected children with normal CD4+ counts. Twenty-one percent of HIV-infected children received tympanotomy tubes, compared with 6% of seroreverted children.

The prevalence of OM and its complications were examined in a retrospective study of 37 children with perinatally acquired HIV infection (15). Approximately half (18) of the children had an AIDS-defining illness. Episodes of OM were documented by the primary care physician and complications, including tympanic membrane perforations and otorrhea, were noted. Tympanotomy tube placement also was recorded. The history of OM was similar in children with perinatally acquired HIV, regardless of whether they had an AIDS-defining illness. However, children with AIDS-defining illnesses underwent tympanotomy tube placement twice as often as did HIV-positive children without AIDS. In addition, the children with AIDS-defining illnesses had twice as many tympanic membrane perforations as did HIV-positive children without an AIDS-defining illness.

The increased incidence of recurrent OM in pediatric AIDS patients is probably multifactorial. The lymphadenopathy that is common in HIV patients can be associated with adenoidal hypertrophy, with subsequent compromise and obstruction of the eustachian tube. Recurrent adenotonsillitis and hypertrophy have been observed in several pediatric AIDS patients, resulting in obstructive sleep apnea (16). An association between adenoid hypertrophy, HIV-positivity, and secretory OM has been reported in adults (17). In this study, 14 adults (eight men and six women) presented with nasal blockage and mouth breathing. Nine of the 14 patients reported decreased hearing, with evidence of secretory OM on physical examination. Lateral neck radiographs were positive for a nasopharyngeal mass, and examination of the nasopharynx under general anesthesia confirmed adenoidal hypertrophy. Biopsies were remarkable for nonspecific follicular and perifollicular lymphoid hyperplasia. Myringotomies were performed on the nine patients with hearing loss, and fluid was noted in seven patients. All patients were positive for HIV.

The clinical manifestations of OM generally do not differ between children with HIV infections and noninfected children. The otolaryngologist should be suspicious of an underlying immunodeficiency when a child with recurrent or chronic OM also has significant cervical adenopathy, axillary or inguinal adenopathy, oral candidiasis (although this may be secondary to chronic antimicrobial use), or failure to thrive (18). Treatment with routine antimicrobial agents for OM generally results in a satisfactory outcome (19). However, unusually frequent or severe episodes of OM should alert the clinician that the patient may be suffering from an undiagnosed immunodeficiency. In a study by Church (20), eight of 21 children exhibited severe, chronic, or recurrent episodes of OM 4 to 34 months before being diagnosed as HIV-positive. Williams (21) reported that eight of ten children with AIDS had either persistent OME, recurrent OM, or chronic otorrhea. *Staphylococcus aureus, S. pneumoniae,* and *Candida* were noted to be commonly cultured, but no incidence data were presented. One child with chronic *Pseudomonas aeruginosa* otitis developed sepsis. No child developed cholesteatoma.

Principi et al. (22), prospectively followed a cohort of 27 HIV-positive children from Milan, Italy, that were individually matched with paired control subjects that were HIV-negative. The occurrence of acute OM was not modified by HIV infection; however, recurrent acute OM (defined as three or more episodes in 6 mo) was more common in P-2 children. The cure rate with amoxicillin was the same in control and P-1 children but was lower in P-2 versus control children (47.3% v. 100%). Interestingly, CD4− counts and CD4−/CD8− ratios were not significantly different in the HIV-infected children with good response to antimicrobial therapy when compared with those who failed therapy. Treatment failures underwent tympanocentesis, with therapy directed according to culture results, or empiric treatment with amoxicillin and clavulanic acid. Two P-2 children developed chronic otorrhea that was repeated culture-positive for *Streptococcus pyogenes.*

Culture results from middle ear fluid obtained by tympanocentesis from 17 of 19 cases of acute OM in P-2 children were similar to the culture results generally found in Italian children with acute OM. Specifically, *S. pneumoniae* was cultured in six cases (33.5%), *H. influenzae* nontypable in two cases (11.7%), *S. pyogenes* in two cases (11.7%), *Proteus mirabilis* in two cases, (11.7%) and *Escherichia coli* in one case (5.9%). Four cases had no growth. All isolates were sensitive to amoxicillin. Given these data, the authors concluded that HIV infection did not increase the occurrence rate of acute OM but did predispose to recurrence. They also recommended treating episodes of acute OM in P-1 children in the same manner that normal children would be treated. The authors suggested that P-2 children receive prophylactic antibiotics after the first or second episode of acute OM and that therapy be extended for 14 days.

In a later study from the same group (23), the microbiology of acute OM was systematically studied using culture results from tympanocentesis. The microbiology of 60 episodes of acute OM occurring in 21 HIV-positive children was compared with that of 121 episodes occurring in 113 normal children. *Streptococcus pneumonia, H. influenzae* and group A beta-hemolytic Streptococcus were the three most commonly cultured organisms, and there was no difference between the two groups. Interestingly, *S. aureus* was significantly more frequent in children with severe immunocompromise. No penicillin-resistant *S. pneumoniae* was isolated, and beta-lactamase production by *H. influenzae* isolates was unusual, which reflects the overall Italian experience. Children who were HIV-positive also had a higher rate of culture-positive effusions, which the authors believed to be a result of local mucosal immune dysfunction in this group of patients. The low prevalence of *Moraxella catarrhalis* (only one isolate) reflects the low prevalence of this organism in normal Italian children. The authors suggest that, given the similarity of microbiologic results between HIV-positive children and normal children, tympanocentesis is not necessary in all patients but only in those that fail first-line antimicrobial agents. Antimicrobial therapy should be the same as for normal children in the same geographic region. In addition, the empiric choice of antimicrobials for severely immunocompromised children should take into account the increased incidence noted of *S. aureus* in cultures.

In recurrent cases of OM or OME, a nasopharyngeal examination should be considered to evaluate the patient for enlarged adenoid tissue or, in older populations, malignant nasopharyngeal processes such as Kaposi's sarcoma (24).

UNUSUAL ORGANISMS IN OTITIS MEDIA

Infections with unusual and opportunistic organisms is one of the hallmarks of AIDS, and otologic infections with these types of organisms in the adult population have been reported. *Pneumocystis carinii* has been shown to cause OM and mastoiditis (25,26) and generally presents as an aural polypoid mass with conductive hearing loss. Biopsy of the mass will show a foamy, eosinophilic exudate on H&E stain, and staining with methenamine-silver stain demonstrates the cysts of *P. carinii*. The incidence of *P. carinii* otologic involvement in AIDS patients is increasing and can present without concomitant pulmonary disease (27). *Pneumocystis carinii* OM may be the inital manifestation of HIV infection (28,29).

Aspergillus fumigatus has been reported as causing an otomastoiditis in two adult patients (30). In one patient, conservative medical management resulted in a favorable outcome, whereas the other patient, despite aggressive imaging and surgical intervention, the fungus progressed to dural sinus thrombosis with extension into the brain. The authors recommend that early imaging and mastoidectomy be used to manage immunocompromised patients presenting with otomycoses.

TEMPORAL BONE FINDINGS

Several studies on the histopathologic findings in the temporal bones of AIDS patients have been reported. Ten temporal bones from five adult patients, (three men with AIDS, one man with AIDS-related complex, and one woman with AIDS), were obtained and the results of light and electron microscopy examination of seven bones reported (31). Only one patient had a history of otologic symptoms. Most of the pathologic findings were consistent with a severe inflammatory reaction in the middle ear, mastoid, and petrous air-cell systems. Petrositis with marrow replacement, mastoiditis, otitis, and ossicular destruction were noted. Several findings consistent with viral infection also were noted, including endosteal membrane elevation, subepithelial elevation of the neurosensory epithelium of the saccule and utricle, and an inflammatory endolymphatic precipitate in the semicircular canals. The organ of Corti was relatively spared in these specimens, with hypocellularity of the spiral ligament and, in one case, the spiral ligament noted. This is an unexpected finding, given the high incidence of sensorineural hearing loss associated with AIDS.

In another study, 49 temporal bones from 25 patients were examined with light microscopy, immunohistochemistry for fibrin and cytomegalovirus (CMV), and in situ hybridization for CMV (32). The patient population consisted of 24 male homosexuals and one woman, who contracted the disease by heterosexual transmission. The mean age of the population was 40 years, and no children were included. A majority of the patients had sensorineural hearing loss, and many had tinnitus or vertigo. Middle ear findings included severe OM in 16% of the temporal bones, and low-grade OM in 55% of the temporal bones. An exudate was present in the middle ear cavity that was composed of interweaving thread less than 1 μm in length. These stained positive for fibrinogen by immunohistochemistry. Several bones also had a clear, gelatinous material in the middle ear cavity. Two bones contained cholesteatoma, and the middle ear epithelium of one bone had cellular changes with inclusions consistent with CMV.

The inner ears of these patients contained evidence of infection and neoplastic changes associated with AIDS, including cryptococci, CMV, and Kaposi's sarcoma. Cryptococci were present in four temporal bones from two patients with known cryptococcal meningitis. Fungi were present in the subarachnoid space in the internal auditory canal, and invasion of the VIIIth nerve was noted. Histologic changes consistent with CMV were noted in seven bones, but no bones were positive for CMV by immunohistochemical staining. Two bones were positive for CMV by in situ hybridization. These negative results were attributed to decalcification in acid during specimen preparation. Kaposi's sarcoma deposits were noted in the VIIIth nerve of one bone.

SENSORINEURAL HEARING LOSS IN THE PEDIATRIC ACQUIRED IMMUNODEFICIENCY SYNDROME PATIENT

There is a growing awareness that sensorineural hearing loss is present in a large percentage of HIV-positive patients, with estimates ranging from 20.9% to 49.0% (33). Central nervous system and cranial nerve involvement combine to challenge the HIV-positive patient with increased difficulties in hearing with the attendant communication challenges (34). A disproportionate degradation in discriminate language skills may be present secondary to central auditory dysfunction; indeed, AIDS should be considered a new cause of acquired central auditory dysfunction (35).

Brainstem auditory evoked responses (BAERs) may be abnormal in infants and children with AIDS, but increased stimulation rates may be necessary to unmask pathology. In 16 infants and children with AIDS and nine normal control children, increasing the stimulation rate to 50 Hz (from a conventional stimulation rate of 10 Hz) increased the number of differences between the AIDS group and the normal children (36). While there were no significant differences between the interpeak latencies of the two groups, the higher stimulation rates generated significant differences between the two groups in the latencies of waves I, III, and V bilaterally. In a second publication (37), it was noted that two children with an increase of all wave latencies over time had the worst neurologic involvement and that serial BAER studies may be useful in following the progression of CNS involvement in infants and children with AIDS (37).

CONCLUSIONS

Human immunodeficiency virus infection does not appear to cause more episodes of OM in infected children but does increase the recurrence rate. Treatment of mildly immunocompromised children should be the same as that for normal children, but severely immunocompromised children may require tympanocentesis and broader spectrum antimicrobials. Prophylaxis for HIV-positive children should be initiated early. The organisms that cause OM generally do not differ between HIV-positive children and normal children, with the exception of *S. aureus*. The opportunistic otologic infections seen in adults with AIDS do not appear to be present in HIV-positive children, but they should always be suspected in refractory cases.

REFERENCES

1. Schappert SM. Office visits for otitis media: United States, 1975–1900. Hyattsville, MD: National Center for Health Statistics; 1990.
2. Bluestone CD, Klein JO. *Otitis media in infants and children.* Philadelphia: WB Saunders; 1995.
3. Stool SE, Field MJ. The impact of otitis media. *Pediatr Infect Dis J* 1989; 8:S11–14.
4. Teele DW, Klein JO, Rosner B, Greater Boston Otitis Media Study Group. Epidemiology of otitis media during the first seven years of life in children in Greater Boston: a prospective cohort study. *J Infect Dis* 1989;160:83–94.
5. Centers for Disease Control. *Pneumocystis carinii* pneumonia—Los Angeles. *MMWR* 1981;30:250.
6. Centers for Disease Control. Kaposi's sarcoma and *Pneumocystis carinii* pneumonia—New York City and California. *MMWR* 1981;30:305.
7. Centers for Disease Control. Unexplained immunodeficiency and opportunistic infection in infants—New York, New Jersey, California. *MMWR* 1982;31:665–7.
8. Oleske J, Minnefor A Cooper R, et al. Immune deficiency syndrome in children. *JAMA* 1983;249:2345.
9. Centers for Disease Control. 1994 revised classification system for human immunodeficiency virus infection in children less than 13 years of age. *MMWR* 1994;43:1–10.
10. Report of a consensus workshop, Siena, Italy, January 17–18, 1992; Early diagnosis of HIV infection in infants. *J Acquir Immune Defic Syndr* 1992;5:1169–78.
11. Buchman CA, Liederman E, Sirko DA, White GJ, Post JC, Ehrlich GD. Molecular microbiologic analysis of otitis media in adults. Sixth International Symposium on Recent Advances in Otitis Media, Ft. Lauderdale, FL, June, 1995.
12. Centers for Disease Control. Classification system for human immunodeficiency virus in children under 13 years of age. *MMWR* 1987;36:225.
13. Berger BJ, Hussain F, Roistacher K. Bacterial infections in HIV-infected patients. *Infect Dis Clin North Am* 1994;8:449–65.
14. Barnett ED, Klein JO, Pelton SI, Luginbuhl LM. Otitis media in children born to human immunodeficiency virus-infected mothers. *Pediatr Infect Dis J* 1992;11:360–4.
15. Magit AE, Fleming G, Hatch R, Spector S, Dankner W. Complications of otitis media in children with HIV. Presented at the American Society of Pediatric Otolaryngology, Tamaron, CO, May 1995.
16. Chow JH, Stren JC, Kaul A, Pincus RL, Gromisch DS. Head and neck manifestations of the acquired immunodeficiency syndrome in children. *Ear Nose Throat J* 1990;69:416–23.
17. Desai SD. Seropositivity, adenoid hypertrophy, and secretory otitis media in adults—A recognized clinical entity. *Otolaryngol Head Neck Surg* 1992;107:755–7.
18. Sculerati N, Borkowsky W. Pediatric human immunodeficiency virus infection: an otolaryngologist's perspective. *J Otolaryngol* 1990;19:182–188.
19. Shah UK, McGuirt WF, Forsen J, Caradonna D, Jones D. Congenital and acquired immunodeficiency in the pediatric patient. *Curr Opin Otolaryngol Head Neck Surg* 1994;2:462–67.
20. Church JA. Human immunodeficiency virus (HIV) infection at Children's Hospital of Los Angeles: recurrent otitis media or chronic sinusitis as the presenting process in pediatric AIDS. *Immunology Allergy Pract* 1987;9:25–32.
21. Williams MA. Head and neck findings in pediatric acquired immune deficiency syndrome. *Laryngoscope* 1987;97:713–16.
22. Principi N, Marchisio P, Tornaghi R, Onorato J, Massironi E, Picco P. Acute otitis media in human immunodeficiency virus-infected children. *Pediatrics* 1991;88:566–71.
23. Marchisio P, Principi N, Sorella S, Sala E, Tornaghi R. Etiology of acute otitis media in human immunodeficiency virus-infected children. *Pediatric Infect Dis J* 1996;15:58–61.
24. Morris MS, Prasad S. Otologic disease in the acquired immunodeficiency syndrome. *Ear Nose Throat J* 1990;69:451–3.
25. Sandler ED, Sandler JM, LeBoit PE, Wenig BM, Mortensen N. *Pneu-*

mocystis carinii otitis media in AIDS: a case report and review of the literature regarding extrapulmonary pneumocystosis. *Otolaryngol Head Neck Surg* 1990;103:817–21.
26. Park S, Wunderlich H, Goldenberg RA, Marshall M. *Pneumocystis carinii* infection in the middle ear. *Arch Otolaryngol Head Neck Surg* 1992;118:269–70.
27. Wasserman L, Haghighi P. Otic and ophthalmic pneumocystosis in acquired immunodeficiency syndrome. *Arch Pathol Lab Med* 1992;116:500–3.
28. Schinella RA, Breda SD, Hammerschlag PE. Otic infection due to *Pneumocystis carinii* in an apparently healthy man with antibody to the human immunodeficiency virus. *Ann Intern Med* 1987;106:399–400.
29. Gherman CR, Ward RR, Bassis ML. *Pneumocystis carinii* otitis media and mastoiditis as the initial manifestation of the acquired immunodeficiency syndrome. *Am J Med* 1988;85:250–2.
30. Strauss M, Fine E. Aspergillus otomastoiditis in acquired immunodeficiency syndrome. *Am J Otol* 12:49–53.
31. Chandrasekhar SS, Siverls V, Sekhar HKC. Histopathologic and ultrastructural changes in the temporal bones of HIV-infected human adults. *Am J Otol* 1992;13:207–14.
32. Michaels L, Soucel S, Liang J. The ear in the acquired immunodeficiency syndrome: I. Temporal bone histopathologic study. *Am J Otolaryngol* 1994;15:515–22.
33. Lalwani AE, Sooy D. Manifestaciones otologicas y neuro-otologicas del SIDA. *Clin Otorhinolaryngol North Am* 1992;6:1239–54.
34. Madriz JJ, Herrera G. Human immunodeficiency virus and acquired immune deficiency syndrome: AIDS-related hearing disorders. *J Am Acad Audiol* 1995;6:358–64.
35. Strutz J. Non-neoplastic central hearing loss: a review. *HNO* 1991;39:332–8.
36. Frank Y, Vishnubhakat SM, Pahwa S. Brainstem auditory evoked responses in infants and children with AIDS. *Pediatr Neurol* 1992;8:262–6.
37. Frank Y, Pahwa S. Serial brainstem auditory evoked responses in infants and children with AIDS. *Clin Electroencephalogr* 1993;24:160–5.

PART XI
Neoplasms

CHAPTER 32

Posterior Fossa Tumors

Simón I. Angeli and Derald E. Brackmann

Tumors of the posterior cranial fossa encompass a variety of neoplasms of the infratentorial brain parenchyma and adjacent cranial nerves, as well as some inflammatory and neoplastic conditions affecting the bones of the posterior skull base. Just over half of all pediatric brain tumors are infratentorial (1). In contrast to older teenagers and adults, who are more frequently affected by vestibular schwannoma, meningioma and epidermoid, the majority of posterior fossa tumors in younger children are intrinsic brain neoplasms (medulloblastoma, astrocytoma, glioma, ependymoma).

Although the morbidity and mortality for these tumors continues to be significant, recent advances in neuroimaging and therapy have facilitated earlier diagnosis and improved treatment planning. This has resulted in more long-term survivals, and the serious effects of treatment on the developing child are becoming more evident. Since both the disease itself and the treatment approach have formidable impact on the development and quality of life of children with posterior fossa tumors, current therapeutic approaches emphasize both the preservation of function and the eradication of disease when possible.

This chapter addresses the classification, diagnosis, and treatment of posterior fossa tumors in children and discusses specific management strategies for the most common of these tumors. By far, the most common posterior fossa tumor in patients under 18 years of age encountered in our practice is acoustic neuroma in association with neurofibromatosis type II (NF2).

CLASSIFICATION OF POSTERIOR FOSSA TUMORS IN CHILDREN

Table 1 shows an overview of tumors that originate in or invade the posterior fossa in children and teenagers according to their location and histologic appearance. Current neuroimaging techniques afford enough resolution to aid in the differential diagnosis, greatly facilitating subsequent therapeutic planning.

CLINICAL MANIFESTATIONS

In general terms, the clinical manifestations of posterior fossa tumors can be grouped according to the site of origin. Infratentorial, intra-axial brain tumors commonly present with manifestations due to hydrocephalus. Typically, headaches, nausea, vomiting, irritability, failure to thrive, and progressive macrocephaly are present. Infants and younger children are notorious for the unspecificity of their symptoms; focal neurologic findings are more likely in older children. During the initial evaluation, the child's level of consciousness is of critical importance to determine the rapidity of subsequent interventions. Stuporous patients require urgent care, but the awake child can undergo a more detailed preoperative evaluation including cranial nerve function, speech, and so forth.

Involvement of the seventh and eighth cranial nerves is common in tumors of the cerebellopontine angle (CPA), and hydrocephalus tends to be a late finding. Ataxia and unsteadiness of arm movements can occur from cerebellar compression by large CPA tumors, and by intrinsic cerebellar neoplasms. Extradural tumors involving the petrous apex of the temporal bone can be silent or present with retro-orbital pain, otorrhea, and diplopia.

DIAGNOSTIC EVALUATION

The diagnostic work-up is tailored after the results of the initial clinical examination. Computed tomography (CT) and magnetic resonance imaging (MRI) with and without contrast enhancement are used to diagnose a brain tumor. Typical imaging characteristics of the more common posterior fossa tumors are shown in Tables 2 and Table 3 (2). A child who requires sedation to obtain a scan, should be closely monitored because of the risk of hypoventilation with resul-

---

S.I. Angeli and D.E. Brackmann: House Ear Clinic, Los Angeles, California 90057.

TABLE 1. Common posterior fossa tumors in children and teenagers

Location	Type of tumor
Extra-axial	Vestibular schwannoma (neurofibromatosis type 2)
	Meningioma
	Epidermoid and dermoid
	Arachnoid cyst
	Other
Intra-axial	Medulloblastoma (infratentorial primitive neuroectodermal tumor)
	Astrocytoma, cerebellar
	Glioma, brainstem
	Ependymoma
	Other
Extradural	Chordoma
	Rhabdomyosarcoma
	Inflammatory petrous apex lesions
	Cholesterol granuloma
	Mucocele (mucous retention cyst within a petrous air cell)
	Cholesteatoma/epidermoid

tant increase in intracranial pressure and herniation. Use of MRI affords multiplanar images and better soft tissue detail than does CT (3). However, CT is faster and simpler to perform than MR when one is dealing with an obtunded patient in an urgent situation. A combination of MRI and high-resolution CT of the temporal bones is useful in the diagnosis of petrous apex lesions (4). Currently, there is no indication for angiography except to confirm and embolize a hemangioblastoma.

Spinal MRI and cytologic evaluation of the cerebrospinal fluid (CSF) are used for staging for tumors with high incidence of dissemination, such as medulloblastomas and ependymomas. Spinal MRI is also indicated to diagnose spinal cord tumors in NF2.

Audiovestibular evaluation is used for tumors of the CPA and temporal bone. Routine audiological testing sometimes offers the first diagnostic clue of a retrocochlear lesion by revealing the unspecific findings of asymmetric sensorineural hearing loss or impairment of speech discrimination disproportionate to the pure-tone loss. Auditory brainstem response audiometry (ABR) is used to detect CPA tumors in patients with enough hearing to generate a response. The parameters used in our institution for diagnosis of acoustic neuroma are a wave V latency interaural difference of 0.2 msec or greater and an abnormal waveform. The overall diagnostic sensitivity of these ABR parameters is 92% and 83%, respectively, but falls significantly for tumors 1 cm or less in size (5). ABR can also be used to evaluate the degree of brainstem compression and as a preoperative baseline if hearing is to be monitored intraoperatively. Assessment of eighth cranial nerve integrity by audiogram, speech discrimination score, ABR, and electronystagmography is useful when entertaining hearing preservation surgery for vestibular schwannomas. Hypoactive caloric response on electronystagmography, indicating superior vestibular nerve involvement, and an ABR interaural wave V latency difference of less than 0.4 msec are positive prognostic indicators (6).

GENERAL PRINCIPLES OF TREATMENT

For brain tumors of the posterior fossa, the initial management involves surgery to establish the histologic diagnosis and to reduce the tumor burden. Open biopsy and an attempt at extensive microsurgical resection are indicated because the prognosis is affected by the extent of residual disease. Diffuse malignant gliomas of the brainstem are one exception due to their unresectability and characteristic diagnostic features on MRI. Adjuvant modalities such as radiation and chemotherapy are usually needed for tumors with high propensity for dissemination or local invasion.

In the treatment of brain tumors of the posterior fossa, some common preoperative problems are worth reviewing.

TABLE 2. Magnetic resonance imaging features of common infratentorial brain tumors in children

Tumor type	Location	T1	T2	Enhancement (gadolinium)	Cystic component	Calcification	Other
Medulloblastoma	Cerebellum (anterior vermis)	Hypointense	Isointense[a]	+	−	+	May fill 4th ventricle, subarachnoid dissemination
Glioma, brainstem	Pons, medulla	Hypointense	Hyperintense	±[b]	+	−	May displace 4th ventricle posteriorly
Astrocytoma	Cerebellum (posterior vermis or lateral cerebellum)	Hypointense	Hyperintense	±[c]	++[a]	+	May displace 4th ventricle anteriorly or laterally
Ependymoma	4th ventricle	Hypointense–isointense (mixed signal)[a]	Hypointense–hyperintense (mixed signal)[a]	±[c]	+	++[a]	Fills 4th ventricle, extends into contiguous CSF spaces

[a] Most specific sign.
[b] Pontine tumors that do not enhance are more likely malignant.
[c] Enhancing in cystic tumors may be ring-like or absent.
Adapted from Zimmerman et al. (2) and Lizak and Woodruff (3).

TABLE 3. *Imaging features of the three most common CPA tumors*

Characteristic	Vestibular schwannoma	Meningioma	Epidermoid
Location	Centered to IAC	Eccentric to IAC	Antero- or posterolateral to brainstem
Bone changes	May enlarge IAC	Hypertosis	Erosion
Shape	Spherical or ovoid	Hemispherical	Variable, dumbbell
CT density	Mostly isodense	Isodense, some calcified	Hypodense
CT enhancement	+/++ (often inhomogeneous)	++ (homogeneous)	–
T1	Hypointense–isointense	Hypointense–isointense	Hypointense
T2	isointense–hyperintense	Isointense–hyperintense	
MR enhancement	++	+	Hyperintense

IAC, internal auditory canal.
Adapted from Lo (4), with permission.

Peritumoral edema can be quite prominent in some large tumors and also in smaller tumors in critical areas such as the brainstem. Corticosteroids (e.g., dexamethasone, 0.05–0.1 mg/kg body weight, four times daily) are administered 24 to 48 hours before surgical resection. Hydrocephalus is usually treated at the time of craniotomy, and its severity determines the urgency of the procedure. An external ventricular drain is performed immediately before tumor resection. If CSF drainage is reestablished after tumor resection, ventriculostomy can usually be stopped within a few days of surgery. If progressive ventriculomegaly or an enlarging pseudomeningocele develops, a definitive shunting of CSF is required.

The great majority of CPA tumors are benign neoplasms that directly or indirectly involve the seventh and eighth cranial nerve complex. The therapeutic approach is usually based on factors such as tumor size, hearing status, and contralateral involvement (see below). Their general management involves the selection of the most appropriate strategy that allows both tumor resection and preservation of function.

TREATMENT AND OUTCOME OF COMMON ENTITIES

Cerebellopontine Angle Tumors

Neurofibromatosis Type II

Neurofibromatosis type II is an autosomal dominant disorder characterized by bilateral eighth-nerve tumors, or a first-degree relative with NF2 and either unilateral eighth-nerve tumors or one of the following: neurofibroma, meningioma, glioma, schwannoma, or juvenile posterior subcapsular lenticular opacity (7). Table 4 outlines the diagnostic criteria for NF2. Linkage analysis has localized the NF2 gene to chromosome 22 (8), and the tumor suppressor gene (merlin) has been mapped (9,10).

Gadolinium-enhanced MRI is currently the gold standard for preoperative diagnosis of bilateral vestibular schwannomas and has replaced audiologic tests for screening families of patients with NF2 (Fig. 1). Gadolinium-enhanced MRI can detect lesions as small as 2 mm. Presymptomatic identification of patients with NF2 while the tumors are still small allows the greatest chance of tumor removal with hearing preservation.

Our treatment strategies for NF2 have recently been reviewed by Briggs et al (11). Once the diagnosis of NF2 is established, the patient and his or her family are assessed by a multidisciplinary team of physicians and health professionals who are experts in the surgical treatment, rehabilitation, and genetic aspects of the disease. Individualized treatment strategy is necessary because there is a wide variation in presentation and progression of the tumors. The treatment options include:

1. hearing preservation surgery with total tumor removal,
2. observation without surgical intervention,
3. tumor decompression without tumor removal (via middle fossa craniotomy),
4. retrosigmoid craniotomy with partial tumor removal,
5. nonhearing preservation with translabyrinthine total tumor removal,
6. auditory brainstem or cochlear implantation,
7. stereotactic irradiation.

Hearing Preservation Surgery with Total Tumor Removal

Undoubtedly, the widespread use of gadolinium-enhanced MRI and the introduction of several technical modifications to the middle fossa craniotomy approach have resulted in increased numbers of patients with vestibular schwannomas

TABLE 4. *Diagnostic criteria for neurofibromatosis type 2*

Bilateral vestibular schwannomas
A parent, sibling, or child with NF2 plus:
 Unilateral vestibular schwannoma
  Meningioma, glioma, neurofibroma, cerebral calcification, or posterior subcapular lenticular opacities
Unilateral vestibular schwannoma plus one in second entry above
Multiple meningiomas plus unilateral vestibular schwannoma, glioma, neurofibroma, schwannoma, posterior subscapular lenticular opacities, cerebral calcification

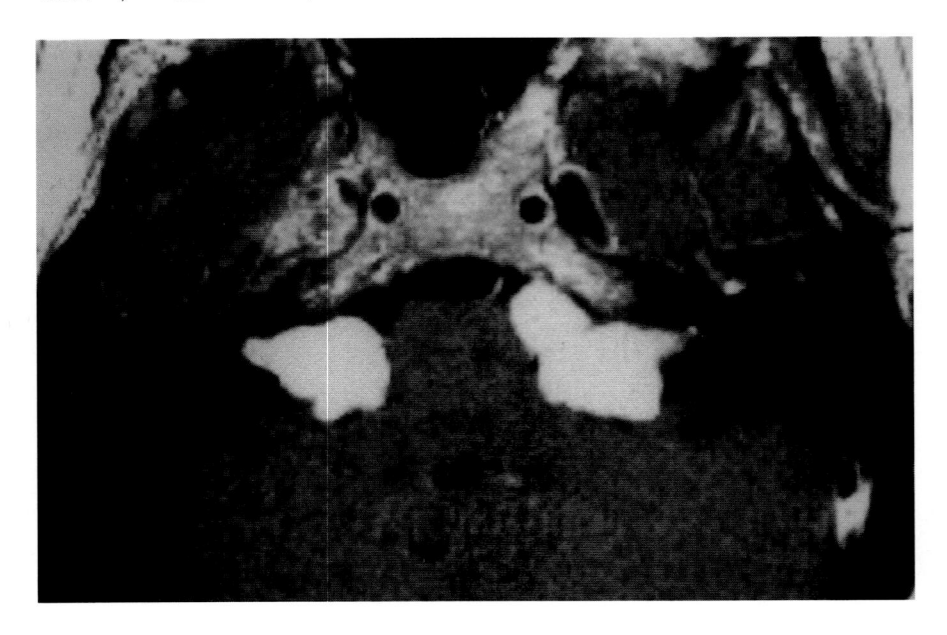

FIG. 1. Gadolinium-enhanced MRI demonstrating bilateral large acoustic neuromas. Reprinted with permission of House Ear Institue.

who successfully undergo a hearing preservation procedure in our center. Brackmann et al. (12) reported that 17 (71%) of 24 consecutive patients had hearing preserved at or near preoperative level. More patients with NF2 are being diagnosed with smaller tumors and better preoperative hearing (Fig. 2). Because of the greater invasiveness of NF2, the rate of hearing preservation is believed to have been worse for these patients than for patients with sporadic unilateral acoustic neuromas. Nevertheless, we feel strongly that total tumor removal with preserved useful hearing is an achievable goal in selected NF2 patients.

Patient selection has become the most critical issue. The potential for hearing preservation after tumor removal is limited by many factors, primarily tumor size. For unilateral tumors, 1.5 cm is the upper limit for hearing preservation with middle fossa removal and 1.5 to 2.0 cm for retrosigmoid-suboccipital removal. For tumors larger than 2 cm, we believe that the chance of hearing preservation is too small to justify surgical removal unless other factors mandate it. Assessment of eighth-nerve integrity by pure-tone average (PTA) audiogram, speech discrimination score (SDS), ABR, and electronystagmography aid in the prediction of successful hearing preservation. The audiometric criteria for hearing preservation in NF2 should probably be less stringent than that used for sporadic acoustic neuromas (50 dB PTA, 50% SDS) since any hearing is useful for these patients. Hypoactive caloric responses (superior vestibular nerve tumor) and an ABR interaural wave V latency difference of less than 0.4 msec are positive prognostic indicators (6). The size and location of the tumor determines the selection of the surgical

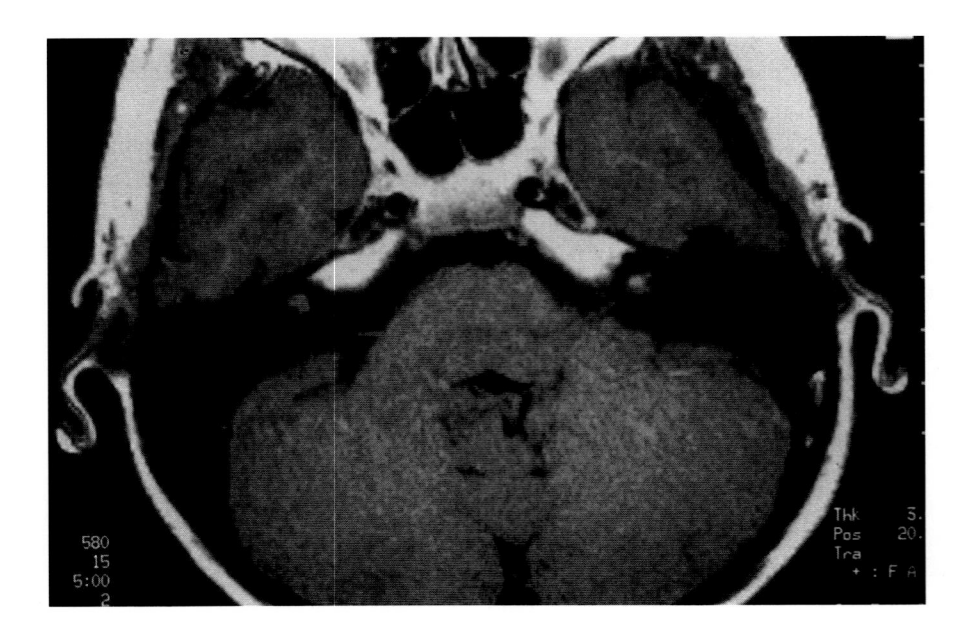

FIG. 2. Gadolinium-enhanced MRI demonstrating small bilateral acoustic neuromas suitable for potential hearing preservation. Reprinted with permission of House Ear Institute.

approach. The middle fossa craniotomy is ideal for intracanalicular tumors that do not extend to 1 cm beyond the porus acousticus into the CPA and it is our preferred approach. The retrosigmoid-suboccipital approach is suitable for tumors with more medial extension (1–2 cm) into the CPA, but access to the lateral aspect of the internal auditory canal (IAC) is limited by the posterior semicircular canal and vestibule.

There is usually some asymmetry in tumor size and hearing levels in patients with bilateral acoustic tumors. Generally, we do not advise attempted hearing-preservation surgery unless there is bilateral serviceable hearing. In patients with favorable prognostic indicators, we recommend total tumor removal with attempted hearing preservation on the side with the larger tumor or greater hearing impairment or both. If hearing is successfully preserved at a serviceable level, we recommend removal of the contralateral tumor after 6 months. The delay is necessary to show that hearing is stable in the operated side. If tumor removal results in loss of hearing, the contralateral tumor is observed and hearing-preservation surgery is not attempted. However, we occasionally treat the smaller tumor first when there is a large discrepancy in tumor size or in ABR responses to improve the chance of long-term hearing. Conversely, others contend that for the best chance of any hearing preservation the smaller tumor should routinely be addressed first in all cases (13).

Observation Without Surgical Intervention

This conservative approach is aimed at maintaining hearing function in selected patients whose tumors do not pose an imminent risk of hydrocephalus or brainstem compression. We recommend expectant observation for small tumors in an only-hearing ear or when there is bilateral hearing but the tumors are too large for a successful hearing-preservation procedure. Patients are followed clinically, audiologically, and with MRI initially at 6 months and then annually, to document hearing level, involvement of other cranial nerves, raised intracranial pressure, and tumor growth. Surgery is then considered if further hearing loss occurs or if the tumor reaches sufficient size (approximately 3 cm) to produce neurological symptoms.

Tumor Decompression Without Removal

For patients who experience progression or fluctuation of their hearing loss while being observed, tumor decompression via middle fossa craniotomy with wide bone removal around the IAC has resulted in stabilization or even improvement of hearing (14). Tumor debulking is not attempted because this procedure markedly increases the chances of hearing loss.

Retrosigmoid Craniotomy

Partial tumor removal by retrosigmoid craniotomy may be considered in a patient with unilateral hearing but whose tumor is large and symptomatic (e.g., hydrocephalus, brainstem compression). Tumor debulking is done and a cuff of tumor capsule is left in an attempt to protect the seventh and eighth cranial nerves. In our experience, even partial tumor removal often results in hearing loss and rapid tumor regrowth.

Translabyrinthine Total Tumor Removal

The translabyrinthine craniotomy is our preferred approach when hearing preservation is no longer possible. The translabyrinthine approach allows safe tumor removal with minimal cerebellar retraction and maximal preservation of facial nerve function (15). In addition, the translabyrinthine approach provides direct access to the lateral recess of the fourth ventricle for placement of an auditory brainstem prosthesis.

Auditory Brainstem or Cochlear Implants

Pioneered by House and Hitselberger, the auditory brainstem implant (ABI) has revolutionized the management of NF2. The current device consists of a multielectrode prosthesis connected to a subcutaneous electromagnetic receiver similar to the Nucleus multichannel cochlear implant (Cochlear Corp., Engelwood, CO). The electrode array is placed directly over the cochlear nucleus in the lateral recess of the fourth ventricle. Most patients perceive auditory stimulation without significant side effects and may even have some speech recognition (16,17). The Food and Drug Administration has approved the use of ABI for patients with NF2 who are undergoing translabyrinthine tumor removal and who have (a) nonaidable hearing or an only-hearing ear with a symptomatic tumor or (b) serviceable hearing in the contralateral ear but a contralateral tumor of sufficient size to indicate that hearing will likely be lost in a short period.

Patients who have an intact cochlear nerve following tumor removal (failed attempted hearing preservation) may be suitable candidates for rehabilitation with a cochlear implant (18). Cochlear implantation may be performed after translabyrinthine tumor removal if the cochlear nerve has been anatomically and functionally preserved (19).

Stereotactic Radiation Therapy

The treatment of choice for acoustic neuromas in patients with NF2 is surgical extirpation (7). Stereotactic radiation has emerged as a treatment option for patients who are unable (medically infirmed) or unwilling to undergo surgery. Stereotactic radiation involves use of a highly focused beam of radiation delivered to the target lesion, which minimizes radiation to adjacent tissue and can be performed in a single session. One large series (20) reported tumor shrinkage in 33% of patients, unchanged size in 43%, and continuous growth in 24% of patients with NF2. Patients need periodic surveillance with MRI scanning to assess the efficacy of treatment because tumor cells and the potential for growth remain. Complications after stereotactic radiation are characteristically delayed in onset, probably due to the effects of radiation on the vasculature of adjacent structures. Facial weakness (15%–34%), facial numbness (18%–32%), progressive hearing loss (62%), progression of tumor growth (4%–24%), and hydrocephalus have been reported (20,21). Because of scarring surgery after stereotactic radiation is more difficult and has fewer chances of preserving facial function (22). In addition, there is a potential risk of radiation-induced malignancies.

Other Issues

All patients with NF2 should undergo a complete brain and spinal MRI to identify accompanying tumors. Ideally, treatment of nonmalignant neoplasms is timed according to the progression of clinical symptoms and when surgery can be performed without significant morbidity. In severe forms of NF2, spinal lesions, not intracranial lesions, are responsible for early mortality.

Meningioma

Meningiomas account for approximately 1.5% of pediatric brain tumors, and 15% of meningiomas occur in the posterior fossa. Meningiomas tend to occur in teenagers in the context of NF2. Most meningiomas in the posterior fossa arise along the petrous ridge or in the CPA (Fig. 3). These tumors are locally aggressive. Clinical manifestations and audiologic findings when these tumors affect the eighth cranial nerve are those of a retrocochlear lesion, without specificity. Meningiomas can grow to a considerable size before the onset of otologic symptoms when arising away from the IAC. Use of MRI can usually help distinguish meningioma by demonstrating its characteristic features (see Table 3). Management of meningiomas in the posterior fossa depends on their location, tumor size, and clinical manifestations. Tumors that are predominately located on the petrous ridge posterior to the IAC can be approached by the retrosigmoid-suboccipital approach or for tumors with extension into the IAC, by the translabyrinthine approach. Tumors originating anterior to the IAC may require a translabyrinthine-transcochlear or petro-occipital transigmoid approach. The translabyrinthine-transcochlear approach offers the most direct access with minimal cerebellar retraction and morbidity but carries the disadvantages of total hearing loss and temporary facial weakness (23). Tumors on the petrous ridge anterior to the IAC or invading the clivus can be reached by an extended middle fossa craniotomy if hearing preservation is to be attempted (24). In this technique, bone is removed medial to the petrous carotid artery and superior to the inferior petrosal sinus for ventral exposure. The superior petrosal sinus, tentorium, and third division of the trigeminal nerve are transected to improve surgical exposure above the tentorial incisura and to the petrous tip. The middle fossa transpetrous approach (extended middle fossa) is not appropriate for tumors located posterior to the IAC. This approach can also be used in cases of recurrences or residual tumors after translabyrinthine or suboccipital removal because it provides a previously unoperated field. In surgery for meningioma, extirpation of the dural attachment is necessary to prevent recurrences. Surgery for meningiomas is fraught with significant morbidity, and treatment should be individualized; in selected cases, surgery may be delayed if there is no evidence of tumor growth or progression of symptoms. Recurrent or residual meningiomas that show clinical progression have also been treated with external beam radiotherapy with improvement of the disease-free interval (25).

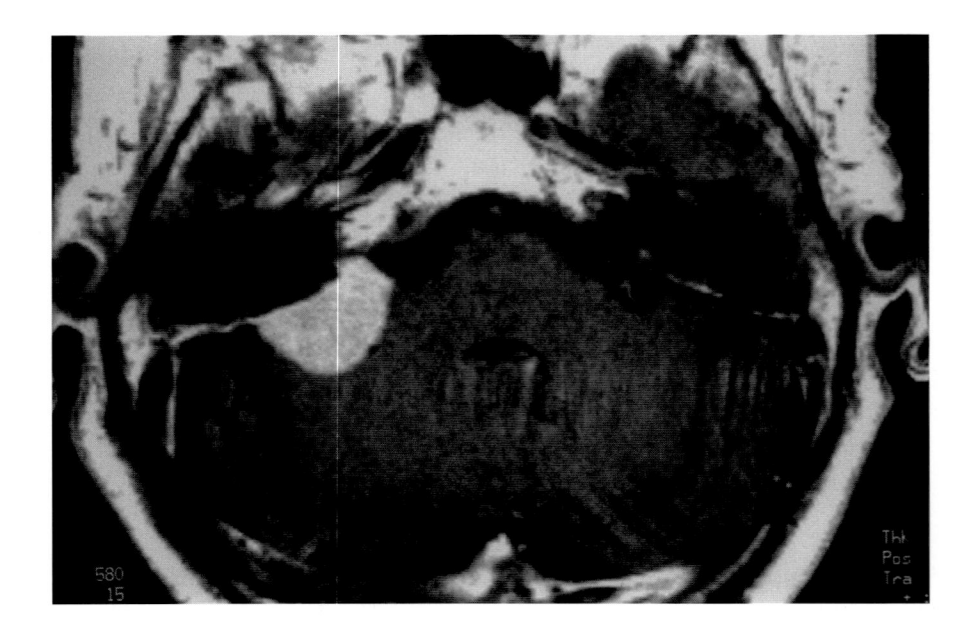

FIG. 3. MRI with gadolinium demonstrating posterior fossa meningioma arising from the posterior ridge of the petrous bone. Reprinted with permission of House Ear Institute.

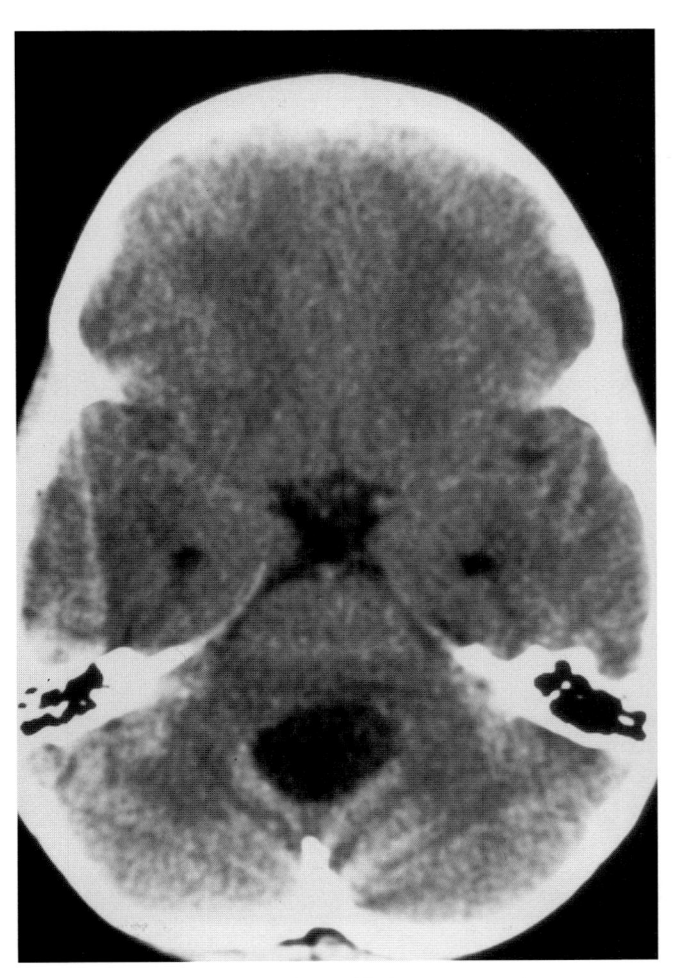

FIG. 4. Fourth ventricle dermoid demonstrated on noncontrast CT. Patient had a dermal sinus tracking into the mass. Courtesy of Dr. Marvin Nelson, Childrens Hospital Los Angeles.

Dermoids and Epidermoids

Dermoid and epidermoid cysts are rare congenital lesions that result from defective closure of the neural tube. Dermoids contain hair, sweat, and sebaceous glands; epidermoids only contain desquamated cells from an epidermal layer. They also differ in their location and clinical presentation; dermoids can be intra- or extradural posterior fossa lesions, usually in or near the midline. Epidermoids are usually extradural and prefer the CPA.

Epidermoids are slow growing, and symptoms do not usually become apparent until the third or fourth decade of life, often with symptoms and signs of a CPA lesion. In contrast, dermoids tend to be symptomatic at an earlier age (26) and present with manifestations of intracranial hypertension or of bacterial meningitis (Fig. 4). Since dermoids are often associated with a sinus or fistula from the intracranial cavity to the skin, they should be suspected and looked for in children with recurrent bouts of meningitis or brain abscess. Careful search for a skin lesion or dimple near the posterior midline may reveal the port of entry of infection. Use of MRI can suggest the diagnosis of dermoid cysts, but high-resolution CT can better delineate a bony skull defect.

The treatment of choice for dermoids and epidermoids is surgical removal of the cyst, its content, and its fistulous tract if present, with preservation of vital or important structures. The surgical approach is selected according to the location of the lesion. Median suboccipital craniotomy is suitable for midline dermoids, and a retrolabyrinthine or retrosigmoid craniotomy is adequate for CPA epidermoids.

Arachnoid Cysts

Arachnoid cysts are thin-walled sacs within the arachnoid and contain CSF. They are considered to be congenital on the basis of their common occurrence in early childhood. However, events that elicit inflammation, such as surgical manipulation, infection, or bleeding, within the arachnoid space can result in acquired arachnoid cysts (27).

Of all arachnoid cysts, 11% occur in the CPA. Their presentation is variable and includes hydrocephalus or CPA syndrome. Symptoms can characteristically be fleeting or fluctuating and reflect changes in the size of the cyst (28). Their appearance is quite typical on CT and MRI: smooth surface lesion, nonenhancing, with intensity signal similar to that of CSF. Treatment of symptomatic lesions is drainage by insertion of a cystoperitoneal shunt. When there is associated hydrocephalus, an additional catheter is placed in the ventricle (27). Diuretic therapy has been used to provide symptomatic relief in a minority of patients (28).

Intra-Axial Tumors

Approximately 60% of pediatric brain tumors are located within the posterior fossa. The most common types arise from the brainstem (gliomas), the cerebellum (medulloblastoma, astrocytoma), and the fourth ventricle (ependymoma). They typically present with symptoms and signs of hydrocephalus, and approximately 10% of cases manifest secondary to intratumoral hemorrhage. They occasionally invade the CPA and their symptoms are indistinguishable from other primary CPA lesions. Imaging features of most of these tumors are quite characteristic (see Table 2) and aid in the preoperative diagnosis. In general terms, treatment consists of removal of as much tumor as is safely possible (usually via median suboccipital craniotomy) with or without adjuvant therapy (radiation, chemotherapy) (1).

Medulloblastoma

Medulloblastomas (primitive neuroectodermal tumors) of the posterior fossa are the most common malignant neoplasms of the central nervous system in children, comprising approximately 20% to 25% of all pediatric brain tumors (Fig. 5). This malignancy has a propensity for disseminating within the CSF, and a complete neuraxis staging is required upon diagnosis.

Survival for children with medulloblastomas has changed dramatically in the last few years. Overall, the 5-year disease-free survival is greater than 50%. This improved outcome is largely secondary to advances in diagnosis, surgery, postoperative care, the addition of craniospinal radiation and, for some patients, chemotherapy. Among patients without evidence of metastasis, complete or nearly complete tumor removal improves the chances of cure. Complete radical resection should be limited by the potential morbidity. The most important factors associated with an increased risk of recurrence are the presence of disseminated disease, age younger than 2 years, and extensive residual disease after surgery. The goal is to reduce treatment-induced morbidity while attaining long-term survival. Low-risk patients are treated with craniospinal radiation following surgery. High-risk patients may benefit from the addition of chemotherapy. In patients 3 years of age or younger without residual intracranial or spinal disease, radiotherapy may be delayed 1 or 2 years in lieu of chemotherapy to avoid the significant effects of radiation on the developing brain. These children are followed with serial MRI and if there is growth or recurrence of tumor, radiation is given. Treatment of recurrent medulloblastoma after surgery and radiation has very poor results. The impact of intensive chemotherapy and bone marrow transplant on these cases has yet to be determined (29–32).

Astrocytoma

Astrocytomas account for 30% of intra-axial posterior fossa tumors in childhood. Most are low-grade cerebellar astrocytomas. There are two types of benign cerebellar astrocytomas: mycrocystic, astrocytoma type A (juvenile pilocytic astrocytoma) and diffuse, or type B (Figs. 6,7,8). Juvenile pylocytic astrocytomas are usually amenable to surgical resection and their prognosis is excellent. If residual or recurrent disease is noted on postoperative scanning, reoperation may be indicated. If the risks of reoperation are unacceptable

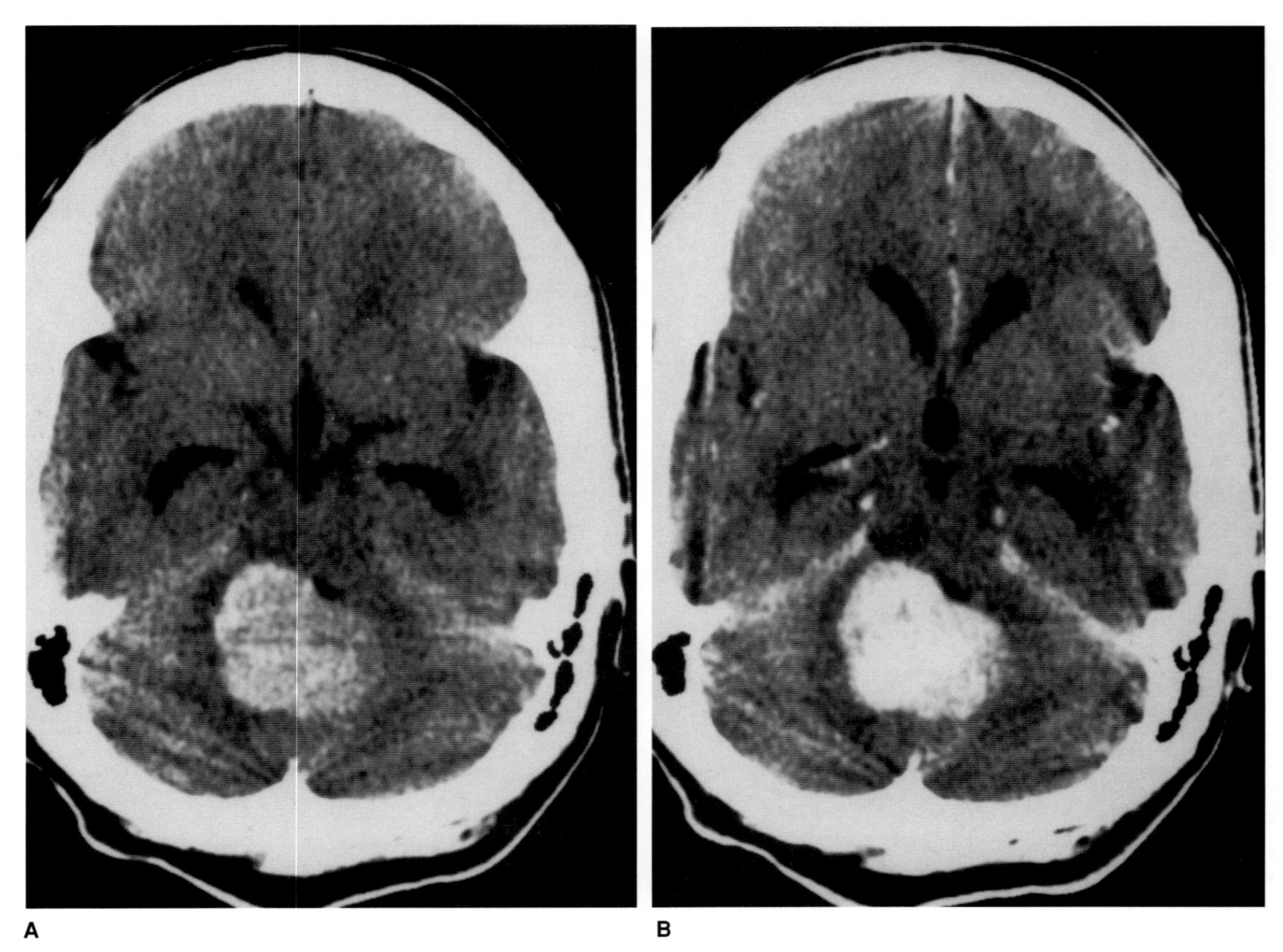

FIG. 5. A: Noncontrast CT scan of medulloblastoma. **B:** Postcontrast CT scan of medulloblastoma. Courtesy of Dr. Marvin Nelson, Childrens Hospital Los Angeles.

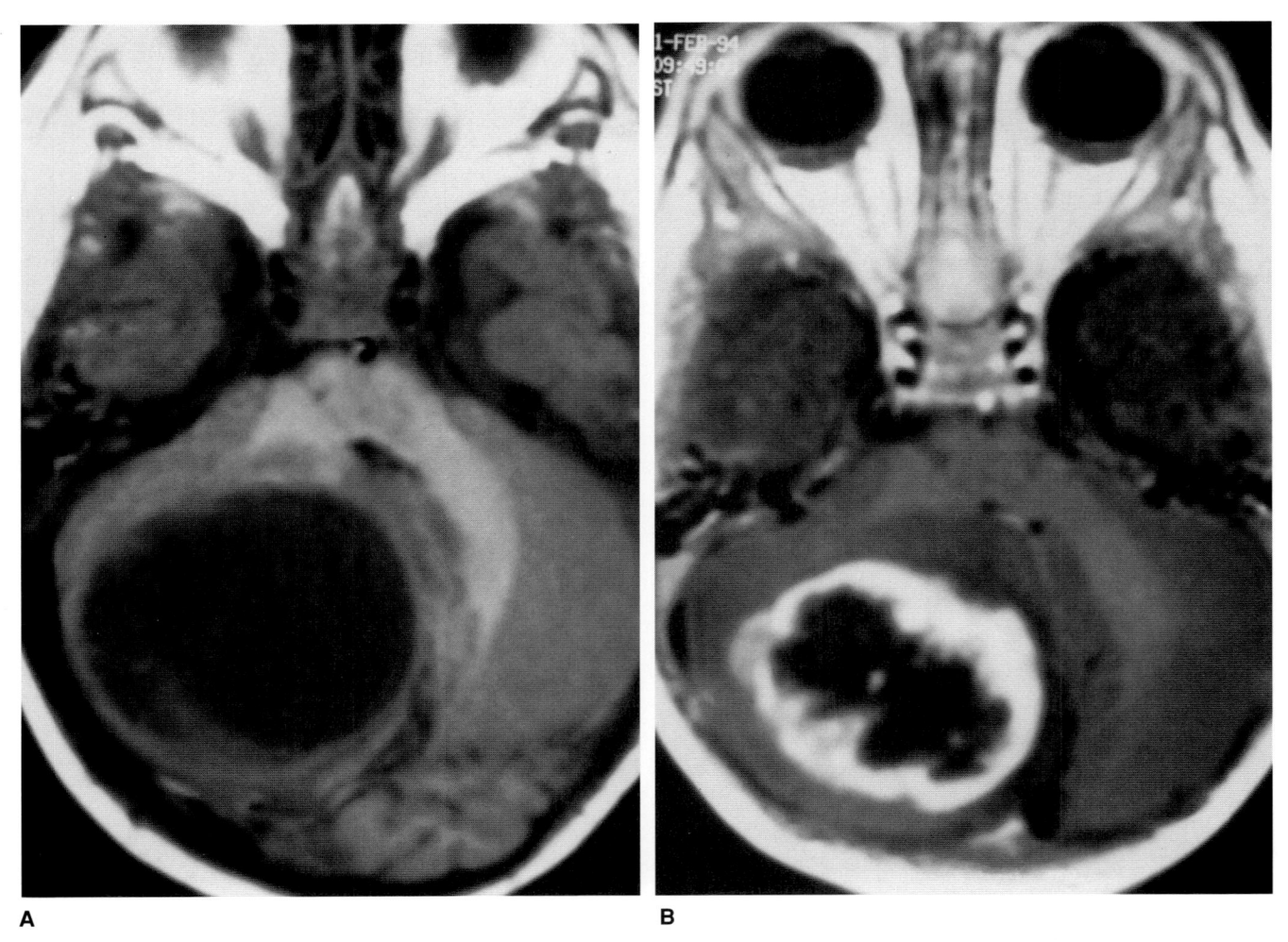

FIG. 6. A: T1 MRI without contrast of cystic astrocytoma of the cerebellum. **B:** T1 MRI with contrast. Contrast demonstrates cystic component. Courtesy of Dr. Marvin Nelson, Childrens Hospital Los Angeles.

and there is evidence of tumor regrowth, limited-field, external-beam irradiation or stereotactic irradiation may be used. Anaplastic astrocytomas require postoperative irradiation and intensive chemotherapy (31,33).

Brainstem Gliomas

Infratentorial malignant gliomas account for 3% to 9% of all brain tumors in children. They are usually very infiltrative and unresectable brainstem lesions. Features seen on MRI are quite characteristic, and biopsy is usually not needed, but when the diagnosis is in doubt, stereotactic biopsy has been attempted (Fig. 9) (34).

Radiotherapy is the treatment of choice, but few patients survive more than 1 year after diagnosis. Clinical trials using high-dose hyperfractionated radiation and intensive chemotherapy are being performed. Of note is the distinctive benign behavior and indolent course of brainstem gliomas in children with neurofibromatosis, in whom symptomatic treatment of hydrocephalus with a ventriculostomy may suffice (32).

Ependymoma

Ependymomas are neoplasms that originate from ependymal cells in the fourth ventricle. They account for 4% to 8% of all pediatric brain tumors (32). They show a propensity to extend into the subarachnoid space by projecting through the apertures of the fourth ventricle (Fig. 10). According to their origins and extensions, ependymomas can be classified into three types: (a) tumors originating from the ventricular floor and extending downward into the upper cervical canal through the foramen of Magendie, (b) tumors arising laterally and extending through the foramen of Luschka into the lateral recess and CPA, and (c) tumors originating from the roof of the fourth ventricle. Although ependymomas are histologically benign, they are difficult to eradicate surgically without significant morbidity (Fig. 11). Among the

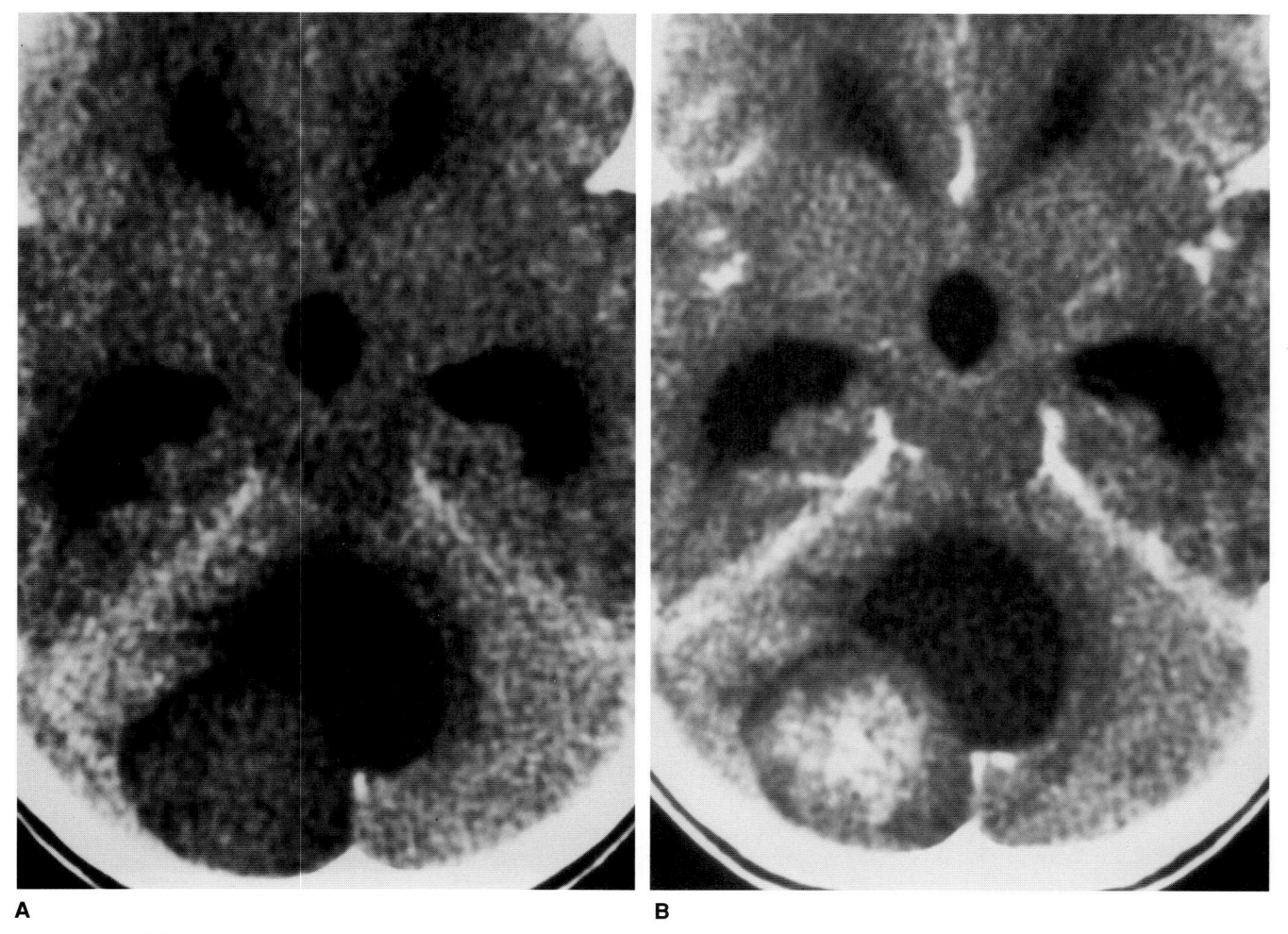

FIG. 7. A: Noncontrast CT of pilocystic astrocytoma of the cerebellum. **B:** Postcontrast CT of pilocystic astrocytoma of the cerebellum demonstrating the cyst with enhancing mural nodule. Courtesy of Dr. Marvin Nelson, Childrens Hospital Los Angeles.

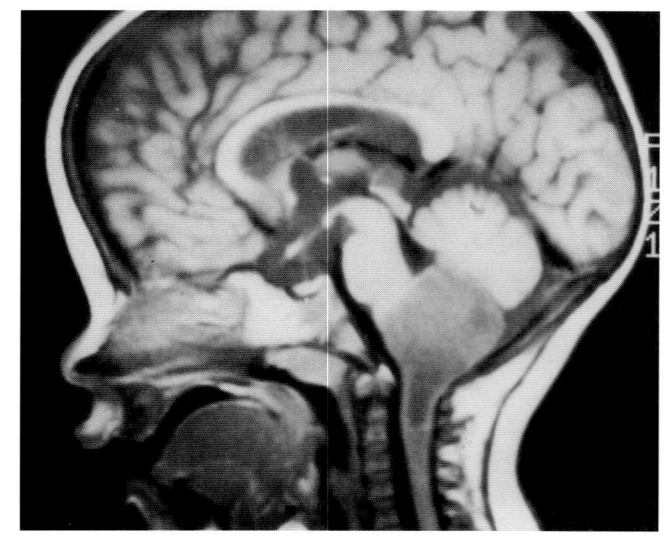

FIG. 8. Cervical medullary astrocytoma noncontrast T1-weighted MRI. Courtesy of Dr. Marvin Nelson, Childrens Hospital Los Angeles.

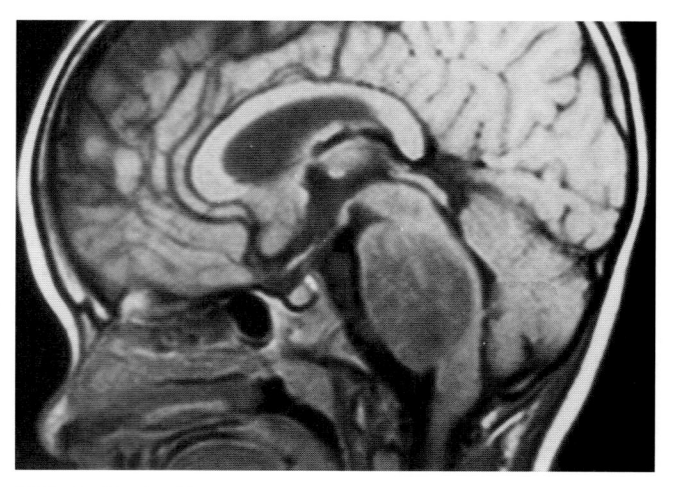

FIG. 9. Sagittal T1-weighted noncontrast MRI demonstrating a pontine glioma. Courtesy of Dr. Marvin Nelson, Childrens Hospital Los Angeles.

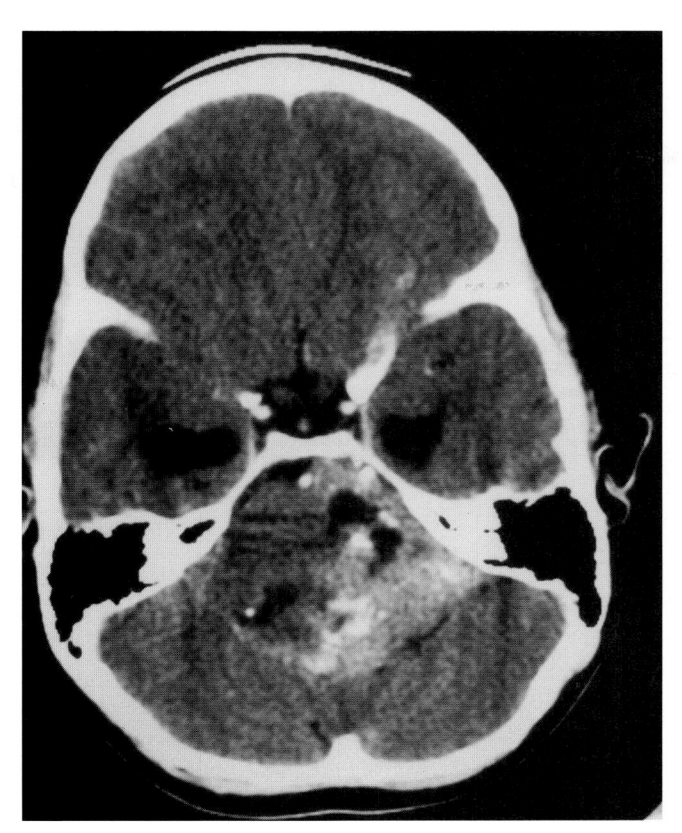

FIG. 10. Postcontrast CT of posterior fossa ependymoma with projection into the fourth ventricle. Courtesy of Dr. Marvin Nelson, Childrens Hospital Los Angeles.

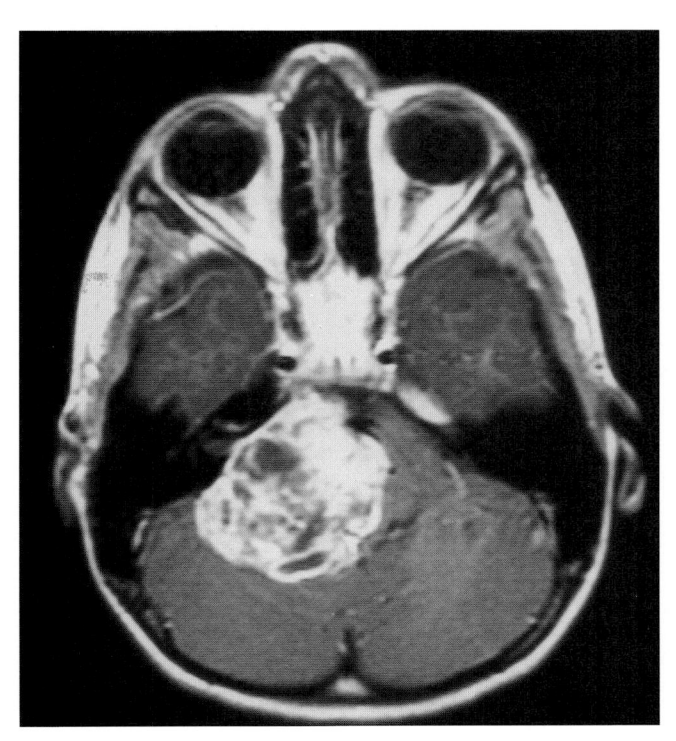

FIG. 11. Anaplastic ependymoma demonstrated on postcontrast T1-weighted MRI scan. Courtesy of Dr. Marvin Nelson, Childrens Hospital Los Angeles.

several prognostic indicators for ependymomas (age of patient, histology, cranial nerve deficits), one of the most significant is extent of tumor removal. The 5-year disease-free survival rate after total resection is 60% to 80%, but after incomplete resection the rate is less than 30%. Roof-type tumors have the best chance of total removal, whereas those tumors extending laterally into the CPA are often intermingled with neighboring structures (lower cranial nerves, posterior inferior cerebellar artery, anterior inferior cerebellar artery) and make total removal difficult (35). Posterior fossa ependymomas are approached through a midline suboccipital craniectomy. Postoperative staging is then performed because there is an incidence of seeding of 3% to 15%. Disseminated disease is treated with craniospinal radiation. However, since most recurrences are local, limited-field radiotherapy or stereotactic radiation are often used. Residual ependymomas do not respond well to radiation or chemotherapy and tend to lead to a fatal outcome. Residual or recurrent tumor in the CPA may be surgically accessed by a laterally based approach (e.g., retrosigmoid or translabyrinthine craniotomy), although the value of reoperation for ependymomas has not been evaluated.

Extra-Dural Tumors

Chordoma

Chordomas are congenital tumors that arise from cell rests of the notochord. Intracranial chordomas usually originate from the region of the clivus and basiocciput. Although they are histologically benign and slow growing, they are locally aggressive and have high rates of recurrence (Fig. 12). Their symptomatology is variable and depends on their location and their direction and rapidity of growth. Headaches, progressive cranial nerve palsies, and long-tract signs without increased intracranial pressure are typical presentations of chordomas. A sixth cranial nerve palsy is a common presenting sign; rarely, initial symptoms may reflect extension into the CPA. Although chordomas are usually slow growing and present in the third and fourth decade, younger children can occasionally be affected. Infants and children tend to have a more rapid clinical course and a higher incidence of metastatic disease at presentation than that in adults (36). The imaging features of chordomas are quite distinctive. Use of CT shows a homogeneous mass, which destroys bone and has irregular contrast enhancement. On MRI, the extent of intracranial invasion and brainstem displacement is readily apparent, and the lesion demonstrates isointense T1-weighted and hyperintense T2-weighted signals. The treatment combination that appears to offer the best survival is surgical resection and postoperative irradiation, although the role of radiation is not proven. Because complete resection of chordomas is a formidable task and is rarely feasible, and a multidisciplinary team and a variety of surgical approaches may be needed (37).

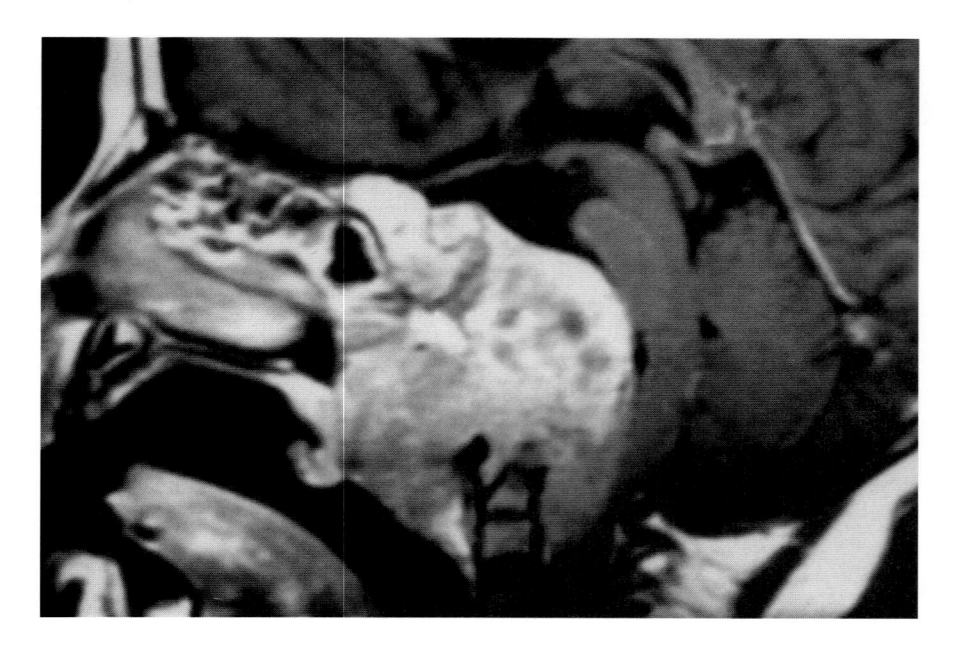

FIG. 12. Sagittal T1-weighted MRI with gadolinium of clival chordoma. Courtesy of Dr. Marvin Nelson, Childrens Hospital Los Angeles.

Petrous Apex Lesions

Lesions that originate from the petrous portion of the temporal bone in the skull base occasionally afflict children. The first step in diagnosis is to identify lesions that require extirpative procedures and lesions that can be treated by surgical drainage. Rhabdomyosarcoma and other neoplastic lesions of the petrous skull base are treated with surgical extirpation (discussed in other chapters of this textbook). Cystic lesions of the petrous apex, such as cholesterol granuloma and mucocele, are amenable to more conservative management by drainage.

Cholesterol granuloma is an inflammatory lesion resulting from foreign-body reaction to hemorrhage within the air cell system of the petrous apex. The lesions are expansible masses that may extend into the CPA and IAC and produce symptoms in seventh and eighth cranial nerves. The complementary use of high-resolution CT scan of the temporal bone and MRI reliably help in the preoperative diagnosis. On CT, cholesterol granuloma appears as a well-delineated, round, rim-enhancing lesion in the petrous apex (Fig. 13). Both T1- and T2-weighted images are hyperintense, contrasting with the typical hypointense signal on T1-weighted images of epidermoid and mucocele (Fig. 14) (4). In our experience, cholesterol granulomas are much more common than epidermoids.

Controversy exists on the surgical management of cholesterol granuloma. We believe that complete excision carries significant operative morbidity and is usually not necessary. The transcranial, infracochlear approach provides a direct,

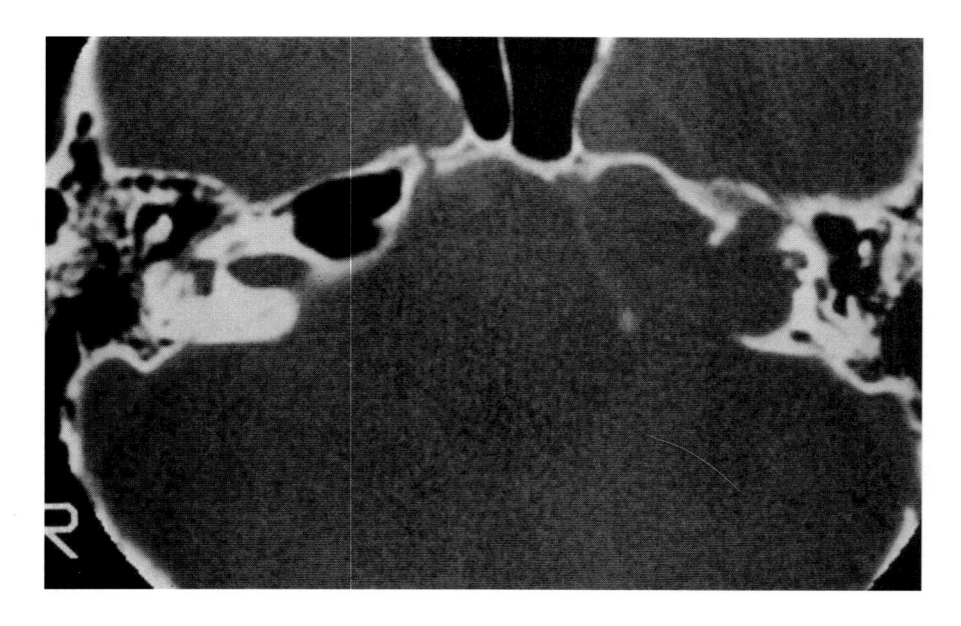

FIG. 13. Noncontrast CT of cholesterol granuloma. Slow expansion of the cyst produces a smooth, round mass. Reprinted with permission of House Ear Institute.

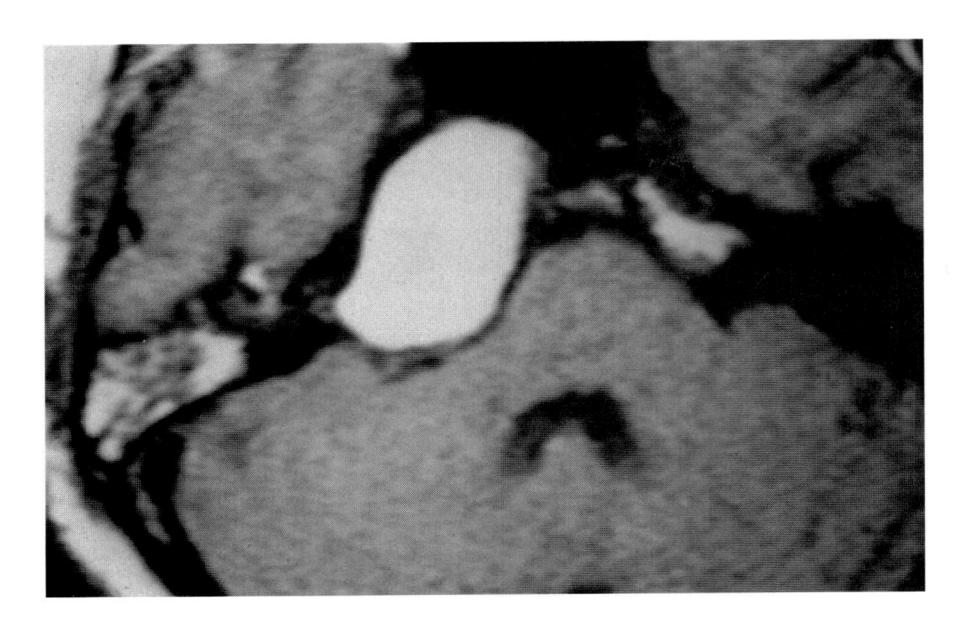

FIG. 14. MRI demostrating hypertense lesion of the petrous apex. Cholesterol granulomas are hyperintense on both T1- and T2-weighted images. Reprinted with permission of House Ear Institute.

technically simple route that affords long-term, dependable drainage; it is our preferred surgical option for drainage of petrous apex cholesterol granulomas or symptomatic mucoceles (38). Transsphenoidal drainage of the petrous apex and extirpative procedures via transcochlear, middle fossa craniotomy, or subtotal petrosectomy are alternative options (39,40).

EARLY COMPLICATIONS AND LATE SEQUELAE OF TREATMENT

Depending on the type of the operative approach one uses, the complications from surgery of posterior fossa tumors can be general or specific. General complications to posterior fossa craniotomy (median, retrosigmoid, and translabyrinthine) include leakage of CSF, chemical meningitis, bacterial meningitis (rare), intracranial hemorrhage, wound infection, neurologic deficits, and death. In surgery for benign tumors, failure to achieve gross total tumor removal is also considered a complication if it is secondary to a poorly performed operative approach, technique, or both, particularly if the patient required reoperation.

In the early postoperative period, a patient with deteriorating mental status and focal neurologic signs must be considered to have an intracranial hemorrhage until proved otherwise. This can be shown by CT scan, but in the rapidly deteriorating patient, the wound is opened and the clot evacuated at the bedside to relieve brainstem compression. The patient is then taken to the operative room for control of the bleeding site.

Leakage of CSF can be treated conservatively with pressure dressings, bed rest, diuretics (acetazolamide), and external drainage with a lumbar catheter or may require reintervention and closure of the dural defect. Prolonged leakage of CSF carries a risk of bacterial meningitis.

Aseptic or chemical meningitis is characterized by fever and meningismus in as much as 30% of patients undergoing craniotomy for posterior fossa tumors. There is pleocytosis, mild hypoglycorrhachia, and elevation of protein in the CSF. The clinical picture can help in differentiating bacterial from aseptic meningitis, because a more severe clinical picture usually accompanies the infected cases: headache, fever, nausea, vomiting, altered mental status, presence of leakage of CSF, and development of a new focal deficit. Aseptic meningitis is still a diagnosis of exclusion, and multiple CSF cultures must fail to show bacterial growth. Treatment with high-dose steroids has been found helpful for control of symptoms, but most patients recover by the second or third postoperative week (41). Bacterial meningitis must be treated promptly with systemic antibiotics and culture guidance.

Postoperative hydrocephalus and pseudomeningocele have been reported with some frequency after medial suboccipital craniotomy for intra-axial tumors. The treatment for these two entities include some form of ventricular and lumbar shunting. Perioperative or prolonged ventricular shunting carries risks of infection, upward cerebellar herniation, hemorrhage, and shunt malfunction (42). Placement of a permanent shunt in patients with symptomatic hydrocephalus may be avoided by the use of preoperative external ventricular drainage and corticosteroids. Risk factors of permanent ventriculoperitoneal shunting in children undergoing median suboccipital craniotomy for intra-axial neoplasm include young age at diagnosis, subtotal tumor resection, CSF infection, pseudomeningocele formation, prolonged use of an external ventricular drain, and the use of cadaveric dural grafts (42).

Postoperative neurologic deficits have a significant and usually permanent impact on the patient's quality of life. Cranial nerve palsies, cerebellar dysfunction, bulbar dysfunction, mutism, apnea, hemiparesis, and seizures are reported after surgery for posterior fossa tumors. The critical issue confronting the surgeon is the balance of surgical and natural morbidity with operative and long-term mortality. Long-term survivors are usually plagued with cognitive and neurologic sequelae, some of which have been attributable to whole-brain irradiation, but other preoperative and postoperative factors are also implicated (43–45).

In terms of surgery for CPA tumors, deafness, facial nerve dysfunction, and balance disorders are the most commonly observed neurologic sequelae. The size of the vestibular schwannoma is directly correlated with results in facial nerve fuction and in hearing. Our results show that in vestibular tumors of 2 cm or less, long-term facial nerve function is normal or nearly normal in 85% of patients (46), and we have been able to maintain preoperative hearing in 70% of patients in whom we attempted preservation of hearing (12). However, a significant group of patients that requires rehabilitation for neurologic deficits.

SUMMARY

Tumors of the posterior fossa encompass a variety of neoplasms of the infratentorial brain parenchyma, cranial nerves, as well as tumors and inflammatory conditions of the adjacent structures of the posterior skull base. Current imaging techniques, in particular MRI, are of great help in diagnosis. Infratentorial, intra-axial brain tumors encompass more than half the pediatric brain tumors. Neurosurgical treatment involves attempted gross total removal via median suboccipital craniotomy, followed by craniospinal radiation. Neuro-otological consultation may be required when there is involvement of the CPA. The most common pediatric CPA tumor seen in our practice is acoustic neuroma in the context of NF2. Hearing preservation via middle fossa craniotomy is attempted in selected patients with small tumors (2 cm or less) and bilateral hearing. When there is no preoperative hearing or no chance to save it, the tumor is removed via a translabyrinthine procedure and an ABI is placed. Patients whose hearing has not been preserved may be rehabilitated with a cochlear implant. Management of patients with NF2 goes well beyond treatment of their CPA tumors to include hearing rehabilitation, genetic counseling, treatment of other tumors, and psychological support.

Current advances in the disciplines involved in the treatment of posterior fossa tumors have resulted in improved survival, and the long-term effects of treatment and disease have become evident. Children who survive their disease often live with neurologic and cognitive deficits that greatly affect their quality of life. Treatment- and disease-related morbidity must be balanced against preservation of function, if possible, and appropriate rehabilitative options must be made available to the patients and their relatives.

REFERENCES

1. Rorke LB, Schut L. Introductory survey of pediatric brain tumors. In: McLaurin RL, Schut L, Venes JL, Epstein F, eds. *Pediatric neurosurgery: surgery of the developing nervous system.* 2nd ed. Philadelphia: WB Saunders; 1989:335.
2. Zimmerman RA, Bilaniuk LT, Rebsamen S. Magnetic resonance imaging of pediatric posterior fossa tumors. *Pediatr Neurosurg* 1992;18:58.
3. Lizak PF, Woodruff WW. Posterior fossa neoplasms: multiplanar imaging. *Semin Ultrasound CT MRI* 1992;13:182.
4. Lo WM. Tumors of the temporal bone and cerebellopontine angle. In: Som PM, Bergeron RT, eds. *Head and neck imaging.* St Louis: Mosby; 1991:1055.
5. Chandrasekhar SS, Brackmann DE, Devgan KK. Utility of auditory brainstem response audiometry in diagnosis of acoustic neuromas. *Am J Otol* 1995;16:63.
6. Shelton C, Brackmann DE, House WF, Hitselberger WE. Acoustic tumor surgery: Prognostic factors in hearing conservation. *Arch Otolaryngol Head Neck Surg* 1989;115:1213.
7. National Institute of Health. Acoustic neuroma. NIH Consensus Development Conference Consensus Statement, 1991.
8. Rouleau GA, Wertelecki W, Haines JL, et al. Genetic linkage of bilateral acoustic neurofibromatosis to a DNA marker on chromosome 22. *Nature* 1987;329:246.
9. Trofatter JA, MacCollin MM, Rutter JL, et al. A novel moesin-, ezrin-, radixin-like gene is candidate for the neurofibromatosis 2 tumor suppressor. *Cell* 1993;72:791.
10. Rouleau GA, Merel P, Lutchman M, et al. Alteration in a new gene encoding a putative membrane-organizing protein causes neuro-fibromatosis type 2. *Nature* 1993;363:515.
11. Briggs RJS, Brackmann DE, Baser ME, Hitselberger WE. Comprehensive management of bilateral acoustic neuromas: current perspectives. *Arch Otolaryngol Head Neck Surg* 1994;120:1307.
12. Brackmann DE, House JR, Hitselberger WE. Technical modifications to the middle fossa craniotomy approach in removal of acoustic neuromas. *Am J Otol* 1994;15:614.
13. Glasscock ME III, Hart MJ, Vrabec JT. Management of bilateral acoustic neuroma. *Otolaryngol Clin North Am* 1992;25:449.
14. Gadre AK, Kwartler JA, Brackmann DE, House WF, Hitselberger WE. Middle fossa decompression of the internal auditory canal in acoustic neuroma surgery: a therapeutic alternative. *Laryngoscope* 1990;100:948.
15. House JW. Translabyrinthine Approach. In: Brackmann DE, Shelton C, Arriaga M, eds. *Otologic surgery.* Philadelphia: WB Saunders; 1994:605.
16. Shannon RV, Fayad J, Moore J, et al. Auditory brainstem implant. II: Postsurgical issues and performance. *Otolaryngol Head Neck Surg* 1993;108:634.
17. Brackmann DE, Hitselberger WE, Nelson RA, et al. Auditory brainstem implant, I: Issues in surgical implantation. *Otolaryngol Head Neck Surg* 1993;108:624.
18. Hoffman RA, Kohan D, Cohen NL. Cochlear implants in the management of bilateral acoustic neuromas. *Am J Otol* 1992;13:525.
19. Zwolan TA, Shepherd NT, Niparko JK. Labyrinthectomy with cochlear implantation. *Am J Otol* 1993;14:220.
20. Noren G, Greitz D, Hirsch A, Lax I. Gamma knife radiosurgery in acoustic neurinomas. In: Tos M, Thomsen J, eds. *Acoustic neuroma. proceedings of the First International Conference on acoustic neuroma.* Amsterdam: Kugler; 1991:289.
21. Lunsford LD, Linskey ME. Stereotactic radiosurgery in the treatment of patients with acoustic tumors. *Otolaryngol Clin North Am* 1992;25:471.
22. Slattery WH, Brackmann DE. Results of surgery following stereotactic irradiation for acoustic neuromas. *Am J Otol* 1995;16:315.
23. Arriaga M, Shelton C, Nassif P, and Brackmann DE. Selection of surgical approaches for meningiomas affecting the temporal bone. *Otolaryngol Head Neck Surg* 1992;107:738.
24. Hitselberger WE, Horn KL, Hankinson H, Brackmann DE, House WF. The middle fossa transpetrous approach for petroclival meningiomas. *Skull Base Surg* 1993;3:130.
25. Miralbell R, Linggood RM, de la Monte S, Convery K, Munzenrider JE, Mirimanoff RO. The role of radiotherapy in the treatment of subtotally resected benign meningiomas. *J Neurooncol* 1992;13:157.
26. Lunardi P, Missori P, Gagliardi FM, Fortuna A. Dermoid and epidermoid cysts of the midline in the posterior cranial fossa. *Neurosurg Rev* 1992;15:171.
27. Krisht AF, O'Brien MS. Acquired mirror-image cerebellopontine angle arachnoid cysts: Case report. *Neurosurgery* 1992;30:798.

28. Haberkamp TJ, Monsell EM, House WF, Levine SC, Piazza L. Diagnosis and treatment of arachnoid cysts of the posterior fossa. *Otolaryngol Head Neck Surg* 1990;103:610.
29. Packer RJ, Sutton LN, D'Angio G, Evans AE, Schut L. Management of children with primitive neuroectodermal tumors of the posterior fossa/medulloblastoma. *Pediatr Neurosci* 1986;12:272.
30. Jenkin D, Goddard K, Armstrong D, et al. Posterior fossa medulloblastoma in childhood: Treatment results and a proposal for a new staging system. *Int J Radiat Oncol Biol Phys* 1990;19:265.
31. Albright L. Posterior fossa tumors. *Neurosurg Clin N Am* 1992;3:881.
32. Pollack IF. Brain tumors in children. *N Engl J Med* 1994;331:1500.
33. Schneider JH, Raffel C, McComb JG. Benign cerebellar astrocytomas of childhood. *Neurosurgery* 1992;30:58.
34. Munari C, Musolino A, Rosler JR, et al. Stereotactic approach to space-occupying lesions in the posterior fossa. *Appl Neurophysiol* 1987;50:200.
35. Ikezaki K, Matsushima T, Inoue T, Yokoyama N, Kaneko Y, Fukui M. Correlation of microanatomical localization with postoperative survival in posterior fossa ependymomas. *Neurosurgery* 1993;32:38.
36. Kaneko Y, Sato Y, Iwaki T, Shin RW, Tateishi J, Fukui M. Chordoma in early childhood: A clinicopathological study. *Neurosurgery* 1991;29:442.
37. Handa J, Suzuki F, Nioka H, Koyama T. Clivus chordoma in childhood. *Surg Neurol* 1987;28:58.
38. Giddings NA, Brackmann DE, Kwartler JA. Transcanal infracochlear approach to the petrous apex. *Otolaryngol Head Neck Surg* 1991;104:29.
39. Thedinger BA, Nadol JB, Montgomery WW, et al. Radiographic diagnosis, surgical treatment, and long term follow-up of cholesterol granulomas of the petrous apex. *Laryngoscope* 1989;99:896.
40. Fisch U, Mattox D. *Microsurgery of the skull base.* New York: Thieme; 1988:242.
41. Carmel PW, Greif LK. The aseptic meningitis syndrome: a complication of posterior fossa surgery. *Pediatr Neurosurg* 1993;19:276.
42. Culley DJ, Berger MS, Shaw D, Geyer R. An analysis of factors determining the need for ventriculoperitoneal shunts after posterior fossa tumor surgery in children. *Neurosurgery* 1994;34:402.
43. Packer RJ, Sposto R, Atkins TE, et al. Quality of life in children with primitive neuroectodermal tumors (medulloblastoma) of the posterior fossa. *Pediatr Neurosci* 1987;13:169.
44. Cochrane DD, Gustavsson B, Poskitt KP, Steinbok P, Kestle JRW. The surgical and natural morbidity of aggressive resection for posterior fossa tumors in childhood. *Pediatr Neurosurg* 1994;20:19.
45. LeBaron S, Zeltzer PM, Zeltzer LK, Scott SE, Marlin AE. Assessment of quality of survival in children with medulloblastoma and cerebellar astrocytoma. *Cancer* 1988;62:1215.
46. Kwartler JA, Luxford WM, Atkins J, Shelton C. Facial nerve monitoring in acoustic tumor surgery. *Otolaryngol Head Neck Surg* 1991;104:814.

CHAPTER 33

Tumors of the Temporal Bone

Karen J. Doyle

Tumors of the temporal bone comprise a small percentage of head and neck tumors in both children and adults. However, the two populations differ in the types of neoplasms affecting the temporal bone (Table 1). In adults, squamous-cell carcinoma of the external canal is the most common malignancy of the temporal bone; this disease is essentially unknown in the pediatric population. The most frequent pediatric temporal bone malignancy is rhabdomyosarcoma, which is almost exclusively a disease of children. Compared with rhabdomyosarcoma, the other pediatric temporal bone malignancies, such as leukemia, fibrosarcoma, Ewing's sarcoma, aggressive papillary adenoma, and others, are exceedingly rare.

In contrast, the benign neoplasms of the temporal bone occur in both adults and children, although less commonly in pediatric patients. These tumors, all of which are unusual, include adenomatous tumors of the middle ear and mastoid, glomus tumors, dermoid tumors, and teratomas. Langerhans' histiocytosis is not a tumor but an idiopathic proliferation of histiocytes that can involve the temporal bone. It is included in this chapter because it is treated as a neoplasm. In this chapter, the malignant and benign tumors of the temporal bone found in children are described, as well as their clinical presentation, diagnosis, and treatment.

MALIGNANT TUMORS

Rhabdomyosarcoma

Despite being the third most common sarcoma overall, rhabdomyosarcoma is the most common soft tissue sarcoma in children (1). It represents 5 to 15% of childhood neoplasms. It affects males more than females (1.37–1.5 : 1.00). The ear is the third most common site for rhabdomyosarcoma of the head and neck, after the orbit and nasopharynx (1). There are two subgroups of rhabdomyosarcomas: pleomorphic, which is more common in adults, and juvenile, which is comprised usually of embryonal, and less often, alveolar and botryoid elements. Rhabdomyosarcoma tumors contain cells resembling developing skeletal muscle (1). Pleomorphic rhabdomyosarcoma represents dedifferentiation of normal muscle, producing a spindle-cell tumor. The cells in embryonal rhabdomyosarcoma resemble those of normally developing skeletal muscle of a 7 to 10-week fetus, with long, thin, spindle-shaped cells having centrally located nuclei and prominent mitoses. Alveolar rhabdomyosarcoma resembles the hollow tube stage of fetal muscle development normally seen at 10 to 12 weeks. The appearance is that of a pulmonary alveolus surrounded by small, round rhabdomyosarcoma cells. Finally, botryoid rhabdomyosarcoma differs grossly from embryonal tumors in that its appearance is like a cluster of grapes. Histologically, it contains a surface layer of spindle cells parallel to the mucosal surface below which occurs a loose arrangement of tumor cells. The origin of temporal bone rhabdomyosarcoma cells may be the muscles of the eustachian tube or tympanic muscles, or they may originate from primitive mesenchyme predating temporal bone development.

Diagnosis

Prat and Gray (2) presented the presenting symptoms and signs of rhabdomyosarcoma of the ear in 50 patients: 56% had a mass in the ear region, 54% had an aural polyp, 40% had ear discharge, 30% had bleeding from the ear, 22% had ear pain, 14% had hearing loss, and 14% had facial paralysis. They found that the average age at presentation was 4.4 years. Canalis and Gussen (3) outlined the clinical course of rhabdomyosarcoma of the ear in three stages: (a) neoplasm limited to the middle ear, producing symptoms similar to otitis media; (b) intratemporal bone expansion resulting in increased pain, hearing loss, and facial nerve paralysis; (c) the terminal stage, characterized by brain, neck, and infratemporal and parapharyngeal space invasion with or without

---

K.J. Doyle: Department of Neurology, University of California/Irvine, Orange, California 92868, and Hearing and Balance Services, Newport Beach, California 92663.

TABLE 1. *Adult and pediatric types of neoplasms that affect temporal bone*

Adult temporal bone tumors		Pediatric temporal bone tumors	
Benign	Malignant	Benign	Malignant
Glomus tumor	Squamous-cell carcinoma	Histiocytosis	Rhabdomyosarcoma
Adenomatous tumor	Basal-cell carcinoma	Adenomatous tumor	Adenocarcinoma
Hemangioma	Adenocarcinoma	Dermoid/teratoma	Leukemia
Eosinophilic granuloma	Chondrosarcoma	Glomus tumor	Ewings sarcoma
Hemangiopericytoma	Rhabdomyosarcoma		Chondrosarcoma
Chondroblastoma	Ceruminoma		Fibrosarcoma
Osteogenic sarcoma			Endodermal sinus
Tumor—leukemia			
Giant-cell tumor			

metastases (3). They also emphasized that rhabdomyosarcoma originating from the petrous temporal bone did not usually become evident until the third stage of the disease, when headaches and cranial nerve palsies occur. They estimated that 25% of temporal bone rhabdomyosarcomas originated in the petrous temporal bone.

The work-up for rhabdomyosarcoma starts with a careful neurotologic examination. Computed tomography (CT) has been recommended for evaluation of the primary tumor, to determine its size, anatomic site, bony destruction, and extent of disease (4). Little has been written about the role of magnetic resonance imaging (MRI) in the work-up of rhabdomyosarcoma of the temporal bone. This author strongly recommends MRI in cases of rhabdomyosarcoma involving the petrous temporal bone or in cases of suspected dural involvement. While CT should always be performed, MRI is useful in evaluating involvement of the internal carotid artery, cavernous sinus, or temporal lobe (Figs. 1, 2).

Intraoperative tissue biopsy provides the diagnosis of rhabdomyosarcoma of the ear. Wiatrak and Pensak (4) recommend thorough metastatic evaluation, including CT of the chest, bone scan, and lumbar puncture. Bone marrow biopsy is indicated when skeletal lesions are suspected.

Treatment

The Intergroup Rhabdomyosarcoma Study (IRS) was started in 1972 to determine the most effective treatments for rhabdomyosarcoma. Maurer (5) introduced the IRS classification system: group I: localized disease, completely resected; group II: grossly resected tumor with microscopic residual disease with or without lymph nodes; group III: gross residual disease; and group IV: metastatic disease. Therapeutic randomized trials were designed to determine optimal treatment for each group. Generally, temporal bone rhabdomyosarcoma falls into group III or IV. For these groups, the IRS uses intensive therapy consisting of radiotherapy and chemotherapy, and the trials are aimed at comparing chemotherapy regimens. The first IRS study, published in 1978, reviewed the results of treatment of 141 patients with embryonal rhabdomyosarcoma of the head and neck (6). Of the 57 patients with parameningeal-site tumor (including the temporal bone), 90% died. It was determined that radiation therapy needed to be administered earlier in such patients, and in higher doses. Outcome of temporal bone rhabdomyosarcoma was noted to be dismal by other authors. Deutsch and Felder (7) found that rhabdomyosarcoma of the ear or mastoid was usually rapidly fatal. Their review of the world literature prior to 1973 revealed 73 cases, with only five long-term survivors, all of whom received a minimum of 5,200 rads to the tumor over 6 weeks. Twenty-four cases developed distant metastases, most often bone and lung. The majority died with uncontrollable disease in the head and neck region. The authors recommended more

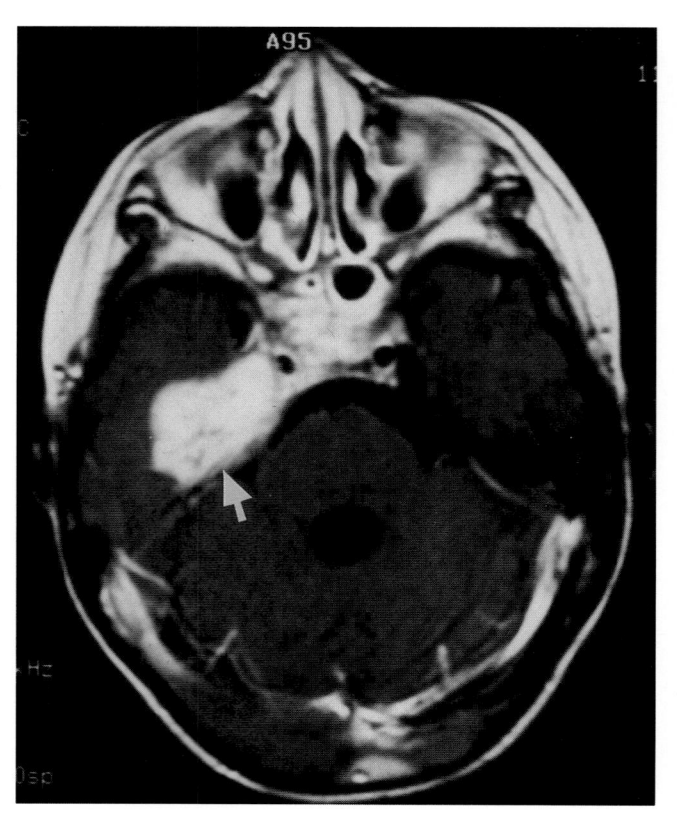

FIG. 1. Axial T1-weighted MRI with gadolinium contrast of large right petrous temporal bone rhabdomyosarcoma *(arrow)*.

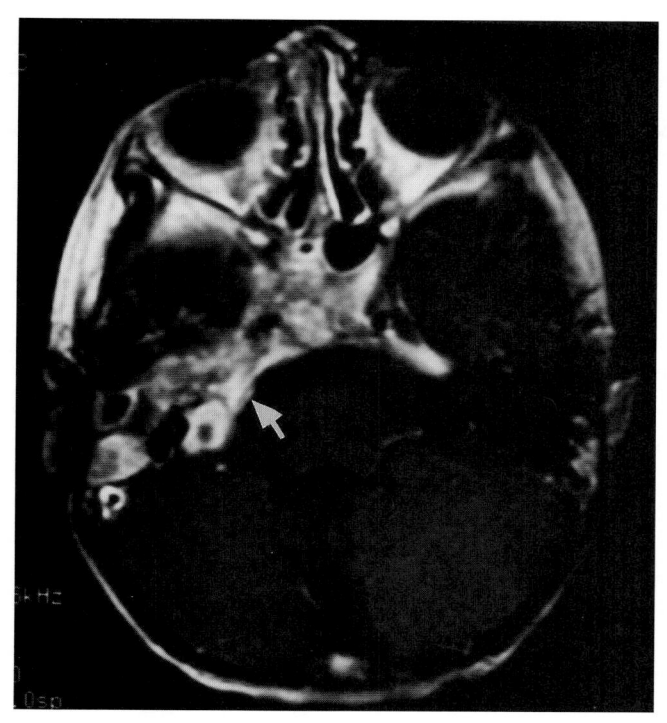

FIG. 2. Postchemotherapy axial MRI demonstrating decrease in tumor size.

aggressive radiation, extirpative surgery when feasible, and adjuvant chemotherapy.

Liebner (8) noted that the orbit, facial soft tissues, and larynx were favorable sites for survival if treated with radiation and single-agent chemotherapy. He included three cases of middle ear rhabdomyosarcoma in his series. Only one of the three children was alive and well at 3 years. Schuller, Lawrence, and Newton (9) had two patients with temporal bone rhabdomyosarcoma in their series of 35, neither of whom survived. Anderson et al. (10) found that the overall death rate for 60 children with head and neck rhabdomyosarcoma of 50% from 1970 to 1979 decreased to 23% from 1980 to 1987. There were six patients with rhabdomyosarcoma of the ear (10%). All patients had multiagent chemotherapy, usually vincristine, cyclophosphamide, actinomycin D, and/or doxyrubicin. Radiation therapy was given to 58 of the 60 patients. Despite this aggressive regimen, the improvement in survival noted in rhabdomyosarcoma in other regions did not extend to the temporal bone. Mortality was 100% for cases involving the temporal bone during both time periods.

In the last decade, the outlook for patients with otic rhabdomyosarcoma has improved slightly. In 1987, Raney et al. (11) reported on outcome in IRS trials in patients having meningeal involvement. Of 32 patients with rhabdomyosarcoma of the temporal bone, survival was only 35% in the group not receiving intensive radiation therapy, as compared with 73% 3-year survival after intensive meningeal radiotherapy and intrathecal chemotherapy consisting of vincristine and actinomycin D. Wiatrak and Pensak (4) feel that rhabdomyosarcoma of the ear and temporal bone is now, for the first time, a potentially curable disease due to multiagent chemotherapy, high-dose–high-volume radiation therapy, and surgical resection. They had two 5-year survivors among 12 patients with rhabdomyosarcoma of the temporal bone. It is important to emphasize that in group IV (metastatic) disease, and recurrent disease, patient outcome remains poor (in the range of 20% 5-yr survival) (12).

Adenocarcinoma

Adenocarcinoma of the temporal bone is rare; Glasscock et al. (13) found only 40 cases in the English language literature. Although the disease typically occurs in adults of approximately 50 years, these tumors have been reported in older pediatric patients (ages 17–19 yrs). Three types of middle ear and mastoid adenocarcinoma have been described: low grade, high grade, and the so-called aggressive papillary adenomas. Low-grade adenocarcinoma contains irregular tubular or glandular structures that are lined by epithelial cells (14). They exhibit some mitotic activity and nuclear pleomorphism. In contrast, high-grade adenocarcinomas contain less well differentiated glands and solid sheets of cells that produce mucin. Schuller et al. (15) described a third type of tumor composed of multiple follicles lined by columnar cells with other areas of papillary proliferation of cells. Benecke et al. (16) described two more cases of papillary adenoma of the temporal bone. This tumor was more common in female patients. They argued that it was a usually benign histology, but it behaved aggressively, with extensive bone involvement. In a few of their cases of papillary adenomatous tumor, there were histologic signs of malignancy, such as mitotic figures and nuclear atypia. Gaffey et al. (17) called these lesions agressive papillary middle ear tumor to distinguish them from benign middle ear adenoma. Heffner (18) first guessed that these tumors were actually low-grade adenocarcinomas derived from the endolymphatic sac. Li et al. (19) determined that these lesions were typically centered in the location of the endolymphatic sac between the sigmoid sinus and internal auditory canal, with early dural involvement and late mastoid involvement, supportive of endolymphatic sac origin. Two case reports in the literature link these agressive papillary adenomas to von Hippel-Lindau disease, an autosomal dominantly inherited syndrome associated with retinal angiomata, hemangioblastoma of the CNS, renal-cell carcinoma, and pheochromocytoma (20,21).

Diagnosis

Amble et al. (22) found that hearing loss was the most common initial symptom of adenocarcinoma of the middle ear, followed by tinnitus, pressure, otalgia, and otorrhea. When diagnosis was delayed, as it usually was in these tumors, pain and facial weakness became more common at presentation. In the tumors described by Glasscock et al. (13), benign tumors presented with aural fullness and conductive hearing loss, while patients with adenocarcinoma had sensorineural hearing loss, vertigo, and cranial nerve signs.

The diagnostic work-up for adenocarcinoma of the ear includes careful neurotologic examination, audiogram, and selected imaging studies. Because the signs may be similar to cholesteatoma or glomus tumor, computed tomography should be performed first. CT findings include bone erosion in the middle ear, mastoid, and external auditory canal for low-grade adenocarcinomas, and petrous, posterior fossa, or middle fossa involvement in more advanced tumors. Endolymphatic sac tumors would be expected to show posterior fossa bone erosion without middle ear involvement (19). If tumor is suspected on the basis of CT findings, MRI should follow. Magnetic resonance imaging with gadolinium differentiates contrast-enhancing tumor from non-enhancing cholesteatoma, soft-tissue reaction, and infection. The combination of CT and MRI aids in surgical planning for tumor margins. Preoperative arteriography is helpful if there is suspicion of vascular tumor.

Treatment

Adenocarcinoma of the temporal bone is treated with transtemporal removal, with infratemporal and suboccipital extensions when necessary (16). With malignant lesions, surgical resection must include a margin of normal tissue. Frequently, dural resection and grafting is necessary (19). Postoperative radiation is controversial; cures of even large tumors have been effected with surgery alone (19,22). Glasscock et al. (13) recommend individualization of therapy; when feasible, total temporal bone resection is undertaken to remove disease with margins. With adequate surgical removal, the decision to irradiate must be based on the age of the patient and the grade of the tumor.

Survival of adenocarcinoma of the temporal bone depends on the extent of disease, the tumor grade, and the adequacy of resection. The three patients with high-grade adenocarcinoma of Dehner and Chen (14) all died within 1 year. The overall mortality in the literature reported by Glasscock et al. (13) was 18%, with most patients succumbing to local invasion.

Leukemia

The acute leukemias—acute myelogenous leukemia—and acute lymphocytic leukemia can affect younger age groups. Acute lymphocytic leukemia, in particular, is more common in the pediatric population. In 1885, Politzer (23) was the first to discover the otologic complications of leukemia, when he discovered leukemic cells in the endolymphatic spaces of a patient with leukemia and sudden deafness. Since that time, many authors have found a significant incidence of otologic complications secondary to leukemia. Druss (24) found that 16.8% of patients with leukemia had otitis media, sensorineural hearing loss, nystagmus, vertigo, vestibular hypofunction, or facial paralysis.

Zechner and Altmann (25) found leukemic infiltrates in the middle ear and mastoid mucous membranes and the marrow spaces of the temporal bone. In four cases, the mucous membranes were so heavily infiltrated that the middle ear and eustachian tube lumens were almost obliterated. The temporal bone infiltration sometimes produced osteoclastic bony erosion of the ossicles, promontory, and in one case, the carotid canal. Infiltration was also seen of the perineural sheath and endoneurium of the facial and cochleovestibular nerves. Hemorrhage of the middle ear and mastoid is also common.

Paparella et al. (26) presented the clinical findings and temporal bone histology of 25 patients with leukemia. Forty-eight percent of the patients had otologic symptoms or signs, and 20% of the patients had otologic problems that could be ascribed to the leukemia process involving the ear. Acute lymphocytic leukemia produced otologic complications more frequently than the other types of leukemia. In 36% of patients, the middle ear was infiltrated by leukemia cells, and infrequently the inner ear also was. Patients who evidenced suppuration had moderate to marked tympanomastoid infiltrates, while leukemic infiltrations judged mild to moderate were never associated with clinical ear disease. Middle ear hemorrhage with hemotympanum was also more common in ALL.

Diagnosis

On the basis of these studies, patients with acute leukemia have a significant chance of developing otologic disease. Therefore, otoscopic examination should be performed periodically in patients having leukemia, and audiologic examination in patients complaining of hearing loss. Computed tomography of the temporal bones should be reserved for patients in whom cholesteatoma is suspected, because surgery is unlikely to be required for most otologic complications of leukemia.

Treatment

Treatment of the leukemic infiltrates is simply the recommended oncologic treatment for leukemia. Suppurative otitis media should be cultured for unusual organisms, with myringotomy to provide drainage and appropriate antibiotics (26). If antibiotic treatment is ineffective for acute mastoiditis, antrotomy or mastoidectomy may be performed.

Ewing's Sarcoma

Ewing's sarcoma, which is most frequently seen in the long bones or pelvis, is rarely found in the temporal bone. While 90% of Ewing's sarcoma patients are under 30 years of age, and it is the second most common primary bone malignancy in children, only ten cases of primary Ewing's sarcoma of the cranium were reported up to 1990 (27). Three of these ten were in the temporal bone, all in young patients aged 4 to 19 years. The male–female ratio is 1.6:1. The tumor is histologically highly anaplastic, with solidly packed small round cells that stain positive for glycogen (28).

Diagnosis

In two of the three pediatric cases of Ewing's sarcoma reported, solid bony masses were noted in the temporal region: one painless and the other tender (27,29). The third patient presented with a long history of recurrent otitis media requiring tympanostomy tubes, followed by severe right otalgia and facial nerve paralysis (28). In the first two patients, the tumors were partially extracranial, while the third tumor had its origin in the petrous temporal bone.

Imaging should include both CT and MRI. Computed tomography reveals a well-circumscribed mass isointense with brain, surrounded by a hypointense area and hyperostosis and remodeling of the bone surrounding the tumor. The soft-tissue mass of Ewing's sarcoma does not ossify, in contrast with osteogenic sarcoma (28). Magnetic resonance imaging demonstrates hypointensity on T1-weighted images and mixed intensity on T2-weighted images, with gadolinium contrast enhancement. Fitzer and Steffey (28) recommended bone scan to delineate bone metastases. Chest CT should be performed to rule out pulmonary metastases.

Treatment

The prognosis of Ewing's sarcoma is often poor because 20% of patients have metastases to lung or other bones present at the time of diagnosis (27). However, in those patients with lesions with an extracranial mass that enables early diagnosis, metastases are rare, and outcome is better. Watanabe et al. (27) found good outcome at 1 year for patients with local swelling as the presenting symptom (27). Few long-term data are published. The recommended treatment is complete surgical excision, followed by wide-field radiation therapy and chemotherapy.

Other Rare Malignancies

Other temporal bone malignancies have been very rarely reported in the pediatric population. Squamous-cell carcinoma of the external auditory canal has been noted only in adults. Several other malignancies have been very rarely reported in children. Chondrosarcoma is a malignancy that typically occurs between the ages of 30 and 50 years and involves the long bones or ribs. Chondrosarcoma of the temporal bone has been usually reported in adults; however, Eggston and Wolff (30) found a chondromyxosarcoma in the temporal bone of a 9-year-old child. Naufal (31) hypothesized that the origin was in the cartilaginous rests of the temporal bone. Fibrosarcoma is another malignant tumor that has very rarely occurred in the temporal bone of children (32,33). It is a mesenchymal tumor arising from fibroblasts that is usually found in the extremities of patients ages 50 to 55. The histologic appearance is of closely packed bands and bundles of elongated spindle cells with numerous mitotic figures and hyperchromatic nuclei. In the two reported cases of pediatric fibrosarcoma of the temporal bone, the tumor was very large, inoperable, and essentially replaced the temporal bone (32,33). Finally, a single case of endodermal sinus tumor of the ear in an infant was reported by Stanley et al. (1987) (34). These are malignant germ-cell tumors in which neoplastic germ cells differentiate into extraembryonic structures and may contain cysts resembling yolk sac vesicles. They usually arise in the ovary or testis or other midline sites. The reported case of an infant with a yolk sac tumor of the ear was a 1-year-old with unilateral facial paralysis and a polypoid mass of the external canal. The prognosis of yolk sac tumors is dismal, and the recommended treatment is chemotherapy.

BENIGN TUMORS

Langerhans' Cell Histiocytosis

Lichtenstein (35) coined the term *histiocytosis X* to designate several clinical syndromes characterized by a nonneoplastic proliferation of unique histiocytes that contain "X" bodies, known as Langerhans' cells. The term *histiocytosis X* includes three disorders: eosinophilic granuloma, Hand-Schuller-Christian disease, and Letterer-Siwe disease. The cause of these syndromes is unknown. Some authors prefer to replace the term *histiocytosis X* with *Langerhans' cell histiocytosis* (LCH). *Eosinophilic granuloma* is defined as a single osseous lesion, usually in the skull, that contains necrosis and Langerhans' cells. Eosinophilic granuloma occurs before age 20 years 75% of the time. Hand-Schuller-Christian syndrome is characterized by multifocal bone lesions and limited extraskeletal involvement of skin, lymph nodes, or viscera. The disease usually occurs in early childhood, though young adults may be affected. Letterer-Siwe disease is disseminated histiocytosis that occurs before age 3 years, with multiorgan involvement and a rapid, severe course.

All three types of LCH may present with temporal bone lesions. The histopathology of the lesions of all three manifestations is alike: sheets and strands of large, round histiocytes, with giant cells, eosinophils, and neutrophils. Areas of necrosis and hemorrhage are common (36).

The incidence of LCH in the pediatric population is 3 per million per year. The male–female ratio is 2:1. Of patients with the different types of LCH, 21% have aural disease (37).

Diagnosis

The presentation of eosinophilic granuloma of the temporal bone is usually that of an aural polyp when the external canal, middle ear, or mastoid is involved (38). Other cases have presented with subcutaneous postauricular or temporal masses (39). Conductive or sensorineural hearing loss may be present, depending on the site of involvement. Because the lesions are osseous, CT scan of the temporal bones is the imaging study of choice; it would show an erosive, punched-out lesion in the involved temporal bone. Biopsy specimens are obtained to make the pathologic diagnosis. Bone survey should be carried out to determine whether there are multiple lesions.

Hand-Schuller-Christian disease consists of multifocal eosinophilic granulomas, usually in the skull or long bones and sometimes in the viscera. The presentation of temporal bone lesions is the same as in solitary eosinophilic granuloma. Jones and Pillsbury (40) noted that temporal bone lesions in histiocytosis were bilateral approximately 30% of the time. In multifocal LCH, involvement of the pituitary is common, and these patients develop diabetes insipidus, so urine osmolality should be measured. Another key to diagnosis is the development of loose teeth, because osseous lesions occur commonly in the mandible and maxilla (40). Facial nerve involvement is rare in LCH (41).

Letterer-Siwe disease is an acute variety of LCH, and the patients succumb rapidly to their disease. Therefore, otologic involvement is not usually emphasized. However, multiple cranial nerve palsies and inner ear involvement have been reported in this syndrome (42,43).

McCaffrey and McDonald (44) summarized the presenting symptoms of all three types of histiocytosis X in 22 patients with temporal bone involvement (15% of all patients with histiocytosis X). The most frequent otologic symptom was aural discharge (15 patients), followed by swelling in the temporal region (11 patients), vertigo (6 patients), and deafness (5 patients). Examination was consistent with otitis media in 13 patients, otitis externa in 10, and temporal bone lesions in 9.

Treatment

The treatment of LCH involving the temporal bone varies, depending on its location. Some lesions have been cured with curettage; others have been cured with mastoidectomy technique. Lesions of LCH respond well to low-dose radiation (100–1,000 rad) (45). Cunningham et al. (46) recommend using CT to precisely define radiotherapy portals. Cure rates for unifocal disease are better than 90%. Chemotherapy has been recommended for multiple lesions. Letterer-Siwe disease has been treated with different chemotherapy regimens, without improvement in survival.

The outcome of LCH was studied in 24 cases by Anonsen and Donaldson (1987) (47). In children with one or more sites of involvement (diabetes insipidus, teeth, lymph nodes, skin, mild pulmonary involvement, or focal bone marrow involvement), there was 86% survival, which was enhanced by the addition of chemotherapy to their radiation therapy. Morbidity was high, however, due to persistent diabetes insipidus, chronic pain, anemia, or growth hormone deficiency resulting in short stature. Angeli et al. (48) reported outcome of LCH. Of their four cases with temporal bone involvement, all of which were multifocal, none of the four patients were free of disease at greater than 5-year follow-up, despite treatment with radiation therapy or chemotherapy. They warned that complete eradication of disease was unusual in multifocal disease, and significant morbidity resulted regardless of the treatment given.

Adenomatous Tumors

Over 100 case reports of benign glandular tumors of the middle ear have been published, but the vast majority of these neoplasms occur in adults (49). However, they have been infrequently reported in children (22,50). They originate from the middle ear mucosa and are locally invasive. There is no sex predilection. Their histologic appearance is uniform, cuboidal-to-columnar cells with round nuclei, eosinophilic cytoplasm, and no mitoses. The cells may be arranged as closely packed glands or solid sheets. In the first part of this chapter, malignant adenomatous tumors of the middle ear were discussed. Some authors have discussed the difficulty of classifying adenomas, because some benign-appearing adenomas behave aggressively (22). There is some controversy as to whether middle ear adenomas originate from neural crest cells rather than mucosal cells. Bold et al. (51) used neuroendocrine immunohistochemical markers to differentiate the types of adenomatous lesions of the temporal bone. Of two glandular tumors they analyzed, they found positive immunohistochemistry for the neuroendocrine markers synaptophysin and neuron-specific enolase. They theorized that some temporal bone adenomas could be derived from the neural crest, rather than from the endoderm, as previously thought.

Diagnosis

Middle ear adenomas usually present with unilateral conductive hearing loss, ear fullness, and tinnitus (52). Others are asymptomatic and present as a mass behind the tympanic membrane. Symptoms may last for years before diagnosis. On CT, the mastoid air cells are opacified, there is little bone erosion, and the ossicles are often encased by a mass (49).

Treatment

Jahrsdoerfer et al. (52) described the treatment of middle ear adenoma. When the tumor is small and confined to the middle ear, exploratory tympanotomy may be used to excise it. For tumors filling the middle ear space, a facial recess mastoidectomy is performed. Radiation therapy is not necessary for these benign lesions.

Glomus Tumors

While glomus tumors or paragangliomas of the temporal bone are the most common benign middle ear neoplasms in adults, they are extremely rare in infants and children (53). They arise along the course of Jacobsen's nerve from the jugular fossa to the promontory in the middle ear, or along Arnold's nerve from the jugular fossa to the descending facial nerve. Paragangliomas located in the jugular fossa are called glomus jugulare tumors, and those originating in the middle ear are called glomus tympanicum tumors. Bartels and Gurucharri (54) reviewed the English language literature and found only seven case reports of pediatric glomus tumors among more than 1,000 reports of adult glomus jugulare tumors. They reported three more cases, and Jacobs and Potsic (55) brought the number of reported pediatric glomus tumors of the temporal bone up to 11. Of these 11 cases, six occurred in girls and four in boys (one not specified). The youngest child was age 6 months, and most of the others were in the age range of 10 to 14 years. While glomus tumors secrete vasoactive substances, such as vanillylmandelic acid and metanephrine only 3% of the time in adults, three of the 11 cases in children (33%) have been secreting tumors.

Diagnosis

While the glomus tumor in adults typically presents with pulsatile tinnitus, conductive hearing loss, and a red mass behind the eardrum, the diagnosis in children has been more difficult. In five of the reported cases, the children were initially treated for chronic otitis media. Four patients had glomus tympanicum tumors that presented with red masses behind the tympanic membrane (three) or in the ear canal (one). Two of these children had bilateral tumors. The other seven patients had glomus jugulare tumors (one bilateral); four of these had cranial neuropathies at presentation. Cranial nerve involvement of nerves V through XII were reported, though facial weakness was the most common deficit. Bartels and Gurucharri (54) noted that glomus tumors in infants were more likely to be tympanicum tumors, while those diagnosed in adolescents were more often jugulare tumors.

Radiologic imaging permits definitive diagnosis of glomus tumors. Magnetic resonance imaging shows intense signal on T1-weighted images, T2 isointense with brain, and gadolinium contrast enhancement. Flow voids are common with paragangliomas and specify the diagnosis. Intracranial extension of tumor is accurately demonstrated, which aids in surgical planning. High-resolution CT with iodine contrast permits differentiation of the jugulare tumor from the tympanicum tumor, which is separated from the jugular bulb by the normal hypotympanic bone that covers the bulb. Computed tomography enables identification of the inferior extent of tympanicum tumors that extend inferior to the tympanic annulus. Finally, CT demonstrates bony erosion of the jugular foramen, mastoid, tegmen, and posterior fossa in extensive tumors. Magnetic resonance venography combined with spin-echo MRI allows differentiation between glomus jugulare tumor and blood flow in the venous sinuses (56). Magnetic resonance venography shows the position of the jugular bulb or thrombus of the jugular bulb, sigmoid sinus, or transverse sinus. However, CT is more useful to differentiate a high-riding jugular bulb from a small glomus jugulare tumor. Carotid angiography is used to identify and preoperatively embolize the feeder vessels of larger tumors.

Treatment

Surgery is the recommended treatment for glomus tumors. Small tympanicum tumors that can be visualized in total through the tympanic membrane can be excised via a transcanal approach. Larger tympanicum tumors that are confined to the middle ear may be removed via a postauricular approach, with limited drilling of the inferior tympanic annulus for additional exposure. Tumors with mastoid or hypotympanum extension require the extended facial recess approach (57). The infratemporal fossa approach is used for extensive lesions (58). Radiation therapy has been used in four pediatric cases with extensive disease; two of these children died, and no follow-up information was available for the other two. Choa and Colman (59) described a large glomus tympanicum tumor that invaded the temporal lobe on autopsy, which was treated with radiation therapy without success (59). Radiation therapy is not recommended for pediatric glomus tumors because no positive outcomes have been reported and because surgical treatment provides the best chance for cure.

Dermoids and Teratomas

Dermoids are tumors that derive from both ectoderm and mesoderm. The head and neck is the site of only 7% of all dermoids (60). Of these, half appear in the orbital region, one-fourth in the oral cavity, and 13% in the nasal cavity (61). Only 24 cases of dermoids involving the temporal bone have been recorded (60). The age range was 14 months to 67 years, with no sex preponderance. Only four cases occurred in patients older than 20 years.

The pathologic appearance of dermoids usually consists of keratinizing epithelium, hair follicles, smooth muscle, and sweat and sebacious glands. It is theorized that they are embryonic rests persisting from early development and are the points of fusion of the first branchial cleft and groove. They usually occur in the midline.

Teratomas derive from all three germ-cell layers. According to Vrabec and Schwaber (60) only six teratomas have been found in the temporal bone. There is a 6:1 female preponderance, and they are usually evident at birth.

Diagnosis

The most common presentations of temporal bone dermoids are otorrhea, hearing loss, middle ear mass, and serous

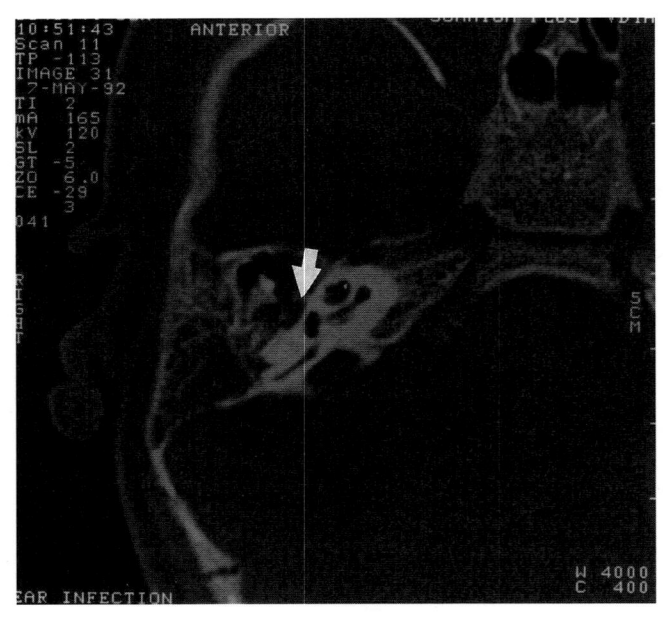

FIG. 3. CT scan demonstrating middle ear and epitympanic dermoid that involved the ossicles *(arrow)*.

effusion. Of the 24 reported cases of temporal bone dermoids, 11 were in the middle ear, and the rest were in the mastoid, eustachian tube, and petrous apex (62). Temporal bone teratomas have been found in the eustachian tube, external canal, middle ear, and mastoid (63). A single case of internal auditory canal teratoma has been reported in a child with multiple anomalies (64).

Dermoids and teratomas are diagnosed after biopsy, but preoperative examination should include microscopic examination to identify a middle ear mass, with biopsy if the mass is exposed in the external auditory canal. Temporal bone CT should be performed if tumor is suspected, to determine the anatomic extent of disease (Fig. 3). An audiogram should be performed preoperatively.

Treatment

Treatment is complete excision. Surgery is tailored to the location of the lesion. Javaheri and MacArthur (65) described transcanal excision of a middle ear dermoid that was visible as a mass behind an intact tympanic membrane. Fried and Vernick (61) described a tympanomastoid approach to a dermoid that filled the middle ear and extended into the attic and antrum. The ossicles were reconstructed. Vrabec and Schwaber (60) encountered a more extensive dermoid that filled the eustachian tube, middle ear, and antrum. Behnke and Schindler (62) used the infralabyrinthine approach to decompress a large dermoid involving the petrous apex. There is no role for radiotherapy or chemotherapy in the treatment of temporal bone dermoids.

CONCLUSIONS

This chapter has outlined the different malignant and benign tumors that involve the temporal bone. In malignant disease, treatment is aimed at cure whenever possible, with a secondary emphasis on preservation of function. In benign disease that carries risk of mortality, such as large glomus tumors or CH, the goal of treatment is control of the disease to ensure long-term survival. In benign tumors of the temporal bone, complete removal of disease and preservation of function with low morbidity are often attainable.

REFERENCES

1. Feldman BA. Rhabdomyosarcoma of the head and neck. *Laryngoscope* 1982;92:424–40.
2. Prat J, Gray GF. Massive neuraxial spread of aural rhabdomyosarcoma. *Arch Otolaryngol* 1977;103:301–3.
3. Canalis R, Gussen R. Temporal bone findings in rhabdomyosarcoma with predominantly petrous involvement. *Arch Otolaryngol* 1980;106:290–3.
4. Wiatrak BJ, Pensak ML. Rhabdomyosarcoma of the ear and temporal bone. *Laryngoscope* 1989;99:1188–92.
5. Maurer HM, The Intergroup Rhabdomyosarcoma Study (NIH): Objectives and Clinical Staging Classification. *J Pediatr Surg* 1975;10:977–8.
6. Tefft M, Fernandez C, Donaldson M, Newton W, Moon TE. Incidence of meningeal involvement by rhabdomyosarcoma of the head and neck in children. *Cancer* 1978;42:253–8.
7. Deutsch M, Felder H. Rhabdomyosarcoma of the ear-mastoid. *Laryngoscope* 1974;84:586–92.
8. Liebner EJ. Embryonal rhabdomyosarcoma of head and neck in children. *Cancer* 1976;37:2777–86.
9. Schuller DE, Lawrence TL, Newton WA. Childhood rhabdomyosarcomas of the head and neck. *Arch Otolaryngol* 1979;105:689–94.
10. Anderson GJ, Tom LWC, Womer RB, Handler SD, Wetmore RF, Potsic WP. Rhabdomyosarcoma of the head and neck in children. *Arch Otolaryngol Head Neck Surg* 1990;116:428–31.
11. Raney RB, Tefft M, Newton WA, et al. Improved prognosis with intensive treatment of children with cranial soft tissue sarcomas arising in nonorbital parameningeal sites. *Cancer* 1987;59:147–55.
12. Maurer HM, Gehan EA, Geltangady M, et al. The intergroup rhabdomyosarcoma study-II. *Cancer* 1993;71:1904–22.
13. Glasscock ME, McKennan KX, Levine SC, Jackson CG. Primary adenocarcinoma of the middle ear and temporal bone. *Arch Otolaryngol Head Neck Surg* 1987;113:822–4.
14. Dehner LP, Chen KTK. Primary tumors of the external and middle ear. *Arch Otolaryngol* 1980;106:13–9.
15. Schuller DE, Conley JJ, Goodman JH, Clausen KP, Miller WJ. Primary adenocarcinoma of the middle ear. *Otolaryngol Head Neck Surg* 1983;91:280–3.
16. Benecke JE, Noel FL, Carberry JN, House JW, Patterson M. Adenomatous tumors of the middle ear and mastoid. *Am J Otol* 1990;11:20–6.
17. Gaffey MJ, Mills SE, Fechner RE, Intemann SR, Wick MR. Aggressive papillary middle ear tumor. *Am J Surg Pathol* 1988;12:790–7.
18. Heffner DK. Lowgrade adenocarcinoma of probable endolymphatic sac origin: a clinicopathologic study of 20 cases. *Cancer* 1989;64:2292–2302.
19. Li JC, Brackmann DE, Lo WM, Carberry JN, House JW. Reclassification of aggressive adenomatous mastoid neoplasms as endolymphatic sac tumors. *Laryngoscope* 1993;103:1342–8.
20. Eby TL, Makek MS, Fisch U. Adenomas of the temporal bone. *Ann Otol Rhinol Laryngol* 1988;97:605–12.
21. Palmer JM, Coker NJ, Harper RL. Papillary adenoma of the temporal bone in von Hippel-Lindau disease. *Otolaryngol Head Neck Surg* 1989;100:64–8.
22. Amble FR, Harner SG, Weiland LH, McDonald TJ. Middle ear adenoma and adenocarcinoma. *Otolaryngol Head Neck Surg* 1993;109:871–6.
23. Politzer A. Pathologische Veranderungen im Labyrinthe bei leukamischer Taubheit. *Cong Int Otol* 1885;3:139.
24. Druss J. Aural manifestations of leukemia. *Arch Otolaryngol* 1945;42:267–85.
25. Zechner G, Altmann F. The temporal bone in leukemia: histological studies. *Ann Otol Rhinol Laryngol* 1969;78:375–87.

26. Paparella MM, Berlinger NT, Oda M, Fiky FE. Otological manifestations of leukemia. *Laryngoscope* 1973;83:1510–26.
27. Watanabe H, Tsubokawa T, Katayama Y, Koyama S, Nakamura S. Primary Ewing s sarcoma of the temporal bone. *Surg Neurol* 1992;37:54–8.
28. Fitzer PM, Steffey WR. Brain and bone scans in primary Ewing's sarcoma of the petrous bone. *J Neurosurg* 1976;44:608–12.
29. Carroll R, Miketic LM. Ewing sarcoma of the temporal bone: CT appearance. *J Comput Assist Tomogr* 1987;11:362–3.
30. Eggston AA, Wolff D. Neoplasms of the ear. In: *Histopathology of the ear, nose and throat.* Baltimore: Williams & Wilkins; 1947:476.
31. Naufal PM, Primary sarcomas of the temporal bone. *Arch Otolaryngol* 1973;98:44–50.
32. Proctor B, Lindsay JR. Tumors involving the petrous pyramid of the temporal bone. *Arch Otolaryngol* 1947;46:180–94.
33. Singh PK, Singh RK, Agarwal A, Rajvanshi VS. Fibrosarcoma of the middle ear. *Ear Nose Throat J* 1989;68:479–80.
34. Stanley RJ, Scheithauer BW, Thompson EI, Kispert DB, Weiland LH, Pearson BW. Endodermal sinus tumor (yolk sac tumor) of the ear. *Arch Otolaryngol Head Neck Surg* 1987;113:200–3.
35. Lichtenstein L. Histiocytosis X: integration of eosinophilic granuloma of bone, Letterer-Siwe disease, and Schuller-Christian disease as related manifestations of a single nosological entity. *Arch Pathol* 1953;56:84–102.
36. Hudson WR, Kenan PD. Otologic manifestations of histiocytosis X. *Laryngoscope* 1970;80:678–93.
37. Smith RJ, Evans JNG. Head and neck manifestations of histiocytosisX. *Laryngoscope* 1984;94:395–9.
38. Toohill RJ, Kidder TM, Eby LG. Eosinophilic granuloma of the temporal bone. *Laryngoscope* 1973;83:877–87.
39. Martin TH. Solitary eosinophilic granuloma of the temporal bone. *Laryngoscope* 1969;79:2165–71.
40. Jones RO, Pillsbury HC. Histiocytosis X of the head and neck. *Laryngoscope* 1984;94:1031–5.
41. Sweet RM, Kornblut AD, Hyams VJ. Eosinophilic granuloma in the temporal bone. *Laryngoscope* 1979;89:1545–52.
42. Cohn AM, Sataloff J, Lindsay JR. Histiocytosis X (Letterer-Siwe disease) with involvement of the inner ear. *Arch Otolaryngol* 1970;91:24–9.
43. Tos M. A survey of Hand-Schuller-Christian's disease in otolaryngology. *Acta Otolaryngol* 1966;62:217–28.
44. McCaffrey TV, McDonald TJ. Histiocytosis X of the ear and temporal bone: Review of 22 cases. *Laryngoscope* 1979;89:1735–42.
45. Kimmelman CP, Nielsen E, Snow JB. Histiocytosis X of the temporal bone. *Otolaryngol Head Neck Surg* 1984;92:588–90.
46. Cunningham MJ, Curtin HD, Jaffe R, Stool SE. Otologic manifestations of Langerhans cell histiocytosis. *Arch Otolaryngol Head Neck Surg* 1989;115:807–13.
47. Anonsen CK, Donaldson SS. Langerhans cell histiocytosis of the head and neck. *Laryngoscope* 1987;97:537–42.
48. Angeli SI, Alcalde J, Hoffman HT, Smith RJ. Langerhans cell histiocytosis of the head and neck in children. *Ann Otol Rhinol Laryngol* 1995;104:173–80.
49. Woods RH, Moses B, Roa A, Lumpkin S, Pearlman S. Middle ear adenoma: Report of two cases. *Otolaryngol Head Neck Surg* 1993;108:754–9.
50. Hyams VJ, Michaels L. Benign adenomatous neoplasm (adenoma) of the middle ear. *Clin Otolaryngol* 1976;1:17–26.
51. Bold EL, Wanamaker JR, Hughes GB, Rhee CK, Sebek BA, Kinney SE. Adenomatous lesions of the temporal bone: Immunohistochemical analysis and theories of histogenesis. *Am J Otol* 1995;16:146–52.
52. Jahrsdoerfer RA, Fechner RE, Moon CN, Selman JW, Powell JB. Adenoma of the middle ear. *Laryngoscope* 1983;93:1041–4.
53. Busby DR, Hepp VE. Glomus tympanicum tumor in infancy. *Arch Otolaryngol* 1974;99:377–8.
54. Bartels LJ, Gurucharri M. Pediatric glomus tumors. *Otolaryngol Head Neck Surg* 1988;98:392–5.
55. Jacobs IN, Potsic WP. Glomus tympanicum in infancy. *Arch Otolaryngol Head Neck Surg* 1994;120:203–5.
56. Vogl TJ, Juergens M, Balzer JO, et al. Glomus tumors of the skull base: combined use of MR angiography and spin-echo imaging. *Radiology* 1994;192:103–10.
57. House WF, Glasscock ME. Glomus tympanicum tumors. *Arch Otolaryngol* 1973;97:43–8.
58. Fisch U, Pillsbury HC. Infratemporal fossa approach to lesions in the temporal bone and base of skull. *Arch Otolaryngol* 1979;105:99–107.
59. Choa DI, Colman BH. Paraganglioma of the temporal bone in infancy. *Arch Otolaryngol Head Neck Surg* 1987;113:421–4.
60. Vrabec J, Schwaber MK. Dermoid tumor of the middle ear: case report and literature review. *Am J Otol* 1992;13:580–1.
61. Fried MP, Vernick DM, Dermoid cyst of the middle ear and mastoid. *Otolaryngol Head Neck Surg* 1984;92:594–6.
62. Behnke EE, Schindler RA. Dermoid of the petrous apex. *Laryngoscope* 1984;94:779–83.
63. Silverstein H, Griffin WL, Balogh K. Teratoma of the middle ear and mastoid process. *Arch Otolaryngol* 1967;85:243–8.
64. Maniglia AJ, Wolff D, Herques AJ. Congenital deafness in 13-15 trisomy syndrome. *Arch Otolaryngol* 1970;92:181–8.
65. Javaheri S, MacArthur C. Dermoid cysts of the middle ear. *Otolaryngol Head Neck Surg* 1994;111:P197.

PART XII

Surgical Considerations and Reconstructive Surgery

CHAPTER 34

Congenital Auricular Deformities

Dysmorphic and Dysplastic Ears

Robert O. Ruder

Microtia is a malformation of the auricle ranging from a small external ear with minimal structural abnormality, to an ear with major external, middle-, and inner-ear structural aberrations. It occurs in 1 in 7,000 births. Management of patients with microtia may be one of the most satisfying or frustrating experiences encountered by otolaryngologists. Reconstruction of the auricle and associated atretic external canal requires a sound understanding of the normal anatomy and supporting elements of the pinna. Close communication between the otologist and facial plastic surgeon is paramount for proper timing, sequence, and positioning of this multistage reconstructive problem.

Children with any craniofacial deformity often bring overwhelming devastation to the family. Parental guilt, anger, hostility, and depression must be delicately handled. The young patients must also be approached and counseled before peer-group teasing and ridicule becomes an obstacle to their emotional growth and development (1).

The literature is replete with descriptions of numerous malformations and techniques, which are often confusing to understand and frustrating to implement (2) The terms prominent, protruding, cupped, hooded, lidded, cryptotic, constricted, and ''peanut'' ears have been used interchangeably for very different developmental problems. Auricular reconstruction requires a thorough understanding of the anatomy and the supporting elements of the normal ear. The surgeon needs to recognize and differentiate *dysmorphic* (deformational) development from *dysplastic* (arrested) development.

ANATOMY

Microtia is the consequence of arrested development of the six swellings (hillocks) of mesodermal and epidermal tissue around the first and second branchial arches. These hillocks surround the pharyngeal groove lying between them (Fig. 1).

The grooves and arches represent what were originally the primordial gill slits of a fish. The anlage of the external ear is first seen beneath the developing mandible by the fourth week of gestation (3). By the second month, the primordial ear tissue begins its migration from an inferior medial position beneath the mandible to a posterior superior location on the mastoid. The pinna reaches its adult configuration by the beginning of the second trimester.

The pinna consists of an internal skeleton of fibroelastic cartilage and a fibroadipose lobule. Measurements and relationships between various parts of the auricle have been described (4). It is perhaps best to conceptualize the ear as a flap-like structure attached to the head, which is composed of three layers (Fig. 2). The internal layer is the *concha*, which surrounds the opening of the ear canal. The second layer is the *scapha*, the main buttress and the site at which most anomalies occur. The *helix* is the outer layer, which defines the boundary and configuration of the auricle.

EPIDEMIOLOGY

Late gestational mechanical forces may also affect auricular shape and form. Abnormal intrauterine fetal positioning because of intrauterine masses such as cystic hygromas may displace the ear and cause excessive protrusion or constriction. At birth, the ear is still at a lower position on the face than that of the adult ear, is rounder (less oval-shaped), and is almost two thirds the size of the adult auricle.

Subtle adverse genetic, ototoxic, or environmental factors can interfere with the rapid sequence of developmental changes and cause catastrophic abnormalities. Microtia can occur either as an isolated defect or in association with other abnormalities (4,5). In only a few patients has a genetic or

---

R.O. Ruder: Head and Neck Surgery, Cedars Sinai Medical Center, Los Angeles, California 90048; and Department of Head and Neck Surgery, UCLA Medical Center, Beverly Hills, California 90024.

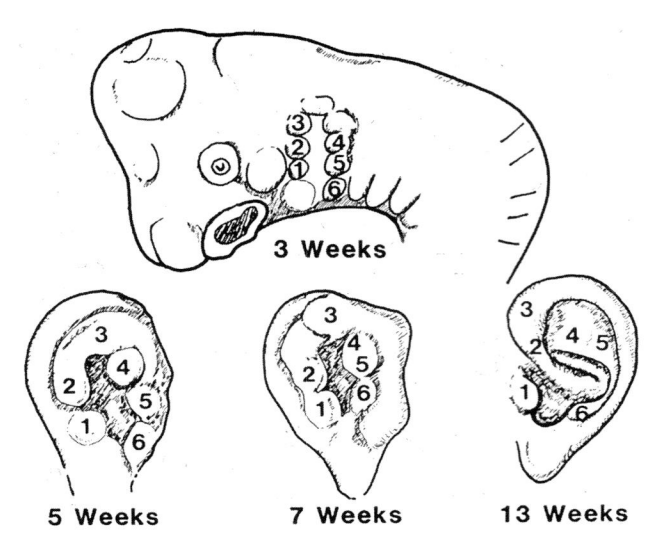

FIG. 1. The auricle develops from six hillocks of the first and second branchial arches. It is first seen in the third week of gestation and reaches adult configuration by the end of the first trimester.

environmental cause been found. In these patients, microtia is usually part of pattern of several other congenital anomalies. Microtia is an essential component of thalidomide and isotretinoin embryopathies. It can also be a part of the fetal alcohol syndrome and maternal diabetes embryopathy. It has been reported in number of gene disorders, such as Treacher Collins syndrome, and in chromosomal syndromes such as trisomy 18.

Because of the close association of ear anomalies with a variety of specific pattern of defects (syndromes), careful evaluation of all patients for associated anomalies is mandatory and is usually most effective if accomplished by an experienced dysmorphologist or clinical geneticist. More than 50% of children with severe ear anomalies have associated preauricular appendages, facial asymmetry, facial paresis or paralysis, deafness, and cervical vertebral anomalies (6–8). More distal concomitant anomalies can be seen in the kidneys and in the conductive system of the heart. These infants should all be carefully evaluated early; but it is critical to evaluate for hearing loss in the unaffected ear within the first 2 months of life. Brainstem-evoked-response audiometry (BSERA) is the most reliable test for hearing evaluation at this age. This noninvasive test can be administered without sedation if it is given before the infant is 3 months old (9,10).

CLASSIFICATION

Auricular anomalies have been categorized and graded in numerous, often confusing, ways. I use a grading system based on three levels of severity.

Grade I

Grade I deformities (dysmorphic) include ears with all anatomic subunits present, but the ears are misshapened (Fig. 3). These seemingly severe deformities can often be corrected at birth with nonsurgical methods because of the excessive plasticity of the auricles within the first days after birth. During the first few days of life, the large amounts of maternal estrogen still circulating in the neonate cause the hyaluronic acid content and the mucopolysaccharide matrix of the ear cartilage to remain soft and pliable (11). If all anatomic subunits of the pinna are present, even strikingly dysmorphic deformities can be resculptured with tape and molding (12–15).

The protruding or prominent ear presents a special problem. Although many minor anomalies spontaneously improve during the infant's first year, excessive ear protrusion can be an acquired deformity and may become more accentuated at 1 year. Two different mechanisms may explain the excessive unfurling of the anthelical fold and the increased

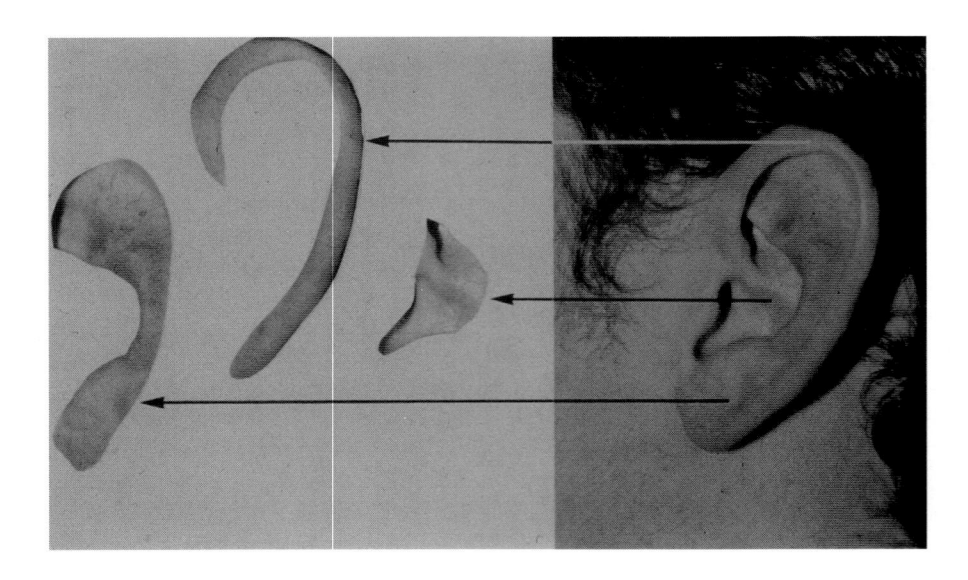

FIG. 2. The auricle can be conceptualized as three layers: concha, scapha, and helix. The scapha is the main buttress and structural support.

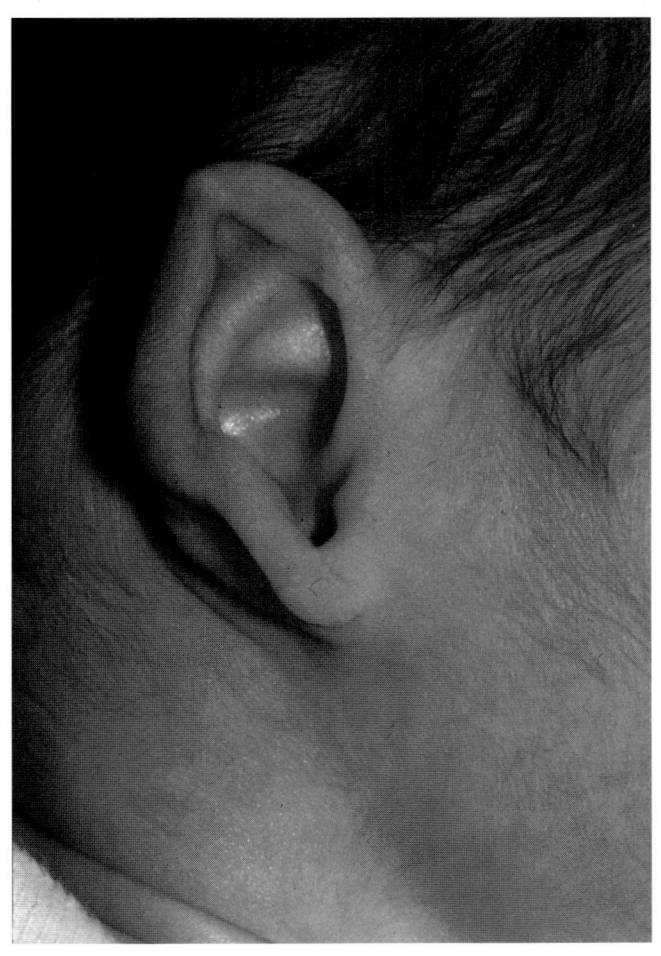

FIG. 3. Dysmorphic ear anomalies result from abnormal intrauterine positioning, which causes pressure on the developing auricle.

velop. The deformed (dysplastic) ears are small and constricted in configuration. Such defects do not respond to the molding approaches that are successful with the dysmorphic ear (17,18).

Grade II anomalies result from dysplastic or aplastic development of the auricular hillocks of the first two branchial arches. One or more anatomic subunits of the three-layered auricle fails to develop (Fig. 4). Unlike overly prominent protruding ears, dysplastic or constricted ears do not worsen after birth. Most commonly, the scapha (the main supporting buttress of the ear) is weak and deficient. Without its support, the superior aspect of the pinna appears to fall over on itself, thus causing lidding and foreshortening (Fig. 5). These defects must be surgically reconstructed with grafts of cartilage and skin, usually at age 6 years (Table 1).

The microtic auricle (grade III) results from arrested development of the first two branchial arches before the fifth gestational week. Classically, the microtic ear (Fig. 6) is a vestigial anlage of the six hillocks represented as a vertically oriented flap of tissue with cartilage remnants superiorly and a fibroadipose nubbin inferiorly. In most patients, the external canal also fails to develop. Such atretic ear canals

angulation of the concha present in the prominent ear: (a) weakness of the intrinsic auricular muscles or (b) the forward displacement of one ear when the infant lies with the head turned to one side for an excessive length of time (e.g., plagiocephaly-torticollis deformation sequence) (16). Whenever the rim of the helix protrudes more than 2 cm from the mastoid, one should consider placing a tubular elastic headband over the pinna when the child is lying supine. Such "head banding" must be continued throughout the infant's first year. However, if ear molding is begun immediately after birth, prolonged head banding may be unnecessary for some patients.

Remolding prominent ears *after* the first year without surgery has not been successful. The children must wait until age 5 or 6, when the auricle attains 80% of its adult size. At this age, formal surgical otoplasty can readily improve both types of problems causing protrusion.

Grades II and III

The more severe types of congenital anomalies result when the primordial tissues that form the auricle fail to de-

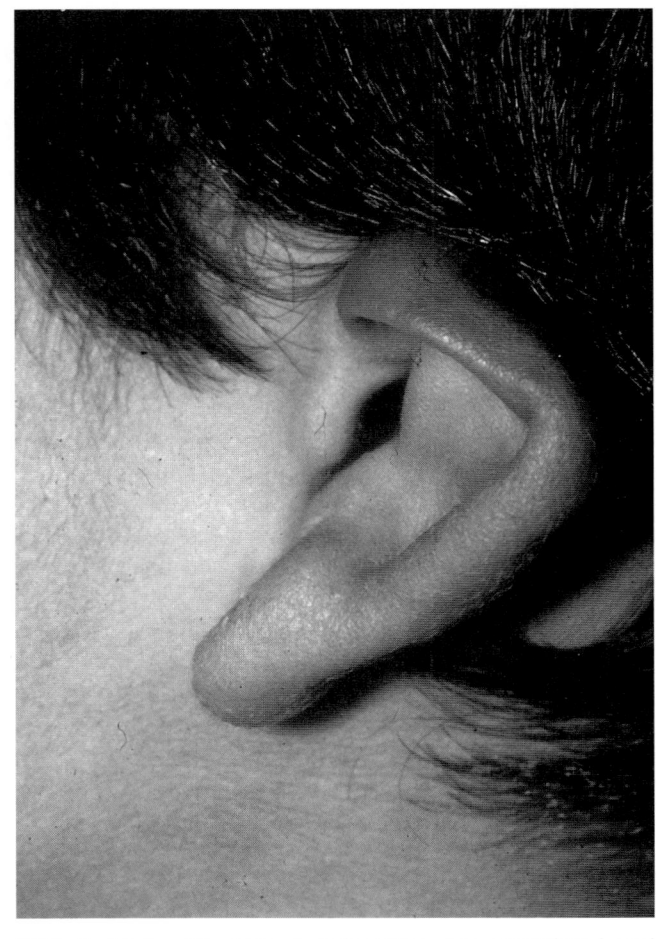

FIG. 4. Ears with class II deformities are constricted and small, and they lack anatomic subunits.

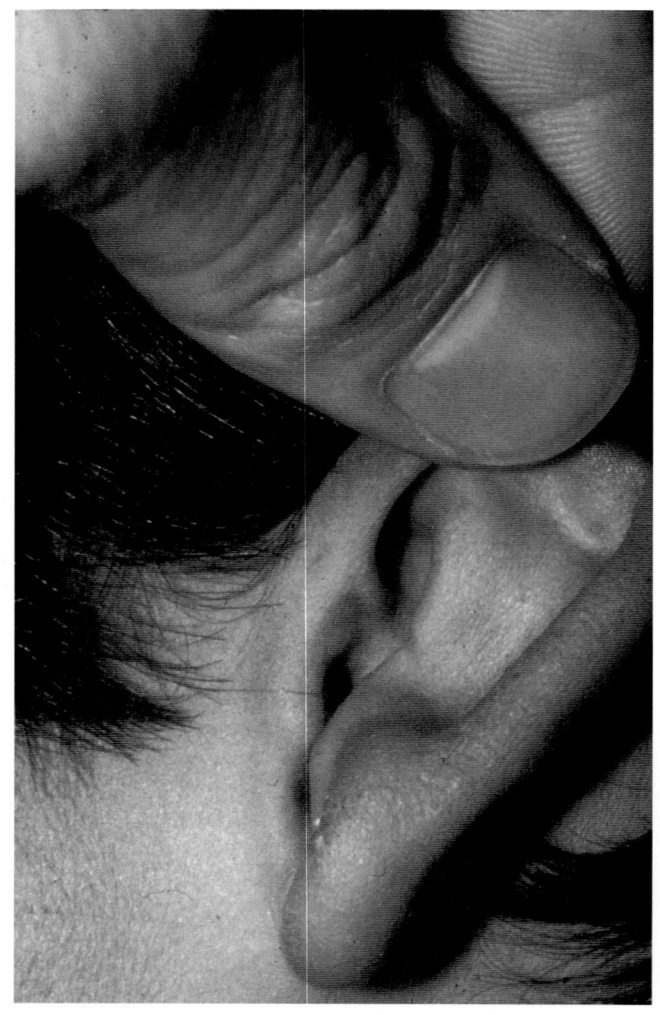

FIG. 5. The constricted ear often seems to fold over on itself. When the fold is elevated, deficient units are easily seen.

with microtia should be screened for heart and urinary tract anomalies. However, syndromes in which the ear and renal anomalies are associated together on a genetic basis (e.g., branchio-otorenal syndrome) are rare, considerably less common than the isolated association of external and middle-ear (conductive hearing loss) deformities. The National Collaborative Perinatal Project followed more than 50,000 mothers from pregnancy and their children through 8 years. Data collected by the Italian Multicenter Birth Defects Registry encompassed 1,173,794 births from 1983 to 1992. Of these combined groups, 1.46 in 10,000 children had at least one malformed auricle. Of infants with microtia, 31% had congenital heart abnormalities, 17% had cleft palate, 15% had esophageal atresia, 13% had vertebral defects, but only 6% had renal anomalies. Of the patients with isolated ear malformations, 6% had sensorineural hearing loss. These data suggest that evaluation for hearing loss and heart defects is much more important in this group of patients than is evaluation for urinary tract anomalies (20).

are often associated with a moderate to profound unilateral conductive hearing loss. These patients require early hearing evaluation with brainstem audiometry (ABR) before 3 months of age. Infants with bilateral profound hearing loss should be fitted with hearing amplification by age 3 months to enhance processing in the auditory nuclei and in the cerebral cortex (19). Previously, many clinicians felt that patients

TABLE 1. *Common anatomic auricular deformities*

Unfurling of anthelical fold
Increased angulation of vertical portion of concha
Protrusion of ear
Flattening of helical fold
Low-lying crus helicis
Absent fossa triangularis
Inadequate support of scapha, causing lidding of helical rim
Inadequate cartilage framework
Lack of adequate skin envelope

Deformities are listed in order of increasing severity.

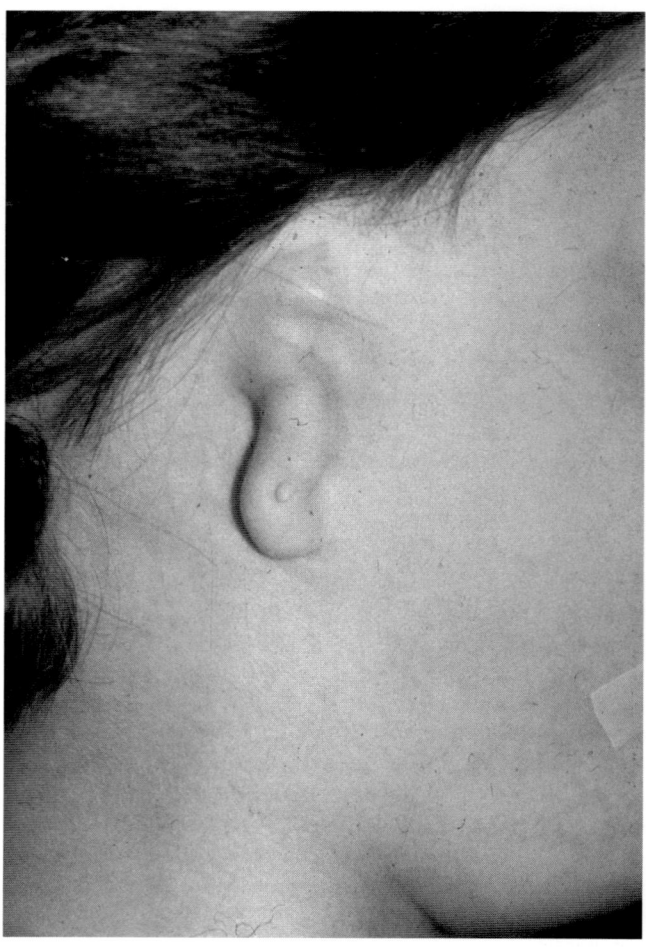

FIG. 6. Ears with grade III deformities have an inferior fibroadipose lobule and a nubbin of cartilage in the superior remnant.

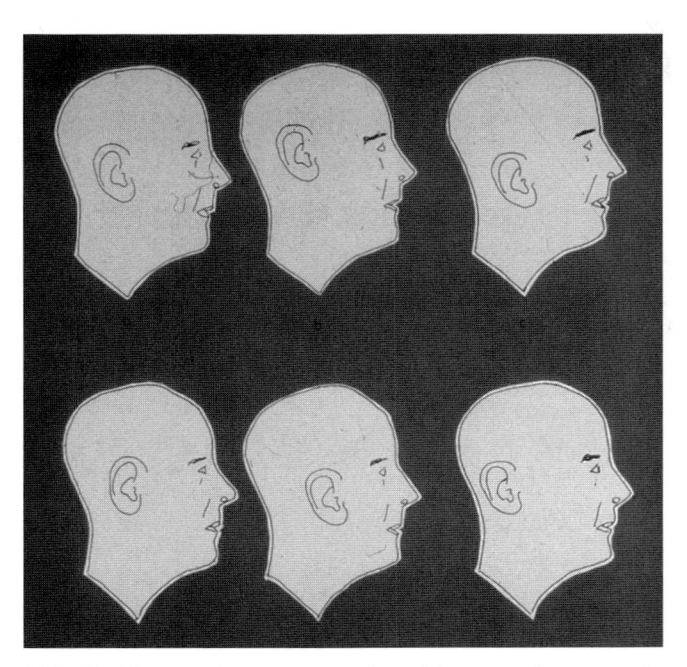

FIG. 7. The newly constructed auricle must be properly placed. It should lie between the eyebrows and the base of the columella. The ideal lateral position is 6 cm (the vertical height) from the lateral canthus. A pinna positioned too inferiorly, superiorly, anteriorly, or posteriorly should signal that something is wrong.

CLINICAL MANIFESTATIONS AND DIAGNOSIS

The microtic deformity is only one part of a multifaceted problem. Most (85%) of the afflicted patients have unilateral microtia. Of the 15% with bilateral microtia, the severity was not the same on the two sides. Bilaterality was more common (50%) with syndromic cases than with non-syndromic cases 12%. Four common syndromes with bilateral involvement are Fraser syndrome, Nager syndrome, Goldenhar syndrome, and Treacher Collins syndrome. Of patients with nonsyndromic microtia, 50% have other associated congenital deformities. A well-coordinated team approach of otologists, facial plastic surgeons, social workers, geneticists, pediatricians, audiologists, nurses, and dentists is essential to adequately assist both the afflicted infant and the emotionally (and financially) affected family.

Farkas assessed ear morphology and presented a detailed, uniform standard of measurements for planning ear reconstruction (21). The many descriptions of proper placement, positioning, and configuration are often confusing to the less experienced surgeon. It is perhaps best to use one's fingers and eyes to make a proper diagnosis and to integrate the "formulas" with aesthetic guidelines. The position of the auricle is the most important aesthetic landmark. A malpositioned pinna should bring immediate attention that something is wrong (Fig. 7). The newly constructed ear should lie between the eyebrow and the base of the columella. It should not be vertical, but slightly inclined, similar to the angulation of the nose. The normal auricle lies the vertical height of a normal ear (5½ cm) from the lateral orbital rim. In patients with unilateral microtia, the surgeon can use the unaffected side as a template for proper position, size, and configuration. However, with bilateral microtia, one needs a sounder knowledge of facial proportions, shape, and orientation.

The *flap-like* structured ear is slightly oval and positioned slightly posterior to the vertical axis in relation to other facial structures. The ear must not be flat against the skull, but have some protrusion. Grafts of rib cartilage must be sculptured into a three-layered framework with enough definition to simulate the convolutions of the scapha and conchal subunits.

The classic microtic ear is "peanut shaped" with a small nubbin of fibroelastic cartilage superiorly and a well-developed lobule of fibroadipose tissue inferiorly. If the auricle fails to migrate from the mandible toward the mastoid during gestation, it can lie anywhere along the pathway of migration and lie anteriorly, posteriorly, and inferiorly beneath the mandible (Fig. 8). Remnants of auricular skin tags and ear

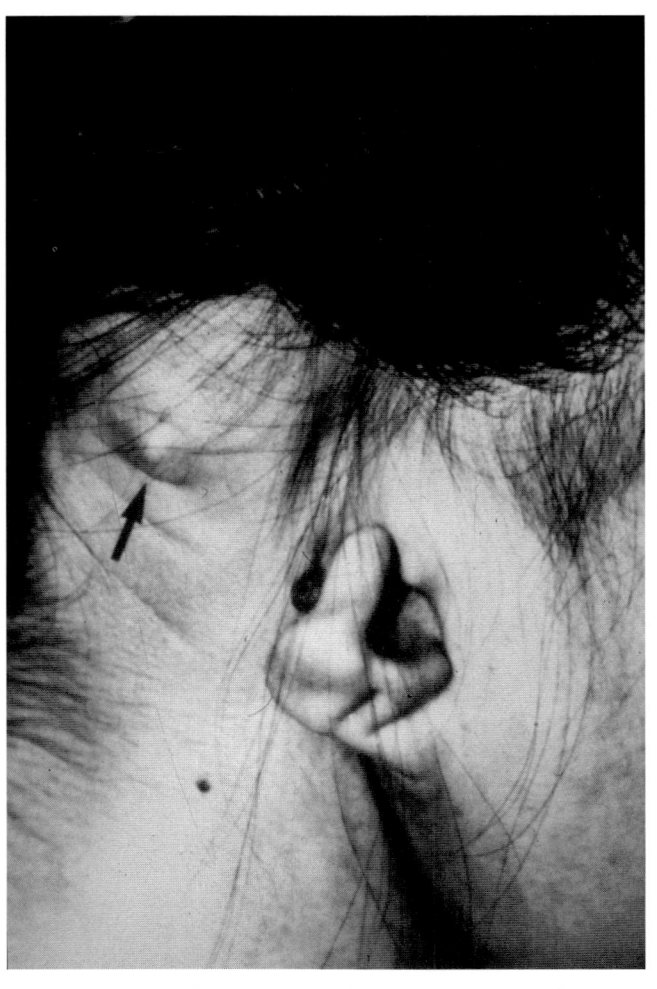

FIG. 8. The developing auricle failed to migrate to the mastoid, and is lying on the mandible.

"pits" are often seen along this path of migration. Reconstruction must address problems with a lack of auricular cartilage, inadequate skin envelope, and the abnormally positioned remnant of microtic tissue.

MANAGEMENT GOALS

My method of microtia reconstruction usually involves four surgical stages separated by 3-month intervals. The first procedure entails harvesting and sculpturing of rib cartilage and placement in a thin skin pocket. During the second stage, the inferior third of the pinna is constructed by rotating the fibroadipose remnant into a lobule. Stage three consists of constructing a tragus and neointroitus of the canal. In the final setting, the neoauricle is elevated and separated from the skull with a scalp advancement flap and skin graft.

Reconstruction usually begins when the child is 6 or 7 years. Although age 8 or 9 may be more ideal, by age 6 the chest wall is of adequate size for harvesting ribs without leaving a significant cosmetic deformity (22). By this age, the normal auricle is almost 85% of adult size, and the patient is often asking for help. By age 5, children are extremely sensitive to their body image. Their deformity becomes an object of curiosity to kindergarten playmates. The emotional impact of this undue attention and ridicule often causes intense shame and devastating anguish.

Children with bilateral microtia have compounded problems. In addition to the heightened incidence of other syndromic deformities, which also need investigation and treatment, hearing must be restored as early as possible. If adequate hearing restoration cannot be achieved with amplification, the conductive component should be addressed surgically by the time the child is age 4.

Alternative Approaches

The two most important decisions in microtia reconstructions concern the skin coverage and the underlying sculptured framework. Several different implant materials have been used to create the framework. Gilles first popularized cartilage allografts in the 1920s (23). Although these grafts were soon absorbed, they were the most common grafts used until the late 1950s. Cronin described silicone framework auricular grafts in 1961 (Fig. 9) (24,25). Because these grafts were preformed, they eliminated the work and morbidity of harvesting and sculpturing rib grafts; however, high infection and rejection rates curtailed use of this material. Ohmori believed he could reduce rejection and infection of the silastic implants by covering the framework with polyethylene mesh, (26) but the high infection rate (30%), and extrusion rate (25%) persisted.

Tanzer gained considerable experience with autogenous cartilage grafts during the 1960s (27). He sculptured a three-layered auricular framework to create the concha, scapha, and helix. In the 1980s, Brent expanded Tanzer's techniques with autogenous grafts by first creating an open framework

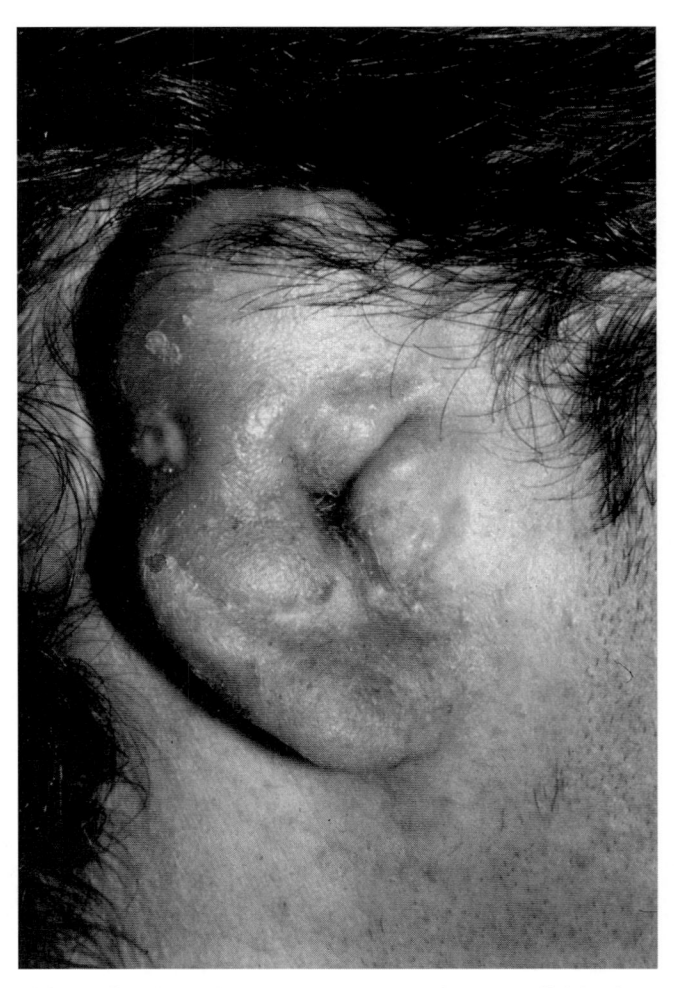

FIG. 9. Synthetic frameworks have not been a reliable alternative because they are too often rejected and become infected, even with minor trauma.

(28). Howver, this sutured graft technique was unstable and separate pieces of cartilage often become detached and absorbed. In the mid-1980s Brent changed his sculpturing technique by constructing a less delicate cartilage framework consisting of three layers (29). I have used this technique for the past 10 years (29).

Gorney described use of autogenous ear cartilage from the normal unaffected side (30). This technique is extremely demanding and requires experience and unique skill. Reinish is now using prefabricated auricles made of Medpor (manufacturer, city) (30). The graft is covered with a temporoparietal fascia flap. Although Reinish's patients have had exposure of the underlying Medpor framework, no rejection of the grafts has yet occurred. However, the resutls are still preliminary (J. Reinish, *personal communication,* 1995).

The overlying skin is often the most compelling problem with successful reconstruction. Ideally, the mastoid skin should be well vascularized, unscarred, elastic, and not deformed from the convolutions of the underlying microtia nubbin. The lack of any of these parameters compromises the outcome. Scarring from prior atresia canalplasty and craniofacial reconstruction must be removed and replaced with temporoparietal fascia and skin grafts. It is therefore better to coordinate teams handling auricular repair and atresia reconstruction to prevent excessive and abnormally placed scars. If possible, auricular repair should precede canalplasty.

Recommended Approach

Treatment begins during the initial consultation with the family. Often the parents feel unjustified guilt that their genetic pool or behavior during pregnancy caused their child's deformity. Every child should be evaluated by geneticists, social workers, and craniofacial teams to help resolve these anxiety-provoking questions. The family must be comforted and introduced into a secure relation with their surgeon for optimal patient compliance during the multistaged postoperative periods.

Development of the reconstructed ear should parallel the growth of the normal side; thus, one should lengthen the lobular soft tissue. Brent's series suggested that 48% of constructed ears grew at an even pace with the opposite normal side. Only 10% of his patients had disparity of growth between the two sides (31). In the youngest patients, I make the ear the same size or slightly smaller than the normal ear in the youngest patients.

Proper placement of the neoauricle is critical. One should use landmarks from the normal side to ensure proper positioning, size, and configuration. Templates of exposed x-ray film are used to draw the proper distances from the lateral canthus, lip commissure, and nasal alae (Fig. 10). The tem-

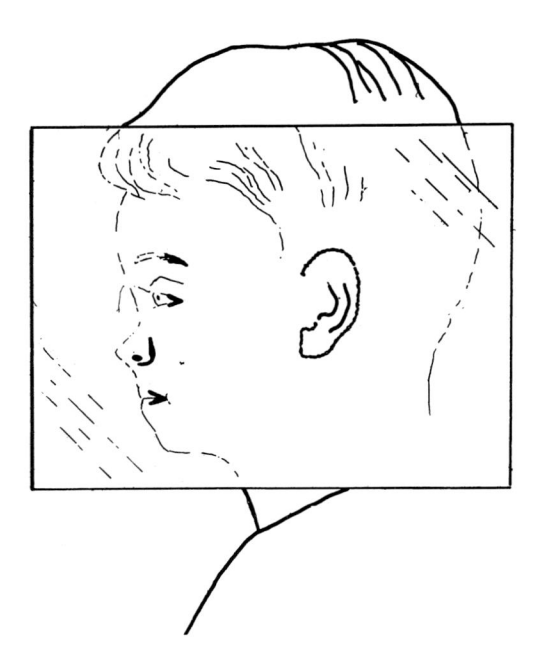

FIG. 10. A template of x-ray film from the normal pinna, drawn slightly smaller to allow for skin thickness, is made for size and configuration of the microtic ear.

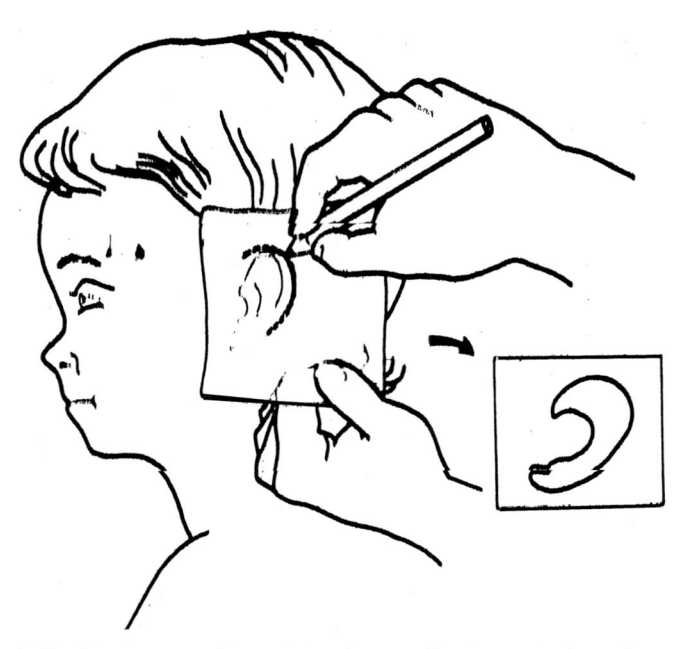

FIG. 11. A second template of x-ray film is made from the normal side using the eyebrow, lateral canthus, nostril, and lip as landmarks to ensure proper positioning.

plate is reversed and tattooed into the skin of the microtic ear with methylene blue. A second template of x-ray film is then placed over the normal ear, and the ear's outline is drawn 2 mm smaller in all dimensions to allow for the thickness of the overlying skin (Fig. 11). This template is cut for later use when one creates the shape and size of the cartilage framework.

Patients with severe craniofacial asymmetry present additional problems in placement of the neoauricle. Differences in facial height and other dimensions may require positioning at slightly different levels, and the new ear may need to be larger or smaller than the unaffected side (32). The neoauricle must not be placed too close to the eye nor too posteriorly on the mastoid. When both auricular reconstruction and craniofacial bony repairs are necessary, the surgical teams need to be integrated and well coordinated. Ideally, the auricular reconstruction should be done first to avoid scarred unusable skin. If the craniofacial reconstruction is started first, incisions should be made peripherally to the mastoid skin.

Low-lying hairline is often troublesome. One should not avoid a low-lying hairline by placing the graft too low or anteriorly; a few options that do not compromise correct position are available. Depilation and electrolysis are helpful in light-skinned patients (33). Dark-skinned patients with thick hair may need to have the overlying hairline removed and replaced with temporoparietal fascia and a nonpilous skin graft. The reconstructed ear may have to be made smaller to avoid hair and the size of the normal ear later reduced for symmetry.

OPERATIVE TECHNIQUE

Rib cartilage is taken from the *contralateral* chest wall because its curvature allows better configuration of the sculptured framework. An incision is made above and parallel to the inferior border of the rib cage. The rectus abdominis muscle and the rectus sheath are divided and dissected until the ribs are visualized. The previously made x-ray template is used to estimate the amount of costal cartilage necessary (Fig. 12). All perichondrium should be carefully preserved in this *extraperichondrial* dissection. Iatrogenic tears in the pleura must be identified and can be repaired without chest tubes if intrathoracic air is suctioned with a red rubber catheter and syringe while the anesthesiologist is hyperinflating the lungs. The syndrotic region of ribs 7 and 8 are usually adequate for the framework. The ninth rib is separately dissected to create a helix.

Construction of the Auricle

While the co-surgeon is repairing the donor site, the cartilage grafts are taken to a separate "carving" table. A three-layered auricle (concha, scapha, and helix) is created by sculpturing and suturing the cartilages with 4-0 stainless steel wire (Fig. 13). The cartilage should be made 2 to 3 mm smaller than the opposite (normal) ear to allow for the thickness of the covering skin pocket. A common error is to make the framework too wide rather than too long. The shape and natural curvature of the ninth rib make it ideal for a helical rim. The helix is created by delicately removing perichondrium and cartilage from the *convex* side only, which allows the rib to bend away from the side of dissection. The rim must be gently thinned to create adequate curvature but maintain enough height to exaggerate the ridge.

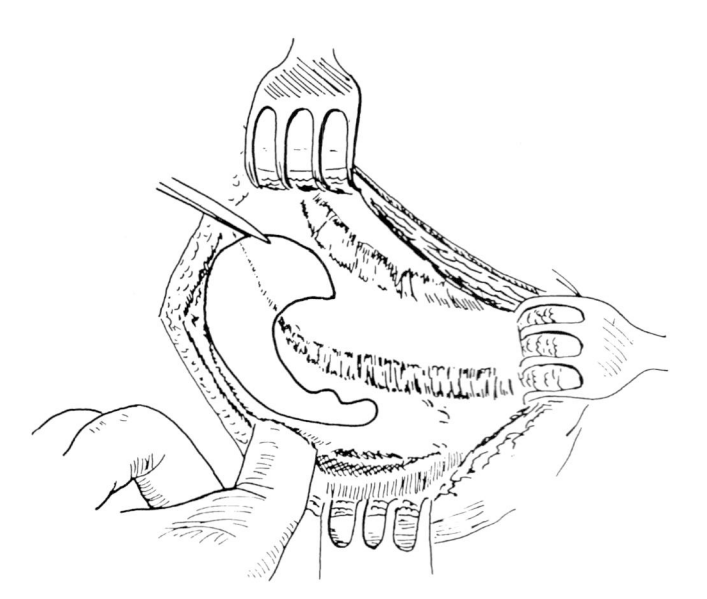

FIG. 12. The x-ray template is placed over the dissected seventh and eighth cartilaginous ribs.

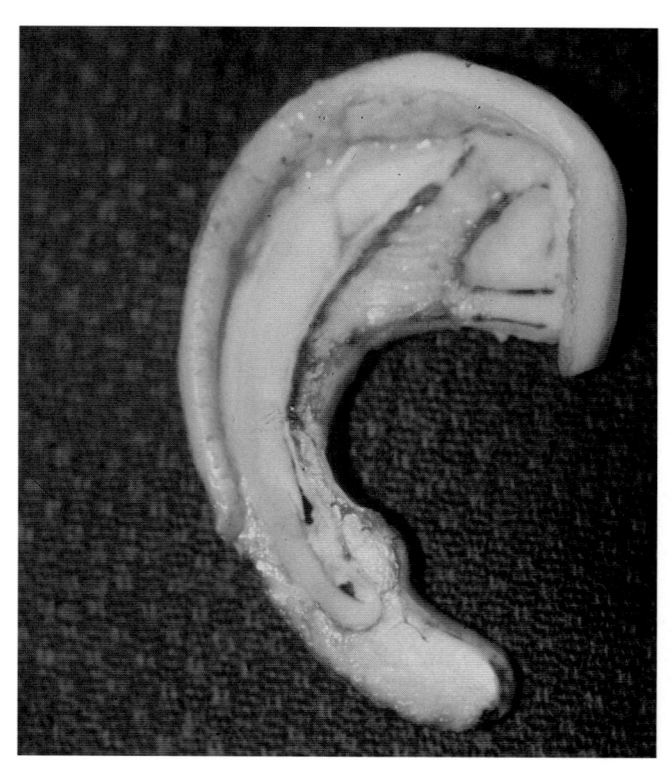

FIG. 13. A three-layered auricular framework is sculptured to create a concha, scapha, and helix.

It is secured to the base plate of cartilage with 4-0 and 5-0 wire. The rim should be placed a few millimeters beyond the base anteriorly to simulate the helical crus and should reach the level of the antitragus inferiorly to resemble a cauda helix. The convolutions of the fossa triangularis and scapha are excavated into the framework with carving tools. This three-layered framework has been more reliable, more sturdy, and more resistant to infection than have "expansile" and monoblock frameworks, which tend to flatten with time (34,35).

An incision is placed anterior to the microtia nubbin and a thin, well-vascularized subdermal pocket is created. It is imperative not to infiltrate this area with adrenalin. Any blanching of the skin pocket suggests excessive tension and forebodes skin necrosis. However, skin blanching must not be confused with the vasospastic effects of the infiltrate. The pocket is dissected 2 cm superior and 10 mm inferior to the skin markings to gain enough skin laxity to lie within the sculptured crevices. Vestigial microtic cartilage in the superior aspect is removed. The graft is inserted into the pocket and rotated into position (Fig. 14). Two Jackson-Pratt drains are inserted below the graft and are attached to continuous wall suction 80 mm Hg for 3 days to remove inevitable accumulation of serum and prevent disastrous formation of hematoma (Fig. 15). Use of suction avoids bolsters and mattress sutures, and maintains adequate cooptation of the skin against the cartilage graft. The newly created sulci are

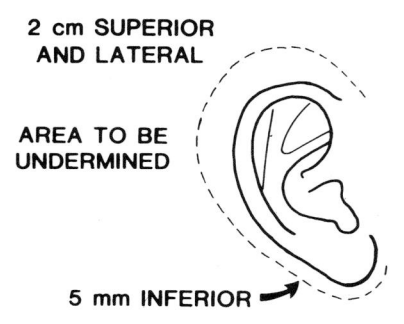

FIG. 14. A subdermal pocket is dissected 2 cm superiorly and 5 mm inferiorly beyond the tattooed outline framework to gain skin laxity to lie in the newly created convolutions without tension.

packed with petrolatum gauze for 1 week. Antibiotics are also given until the packing is removed.

Reconstruction of the Lobule

Construction of the ear lobe can begin after 3 months. The inferior remnant of fibroadipose tissue is transposed into

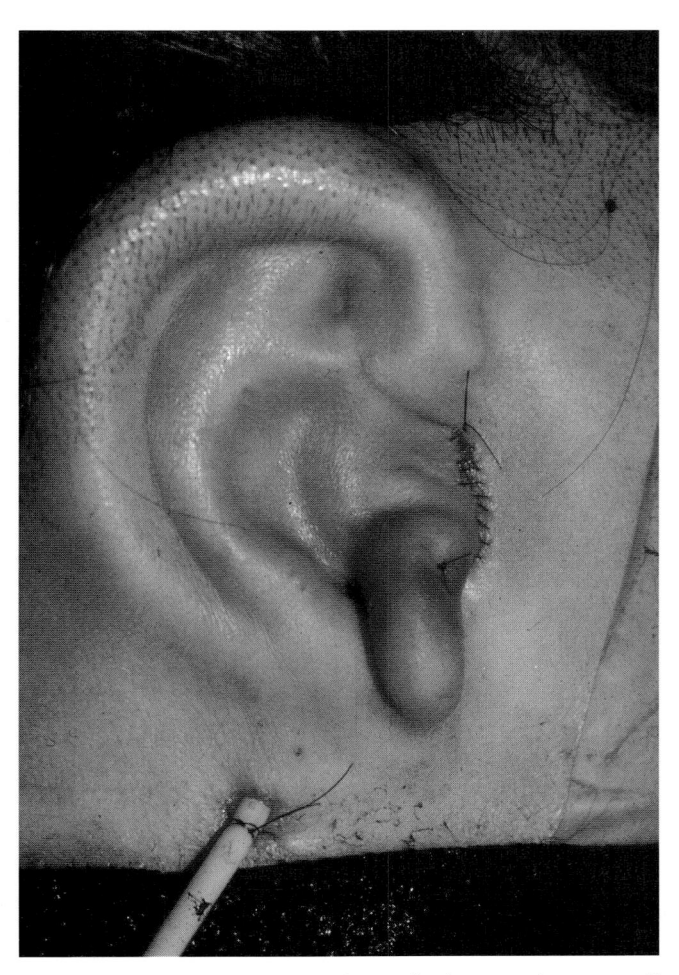

FIG. 15. Drains are used and attached to continuous wall suction to help coapt the skin against the cartilage framework.

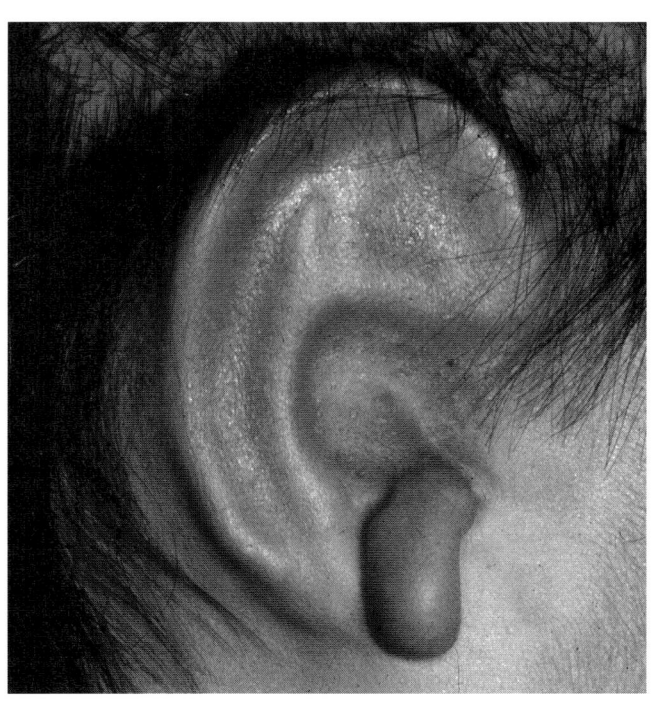

FIG. 16. Inferior fibroadipose lobular remnant remains in an abnormal vertical axis. The lobule is rotated posteriorly and inferiorly to follow the delicate curvature of the helix.

a lobule by creating an inferiorly based flap (Fig. 16). The delicate flap is defatted and sculptured. The skin overlying the framework is carefully elevated so that the underlying cartilage is not exposed. The lobular fibroadipose flap is sutured to the inferior border of the framework, thus creating the lobe. If skin tension is avoided, no internal support is necessary to prevent retraction and shrinkage of the flap. Redundant skin is redraped over the conchal area and extra amounts are removed. Steri-Strips are placed over the absorbable 5-0 catgut sutures (Fig. 17).

Creation of the Tragus and Evacuation of the Concha

The neoauricle now more closely resembles the opposite pinna. There is still no canal and there is asymmetry because of relative protrusion of the opposite ear compared to the microtic side. A composite graft of chondrocutaneous tissue is taken from the concha of the normal side. A full-thickness skin graft 2 cm in diameter is also harvested from the postauricular area. Closure of these donor sites brings the normal ear closer to the skull, thus improving asymmetry.

A J-shaped incision is made in the conchal area of the neoauricle where the tragus will be created (Fig. 18). Only anterior facial skin is elevated. The composite graft is sutured to the elevated facial skin anteriorly and to the full-thickness skin graft posteriorly. The three tissues (anterior skin, composite graft, and skin graft) are folded on themselves in an accordion-like fashion with the supporting composite graft on the under surface of the facial skin (36,37).

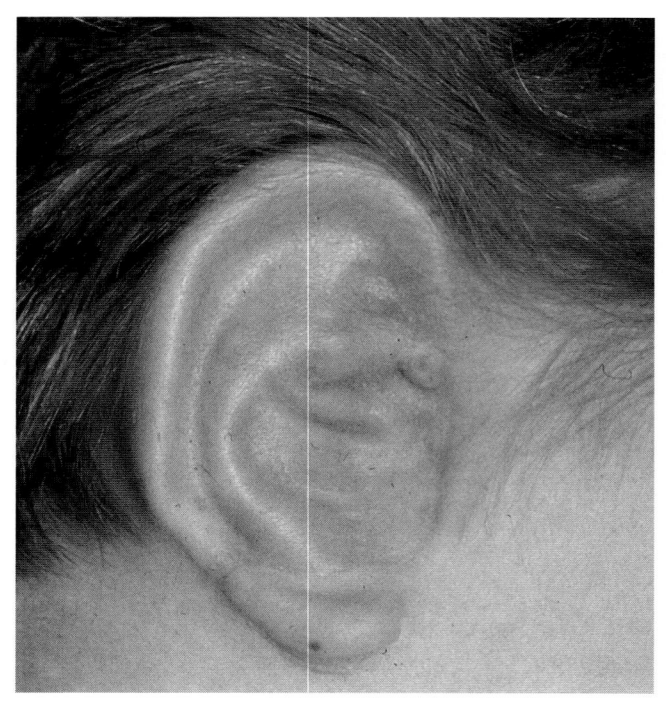

FIG. 17. The lobule has been transposed to its proper location. No internal skeletal support is necessary to prevent contraction of the soft tissue.

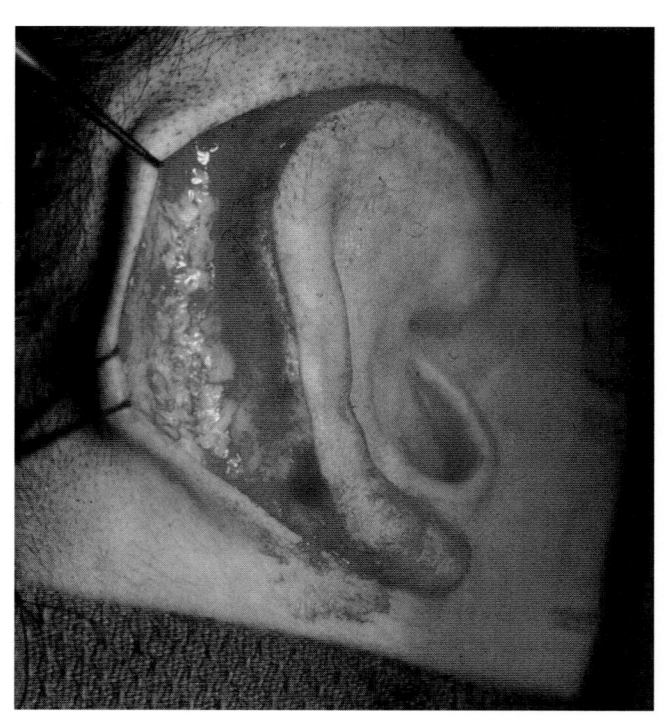

FIG. 19. Additional protrusion is obtained through a scalp advancement flap and a skin graft.

The created bowl is packed with bismuth tribromophenate (Xeroform) for 1 week to prevent blunting. This tragus and concha resembles a meatus. I have not observed the shrinkage problems seen with other techniques that do not use a supporting cartilage graft. Patients with bilateral microtia have no available cartilage for grafting and may need to have their tragus reconstructed with less reliable soft-tissue flaps.

Elevation of the Auricle

The neoauricle is adherent to the mastoid and may still lack adequate projection (Fig. 19). Formation of a postauricular sulcus can cosmetically improve protrusion and also create a "shelf" for a hearing aid. An incision is placed 5 mm outside the peripheral margin of the pinna. A subgaleal retroauricular scalp flap is elevated 6 cm superiorly and posteriorly. The cartilage framework is elevated above the mastoid periosteum to the level of the concha, with care taken so that its soft-tissue covering is not violated. If the framework is elevated beyond the concha, it may become floppy and the superior pole may shift forward. Exposure of any cartilage must be covered with soft tissue. If excessive cartilage is exposed, the procedure should be terminated because the skin graft will not adhere to denuded cartilage. The scalp flap is advanced under tension anteriorly under the cartilage framework. The flap is secured with 2-0 polyglactin sutures to the mastoid periosteum. The denuded posterior surface of the auricle is covered with a full-thickness skin graft from the groin (color match is not essential) (Fig. 20). Xeroform packing is placed for 10 days to prevent formation of hematoma and blunting of the sulcus. This elevation gains additional protrusion and harmony with the normal ear.

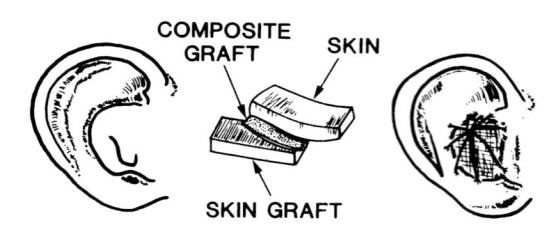

FIG. 18. A J-shaped incision is made at the proposed site of the tragus. The chondrocutaneous graft is sutured to the facial skin anteriorly and the free skin graft is sutured posteriorly. The grafts are folded in an accordion-like fashion to create a tragus.

ATYPICAL MICROTIA

Patients with grade II dysmorphic ears or with prior auricular or canalplasty surgery often have nonpliable skin. If the skin pocket is scarred, it will not conform to the sculptured convolutions in the cartilage framework. Detail will be lost and the neoauricle will be appear thick and amorphous. All scarred skin should be removed and replaced with a thin skin graft. Well-vascularized tissue must be interposed to accept the grafted skin. The thin, well-vascularized, hairless superficial temporoparietal aponeurotic fascia (STAF) has been a reliable bed to nourish a covering skin graft (38).

The durable STAF is readily harvested as a thin flap with minimal donor-site morbidity. It is continuous with the superficial musculoaponeurotic fascia that inserts on the zygomatic arch. This fascia must not be confused with the underlying, less vascular, temporalis fascia, which inserts more interiorly to the zygomatic arch and on the mandibular condyle. The STAF is supplied by the superficial temporalis and the posterior auricular arteries and veins. These vessels lie within the fascia and beneath the subcutaneous fat and hair follicles. This tedious dissection is often bloody because epinephrine injections may damage the fragile microcirculation and therefore cannot be used. The STAF extends 12 cm above the ear, where it becomes superficial and fuses with the subdermal plexus. This is the superior boundary of its vascularity and the superior limit of dissection (Fig. 21). The anterior border is limited by the temporal branch of the facial nerve where it crosses the zygomatic arch. Posteriorly the flap should include the posterior branches of the temporal artery and vein (39).

Inferiorly, a similar thin subdermal pocket is created similar to that in an unscarred microtic ear. The framework is placed in the skin pocket and unusable scarred tissue is excised (Fig. 22). An incision is made in the parietal scalp just through the bulbs of the hair follicles. Too superficial dissection causes alopecia, and too deep dissection injures the axial arrangement of vessels within the flap. The STAF is measured to adequately cover the exposed framework and to lie with the convolutions and sulci without tension. A 6-cm transverse incision made at its superior limit is connected to two vertical incisions to free the STAF from the temporalis fascia. The flap is elevated from the underlying temporalis fascia and rotated downward to cover the framework (Fig. 23). It is sutured to the undersurface of the skin pocket in a "vest-over-pants" fashion. One drain is inserted under the fascial graft. A 0.0018-inch skin graft from the buttocks is placed over the STAF, ecured with Xeroform, and tied over bolsters. A second, closed, suction drain is placed under the posterior aspect of the scalp and attached to continuous wall suction at 80 mm Hg for 3 days.

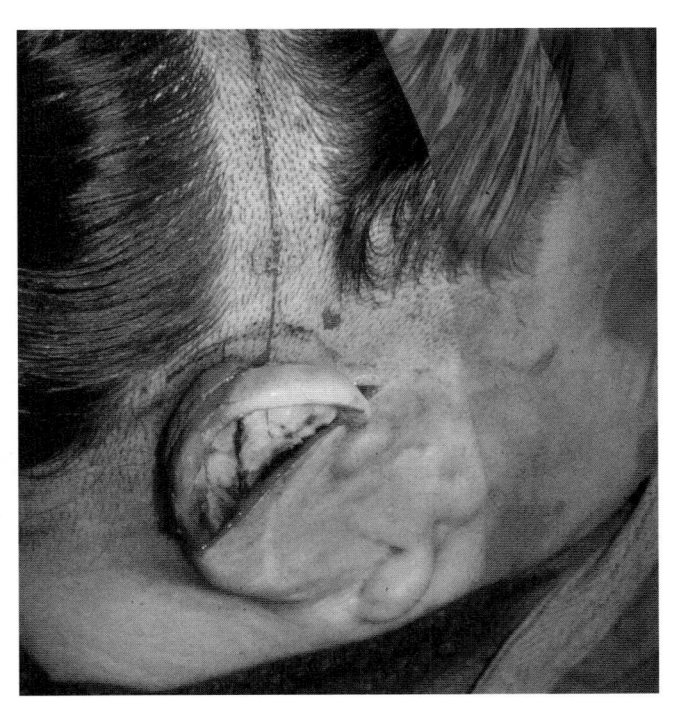

FIG. 21. The temporoparietal aponeurotic flap is contiguous with the superficial musculoaponeurotic flap inferiorly. It extends almost 12 cm superiorly and is limited anteriorly by the facial nerve.

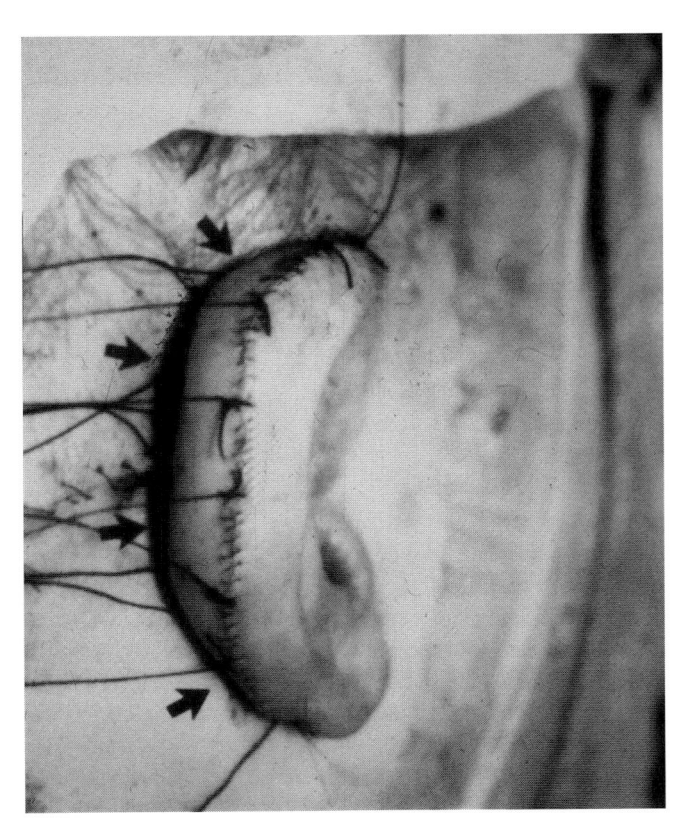

FIG. 20. A full-thickness skin graft covers the denuded postauricular surface and is secured with Xeroform packing.

COMPLICATIONS AND POTENTIAL PITFALLS

Hematoma

I have had no problems with formation of hematoma or seroma since I began using *two* continuous suction drains during the first stage when the framework is placed within the subdermal pocket. No drains are necessary with any other stages if meticulous hemostasis is achieved intraoperatively. If hematoma does occur, the area must be evacuated soon to prevent skin breakdown and cartilage graft exposure.

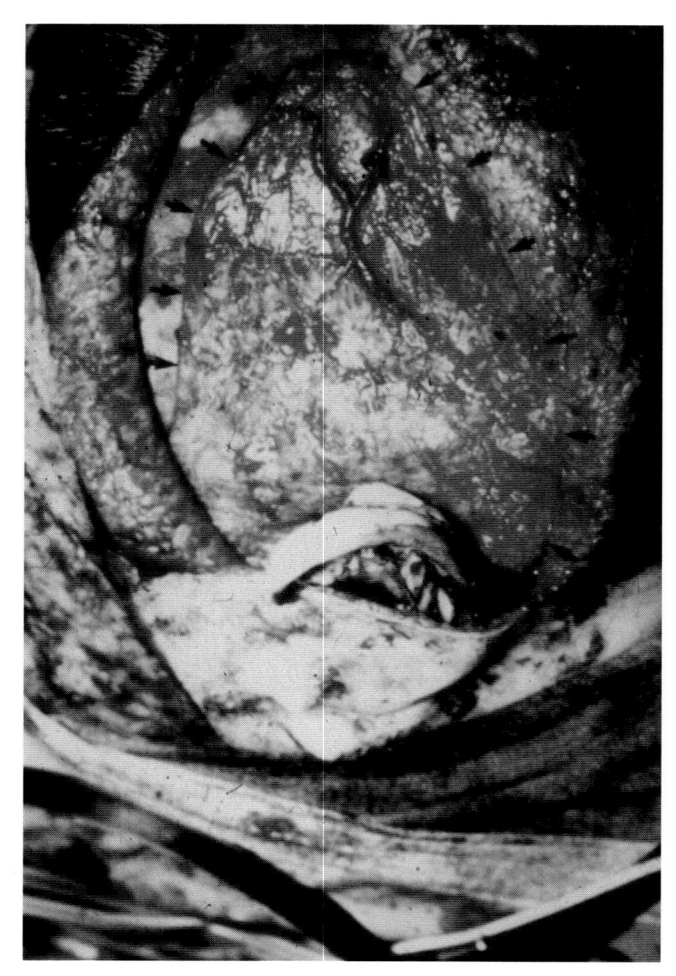

FIG. 22. The framework is inserted into a subdermal pocket. Nonusable scarred skin is discarded. The temporoparietal fascial flap is measured for adequate coverage and elevated.

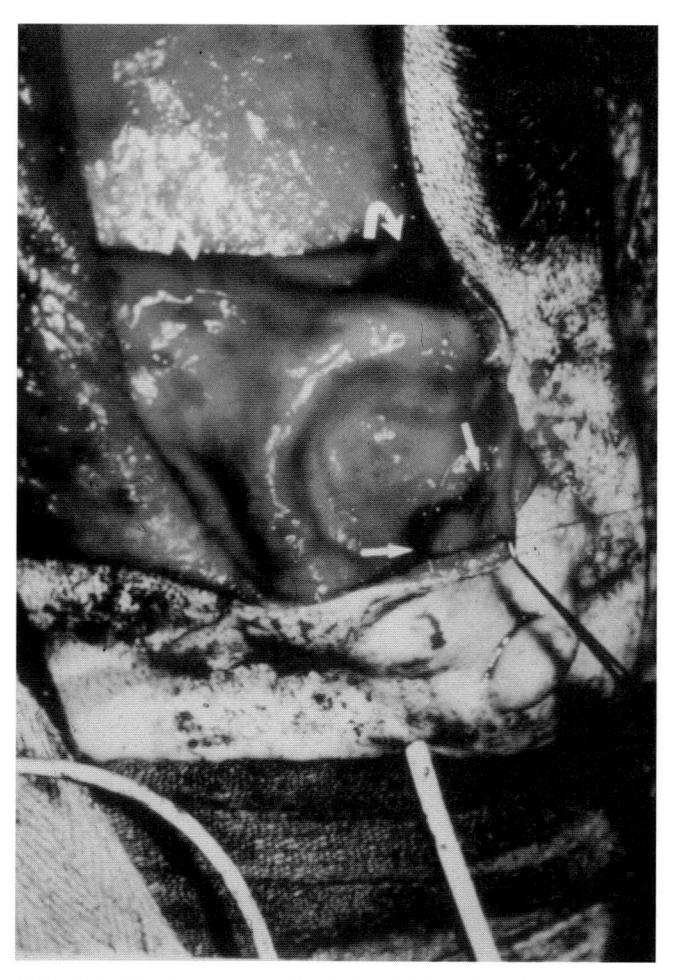

FIG. 23. The temporoparietal fascial flap is folded over to cover the exposed cartilage framework.

Infection and Tissue Necrosis

The most common factors causing infection and skin necrosis are inadequate vascularity from too superficial dissection of the subdermal pocket and excessive tension on the overlying skin. Exposure of the cartilage is also a problem when the neoauricle is elevated and the postauricular skin graft fails to survive. Again, any exposure of the cartilage framework must be covered to have adequate nourishment for the skin graft. The most prevalent cultured organisms have been *Pseudomonas aeruginosa* and *Staphylococcus aureus*. Antibiotic coverage with ciprofloxacin for infection and bacitracin ointment to prevent desiccation of the exposed cartilage helps avoid rapid resorption of the graft and encourages granulation tissue. If skin necrosis exposes more than 5 mm of the cartilage graft, the defect should be covered with a local advancement scalp flap. However, if no cartilage is exposed, a more conservative approach with antibiotics and local irrigations of 0.25% acetic acid has been successful (39).

Patients with prior canalplasty often have a moist, weeping canal cavity contaminated with *Pseudomonas* (Fig. 24). It is imperative to create good vascular coverage with the temporoparietal fascia flap for these patients. Auricular reconstruction should not begin until all signs of infection and inflammation have been resolved for several months preoperatively.

Detachment of the Cartilage Framework

Early in my experience I encountered displacement of the helix (ninth rib) onto the scaphal subunit of the framework. This problem was resolved by more aggressive thinning of the ninth rib helical rim on its convex side. Minimal tension in the helix lessens the "spring" of tension, thus allowing it to conform to the curvature of the framework, and helps prevent its detachment.

Lateralization of the neotragus can be minimized by obtaining an adequately large chondrocutaneous graft, which can be folded onto the framework inferiorly and act as a stable skeletal support for the skin graft. If the chondrocutaneous graft is placed too anteriorly and not within the neoconchal bowl, it migrates excessively.

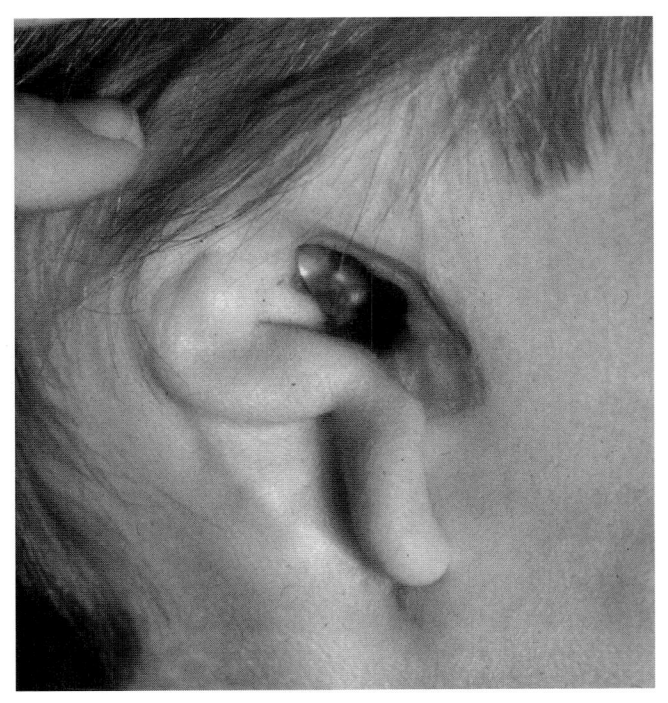

FIG. 24. Patients with prior canalplasty often have large, infected, weeping cavities. Cartilage necrosis soon develops if infection is not controlled preoperatively and the cavity covered with well-vascularized tissue.

Hypertrophic Scarring and Chest Wall Deformities

Healing of the chest wall determines whether mastoid scarring will be problematic. Excessive hypertrophic and keloid scarring of the chest will prohibit further surgeries to create a tragus and a postauricular sulcus. In these patients, completion of the reconstruction has had to be delayed until after the patient had attained puberty, when hypertrophic scarring appears to lessen.

Deformity of the chest-wall donor site has not been a problem when reconstruction is delayed until the patient is age 6. I have not experienced severe retraction deformities in more than 200 patients. Other authors have noted significant long-term chest-wall retractions in 20% of patients who had rib grafts taken before age 5.

ILLUSTRATIVE CASES

The Dysmorphic Auricle

History and Diagnosis

A.J. was born at 39 weeks of gestation via cesarean section because of a breech presentation. The patient's bilaterally deformed ears appeared to have all of their anatomic components present, thus representing a dysmorphic ear caused by intrauterine malpositioning (Fig. 25). The high concentration of circulating maternal estrogens in the first post partum week kept the cartilage pliable, which allowed sculpting the auricles without surgery. The estrogen level prevents tight binding of the chondroitin sulfate in the mucopolysaccharide cartilage matrix for several days after birth.

Reconstruction

The ears were properly positioned (using fingers), and moistened cotton was secured into each deformed area for 1 week. The ears were then retaped for an additional seven days (Fig. 26).

Dysplastic Constricted Auricle

History and Diagnosis

R.M., an 8-year-old boy, presented with a constricted dysplastic right pinna (Fig. 27). Several anatomic subunits were lacking. There was maldevelopment of the supporting scaphal layer with foreshortening of the fossa triangularis, folding over and flattening (lidding) of the superior aspect of the helix, unfurling of the anthelical fold, abnormal positioning of the crus helicis, and an inadequate skin pocket.

Reconstruction

The crus helicis was detached and repositioned superiorly utilizing V to Y advancement, which opened the constricted portion of the superior scapha. Radial incisions were made in the scapha cartilage to allow it to open in a fan-like manner. The unfurled anthelical fold was corrected with 4-0 clear nylon sutured using a Mustarde technique. A postauricular skin graft was placed over the exposed scaphal cartilage and secured with Xeroform gauze and tie-over bolsters for 5 days (see Fig. 27).

Left Microtia

History and Diagnosis

B.G. was born with left microtia, grade III. She had a classic "peanut-shaped" appendage with a superior nubbin of cartilage and an inferior fibroadipose lobule. The auricular remnant was lower than her normal ear. There was complete atresia of the canal with conductive hearing loss (speech reception threshold of 50 dB). Mild canting of the mandible was noted with left hemifacial microsomia. No cardiac, renal, or cervical abnormalities were found.

Reconstruction

Costal cartilage rib grafts were harvested from the opposite chest wall and sculptured into a three-layered auricular framework. Four stages of reconstruction were completed during an 18-month period. No canalplasty was performed because the facial nerve was too anteriorly displaced and the middle ear cleft was too shallow (Fig. 28).

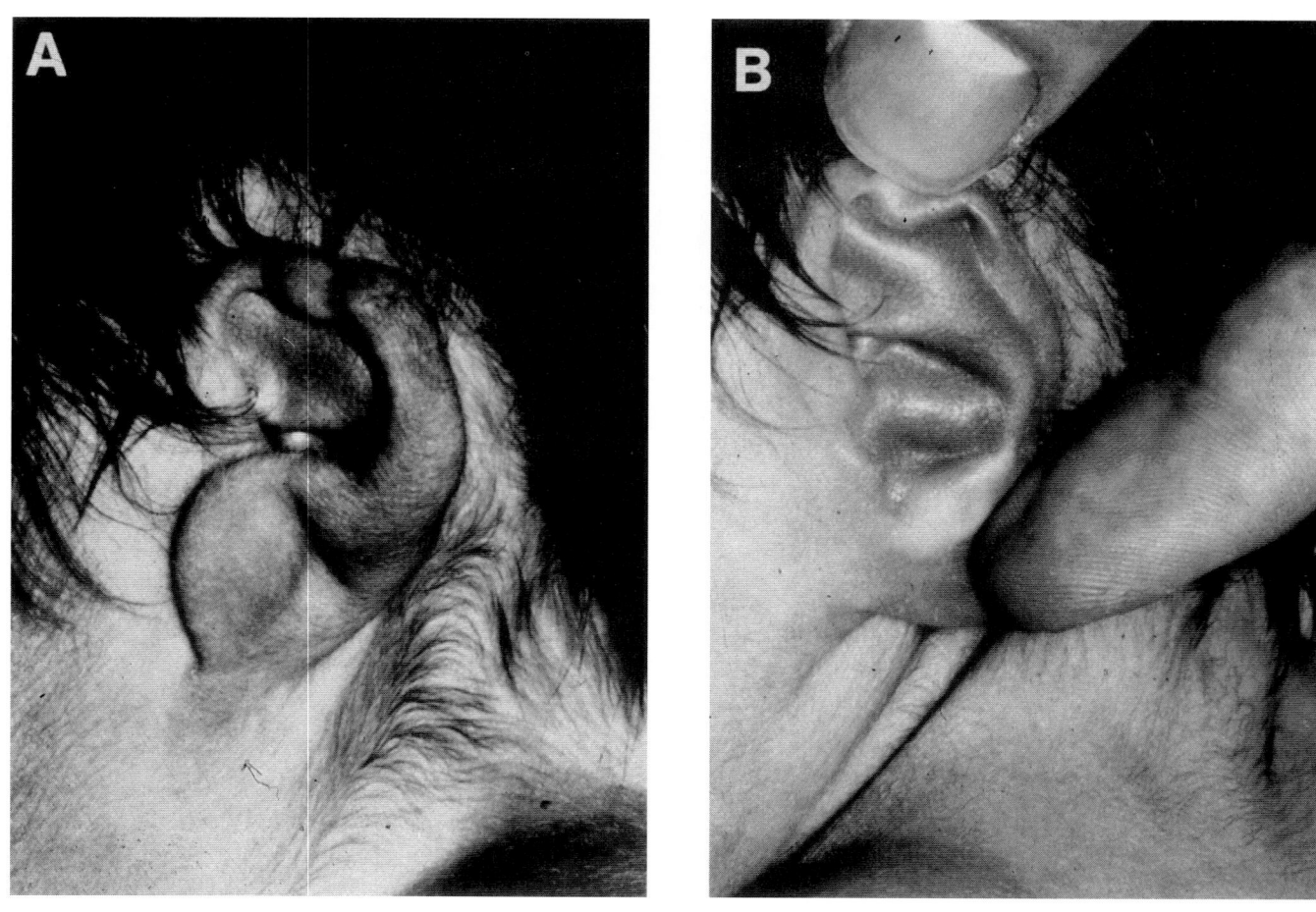

FIG. 25. A and **B:** Using one's fingers to open the ear reveals that all anatomic subunits are present.

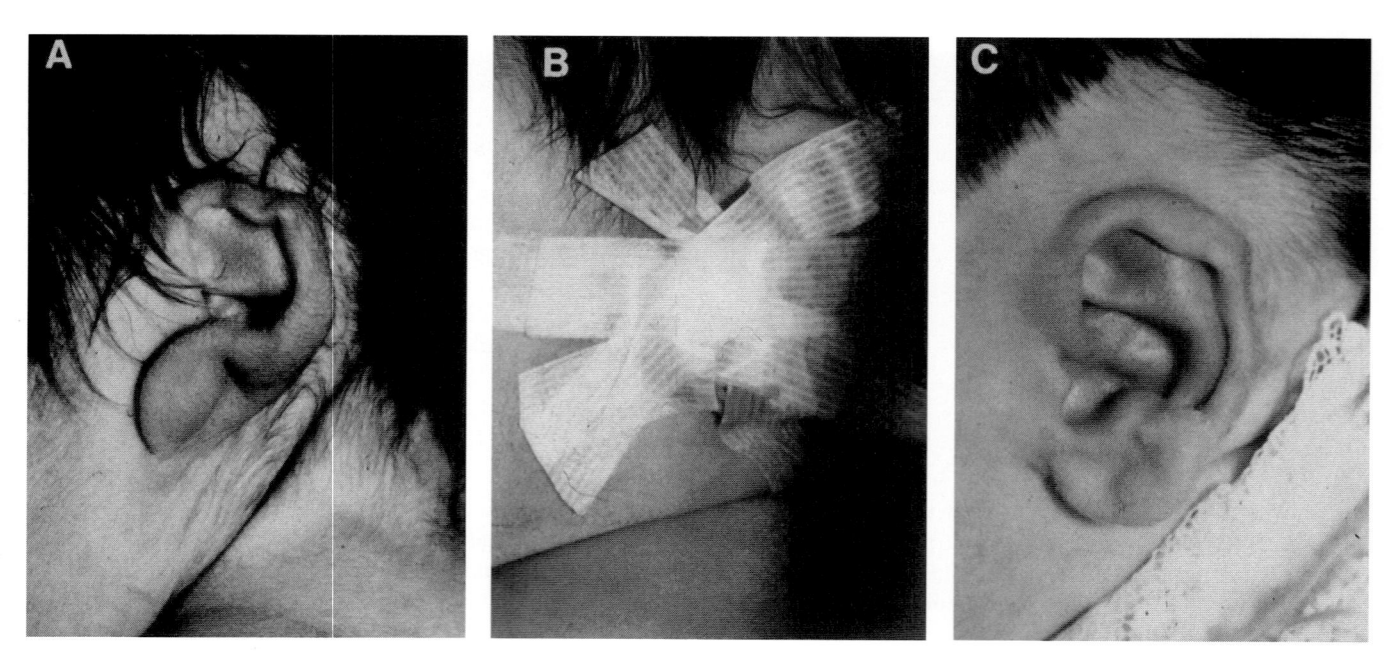

FIG. 26. A: Moistened cotton is placed in the appropriate areas and **B:** taped for 1 week. **C:** Pre- and postmolding was done for 10 days after sculpturing by use of a nonsurgical technique.

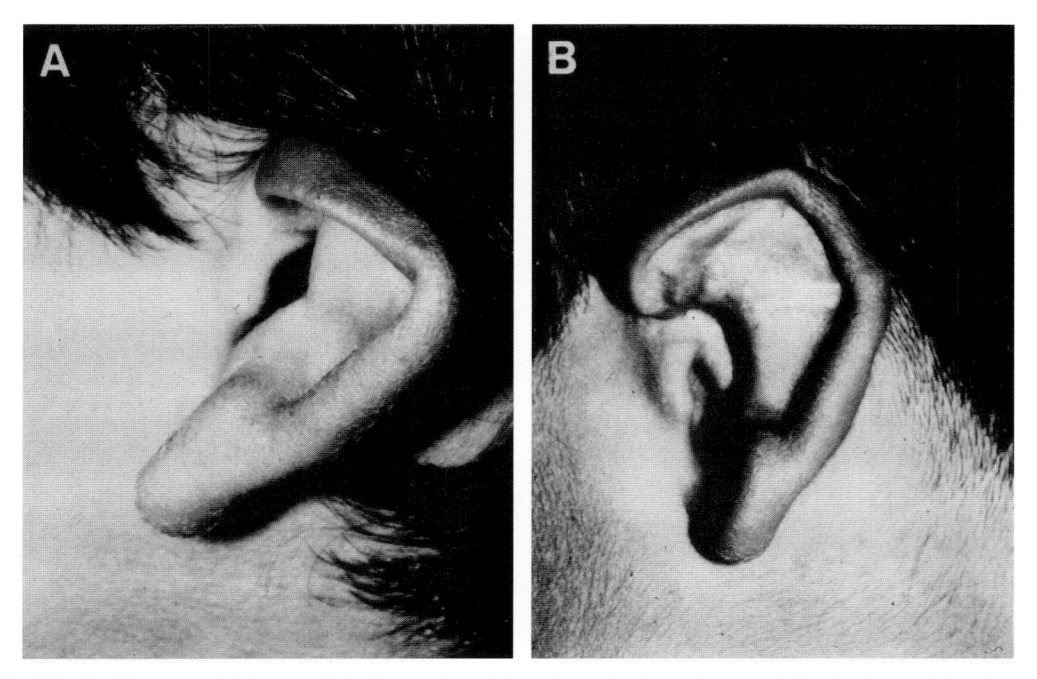

FIG. 27. **A:** The constricted auricle has a low-lying, foreshortened crus of the helix and inadequate scaphal support. **B:** Repositioning of the helix and composite chondrocutaneous grafts to the deficient scapha were completed.

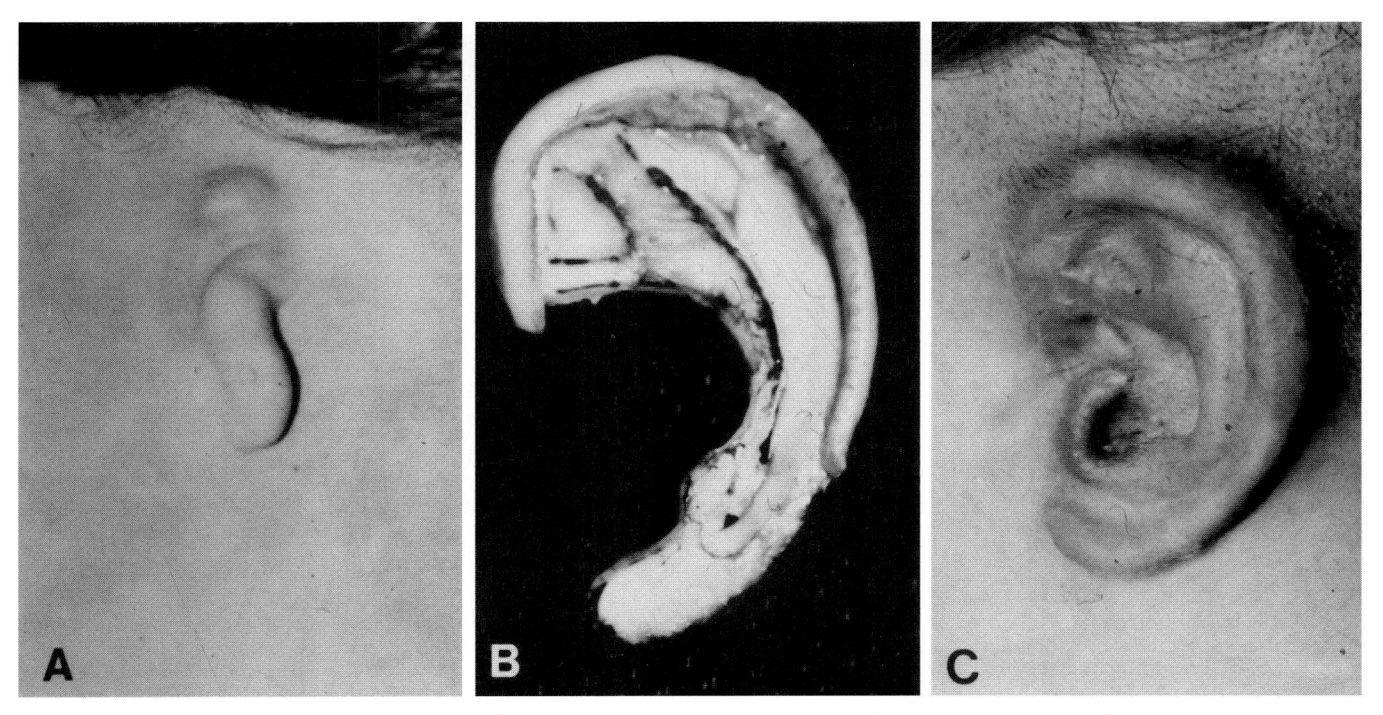

FIG. 28. **A, B,** and **C:** This microtic ear was reconstructed with sculptured rib cartilage.

SUMMARY AND CONCLUSIONS

Reconstruction of congenitally malformed ears requires a thorough understanding of head and neck embryology, auricular anatomy, and the techniques available for reconstruction. Awareness and early recognition of dysmorphic anomalies by the pediatric team can often avoid extensive surgery. The unique pliability of the dysmorphically deformed neonatal ear cartilage lends itself to nonsurgical correction. Simple sculpturing with cotton and tape can correct severely cupped, folded, or protruding ears if performed early and all anatomical subunits are present.

Dysplastic deformities require surgical intervention. Constricted ears can be improved with expansion techniques, composite grafts, and rib cartilage. The microtia or anotia deformity lacks a adequate skin envelope and cartilage framework. Improvements with delicate dissection, rib cartilage, and temporoparietal fascial flaps have enabled us to attain more consistent and lasting results. However, there no implant is ideal (40,41). External prosthesis, silastic implants, and heterologous cartilage grafts have fallen off, resorbed, or have been extruded. Ongoing work with Medpor or developing methods to grow one's own cartilage into an auricle may enable construction of a more aesthetic, translucent, and delicately pliable ear. Nevertheless, understanding and preventing the embryopathy of microtia is our ultimate goal.

REFERENCES

1. MacGregor FC. Ear deformities: Social and psychological implications. *Clin Past Surg* 1978;5:347–350.
2. Berghaus A, Toplak F. Surgical concepts for reconstruction of the auricle: History and current state of the art. *Arch Otolaryngol Head Neck Surg* 1986;112:338.
3. Anson B, Blast T. Developmental anatomy of the ear. In: Shambaugh G Jr, Glasscock M, eds. *Surgery of the ear,* 3rd ed. Philadelphia: WB Saunders; 1988.
4. Tolleth H. AF Hierarchy of values in the design and construction of the ear. *Clin Plast Surg* 1990;17:193–7.
5. Graham, JM Jr. In: Smith's *Recognizable patterns of human deformation.* Philadelphia: WB Saunders; 1988.
6. Mastroiacovo P, Corchia C, Botto. Epidemiology and genetics of microtia: a registry based study on over one million births. *J Med Genet* 1995;32:453–7.
7. Zoltogora J, Cohen T. Krabbe disease and protruding ears. *Am J Med Genet* 1987;28:759–60.
8. Crabtree JA. Congenital atresia: case selection, complications, and prevention. *Otolaryngol Clin North Am* 1982;15:755–62.
9. Derlacki EL. The role of the otologist in the management of microtia and related malformations of the hearing apparatus. *Arch Otolaryngol* 1969;72:980.
10. Crabtree JA. The facial nerve in congenital ear surgery. In: Graham MD, House WF, eds. *Disorders of the facial nerve.* New York: Raven; 1982.
11. Brown FE, Colen LB, Addante RR, Graham JM Jr. Correction of congenital auricular deformities by splinting in the neonatal period. *Pediatrics* 1986;78:406-11.
12. Millay DJ, Larrabee WF, Dion FR. Nonsurgical correction of auricular deformities, *Laryngoscope* 1990;100:910–3.
13. Ruder RO, Maceri D, Crockett D. Congenital aural atresia and microtia. In: Meyerhoff W, Rice D, eds. *Otolaryngology—head and neck surgery.* Philadelphia: 1992.
14. Smith DW, Takashima H. Protruding auricle: a neuromuscular sign. *Lancet* 1978;1:747–9.
15. Zerin M, Van Allen MI, Smith DW. Intrinsic auricular muscles and auricular form. *Pediatrics* 1982;69:91–3.
16. Kurozumi N, On S, Ishida H. Nonsurgical correction of a congenital lop ear deformity by splinting with reston foam. *Br J Plast Surg* 1982;35:181–2.
17. Ono I, Gunji H, Suda K. A new operative method for treating severe cryptotia. *Plast Reconstr Surg* 1995;96:461–8.
18. Cosman B. The constricted ear. *Clin Plast Surg* 1988;5:389–94.
19. Rousch J, Rauch SD. Clinical application of implantable bone conduction hearing device. *Laryngoscope* 1990;100:281–5.
20. Melnick M. The etiology of external ear malformations and its relation to abnormalities of the middle ear, inner ear, and other organ systems. *Birth Defects Orig Art Seri* 1980;16:303–31.
21. Farkas LG Anthropometry of the normal and anomalous ear. *Clin Plast Surg* 1978;5:401.
22. Thompson HG, Kim T. Residual problems in chest donor sites after microtia reconstruction: a long-term study. *Plast Reconstr Surg* 1995;95:961–8.
23. Gilles H. *Plastic surgery of the face.* London: Frowde, Hodder, and Stoughton; 1920.
24. Cronin TD, Ascough BM. Silastic ear construction. *Clin Plast Surg* 1978;5:375.
25. Cronin T. Use of a silastic frame for total reconstruction of the external ear: preliminary report. *Plast Reconstr Surg* 1966;37:399.
26. Ohmori S, Sekiguchi H. Follow-up of the reconstruction of microtia using a silastic frame *Aesthetic Plast Surg* 8:1, 1984.
27. Tanzer RC. Reconstruction of microtia a long term follow-up. In: Goldwyn RM, Murray JE, eds. *Long term results in plastic and reconstructive surgery.* Boston: Little Brown; 1980.
28. Brent B. Ear reconstruction with an expansible framework of autogenous rib cartilage. *Plast Reconstr Surg* 1978;5:351.
29. Brent B. Auricular repair with autogenous rib cartilage grafts: two decades of experience with 600 cases. *Plast Reconstr Surg* 1993;90:355–74.
30. Gorney M. Ear cartilage. In: Davis J. *Aesthetic and reconstructive otoplasty.* New York: Springer-Verlag; 1987.
31. Brent B. Cartilage and perichondrial grafting. In: McCarthy JC, ed. *Plastic surgery.* Philadelphia: Saunders; 1990.
32. Lauritzen C, Munro IR, Rose RB. Classification and treatment of hemifacial microsomia. *Scand J Plast Surg* 1985;19:33.
33. Richards RN, McKenziee MA, Meharg G. Electroepilation (electrolysis) in hirsutism: 35,000 hours experience on the face and neck. *J Am Acad Dermatol* 1986;15:693.
34. Ruder RO, Maceri D, Crockett D. Management of congenital aural atresia and microtia. In: Johnson J, Mandel-Brown M, Newman R, eds. *Instructional Courses.* Vol 4. St. Louis, Mosby; 1991.
35. Ruder O. New concepts in micotia repair. *Arch Otolaryngol Head Neck Surg* 1986;114:1016–9.
36. Distant F, Morgan A. Correction deux microtus e deux temps, *Pediatrie* 1993;48:407.
37. Ruder RO. Microtia reconstruction. In: Papel I, Nachlas N, eds. *Facial plastic surgery.* St. Louis: CV Mosby Co; 1992.
38. Brent B, Byrd HS. Secondary ear reconstruction with cartilage grafts covered by axial, random, and free flaps of temporoparietal fascia. *Plast Reconstr Surg* 1983;72:141.
39. David S, Cheney M. An anatomical study of the temporoparietal flap. *Arch Otolaryngol Head Neck Surg* 1995;121:1153–6.
40. Ruder RO. Injuries of the pinna. In: Gates G. Current therapy in otolaryngology. *Head Neck Surgery.* St. Louis: CV Mosby Co; 1993.
41. Ruder RO. Evaluation and treatment of the deformed and malformed auricle. *Clin Pedriatr* 1996;461–5.

CHAPTER 35

External Auditory Canal Atresia

Robert A. Jahrsdoerfer

Surgery for the correction of congenital aural atresia is one of the most challenging operations an otologist may attempt. It is also one of the most difficult. There is a genuine risk of facial nerve injury, and the hearing may be made worse. These two conditions should give the inexperienced surgeon pause in deciding whether to undertake atresia surgery.

This chapter is written from personal experience, in which over 1,700 patients with a congenital ear malformation have been evaluated and 800 patients have been operated. In the past year (1994–1995), 90 patients with atresia were operated. Approximately two new patients are seen weekly. From this experience, I have developed a philosophy on the treatment of aural atresia which, I believe, will enable the reader to refine decision making concerning these patients.

In the initial evaluation of patients with aural atresia, it is important to take a thorough family history. Approximately 15% of patients will have a positive family history for a congenital malformation involving the ear and/or other body organs or sites. Although atresia secondary to a teratogen accounts for only 0.05% of patients in this series, it is still important to gather information about the use of drugs during pregnancy. It is not unusual for a woman to be unaware that she has recently become pregnant, and continue to take fertility medication. Progesterone derivatives are strongly suspected of contributing to the congenital ear malformation under these circumstances.

A careful physical examination is mandatory. While microtia and atresia may be obvious on routine examination, patients with a well-formed auricle may have their atresia go undiagnosed for years, or even decades. This is particularly true when the patient is seen by a primary care physician untrained in the subtleties of abnormal ear anatomy. A patient with unilateral atresia should have a careful microscopic examination of the contralateral ear, particularly if a conductive hearing loss is present. The examiner may find subtle clues to suggest that a middle ear malformation is present in an ear previously thought to be without flaw. The presence of skin tags or a preauricular fistula on the lateral face, is an alerting sign, as is paresis of the mandibular branch of the facial nerve. When using the operating microscope, the normal-appearing external ear should be carefully inspected for ossicular defects. Does the malleus handle curve anteriorly? Does it crowd the anterior bony annulus? Does it appear to be suspended within the substance of the ear drum? Is it angulated in a peculiar fashion? These are all physical findings that should alert the examiner to the possible presence of a congenital ear malformation.

CLINICAL MANIFESTATIONS AND DIAGNOSIS

When Should the Patient Be Evaluated?

When a neonate is found to have a malformed ear on initial evaluation, it is imperative to assess the hearing. This is important, whether the malformation is unilateral or bilateral. Most neonates who are diagnosed at birth with this condition or other dysmorphic craniofacial problems will usually be consigned to a high-risk registry wherein the investigation of hearing acuity is automatic. Nonetheless, one cannot assume that a newborn with an ear malformation limited to only one side has normal hearing in the contralateral ear.

Auditory brain-stem response (ABR) testing is the procedure of choice to determine the presence or absence of cochlear function. Auditory brainstem response testing should be performed in the newborn nursery in both air conduction and bone conduction modes. If there is any doubt concerning the hearing, a bone conduction hearing aid should be placed early on. Thereafter, ABR testing should be repeated as often as necessary until an accurate assessment of the hearing is made.

Once it has been established by ABR and behavioral audiometry that the child with unilateral congenital aural atresia hears normally in the contralateral ear, nothing more needs

---

R.A. Jahrsdoerfer: Department of Otolaryngology—Head and Neck Surgery, University of Virginia Health Medical Center, Charlottesville, Virginia 22908.

TABLE 1. Grading system of candidacy for surgery of congenital aural atresia

Parameter	Points
Stapes present	2
Oval window open	1
Middle ear space	1
Facial nerve	1
Malleus/incus complex	1
Mastoid pneumatized	1
Incus–stapes connection	1
Round window	1
Appearance external ear	1
Total available points	10

to be done until age 5 years. At that time, a consultation should be had with an otologist knowledgeable with, and experienced in, congenital atresia surgery. High-resolution computed tomography (CT) of the temporal bone also should be done at that time. Magnetic resonance imaging (MRI) is not the study of choice because it fails to image bone. Because one is primarily interested in the bony structures within the temporal bone (i.e., ossicles, labyrinthine windows, atretic plate, etc.) MRI is of little utility. High-resolution CT scanning is done in the 105° coronal and 30° axial views. The coronal view will show the relationship of the fused incus/malleus to the atretic plate, the status of the labyrinthine windows, the position of the horizontal and vertical facial nerve segments, and the size of the middle ear cavity. The coronal view is also essential in plotting the direction of drilling through the temporal bone. The axial view tracks the labyrinthine and middle ear course of the facial nerve, as well as depicts the exit of the facial nerve from the temporal bone by serial tomographic slices. I routinely review the CT scan in the operating room prior to surgery.

Grading

A grading scheme was developed a few years ago in an effort to select those patients for surgery who would have the best chance of success (1). This scheme was based primarily on the preoperative CT scan, and points were assigned according to the degree of development of vital temporal bone structures. The presence of a well-defined stapes rated 2 points, while all other parameters were assigned 1 point each (Table 1). The appearance of the external ear was factored in because this was found to correlate well with the development of the middle ear (2). The best possible score is 10 points, although it is my conservative nature to grade no higher than 9. Most patients selected for surgery will usually grade 7 or 8. A grade of 5 or below disqualifies the patient for surgery, because the risk of the operation outweighs the potential benefits. The significance of the grading system is that it allows a prediction of surgical outcome. For example, a grade of 8 out of 10 translates to an 80% chance of restoring hearing to normal or near normal levels (15–25 dB) postoperatively.

It is noteworthy that only one half of all patients seen and evaluated qualify for surgery. In patients with a craniofacial syndrome, the percentage is even less: only 25% with Treacher Collins syndrome and 15% for patients with hemifacial microsomia. This does not imply that the development of the temporal bone is poorer in hemifacial microsomia than in Treacher Collins syndrome. In Treacher Collins syndrome, the problem is bilateral, while in hemifacial microsomia, usually only one ear is involved, although both may be affected. In bilateral congenital ear atresia, the criteria for surgery are sometimes relaxed in an effort to restore hearing in at least one ear prior to the beginning of school.

Two absolute criteria must be met to consider the patient for surgery: (a) There must be good cochlear function, and, (b) there must be no imaging evidence of a malformed inner ear. Additionally, if the mastoid and middle ear are not aerated, surgery is deferred and high-resolution CT is repeated in 1 year.

Timing of Operation

Although timing of operation has generated controversy in the past, there should be none now. Microtia repair should precede atresia repair. The plastic surgeon should complete surgery before the otologist operates. This allows for the best chance of achieving improvement in both form and function. It also allows the plastic surgeon to operate in a virgin field, unencumbered by scar tissue and a compromised blood supply. There is no rationale for making a hole in the side of the head independent of external ear reconstruction. The only exception to this statement is the presence of cholesteatoma or a patient who is not interested in having the auricle reconstructed.

The age at which a child undergoes auricular reconstruction depends largely on the size of the rib cage. Because the external ear framework is sculpted from rib cartilage, there must be sufficient cartilage with which to work. This usually means that the child should be age 6 or older before microtia repair begins. Because there are four stages of microtia repair, each at least 3 months apart, the otologist usually does not operate until the child is about 8 years of age. However, in cases of bilateral microtia/atresia, the plastic surgeon should be encouraged to operate earlier (age 5) so atresia repair can be done sooner and the child will have the benefit of hearing in one ear in the early school years.

There is still some controversy concerning whether to operate in cases of unilateral atresia. While this dispute is not as heated as it was years ago, even today there are prominent otologists who are critical of operating on patients with unilateral atresia. Because the hearing results are usually predictable, it is immaterial if the malformation involves one or both ears.

GOALS FOR MANAGEMENT, SPECIFIC OUTCOME SOUGHT

It should never be forgotten that the operation is done to improve hearing. If there is a poor likelihood of achieving this outcome, surgery is not indicated. Serviceable hearing is described as a threshold of 30 dB or better. A postoperative speech threshold of 15 to 25 dB allows the patient with unilateral atresia to have binaural hearing. If the postoperative speech threshold is 35 dB or greater, the patient probably has not been helped. An advantage of the grading system is that it allows the surgeon to avoid operating on impossible cases. By this, I mean those cases in which the middle ear is so poorly developed that there is little chance of restoring hearing to serviceable levels.

Risks

The risks of the operation should be discussed carefully preoperatively with the patient or parents. The two greatest risks are, (a) facial nerve injury and (b) hearing being made worse. A high-frequency sensorineural hearing loss can be expected in 15% of cases. While some high frequency losses improve with time, most are permanent. However, while the loss is commonly at 6 to 8 kHz, the hearing through the speech range is often improved to a significant extent. Moreover, the high-frequency sensorineural hearing loss may be found despite an excellent discrimination score. The etiology of the loss is presumably related to vibratory energy from drilling being transferred to the inner ear. This does not necessarily incriminate the drill brushing the ossicles; rather, it is sufficient that dense atretic bone conduct acoustic energy to the cochlea. This statement should not be construed as condoning inexact drilling around the ossicles. Brushing the fixed incus/malleus with a rotating burr is poor technique. It is bad enough if the offending burr is a diamond, and worse yet if it is a cutting burr with fluted grooves. In addition to a high risk of sensorineural hearing loss from this maneuver, the surgeon also must be alert to a disruption of the ossicular chain, either by a subluxation of the incus/malleus complex or a separation of the incudostapedial joint, or from a fracture of the stapes crura at the level of the footplate. If the chain becomes discontinuous, routine methods of ossicular repair may be performed to reconstruct it. If the stapes footplate is fractured or partially subluxed, the surgeon should attempt to restore the stapes to its original anatomic position and block any perilymphatic leak with soft tissue such as temporalis fascia. If the stapes is entirely dislodged from the oval window, it is best to place a soft-tissue seal (fascia) over the oval window and terminate the procedure. It is unwise to insert a stapes prosthesis, or total ossicular replacement prosthesis, when one has unstable membranes (oval window graft neotympanum) at both ends of the prosthesis.

The parents are routinely informed that the operation takes 5 hours. I have completed atresia repair in as little as 3 hours and as long as 6 hours. It is my preference not to render periodic updates to the parents or family during the surgery. Rather, they are told that they will be met after the operation has been completed. The only exception to this is when the procedure is aborted due to an unexpected finding (infection) or if there is a surgical mishap (facial nerve injury).

SURGICAL TECHNIQUE AND RECOMMENDED APPROACH

Positioning the Patient

The operation is done with the patient in the supine position with the involved ear up. The head is turned away from the surgeon, as in standard ear surgery. I prefer a patient position that is slightly in the reverse Trendelenburg mode to allow for decreased venous pressure in the head and neck area. The hair is shaved for only a short distance above and behind the ear (<1 in.). The postauricular area is infiltrated with lidocaine 1%, with epinephrine 1:50,000. I also inject deep and inferior to where the new external ear canal is to be drilled. This maneuver may occasionally produce a transient facial nerve paresis from a conduction block, particularly if the operation lasts for less than 2 hours. It is not a problem in cases lasting 4 to 5 hours because the local anesthetic will wear off.

The donor site for the skin graft, the medial aspect of the ipsilateral arm, is not prepped preoperatively. Rather, the arm is mobilized at that point in the operation when the skin graft is needed.

Facial nerve monitoring is not routinely done. I reserve the use of monitoring for those cases in which I know preoperatively that the nerve is significantly displaced, or for those cases in which I intend to reroute the nerve or the patient has had a previous facial nerve injury. I have no objection to the otologic surgeon using facial nerve monitoring in any surgical procedure on the ear as befits his or her level of security. It is important to be in synchrony with the anesthesiologist and not to be surprised by the sudden revelation intraoperatively that paralytic agents are being used, particularly when the surgeon had assumed they were discontinued following induction.

SURGICAL APPROACH

Because I operate only after the reconstructive surgeon has completed surgery on the external ear, there already should be an adequate postauricular sulcus. The incision for atresia surgery should be made in the postauricular crease to avoid postoperative scarring and narrowing of the sulcus. While this may require some additional time and skill in closure, particularly when the external ear is immobile, it is worth the effort. If the postauricular sulcus is obliterated by the atresia operation, one loses the ability to wear glasses or use a behind-the-ear hearing aid. Moreover, the patient or parents would be unhappy with the outcome.

Temporalis fossa is harvested, placed on a Petrie dish,

scraped to remove muscle tissue, and allowed to dry for later use. The periosteum over the mastoid is incised elliptically at the posterior wall of the temporomandibular fossa (anterior wall of the mastoid) and horizontally along the inferior border of the temporalis muscle (temporal line). The periosteum is elevated to expose the lateral surface of the temporal bone. The posterior extent of the glenoid fossa is identified by elevating soft tissue medially for a short distance. Deep dissection into the temporomandibular fossa should be avoided to prevent injury to a shallow facial nerve that may have exited the temporal bone into the temporomandibular joint. A tympanic bone remnant should be sought for on the lateral surface of the mastoid because this will point to the middle ear, which is usually directly medial. If no bony remnant is found, drilling should begin over the cribriform area. A word of caution is necessary here. Patients with hemifacial microsomia or Treacher Collins syndrome may have a cleft in the temporal bone or a failure of the zygomatic arch to fuse to the temporal bone. The arch may be free floating and obstruct the surgeon's access to the temporal bone. These bony malformations should be noted preoperatively from the high-resolution temporal bone CT scan or from three-dimensional CT imaging (3). In straightforward aural atresia, a well-demarcated cribriform area is usually found. Drilling should begin in that area, and the direction of the drilling should be superior and anterior. The surgeon should be extremely cautious of those cases in which a cleft is found in the lateral surface of the temporal bone. While clefts are commonly filled with soft tissue, the facial nerve may course through it. In this location, it is subject to injury from careless dissection.

Do not drill out the mastoid. This maneuver may soothe the anxiety of an insecure surgeon but does nothing for the patient except create a large unsightly cavity with all its attendant long-term problems. If the tegmen is low, it can be followed medially to the epitympanum. If the tegmen is high, it is best to follow atretic bone medially to the atretic plate. Do not follow mastoid air-cell tracts, because these will lead into the antrum, and the surgeon will soon realize that the approach is too far posterior.

The atretic plate is usually found at a depth of about 1.5 cm. The atretic plate is that medial portion of the dense atretic bone contiguous to the middle ear (Fig. 1A). The plate is thinned to eggshell thickness by drilling with a diamond burr and then is carefully picked away with a dental excavator or right-angle pick. At this junction, the first ossicular landmarks will be noted. The superior aspect of the fused incus/malleus is now seen in the epitympanum (Fig. 1B). We have named the appearance of the ossicles in this first encounter the buttock sign because of the close resemblance to the derriere of a newborn (4). Additional atretic bone is thinned and picked away to expose more of the middle ear and its contents.

No attempt is made to completely mobilize the ossicular chain at this point. The attachment of the chain will be either bony or periosteal from the atretic plate to the neck of the malleus (Fig. 1C). (Remember that the handle of the malleus is commonly absent). This attachment should be the last bridge to be drilled away (Fig. 1D). If it is bony, drilling should proceed at a slow speed, and if the attachment is periosteal, it should be incised with great care or vaporized with the laser according to De la Cruz (5). Prior to mobilizing the chain, bone peripheral to the ossicular mass is drilled away in a circumferential fashion to center the ossicles in the approximate middle of the new tympanic membrane (Fig. 2). Only a finite amount of bone can be drilled away, because the surgeon is constrained anteriorly by the temporomandib-

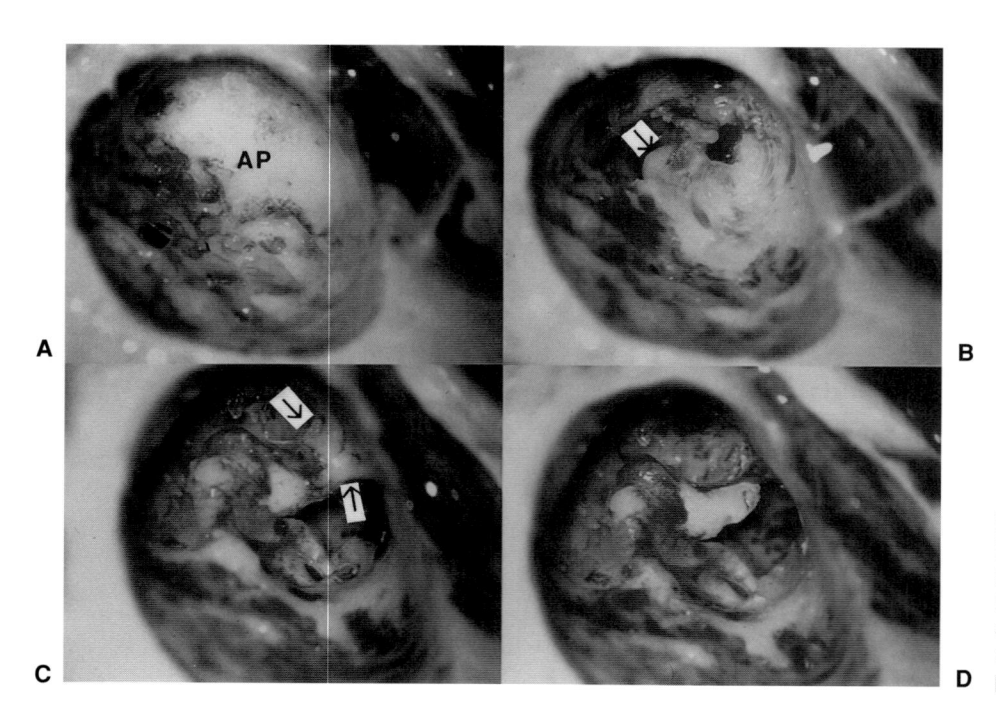

FIG. 1. A: Atretic plate (*AP*) overlying right middle ear. **B:** First appearance of ossicles in epitympanum (*arrow*). **C:** Bony bridge between atretic plate and neck of malleus (*arrows*). **D:** Ossicles free of bony or periosteal attachments.

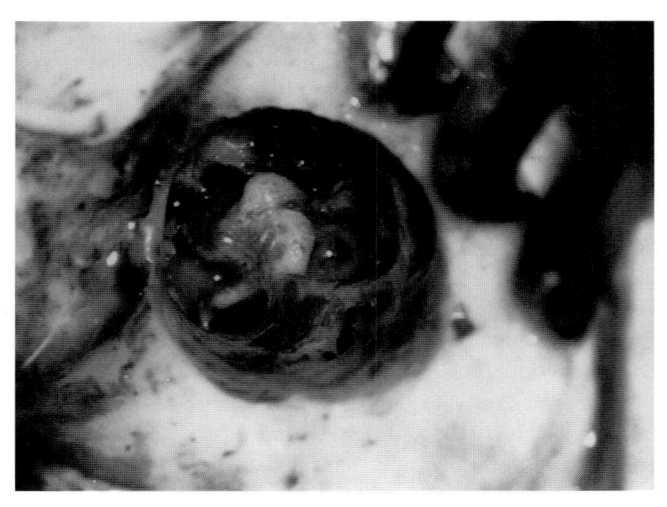

FIG. 2. Ossicular mass centered, and ready for lateral fascia graft.

ular joint, superiorly by the middle fossa dura, inferiorly by the facial nerve, and posteriorly by the mastoid air cells. The middle ear is carefully appraised. The attachment of the incus to the stapes is assessed. This connection is highly variable. It may be discontinuous or connected by soft tissue only (Fig. 3A). If only a fibrous connection is present, and challenge of the incus malleus complex fails to evoke movement of the stapes, then alternate methods of ossicular reconstruction should be considered (Fig. 3B).

The status of the stapes is now investigated. The stapes is often smaller, usually two-thirds normal size, and commonly without a well-defined head. It may not be possible to see the crural attachments to the footplate, particularly in a tight middle ear space. It is absolutely essential, however, that the mobility of the footplate be evaluated. Four percent of atresia patients in my series were found to have a fixed stapes. This occurs either from the annular rim of the footplate failing to differentiate or from an anomalous bony strut from the crura to contiguous bony structures. If the footplate has failed to differentiate, but only nearly so, the annular margin may be scraped with a fine, sharp, straight pick in an attempt to mobilize the stapes. Remember that one is not dealing with otosclerosis and that the labyrinthine bone (endochondral) will not regenerate well. On the other hand, if there is little or no demarcation of a footplate margin, it is best to avoid a stapedectomy or stapedotomy at this stage. Rarely will the incus long arm be developed to a degree that it can accommodate a wire stapes prosthesis. It is not uncommon for the incus long arm to be perpendicular to the footplate, rather than in the same (horizontal) plane. In this anatomic variation, only a bucket-type stapes prosthesis can be used. The main reason for avoiding a stapedectomy at the initial stage of the atresia repair is that there would then be two unstable membranes at either end of the ossicular repair. Laterally, there would be the new tympanic membrane, and medially, the tissue graft over the oval window. From experience, I can state that this unstable situation would very likely cause vertigo from pressure on vestibular structures in the vestibule. It is best to stage the operation under this condition. A new tympanic membrane, external ear canal, and meatus are constructed initially, and a second-stage stapedectomy or stapedotomy performed at a later date.

ANESTHESIA GASES AND MIDDLE EAR PRESSURE

As mentioned previously, nitrous oxide is not used except in the induction phase of anesthesia, if required. The reason for curtailing the use of nitrous oxide is well known—namely, that it is released into the middle ear space by mucosal capillaries, thereby increasing the middle ear pressure and ballooning the tympanic membrane graft.

This is also true of oxygen. If the partial pressure of expired oxygen is 30% or greater, there will be an increase of oxygen being released into the middle ear. While this may

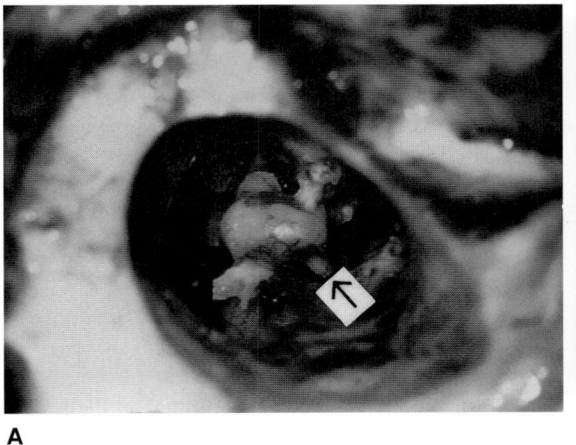

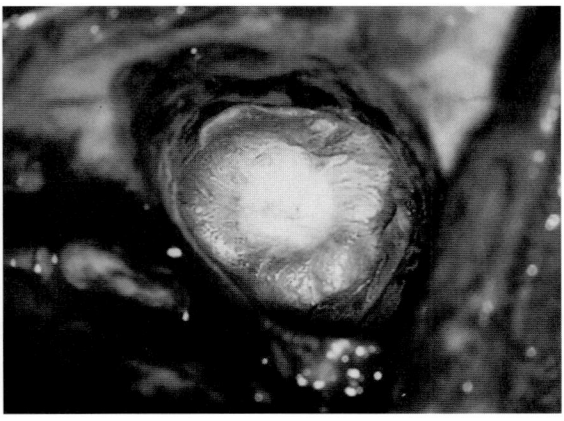

FIG. 3. A: Separated incudostapedial joint (*arrow*). **B:** Flange of partial ossicular replacement graft seen through new fascia tympanic membrane.

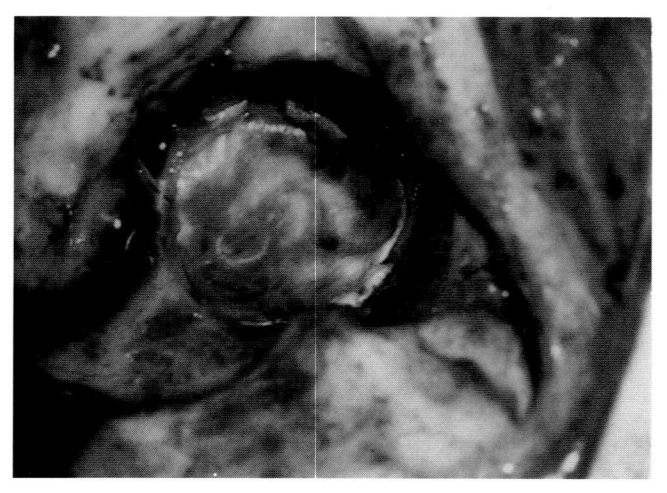

FIG. 4. Ossicular mass clearly seen through thin fascia eardrum (same ear as in Fig. 2).

be inconsequential in straightforward tympanoplasty surgery, in total tympanic membrane reconstruction, atresia patients or otherwise, the graft will balloon. Remember that the new tympanic membrane is a lateral graft onto a fused incus/malleus complex. Ballooning, therefore, will lateralize the graft off of the ossicles, and reattachment may not occur. To circumvent this potential problem, I ask the anesthesiologist to lower the expiratory PO^2 to 25% before proceeding with placement of the fascia graft tympanic membrane.

The fascia graft is cut to size and placed in the new external ear canal to cover the ossicles and middle ear cavity (Fig. 4). The edges of the graft are reflected onto the walls of the new bony ear canal for a short distance (2–3 mm). No attempt is made to carve a new bony annulus by drilling, because this is unnecessary. The incus/malleus complex should protrude the graft slightly in its center portion. If contact is maintained between the graft and the ossicles, a bond will develop that will prevent lateralization.

THE SKIN GRAFT

A thin, split-thickness skin graft is now harvested. I prefer to use the medial aspect of the ipsilateral upper arm. The graft is taken at the time it is needed and not at the inception of the operation. The circulating nurse extracts the arm from beneath the drapes and positions it on an arm board with the elbow flexed and the medial arm up. The upper arm is prepped with Betadine and draped in a sterile fashion. Sterile mineral oil is liberally swabbed on the arm, and a marking pen used to demarcate the length of the graft to be harvested. My dermatome preference is an air-driven Zimmer model. The 2 in. width template is used, and the thickness is set at 10 (0.01 in.). Gentle traction is placed inferiorly on the skin, and a piece of skin measuring about 5 × 7 cm is harvested. The graft is examined for size and appropriate thickness before dressing the arm. If the graft is not satisfactory (i.e., too thick, too thin), an additional graft is harvested. The arm is dressed with scarlet red gauze, Telfa, 4 × 4 surgical dressing, and wrapped with Kling. It is repositioned at the patient's side, and the surgical area is covered with additional sterile towels. The harvested skin is placed on a smooth cutting board and shaped to fit the new bony external canal. Usually, one side of the graft is thinner than the other, and this side is chosen to be used at the level of the eardrum. Four notches are cut in the thin side to form five skin tabs. The graft is placed in the bony external ear canal, with the vertical slit facing anteriorly. This will prevent skin edges from migrating into the mastoid air-cell system. The skin tabs are systematically positioned over the fascia graft, starting anteriorly and proceeding in a clockwise direction. This is the most difficult and demanding part of the operation and requires patience and perseverance on the part of the surgeon. The skin tabs should cover the entire fascia graft. If the skin graft is thick, the edges will tend to curl and will be difficult to position.

Once the skin graft is in place, an oval silastic button, 0.04 or 0.05 in. thick, is cut to size and inserted into the external canal over the new tympanic membrane. The button secures the tabs of the skin graft in place and creates a sulcus anteriorly and inferiorly. Proper placement of the skin graft and silastic button is key to the success of the operation.

Next, Merocel ear wicks (Pope), four in number, are inserted into the new bony ear canal and hydrated with an eardrop preparation. The lateral edges of the skin graft are reflected over the Merocel packing, and attention is turned to the meatus.

Careful inspection will indicate whether the area of the new meatus aligns with the new ear canal. In approximately one half of the cases, the alignment is poor, and the external ear needs to be repositioned. This is almost always in a superior or posterosuperior direction. Because there is no preexisting ear canal to tether the external ear, the auricle can be moved about with few sequelae. This is done by undermining the ear anteriorly to free it from its preauricular attachments. If the ear needs to be elevated, an ellipse of skin measuring about 1 cm in its greatest width is excised from the superior aspect of the incision. A skin hook is used to hold the ear in its approximate new position, where alignment is good with the meatus, and a marking pen is used to outline the new opening. Holding the ear in this position, a no. 11 scalpel blade is used to sharply excise an oval of skin and cartilage. The new meatus should be twice the normal size if there is only soft tissue in the area, or 1.5 times the normal size if there is conchal cartilage present. The alignment of the ear canal with the meatus is then rechecked and the external ear tacked in place subcutaneously with 3-0 interrupted vicryl sutures. Thereafter, all work is done through the meatus.

The edges of the skin graft are identified, brought to the edges of the meatal skin, and sutured in place at four quadrants with 5-0 vicryl suture material. Once these four points are secured, a running nonabsorbable suture is used circumferentially to coapt the skin graft to the meatal skin. Additional Merocel packing is inserted in the soft-tissue lateral end of the new ear canal and hydrated with an eardrop preparation. Bacitracin ointment is applied over the Merocel packing and sterile cotton is used to cover the meatus. The postauricular incision is sutured with a running nylon suture. (The subcutaneous suture used previously was to stabilize the auricle while the meatus was sutured.) A mastoid dressing is applied, and the patient is sent to the recovery room.

Because the operation typically takes 4 to 5 hours, the patient stays in the hospital overnight. The following morning, the mastoid dressing is removed, and the arm bandage is also removed, with the exception of the scarlet red gauze dressing, which remains on until it spontaneously sloughs in about 2 weeks. The patient and or parents are cautioned not to allow water in the ear or on the arm. Assuming everything else is satisfactory, the patient is discharged the morning following the surgery.

If the patient lives beyond easy driving distance (400–500 mi), I request that he or she remain in the area for 1 week, at which time all packing and sutures are removed. Otherwise, the patient may return home. Discharge medications include prophylactic antibiotics, until the packing is removed, and analgesics as necessary.

When seen back in 1 week, the canal packing, silastic button, and meatal and postauricular sutures are removed. The new canal is flooded with a steroid/antibiotic eardrop preparation for 5 minutes, after which it is aspirated or allowed to drain out by tilting the head toward the ipsilateral shoulder. It is at this junction that one gets the first indication of the postoperative hearing. A tuning fork may be used to grossly assess hearing threshold, or the patient may be asked to repeat numbers spoken by the doctor in a progressively softer voice. Although a rough estimate of the hearing threshold may be obtained, no attempt is made to do a formal audiogram. The patient is placed on antibiotic/steroid eardrops for 1 week, after which the medication is discontinued and the new ear canal is left exposed to the air.

A second postoperative visit takes place 4 weeks after surgery or 3 weeks after the first visit. Ideally, on this visit, the skin graft will have desquamated its outer layer, which presents as a thick, brownish-black crust in the ear canal. This is carefully removed, in the office, under the operating microscope. If possible, one should try to remove the crust intact, much like a cast. Beneath will be healthy pink skin, indicating a good take of the graft.

At the second postoperative visit, the new tympanic membrane, ear canal, and meatus are inspected carefully. One now has the opportunity of salvaging a potentially bad result. For example, a hematoma or seroma may be incised and evacuated, early epithelial cysts may be unroofed or marsupialized, and excess or redundant skin folds may be excised with fine alligator scissors. If there is early meatal stenosis, the meatus may be injected with triamcinolone 40 mg/ml. I prefer to first inject Xylocaine 1% through a short 30-gauge needle followed by 0.5 ml of triamcinolone administered through a short 27-gauge needle. Thereafter, the patient is seen in 2 to 3 months by an otologist or otolaryngologist close to the patient's home or by the surgeon if the patient lives nearby. A number of patients will prefer to return to the surgeon for continuing postoperative care, regardless of the distance.

It is important that the patient or family be aware that the reconstructed ear canal will require periodic debridement every 6 to 12 months indefinitely. Because the skin graft is viable but lacks memory, compared with normal external ear canal skin, it will not migrate and, therefore, will not be self-cleaning. The desquamated skin will accumulate in layers, which can affect both the hearing and hygiene of the ear canal. Unless there is periodic removal of the skin, there will be a heightened chance of infection.

The first postoperative audiogram is obtained at 4 weeks. The hearing threshold usually correlates well with the preoperative grade (i.e., a 7 of 10 candidate having a 70% chance of obtaining a postoperative hearing result of 15- to 25-dB speech reception threshold). If the patient has bilateral atresia, and normal thresholds are obtained in the operated ear, the patient response is dramatic. The patient now hears environmental sounds unaided for the first time—the hum of the air conditioner, a cat purring, a rooster crowing, and so on. If the patient has normal hearing in one ear, and a 15- to 25-dB speech threshold is obtained in the operated ear, the response is less ebullient. However, the benefits of the operation are subtle. There is an immediate improvement in discrimination (6)—the ability to understand speech in the presence of other noise. Improvement in sound localization is not immediate but shows a tendency to improve with time. The early postoperative hearing usually endures with minor fluctuations.

The patient is placed on no restrictions regarding activities. If the new ear canal is fully epithelialized, swimming is allowed with the condition that 1 to 2 drops of an alcohol ear preparation will be used after each swimming outing. Commonly, I advise the patient to use 1 to 2 drops of alcohol every Saturday night at bedtime. This will have a salutary effect, because it will dry the ear. Do *not* use 6 to 7 drops of alcohol as recommended in the accompanying literature. This is excessive and will give the ear canal skin a chronic, thickened appearance.

COMPLICATIONS

The major risks of the operation are facial nerve injury and hearing being made worse. Although facial nerve injury was rare in the author s series, there is no substitute for careful tracking of the facial nerve on the preoperative CT scan. Moreover, facial nerve monitoring may be used intraoperatively. I do not routinely monitor every atresia patient but reserve it for those cases in which the nerve is significantly displaced, a nerve rerouting procedure is planned, or the patient has had a previous nerve injury elsewhere.

A high-frequency sensorineural hearing loss will occur in approximately 15% of cases. This has been addressed previously in this chapter in the section entitled, "Risks."

Postoperative meatal stenosis will recur in fully one half of those surgical patients who initially had grade III microtia. If the patient is lacking conchal cartilage, and there is only soft tissue in the area, the chance of stenosis is greater. Grades I and II microtia have conchal cartilage, and stenosis is not a problem. To thwart this tendency for stenosis, I deliberately make the meatus larger than normal, about 1.5 to 2.0 times normal size, and inject triamcinolone into the meatal soft tissue at the end of the operation. No stents or molds are used, because I believe this is counterproductive. Intraluminal pressure at the meatus has a tendency to encourage a counterpressure with robust soft-tissue scarring. The meatus is carefully watched postoperatively and injected with triamcinolone as indicated. Multiple injections may be required. Despite this treatment protocol with steroids, approximately 10% of patients with grade III microtia who develop meatal stenosis will require subsequent revision. Late complications (5 to 10 yr) include new bone growth within the reconstructed ear canal. Although this rarely closes off the ear canal, it may obstruct access to the deeper portions of the ear canal and may trap epithelium behind bony protuberances. Careful cleaning of the ear canal may be impossible, and revision surgery is indicated.

SUMMARY

While the surgical correction of congenital atresia is difficult and challenging, it has the potential to achieve a level of patient and doctor satisfaction unparalleled in other types of ear surgery. Nothing compensates the surgeon more for his or her efforts than a good hearing result and a grateful patient.

REFERENCES

1. Jahrsdoerfer RA, Yeakley JW, Aguilar EA, Cole RR, Gray LC. Grading system for the selection of patients with congenital aural atresia. *Am J Otol* 1992;13:6.
2. Kountakis SE, Helidonis E, Jahrsdoerfer RA. Microtia grade as an indicator of middle ear development in aural atresia. *Arch Otolaryngol Head Neck Surg* 1995;121:885.
3. Jahrsdoerfer RA, Garcia ET, Yeakley JW, Jacobson JT. Surface contour three-dimensional imaging in congenital aural atresia. *Arch Otolaryngol Head Neck Surg* 1993;119:95.
4. Jahrsdoerfer RA, Cole RR, Gray LC. Advances in congenital aural atresia. *Adv Otolaryngol* 1991;5:1.
5. Chandrasekhar SS, De La Cruz A, Garrido E. Surgery of congenital aural atresia. *Am J Otol* 1995;16:713.
6. Wilmington D, Gray LC, Jahrsdoerfer RA. Binaural processing after corrected congenital aural atresia. *Hear Res* 1994;74:99.

CHAPTER 36

Stapedectomy

Charles A. Syms, Antonio De la Cruz, and Simón I. Angeli

The repair of non-otitis media conductive hearing impairment is elective. Although some advocate delaying surgery until adulthood, we believe surgery is indicated in certain circumstances. With the advent of modern stapedectomy techniques, several generations of otolaryngologists have been trained with a surgical armamentarium including the operative correction of conductive hearing impairment. Our stapedectomy technique in children is similar to that used in adults. This chapter discusses the evaluation and management of children who have conductive hearing impairment and who have an intact tympanic membrane and no middle-ear effusion or cholesteatoma and includes children with stable, congenital hearing loss and those with a progressive loss due to otosclerosis.

Ankylosis of the stapes was first described by Antonio Valsalva in 1735 (1). Politzer first called the condition "otosclerosis" in 1893 and, more important, stated that the condition was not secondary to middle-ear inflammation (2). Ménière reported in 1842 the first case of a patient performing stapes mobilization on himself (3). Kessel first reported in 1878 the successful surgical correction of stapes fixation (4). In 1897, Passow described fenestration of the labyrinth with subsequent improvement in hearing (5). The problem was maintenance of the fenestra, which frequently closed. Sourdille, more than 30 years later, is generally credited with refining the technique of fenestration to enable the long-term preservation of an open fenestra (6). Shea, in 1958, reported on stapedectomy initiating the age of modern surgical treatment of otosclerosis (7).

CLASSIFICATION

Two categories of conductive hearing impairment are not due to otitis media: congenital stapes fixation and juvenile otosclerosis. Congenital stapes fixation can be further subdivided into idiopathic stapes fixation or stapes fixation associated with known syndromes. Treacher Collins, Klippel-Feil, Pfeiffer, and cervico-oculoacoustic syndromes, branchio-otorenal, earpits-deafness, Crouzon's disease, X-linked progressive mixed deafness with perilymphatic gusher, osteogenesis imperfecta, and various other diseases are well known to be associated with stapes anomalies and occasionally other ossicular anomalies (8).

EPIDEMIOLOGY

Clinical otosclerosis develops in approximately 1% of Caucasians and histologic evidence of disease purportedly occurs in 10% to 12% of Caucasians. Asians, blacks and Native Americans have a much lower incidence of otosclerosis, although racial admixture makes it possible to see this disease in any population. Of patients who have stapedectomies for otosclerosis, 2% (9) to 15% develop hearing loss before 20 years of age. Congenital malformations of the middle ear are considered as rare, but both older and recent reviews from our institution (11,12) revealed that congenital malformations were more common than otosclerosis in pediatric patients undergoing stapedectomy. In these series, congenital malformations comprised 53% (11) and 59% (12) of the patient population. In reviews that evaluated proportions by gender (9–11), girls predominated 54% (11) to 66% (10).

PATHOPHYSIOLOGY

It is generally accepted that otosclerosis is an autosomal dominant disease with variable (40%) penetrance (8). There is convincing evidence that otosclerosis is an immunologically mediated disease (13), possibly associated with a virus (14), an inherited systemic defect of the collagen remodeling system (15), or a combination of these causes. Although the exact etiology remains unclear, it is obvious from clinical experience that when the disease presents in childhood, the course is more aggressive. In these studies, compared to that in adult series there was a much higher incidence of bilateral

---

C.A. Syms: Uniformed Services University of the Health Sciences, San Antonio, Texas 78236-5000.
A. De la Cruz, and S.I. Angeli: House Ear Clinic, Los Angeles, California 90057.

disease (92%–100%) (9–12) and obliterative disease (27%–42%) (9,10).

Recently there has been an explosion of knowledge of the exact gene loci for diseases that can cause hearing impairment. Multiple molecular biology tools were instrumental in enabling these developments; a single example is reviewed here. Although for some time, the region of the gene for X-linked mixed deafness has been localized to a 500-kb segment of Xq21 (16) the exact gene locus, brain 4 (POU3F4), which encodes for a transcription factor, has recently been reported (17). Mutations that resulted in an abnormal protein product from this region were found in five unrelated patients with the syndrome but not among 50 normal controls. Breakthroughs such as these may enable noninvasive therapies to eventually become a reality.

CLINICAL MANIFESTATIONS

The most likely etiology of the hearing loss can sometimes be determined from the history. The chief complaint of a child with congenital stapedial fixation is usually hearing loss, although speech delay or impairment may be the first symptom. The hearing loss is not progressive and the age of detection averages around 3 years (11). The hearing defect is bilateral in 75% of the patients. Children with juvenile otosclerosis, on the other hand, develop a progressive hearing impairment much later. The average age of onset at our institution was 10 years, the loss was bilateral 90% of the time, and there was a family history of otosclerosis in half the patients (11).

The physical examination is generally normal, though one should be constantly vigilant for the sometimes subtle signs of the syndromes associated with a congenital hearing impairment. In our experience, a Schwartze's sign is not common but, if present, would greatly influence the diagnosis of juvenile otosclerosis.

In addition to routine audiometry, the use of impedance audiometry is valuable. We do recommend high-resolution computerized tomography of the temporal bone in all children with a conductive hearing loss. The imaging should be in axial and coronal planes and in overlapping 1.5-mm sections. We evaluate the films for the status of the oval window, the inner ear, the internal auditory canal, the vestibular and cochlear aqueducts, the ossicles, and the relationship of the facial nerve to the oval window.

MANAGEMENT GOALS

The goal in children with bilateral hearing impairment is to boost their hearing as close to normal as possible. Figure 1 outlines our protocol for evaluation and treatment of hearing loss in children. We use hearing aids, speech rehabilitation, and preferential seating until the child is deemed a surgical candidate, or continue these measures indefinitely if that is the preference of the child and the parents.

We classify the results of surgical intervention by the results of air-bone gap (ABG) testing :excellent (ABG ≤ 10 dB), good (ABG ≤ 20 dB), acceptable (ABG ≤ 30 dB), and serviceable (ABG ≥ 31 dB). This categorization is based on the classification scheme proposed by the American Academy of Otolaryngology—Head and Neck Surgery (18).

RECOMMENDED APPROACH

A persistent bilateral conductive hearing impairment greater than 30 dB in a child less than 5 years of age, not due to effusion or cholesteatoma, should be treated with binaural hearing aids. We recommend that prior to amplification, a painstaking search for otitis media and congenital cholesteatoma be undertaken. In patients with unilateral hearing loss, a hearing aid is not absolutely necessary, and it is rarely accepted. Surgical intervention is preferred but is completely elective and can be delayed until the family is ready to proceed. How the child functions at school, at home, and the presence or absence of other disabilities needs to be addressed (12). If possible, we delay surgical intervention until after the child's fifth birthday to minimize the chance of complications from otitis media. In children presenting after 5 years of age with bilateral hearing impairment, for example a speech reception threshold of 35 dB or more, we recommend either stapedectomy or hearing aids. In patients with bilateral congenital hearing impairment, we obtain high-resolution computerized tomography in both the axial and coronal views. Patients with a history suggestive of otosclerosis and abnormal impedance audiometry need not necessarily be imaged. We defer surgery on any individual in whom the inner ear or facial nerve appears to be unfavorable to elective surgical intervention.

Surgeons must have in their surgical armamentarium the full spectrum of tympanoplasty techniques when they approach congenital stapes fixation or revision surgery for otosclerosis. When the malleus-incus complex is not suitable for stapedectomy, we prefer a Sheehy total ossicular prosthesis over a connective tissue seal to the oval window and under tragal cartilage. Our series revealed that 15% of pediatric patients undergoing primary surgeries and 45% of patients having revision stapes surgery had concomitant malleus-incus abnormalities. The facial nerve was dehiscent in 16% of primary cases and 18% of revisions. An abnormal position of the facial nerve was reported in 11% and 27% of primary and revision cases, respectively (11).

Robinson first pointed out that the longer the hearing loss is followed in a child with otosclerosis, the higher the risk of obliterative disease (10). Although the hearing results in our patients undergoing a "drillout" did not reveal any difference from uncomplicated cases, the procedure is certainly more technically demanding and stressful (11).

Our present technique is a transcanal approach, which emphasizes maximal exposure and minimal bleeding. The major difference in our techniques for children and adults is that we perform almost all our operations with use of general anesthesia in children, but we do operations on adults

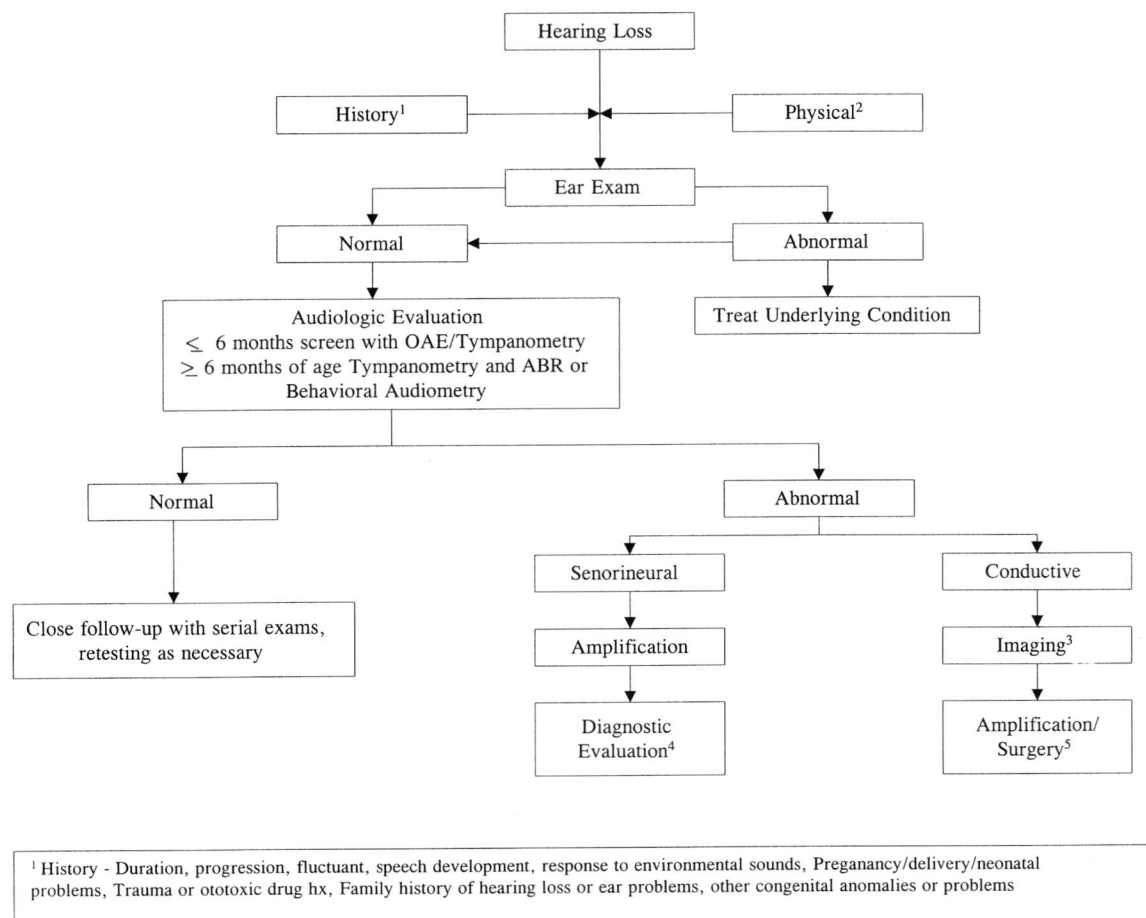

```
                        ┌─────────────┐
                        │Hearing Loss │
                        └─────────────┘
              ┌──────────────┼──────────────┐
         ┌─────────┐                   ┌──────────┐
         │History¹ │                   │Physical² │
         └─────────┘                   └──────────┘
                        ┌─────────────┐
                        │  Ear Exam   │
                        └─────────────┘
                   ┌─────────┴─────────┐
              ┌─────────┐          ┌──────────┐
              │ Normal  │◄─────────│ Abnormal │
              └─────────┘          └──────────┘
                   │                    │
    ┌──────────────────────────┐  ┌──────────────────────────┐
    │  Audiologic Evaluation   │  │Treat Underlying Condition│
    │≤ 6 months screen with    │  └──────────────────────────┘
    │  OAE/Tympanometry        │
    │≥ 6 months of age         │
    │  Tympanometry and ABR or │
    │  Behavioral Audiometry   │
    └──────────────────────────┘
              ┌─────────┴───────────────────────┐
         ┌─────────┐                      ┌──────────┐
         │ Normal  │                      │ Abnormal │
         └─────────┘                      └──────────┘
              │                      ┌─────────┴─────────┐
    ┌──────────────────────┐   ┌──────────────┐   ┌──────────────┐
    │Close follow-up with  │   │Senorineural  │   │  Conductive  │
    │serial exams,         │   └──────────────┘   └──────────────┘
    │retesting as necessary│          │                  │
    └──────────────────────┘   ┌──────────────┐   ┌──────────────┐
                               │Amplification │   │  Imaging³    │
                               └──────────────┘   └──────────────┘
                                      │                  │
                               ┌──────────────┐   ┌──────────────┐
                               │  Diagnostic  │   │Amplification/│
                               │ Evaluation⁴  │   │  Surgery⁵    │
                               └──────────────┘   └──────────────┘
```

¹ History - Duration, progression, fluctuant, speech development, response to environmental sounds, Preganancy/delivery/neonatal problems, Trauma or ototoxic drug hx, Family history of hearing loss or ear problems, other congenital anomalies or problems

² Physical - General head and neck exam, Otoscopic exam with the microscope including pneumotoscopy, tuning fork exam (for children six years of age or older)

³ Imaging - For patients with conductive hearing losses, High resolution computerized tomography (HRCT) in the axial and coronal planes

⁴ Diagnostic Evaluation consisting of:
- Ophthalmologic evaluation
- Lab testing CBC, UA, TFT's (T_4, T_3, TSH), EST. FTA-ABS, Consider additional testing Lyme disease titres, Western blot for T. pallidum (IgG, IgM), electrocardiogram, HIV, TORCH
- Imaging - MRI if T_2 Fast Spin Echo technique if available, otherwise obtain HRCT

⁵ See Text for explanation of choice of therapy

FIG. 1. Protocol for evaluation and treatment of hearing loss in children.

almost universally with use of local anesthesia and intravenous sedation. We prefer the use of a "no touch technique" with the CO_2 laser, but frequently use the microdrill and instruments when necessary. Mobility of the stapes is checked by direct palpation of the anterior aspect of the footplate because the stapes can appear to be mobile when the crura are malformed. In congenital stapes fixation, when the footplate appears to be cartilaginous, we prefer stapes mobilization alone because the footplate in these patients does not tend to refix. For in otosclerosis, we prefer a microfenestra technique.

In a patient with a mobile incus and malleus, our prosthesis of choice is the De la Cruz Teflon-platinum-piston (Fig. 2A). This prosthesis allows the surgeon to see the relationship between the footplate and piston with the prosthesis in place and to make an accurate determination of the depth of penetration into the vestibule (its greatest advantage). The prosthesis can never be too long nor too short (Fig. 2B). If an obliterative oval window or a biscuit footplate is detected, a wide area of drilling must be started laterally and made cone-shaped down to the fenestration. The surgeon must constantly keep in mind that the plane of visualization is different from the plane in which the prosthesis will lie (Fig. 3).

Our results show the efficacy of surgical intervention in experienced hands. We define improvement as a decrease

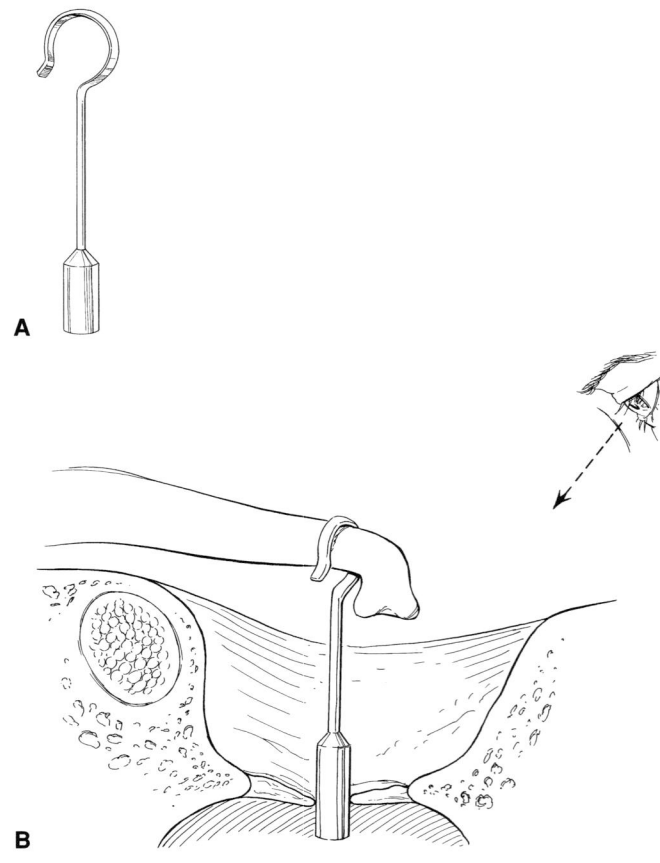

FIG. 2. A: The De la Cruz Teflon-platinum piston. **B:** The De la Cruz prosthesis in the oval window demonstrating excellent visualization of the penetration of the prosthesis.

in the pure-tone average of greater than 10 dB or an increase in the speech discrimination score of more than 15%. Of patients with congenital stapes fixation, 76% improved and 83% of patients with juvenile otosclerosis improved by using this definition. Of patients with congenital stapes fixation, 45% had closure of their air-bone gap to within 10 dB, and 82% of those with otosclerosis had similar results (11). These results must be interpreted with the knowledge that 13% of the cases were revision stapedectomies and that there was a much higher incidence of accompanying ossicular problems in these patients.

MANAGEMENT ALTERNATIVES

When a patient is diagnosed as having a correctable conductive hearing impairment, there are always three options. The first option is to do nothing. This option is not desirable for a school-age child because academic performance, language acquisition, and social development may be impaired. The same loss that would be an annoyance in an adult may have serious consequences in a child. The second, more reasonable, option is hearing amplification. Properly fitted hearing aids that are optimal for the loss should be the first option for any child with bilateral impairment. Even if surgery is desired, hearing aids should be used until such time that the hearing is restored. The child should be provided with hearing aids as soon as the loss is detected. The third option, surgery, is the eventual preferred treatment, provided the indications outlined above are met.

CONTROVERSIES IN MANAGEMENT

Stapedectomy on a child? Never! was the opening statement of the classic review from our institution in 1980 (12). House, Sheehy, and Antunez, however, believed then, as we do now, that there are situations that indicate surgical intervention (12). Many otolaryngologists argue that surgery should be reserved until the child reaches adulthood, because properly fitted hearing aids enable normal auditory and

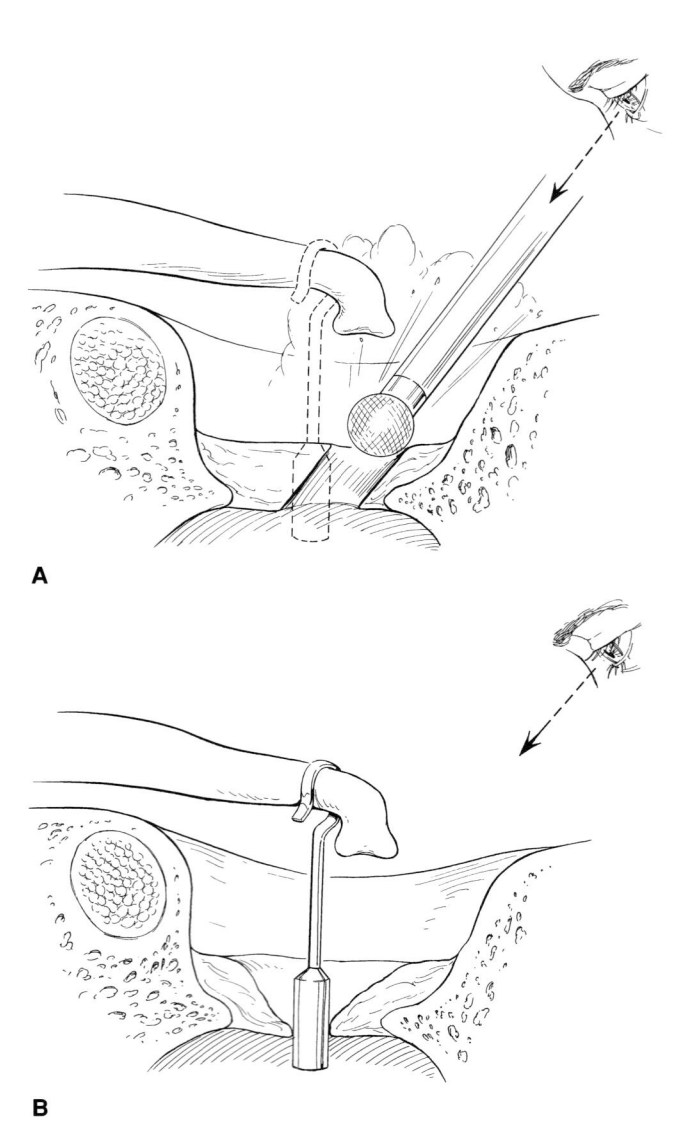

FIG. 3. A: Fenestration of an obliterated footplate along the plane of the visualization results in an inadequate opening into the vestibule. **B:** A wide trough fenestration of the obliterated footplate results in proper prosthesis placement.

speech development and thus assist academic performance. We agree that the risk of otitis in the perioperative period is sufficient reason to delay surgery in most patients until after the age of 5 years. Most otitis-prone children reveal the tendency by 5 years of age. We consider the results of surgery in children comparable to the results in adults for the same disease process. We have no illusions that children, with a higher incidence of ossicular and facial anomalies, do not present the otologist with a very great surgical challenge. We feel that the benefits of unencumbered hearing improvement in a child far outweigh the risks.

Any woman who reaches childbearing age with otosclerosis should be educated about the potential for accelerated otosclerosis and advised to avoid oral hormonal contraceptives. Although some authors advocate the use of sodium fluoride in children and pregnant women (19), we believe it is best to withhold fluoride in these patients until it can be used safely (after delivery and breast feeding or after puberty).

COMPLICATIONS

The most dreaded complication of pediatric stapedectomy is total hearing loss. This occurred in two patients in our first series of 34 patients (12). One patient had undergone a drillout for a congenital absence of an oval window. Our most recent review of 93 ears revealed no cases of profound hearing loss, tinnitus, facial palsy, or tympanic membrane perforation (11). One patient had persistent taste disturbance, and five patients complained of transient vertigo.

The much feared "gusher" was present in two patients, as was an "oozer." Computed tomography obtained several years after surgery on one of the patients with a "gusher" revealed abnormalities of the lateral internal auditory canal allowing abnormal communication of cerebrospinal fluid with perilymph. In none of these four patients was there a sensorineural loss; their bone conduction and speech discrimination remained stable. Unfortunately, none of them showed improvement in their conductive losses (11). We believe these four cases and the four cases from the earlier series represent an inner-ear conductive loss (11). We are not sure of the etiology, but it is possible that high hydraulic pressure in the vestibule may prohibit normal sound transduction. If high pressure is detected preoperatively, we do not advocate surgery for any patient with a bone deficiency at the lateral end of the internal auditory canal because all separation from the cochlea is lost. Phelps (20) first indicated that this bony deficiency, not the widened internal auditory canal, represents the essential defect of X-linked progressive deafness with stapes gusher.

CASE HISTORIES

Case History 1

A 9-year-old girl presented to the House Ear Clinic with a 1-year history of progressive hearing loss. There was a family history of otosclerosis. The girl's tympanic membranes moved well, and the remainder of the physical examination was normal. The patient s audiogram showed a four-frequency bone conduction pure-tone average (BCPTA) of 24 dB and a four-frequency air conduction pure-tone average (ACPTA) of 35 dB in the right ear, and the left ear had a BCPTA of 10 dB and an ACPTA of 15 dB. The speech discrimination was 100% in both ears. Impedance audiometry reveled a type A pattern and absent reflexes bilaterally. The diagnosis was otosclerosis. After discussing options with the child and parents, it was elected to follow the patient s hearing with annual audiograms. The only treatment administered was preferential seating in school and educating the family on difficult hearing environments. Two years later, the child's right ear had a progressive hearing loss, with the BCPTA now at 26 dB and the ACPTA at 56 dB; the left ear remained unchanged. The child was having increasing difficulty at school, and it was decided that an elective stapedectomy would be performed.

At surgery, under general anesthesia, an obliterative oval window was encountered. This was drilled out with a wide area laterally, narrowing down to a smaller area as the drill out proceeded medially. The facial nerve was encountered overhanging into the oval window. A microfenestration was created, and a 4.0 mm × 0.6 mm De la Cruz piston prosthesis was placed. The patient's postoperative course was uneventful, and her facial nerve was normal after the operation. Her postoperative hearing revealed an ACPTA of 20 dB, which has remained stable over the subsequent 7 years. The hearing in her left ear has had progression of sensorineural loss to an ACPTA of 35 dB, but her air-bone gap has remained at less than 10 dB. She was started on a combination of calcium carbonate and sodium floride (Florical) three times a day at 17 years of age.

This case demonstrates a common intraoperative difficulty in this group of patients; obliterative otosclerosis. The techniques of management are no different from those used for adults, with the exception that there is an increased likelihood that a congenital abnormality (in this case, the facial nerve) will be encountered. In this patient, the ideal goal of closure of the ABG (≤10 dB) was achieved, in fact "overclosure" was obtained. The patient also illustrated the need for long-term follow-up. She developed cochlear (labyrinthine) otosclerosis in the other ear. We do not advocate using fluoride therapy in any child while bone growth is still occurring, but others do (19).

Case History 2

An 8-year-old boy presented to the House Ear Clinic with a 6 year (or possibly longer) history of severe mixed hearing loss in both ears. He had a 36 dB and 33 dB ABG in the right and left ears, respectively. His speech discrimination was 68% in both ears. He had been wearing hearing aids for 6 years with good results. The parents desired to proceed with surgery. Impedance audiometry revealed type A tympanograms and absent reflexes in both ears. The child was taken to surgery, under general anesthesia, and the case appeared to be routine, with the exception that the long process of the incus was abnormally thin (approximately the size of the stapes crus). On down fracture of the stapes (which appeared slightly thickened), the entire stapes mobilized and a "gusher" of fluid filled the speculum several times. The patient was placed in a semisitting position. The oval window was sealed with soft tissue, a 4.5 mm De la Cruz piston was placed, and the middle ear was packed. The leak was not present at the end of the procedure. The patient was maintained in a sitting position for 2 weeks at all times and was started on antibiotics. His ACPTA, BCPTA, ABG, and speech discrimination remained stable, without improvement or deterioration.

This patient demonstrates a failure to improve hearing, but the preoperative cochlear reserve was still maintained and aided. These intraoperative steps represent our standard technique of managing a stapes gusher.

CONCLUSION

The decision to proceed with a stapedectomy in a child is a difficult one. We use hearing aids in any child with bilateral losses, explain the risks of surgery, and ask the parents and child to let us know when they are ready to proceed with surgical intervention. In children with unilateral losses, we use preferential seating in academic settings and proceed with surgery when the family is ready and the patient can tolerate surgery under local anesthesia. Imaging is used judiciously and only for children in whom surgery is being considered. Counseling prior to surgery explains that although the results have been shown to be good and that the complications are infrequent, there are greater surgical challenges for this group of patients. We believe that stapedectomy in children is a reasonable option in patients with congenital stapes fixation and juvenile otosclerosis.

REFERENCES

1. Valsalva AM. *Opera, hoc est, tractatus de aure humana.* Venice: Pitteri 1741.
2. Politzer A. Üeber primäre erkrankung der knöchernen labyrinthkapsel. *Z Ohrenheilkd Kr Luftwege* 1893;25:309.
3. Ménière P. De I exploration de I appareil auditif, ou recherches sur les moynes propes àconduire auditory diagnostic des maladies device l oreille. *Gaz Med Fr* 1842;10:114.
4. Kessel J. Über das Mobilisieren des Steigbügels durch ausschneiden des Trommelfelles. Hammers und Ambosses bei undurchgangigkeit der Tuba. *Arch Ohrenheilkd* 1878;13:69.
5. Passow KA. Operative anlegung einer Offnung die mediale Paukenhohlenwand bei Stapesankylose. *Verh Dtsch Otol Ges Versamml* 1897;6:141.
6. Sourdille J. Résultats primitifs et secondaires de quatorze cas de surdité par otospongiose operés. *Rev Laryngol* 1930;51:595.
7. Shea JJ Jr. Fenestration of the oval window. *Ann Otol Rhinol Laryngol* 1958;67:932.
8. Konigsmark BW, Gorlin RJ. *Genetic and metabolic deafness.* Philadelphia: WB Saunders; 1976.
9. Cole JM. Surgery for otosclerosis in children. *Laryngoscope* 1982;92:859.
10. Robinson M. Juvenile otosclerosis. A 20-year study. *Ann Otol Rhinol Laryngol* 1983;92:561.
11. De la Cruz A, Angeli S. Stapedectomy in children. *Otolaryngol Head Neck Surgery* [Submitted].
12. House JW, Sheehy JL, Antunez JC. Stapedectomy in children. *Laryngoscope* 1980;90:1804.
13. Yoo TJ. Etiopathogenesis of otosclerosis: a hypothesis. *Ann Otol Rhinol Laryngol* 1984;93:28.
14. McKenna MJ, Mills BG. Immunohistochemical evidence of measles virus antigens in active otosclerosis. *Otolaryngol Head Neck Surg* 1989;101:415.
15. Gordon MA, McPhee JR, Van de Water TR, Ruben RJ. Aberration of the tissue collagenase system in association with otosclerosis. *Am J Otol* 1992;13:398.
16. Brunner HG, van Bennekom A, Lambermon EM, et al. The gene for X-linked progressive mixed deafness with perilymphatic gusher during stapes surgery (DFN3) is linked to PGK. *Hum Genet* 1988;80:337.
17. de Kok YJ, van der Maarel SM, Bitner-Glindzicz M, et al. Association between X-linked mixed deafness and mutations in the POU domain gene POU3F4. *Science* 1995;267:685.
18. Committee on Hearing and Equilibrium of the American Academy of Otolaryngology-Head and Neck Surgery. Draft guidelines for the evaluation of results of treatment of conductive hearing loss. *AAOHNS Bull* 1994;13:14.
19. Causse JR, Causse JB. Otospongiosis as a genetic disease. Early detection, medical management, and prevention. *Am J Otol* 1984;5:211.
20. Phelps PD, Reardon W, Pembrey M, Bellman S, Luxom L. X-linked deafness, stapes gushers and a distinctive defect of the inner ear. *Neuroradiology* 1991;33:326.

CHAPTER 37

Ossicular Reconstruction

Robert A. Goldenberg

Improving and maintaining hearing are two of the primary goals of the otologist. To these ends, microscopic reconstruction of the middle ear has been possible for almost half a century. Although techniques have been modified over the years and newer biomaterials have been exchanged for existing ones, the basic principles of ossicular reconstruction have remained the same.

Despite advances in technology, optics, technique, and biomaterials, the ability to reconstruct hearing depends primarily on the type and degree of disease present. It should be relatively obvious that the more normal the anatomy, the better the hearing results. The amount of improvement in hearing from reconstruction of the ossicles will depend largely on the presence or absence of the stapes, the mobility of the stapes, the presence or absence of the long process of the malleus, and the underlying pathology of the middle ear.

Reconstruction of the hearing mechanism must always be attempted realistically. Each surgeon must interpret and analyze published results with a keen understanding and appreciation of reporting methods. Enthusiastic reports of a small number of patients followed for a short time should be tempered with a larger series based on long-term follow-up. As is true with any technique, each surgeon is obligated to evaluate his or her own results. While these may be based on the experience of others, self-evaluation of personal experience is critical to accurate preoperative counseling of patient and parents. With children in particular, each surgeon must attempt reconstruction with an ever-watchful eye toward the future. Each surgical procedure, usually performed with consent of the parents but without clear understanding from the patient, will obligate that child to a lifetime of consequences based on the outcome of surgery. Yet unknown techniques of the future may readily solve problems that present a struggle for the expert of today.

Despite beginning with a rather somber plea for conservatism, there are nonetheless many exciting and rewarding opportunities for hearing reconstruction in the child who has a middle ear abnormality with a conductive hearing loss. This chapter discusses patient selection, patient and parent counseling, diagnostic methods, and indications for surgery. Technical aspects of reconstruction, controversies, and complications are presented. Two case reports illustrate many of the key points of this chapter.

CLASSIFICATION

In this chapter, four basic causes of conductive hearing loss in children are discussed: congenital, otitis media, trauma, and otosclerosis. Because the possibility of a coexisting sensorineural hearing loss must always be considered, accurate audiometric evaluation is critical to assess the patient as a surgical candidate.

Congenital

There is great variety of ossicular malformation with congenital conditions. The embryology of the middle ear is quite complex and has been well discussed previously. Most congenital anomalies have association with known syndromes such as Treacher Collins or Goldenhar's, metobolic disorders such as the mucopolysaccharidoses, or even complete atresia of the pinna and external auditory canal. Bergstrom (1) has reviewed middle ear abnormalities with their known associations. She found that 17 percent of children with congenital hearing loss were eventually noted to have defects of the conductive mechanism; however, only 1.2% had a conductive hearing loss without pathology of the outer or inner ear or other systemic abnormalities. Stewart and Downs (2) identified 9.5% of hearing-impaired children as having a conductive impairment not related to otitis media. Of these children, the overwhelming majority had associated syndromes, and only 0.5% had an isolated middle ear anom-

R.A. Goldenberg: Department of Otolaryngology, Wright State University School of Medicine, Children's Medical Center, Dayton, Ohio 45402.

aly. Teunissen and Cremers (3) studied 104 patients with congenital middle ear anomalies; there were 27 patients with a mobile stapes. In eight of these patients, there was a discontinuity of the ossicular chain, and in 19 patients, there was an epitympanic fixation of the ossicles. There were 13 unilateral and 14 bilateral cases in this series. It was noted that the hearing gain was much better if the stapes superstructure was not malformed. In another study, Teunissen and Cremers (4) evaluated the same 104 patients and found that 32 patients had a congenital stapes fixation as well as a congenital abnormality of other ossicles. One third of these patients had an associated syndrome. On these patients, 26 stapedectomies were performed, but only two stapes mobilization procedures and four exploratory tympanotomies were done. The hearing results were somewhat poorer than when the stapes was mobile.

Ossicular malformation in the middle ear is often associated with a smaller than normal external auditory canal. In the middle ear, the malleus and incus may be totally fused or severely fixed. The malleus and incus may be formed normally and mobile but with an absent or fibrous inendostapedial connection. The stapes superstructure may be malformed, partially or totally absent, and/or fixed.

There are miscellaneous structural abnormalities as well, all of which have been well described in the otologic literature. The facial nerve may be malpositioned, dehiscent, severely overhanging the stapes, or positioned inferiorly to the oval window. There may be associated abnormalities of the chorda tympani tendon, abnormality or absence of the middle ear muscles, a persistent stapedial artery, or a complete absence of the round window. It is possible to have complete absence of the oval window with the facial nerve in an abnormal position.

While not usually associated with an abnormality of the ossicular chain, a congenital cholesteatoma as a cause for conductive hearing loss in the middle ear must be mentioned. This clinical entity has been well described by Levenson, Michaels, Parisier (5). When found early, the ossicular chain is usually intact, and complete removal of the cholesteatoma is possible without the need for ossicular reconstruction. In extensive or advanced cases of congenital cholesteatoma, when the ossicular chain has been disrupted, reconstruction can be accomplished much as in cases of acquired cholesteatoma.

Chronic Otitis Media

Discontinuity of the ossicular chain due to erosion of the ossicle itself is the most common cause of conductive hearing loss in chronic otitis media. A destroyed incudostapedial joint or long process of the incus is the most common site of discontinuity. This may be associated with destruction of the stapes superstructure and, occasionally, the stapes footplate as well. There may be erosion of the long process of the malleus; advanced cases exhibit more complete necrosis of all of the three ossicles. Even without complete necrosis, involvement of the ossicles by the infectious process, particularly cases with cholesteatoma, often requires removal of all or part of the ossicles in order to eradicate the primary disease.

Tympanosclerosis of the tympanic membrane, middle ear, and/or stapes itself may cause loss of mobility of the vibratory action of the ossicular chain from the tympanic membrane to the oval window. There may be a fixation of the malleus head, fixation of the stapes, and/or obliteration of the oval and round window.

Although this chapter focuses on ossicular reconstruction, the coexistence of pathologic conditions of the middle ear discussed elsewhere (e.g., a perforation, mucosal disease, and cholesteatoma) will affect the method by which hearing reconstruction is accomplished. Brackmann (6) has noted that there is a tendency for a greater degree of ossicular destruction and greater incidence of residual cholesteatoma in children. However, he did not notice any significant difference in the extent of cholesteatoma between children and adults. Arriaga (7) describes more aggressive involvement of the ossicles with cholesteatoma in children as well. The epitympanic area is particularly vulnerable for residual cholesteatoma, and consideration of hearing improvement should be secondary to the total removal of cholesteatoma in all cases.

Trauma

Trauma is an infrequent cause of conductive hearing loss in children, but nonetheless a significant one. A history of head injury, basilar skull fracture, and/or concussion is the key factor. Some cases of head trauma may have an associated perilymph fistula present and certainly carry the risk of sensorineural hearing loss. Often, patients with a traumatic type of hearing loss in childhood will not seek help until they are adults. When a specific history of head trauma and a documented conductive hearing loss present themselves, exploration of the middle ear for ossicular dislocation or discontinuity is indicated.

Otosclerosis

Although otosclerosis classically presents in the second and third decades of life, it is recognized that otosclerosis can occur in children. Children with a strong family history of otosclerosis, no other history or physical findings, and a well-documented conductive hearing loss confirmed with tuning forks should be suspected of having this disease. Differentiation from congenital fixation of the stapes is often impossible preoperatively and can be made only on inspection of the oval window. Although distinction between these two disease entities may be difficult, stapedectomy or stapedotomy is the procedure of choice, and excellent results have been reported in the literature (8,9).

CLINICAL MANIFESTATIONS AND DIAGNOSIS

In this section, we examine the pertinent points from the patient's history, physical examination, audiologic evaluation, and radiograph assessment.

History and Physical Examination

Often, a child with a mild or moderate hearing loss in one or both ears is not aware of the condition, particularly if it is of long-standing duration. A child born with a total loss in one ear may simply consider this a normal situation and may not recognize the problem until a telephone receiver is held against the nonhearing ear. Even observant and involved parents may simply feel their child is not paying attention. Screening hearing tests performed early in childhood and/or with school-age children are often the initial method of diagnosis. *If a parent questions a child's hearing ability, accurate audiometric assessment should be performed.* Information regarding family history of hearing loss, previous ear infections (particularly the use of ventilation tubes), trauma, and/or other coexisting medical conditions should be noted.

If hearing loss has been established by audiometric testing, further assessment of the patient's performance in school, as well as of social and communicative skills is important in determining how the hearing loss affects this particular child. Decline in grades, difficulty with verbal skills such as spelling and reading, and inattention in class are key points to question. Other associated factors, such as learning disabilities, perceptual problems, and/or psychomotor abnormalities, should be noted as well. Lack of response to parental requests, inattention, and "just not listening" are much more subtle and difficult to assess; a worsening condition might indicate a more serious problem. Because these concomitant conditions will place the hearing impairment into perspective for each individual patient, the decision between surgical intervention and watchful waiting can be made on an informed and realistic basis.

During the physical examination, cases of congenital hearing loss may not show any abnormality of the tympanic membrane. However, the external auditory canal may be somewhat smaller in diameter than normal, very stenotic, and/or completely atretic. There may be other associated physical abnormalities, particularly with specific congenital syndromes. Preauricular cysts and/or fistulae, for example, may be present. A smooth white mass in the anterior superior quadrant, visualized behind an intact and normal tympanic membrane, is indicative of a congenital cholesteatoma. In cases of chronic otitis media, the tympanic membrane may exhibit any of the known findings of chronic ear disease—perforation, middle ear fluid, cholesteatoma, tympanosclerosis, granulation tissue, and the like. A total tympanic membrane perforation, severe middle ear mucosal disease, and/or an atelectatic tympanic membrane are often indications of more severe eustachian tube dysfunction and should make the surgeon less optimistic regarding successful ossicular reconstruction, particularly in the long term. In particular, the condition of the middle ear mucosa is an extremely significant factor in predicting the success of reconstructive results of the hearing mechanism.

In cases of trauma, the otoscopic evaluation may be perfectly normal or the ossicular discontinuity may be obvious through the tympanic membrane. Occasionally, a fracture line through the posterior–superior exterior auditory canal may be visualized. In cases of otosclerosis, the physical evaluation is almost always normal.

Audiometry

Although audiometric assessment has been covered elsewhere in this textbook, a few comments are critical regarding the indications for surgical intervention. Assessment of hearing levels in children depends largely on the child's age and ability. If the patient is 4 years of age or older, pure tone audiometry with masked air and bone conduction levels should be obtained along with speech reception thresholds and speech discrimination scores. Children between 2 and 4 years of age should be tested using play audiometry. In selected cases, masked air and bone conduction thresholds can be obtained if the child will tolerate headphones and the bone conductor. In children under 2, conditioned audiometry can usually give a fair assessment of air conduction thresholds, either monaurally or binaurally. Repeated assessments should continue until the patient is fully conditioned and a reliable audiogram has been obtained. Several appointments may be required, particularly with younger children and those with physical and/or intellectual disabilities or attention-deficit disorders (10).

Where conventional audiometry has been impractical or unsuccessful, threshold auditory brainstem response testing (ABR) should be performed. However, ABR testing is never a replacement for conventional audiometry. Tympanometry may be useful in testing for middle ear effusion. If the tympanic membrane is normal, low compliance often suggests fixation, and high compliance of the tympanic membrane generally indicates discontinuity of the ossicular chain. Absence of a stapedial reflex may indicate an ossicular abnormality or fixation of the stapes.

Because surgery is rarely contemplated in children under 5 or 6 years old, obtaining accurate masked air and bone conduction thresholds at a younger age is not urgent, although this does make early diagnosis more accurate and may allow for the selection of a hearing aid prior to surgical intervention.

Medical Imaging

High-resolution computed tomography scans (CT) should be obtained in children prior to surgical intervention for conductive hearing loss. Axial and coronal images allow precise identification of the structures of the middle and inner ear.

Classic inner ear anomalies, such as a Mondini's defect or Michel's aplasia, are associated with severe sensorineural hearing loss; however, a large vestibule or widened internal auditory canal may temper the decision to recommend surgery for conductive hearing loss. A large cochlear aquaduct may indicate the presence of a "gusher" if stapedectomy is contemplated. The incus and malleus should be readily identified, although the stapes often may not be fully visualized. Presence of a round window niche should be noted, and the course of the fallopian canal should be demonstrated.

Inner ear anomalies can be associated with ossicular malformations and should be readily noted on CT scanning images; correlation must be made between audiometry and the imaging studies. Magnetic resonance imaging is not as useful as CT scanning techniques, unless a soft-tissue abnormality or tumor mass is suspected.

Other Tests

Tuning fork tests have limited value in younger children but may help validate a conductive loss in the older child.

Previous medical or surgical records may be helpful but are not essential for preoperative evaluation. Formal assessment of psychomotor behavior, learning, and/or perceptual problems should be accomplished in those children with a suspected history of these problems. Information from a parent–teacher conference can be quite helpful in determining the impact of the child's hearing loss on the educational progress. Occasionally, psychological testing also may be indicated. These additional tests will allow the child's hearing impairment to be put into proper context regarding the degree of handicap present in order to fully determine the need for surgical intervention.

GOALS FOR MANAGEMENT

Degree of Impairment

Information from the parents' (or patient's) history combined with the audiometric assessment should be used to fully assess the degree of hearing impairment present in the child. Generally, a child with a hearing impairment less than 20 dB air–bone gap or a 30 dB speech reception threshold should not be considered a surgical candidate. This rule of thumb obviously depends on whether the hearing loss is unilateral or bilateral and the age of the patient. However, the patient's educational and social abilities also should be taken into account. There is a world of difference between an 8 year-old child with a unilateral 30-dB conductive hearing loss who has excellent reading and social skills and a similar child with a learning disability who is failing in school. Parents understandably are anxious to "have something done," and it is important to resist this temptation to "fix something" when surgical intervention is not fully indicated.

Reconstruct Realistically

There is an old saying that it is just as important to know what you cannot do as what you can do. Reconstruction of the middle ear in general, but particularly in children, should follow this axiom. Over the years, the tendency toward overenthusiastic reporting of hearing results has been noted by Smyth and Patterson (11). They caution surgeons to accurately assess and report hearing results in a more stringent manner, with particular attention to long-term follow-up.

Kessler, Potsic, and Marsh (12) reported that ossicular reconstruction in younger children may carry a greater risk of failure than in adults. Arriaga (7) equivocally stated that parents and children should understand that reconstructive surgery in the presence of cholesteatoma is almost always associated with some degree of permanent conductive hearing loss. He also cautioned about reporting hearing results expressed as improvement in air–bone gap alone when patients and parents are ultimately more interested in the air conduction level and prospects for long-term hearing improvement.

Postoperative Follow-up

Although the principle of long-term follow-up for chronic ear disease has been well established, the need for long-term follow-up in children is critical and should be emphasized. Opportunities exist for recurrent and/or residual cholesteatoma, malposition or extrusion of the prostheses, recurrent infections in the middle ear, and, most importantly, retraction and atelectasis of the tympanic membrane and/or graft. Each of these conditions alone or in combination can result in later failure of an initial success. Patients and parents should be counseled preoperatively regarding the probability of staged procedures, the need for long-term follow-up, and the possibility for repeated procedures over time. Telling a child's parents that the ear must be examined at least once a year "forever" is not inappropriate, particularly in cases involving cholesteatoma or severe eustachian tube dysfunction. The possibility of newer technology in the future should always be reinforced following the initial procedure.

RECOMMENDED APPROACH

This section discusses a method used to assess and solve the various types of reconstructive problems encountered in the middle ear. It is not intended to be comprehensive: A myriad of techniques and approaches for reconstruction of the hearing mechanism have been developed over the years. It is not intended to be dogmatic; there is always more than one way to solve a problem. It is intended to represent the author's systematic approach to ossicular reconstruction, an approach that has been successful over many years.

The author has developed his own implant system using prostheses, constructed from hydroxylapatite and Plastipore, that can be used in almost every type of middle ear situation. The surgical techniques are similar regardless of the type of implant used, and the basic techniques can be readily adapted to other biomaterials. Similar techniques have been used by the author with many other prostheses prior to development of these particular implants. The techniques and results of this implant system have been reported previously in the literature (13–16).

Because this chapter is limited to ossicular reconstruction, several assumptions about the condition of the middle ear have been made. The first is that no cholesteatoma is present. In many cases, this means the procedure has been staged and follows an initial procedure to remove cholesteatoma. If cholesteatoma is not present or has been fully removed, obviously a one-stage procedure is all that is required. The second assumption is that there is no evidence of mucosal disease; if this were encountered, the procedure would also have been staged. If there is normal middle ear mucosa at the initial procedure, staging, again, would not be necessary. The third assumption is that the tympanic membrane is intact, having been normal to begin with or grafted at this or a primary procedure. In unusual cases, a persistent perforation or even ventilation tube may be present at the time of ossicular reconstruction.

It is assumed that the external auditory canal is patent, although it may be smaller than normal. The techniques of canal wall up, canal wall down, canal wall reconstruction, and/or obliteration of the mastoid cavity make little difference regarding the technique of ossicular reconstruction. There may be some difference in the position of the tympanic membrane or tympanic membrane graft related to the presence or absence of a posterior bony canal wall or replacement.

Initial Assessment

The initial approach to the middle ear may be through a transcanal, endaural, or postauricular incision. A small external auditory canal, a suspected or actual cholesteatoma, the size of a perforation, and the general anatomic configuration of the middle ear will dictate the need for a particular approach. Use of the middle ear endoscope, as described by Poe and Bottrill (17), to inspect the epitympanum and mastoid cavity may obviate the need for a postauricular approach in some cases. In most cases of ossicular reconstruction of the middle ear, a tympanomeatal incision through the ear canal can afford satisfactory exposure.

Once the tympanic membrane has been reflected from the posterior sulcus, the entire middle ear must be inspected in a methodical fashion. Visualization must include the eustachian tube orifice, hypotympanum, round window membrane, long process of the malleus, long process of the incus, stapes, stapes superstructure, and footplate. The course of the facial nerve should be determined, and presence or absence of middle ear muscles should be noted. The condition of the middle ear mucosa must be observed and noted. Any erosion or necrosis of the ossicles should be noted. In addition to visual inspection, palpation of all structures (particularly the ossicular chain) yields much information. Presence or absence of a round window reflex can provide invaluable information at this initial assessment.

There will be some cases in which the ossicular chain appears intact and mobile but is stiff to direct palpation. This may be caused by a partially fixed stapes, malleus, and/or other partial immobility of the ossicular chain. In this case, the preoperative audiogram should be reevaluated intraoperatively and the amount of air–bone gap present compared to the degree of stiffness of the ossicular chain. Conservatism should be the rule: The smaller the air–bone gap, the less indication to remove any portion of the ossicular chain. Mobilization of the ossicles with repeated audiometric evaluation postoperatively might be better than removing an ossicle and creating an irreversable defect in the ossicular chain. Often, a congenitally fixed stapes can be mobilized without disrupting the ossicular chain, and excellent hearing will result without refixation of the stapes (9).

In cases in which the horizontal portion of the facial nerve is dehiscent, assessment of the amount of overhang is critical. If the oval window is readily visible and the prosthesis can be placed into the oval window niche without compressing the facial nerve, there should be no disruption of facial nerve function. When the facial nerve overhang is extreme, there can be a risk of injury to the facial nerve due to placement of the prosthesis during surgery. If the prosthesis places undue pressure on or indentation of the dehiscent facial nerve, an alternative method of treatment should be considered. Also, the prosthesis may extend into the oval window at such an inefficient angle as to decrease the efficiency of normal vibratory energy and thus reduce the amount of hearing gain from reconstruction.

Occasionally, extensive tympanosclerosis of the middle ear will be found to cause immobility of the stapes and stapes footplate. In these cases, the tympanosclerotic plaque can be removed from the oval window and the stapes mobilized. Often this will be enough to achieve an excellent closure of the air–bone gap. If stapes mobilization cannot be performed, a stapedectomy or stapedotomy can also result in hearing improvement. Once again, conservatism should prevail; mobilization with postoperative evaluation of hearing may be a better choice than opening the vestibule and risking a decrease in cochlear reserve. Tympanosclerosis that causes the malleus to be fixed can be dealt with in a relatively straightforward fashion with an incus prosthesis, as will be described. This prosthesis gives excellent hearing results. Tympanosclerosis confined only to the tympanic membrane must be assessed with respect to the level of hearing impairment present. There should be enough of an air–bone gap to consider replacement of a tympanosclerotic membrane with a graft, certainly at least 30 dB or greater.

One of the most difficult conditions for ossicular reconstruction occurs when cholesteatoma involves an intact ossicular chain with normal hearing. In this instance, the cholesteatoma must be totally removed. In addition, disarticulation of the incudo-occipital joint and removal of the incus, possibly the stapes superstructure, and occasionally the malleus may be required. If the cholesteatoma extends aggressively into the oval window niche, complete removal may

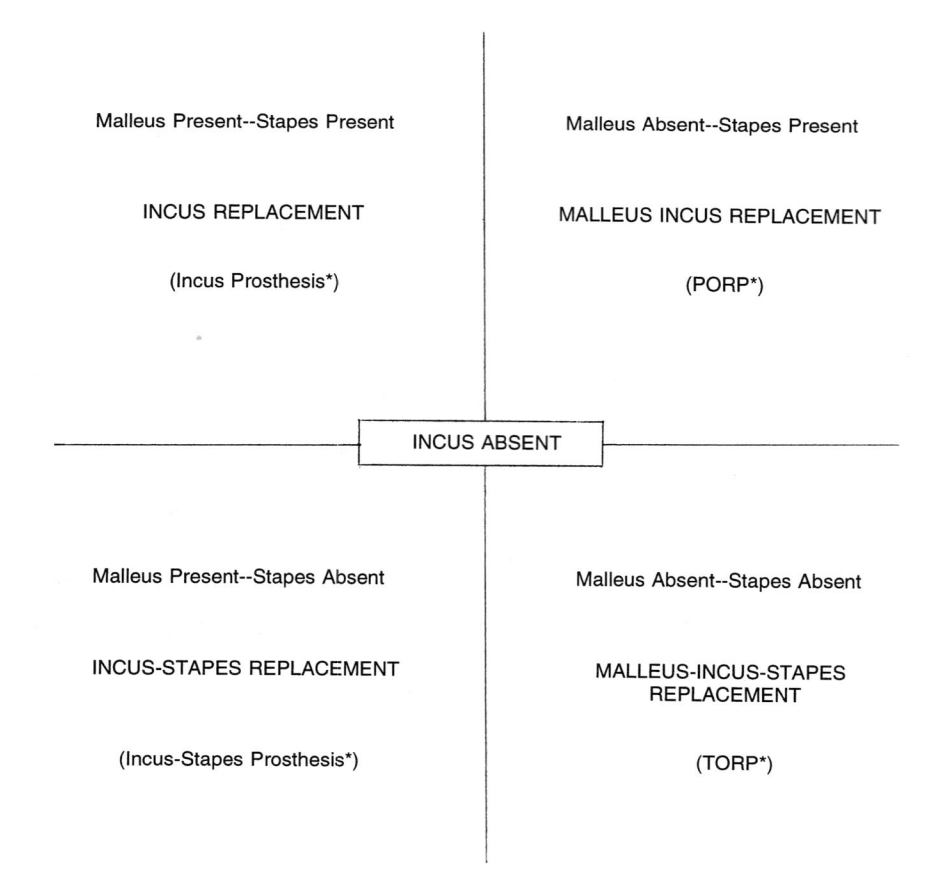

```
                    |
Malleus Present--Stapes Present    |   Malleus Absent--Stapes Present
                    |
    INCUS REPLACEMENT              |   MALLEUS INCUS REPLACEMENT
                    |
     (Incus Prosthesis*)           |          (PORP*)
                    |
─────────────────────────── INCUS ABSENT ───────────────────────────
                    |
Malleus Present--Stapes Absent     |   Malleus Absent--Stapes Absent
                    |
 INCUS-STAPES REPLACEMENT          |    MALLEUS-INCUS-STAPES
                    |                      REPLACEMENT
  (Incus-Stapes Prosthesis*)       |          (TORP*)
```

FIG. 1. Paradigm for ossicular reconstruction. The appropriate Goldenberg implant is noted by asterisk. *PORP,* partial ossicular replacement prosthesis; *TORP,* total ossicular replacement prosthesis. Modified from Austin (18).

not be possible at the first stage, and a planned second stage is obligatory. Although this condition is infrequent, it reinforces the need for preoperative explanation of the possibility for a staged procedure.

Once the condition of the middle ear has been fully evaluated, there is usually a fairly straightforward way of dealing with the different defects in the hearing mechanism. Figure 1 displays the four basic conditions that require reconstruction of the ossicular chain (18). The four basic prostheses in the author's implant system are denoted with an asterisk. These have been arbitrarily divided into cases of ossicular discontinuity, ossicular fixation, and the rare case of absence of the oval window. A brief but important comment about staging concludes this section.

Ossicular Discontinuity

One of the most common conditions encountered in middle ear reconstruction occurs with absence of the long process of the incus or the incudostapedial joint. The malleus and stapes are mobile and normal; a round window reflex is observed with palpation of the stapes. If present, the remainder of the long process and body of the incus should be removed by means of a right-angle hook.

An incus prosthesis can be used to reconstruct hearing in this case. A standard measuring rod is used to measure the distance from the stapes capitulum to either a point midway between the long process of the malleus and the scutum, if the canal wall is up, or the lateral semicircular canal, if the canal wall is down (Fig. 2). This point represents the position of the tympanic membrane when replaced in its normal anatomic position and is the point where the lateral surface of the prosthesis will contact the tympanic membrane. The Plastipore® shaft of the prosthesis is then trimmed to the appropriate length (average 2.5 mm) on a cutting block marked in millimeter increments (Fig. 3). A small notch is made in the posterior aspect of the Plastipore shaft to allow for insertion of the stapedius tendon (Fig. 4). The long hook of the hydroxylapatite head is then introduced underneath the long process of the malleus (Fig. 5); the Plastipore shaft is placed onto the capitulum of the stapes with the notch straddling the stapedius tendon (Fig. 6). The hydroxylapatite head can be adjusted in an inferior or superior direction to allow for the vagaries of middle ear anatomy. Because of the stability of the prosthesis on the stapes capitulum and the stapedius tendon, middle ear packing may not be necessary. However, Gelfoam® packing is usually used in the middle ear to stabilize the prosthesis (Fig. 7). After notation of the presence or absence of a round window reflex, the tympanic membrane is replaced into its normal anatomic position, and the external canal is packed with Gelfoam®.

In this next case, the stapes superstructure and the incus are absent, but the malleus and stapes footplate are present and normal. The same technique of reconstruction may be

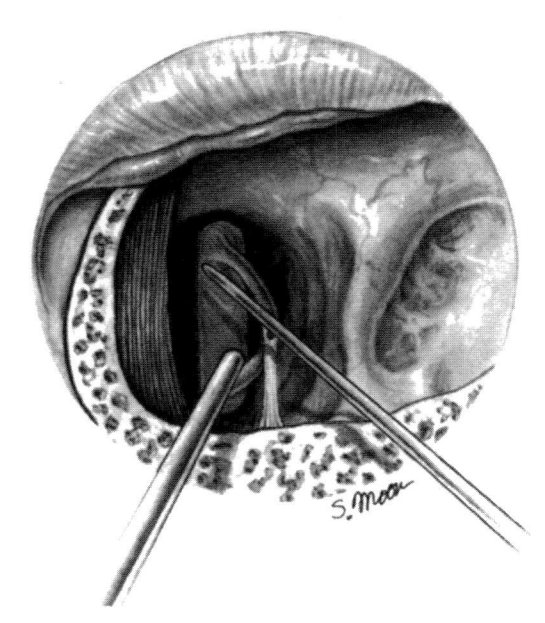

FIG. 2. Measurement for Goldenberg incus prosthesis (incus missing). From Goldenberg RA (32) with permission.

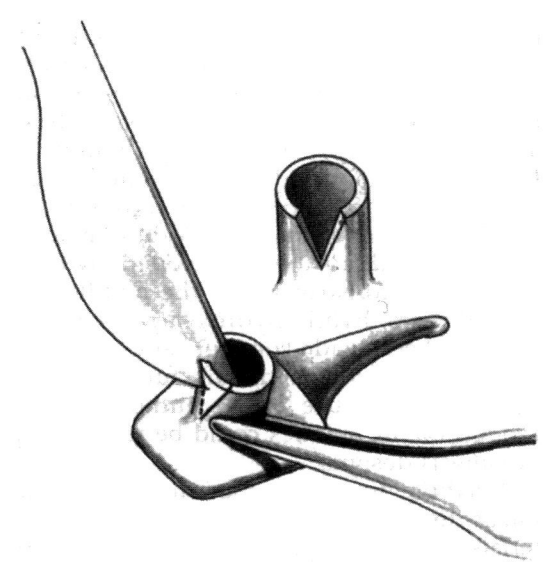

FIG. 4. Making notch for stapedius tendon. From Goldenberg RA (32) with permission.

used if the stapes footplate is absent, but an oval window graft of fascia, vein, or perichondrium must be used. If cholesteatoma or otitis media involve the oval window, this graft should have been placed at a planned second-stage procedure because of increased risk of hearing loss from opening the oval window at the time of the initial operation. However, if the footplate problem is from trauma, congenital abnormality, or a noninfectious process, the footplate may be removed and the graft placed at the time of ossicular reconstruction in one stage. In either case, the technique of ossicular reconstruction is the same. Measurement is taken from the footplate or graft to the same midpoint on the tympanic membrane, as previously described (Fig. 8). An incus-stapes prosthesis is trimmed to an appropriate length (average 4.5 mm) on a cutting block (Fig. 9). The hook of the hydroxylapatite head is directed anteriorly and placed underneath the long process of the malleus. The Plastipore® shaft is then centered in the oval window niche and checked for mobility. A hydroxylapatite shoe can be fitted over the end of the Plastipore® shaft in cases in which this is desirable for stability or to avoid the use of Plastipore® directly on the footplate or graft material (Fig. 10). A round window reflex should be observed, Gelfoam® packing may or may not be used, and the tympanic membrane is returned to its normal position, as previously described. If the anomaly is

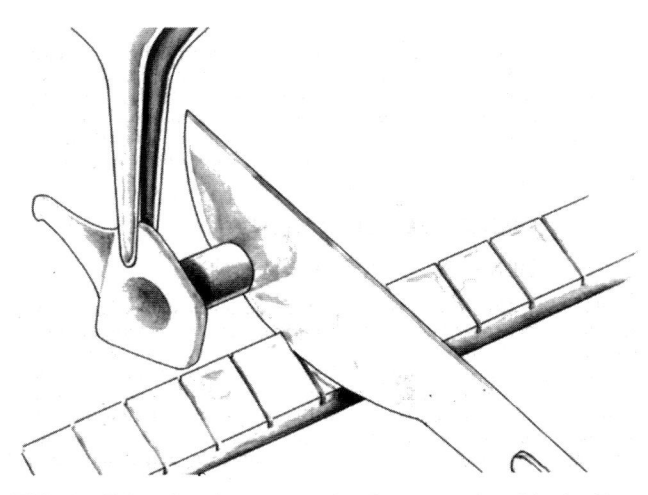

FIG. 3. Trimming incus prosthesis on cutting block. From Goldenberg RA (32) with permission.

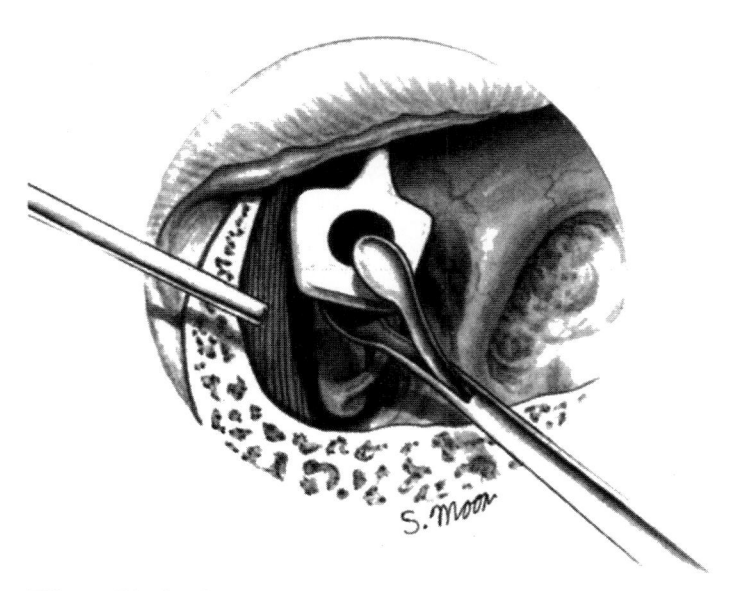

FIG. 5. Placing incus prostheses with hook under malleus. From Goldenberg RA (32) with permission.

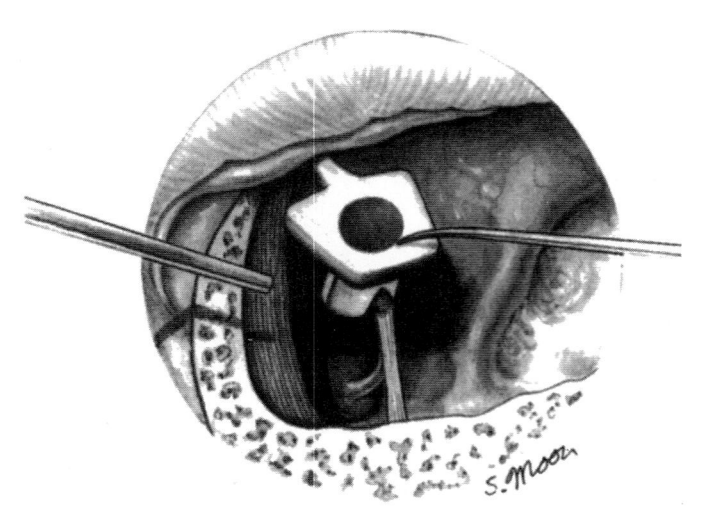

FIG. 6. Placing notched shaft over stapedius tendon. From Goldenberg RA (32) with permission.

congenital and not infectious, a wire incus replacement prosthesis (IRP), as initially described by Sheehy and Powers (19), may give better hearing results. Obviously, the wire cannot be used in cases involving chronic infection of the middle ear.

The third example of ossicular discontinuity is characterized by absence of the incus and malleus presence of a normal stapes and footplate. The distance between the capitulum of the stapes and midpoint of the tympanic membrane is measured, as previously described (Fig. 11). A partial ossicular replacement prosthesis (PORP®) is trimmed to the appropriate length (Fig. 12) and a notch made for the stapedius tendon (average length for the prosthesis is 1.5–3.5 mm depending on whether the posterior canal wall is present or absent). The PORP® is then placed into position (Fig. 13) and the triangular head rotated to achieve maximal contact against the tympanic membrane. After inspection for a round window reflex, Gelfoam® packing may be used for stability

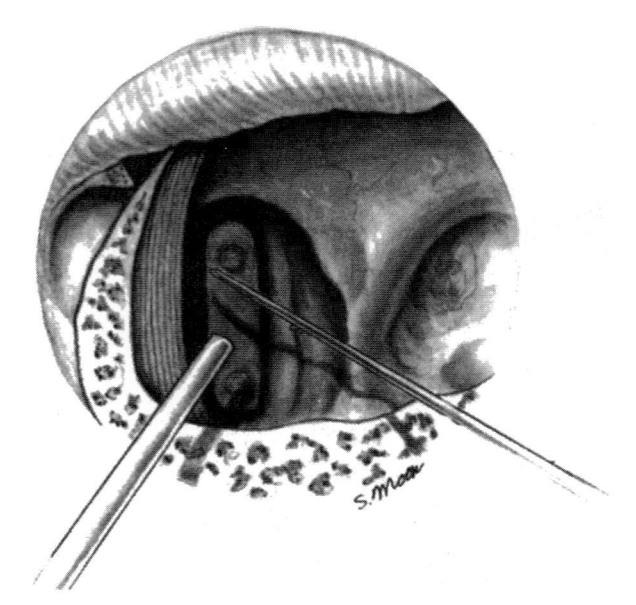

FIG. 8. Measuring for Goldenberg incus-stapes prosthesis (incus and stapes superstructure missing). From Goldenberg RA (32) with permission.

of the prosthesis, particularly in cases in which the posterior canal wall is absent.

The fourth example of ossicular discontinuity is characterized by absence of the malleus, incus, and stapes and/or stapes superstructure. The stapes footplate or oval window graft is present, as previously described. The distance between the stapes footplate or oval window graft and the midpoint of the tympanic membrane is measured, and a total ossicular replacement prosthesis (TORP)® is trimmed to the appropriate length (average 4–7 mms) and placed into the middle ear (Fig. 14). A hydroxylapatite shoe may or may not be used on the end of the Plastipore® shaft. The shaft of the TORP® is centered in the oval window niche, and the TORP® is rotated perpendicularly to the level of the tym-

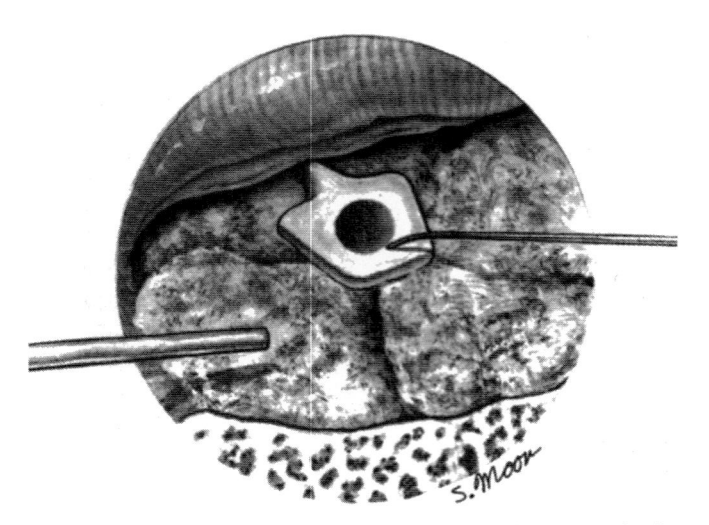

FIG. 7. Looking through cannulation with middle ear packed. From Goldenberg RA (32) with permission.

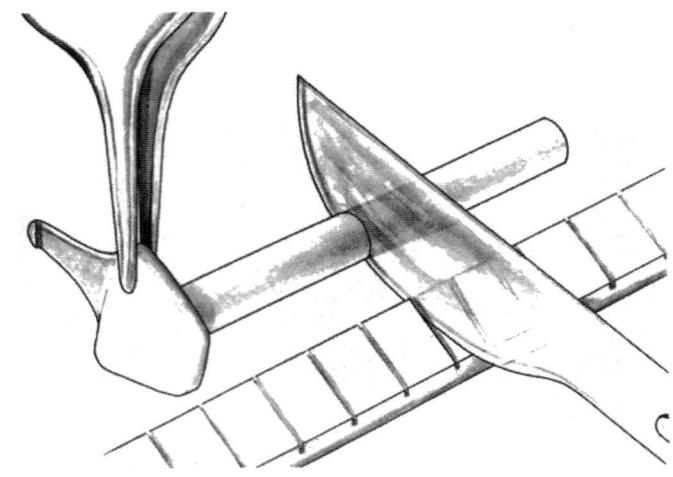

FIG. 9. Trimming incus stapes prosthesis (cut wire against metal surface). From Goldenberg RA (32) with permission.

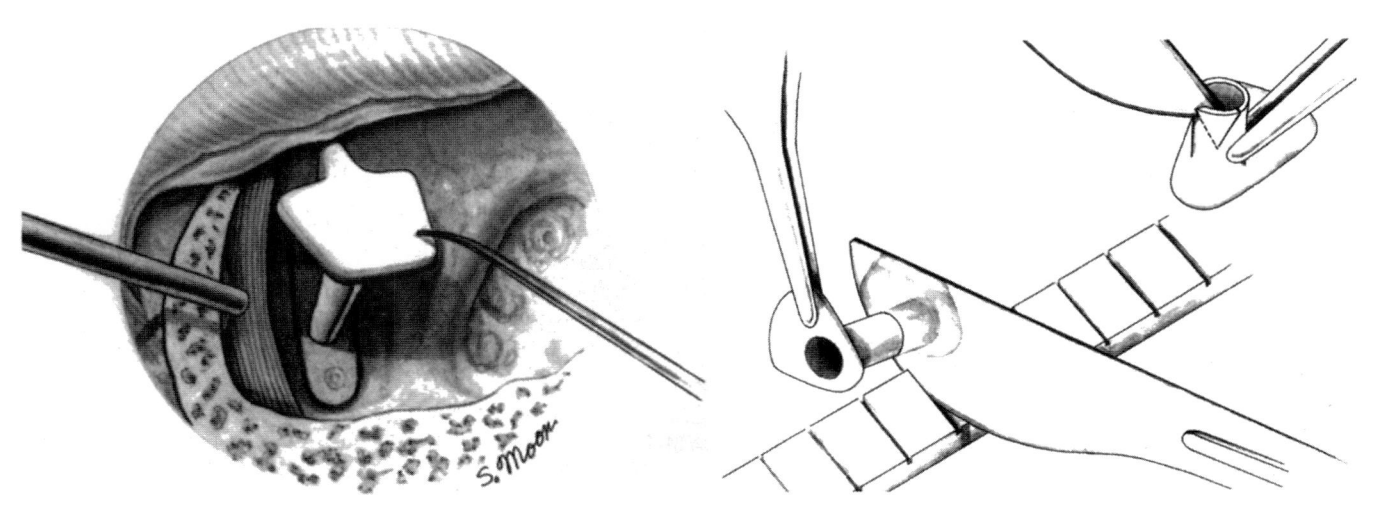

FIG. 10. Placing incus stapes prosthesis with hook under malleus. From Goldenberg RA (32) with permission.

FIG. 12. Trimming and notching shaft of PORP. From Goldenberg RA (32) with permission.

panic membrane. The triangular head may then be rotated to achieve optimal contact with the undersurface of the tympanic membrane. After inspection for a round window reflex, the middle ear may or may not be packed with Gelfoam®, and the tympanic membrane graft is replaced in its normal position.

In certain cases, initial assessment of the middle ear will demonstrate that the long process of the malleus is extremely anterior. Using the incus or incus stapes prosthesis previously described will result in instability of the prosthesis and/or loss of direct downward motion on the capitulum of the stapes, thus reducing the vibratory energy required for optimal hearing results. In these cases, a PORP® or TORP® may be used. The triangular-shaped head demonstrated in this chapter allows the prosthesis to be positioned so that one side of the head lies directly against the posterior portion of the malleus handle for increased stability and maximal surface contact with the tympanic membrane (Figs. 15, 16).

In some cases of ossicular discontinuity, incus erosion is minimal and only the lenticular process of the incus is missing. In these cases, the Applebaum (20) hydroxylapatite prosthesis can be used to reconstruct the attachment between the long process of the incus and the capitulum of the stapes (Fig. 17).

The techniques described in this section are used in a planned second-stage procedure and/or when the tympanic membrane is intact. If the tympanic membrane must be reconstructed at the same time as the ossicles are reconstructed, graft material should be placed prior to insertion of the prosthesis in most cases. In certain cases, the graft

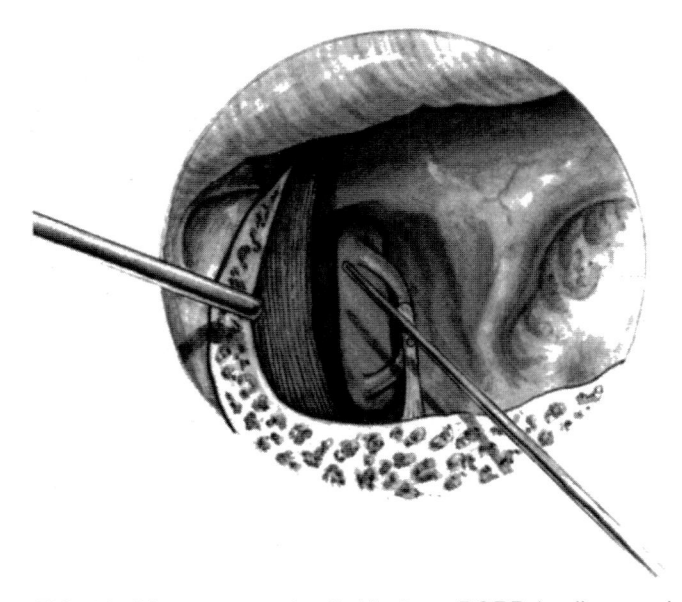

FIG. 11. Measurement for Goldenberg PORP (malleus and incus missing). From Goldenberg RA (32) with permission.

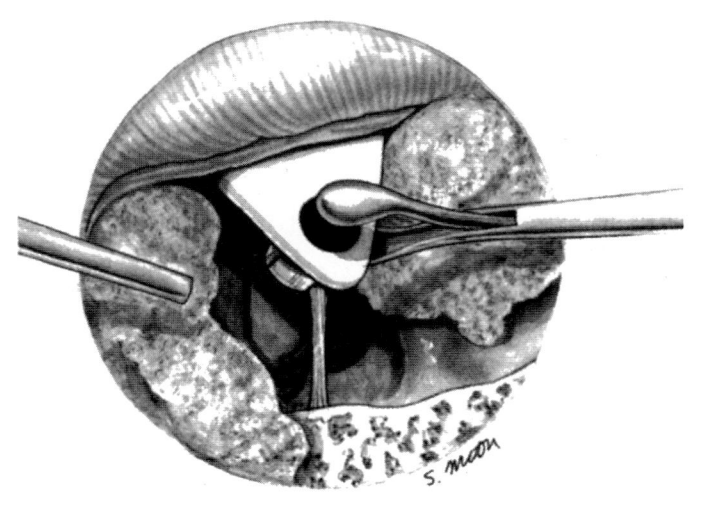

FIG. 13. Placing PORP with larger portion of head anteriorly. From Goldenberg RA (32) with permission.

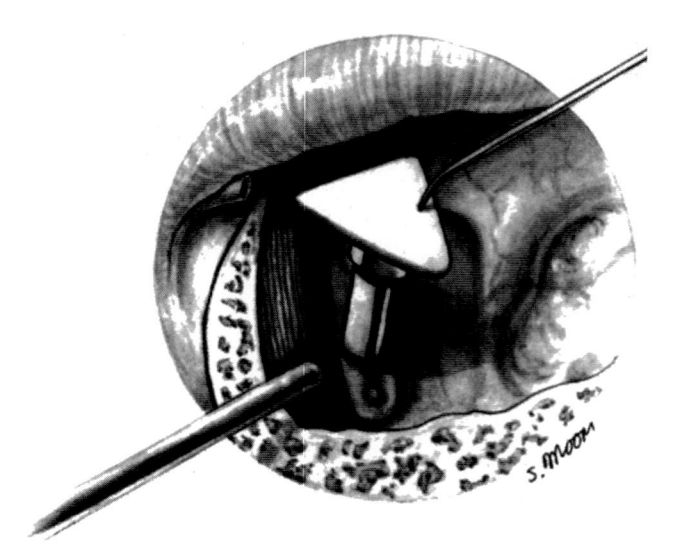

FIG. 14. Placing Goldenberg TORP with larger portion of head anteriorly (malleus, incus, and stapes superstructure missing). From Goldenberg RA (32) with permission.

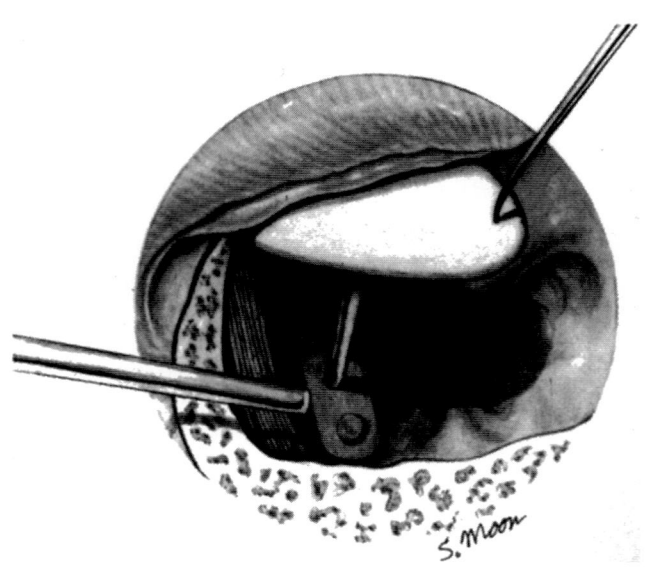

FIG. 16. Placing Goldenberg TORP, head posterior to anteriorly rotated malleus. From Goldenberg RA (32) with permission.

may be placed on top of the prosthesis, which is already in position.

This particular implant system has the advantage of having a hydroxylapatite head, which may be placed directly against the tympanic membrane or tympanic membrane graft without the need for cartilage interposition. Cartilage can be used to reinforce the tympanic membrane or to reconstruct the posterior canal wall as dictated by the pathologic condition, but it is not necessary to prevent extrusion of the prosthesis. The extrusion rate for this particular prosthesis is approximately 5% (16). The Plastipore® shaft of this implant system can be easily trimmed to the appropriate length, which precludes the need for using a drill to shape the prosthesis.

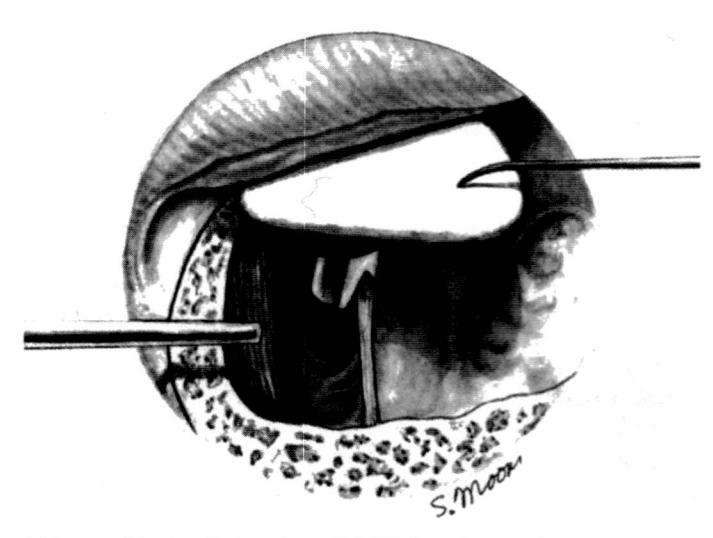

FIG. 15. Placing Goldenberg PORP, head posterior to anteriorly rotated malleus. From Goldenberg RA (32) with permission.

Ossicular Fixation

Immobility of an intact ossicular chain can be caused by fixation of the malleus head to the surrounding bone of the epitympanum. This may be due to tympanosclerosis, bony fixation, or a congenital defect. Diagnosis is made when palpation of the malleus and/or incus demonstrates immobility, and palpation of the stapes reveals good mobility. This may be demonstrated before disarticulation of the incudostapedial joint, because the mobility of the stapes increases after disarticulation and should be readily and easily observed. The presence of a round window reflex confirms stapes mobility. After separation of the incudostapedial joint, the incus can be delivered from the epitympanum with a right-angle hook. The malleus is divided just superior to the short process; and care must be taken not to tear the tympanic membrane by overmanipulation of the malleus. Ossicular reconstruction can then be accomplished by using an incus prosthesis in the manner previously described.

Fixation of the stapes most commonly occurs wtih otosclerosis, congenital abnormalities, and/or tympanosclerosis. Hearing restoration can be achieved by stapes mobilization, stapedectomy, or stapedotomy. These procedures are described in another chapter, but several key points are discussed here.

A wire prosthesis should not be used to replace a stapes fixed by chronic otitis media. One of the other non-wire implants should be selected. When tympanosclerosis causes fixation, the stapes should be isolated by removing the plaque of tympanosclerosis that surrounds it. This can readily be accomplished by use of a surgical laser in a more atraumatic fashion than can removal with a microdrill or mechanical techniques. After the stapes has been isolated, the mobility should be determined. If a round window reflex

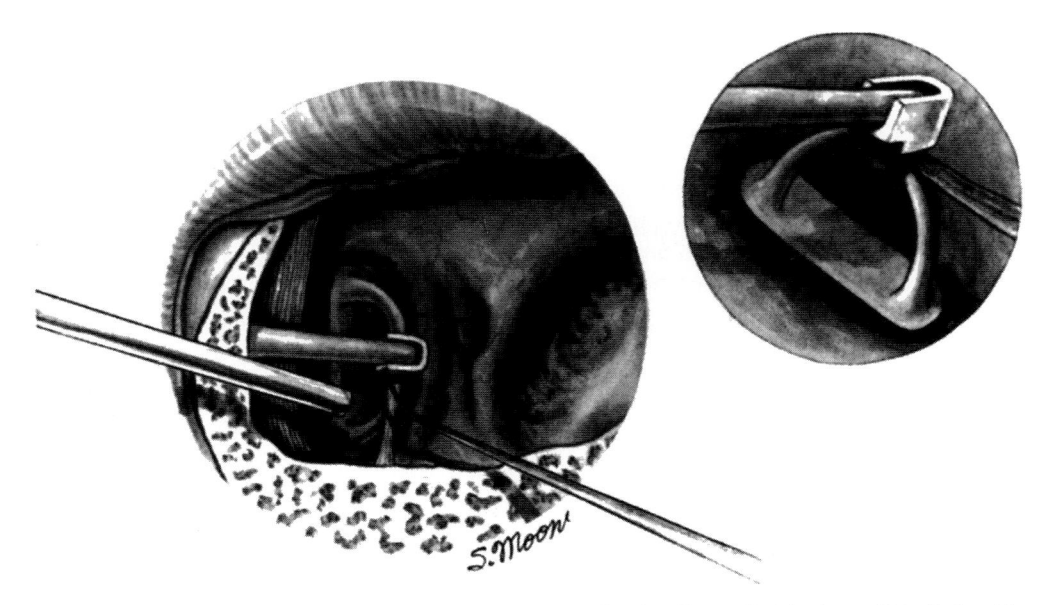

FIG. 17. Placing Applebaum incudostapedial joint prosthesis. From Goldenberg RA (32) with permission.

is noted, the procedure can be terminated and postoperative hearing evaluated. If the hearing does not improve, or if the stapes refixes after an initial period of improved hearing, a secondary stapedectomy or stapedotomy can be performed.

In cases of congenital fixation of the stapes, the procedure should be performed with caution by initially making a very small control hole in the footplate of the stapes to diagnosis a "gusher." Although there is a very high incidence of severe or total sensorineural deafness in these cases, this incidence can be greatly reduced by packing the control hole with tissue immediately if a "gusher" is found. With congenital fixation of the stapes, simple mobilization may be successful, thus eliminating the need for a stapedectomy or stapedotomy. If postoperative hearing does not improve or hearing drops subsequent to initial improvement, a secondary stapedectomy or stapedotomy may be performed. When the incus is shortened or malformed along with a congenital anomaly of the stapes, the use of an incus replacement prosthesis (IRP) or incus-stapes prosthesis (rather than the regular stapes prosthesis) should be considered (19).

Dislocation of the ossicles occurs in cases of trauma—either head trauma from a concussion or basilar skull fracture or direct surgical trauma from a previous procedure. In every case, cochlear reserve must be fully assessed preoperatively. If there is a minimal fracture or dislocation of the incudostapedial joint, the incudostapedial joint prosthesis, as previously described (20), may be used. If the dislocation is more extensive, the incus can be totally removed and an incus prosthesis used. Attempts at repositioning the incus into its normal anatomic position usually result in unsatisfactory hearing improvement. If the stapes superstructure has been fractured or dislocated, a wire prosthesis from the stapes footplate to the incus or malleus usually gives the best results. If both the stapes superstructure and incus have been dislocated, an incus-stapes prosthesis, as previously described, can be used.

Absence of Stapes and/or Oval Window

In cases of congenital absence of the stapes and/or oval window, a preoperative radiographic evaluation can often show normal inner ear anatomy. The audiogram usually shows a complete air–bone gap with excellent cochlear function. The facial nerve may lie in a variety of abnormal positions. Sterkers and Sterkers (21) have reported successful hearing results by performing a vestibulotomy and reconstructing the ossicular chain. Lambert (22) has noted that if hearing improves, it tends to diminish over time; he recommends a much more conservative approach. Briggs and Luxford (10) recommend the use of a hearing aid until the patient is older and can participate in an informed decision regarding surgical intervention. Because results of hearing improvement from surgery involving this condition are not encouraging, it seems as if use of a hearing aid is more prudent at this time.

Staging

The concept of a planned second-stage procedure for ossicular reconstruction, primarily utilized in cases involving chronic otitis media with or without cholesteatoma, has been well established over the years. Brackmann (6) has described a much higher incidence of residual cholesteatoma in children and suggests that nearly all cases of cholesteatoma in children should be staged. Schuring et al. (23) have reported that children have more recurring cholesteatomas, greater ossicular necrosis, and poorer hearing results. For these reasons, they strongly recommend staged techniques in children. Arriaga (7) also supports the principle of performing staged procedures in children. When a staged technique is used, there is little question that the tympanic membrane graft is stable and in a fixed position, that the middle ear mucosa has reverted to a more normal condition, and that the technical aspects of ossicular reconstruction are easier to accomplish at a second stage. Although staging is always an option in performing surgery for chronic otitis media, it is highly recommended in children.

ALTERNATIVES FOR MANAGEMENT

The techniques and instrumentation for middle ear reconstruction have evolved over the past four decades. Improved illumination and optics have increased visualization of middle ear structures. The use of a surgical laser, particularly for operations involving the stapes, may reduce the incidence of inner ear trauma. It is beyond the scope of this chapter to describe the multitude of surgical techniques and biomaterials for ossicular reconstruction that have been reported. However, several of the more frequently used methods are discussed.

Cartilage has been used to reconstruct the sound-conducting mechanism. Autograft or homograft cartilage from the auricle, tragus, or septum can be shaped into an ''L'' or ''T'' configuration (24). Presculpted banked cartilage is commercially available in several designs and can be further sculpted intraoperatively as required (25).

Bone, most often an ossicle, is an excellent implant material. Wehrs (26) has described a technique for shaping a homograft incus to fit between the malleus and stapes capitulum, or another to fit between the malleus and stapes footplate. If free of disease, an autograft incus can be used at a primary procedure, stored in a tissue pocket in the patient, or stored in alcohol for use in a planned second stage.

Shea (27) was one of the first to use Plastipore® as a PORP® or TORP® to bridge an ossicular defect; Brackmann, Sheehy, and Luxford (28) reported results of the use of this material in a large series of patients. Kartush (29) has developed a total hydroxylapatite implant, and McElveen (30) has described his experience with polymaleinate ionomeric prostheses.

A final alternative for management in cases of ossicular reconstruction is to advise against surgery altogether. The use of a hearing aid often may be a quite satisfactory alternative to an invasive procedure, particularly in a multihandicapped and/or medically compromised child. Amplification also may be preferable when the social or educational benefits of improved hearing may be questionable.

CONTROVERSIAL ASPECTS OF MANAGEMENT

As with any procedure, there are several controversies regarding ossicular reconstruction in children. These relate to patient selection, technical considerations, and even who should perform surgery.

Patient Selection

What degree of hearing loss creates an impairment for one child and not another? In the case of a unilateral 30-dB loss, which is the better choice: operate or observe? Should the parents be allowed to make a lifetime decision for a child? These questions have different answers for different patients but obviously are important factors to consider when considering surgical intervention. Audiometric assessment of children under 5 years of age can be difficult, particularly in the multihandicapped and/or educationally compromised child. Hearing is critical to academic and social achievement, and in cases in which coexisting perceptual and/or psychomotor impairment exists, maximal hearing levels are absolutely critical to the full developmental potential of a child. Therefore, accurate and complete assessment of the child—not only from an audiometric, but also from a psychosocial viewpoint—is quite important.

Technical Considerations

The choice of technique or implant depends entirely on the surgeon performing the procedure. It is essential that each surgeon assesses his or her personal results realistically. Continual reevaluation of surgical skills, as well as newly emerging techniques, will optimize results in reconstruction of the hearing mechanism.

Who Should Perform Surgery

The decision of whether to perform otologic surgery is one that should be made after a great deal of honest introspection. Reconstruction of the hearing mechanism requires an exacting and precise technique. In an era of changing healthcare delivery systems, increasing emphasis on primary care, decreasing emphasis on the specialist, decreasing numbers of otologic cases, and increasing difficulty in providing surgical experience during residency training, there is understandably much confusion about the best answer to this question. Knowing one's own limitations—because of either technique or pathology—is often more important than knowing what is expected. Each surgeon must make this choice individually and personally.

COMPLICATIONS

The most significant and common pitfall in ossicular reconstruction results when the expected closure of the air–bone gap is not obtained. This can be quite frustrating, particularly when the technical aspects of the case did not present any particular problem. As discussed previously, hearing results tend to be somewhat poorer in children as opposed to adults. In cases in which the air–bone gap does not close as expected, there are three choices. These are reoperation, use of a hearing aid, and/or simple acceptance of the hearing impairment. Every situation is different and must be evaluated on an individual basis.

Extrusion and rejection of a prosthesis is an unwanted but accepted fact of middle ear reconstruction. Kessler, Potsic, and Marsh (12) reported a 13% extrusion rate in children for their series, and Silverstein, McDaniels, and Lichtenstein (31) reported a 17% extrusion rate for Plastipore® prostheses in children. This is higher than the reported results in the author's series 5% (16), which included children and adults. The extrusion of a middle ear implant, particularly when used in cases of chronic otitis media, may be caused by a true foreign body reaction and/or by the disease process itself. This is particularly true in cases of severe eustachian tube dysfunction. The higher incidence of extrusion in children may relate to the expected poor eustachian tube function in this age group.

Other complications involve worsening hearing (either conductive or neural) and total sensorineural deafness. Facial paralysis (temporary or permanent), postoperative vertigo, infection, hemorrhage, and chorda tympani nerve symptoms complete the list of possible complications.

Patient and parents should be cautioned that postoperative care and follow-up is more difficult with a younger and/or apprehensive child. Postoperative dressing changes, removal of packing from the external auditory canal, and/or topical treatment of healing skin are procedures that can become extremely difficult with children. Rarely, general anesthesia is required for routine postoperative care. Usually, however, the amount of postoperative pain and discomfort does not require much use of analgesics.

CASE HISTORIES

Case History One

A 7-year-old boy is referred for a left-sided hearing loss after failing a second grade screening audiogram. He is doing quite well in school, and his parents are totally unaware that a hearing loss exists. They are very concerned, however, about future school performance and grades. His audiogram confirms a 30-dB conductive hearing loss in the left ear, with a speech reception threshold (SRT) of 35 dB and a word discrimination score (WDS) of 100%. Hearing in his right ear is perfect. The physical examination is normal, except for the left external auditory canal, which is noticeably smaller than the right. A CT scan demonstrates normal middle and inner ear structures.

A surgical procedure was recommended. Because of the small external auditory canal, the middle ear was approached through a postauricular incision. Inspection of the middle ear revealed all ossicles to be present, but there was an overall stiffness of the ossicular chain. A round window reflex was questionable. The stapes appeared mobile prior to division of the incudostapedial joint; after disarticulation, the stapes was very mobile and an excellent round window reflex was observed. The malleus and incus moved poorly with direct palpation, leading to an intraoperative diagnosis of a fixed malleus. Attempted delivery of the incus with a right-angle hook was impossible and resulted in a slight tear of the tympanic membrane just anterior to the short process of the malleus. Because the incus could not be delivered, the neck of the malleus was divided, and a single bony mass (which represented a fused malleus head and body of the incus) was delivered from the epitympanum. Following removal of this mass, the long process of the malleus was freely mobile. A small piece of perichondrium was used to reinforce the tear in the tympanic membrane, and an incus prosthesis was positioned between the long process of the malleus and the capitulum of the stapes. An excellent round window reflex was noted on direct palpation of the malleus handle. The postoperative audiogram demonstrated a 25-dB conductive component with a 30-dB SRT and a 96% WDS.

The child did not volunteer that the hearing had improved but noted that the ear did not feel quite as full as it did prior to surgery. The child has continued to do well in school; and the hearing has been stable for the past 2 years.

While this patient conformed to the accepted indications for surgical intervention, the fact that the child was doing well in school could have delayed surgery into the future. Pressure from parents who want their child to be as normal as possible should not be a factor in determining proper surgical indications. The potential for a surgical misadventure should lead the surgeon down a more conservative road. Was this procedure a failure or a success? Although this surgeon skillfully achieved excellent hearing results and avoided several major intraoperative problems, in this case it seems that the benefits did not outweigh the risks.

Case History Two

A 10-year-old girl with Down syndrome has had a history of recurrent otitis media since birth. She has had five sets of pressure equalization tubes placed and presently has a moderately severe mixed hearing loss in both ears (air average 70 dB, bone average 30 dB right; air average 55 dB, bone average 25 dB left). She has fairly good communication skills, and her parents are actively involved and motivated with respect to her education and development. She has a large perforation of the right tympanic membrane with obvious cholesteatoma, mucosal disease, and severe otorrhea. The left tympanic membrane is intact but quite atelectatic; there is a small amount of middle ear fluid present but no obvious cholesteatoma. The parents have noticed a definite decrease in communication skills during the past year. Otorrhea of the right ear is worse than the left but can be intermittently cleared with topical and systemic antibiotic treatment. This has been required on a much more frequent basis in the past year.

Surgery for the right (poorer) ear was recommended because of the obvious cholesteatoma and perforation, the persistent and worsening otorrhea, the degree of hearing loss, and the increasing difficulty in communication skills. Although amplification may also be required, the presence of active otorrhea could cause a potential problem for the use of a hearing aid. A postauricular approach to the middle ear was performed. Inspection of the middle ear revealed extensive damage to the middle ear mucosa. There was no long process of the incus present, and the malleus was normal. On trying to remove mucosa and cholesteatoma from the oval window, a thin footplate was partially mobilized and cracked. An intact canal wall mastoidectomy was performed to remove cholesteatoma from the mastoid portion of the temporal bone. A small fascia graft was placed onto the cracked footplate in the oval window, thick Silastic was placed into the middle ear, and a fascia graft was used to close the perforation. The 3-month postoperative audiogram demonstrated a slight drop in the cochlear reserve (air average 80 dB; bone average 40 dB).

Postoperatively the tympanic membrane appeared well healed, with no obvious fluid present. At a second-stage procedure, a postauricular approach was used to examine the middle ear and mastoid; no cholesteatoma was observed. Palpation of the oval window graft demonstrated an excellent round window reflex. An incus-stapes prosthesis with hydroxylapatite shoe was used to connect the malleus long process to the stapes footplate. The postoperative course was uneventful, and the audiogram confirmed that hearing improved to a 60-dB level despite the slight decrease in cochlear reserve. A hearing aid was recommended for the right ear. The parents report that the patient s hearing seems to be better than before the initial operation and that there has been an increase in her communication skills. Because of continued otorrhea on the left, a hearing aid cannot be used.

Despite the surgical misadventure in this case involving the cracked footplate, a two-stage procedure resulted in an improved situation for the patient. The right ear is now dry, and a hearing aid can be used satisfactorily. The left ear will be watched carefully and surgery performed only if the hearing worsens on that side. Despite the fact that a difficult pathologic condition was anticipated preoperatively, the potential benefits of the surgery far outweighed the risks and complications that could have occurred.

SUMMARY

This chapter has described the pathologic findings in four basic causes of conductive hearing loss in children: congenital, chronic otitis media, trauma, and otosclerosis. Audiometric evaluation may not be able to accurately document the conductive component and cochlear reserve until the age of 4 or 5 years. A detailed history from the parents should reveal how much of a handicap exists because of the hearing impairment. This is a critical factor in determining the need for surgical intervention. Medical imaging will demonstrate any abnormality of the inner ear that might preclude successful surgical results.

Once the degree of impairment and its effect on the individual child have been determined, the surgeon must consider his or her personal experience in ossicular reconstruction. A realistic appraisal of one's own experience is critical for successful results.

A systematic approach to middle ear reconstruction was outlined, beginning with the need for thorough assessment of the middle ear prior to any removal or rearrangement of existing anatomy. The author's techniques of dealing with ossicular discontinuity, fixation, or absence were presented. Emphasis on a two-stage approach to hearing reconstruction in children was stressed. Alternatives of technique and biomaterials were discussed, as well as some controversial aspects of management and possible complications of surgery. Two case presentations illustrated the need for deciding whether benefits outweigh risks in a planned surgical intervention.

Reconstruction of the ossicular chain resulting in improved hearing can be extremely rewarding in children whose educational, social, and language skills are still in the developmental stages. The risk of creating increased impairment, particularly in cases involving opening of the vestibule, must always be considered. With a lifetime of technologic advances ahead, each child must be evaluated with an eye to the future. Prudent judgement, along with realistic goals, will allow for successful results in the majority of surgical cases.

REFERENCES

1. Bergstrom L. Assessment and consequences of malformation of the middle ear. *Birth Defects* 1980;16:217.
2. Stewart JM, Downs MP. Congenital conductive hearing loss: the need for early identification and intervention. *Pediatrics* 1993;91:355.
3. Teunissen E, Cremers CWRJ. Surgery for congenital anomalies of the middle ear with mobile stapes. *Eur Arch Otorhinolaryngol* 1993;250:327.
4. Teunissen E, Cremers CWRJ. Surgery for congenital ankylosis with an associated congenital ossicular chain anomaly. *Int J Pediatr Otorhinolaryngol* 1991;21:217.
5. Levenson MJ, Michaels L, Parisier SC. Congenital cholesteatomas of the middle ear in children. *Otolaryngol Clinics North Am* 1989;22:941.
6. Brackmann DE. Tympanoplasty with mastoidectomy: canal wall up procedures. *Am J Otol* 1993;14:380.
7. Arriaga MA. Cholesteatoma in children. *Otolaryngol Clin North Am* 1994;27:573.
8. Cole JM. Surgery for otosclerosis in children. *Laryngoscope* 1982;92:859.
9. House WJ, Sheehy JL, Antunez JC. Stapedectomy in children. *Laryngoscope* 1980;90:1804.
10. Briggs RSJ, Luxford WM. Correction of conductive hearing loss in children. *Otolaryngol Clin North Am* 1994;27:607.
11. Smyth GDL, Patterson CC. Results of middle ear reconstruction: do patients and surgeons agree. *Am J Otol* 1985;6:276.
12. Kessler A, Potsic WP, Marsh RR. Total and partial ossicular replacement prostheses in children. *Otolaryngol Head Neck Surg* 1994;110:302.
13. Goldenberg RA. Hydroxylapatite ossicular replacement prostheses: preliminary results. *Laryngoscope* 1990;100:693.
14. Goldenberg RA. Hydroxylapatite ossicular replacement prostheses: a four year experience. *Otolaryngol Head Neck Surg* 1992;106:261.
15. Goldenberg RA. Hydroxylapatite ossicular replacement prostheses: results in 157 consecutive cases. *Laryngoscope* 1992;102:1091.
16. Goldenberg RA. Ossiculoplasty with composite prostheses: PORP and TORP. *Otolaryngol Clin North Am* 1994;27:727.

17. Poe DS, Bottrill ID. Comparison of endoscopic and surgical explorations for perilymph fistulas. *Am J Otol* 1994;15:735.
18. Austin DF. Reporting results in tympanoplasty. *Amer J Otol* 1985;6:85.
19. Sheehy JL, Powers WH. Incus replacement prosthesis in otosclerosis surgery. *Arch Otolaryngol* 1969;89:209.
20. Applebaum EL. An hydroxylapatite prosthesis for defects of the incus long process. *Laryngoscope* 1993;103:330.
21. Sterkers JH, Sterkers O. Surgical management of absence of the oval window with malposition of the facial nerve. *Adv Otorhinolaryngol* 1988;40:33.
22. Lambert PR. Congenital absence of oval window. *Laryngoscope* 1990;100:37.
23. Schuring AG, Rizer FM, Lippy WH, Schuring LT. Staging for cholesteatoma in the child, adolescent and adult. *Ann Otol Rhinol Laryngol* 1990;99:256.
24. Jansen C. Methods of ossicular reconstruction. *Otolaryngol Clin North Am* 1972;5:97.
25. Chole RA. Use of presculpted banked cartilage transplants in ossicular reconstruction. *Arch Otolaryngol* 1987;113:145.
26. Wehrs RE. Homograft ossicles in tympanoplasty. *Laryngoscope* 1982;92:540.
27. Shea JJ. Plastipore total ossicular replacement prostheses. *Laryngoscope* 1976;86:239.
28. Brackmann DE, Sheehy JL, Luxford WM. TORPs and PORPs in tympanoplasty: a review of 1042 operations. *Otolaryngol Head Neck Surg* 1984;92:32.
29. Kartush JM. Ossicular chain reconstruction. *Otolaryngol Clinics North Am* 1994;27:689.
30. McElveen JT. Ossiculoplasty with polymaleinate ionomeric prostheses. *Otolaryngol Clin North Am* 1994;27:777.
31. Silverstein H, McDaniel AB, Lichtenstein R. A comparison of PORP, TORP, and incus homograft for ossicular reconstruction in chronic ear surgery. *Laryngoscope* 1986;96:159.
32. Goldenberg RA. Hydroxylapitite prosthesis. *Otolaryngol Head Neck Surg* 1992;3:225–231.

CHAPTER 38

Reconstruction after Mastoidectomy

Juan J. Garro

Since the development of reconstructive ear surgery by Zöllner and by Wullstein in the early 1950s (1–3), there have been many attempts to reconstruct middle ears that had previously undergone various radical operations. Betow (3–5) described these early efforts. Marquet (6) reviewed much of the history of the use of homografts in tympanoplasty. Efforts at middle ear reconstructive surgery have also been described in a text (7), monographs (8–11), at symposia (12–14), in issues of *Otolaryngologic Clinics of North America* (15–17), an issue of *Acta Otorhinolaryngologica Belgica*, in a review (18), in a techniques manual (19), panel discussions (20, 21), and in journal articles (22–38).

In 1959, Betow introduced his pioneering work on homograft transplantation en bloc (3–5). Initially, he tested the procedure on rabbits. These experiments showed that healing progresses normally, as seen by visual and microscopic examination. By the 18th day after surgery, the transplanted eardrum looks smooth, transparent, and mobile. Later follow-up confirmed these findings. The transplanted eardrum is vascularized, and there are no signs of inflammation or degradation. Betow extended his work to human patients, pointing out that an advantage of using homografts is that transplant materials can be stored and used as needed.

From his experience, Betow concluded that the best healing and functional results are obtained with homograft en bloc by the anterior-posterior approach and by preparing the tympanic cavity for homograft implantation. Betow acknowledged that the results did not fully meet expectations. Use of homografts led to good functional results; however, because of the loss of middle ear muscles and ossicular ligaments, there was always a difference of at least 5 to 10 dB between bone and air conduction. In cases in which the middle ear had been completely destroyed by inflammation and in which only the stapes footplate remained, Betow added that it was very difficult to totally restore a tympanic cavity with a good mucosal covering.

The procedure described in this chapter represents extensive modifications of those of Betow and of others. The procedure combines the use of homograft eardrum and ossicles with the use of autologous cortical bone and temporalis fascia. Thus, the procedure reconstructs both the container, the surroundings of the middle ear, such as the mastoid and the external auditory canal (EAC), and the contents, the eardrum and ossicles (32).

Using this procedure to treat children and adolescents represents more than 25 years of surgical experience in reconstructing middle ears and mastoid cavities. The patients had canal wall down mastoidectomies because of chronic ear disease with or without cholesteatoma (39).

The key change distinguishing my procedure from those of Betow and others is that I disarticulate the homograft ossicular chain before transplantation. This entails the separation of the incus and the removal of the head of the malleus. These steps prevent progressive ossicular fixation after transplantation, and enable the restoration and maintenance of normal hearing. Cutting off the head of malleus prevents adhesions to the wall of the cavity. Transplantation with an intact ossicle can lead to the malleus adhering to the cavity, ossicular fixation, and loss of hearing. Thus, the outcome using disarticulated ossicles is superior to the outcome using a homograft en bloc.

Furthermore, the incus homograft can be used to ensure the continuity of the ossicular chain between the long handle of the malleus homograft and the head of the stapes in patients in whom the stapes superstructure can be preserved. Alternatively, when the stapes superstructure cannot be preserved, such as in the complete absence of the ossicular chain, the incus homograft can be reshaped and interpositioned as a columella between the malleus homograft and the stapes footplate.

Most of my early patients were adults, although I occasionally performed the procedure on children and adoles-

---

J.J. Garro: Department of Otolaryngology, Children's National Medical Center, Washington, DC 20010; and Georgetown University Hospital, Washington, DC 20007.

cents. Early efforts included the use of skin from inner portion of the patient's upper arm to replace the eardrum. The appearance of the eardrum and functional results were not satisfactory. Later use of synthetic materials to replace ossicles was also not satisfactory because these materials are easily displaced. Most are extruded and expelled by 1 year after implantation.

Similarly, my early efforts included use of cartilage to reconstruct the posterior wall. The cartilage was reabsorbed. Use of hydroxyapatite to reconstruct the mastoid cavity was unsuccessful because it resulted in formation of granulation tissue. Osteointegration of hydoxyapatite was incomplete. Fragments of hydroxyapatite were rejected and came through an ear canal fistula. Fat, muscle pedicle, and bone paté were also tried for mastoid cavity reconstruction but were reabsorbed and disappeared.

As shown in this chapter, reconstruction of middle ear, mastoid, and posterior canal after canal wall down mastoidectomy is a valid choice for children and adolescents. Normal anatomic structures and the conductive hearing mechanism are restored, and complications and risks are acceptable. Although others (34–37) have described techniques that include remodeling the incus, to the best of my knowledge this chapter represents the only description of the surgical procedures applied to the treatment of children and adolescents.

SELECTION CRITERIA

Canal wall down mastoidectomy can result in various consequences to ear structure. Sometimes the tympanic cavity is well healed, containing remnants of the eardrum and ossicles, but sometimes there are no remnants. There might be false membranes, representing the formation of fibrous bands that obscure components of the middle ear, such as the mucosa (if it still exists), the eustachian tube opening, and the oval and round windows.

These differences are primarily due to the initial diagnosis (e.g., as cholesteatoma or chronic granulating mastoiditis); previous surgery (e.g., high or low facial ridge and extent of meatoplasty, if any); recurrence of cholesteatoma; and dry or actively draining middle ear and mastoid cavity.

To be a candidate for total ear reconstruction, the child must have an affected ear that is clean and dry. The ear must show no signs of active disease, such as drainage or purulent discharge, for about 1 year before surgery. In most patients, surgical revisions had been performed to eradicate completely any signs of active disease, such as drainage or purulent discharge. In other respects, the child should be generally healthy.

The middle ear and the radical cavity are examined under the operating microscope. This enables evaluation of the condition of the middle-ear mucosa (promontory, facial recess, epitympanum, hypotympanum). Inflammation requires preoperative treatment. Small residual pearls of cholesteatoma or layers of keratinized squamous epithelium should be removed at surgery. There must be no evidence of large residual or recurrent cholesteatomas. The presence of large cholesteatomas contraindicates reconstructive ear surgery.

Examination of the middle ear reveals the condition of the eustachian tube opening and of the oval and round windows. Patency of the eustachian tube, mobility of the footplate of the stapes in the oval window, and mobility of the round window membrane are essential before one attempts middle ear reconstruction. However, eustachian tube functions are not investigated because I believe that testing methods are unreliable.

The sizes of the external auditory cavity meatus and of the mastoid cavity are assessed. This enables planning for the amount of cortical bone fragments and the size of the temporalis fascia that will be needed for mastoid and posterior wall reconstruction.

Examination of ear s structure indicates the extent of bony dehiscence over the facial nerve, lateral sinus, and dura mater. This enables precautions to avoid surgical injury.

Preoperative computed tomography of the axial and coronal views of the temporalis bones is important. This reveals the integrity of the tegmen tympani, fallopian canal, and the bony coverage of the lateral sinus. Often it is impossible to microscopically visualize abnormalities in these structures. Fibrous bands and false membranes secondary to previous surgery can obscure microscopic examination. Preoperatively, only computed tomography can reveal the abnormalities.

Audiometric examination is done to confirm a conductive type of hearing loss. Bone conduction must be normal. The child must have good hearing in the unaffected ear; in other words, the affected ear is not an "only hearing ear." Reconstructive surgery is contraindicated in an only hearing ear.

Whether the patient fully meets the criteria is not known until surgery, when complete debridement is accomplished. Then it is possible to note contraindications for continuing, such as blocked windows or eustachian tube.

SURGICAL INTERVENTION

Materials for Surgery

Various special material are used for the surgery. One is the tympanic membrane with malleus-incus (en bloc) with skin canal cuff. Homografts can be ordered en bloc, or eardrums and ossicles can be ordered separately. It is preferable that the homografts originate from the same-side (left or right) ear that is being treated.

Homografts are packed and shipped in 0.5% buffered formaldehyde solution. Before use, homografts are rinsed in sterile saline solution according to the instructions from the provider. Then the homografts are ready for use.

Eardrum homografts that are dark upon removal of buffered formaldehyde should not be used because the dark color signifies blood stasis at the moment of harvest from the cadaver. Such homografts should be discarded because they have a poor survival prognosis; they tend to necrotize.

Other special materials include processed human allograft tissue (30 cc of freeze-dried, not demineralized, cancellous chips (4 to 10 mm) rehydrated according to provider's instructions; a polymeric silicone sheet (0.010-inch thick); gauze dressings (initial size, 3 inches by 8 inches) neatly trimmed into narrow and wide strips with smooth edges; and cellulose sponges (photographer sponge) sterilized by autoclavingand cut into small square pieces as necessary for packing.

Surgical Procedure

The surgical procedure for reconstructing the middle ear, posterior bony canal, and mastoid cavity after a canal wall down mastoidectomy has three main steps: preparing the middle ear and the mastoid cavity; preparing and transplanting the homograft, and reconstructing the posterior ear canal and the mastoid cavity.

As long as standard presurgical procedures are followed, surgery can be performed on the same day as the patient's admission. Initially, the procedure took 6 hours, but with experience it takes 3 hours. After surgery the child is kept overnight and then discharged the next day. Postoperatively, the child hears normally in the reconstructed ear.

Preparing the Middle Ear and the Mastoid Cavity

Preparing the middle ear and the mastoid cavity must be performed with great care and deliberation. Because of disease and previous surgery, familiar landmarks are distorted or missing. Patients have often had previous surgery performed by other surgeons, adding to the lack of familiarity. Therefore, considerable effort must be made to understand the anatomic orientation. This reduces the risk of inadvertent damage to the facial nerve. In most cases, the facial nerve is exposed because of dehiscence of the fallopian canal secondary to chronic ear disease. The tegmen tympany might be absent, causing the risk of opening the dura and leakage of spinal fluid, resulting in meningitis. Another risk is entering the lateral sinus, causing massive hemorrhage.

The patient is placed on the operating table in the supine position and prepared and draped in the usual way. General endotracheal anesthesia is induced. Lidocaine (1%) with 1:100,000 parts of epinephrine is injected into the postauricular crease.

The middle ear and the mastoid cavity are examined under the operating microscope to assess their status and the extent of damage from disease or previous surgery. This provides an idea of how much temporalis fascia and cortical bone need to be harvested.

A postauricular incision is made sharply and deepened with the electrocautery. From the mastoid tip up to the temporalis line, the incision is carried down to bone. Then, superior to the temporalis line, the incision is carried down to the temporalis fascia. A periosteal elevator is used to reflect the pinna forward. The scalp is undermined, overlying the temporalis fascia.

Chips of cortical bone are harvested from the remaining cortex of the mastoid bone by use of a light mallet and a curved osteotome. It is particularly important to use a curved osteotome for this purpose. Use of a straight osteotome entails the hazard of penetrating the dura. Furthermore, care must be taken in removing cortical bone to obtain large bone chips with curvature that will be suitable for the reconstruction of the bony ear canal. If necessary, cortical bone can also be harvested from the bone of the mastoid cortex of the other ear. If bone chips are used within in a few minutes, they can be stored dry in a sterile cup; otherwise, they are submerged in sterile saline until use.

A 4 cm by 4 cm square piece of temporalis fascia is harvested, pressed, and set aside to dry. The skin of the anterior bony canal is reflected forward the mastoid cavity is revised. This includes removal of any residual cholesteatomas. A diamond burr is used to saucerize the mastoid cavity, removing all traces of the mucosa, epithelial debris, and granulation tissue.

Preparing and Transplanting the Homograft

Reconstruction of the ossicular chain is completed before mastoid reconstruction to enable easier accessibility to the middle ear during reconstruction of the ossicular chain.

The rinsed homograft (Fig. 1A) is prepared for transplant. When one handles the eardrum, care must be taken not to perforate it.

The incus is disarticulated from the malleus (Fig. 1B) and set aside. By use of a malleus nipper instrument, the malleus is transected at its neck (Fig. 1C, D), and the malleus head is removed and discarded. These are key steps characteristic to this technique.

Blood clots, if present, are suctioned. Clots have to be resolved because plasma diffusion is impaired in the inserted homograft (8). Just before the eardrum homograft is inserted, a 0.010-inch thick polymeric silicone sheet is often inserted in the middle ear cavity to prevent adhesions in the middle ear. Adhesions are particularly of concern when disease has compromised the middle-ear mucosa. This necessitates the removal of the mucosa on reconstructive surgery, leaving the promontory bone bare.

The eardrum homograft is transplanted with a small skin cuff anteriorly and a long one posteriorly. By use of Bellucci scissors, radial incisions are made in the skin cuff (Fig. 1E, F) to facilitate positioning the eardrum homograft. Then the eardrum homograft is positioned in the sulcus tympanicum, if it still exists. If the sulcus tympanicum no longer exits, the eardrum homograft is positioned in the bony surface of the ear canal.

The annulus fibrosis fits into the groove of the sulcus tympanicum. The anterior skin cuff of the eardrum homograft should be in contact with the anterior bony canal. The posterior skin cuff of the eardrum homograft should be in contact with temporalis fascia used in the reconstruction of the poste-

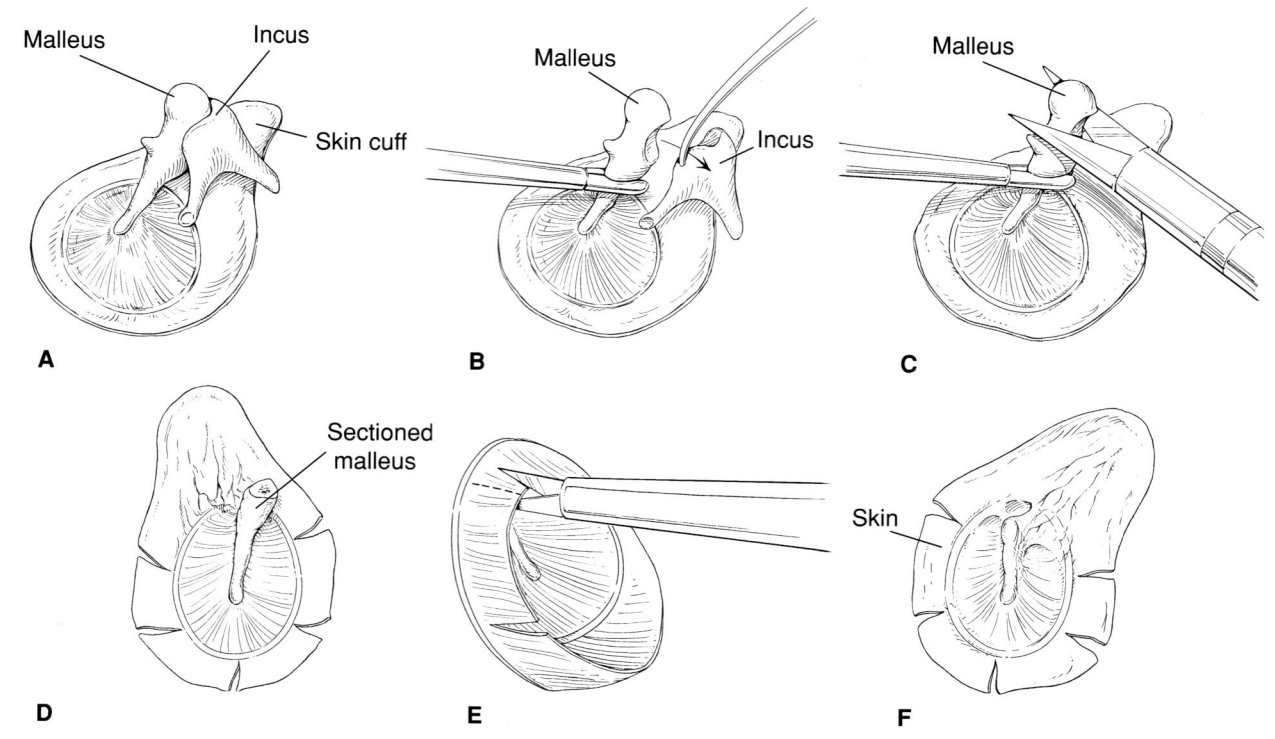

FIG. 1. A: Appearance of eardrum-malleus-incus homograft before remodeling; **B:** as the incus is disarticulated; **C:** after the head of the malleus is being removed; **D, E, F:** after incisions are made around the cuff.

rior bony canal, which will favor rapid vascularization of the posterior aspect of the eardrum homograft (Fig. 2).

The incus homograft is reshaped with a diamond burr to a size that fits the gap from the stapes footplate (or superstructure, if present) to the underside of the malleus manubrium (Fig. 3). The reshaped incus is diminished by drilling its surface to at least one third its original size. Then the incus homograft is fitted into position between the head (or footplate) of the stapes and the remnant of the malleus homograft (see Fig. 7A, 7B on page 569).

Reconstructing the Posterior Ear Canal and the Mastoid Cavity

The temporalis fascia is inserted on the epitympanic area, facial ridge, and mastoid cavity as a basket to receive the

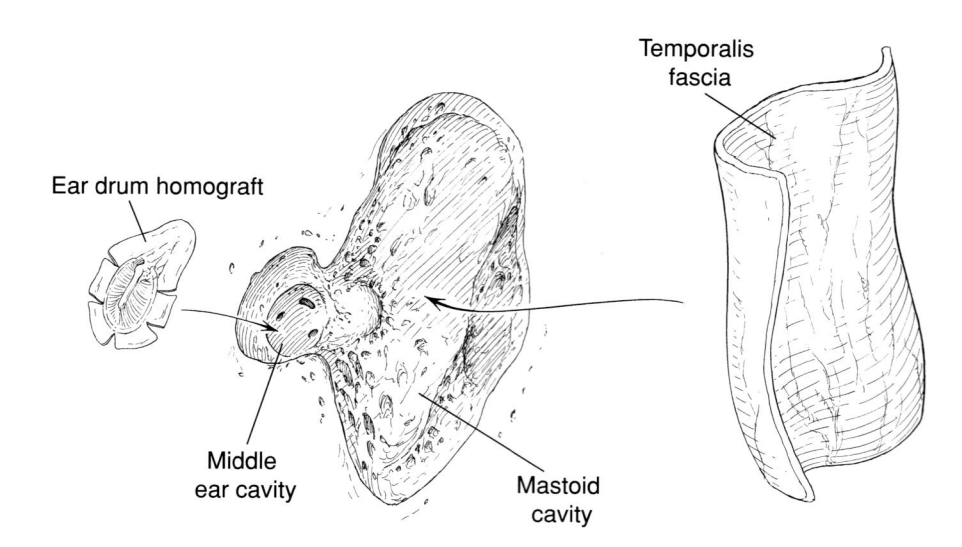

FIG. 2. Exploded view of the alignment of the eardrum/malleus homograft and of the temporalis fascia.

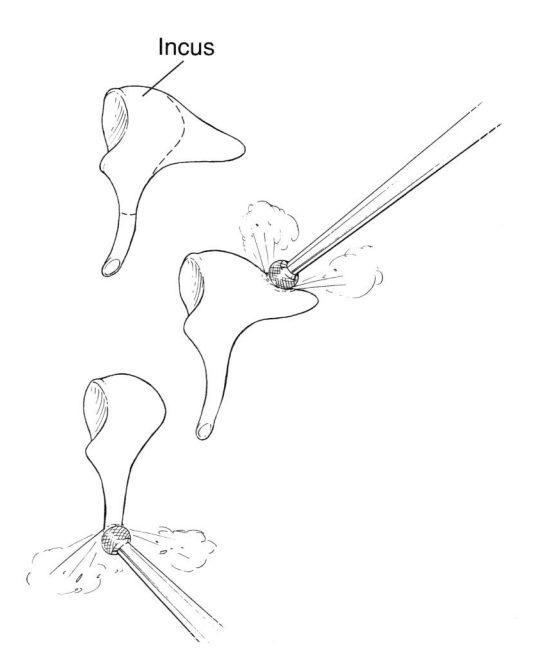

FIG. 3. Remodeling of the incus homograft in preparation for transplantation.

curved fragments of cortical bone. The temporalis fascia should be in contact with the posterior superior aspect of the homograft eardrum to facilitate the eardrum's rapid vascularization (Fig. 4). Then the harvested bone chips are layered to form the reconstructed bony portion of the posterior-superior EAC (Fig. 5A). The mastoid cavity is filled with cortical bone, and if necessary, with freeze-dried cancellous bone chips (Fig. 5B).

The temporalis fascia is reflected over the bony fragments used to reconstruct the mastoid (Fig. 5C). Thus, the mastoid cavity is reconstructed with bony fragments covered by harvested temporalis fascia. The temporalis fascia is also used to seal the middle ear. The covering with temporalis fascia inhibits the migration of skin into the mastoid cavity and eliminates the possibility of growth of a cholesteatoma.

The reconstructed EAC and eardrum can now be observed (Fig. 6). The skin of the anterior bony canal, which had been reflected outward, is put back in place, overlapping the skin cuff of the eardrum homograft. Continuity, stability, and mobility of eardrum and ossicles are checked by touching with a straight pick. The eardrum and ossicles should remain undisplaced.

Packing is important because it helps secure the homograft in position. Gauze dressing is preferred because is does not adhere to tissue. The gauze (initial size, 3 inches by 8 inches) is neatly trimmed into narrow strips for internal packing of the EAC and into wide strips for external packing of the EAC. Care is taken to leave smooth edges. Ragged edges can attach to the wound and cause inflammation and production of granulation tissue, thus making it difficult to remove the packing.

Before the postauricular incision is closed, rosebud packing with a gauze dressing is placed in the EAC. The narrow strips for inner packing are placed in such a way as to form a basket for cotton balls that are treated with antibiotic ointment. The packing also helps secure the homograft.

Some investigators recommend placing a sponge saturated with nutrients in the middle ear or also placing a piece of temporalis fascia over the surface of the eardrum homograft. For example, Wullstein and Wullstein (1) described the use of gelatin sponge saturated with a nutrient solution to facilitate the early nutrition of the eardrum homograft. Use a commercially available, absorbable gelatin sponge soaked with Ringer's lactate for this purpose.

After the postauricular incision is closed, the outer part of the EAC is lined with the wide gauze strips and then with cellulose sponge. Use of this procedure helps prevent stenosis of the EAC.

Postoperative Course and Care

After surgery, the patient (and the patient's parents or guardian) are cautioned about not getting the ear wet. The patient is checked every 3 days until the packing is removed.

Two weeks after surgery, with the patient's ear under the microscope, the external and internal packings are removed. Children are uncomfortable during this procedure, so it is often necessary to remove the packing in the operating room while the child is under mild general anesthesia. Care is taken not to disturb the canal and eardrum, which are healing. Intense vascularization of the temporalis fascia and of the newly reconstructed posterior wall and early vascularization of the eardrum are observable. Even if there is a clot behind the homograft eardrum, the ear canal and the homograft are not suctioned to avoid disturbing healing. Healing is uneventful and takes about 3 months.

Skin is obtained from the inner portion of the upper arm and grafted to the temporal fascia on the reconstructed poste-

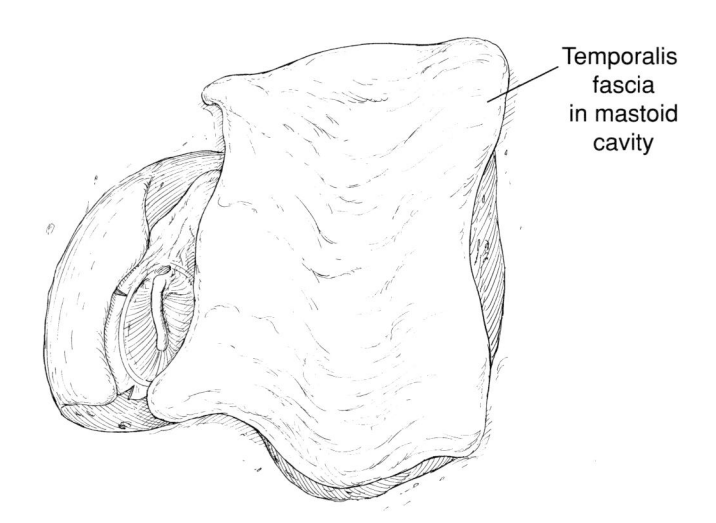

FIG. 4. Temporalis fascia placed on surface of facial ridge and mastoid cavity.

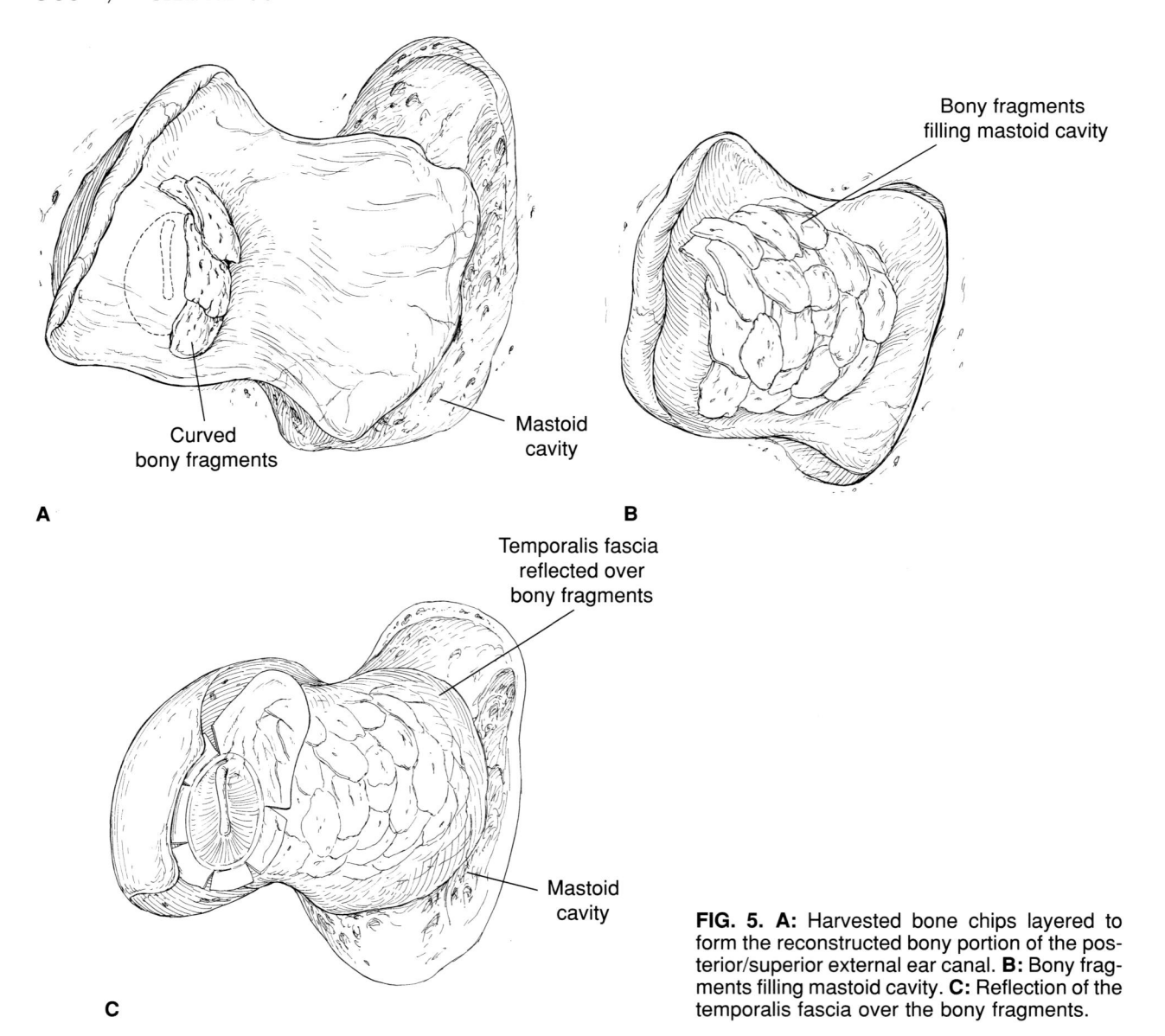

FIG. 5. A: Harvested bone chips layered to form the reconstructed bony portion of the posterior/superior external ear canal. **B:** Bony fragments filling mastoid cavity. **C:** Reflection of the temporalis fascia over the bony fragments.

rior wall. The graft is covered with a piece of gauze dressing, which is left in place for 3 weeks before removal. A skin graft facilitates epithelial regrowth and healing of the reconstructed posterior ear canal wall. It also prevents formation of granulation tissue, retraction of the temporalis fascia, infection, and, often, stenosis of the canal. All children described in this chapter received a skin graft, except for one child who had congenital middle ear deformity. This patient received a skin graft in the newly created bony canal.

Many changes occur in the homograft eardrum and ossicles after they are transplanted. During the first 6 days after transplantation, plasma diffusion from the middle ear nourishes the eardrum. The eardrum vascular channels that had been preserved by buffered formaldehyde become revascularized by capillaries from the bony canal.

When the packing is removed 2 weeks after surgery, plasma is observed covering the eardrum. The plasma is left unsuctioned or otherwise undisturbed because it provides nutrients for the homograft eardrum. The eardrum is substantially revascularized by 3 weeks postoperatively and fully revascularized by 1 to 2 months postoperatively. The posterior canal wall should display epithelial regrowth by 3 weeks postoperatively. The transplanted ossicles are covered by mucosal membrane, and dead bone is gradually replaced by living bone.

The autograft temporalis fascia and cortical bone used in the posterior canal wall and mastoid reconstruction experience changes in ways similar to those in the homograft eardrum and ossicles. The fragments of cortical bone ossify in time. Trabeculae appear with spaces between and enable ventilation of the reconstructed mastoid cavity.

Frequent follow-up is important to detect and manage early complications such as infection, formation of granulation tissue, stenosis of the canal, and necrosis of the eardrum

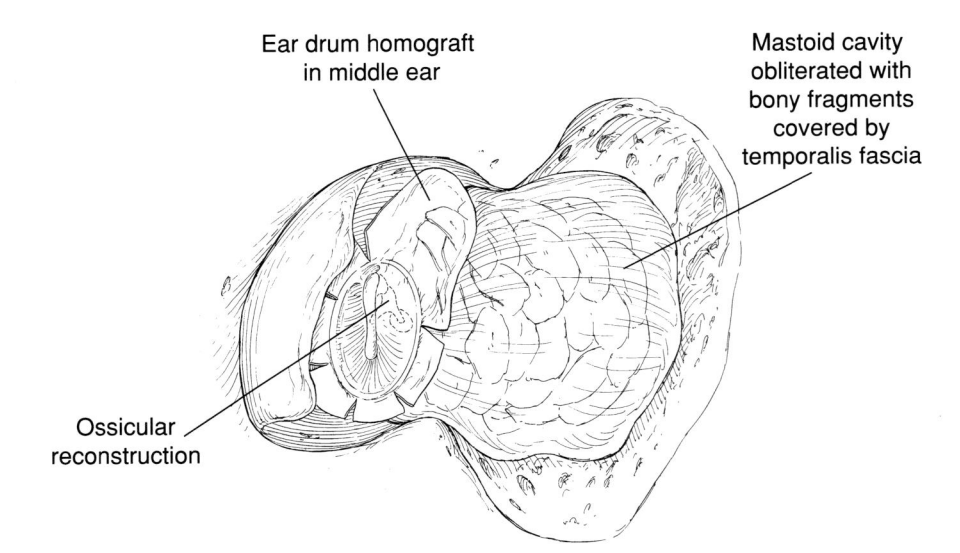

FIG. 6. Appearance of reconstructed EAC and eardrum.

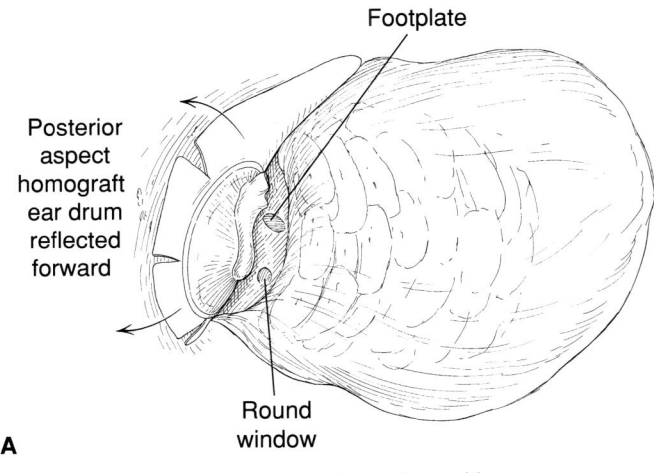

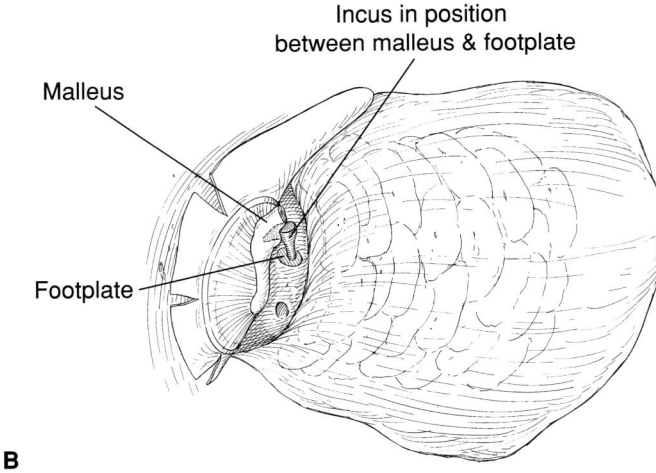

FIG. 7. Appearance of totally reconstructed open mastoid cavity.

homograft. Patients are seen every 3 days for the first 15 days, After the packing is removed at 15 days, patients are seen weekly for 1 month, every 2 weeks for 2 months, and then once every 6 months.

OUTCOME

Table 1 summarizes the surgeries of 18 children and adolescents who underwent reconstruction of the middle ear, mastoid, and EAC. These patients included 14 boys and 4 girls, ranging in age from 4 to 18 years. Except as noted, all had cholesteatomas in the middle ear and in the mastoid, had mastoiditis, and had undergone canal wall down radical mastoidectomy before reconstructive surgery. One patient had congenital middle ear disease. I performed these procedures on other children with similar medical histories, but they have been lost to follow-up, and therefore are not included here.

Eleven patients had the incus homograft interpositioned between the malleus manubrium and the stapes footplate, and six had the incus interpositioned between the malleus and the stapes head. One patient had the incus interpositioned between the malleus manubrium and a vein graft in the oval window.

All patients have been followed up for at least 1 year; one patient has been followed for 20 years. Audiometric results showed marked improvement ($+20$ or -20 speech reception threshold) in 11 patients, and moderate improvement ($+35$ or -35 speech reception threshold) in six patients. One patient had no improvement, probably because of stapes fixation noted during surgery.

COMPLICATIONS

Most complications (see Table 1) have been related to homograft survival, ossicular discontinuity, recurrence of

TABLE 1. *Results of reconstructive surgery in children and adolescents[a]*

Patient (date of first surgery)	Special features of first surgery	Complications of first surgery[b]	Subsequent procedure(s)	Audiometric results SRT	Audiometric results Gain dB	Length of follow-up (yr)
9-yr-old boy (1971)	Incus interposition to stapes footplate; use of temporalis muscle pedicle for mastoid cavity reconstruction	Reabsorption of muscle from mastoid; recurrent cholesteatoma in mastoid; small perforation in eardrum; open mastoid cavity	1982—revision mastoidectomy; removal of cholesteatoma 1991—tympanoplasty of eardrum homograft; reconstruction of posterior wall and mastoid cavity	15	15	20
6-yr-old boy (1985)	Incus interposition to stapes footplate	Ossicular discontinuity due to separation of incus homograft from footplate; eardrum elevated; large separation between eardrum and footplate (unable to find bone long enough to fill gap)	1993—exploratory tympanotomy; incus replacement with artificial prosthesis	20	25	9
9-yr-old boy (1989)	Incus interposition to stapes head	Ossicular discontinuity due to separation of incus homograft from head of stapes caused by multiple adhesions; ossicular discontinuity due to separation of incus homograft from head of stapes	1991—exploratory tympanotomy; repositioning of incus; insertion of polymeric silicone sheet 1992—exploratory tympanotomy; incus left attached to eardrum; gap between incus and stapes head filled by insertion of head of a malleus homograft	15	30	6
5-yr-old boy (1990)	Incus interposition to stapes head	Small recurrent cholesteatoma in middle ear	1991—exploratory tympanotomy and removal of cholesteatoma	15	50	5
16-yr-old boy (1992)	Incus interposition to stapes footplate; use of hydroxyapatite in posterior wall and mastoid reconstruction	Recurrent cholesteatoma in middle ear	1993—removal of cholesteatoma; removal of hydroxyapatite; tympanoplasty of eardrum homograft	20	20	3
12-yr-old boy (1992)	Incus interposition to stapes footplate	None	None	35	25	3
17-yr-old boy (1992)[c]	Retention of patient's eardrum; incus interposition to stapes footplate	None	None	15	60	3
11-yr-old girl (1992)	Incus interposition to stapes footplate	Total reabsorption of eardrum	1993—eardrum-malleus homograft replacement	35	10	3
12-yr-old girl (1992)	Incus interposition to stapes head	Stapes fixation noted during first surgery; ossicular discontinuity due to separation of incus homograft from vein graft covering oval window; adhesions of incus	1993—exploratory tympanotomy; stapedectomy; vein graft from dorsum of hand to cover oval window; remodeling of existing incus homograft and repositioning between malleus manubrium and vein graft covering oval window 1993—exploratory tympanotomy; incus replacement	10	20	6

TABLE 1. Continued

Patient (date of first surgery)	Special features of first surgery	Complications of first surgery[b]	Subsequent procedure(s)	Audiometric results SRT	Audiometric results Gain dB	Length of follow-up (yr)
18-yr-old female (1992)	Incus interposition to stapes footplate	Extrusion of incus homograft	Repair planned	[d]		3
9-yr-old boy (1992)[e]	Incus interposition to stapes head	None	None	15	25	6
13-yr-old boy (1993)	Incus interposition to stapes head	None	None	20	35	5
16-yr-old boy (1992)	Incus interposition to stapes footplate	None	None	14	40	3
13-yr-old boy (1993)	Incus interposition to stapes footplate	None	None	20	25	2
10-yr-old boy (1993)	Incus interposition to stapes footplate	Stapes fixation noted during surgery	None	45	None	2
10-yr-old boy (1993)	Incus interposition to stapes head	None	None	15	50	3
9-yr-old female (1994)[f]	Incus interposition to stapes head; canalplasty; did not have skin graft; no mastoidectomy	None	None	30	25	1
13-yr-old boy (1994)	Incus interposition to stapes footplate	None	None	35	30	1

dB, decibels; SRT, speech reception threshold.
[a] Except as noted, all patients initially had cholesteatoma in the middle ear and in the mastoid, had mastoiditis, and had undergone radical mastoidectomy before reconstructive surgery.
[b] All complications were resolved surgically, except for one 10-yr-old boy (1993) who was not operated on again, and one 17-yr-old boy (1992) for whom surgery was planned.
[c] Patient had cholesteatoma in the middle ear (but not in the mastoid), had mastoiditis, and had undergone radical mastoidectomy before reconstructive surgery.
[d] Audiometric results pending outcome of planned surgery.
[e] Patient had cholesterol granuloma in the middle ear and in the mastoid, had mastoiditis, and had undergone radical mastoidectomy before reconstructive surgery.
[f] Patient had atretic plate ossicle deformation, atrophy of the lenticular process, but less than total stenosis of the EAC before reconstructive surgery.

cholesteatoma, and surgical technique resulting in insufficiently close contact of the homograft eardrum skin cuff with the reconstructed bony canal. Postoperative scarring can cause ossicular discontinuity. Occasionally, eardrum retraction occurs, with apparently poor function of the eustachian tube. In one patient, the incus homograft completely extruded and hearing diminished. Tympanoplasty and reconstruction are planned. Retraction also occurred in a child who was lost to follow-up and is therefore not included in Table 1. My impression is that children have fewer complications and better acceptance of the homografts than do adults.

CASE HISTORIES

Case History 1

A 5-year-old boy who had visited my office in 1990 had a long history of recurrent ear infections. At age 3, he had undergone bilateral myringotomies, and tympanostomy tubes had been inserted. After the tubes were removed a year later, he experienced continual, purulent, foul-smelling discharge from his right ear. Audio metric examination showed severe hearing impairment in the right ear (Fig. 8A).

Microscopic examination revealed a white discoloration of the right eardrum, and a perforation of the attic through which a large aural polyp emerged. Audiometric studies revealed severe conductive hearing loss with a speech reception threshold (SRT) of 50. Computed tomography of the temporalis bones showed complete opacification of the middle ear and of the mastoid cavities and erosion of scutum.

A right radical mastoidectomy and a large meatoplasty were performed. Operative findings revealed invasive cholesteatomas of the middle ear and mastoid cavity, erosion of the lenticular process of the incus, and engulfment of the remaining part of the incus and of the malleus by cholesteatomas. The stapes was intact.

Follow-up examination of the mastoid and middle ear cavities revealed clean, dry mucosa and no evidence of cholesteatoma. I decided to continue with reconstructing the right middle ear, posterior canal wall, and mastoid cavity. Figure 8C shows the appearance at the start of reconstructive surgery.

572 / Chapter 38

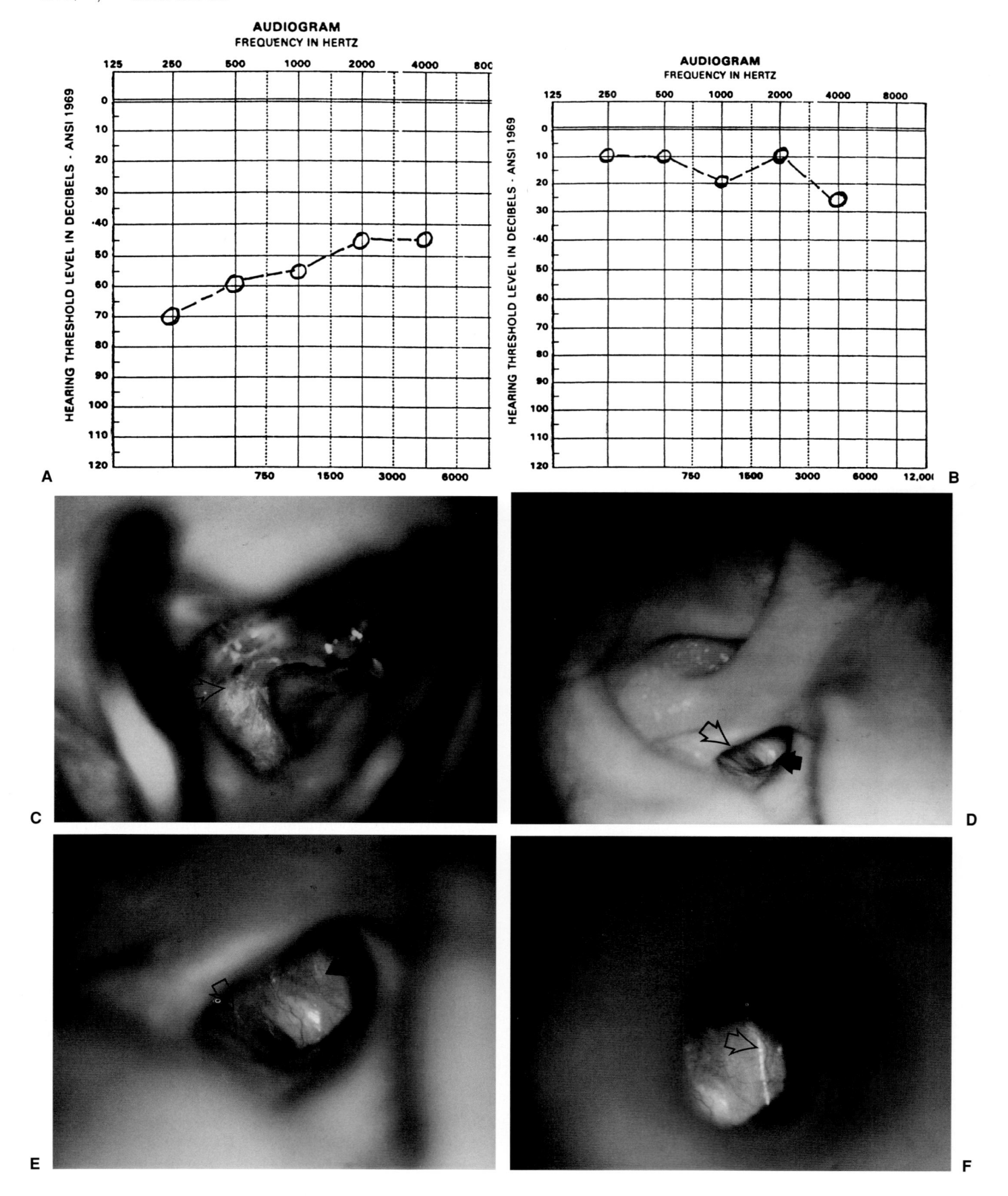

After fibrous tissue was carefully debrided, two small, pearl-like cholesteatomas were found in the anterior epitympanum. The cholesteatomas were eradicated, and the bony surface of the mastoid cavity was saucerized with a diamond burr. There was no other evidence of disease.

Reconstruction then proceeded. In this instance, however, after the incus was disarticulated and the head of the malleus was removed, the remnant of the tendon of the tensor tympani muscle was excised. This was done to prevent difficulties arising from potential interference with the ossicular chain reconstruction.

Fifteen days after reconstruction, the external canal packing was removed and a skin graft was placed in the posterior canal. On follow-up a year later, an exploratory right myringotomy was performed in a second-look procedure. Small cholesteatomas found in the anterior area of the sulcus tympanicum were removed.

Figure 8D, E, F shows the appearance of the right EAC and eardrum after surgery. The right posterior canal wall is observable. It was covered by smooth, pink, healthy skin. His right eardrum was intact, transparent, and well vascularized, and the ossicular chain was stable. The boy remains well, has good hearing in his right ear (Fig. 8B), and enjoys participating in several sports, including swimming. He has had no further recurrence of cholesteatomas and no evidence of recurrent middle-ear disease.

Case History 2

An 8½-year-old boy visited my office in 1985. At that time he had a long history of recurrent otitis media in his left ear, with chronic purulent discharge. Multiple myringotomies with tube insertions had been performed.

Examination of the left ear revealed a large, posterior perforation of the eardrum, with cholesteatomas filling the middle ear, and profuse exudate. Axial and coronal views by computed tomography of the temporalis bones showed invasion of the middle ear and mastoid cavity by soft tissue mass. Audiometric examination demonstrated severe conductive hearing loss in the left ear (Fig. 9A).

A left radical mastoidectomy was performed. Extensive cholesteatomas were removed from the middle ear and from the mastoid cavity. The lenticular process of the incus was found to be completely eroded. Cholesteatomas engulfed the remaining ossicles and invaded the eustachian tube, oval window, mesotympanum, and hypotympanum. Two months later a revision mastoidectomy was performed to remove granulation tissue from the mastoid cavity, and an exploratory tympanotomy was performed to remove residual cholesteatomas from the facial recess and around the stapes superstructure. Granulation tissue from the hypotympanum and eustachian tube was also removed.

One year later partial reconstruction of the middle ear cavity and mastoid reconstruction were attempted. The middle ear was found to be covered by a false membrane eardrum. No cholesteatomas were observed in the mastoid cavity. An incus homograft was inserted between the false membrane and the head of the stapes to restore the ossicular chain. The posterior bony canal was reconstructed with temporalis fascia and curved chips of cortical bone, and the mastoid cavity was reconstructed with cortical bone. However, audiometric results were unsatisfactory because the false eardrum precluded good hearing.

Two years later total middle ear reconstruction was performed. Figure 9C shows the appearance of the middle ear before surgery. The false membrane covering the middle ear was removed. Small, localized cholesteatomas were removed from the anterior epitympanic area. A homograft eardrum having an attached malleus manubrium was transplanted, as was an incus homograft that was interposed between the malleus and the head of the stapes (Fig. 9D, E). The boy's hearing improved markedly, but not for long because there was progressive deterioration to moderate to severe hearing loss.

An exploratory tympanotomy was performed 2 years later. Discontinuity of the ossicular chain was observed due to separation of the incus homograft from the head of the stapes caused by multiple ear adhesions. A 0.010-inch thick polymeric silicone sheet was inserted in the middle ear cavity, and the incus was repositioned. No cholesteatomas were observed. Although hearing returned to normal for several months, it again deteriorated.

One year later a left exploratory tympanotomy was performed. The incus homograft was again observed to be separated from the stapes. The incus was attached to the eardrum. The gap between the incus and the head of the stapes was filled by placing the head of a malleus homograft in it. Ordinarily, the head of the malleus homograft is discarded; in this particular instance, the head of the malleus was a small piece of bone particularly suited for another purpose.

The patient's hearing improved markedly and remains normal (Fig. 9B). The ear drum is transparent and well vascularized, the ossicular chain remains stable, and there have been no other problems. Figure 9D, E, F, G, H shows the appearance of the left EAC and eardrum after surgery.

FIG. 8. A: Audiogram taken before surgery. **B:** Audiogram taken after surgery for patient described in Case 1. **C:** Open mastoid cavity prior to total middle ear reconstruction and mastoid obliteration. *White arrow,* open mastoid cavity; *black arrow,* middle ear cavity. **D:** *White arrow,* contour of reconstructed ear canal; *black arrow,* homograft tympanic membrane. **E:** *White arrow,* appearance of reconstructed posterior ear canal. *Black arrow,* homograft tympanic membrane. Well healed and vascularized. **F:** *White arrow,* view of anterior canal and eardrum with preservation of anterior angle.

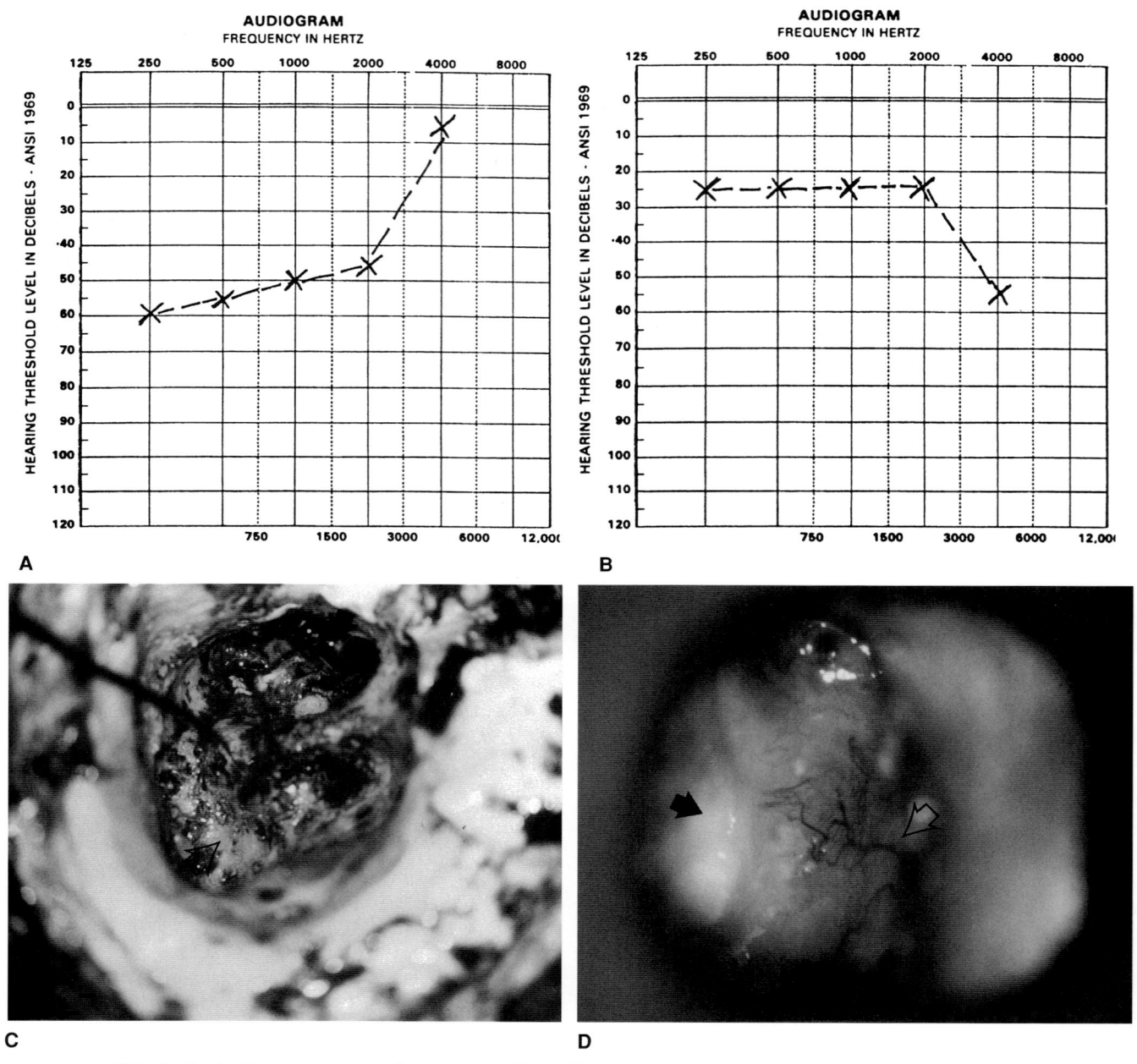

FIG. 9. A: Audiogram taken before surgery; **B:** audiogram taken after surgery for patient described in Case 2. **C:** *White arrow,* mastoid cavity; *black arrow:* middle ear cavity. **D:** Early vascularization of homograft tympanic membrane; *black arrow,* anterior portion of tympanic membrane.

CONTROVERSIES ABOUT OPEN RADICAL CAVITY RESTORATION IN CHILDREN

Are ear homografts safe? The primary concerns have been with potential antigenicity and with virus transmission from donor to recipient.

Homografts and Antigenicity

Many surgeons prefer to use synthetic, biocompatible ossicular prostheses. Consequently, their availability of increasing. In contrast to homografts, synthetics do not depend on donor supply; do not require proper harvest, preparation, and storage; and have a longer storage life. Furthermore, homografts are subject to immunologic rejection by the recipient.

The homografts are shipped and stored in buffered formaldehyde. This destroys epithelial cells, virtually eliminating antigenicity, and maintains the collagenous architecture of the eardrum. The formaldehyde is fixed to the proteins, and the epithelium of Malpighi is destroyed and its removal is facilitated. The eardrum and the annulus fibrosis become fixed, but without retraction.

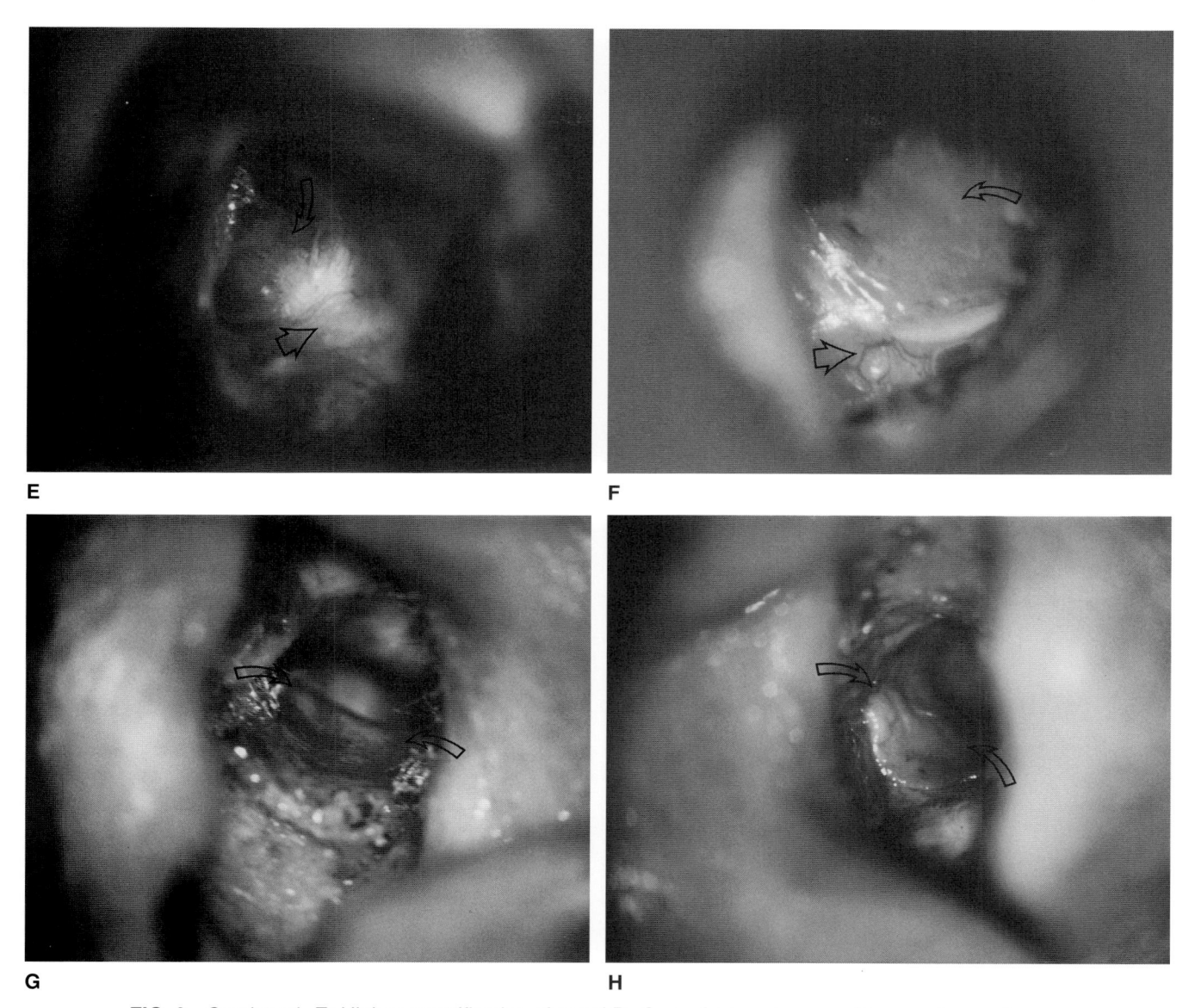

FIG. 9. *Continued.* **E:** Higher magnification of panel D. *Curved arrow,* homograft tympanic membrane; *white arrow,* newly reconstructed posterior wall. **F:** Annulus fibrosis of homograft tympanic membrane in sulcus tympanicum. **G:** Newly reconstructed posterior wall at 14 days postoperatively. Exposed temporalis fascia shows between *curved arrows.* **H:** Skin covering temporalis fascia (between *curved arrows*).

Ossicular new bone formation (4) starts from the periphery and traverse the bone along infiltration of connective tissue within the ossicle. Mesenchymal cells that appear during revascularization are differentiated into osteoclasts that produce the lysis of the dead bone, and into osteoblasts and osteocytes that synthesize new bone. Histologic examination (Fig. 10) of sections of ossicles removed from one of my adult patients 3 years after transplantation shows this process.

In my experience in performing reconstructive middle-ear surgery, homograft eardrum and ossicles and cortical bone from the calvarium have proven to persist in the recipients. There has been little evidence for rejection or reabsorption.

Ear Homografts and the Hazard of Virus Transmission

Use of a homograft comprising the eardrum and ossicles raises concerns about transmitting viruses. Glasscock, Jackson, and Knox (40) assessed the theoretical risk of transmitting human immunodeficiency virus (HIV) and the slow virus that causes Creutzfeldt-Jakob disease (CJD). They concluded that although otologic homografts are not implicated in transmission, the theoretical possibility needs to be strongly considered. Davis (41) also considered the risk.

Because HIV is a fragile virus, it is readily inactivated by 1% (or greater) neutral buffered Formalin, which contains

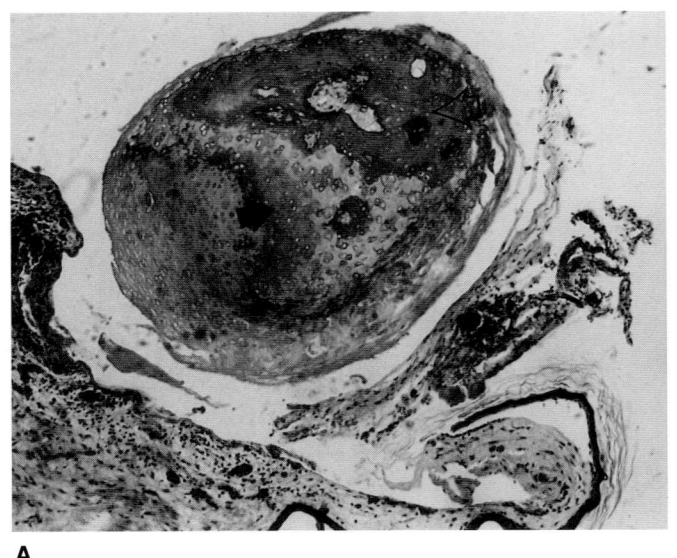

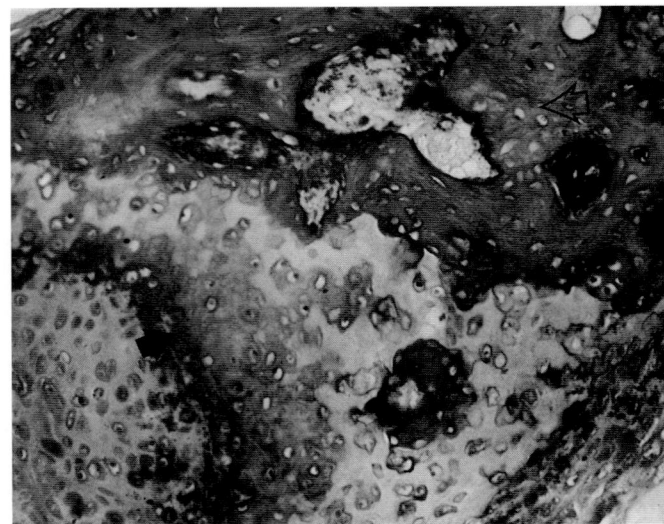

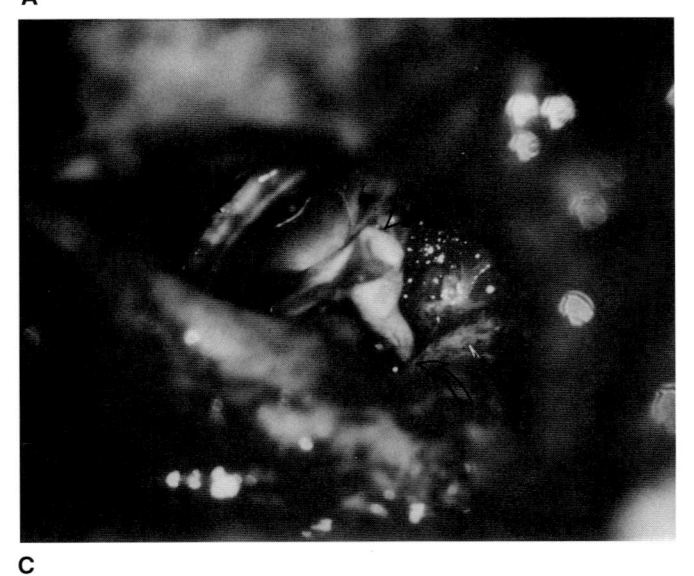

FIG. 10. Histologic sections of ossicles removed from a patient 3 years after transplantation. **A:** Histologic cross section of malleus bone homograft. *Black arrow,* newly regenerated bone; *white arrow,* "dead bone" in process of reabsorption. **B:** Higher magnification of cross section in panel A. **C:** Homograft tympanic membrane with head of malleus removed and connected to footplate of stapes by incus bone homograft. *Straight arrow,* section of neck of malleus; *left curved arrow,* homograft tympanicannulus in position; *right curved arrow,* incus homograft in oval window connected to stapes footplate.

0.4% formaldehyde (41). The Midwest Ear Foundation and Project HEAR use extensive formaldehyde sterilization for the homografts they provide. An unpublished report (SG Lesinski, AIDS virus: sterility of middle ear tissue transplants) from the Midwest Ear Foundation showed that ossicles are completely perfused by formaldehyde within 48 hours of treatment, that formaldehyde fixation does not inactivate the CJD virus, that there is no serologic test for this virus, and that the possibility that the CJD virus is present in the middle ear is remote.

Elaborate donor screening procedures protect against virus transmission. Before the temporal bone is removed, Midwest Ear Foundation prescreens the donor's medical history. Midwest Ear Foundation technicians review medical charts for disqualifying diagnoses, and they draw blood. Midwest Ear Foundation conducts medical and social history screening with next-of-kin as soon as possible after death and before tissue is eligible for transplantation.

Midwest Ear Foundation does not accept donors who have or have had any organic brain disease, such as CJD or other encephalopathy, Alzheimer's disease, dementia (presenile, senile, or praecox), or Parkinson's disease. Also, Midwest Ear Foundation declines donations from those who have received injections of pituitary-derived human growth hormone. Furthermore, Midwest Ear Foundation declines donations if there is a history of other illnesses such as syphilis and rabies.

Midwest Ear Foundation also applies United States Public Health Service criteria for exclusion of high-risk donors. These criteria include, for example, men who have had sex with another man in the preceding 5 years, persons who engaged in sex for money or drugs in the preceding 5 years or who used illegal drugs or substances, and persons who were sexual partners with those who were or are at high risk.

Midwest Ear Foundation obtains gross autopsy reports on all potential donors, declines donations in instances in which request for autopsy has been denied, and declines donors whose bodies are not embalmed within 24 hours after death. If a donor has met the criteria, then the blood is subject to serologic tests for exposure to HIV and other viruses. Positive serologic tests result in rejection of the donation.

Complications in any way associated with virus transmission through homografts comprising the eardrum and ossicles have never been observed in my experience, nor in the experiences of the Midwest Ear Foundation or of Project HEAR. As far as is known, there are no reports of any disease being transmitted from donor to recipient by homograft comprising the eardrum and ossicles. Tange (43) reported a case of CJD in a patient who had received homograft pericardium for tympanic membrane closure.

The use of homograft tissue is part of the risk and benefit of the procedure. This should be should be explained to the patients (or to the patient's parents or guardians, when appropriate) as part of the information for decision making.

ALTERNATIVES FOR MANAGEMENT

Many otologists are reluctant to reconstruct a child s middle ear and mastoid cavity. But middle-ear reconstruction offers the child a much more favorable alternative: a functioning ear.

The presence of chronic cholesteatomas in children has precluded performing reconstructive ear surgery at an early age, perhaps because of the assumption that it is impossible to control and completely eradicate cholesteatoma in children. It is true that children are more likely than adults to have upper respiratory infections with middle ear involvement. However, by closely monitoring the child for years and performing repeated surgery if necessary, it is possible to completely control cholesteatoma.

Cholesteatomas in children generally runs an aggressive course, necessitating a canal wall down mastoidectomy or modified mastoidectomy. These procedures leave the child with an open mastoid bowl, an infection-prone ear, and maximal conductive hearing loss. The child's normal lifestyle is disrupted; for example, the child needs preferential seating at school and cannot participate in water sports. The child is faced with a lifelong disability that requires lifelong care, such as regular cleaning of the mastoid cavity by a physician. Some children become emotionally disturbed.

Middle-ear reconstructions have been performed on children who previously had extensive disease, such as massive middle-ear destruction caused by cholesteatomas. These children have had excellent long-term functional and anatomic results without complications. In considering middle-ear reconstruction, one should be minimally concerned with patient age. Rehabilitative ear surgery can be performed in young children and can offer them a better life.

Others who have reconstructed middle ears in children also advance these views. Perkins (44) described reconstruction after radical tympanomastoidectomy in children age 8 years and older, by using a technique called tympanomastoid reconstruction. Perkins used an autogenous bone paté supported by a homograft dura, combined with reconstruction of the middle ear using a formaldehyde-treated homograft eardrum with en bloc ossicles. The method eliminated the problem of an open mastoid cavity. For improved hearing, however, his procedure also entailed a second stage 1 year later.

Wehrs (45) noted that the eardrum, middle ear, and ossicles are adult size at birth; thus, procedures on these structures in children are the same as procedures in adults. However, he also noted that the eustachian tube and external ear develop more slowly in the child, which might make it necessary to postpone surgery.

Wehrs view was that congenital absence or fixation of the ossicles may be repaired as soon as they are discovered, typically when the child is 4 or 5 years old. In reconstructing ossicular discontinuity due to infection associated with a perforated eardrum, Wehrs preferred to wait until the child was older, unless there was a more urgent indication such as cholesteatoma, because in the younger child, satisfactory results are compromised by poor eustachian tube function, recurrent otitis media, and poor graft intake. Wehrs recommended delaying reconstruction until the child was 7 to 8 years of age for anticipated fascial grafts, and until 15 or 16 years of age for canal skin grafts. Otherwise, Wehrs's methods were the same for children as for adults.

CONCLUSIONS

In my experience, the following assertions regarding reconstruction after mastoidectomy can be made:

1. Reconstruction of middle ear, mastoid cavity, and posterior bony canal after canal wall down mastoidectomy results in good hearing in children who have undergone radical mastoidectomy.

2. Use of homograft eardrum and ossicles are the best materials for middle ear reconstruction, and combination of autologous temporalis fascia and cortical bone are the best materials for reconstructing the posterior bony canal and mastoid.

3. Modification of homograft eardrum and ossicles before transplantation is key to ensuring good, long-term functional results and to preventing ossicular fixation.

4. The benefits of restored structure and function are excellent, and the risk of complications is acceptable.

ACKNOWLEDGMENT

I thank Kenneth M. Grundfast, M.D., for helpful comments on the manuscript.

REFERENCES

1. Wullstein HL, Wullstein SR. *Tympanoplasty: osteoplastic epitympanotomy.* Stuttgart: Georg Thieme Verlag; 1990.
2. Brady DR, Paparella MM. Tympanoplasty and myringoplasty. In: Jaffe

BF, ed. *Hearing loss in children: a comprehensive text.* Baltimore: University Park Press; 1977:516.
3. Betow C. 20 years of experience with homografts in ear surgery. *J Laryngol Otol* 1982;96(Suppl 5):1.
4. Betow K. *Transplantationen von Trommel fell un Gehörknöchelchenkette bei Tympanoplastiken.* Berlin: de Gruyter; 1970.
5. Betow C. Restoration of the conductive system of the middle ear with homograft—evolution. In: Yanagihara N, Suzuki J-I, eds. *Transplants and implants in otology II.* Amsterdam: Kugler; 1992:23.
6. Marquet JFE. Historical notes on homografts. *Otolaryngol Clin N Am* 1977a:10:479.
7. Jaffe BF, ed. *Hearing loss in children.* Baltimore: University Park Press; 1977.
8. Wullstein HL. *Fundamentos y métodos de lacofocirugia.* Barcelona: Ediciones Toray; 1968.
9. Portmann M, Poncet E, Rolleau P, Lacher G. *Leshomogreffes tympanoossiculaires.* Paris: Arnette; 1978.
10. Charachon R, Roulleau P, Bremond G, et al. *Lesossiculoplasties: et at actuel.* Paris: Arnette; 1987.
11. Wayoff M, Chobaut JC, Deguine C, et al. *Les greffes dutympan.* Paris: Arnette; 1994:9.
12. Veldman JE, ed. *Immunobiology, autoimmunity, and transplantation in otorhinolaryngology.* Amsterdam: Kugler Publications; 1985.
13. Babighian G, Veldman JE, eds. *Transplants and implants in otology.* Amsterdam: Kugler & Ghedini; 1988.
14. Yanagihara N, Suzuki J-I, eds. *Transplants and implants in otology* II. Amsterdam: Kugler; 1992.
15. Lesinski SG, ed. Homograft tympanoplasty. *Otolaryngol Clin N Am* 1977;10.
16. Monsell EM, ed. Ossiculoplasty. *Otolaryngol Clin N Am* 1994;27.
17. Goldenberg RA, ed. Implants in otolaryngology. *Otolaryngol Clin N Am* 1995;28.
18. Crabtree JA, Maceri DR. Tympanoplasty and ossicular reconstruction: an update. *Am J Otol* 1988;9:334.
19. Ars B, Ars-Piret N. *Tympano-ossicular allograft tympanoplasty.* Amsterdam: Kugler; 1993.
20. Derlacki EL. Tympanic transplants. *Arch Otolaryngol* 1973;97:67.
21. Tabb HG. Reconstruction of the mastoidectized ear. *Arch Otolaryngol* 1973;97:74.
22. Bergan J. Principles of tissue transplantation as applied to otology. *Arch Otolaryngol* 1973;72:70.
23. Marquet JFE. Twelve years experience with homograft tympanoplasty. *Otolaryngol Clin N Am* 1977b:10:581.
24. Wehrs RE. Results of reconstructive mastoidectomy with homograft knee cartilage. *Laryngoscope* 1978;88:1912.
25. Wehrs RE. Homograft tympanoplasty. *Otolaryngol Clin N Am* 1982; 15:781.
26. Wehrs RE. Hydroxyapatite implants for otologic surgery. *Otolaryngol Clin N Am* 1995;28:273.
27. Robin PE, Clegg RT. Homografts in tympanoplasty: will they be a disaster? An experimental study. *Clin Otolaryngol* 1989;5:311.
28. Lesinski SG. Complications of homograft tympanoplasty. *Otolaryngol Clin N Am* 1982;15:795.
29. Lesinski SG. Homograft (allograft) tympanoplasty update. *Laryngoscope* 1986;966:1211.
30. Lesinski SG. Transplantation in clinical otology. In: Veldman JE, McCabe BF, eds. *Otoimmunology.* Amsterdam: Kugler; 1987:81.
31. Chiossone E. Homograft ossiculoplasty: long-term results. *Am J Otol* 1987;8:545.
32. Portmann M. Results of middle ear reconstruction surgery. *Ann Acad Med Singapore* 1991;20:610.
33. Nissen AJ. Homografts in otologic surgery. *Oper Tech Otolaryngol Head Neck Surg* 1992;3:285.
34. Namyslowski G, Gierek T. Anatomical and functional results of middle ear reconstruction with tympano-ossicular allografts. Part I. Tympanic membrane allograft attached to the handle of malleus. *Otolaryngol Pol* 1993;47:36.
35. Namyslowski G, Gierek T. Anatomical and functional results of middle ear reconstruction with tympano-ossicular allografts. Part II: Total tympano-ossicular allograft. *Otolaryngol Pol* 1993;47:131.
36. Namyslowski G, Gierek T. Evaluation of tympano-ossicular allografts in reconstructive surgery of the middle ear [Polish]. *Otolaryngol Pol* 1994;48:163.
37. Olszewski E, Modrzejewski M, Dobros W. Homograft of incus in tympanoplasty. *Otolaryngol Pol* 1993;47:43.
38. Soushko YA, Borissenko ON, Yalovoi SF. The application of osseous allografts in middle ear surgery: our experience. *Rev Laryngol Otol Rhinol (Bord)* 1993;114:129.
39. Garro, JJ. Reconstruction of middle ear, mastoid, and ear canal, and restoration of hearing after canal-wall down mastoidectomy. Bordeaux, France: Third international symposium on transplants and implants in otology, 1995.
40. Glasscock ME, Jackson CG, Knox GW. Can acquired immunodeficiency syndrome and Creutzfeldt-Jakob disease be transmitted via otologic homografts? *Arch Otolaryngol Head Neck Surg* 1988;114:1252.
41. Davis AE. Homograft materials in otolaryngology: the risk of transmitting human immunodeficiency virus. *Clin Otolaryngol* 1988;13:159.
42. Martin LS, Loskoski SL, McDougal JS. Inactivation of human T-lymphotropic virus type III/lymphadenopathy-associated virus by formaldehyde-based reagents. *Appl Environ Microbiol* 1987;53:708.
43. Tange RA, Troost D, Limburg M. Progressive fatal dementia (Creutzfeldt-Jakob disease) in a patient who received homograft tissue for tympanic membrane closure. *Eur Arch Otorhinolaryngol* 1990;247: 199.
44. Perkins R. Reconstruction following radical tympanomastoidectomy. In: Jaffe BF, ed. *Hearing loss in children: a comprehensive text.* Baltimore: University Park Press; 1977:574.
45. Wehrs RE. Ossiculoplasty. In: Jaffe BF, ed. *Hearing loss in children: a comprehensive text.* Baltimore: University Park Press, 1977:530.

PART XIII

Auditory Habilitation and Rehabilitation

CHAPTER 39

Auditory Amplification

Robert W. Sweetow

Expressive speech and language skills are intrinsically tied to auditory reception. Children learn to speak based largely on what they hear. When an infant's or toddler's hearing is impaired, there is a great likelihood that acquisition of speech and language skills will be delayed. This delay can initiate a chain reaction prompting adverse effects on the child's social, psychological, emotional, and educational development. It also can affect familial relationships.

A growing body of research indicates that auditory impairments occurring during the formative language learning years may precede later learning disorders (1,2). It is thus essential to detect and remediate a hearing loss at the earliest possible age.

Unfortunately, decades have passed during which the age of detection of hearing loss for congenitally impaired children has hovered at an unacceptably high level. In 1980, it was reported that the average detection of hearing loss for a population of severe and profoundly hearing impaired children was nearly 3 years of age (3). Ten years later, the US Department of Health and Human Services indicated that the average age of detection was still an unacceptably late 24 to 30 months of age (4).

In the past decade, there have been great advances in diagnostic testing capabilities. The use of objective measures such as auditory evoked potentials and otoacoustic emissions have equipped audiologists, pediatricians, and otologists with the tools to identify babies with hearing loss from birth. Moreover, the 10% of children who were considered untestable 10 years ago because of our reliance on behavioral assessment techniques has now decreased to the point where virtually no child is truly untestable. Of course, the benefit produced by enhanced ability to identify hearing impairment at an early age can be realized only if there are effective means of habilitation and rehabilitation available. Here, too, we are fortunate that, concurrent with our improved diagnostic test capabilities, there have been significant technologic improvements in hearing aids as well as advances in our knowledge of fitting procedures. Even so, the selection and application of amplification for children is both art and science, quite unique, and in many aspects, different than it is for adults. In this chapter, these principles are discussed.

COMPONENTS OF HEARING AIDS

The discussion begins with a general description of hearing aids. All hearing aids consist of a minimum of three components: a microphone to receive incoming acoustic signals and convert them to electrical energy, an amplifier to increase the amplitude of the electrical signal, and a receiver to convert the amplified electrical signal back to acoustic energy for delivery to the ear (Fig. 1). Hearing aids are powered by a battery. Most (but not all) hearing aids contain a volume control. Additionally, hearing aids utilize various filtering procedures to modify the amount of gain (defined as the difference in intensity between the input to the microphone and the output from the receiver) as a function of the frequency and intensity of the incoming acoustic signal. They also contain output-limiting components to ensure that incoming sounds are not amplified to a degree that could be injurious to the wearer. Plus, some hearing aids contain telecoils (electromagnetic signal receivers, which will be described shortly).

TYPES AND STYLES OF HEARING AIDS

Hearing aids are available in a variety of styles (Fig. 2). Prior to the 1960s, body borne hearing aids (Fig. 2A), consisting of a large microphone-amplifier-battery pack unit worn in the shirt pocket and connected via a cord to a receiver-earmold device were popular. These devices were cumbersome and cosmetically unappealing and produced a relatively low fidelity signal. Fortunately, they are rarely used today, except for some cases of profound hearing loss. The most common type of hearing aids used by children

R.W. Sweetow: Department of Otolaryngology, University of California, San Francisco, San Francisco, California 94143-0340.

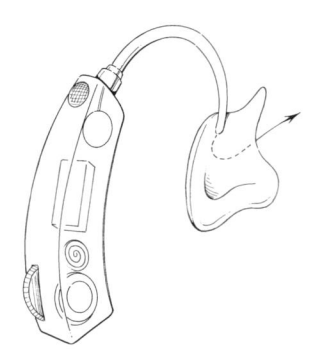

FIG. 1. Behind-the-ear hearing aid showing basic components of hearing aids.

today are the postauricular type (Fig. 2B). These devices have the microphone, amplifier, receiver, and battery housed in the same unit, which fits behind the ear and is coupled to the ear via an earmold made of either a lucite or soft vinyl material. Postauricular, or as they are more often termed, *behind-the-ear* (BTE), hearing aids are available in a variety of sizes and colors. Their shapes are, of course, limited by the contour of the human pinna. Although BTE aids are the most commonly used styles on infants and youngsters, children approximately 9 years old and older may prefer using the in-the-ear (ITE) style (Fig. 2C) Issues such as potential damage to the ear resulting from a fall or a blow to the head should be considered before making this recommendation (5,6). Other current styles, such as the in-the-canal (ITC) (Fig. 2D) or the extremely tiny completely-in-canal (2E) aids, are not appropriate for children.

The specific rationale surrounding the selection of which style is appropriate for a given child also is a function of the degree of loss and possibly the audiometric configuration. In-the-ear or ITC aids are not appropriate for children with severe or profound losses. They lack adequate gain and power and are more likely to produce acoustic feedback. Another major limitation of ITEs for children is that they often lack strong telecoils or direct audio input capability (features that will be discussed shortly). However, for older children who are too vain or intimidated by peer pressure to wear BTEs, it may be better to settle on less than optimal amplification than on no amplification at all.

EARMOLDS

If the hearing aid is a BTE style, an earmold is utilized to couple the instrument to the ear canal. Thus, the earmold is an integral component to the amplification system. A variety of earmolds are available. Some of these are depicted in Fig. 3. Earmolds are typically made out of either a hard lucite or a soft vinyl material. For children, the softer materials are advisable because they are less likely to cause traumatic injury to the canal or eardrum should the child fall or receive a blow to the ear.

Variations to the fit or configuration of an earmold (or the physical configuration of the ITE shell) can significantly alter the acoustic signal delivered to the eardrum. Figure 4 depicts several frequency responses (graphs that plot gain as a function of frequency). Placing a vent in the earmold allows for a reduction in the amount of low-frequency (below 1,000 Hz) gain passing through to the ear canal. Use of a stepped diameter, belled bore or acoustic horn type of earmold (e.g., the Continuous Flow Adaptor, Pacific Coast Laboratories, San Francisco, CA) may increase the amount of acoustic gain above 2500 Hz. In addition, a damping filter appropriately placed in the tubing of the earmold can alter the location of the primary resonant peak and may help to smooth the frequency response. The length and diameter of the tubing as well as the depth of the earmold also can be modified to achieve certain desired effects.

Poorly fitting earmolds can affect the response of the hearing aid in unexpected or unwanted manners. Sharp peaks and valleys can appear in the frequency response and may result in poor transient reproduction, producing an unnatural sound. The amount of low-frequency gain (and the resonant peak) may be altered in an undesired fashion. Perhaps the most serious consequence of a poorly fitting earmold, however, is the likelihood of increasing the presence of acoustic feedback.

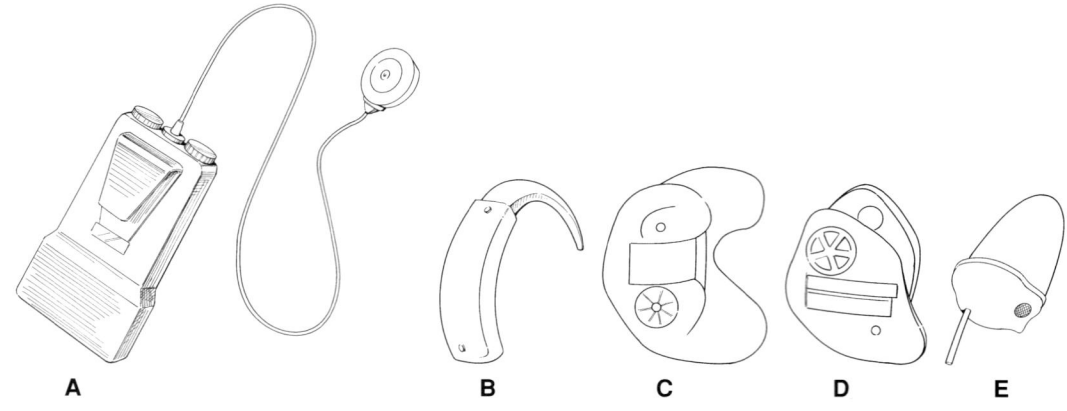

FIG. 2. Hearing aids styles. **A:** body. **B:** BTE. **C:** ITE. **D:** ITC. **E:** Completely-in-canal.

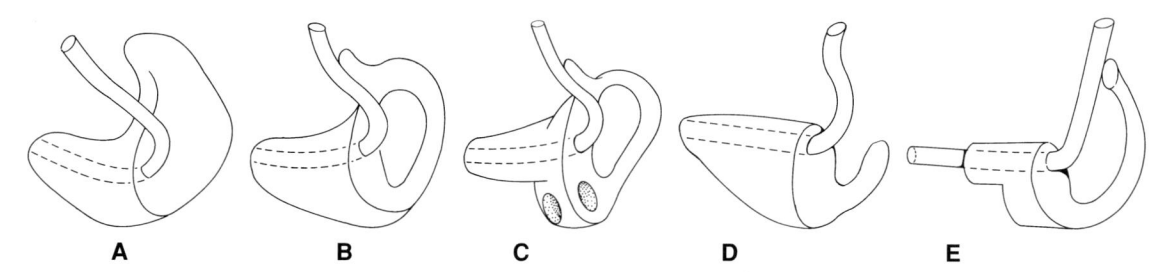

FIG. 3. Variety of earmolds. **A:** Shell. **B:** Silhouette. **C:** Silhouette with vent. **D:** Partial silhouette. **E:** Open (free field).

Acoustic feedback occurs when amplified sound escapes or leaks from the earmold back into the hearing aid's microphone. The resultant whistling sound often forces the child or caretaker to reduce the gain of the hearing aid, effectively minimizing benefit. Generally speaking, the closer the microphone is to the receiver, the greater the likelihood of feedback occurring. Therefore, BTE aids have a clear advantage over smaller ITE or ITC aids. Many manufacturers provide "feedback controls," which are, at the present time, little more than a potentiometer that reduces high frequency amplification. While this does indeed accomplish the desired effect of reducing feedback, it does so at the expense of reducing the audibility of vitally important high-frequency consonants. Thus, this is often not an acceptable trade-off. Certain earmold materials and configuration improvements, such as the use of a Patriot earmold (Entech Laboratories, Roanoke, VA), help to preserve high-frequency gain while minimizing feedback. Electronic advances, such as phase shifting, may someday control feedback problems thus allowing for non-occlusion and full usage of the natural ear canal resonance, which occurs at 2,700 to 3,200 Hz.

Because of pinna growth and changes in the shape of the concha, which occur until the child reaches about 9 years of age, frequent remakes of earmolds are often necessary. Ideally, earmolds and ITE shells should be examined and possibly remade every 3 to 6 months for children below age 5 and every year from ages 5 to 10. As with every other aspect of amplification for the pediatric population, the hearing professional must remain flexible and recognize that, with children, frequent appointments and readjustments are the norm rather than the exception.

TELECOILS

A critically important advantage of BTE aids and some ITE aids is the inclusion of a telecoil (magnetic induction loop). A telecoil circuit consists of a loop placed within the hearing aid that detects electromagnetic signals emanating from telephones, personal neck loops, and audio induction assistive listening systems (such as are currently found in many theatres, churches, and other public places). The electromagnetic signal is converted to electrical current, magnified, and then converted into acoustic energy. Some telecoils operate when the hearing aid microphone is shut off, while others allow the wearer to receive amplified signals via both the microphone and the telecoil.

DIRECT AUDIO INPUT

Hearing aids used on children should contain direct audio input (DAI) capabilities to allow for direct coupling of the hearing aid to a television, radio, or other assistive listening device (ALD). Use of DAI is particularly beneficial because it is not restricted to the power of the electromagnetic field and because the signal can be modified by the hearing aid circuitry, thus adopting the same electroacoustic characteristics as that device.

IMPORTANCE OF BINAURAL AMPLIFICATION

Laboratory-generated psychoacoustic data clearly demonstrate a number of binaural listening advantages. Of these, perhaps the most important advantages are the following.

Elimination of the Head Shadow Effect

Sound intensity is decreased by an average of 6.5 dB as sound crosses the head (the head shadow). However, because of the fluctuating nature of our acoustic environment, listeners find themselves in adverse positions (in which the "good" ear may be closer to the unwanted background

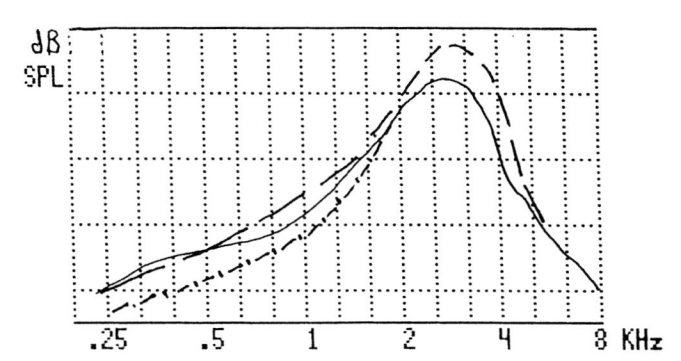

FIG. 4. Frequency responses. ———— closed earmold; —·—·— vented earmold; — — — acoustic horn type earmold.

noise, and the "bad" ear is closer to the desired sound source, i.e., speech) nearly 50% of the time. As a result, the difference between monaural direct listening versus monaural indirect listening may be as much as 13 dB. Furthermore, the head shadow effect is greatest for the high frequencies, those most responsible for speech intelligibility. The use of binaural aids minimizes the probability of being in the adverse monaural indirect location. This is also the principle applied to contralateral routing of sound (CROS) amplification used for patients having only one aidable ear; these aids are used infrequently with children.

Binaural Summation

Absolute binaural thresholds are 2 to 3 dB better than monaural thresholds. At suprathreshold levels, where listeners receive amplified sound, summation increases by as much as 6 to 10 dB. Therefore, a hearing aid user can achieve the same loudness perception from binaural hearing aids set at a lower volume-control setting than with a monaural aid. This may greatly reduce feedback problems.

Release from Masking

Dichotic listening (receiving two separate and distinct signals in each ear) is more tolerable than either monotic (all signals to one ear only) or diotic (the same signal to each ear). A series of classic experiments (7–9) demonstrated the concept of binaural squelch, showing that a significant release from masking could be achieved under certain conditions because of the out-of-phase relations of the signal and noise reaching two ears. The magnitude of this release (termed *masking level differences*) cannot be achieved through monaural listening.

Sensory Deprivation

In a 5-year retrospective study conducted on adults, it was shown that word recognition scores decreased in the unaided but not in the aided ears of monaurally aided patients. In a matched group of binaurally aided patients, however, word recognition scores in both ears remained constant (10). This finding has since been confirmed (11) using different etiologies. Not all scientists agree with the conclusions. In theory, however, the relevance of this finding for children is especially important.

Thus, the general rule is that unless one can demonstrate decreased performance resulting from binaural usage, the standard should be trial with binaural amplification. Rare cases in which monaural amplification would be appropriate include those in which a significant asymmetry exists between the ears in either sensitivity or word recognition ability and, of course, in which there are medical contraindications to placing a hearing aid in one of the ears (i.e., a draining ear or an atretic ear canal). It is interesting to note that the concept of binaural superiority is accepted by nearly all agencies providing third-party payments for children but is yet to be approved by some organizations paying for hearing aids for adults.

DIFFERENCES IN AMPLIFICATION FOR ADULTS VERSUS CHILDREN

Team Members

Although the audiologist is the professional responsible for coordinating efforts to provide amplification for a child, the establishment of a core team of professionals must be instituted early. The basic team should consist of a pediatric audiologist, a pediatric otologist, a pediatrician, an educator of the hearing impaired, and a speech-language pathologist. Additional, adjunct team members might include a social worker, a neurologist, a geneticist, an ophthalmologist, and a psychologist or psychiatrist. Also, remember that the child's family represents one of the most important components of the team.

Diagnostic Capabilities

As options for prescribing electroacoustic parameters increase, the demand for a more specific description of psychoacoustic listening abilities also grows. When testing adults, it is common to obtain a variety of suprathreshold data in addition to measures of threshold sensitivity. For example, assessment of word recognition skills, loudness growth patterns, and ability to function in adverse listening environments contribute to the audiologist's decisions regarding the selection and parameter settings of the amplification system. However, children, particularly infants and those without expressive language, do not readily provide this feedback. Thus, the audiologist often must make decisions based on partial information. A number of alternative approaches have been employed to compensate for this lack of definition. Several of these, which are based on either prescriptive formulas or objective measures, will be discussed later. The important point to remember is that the audiologist must remain flexible and willing to make modifications as a more complete diagnostic description of the child's hearing becomes apparent.

Family Management

Convincing adults to wear hearing aids is often a difficult task. They may not recognize or accept the need for help, they may be concerned about the societal stigma attached to hearing aid use, they may be concerned about cosmetics, or they may be upset about the expense involved. All of these obstacles may be difficult to overcome. Generally speaking, however, the task facing the audiologist is to address the objections of the hearing impaired individual. With children, yet another major hurdle is involved. That barrier is the family of the child. The effects of discovering a child has a disability can be devastating to individual family members and to the family structure itself. They must progress through the normal transitions of mourning. Even then, there may be residual feelings of guilt or blame that could torment the family. Additionally, there may be culturally based reluctance to wearing hearing aids.

Perhaps the biggest difference between ensuring proper usage of amplification for adults versus children is that children are dependent on others (including their parents or caretakers and teachers) to enforce proper usage and maintenance. Thus, an alliance must be formed consisting of an audiologist, otologist, pediatrician, speech/language pathologist, teacher of the hearing impaired, public health or school nurse, and social worker to help the hearing-impaired child's family accept responsibility.

Coordination with Educational and Speech-Language Specialists

For adults, there is a relatively short "break-in" period for adjustment to new hearing aids. For children, however, who are still developing speech and language skills, the introduction of amplification alone is insufficient to guarantee habilitation and/or rehabilitation. These users of hearing aids must be taught to associate newly received sounds with meaning. They require extensive assistance to conjoin sound with speech and language competencies. While the audiologist, pediatrician, and otologist may spend considerable time with the child, the vast majority of a habilitation and/or rehabilitation effort is the task of the teacher and/or speech-language specialist. Thus, helping the family obtain the necessary educational resources is a vital part of the management team's responsibilities.

The educational specialist must assist the management team in determining the proper placement for the child in accordance with Public Law 99-457, the Individuals with Disabilities Education Act. The newly amplified prelingual child must receive auditory stimulation, so some form of organized preschool activity is imperative. This Act allocates monies to states and mandates education from birth to 3 years of age. Once the child enters a preschool or other educational program, a decision must be made for the severe or profoundly hearing impaired child regarding placement in an auditory only (oral) program versus a total (combined manual and oral) communication program. The child with a mild or moderate hearing loss who is wearing proper amplification should receive education in the least restrictive fashion, although it is likely that additional therapy from a speech-language pathologist or an itinerant therapist will be a supplemental necessity.

It is also essential that the audiologist work with the teacher, speech-language pathologist, and parent or caretaker to ensure proper use of the amplification. It was found that only 55% of hearing aids in a school setting were working properly (12). Team members must be aware of the importance of performing daily listening checks of the hearing aids or other ALDs and must accept responsibility for their continued, proper usage. Indeed, they should be aware that the Education for All Handicapped Children Act of 1975 (Public Law 94-142) mandates that public agencies ensure that hearing aids worn in school are functioning properly (13).

Financial Management

Hearing aids and therapy are very expensive. It has been estimated that the annual cost of educating a child in a school for the deaf is more than $35,000, and the cost of educating a hearing-impaired child in the public schools is nearly $10,000 compared with $3,383 for those in regular classes (14). Even if the child qualifies for public school intervention, the cost of hearing aids and/or ALDs alone may run as much as $12,000 during the school years (preschool through college). This financial burden adds to the many other factors that could create hardship for the family of the hearing-impaired child. Fortunately, there are numerous agencies and organizations who may help defray these costs. A list of some these agencies is provided in Appendix C. There are certain financial qualifications associated with most of these organizations, with which the referring specialist should become familiar.

Legal Requirements

Certain laws pertain to fitting hearing aids on children that do not apply to adults. For example, all children must be examined by a physician, preferably an otolaryngologist, prior to wearing amplification. Adults can sign a waiver for this requirement, but children or parents of children under the age of 18 cannot. It is the audiologist's responsibility to ensure that medical clearance has been obtained within 6 months preceding the fitting of a hearing aid. Similarly, children can have hearing aids prescribed only by an audiologist, whereas adults can obtain amplification from a nonaudiologist hearing aid dispenser.

Candidacy for Amplification

The traditional definition of *degree of hearing impairment* has been redefined by the increasing knowledge that what was considered borderline normal hearing in an adult cannot be considered similarly for a child. The traditional classification of normal hearing in an adult listener is 25 dB or better. Yet, in a child of critical language learning age, this "borderline normal" hearing threshold level can produce a significant impact (15,16). One can anticipate that a child with hearing at 25 dB in the better ear will function at least 1 year delayed in language by the time it reaches school age. The child with a 35-dB loss in the better ear will be, on the average, 2 years delayed, and at 45 dB, 3 years delayed (17). Thus, the consideration of candidacy for amplification is somewhat different for a child than it is for an adult. A child who has a permanent hearing loss of greater than an average of 20 dB for the speech frequencies (500–3,000 Hz) should be considered a candidate for hearing aids. A child who has long-standing fluctuating hearing due to otitis media (e.g., the child with otitis media secondary to craniofacial anomalies) should be considered a candidate for either personal amplification (hearing aids) or ALDs.

Also, the child with a unilateral hearing impairment should not be overlooked. There is an an excellent case for using amplification due to the high number (35% fail at least one grade) of educational failures for children with unilateral losses (18). If the impaired ear has sufficient hearing, a monaural ear-level instrument could be provided on a trial basis. If the hearing loss is severe or profound (i.e., as may be found following mumps), a wireless CROS aid can be tried. Not all children, however, will accept amplification. For these children, use of FM systems and other forms of classroom amplification (see page 591) can be invaluable. In addition, the child and parents should be counseled that a unilateral hearing loss will not prevent the child from attending and succeeding in school as well as any other binaurally hearing child; that the teacher should be informed so that special seating arrangements can be made, if necessary; that speech reading is important; and that additional safeguards be taken to prevent deterioration of the good ear. These include, but are not limited to avoiding loud noises (firecrackers, personal headsets), receiving prompt otologic attention for ear infections or ear pain; giving special consideration to the use of potentially ototoxic medication; and obtaining periodic (annual) hearing tests and otologic consultation.

Age of Intervention

It has long been established that there is a critical language-learning period beyond which normal speech and language acquisition is compromised. Thus, the urgency of providing the pediatric patient with amplification at the earliest age possible, in order provide auditory stimulation, is obvious. A professional would be foolhardy, however, to prematurely prescribe amplification before a definitive identification of hearing impairment has been made. A definitive identification, however, differs from a complete description of the psychoacoustic characteristics of the child. If diagnosis of a hearing impairment has been made in the nursery and then confirmed with objective measures, such as auditory brainstem response (ABR) testing and otoacoustic emission testing, it is time to obtain hearing aids. In other words, *no one is too young for amplification.* The audiologist must be prepared to proceed with recommendations for hearing aids, even if a complete picture has not been established. Providing amplification for children is an ongoing process that requires flexibility and modifications in strategy as more information about the child s hearing abilities is obtained. This fact should be clearly explained to all the team members at the outset.

STRATEGIES IN THE SELECTION OF AMPLIFICATION

The first objective in fitting hearing aids is to *make soft sounds audible without making loud sounds uncomfortable.* As recently as 1990, the vast majority of hearing aids dispensed in the United States were of the linear type (19). This meant that the same amount of gain was applied to a low-intensity input as was applied to a high-intensity input. This occurred despite the fact that nearly all sensorineural-impaired listeners demonstrate recruitment (abnormal growth of loudness). In other words, while a hearing-impaired person may not be able to detect soft sounds (sounds below their threshold of audibility), intense sounds (sounds well above their threshold) may be perceived with the same loudness perception as that of the normal-hearing listener. If the normal cochlea was, as was once thought, linear, passive, and broadly tuned, then linear amplification would be appropriate for most hearing losses. However, recent findings indicate that this is certainly not an accurate description of the cochlea. The input–output function of the cochlea is nonlinear. At input sound levels less than 60 dB sound pressure level (SPL), a doubling of amplitude produces far less than a doubling of displacement of the basilar membrane. The active mechanical process of the outer hair cells ''amplifies'' these sounds while also sharpening frequency selectivity. Recruitment results from damage to or loss of the active process in the cochlea that enhances sensitivity for low-input sound levels. Because this process is nonlinear, it results in an amplification of the basilar membrane response to low-level sounds while leaving high-level sounds relatively unamplified. If this active process is compromised, the response to low-input sounds (below 60 dB) is unamplified and absolute threshold is elevated. However, the response to high-level sounds remains nearly the same as in the normal ear (20).

The use of nonlinear (or compression) amplification attempts to solve two important fitting problems. One, it minimizes the likelihood that amplified sound will reach the wearer's loudness discomfort level. If this level is reached, the user will typically lower the volume-control setting, thus causing components of the speech signal to be inaudible. Two, it prevents moderate input levels from driving the aid into saturation. It is believed that the main cause of decreased word recognition of sensorineural-impaired listeners in noisy situations is the presence of harmonic and intermodulation distortion produced by the hearing aid being driven into saturation (21).

An alternative approach to linear amplification that is useful in minimizing distortion and maintaining loudness comfort is compression (sometimes referred to as automatic gain control). In compression circuits, gain is automatically reduced once a predetermined level (either based on the input or the output level) is delivered to the hearing aid, in such a way that the aid never reaches the saturation point. An

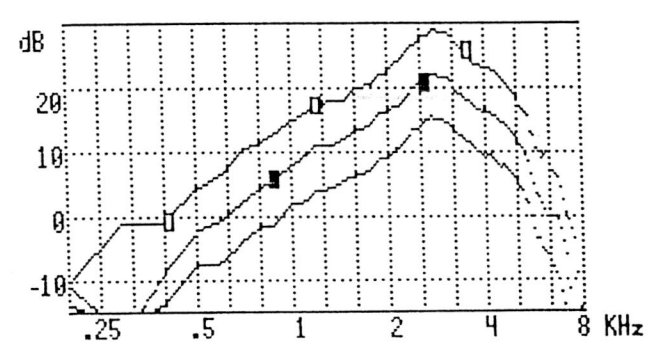

FIG. 5. Single-band compression. Upper curve generated with a 50-dB input, middle curve with a 70-dB input, and lower curve with a 90-dB input. Note progressively decreasing gain resulting as input level increases.

example of input-based compression is shown in Fig. 5. Note that as the input level increases beyond a critical point (the compression kneepoint), the amount of gain produced by the hearing aid decreases. In the past 5 years, compression has replaced linear amplification as the most popular approach to limiting loud sounds. There are some listeners, (e.g., those with conductive losses and those with severe or profound losses), however, who may function better with linear amplification (22). Still, for most children being fit with amplification, some form of compression amplification seems appropriate to ensure that high-input levels to the hearing aid (i.e., other children screaming on the playground) do not drive the hearing aid into distortion and do not exceed uncomfortable loudness levels.

A potential shortcoming of traditional compression circuits is that they are single-channel. Thus, the activating input signal triggers a gain reduction across the frequency range, often reducing the gain of the high frequencies so much that the consonant sounds are not audible. In other words, if the offending, unwanted signal is a low-frequency noise, there is no reason the high-frequency gain of the hearing aid should be compressed. It would be better, in these conditions, to lower only the gain of the unwanted low frequencies. This can be accomplished using multichannel compression. Several hearing aids are now available that incorporate multiple compression circuits acting independently for two or more frequency bands. These circuits are usually found in digitally programmable hearing aids.

Digitally Programmable Hearing Aids

Given the fact that audiologists often must select hearing aids and their specific electroacoustic settings for children based on incomplete patient data, it is always the basic rule to use the most flexible system possible. Current technology has produced a new generation of hearing aids that provide both greater flexibility and advanced compression characteristics. These aids are called digitally programmable. They are not truly digital, in that sound remains processed by analog components, as with conventional amplification, but digital technology is used to *program* the aids. This allows for the audiologist to program dramatic changes to the frequency response, gain, maximum output, and compression characteristics as more specific information becomes available. It also allows for reprogramming should the hearing loss change. Thus, these aids can be particularly useful for small children, children with fluctuating or progressive hearing losses, and children who have low tolerance levels to noise.

Some of these aids feature user-controlled multiple memories, which may be inappropriate for younger children but which can be used to great advantage by older children. It also should be noted that some audiologists advocate remote-controlled multiple memory aids for infants so that the parents can monitor the baby's response using different memories. This also has the always positive effect of increasing parental involvement. Certain hearing aids may not contain volume controls because of their advanced compression characteristics. This can be beneficial to the child who persistently manipulates the volume control in often undesired ways. Of course, conventional (nonprogrammable) hearing aids also can guard against this negative behavior by placing a cap over the volume control.

Unfortunately, despite the greater potential from digitally programmable instruments, many third party agents have not yet recognized their benefits and continue to refuse to reimburse for the added expense. It is hoped that this pattern will be altered in the near future.

Flexibility

When programmable aids cannot be utilized (usually due to financial constraints), it is important that the audiologist use hearing aids that have maximum flexibility. Nonprogrammable hearing aids should contain potentiometers, which allow for a wide range of maximum power (SSPL 90) control, low-frequency reduction, high-frequency roll-off, and compression adjustments.

Establishing the desired frequency response for hearing aids worn by youngsters often requires different philosophies than those typical for adults. For example, adults often prefer low-frequency amplification to be minimized because of upward spread of masking (low frequencies masking high frequencies) as well as amplification of unwanted background noise. Prelingual children, however, may require amplification of the low frequencies because they need to hear the intonation patterns and suprasegmental information found in that range.

FITTING PROCEDURES

Hearing aid selection procedures have undergone numerous and dramatic changes in the past few years. Audiologists no longer choose the "best" system on the basis of which "preselected" hearing aid provides the highest monosyllabic word recognition score (a low face validity task that is rendered impractical in children with limited language skills). Comparative procedures have been replaced largely by the use of prescriptive formulas. Current hearing aid selection procedures begin with the establishment of targets for gain (and ideally, maximum output). These computer-generated targets are based on the individual's threshold data and ear canal resonance.

Real Ear (Probe Microphone) Measures

Although researchers have proposed a variety of formulas to best predict the "ideal" aided response, it was not until the refinement of probe microphone, or real ear, measures that prescriptive techniques really became predominant. Probe microphone (or probe tube) measurements allow for a noninvasive, rapid measurement of the sound received within approximately 5 mm of the tympanic membrane, and thus take into account the effects of the ear canal. It has long been known that the physical characteristics of the external auditory meatus produce a resonance that may vary from ear to ear. Figure 6 depicts an "average" adult Real Ear Unaided Response (REUR) of the unoccluded ear, as well as a real ear aided response (REAR) for the same patient. Modern prescriptive formulas are based on the assumption that a systematic relationship exists between hearing thresholds and judgments of comfort or preference, thereby resulting in specific gain at each frequency. The formula specifies a target goal to which an attempt is made to match the real ear insertion response (REIR), which is simply the difference between the REAR measured at the tympanic membrane and the REUR (Fig. 7). In children, however, the SPL generated at the eardrum can easily exceed the same SPL at the eardrum of an adult by more than 6 or even 12 dB (Fig. 8). This occurs because the average adult has approximately 1.5 to 2.0 cc of airspace between the receiver of the hearing aid and the eardrum, compared with the child, who often has a volume as small as 1.0 cc or even 0.5 cc. For every halving of the volume, there is a 6-dB increase in sound pressure. Thus, if a hearing aid produces 110-dB SPL at the tympanic membrane of an adult with a 2-cc volume, that same hearing aid will deliver 116-dB SPL to the child with a 1-cc volume and 122-dB SPL to an infant having a physical volume of only 0.5 cc. Thus, confirmation with real ear probe microphone measures is critical. Note, too, that the resonant frequency of the ear canal is typically higher for a child than it is for an adult. In fact, a newborn's ear canal resonance can be as high as 7,000 Hz but tends to approach adult resonance by 2 years of age.

Among the more important pieces of information provided by real ear measures are those that relate to the effect of earmold coupling on the hearing aid's response as received at the tympanic membrane. As already stated, the REUR shows the natural resonance produced by the physical characteristics of the external ear. When an ITE or BTE aid coupled to an earmold of any style fully or partially occludes the ear, this natural resonance is altered. The amount of occlusion, vent length and diameter, length of the earmold, bore of the earmold, and so on, all have measurable effects on the natural resonance and ultimately on the REAR. Generally, the larger the vent, the less the low-frequency gain; the longer the canal length, the greater the overall gain. If the coupler contains a belled bore, the greater the high-frequency gain.

It should be noted that specifications of hearing aids are published using hard-walled couplers containing 2 cc of airspace. So, once again, they underestimate the power reaching the ear of a child. Generally, the 2-cc coupler response of a hearing aid overestimates real ear gain between 2,000

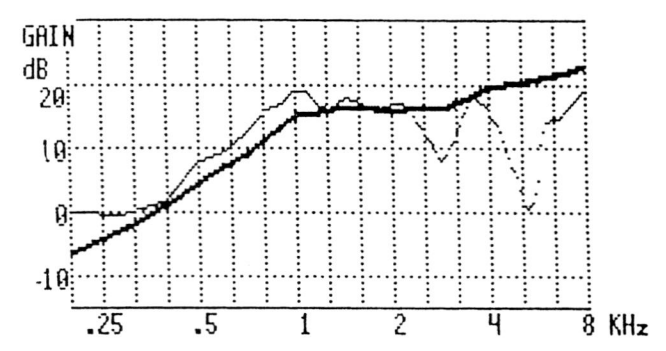

FIG. 7. Match of the REIR and target *(thick line)*.

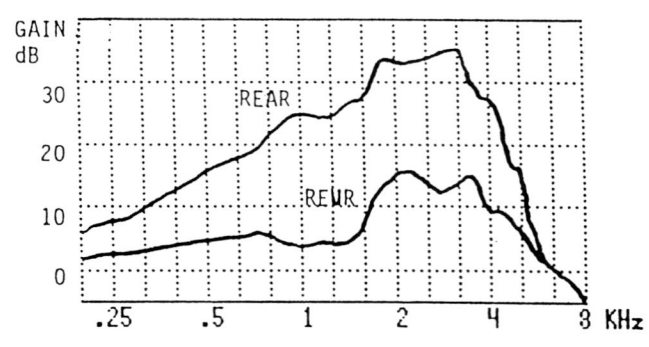

FIG. 6. Normal adult REUR and REAR.

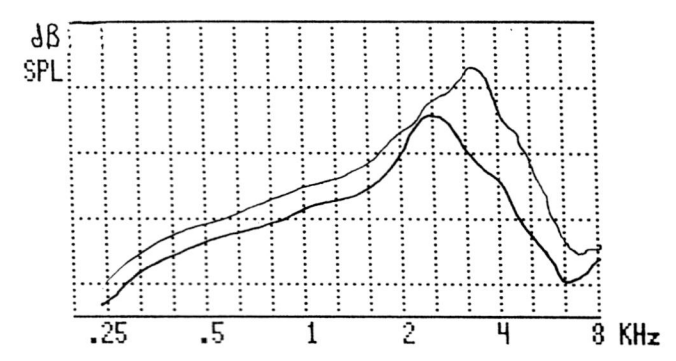

FIG. 8. Real ear aided response of adult *(thick line)* versus that of a 1-year-old child using the same hearing aid.

and 4,000 Hz by 12 to 18 dB and underestimates the real ear gain below 1,500 Hz by 5 to 7 dB.

DETERMINING MAXIMUM OUTPUT OR SATURATION SOUND PRESSURE LEVEL

Because of the increased SPL generated in small ear canals and the measurement uncertainty of the individual child's loudness discomfort levels, perhaps the most important real ear probe microphone measure to be obtained in children is the real ear saturation response (RESR). The RESR is simply the REAR measured with a 90-dB SPL pure-tone input. This input level is sufficient to drive the hearing aid into saturation so that there is a measure of the maximum amount of amplification provided by the hearing aid regardless of further increases in input. The hard-walled coupler equivalent to this procedure formerly was referred to in the literature as the maximum power output and is now commonly termed the *SSPL 90*. It is an essential measure toensure that the individual's loudness discomfort level is not exceeded. It is also crucial to compare the RESR to the REAR to ensure that there is at least a 10- to 20-dB difference so that there is adequate "headroom" present in the hearing aid to minimize distortion for high-input levels.

In addition, it is important to realize that the input SPL generated at the microphone of hearing aids worn by infants often is considerably greater than that for adults. This occurs because the baby may be receiving the parent's voice from a very close distance (i.e. if the baby is held on the parent's shoulder). As a result, both the gain and power requirements may be less for the baby. Thus, the use of conservative maximum power control via compression amplification is prudent in most cases.

The preferable amplification system is one that amplifies the widest possible speech spectrum 10 to 20 dB above the aided threshold. Researchers have proposed using probe tube measures with determination of loudness discomfort levels in children (23). These procedures assume that the child is capable of generating behavioral thresholds and reporting discomfort. Other techniques have been developed that do not rely on subjective test procedures (24).

Desired Sensation Level Approach

The goal of all hearing aid fittings is to package the amplified speech inside of the listener's dynamic range (defined as threshold level to loudness discomfort level) (25). In other words, the amplified signal must be audible across the frequency range but must not be uncomfortably loud for the listener at any frequency. Refined computer software packages, such as the Desired Sensation Level (Auditech, St. Louis, Mo) (26) are available that prescribe the amount of desired gain and output in order to allow conversational speech to fall within these limits. These programs map the amplified level of conversational speech in relationship to the listener's threshold and REAR. Additionally, and of extreme importance, they also map the desired maximum output against the listener's RESR. It is assumed that in order to achieve maximum potential in speech discrimination, it is important to amplify (to a comfortable level) as much of the speech spectrum as possible. It is possible to estimate the average decibel levels above threshold (sensation level) at which the child receives conversational speech by subtracting the aided thresholds (in dB SPL) from the average speech spectrum. The average conversational (70-dB SPL) speech spectrum approximates (for narrow bands of noise) 60 dB at 250 Hz, 61 dB at 500 Hz, 58 dB at 1,000 Hz, 54 dB at 2,000 Hz, and 46 dB at 4,000 Hz (27). The desired sensation level approach determines suprathreshold target levels by using estimates of long-term average speech relative to the child's unaided sound field thresholds. A formula is utilized in which the desired sensation level of amplified speech decreases in an accelerated nonlinear function with increasing levels of hearing loss. Using this formula, the audiologist can determine target levels and then utilize either behavioral techniques or real ear measures to verify the acoustic fit. Formulas also are provided for determining the maximum power output, again based on unaided threshold data.

Despite the proliferation of real ear prescriptive procedures, it is critical that the audiologist view these results merely as "starting off" points. Keep in mind that even though real ear measures are a step in the right direction in tailoring the aid to the individual's external ear canal characteristics, further individual variations in loudness growth, and so on, still need to be accounted for. Therefore, additional fine tuning must be made to suit the individual's preference and verification procedures by using a variety of stimuli including speech.

Alternate Approaches

Some children will not cooperate for real ear probe microphone measures. Because it is often difficult to establish certain psychoacoustic characteristics of the child's hearing loss, alternative approaches have been proposed. One alternative approach uses two of the tests used in the immittance battery to help determine the maximum desirable SPL output level. Recall that the SPL reaching a child's eardrum is increased (relative to that of an adult) because of the reduced cavity of air entrapped between the end of the earmold and the eardrum. By the inverse square law, every halving of the cavity volume (using 2 cc as a reference) increases SPL by 6 dB. It has been demonstrated that this difference is even larger when compared with measures made using a 2-cc coupler (28). As part of the immittance battery, a physical volume test can be performed to rapidly ascertain cavity size. Then, depending on the results, the maximum power of the hearing aid can be adjusted appropriately. In addition, information gleaned from the acoustic reflex thresholds (when present) can be used to estimate the maximum desired output. This is done by ensuring that the maximum power level (SSPL 90) does not exceed the SPL that elicits an aided stapedial reflex. Unfortunately, this technique can be used in only less than half of the cases, because the reflex will be absent in severe and profound losses, as well as in children with middle ear pathology (29).

Some authors have suggested using ABR results to help set the gain of hearing aids for children (30). They recommend that the gain of the aid be adjusted to the level at which further increases in gain no longer produce further decreases in the wave V latency. This technique has been shown to be more effective for a flat audiometric configuration. It is also limited by the fact that use of clicks as the ABR stimulus does not provide frequency specificity, and use of tone pips is not as accurate.

A simple formula for calculating desired SSPL 90 also has been proposed (17).

It specifies setting maximum power as follows:
For preschoolers:

$$100 \text{ dB} + 1/4 \text{ dB HL at } 1,000, 2,000, \text{ and } 4,000 \text{ Hz} - 5 \text{ dB}$$

For infants and toddlers:

$$100 \text{ dB} + 1/4 \text{ dB HL at } 1,000, 2,000, \text{ and } 4,000 \text{ Hz} - 10 \text{ dB}$$

The calculated SSPL 90 should then be confirmed by measurement of the RESR, if possible.

ADDITIONAL CONSIDERATIONS FOR AMPLIFICATION FOR CHILDREN

Because children are curious and unpredictable, certain precautionary safety measures should be taken to prevent potential injuries. For example, although adults know better than to ingest batteries (barring occasional confusion with pills), hearing aids for young children should be ordered with tamper-proof battery compartments. Older children are easily taught how to change batteries when needed, but this mechanism will prevent young children from gaining access to the potentially toxic batteries. Hearing aids for children also can be ordered (or retrofit) with volume-control covers to prevent the child from changing the gain of the hearing aid. Children tend to lose (accidentally or on purpose) their expensive hearing aids. Fabric headbands will help keep BTE products on the young child. Even with such security, there is no guarantee that the resourceful child will not find a way to remove the aids and flush them down the toilet or feed them to the family dog. Thus, it is absolutely essential that all hearing aids ordered for children be accompanied by an extended loss and damage insurance policy.

MAXIMIZING SIGNAL-TO-NOISE RATIO WITH ASSISTIVE LISTENING DEVICES

One of the major goals of amplification strategies is to enhance the signal-to-noise ratio perceived by the listener. The use of aids with automatic low-frequency reduction represents an attempt at this goal. However, despite all the new technologic advances discussed so far in this chapter, a basic problem remains for which wearable amplification falls woefully short. That problem relates to the physical distance between the microphone of the hearing aid and the source of the sound desired to be heard. Intensity decreases by 6 dB for every doubling of the distance, according to the inverse square law. Thus, if the intensity of a speaker standing 3 feet from the listener is 60 dB, that intensity will only be 54 dB if the speaker-to-listener distance is 6 feet. Unfortunately, background noise often surrounds the listener, so while the intensity of the speech decreases with distance, the intensity of the noise may not. Referring to the example just stated; if the original signal to noise ratio was +5 dB (meaning that the speech intensity is 5 dB greater than the noise intensity) at 3 feet, that signal-to-noise ratio could decrease to −1 dB at 6 feet. This is one reason why hearing aids transmit sound so well if the speaker talks directly into the microphone, but at longer, more realistic distances, reception diminishes. It would be ideal to have the sound produced at the source transferred directly to the listener without losing any intensity. It is obviously impractical, however, to ask the speaker to move closer to the listener's ear. One way of achieving this effect is with DAI, in which the speaker holds near his or her mouth a microphone that is hard wired to the hearing aid itself. This is obviously impractical in the classroom, however. An attempt at improving the signal-to-noise ratio has been made using multiple and directional microphones on BTE hearing aids, but these maneuvers still fail to minimize the loss of signal intensity due to distance.

An alternative approach is available through infrared transmission, FM transmission, or inductance loop transmission. These systems are used by many theaters, concert halls, houses of worship, and households. One of the best uses is for television listening. The portable transmitter, usually a box smaller than most cable boxes, and microphone are located near the television's loudspeaker. The sound picked up by the microphone is then transmitted to a receiver, worn by the listener, without any decrease in intensity. These devices can transmit with minimal distortion over a considerable distance (up to 50 ft). Infrared transmissions are limited, in that a direct line of sight is required. Frequency modulation transmission actually can occur around corners and even into different rooms (though occasionally another FM receiver using a similar frequency can cause interference). Inductance loop systems often do not require an expensive receiver, because they are compatible with the telephone coils found in many BTE and some ITE hearing aids. They are sometimes not as popular as infrared and FM systems because they require that a loop be placed around the circumference of the listening area.

Personal FM systems are the preferred choice for maximizing signal to noise ratio. The signal can be coupled directly to the child's ear via earphones, but if the child owns personal hearing aids, it is better to have the signal modified in a manner consistent with the individual's hearing loss characteristics. This is optimally accomplished by having the FM receiver connected directly (via Direct Audio Input (DAI) to the hearing aid. An alternative is to have the signal picked up by a loop worn around the neck that will electromagnetically induce current in the telecoil of the hearing aid. The reason that DAI is preferred is that some hearing aids do not have particularly strong telecoils and that the frequency response of the telecoil may not be the same as that of the hearing aid itself.

Classroom Amplification

Studies have indicated that noise levels in excess of 35 dBA (31) and reverberant conditions (32) can have a deleterious effect on the educational performance of hearing-impaired students. Thus, one might assume that a high priority is placed on classroom acoustics. Unfortunately, while the intention might be there, the funds often are not available to improve classroom acoustics. Average noise levels in schoolrooms range from 55 to 69 dB (33). When this condition is added to the fact that the intensity of the desired signal (presumably the teacher's voice) decreases as a function of distance, the effective signal-to-noise ratio received by the hearing impaired student is often very poor (<0 dB).

Pediatric audiologists must serve as educators and advocates for enhancing room acoustics. Suggestions for inexpensive improvements such as carpeting, fabric, or absorbent material on non-opposing walls; lowering or use of false ceilings; felt fabric on the bottoms of chairs and desks; and so on are all of some help. Many schools place loudspeakers in various locations within the classroom in order to distribute the sound of the teacher s voice evenly in all areas. This is accomplished by having the teacher wear a wireless lavaliere microphone, similar to the arrangement used with FM systems.

It should also be pointed out that an increasing number of advocates propose the use of ALDs for children facing potential educational barriers because of unilateral hearing losses, minimal hearing losses, learning disabilities, central auditory processing disorders, or attention-deficit disorders.

Tactile Devices

Tactile aids transform auditory signals into either vibratory (vibrotactile devices) or electrical (electrotactile devices) patterns on the surface of the skin. The objective of these devices is to supplement or replace acoustic information to the hearing-impaired individual. These devices, while often lacking wide band reproducibility and high power, may be useful in teaching and reinforcing speech production (34). In the future, they may be combined with cochlear implants to increase efficiency.

Wearing Instructions for Children and Parents

Children exhibit a wide variety of responses to wearing amplification. Some are so pleased that they are receiving auditory stimulation that they do not want to take the hearing aids off, even when going to bed. Others are very reluctant to wear the aids in public, and still others refuse to wear them in public or at home. When a child refuses to wear hearing aids, the first question that must be addressed is, "Are the aids set appropriately?" Once the audiologist is satisfied that the aids are not overamplifying at any frequency region for any input intensity, the attention must be turned toward issues regarding physical comfort and then toward emotional reasons for rejection. Additionally, the audiologist should consider whether refusal to wear amplification is a sole decision by the child or whether other family members are contributing to the rejection.

When the child first receives new amplification, the parents (or caretaker) should be supplied with a battery tester, a listening stethoscope, and printed information to augment the instructions given by the audiologist. It is important to recognize when the parents are becoming overloaded with information.

Parents (and older children) should be given detailed instructions regarding insertion and removal of earmolds; setting the volume control; daily cleaning and checking of the earmolds, tubing, and hearing aids; recognizing when feedback is caused by improper insertion versus poor fit; and when and how to change batteries.

Parents should be provided with a stethoscope and taught to perform daily listening checks of the hearing aids. This exercise should include listening to a broad sample of consonant sounds (particularly the high-frequency /s/, /f/, and /th/ sounds), vowels, softly spoken sounds, and sounds spoken loudly. The volume control should be moved slowly so that any nonlinearity, crackling, or dead spots will be detected. After some practice, most parents will be able to recognize distortion and/or insufficient gain. Parents should be encouraged to consult with the audiologist at the first sign of concern regarding the status of the hearing aids, earmolds, or the child's hearing.

Parents must assume responsibility for the child's hearing aid use until such time as the child is capable of doing so. The parents, not the child, should decide when the hearing aids should be removed and put them away. If the child removes the hearing aids, it is important to reinsert them as soon as possible to facilitate the adjustment process. However, as stated earlier, if repeated complaints are expressed, parents should contact the child's audiologist to determine the cause. Hearing aids need to become a part of the child's daily routine, just as glasses would be if the child were visually impaired. Parents must be encouraged to observe the child and note changes in behavior and responsiveness to sound when the hearing aids are worn. This information can be very valuable to the audiologist when modifications are necessary.

Some audiologists prefer a 1-week break-in time, with increased usage each day. Others prefer full usage immediately. Generally speaking, hearing aids should be worn, except when the child is bathing, sleeping, or engaging in rough play.

Follow-up Procedures

Competent audiologic and amplification care does not end with the fitting of the hearing aids. It is essential that excellent follow-up care be directed toward the child, the parents, the educator, the physician, and the speech-language pathologist.

The child and parents should be seen for follow-up counseling, repeat real ear measures, and, when appropriate, aided speech discrimination testing within 2 weeks of the child's being fit with amplification. In addition, children under 3 months of age should receive an unaided and aided hearing retest every 3 months, children under age 7 years should be retested every 6 months, and older children should be retested annually. Earmolds should be checked for the need for tubing changes and possible replacement every year (every 6 months for children under age 5 years).

Teachers and speech-language pathologists should be contacted shortly after the child is fitted so that any questions regarding hearing aid maintenance and room acoustics can be addressed. In addition, schools should provide teachers with battery testers and listening stethoscopes so that daily listening checks can be conducted. This applies not only to personal hearing aids, but also to FM devices and other ALDs.

The child's physician, teacher, and speech-language pathologist should receive reports from the audiologist concerning realistic benefits and limitations of amplification for the individual child with regard to speech-language development and educational prowess.

CAN HEARING AIDS DAMAGE HEARING?

There is no doubt that repeated exposure to extremely high SPLs can cause a temporary or permanent threshold shift. When an individual has a hearing loss, it is obvious that all reasonable precautionary measures should be taken to preserve residual hearing. For example, common sense dictates that it is appropriate to protect the ears from high noise levels, such as gunfire, extremely loud music, and so forth, but what about everyday sounds that are amplified through hearing aids? Can hearing aids cause further damage to hearing? Determining an answer to this question is particularly crucial for pediatric patients, because children may be incapable of reporting changes in their hearing status.

The literature contains numerous references suggesting hearing loss resulting from hearing aid use. A 10-year-old child with a bilateral, moderate sensorineural hearing loss, whose (body-borne) aided ear showed deterioration relative to her unaided ear after 14 months' use (35). After alternating the ear in which the hearing aid was worn, a temporary threshold shift in the aided ear was repeatedly observed. Another study (36) discussed two patients whose hearing temporarily decreased but then returned to baseline following a switch to less powerful amplification. Another researcher found that thresholds of four deaf children improved over a weekend, during which they removed their hearing aids completely, but then decreased again after only 4 hours of hearing aid use (37).

Not all researchers support the notion of decreased hearing following high-gain amplification. Following a review of the records of 120 randomly selected hearing aid patients, one author concluded, on the basis of comparison of hearing loss progression of the aided versus nonaided ear, that changes in hearing as a result of hearing aid use are statistically and clinically nonsignificant (38). These conclusions have been supported by others, as well (39,40).

Regardless of one's conclusion, the serious clinician can not overlook the possibility that high-gain amplification can produce at least a temporary threshold shift. Thus, it appears prudent that the following steps be implemented:

1. Limit the maximum power reaching a child's eardrum to 130 dB SPL (verified via probe microphone measures).
2. Use output-limiting strategies such as compression amplification.
3. Reevaluate hearing after 1 month of high-gain hearing aid use; then check every 3 months for the first year and annually thereafter.

The increasing use of compression in hearing aids, combined with the ability to verify the true acoustic intensity reaching the child's eardrum, signifies that acoustic trauma due to overamplification should never occur for properly fitting hearing aids.

Given all of these precautions, it is equally important that children not be underamplified in an effort to preserve hearing. Underamplification, particularly during the critical language-learning years, is as likely to produce damaging effects on the childs potential as is overamplification.

SUMMARY AND CONCLUSIONS

Fitting amplification on children is an ongoing process, requiring maximum flexibility in thinking. Teamwork is essential. The basic team consists of a pediatric audiologist, a pediatric otologist, a pediatrician, an educator of the hearing impaired, and a speech-language pathologist. Also, remember that the child's family represents one of the most important components of the team. No one is too young for amplification. The audiologist must be prepared to proceed with recommendations for hearing aids, even if a complete picture has not been established.

Whenever possible, children should be fit with binaural BTEs containing telecoils and DAI. Because of the link between hearing and language acquisition, children with unilateral, and even mild, hearing losses should be considered candidates for either personal amplification (hearing aids) or ALDs.

Hearing aids should allow soft sounds to be audible and loud sounds to be comfortable.

Maximum flexibility is essential in hearing aids. This can be best achieved using programmable instruments. Probe microphone measurements should be performed to account for the greater SPL generated at the eardrum in children. The use of conservative maximum power control via compression amplification is prudent in most cases.

Assistive listening devices, such as FM units, should be considered for all hearing-impaired children. The possibility that high-gain amplification can produce at least a temporary threshold shift must be considered; thus, it is wise to limit the maximum power reaching a child's eardrum to 130 dB SPL. It is also essential to not underamplify in an effort to preserve hearing.

Close follow-up care with other team members is crucial. Children under 3 months of age should receive an unaided and aided hearing retest every 3 months, children under age 7 years should be retested every 6 months, and older children should be retested annually.

REFERENCES

1. Dobie RA, Berlin, CI. Influence of otitis media on hearing loss and development. *Ann Otol Rhinol Laryngol* 1979; [Suppl 60]:48–53.
2. Friel-Patti S, Finitzo T. Language learning in a prospective study of otitis media with effusion in the first two years of life. *J Speech Hear Res* 1990;33:188–94.
3. Sweetow R, Barrager D. Quality of comprehensive audiologic care: a survey of parents of hearing impaired children. *Am Speech Hear Assoc J* 1980;22:841–7.
4. US Department of Health and Human Services. *Healthy people 2000: national health promotion and disease prevention objectives.* Washington, DC: Public Health Service; 1990.
5. Sweetow RW. Selecting ITE fittings for the pediatric population. *Hear Instr* 1989;40:10.
6. Sweetow RW. ITEs for children, revisited. *Hear Instr* 1990;41:8.
7. Koenig W. Subjective effects in binaural hearing. *J Acoust Soc Am* 1950;22:61–2.
8. Licklider JC. Influence of interaural phase relations upon the masking of speech by white noise. *J Acoust Soc Am* 1948;20:150–9.
9. Hirsh IJ. The influence of interaural phase on interaural summation and inhibition. *J Acoust Soc Am* 1948;20:536–44.
10. Silman S, Gelfand S, Silverman C. Effects of monaural versus binaural hearing aids. *J Acoustic Soc Am* 1984;76:1357–62.
11. Silverman C, Silman S. Apparent auditory deprivation from monaural amplification and recovery with binaural amplification: two case studies. *J Am Acad Audiol* 1990;1:175–80.
12. Zink G. Hearing aids children wear. *Volta Rev* 1972;74:41–51.
13. *Federal Register.* 1977, August 23; 121a.303.
14. Downs M. The case for detection and intervention at birth. *Semin Hear* 1994;15;76–83.
15. Matkin ND. The role of hearing in language development. In Kavanagh JF, ed. *Otitis media and child development.* Parkton, MD: York Press; 1986:3–11.
16. Bullerdeick K. Minimal hearing loss may not be benign. *Am J Nurs* 1987;87:904–6.
17. Matkin ND. Pediatric hearing aid fittings. Presented at the Academy of Dispensing Audiologists, Las Vegas, October 1989.
18. Bess FH Tharpe AM. Unilateral hearing impairment in children. *Pediatrics* 1984;74:206–16.
19. Hawkins D. Acoustic measures of hearing aid performance. In: Studebaker GF, Bess FH, Beck LB eds. *The Vanderbilt hearing aid report II.* Parkton, MD: York Press; 1991:123–9.
20. Kates J. Modeling normal and hearing impaired hearing: implications for hearing aid design. *Ear Hear* 1991;12[Supp6]:162S–76S.
21. Fabry, DA. Programmable and automatic noise reduction in existing hearing aids. In: Studebaker GA, Bess FH, and Beck LB, eds. *The Vanderbilt hearing aid report II.* Parkton, MD: York Press; 1991: 65–78.
22. Boothroyd A, Springer N, Smith L, Schulman J. Amplitude compression and profound hearing loss. *J Speech Hear Res* 1988;31:362–76.
23. Stuart A, Durieux-Smith A, Stenstrom R. Probe tube microphone measures of loudness discomfort levels in children. *Ear Hear* 1991;12: 140–3.
24. Hawkins D, Morrison T, Halligan P, Cooper W. The use of probe tube microphone measurements in hearing aid selection for children. *Ear Hear* 1989;10:281–7.
25. Skinner M, Pascoe D, Miller J, Popelka G. Measurements to determine the optimal placement of speech energy within the listeners' auditory area. In: Studebaker G, Bess F, eds. *The Vanderbilt report.* Upper Darby, PA: Monographs in Contemporary Audiology; 1982;161–9.
26. Seewald R. The desired sensation level approach for children: selection and verification. *Hear Instr* 1988;39:18–22.
27. Gengel RW, Pascoe D, Shore I. A frequency response procedure for evaluating and selecting hearing aids for severely hearing impaired children. *J Speech Hear Disord* 1971;36:341–53.
28. Jirsa R, Norris TW. Relationship of acoustic gain to aided threshold improvement in children. *J Speech Hear Disord* 1978;43:348–51.
29. Hall JW, Ruth RA. Acoustic reflexes and auditory evoked responses in hearing aid evaluation. *Semin Hearing* 1986;6:251–77.
30. Cox LC, Metz DA. ABER in the prescription of hearing aids. *Hear Instr* 1980;31:12–15
31. Bess FH, McConnell F. *Audiology, education, and the hearing impaired child.* St. Louis: Mosby; 1981.
32. Finitzo-Hieber T. Classroom acoustics. In: Roeser RJ, Downs MP, eds. *Auditory disorders in school children.* New York: Thieme-Stratton; 1982:14.
33. Sanders D. Noise conditions in normal school classrooms. *Except Child* 1965;31.344–53.
34. Friel-Patti S, Roeser RR. Evaluating changes in the communication skills of deaf children using vibrotactile stimulation. *Ear Hear* 1985; 4:31–40.
35. Kasten R, Braunlin R. Traumatic hearing aid usage: a case study. Presented at the American Speech and Hearing Association, Chicago, November 1970.
36. Heffernan HP, Simons MR. Temporary increase in sensorineural hearing loss with hearing aid use. *Ann Otol Rhinol Otolaryngol* 1979;88: 86–91.
37. Macrae JH. TTS and recovery from TTS after use of powerful hearing aids. *J Acoust Soc Am* 1968;44:1445–6.
38. Naunton RF. The effect of hearing aid use upon the user's residual hearing. *Laryngoscope* 1957;67:569–76.
39. Titche LL, Windrem EO, Searmel WL. Hearing aids and hearing deterioration. *Ann Otol Rhinol Otolaryngol* 1977;86:357.
40. Darbyshire JV. A study of the use of high power hearing aids by children with marked degrees of deafness and the possibility of deterioration in acuity. *Br J Audiol* 1976;10:74–8.

CHAPTER 40

Pediatric Cochlear Implantation

Richard T. Miyamoto, Karen I. Kirk, and Amy M. Robbins

Cochlear implants are electronic devices which consist of an electrode array that is surgically implanted into the cochlea, an external unit consisting of a microphone that picks up sound energy and converts it to an electric signal, and a signal processor that modifies the signal according to the processing scheme used. The processed signal is amplified and compressed to match the narrow electrical dynamic range of the ear. The typical response range of a deaf ear to electrical stimulation is only 10 to 20 dB, and even less in the high frequencies. Transmission of the electrical signal across the skin from the external unit to the implanted electrode array is most commonly accomplished by the use of electromagnetic induction or radiofrequency transmission. The various cochlear implant devices differ with respect to processing schemes (feature extraction or analogue), placement of electrodes (intracochlear or extracochlear), stimulation configuration (monopolar or bipolar), and method of transmission of the signal through the skin (transcutaneous or percutaneous).

In the cochlea, the critical residual neural elements stimulated appear to be the spiral ganglion cells or axons. Damaged or missing hair cells of the cochlea are bypassed.

MULTICHANNEL PROCESSING STRATEGIES

Multichannel, multielectrode cochlear implants use place coding to transfer high-frequency information in addition to accurately providing time and intensity information. Two types of multichannel cochlear implants are available in the United States. The Nucleus 22-channel cochlear (Cochlear Corporation, Englewood, CO) implant has received approval from the Food and Drug Administration (FDA) for use in both adults and children and is the most commonly used multichannel system. The Nucleus implantable electrode array consists of platinum-iridium band electrodes placed in a silastic carrier (1).

Several generations of speech processors have been employed with the Nucleus multichannel cochlear implant. Until recently, all the Nucleus speech processors used a feature-extraction scheme in which selected key features of speech were presented to the central auditory system through the implanted electrode array. An early speech processing strategy, the F0F1F2 strategy, primarily conveyed vowel information, including the first and second formant frequencies and their amplitudes, as well as voice pitch. A later coding scheme, the MULTIPEAK strategy, presented these acoustic features along with additional information from three high-frequency spectral bands. The aim of the MULTIPEAK scheme was to present additional cues that would aid in the perception of consonants. The current speech processing strategy provided to all who receive the Nucleus 22-channel implant is the Spectral Peak (SPEAK) strategy implemented in the Spectra 22 processor. This strategy uses a vocoder in which a filter bank consisting of 20 filters covering the center frequencies from 200 to 10,000 Hz is employed. Each filter is allocated to an active electrode in the array. The filter outputs are scanned and the electrodes that are stimulated represent filters that contain speech components with the highest amplitude. Depending on the acoustic input, the number of spectral maxima detected, and thus the number of electrodes stimulated, on each scan cycle can vary from one to ten, with an average of six per cycle. The rate at which the electrodes are stimulated varies adaptively between 180 to 300 pulses per second.

The Clarion multichannel cochlear implant (Advanced Bionics Corporation, Sylmar, CA) has recently received FDA approval for use in adults but remains under investigation for children. The Clarion multichannel cochlear implant has an eight-channel electrode array that utilizes a radial bipolar configuration through electrode pairs positioned adjacent to

---

R.T. Miyamoto and A.M. Robbins: Department of Otolaryngology—Head and Neck Surgery, Indiana University Medical School, DeVault Otologic Research Laboratory; and Riley Children's Hospital, Indianapolis, Indiana 46202.

K.I. Kirk: Department of Otolaryngology—Head and Neck Surgery, Indiana University Medical School, DeVault Otologic Research Laboratory, Indianapolis, Indiana 46202.

the osseous spiral lamina in a 90-degree orientation. Theoretically, the radial bipolar orientation is more beneficial in achieving channel separation (2). The Clarion multichannel cochlear implant offers two types of speech processing strategies: compressed analog (CA) and continuous interleaved sampling (CIS). Both strategies represent the waveform or envelope of the speech signal (3). The Clarion CA strategy first compresses the analog signal into the restricted range for electrically evoked hearing, then filters the signal into a maximum of eight channels for presentation to the corresponding electrodes. Speech information is conveyed via the relative amplitudes and the temporal details contained in each channel. The CIS strategy filters the incoming speech into eight bands, and then obtains the speech envelope and compresses the signal for each channel. Stimulation consists of interleaved digital pulses that sweep rapidly through the channels at about 800 pulses per second. With the CIS strategy, rapid changes in the speech signal are tracked by rapid variations in pulse amplitude. More than 90% of Clarion multichannel cochlear implant recipients use the CIS speech-processing strategy (4).

PATIENT SELECTION

The selection of cochlear implant candidates is a complex and ever-evolving process that requires careful consideration of many factors. Current selection criteria are as follows:

1. Age 2 years or older
2. Profound bilateral sensorineural hearing loss
3. No appreciable benefit from hearing aids
4. No medical contraindications
5. High motivation and appropriate expectations
6. Enrolled in program that emphasizes development of auditory skills

Age Considerations

Because otolaryngologists are increasingly familiar with cochlear implantation in children, a trend toward earlier implantation has emerged in an attempt to ameliorate the devastating effects of early auditory deprivation. Electrical stimulation appears to prevent at least some of the degenerative changes in the central auditory pathways (5).

A lower age limit of 2 years has been applied during the FDA clinical trials. However, because the development of speech perception, speech production, and language competence normally begins at a very early age, implanting congenitally or neonatally deafened children under age 2 years may have substantial advantages over implantation at a later age. As with older children, profound deafness must be substantiated and the inability to benefit from conventional hearing aids demonstrated. The audiologic assessment in children younger than 2 years remains extremely challenging. In addition, when the etiology of deafness is meningitis, progressive intracochlear ossification can preclude standard electrode insertion. A relatively short time window exists during which this advancing process can be circumvented. Impending intracochlear ossification may serve as another incentive to consider implantation before the age of 2 years.

Lowering the age of implantation to less than 2 years requires special consideration of the small dimensions of the temporal bone and the potential problems from postoperative temporal bone growth. However, the feasibility of implantation earlier than the currently accepted age of 2 years is substantiated by developmental anatomy. The cochlea is adult size at birth; (6) by age 1 year, the facial recess and mastoid antrum, which provide access to the middle ear for electrode placement, are adequately developed. For these reasons, extension of implant candidacy to the 1- to 2-year age group is feasible and, in selected patients, is desirable. No upper age limit is applied as long as the patient's health status permits an elective surgical procedure. At the time of this writing, the age at implantation in the Indiana University Cochlear Implant Program spans a range from 16 months to 87 years.

Categories of Recipients

Pediatric cochlear implant recipients can be loosely divided into three main categories that significantly affect the anticipated outcomes when this technology is applied.

1. Postlingually deafened children. Children who become deaf at or after age 5 are generally classified as postlingually deafened. Even though these children have developed many aspects of spoken language before the onset of their deafness, they demonstrate rapid deterioration in the intelligibility of their speech once they lose access to auditory input and feedback. Early implantation can potentially ameliorate the rapid deterioration in speech production and perception abilities. However, a postlingual onset of deafness is an infrequent occurrence in the pediatric population. If this were to be the only category for which cochlear implants positively affected deaf children, there would be limited applicability for this technology in children.
2. Congenitally or early-deafened young children. Congenital or early-acquired deafness is the most frequently encountered type of profound sensorineural hearing loss (SNHL). The acquisition of communication skills is a difficult process for these children. Whether sufficient acoustic input can be provided by cochlear implantation to perceive a speech signal linguistically is currently the focus of a comprehensive longitudinal study.
3. Congenitally or early-deafened adolescents. When one considers cochlear implantation for an adolescent or young adult patient who has had little or no experience with sound because of congenital or early-onset deafness, caution must be exercised because this group has not demonstrated high levels of success with electrical stimulation of the auditory system.

Audiologic Assessment

Audiologic evaluation is the primary means of determining suitability for cochlear implantation. Both unaided and aided thresholds using conventional amplification are determined. A period of experience with a properly fitted hearing aid coupled with training in an appropriate aural rehabilitation program is necessary. Hearing aid performance can then be compared to normative cochlear implant performance.

Children who have been the most obvious candidates for a cochlear implant are those who have demonstrated no response to warble tones in the sound field with appropriate hearing aids, or have responses suggestive of vibrotactile rather than auditory sensation, that is, aided responses at levels greater than 50 to 60 dB in the lower frequencies with no responses above 1,000 Hz.

Not all children with profound SNHL are implant candidates. Many children with pure-tone thresholds between 90 to 105 dB with residual hearing through at least 2,000 Hz demonstrate closed- and open-set speech recognition skills that are superior multichannel implant users.

Sufficient receptive and expressive abilities to allow the child to learn to make a conditioned response assist in accurately estimating the child's auditory potential and, if the child is accepted as an implant candidate, ultimately assist in device setting and permit the child to begin the extensive rehabilitation program.

Medical Assessment

The medical assessment includes the otologic history, physical examination, and radiologic evaluation of the cochlea (7). High-resolution, thin-section computed tomography (CT) of the cochlea remains the initial imaging technique of choice to identify congenital deformities of the cochlea and to determine cochlear patency. Because congenital SNHL is more frequently an indication for cochlear implantation than previously was thought, and because approximately 20% of children with congenital SNHL have some form of cochlear dysplasia, imaging is very important in determining candidacy (8).

Congenital malformations of the cochlea do not contraindicate cochlear implantation, but they do introduce unique complexities. Several reports of successful implantations in children with inner-ear malformations have been published (9–12). A cerebrospinal fluid (CSF) gusher was encountered in several of the reported cases. It is believed that the route of egress of CSF is through a thin cribriform area between the modiolus and a widened internal canal (13). Temporal bone dysplasia may also be associated with an anomalous facial nerve course, and thus may place the nerve at higher risk during surgery.

Intracochlear ossification is not a contraindication to cochlear implantation, but it can limit the type and depth of insertion of the electrode array introduced into the cochlea. Use of CT usually identifies intracochlear bone formation resulting from the labyrinthitis ossificans. However, when obliteration of soft tissue occurs following sclerosing labyrinthitis, CT may not image the obstruction. In these cases, T2-weighted magnetic resonance imaging (MRI) is an effective adjunctive procedure providing additional information regarding cochlear patency. The endolymph-perilymph signal may be lost in sclerosing labyrinthitis.

The precise etiology for the deafness cannot always be determined but is identified whenever possible. However, stimulable auditory neural elements are nearly always present regardless of cause of deafness (14). Two exceptions are (a) the Michel deformity, in which there is congenital agenesis of the cochlea, and (b) the small internal auditory canal syndrome in which the cochlear nerve may be congenitally absent.

Routine otoscopic evaluation of the tympanic membrane is performed. An otologically stable condition should be present prior to consideration of implantation in children. The ear proposed for cochlear implantation must be free of infection and the tympanic membrane must be intact. If these conditions are not met, medical or surgical treatment, or both, prior to implantation is required. Because children are more prone to otitis media than are adults, justifiable concern has been expressed that a middle-ear infection could cause an implanted device to become an infected foreign body requiring its removal. Of even greater concern is infection that might extend along the electrode into the inner ear, resulting in a serious otogenic complication, such as meningitis, or further degeneration of the central auditory system. To date, although the incidence of otitis media in children who have received cochlear implants parallels that seen in the general pediatric population, no serious complications have occurred in our patients.

SURGICAL IMPLANTATION

In both children and adults, cochlear implantation requires meticulous attention to the delicate tissues and small dimensions. Skin incisions are designed to provide access to the mastoid process and coverage of the external portion of the implant package while preserving the blood supply of the postauricular skin. The incision employed at the Indiana University Medical Center has eliminated the need to develop a large postauricular flap (Fig. 1). The inferiorextent of the incision is made well posterior to the mastoid tip to preserve the branches of the postauricular artery. From this point the incision is directed posteriosuperiorly and then directed superiorly without a superior anterior limb. In children, the incision incorporates the temporalis muscle to give added thickness. A pocket is created for positioning the implant induction coil. Well anterior to the skin incision, the periosteum is incised from superior to inferior, and a posterior periosteal flap is developed. At the completion of the procedure, the posterior periosteal flap is sutured to the skin flap to compartmentalize the induction coil from the skin incision (Fig. 2). A bone well tailored to the device being implanted is created and the induction coil is fixed to the cortex with a fixation suture, periosteal flaps, or both.

Following the development of the skin incision, a mastoidectomy is performed (Fig. 3). The horizontal semicircular canal is identified in the depths of the mastoid antrum, and the short process of the incus is identified in the fossa incudis. The facial recess is opened using the fossa incudis

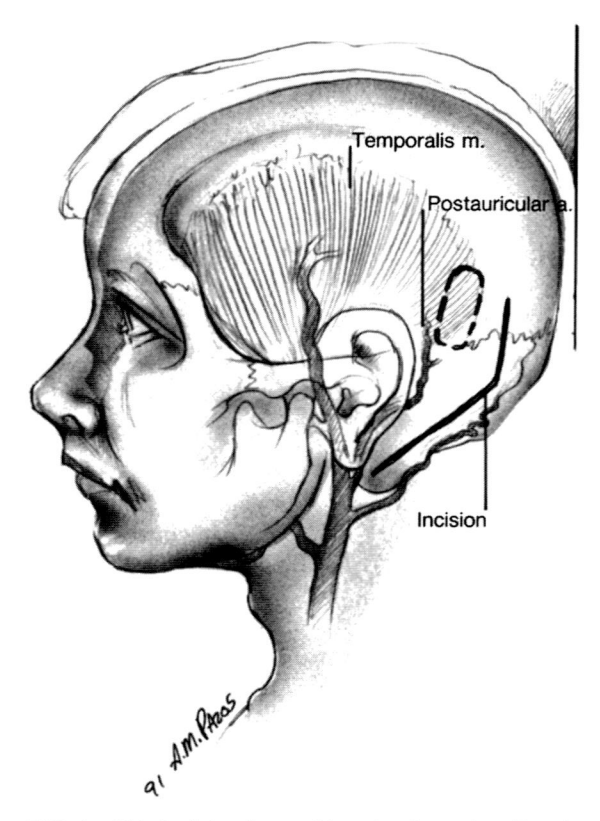

FIG. 1. Skin incision for cochlear implantation. Reprinted with permission from Miyamoto, R.T. (1993) Cochlear Implants. In: B. Bailey, ed. Otolaryngology Head and Neck Surgery, 1850–1858, Philadelphia, Lippincott-Raven Publishers.

Special Surgical Considerations

In patients with cochlear dysplasia, a CSF gusher may be encountered. The authors prefer to enter the cochlea through a small fenestra slightly larger than the electrode to be implanted. Fascia is tightly packed around the electrode at the cochleostomy site to seal the fluid.

In patients with cochlear ossification, the authors prefer to drill open the basal turn and create a tunnel approximately 6 mm in length along the path of scala tympani. A partial insertion of a Nucleus electrode is performed. Usually 10 to 12 active electrodes are implanted. Results quite comparable to full electrode insertion have been achieved (15). Gantz (16) described an extensive drillout procedure to gain access to the upper basal turn. The benefits of this extended procedure remain under investigation. Steenerson (17) described the insertion of the active electrode into the scala vestibuli in patients with cochlear ossification. When possible, this procedure has merit. However, the scala vestibuli is frequently ossified when the scala tympani is completely obliterated.

PERFORMANCE RESULTS IN CHILDREN

The assessment of speech perception abilities in children with cochlear implants has relevance for both clinical and research domains. Speech perception assessment is clinically important because it allows the clinician to monitor progress over time to evaluate whether improvement has occurred. This, in turn, influences decisions about adjustments that are

as an initial landmark (Fig. 4). The facial recess is a triangular area bounded by (a) the fossa incudis superiorly, (b) the chorda tympani nerve laterally and anteriorly, and (c) the facial nerve medially and posteriorly. The facial nerve can usually be visualized through the bone without exposing it. The round window niche is visualized through the facial recess approximately 2 mm inferior to the stapes. Occasionally, the round window niche is posteriorly positioned and thus is not well visualized through the facial recess or is obscured by ossification. Particularly in these situations, it is important not to be misdirected by hypotympanic air cells.

Entry into the scala tympani is best accomplished through a cochleostomy created anterior and inferior to the annulus of the round window membrane. A small fenestra slightly larger than the electrode to be implanted (usually 0.5 mm) is developed. A small diamond burr is used to "blue line" the endosteum of the scala tympani, and the endosteal membrane is removed with small picks. This approach bypasses the hook area of the scala tympani, thus allowing direct insertion of the active electrode array. An electrode is inserted into the basal turn of the cochlea through cochleostomy (Fig. 5). After insertion of the active electrode array, the roundwindow is sealed with small pieces of fascia. Figure 6 demonstrates a typical external system consisting of induction coil, microphone, and speech processor.

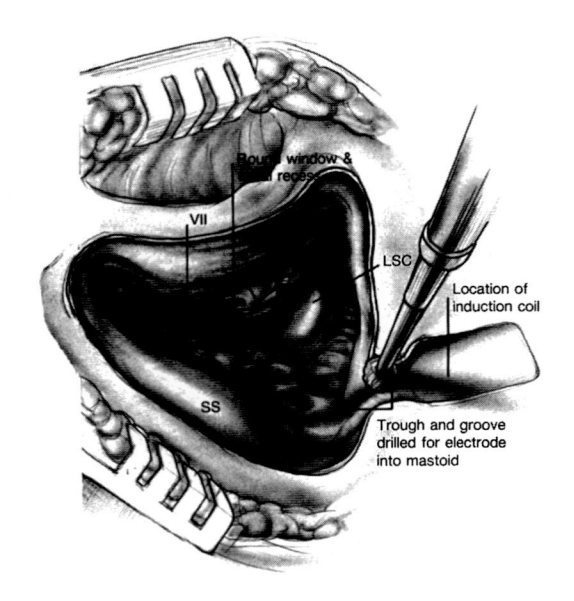

FIG. 2. Mastoidectomy performed to gain access to facial recess. *LSC,* horizontal semicircular canal *SS,* sigmoid sinus; *VII* facial nerve. Reprinted with permission from Miyamoto, R.T. (1993) Cochlear Implants. In: B. Bailey, ed. Otolaryngology Head and Neck Surgery, 1850–1858, Philadelphia, Lippincott-Raven Publishers.

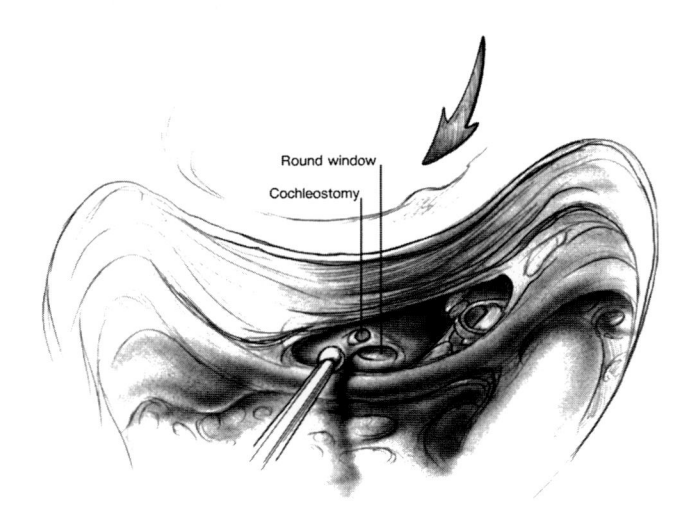

FIG. 3. Facial recess is bounded by the fossa incudis superiorly, the chorda tympani nerve laterally and anteriorly, and the facial nerve medially and posteriorly. A cochleostomy is created anterior and inferior to the round window membrane.

made to the patient's speech-processor program. In addition, the results of assessments provide information that is useful in determining the goals for aural rehabilitation training. From a research standpoint, assessment of speech perception yields empirical data regarding the benefits that can be derived from a cochlear implant and allows comparison of the effectiveness of different sensory aids in this population, which in turn affects candidacy criteria and device selection for cochlear implants.

Unlike postlingually deafened adults who use the information transmitted by a cochlear implant in comparison with previously stored representations of spoken language, pediatric implant users must rely on the same information to develop these representations. Therefore, perceptual skills develop over a relatively long time course in prelingually deafened children (18–20). Substantial improvements in closed-set word recognition usually do not occur in prelingually deafened children until after they use their multichannel implants for more than 1 year, and improvements in open-set speech recognition occur after an even longer period of using the device (21).

Comparison of Single- and Multichannel Implants

Few comparative single- and multichannel implant studies have been conducted with children. Most investigations with children have reported on the performance of either single- or multichannel implant users. A study conducted by Osberger et al. (22) compared the performance of matched groups of children who used either the 3M/House device or the Nucleus multichannel cochlear implant over time. The results revealed that the performance of the Nucleus users was higher than that of the 3M/House users on every speech perception measure, even on those measures that assessed aspects of speech purportedly transmitted the best by the single-channel device (i.e., prosodic information). Thus, the multichannel implant not only permitted better word recognition without speechreading, but it also conveyed better information about the time-intensity cues in speech. Even though some reports have shown that a small percentage of children demonstrated open-set speech recognition with the 3M/House implant (23), the highest level of performance

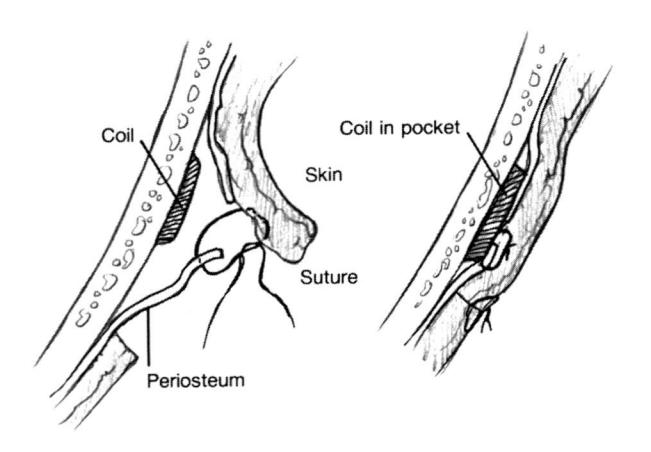

FIG. 4. Posteriorly based periosteal flap is developed anterior to the skin incision and sutured to the anterior skin flap, thus compartmentalizing the induction coil from the skin incision.

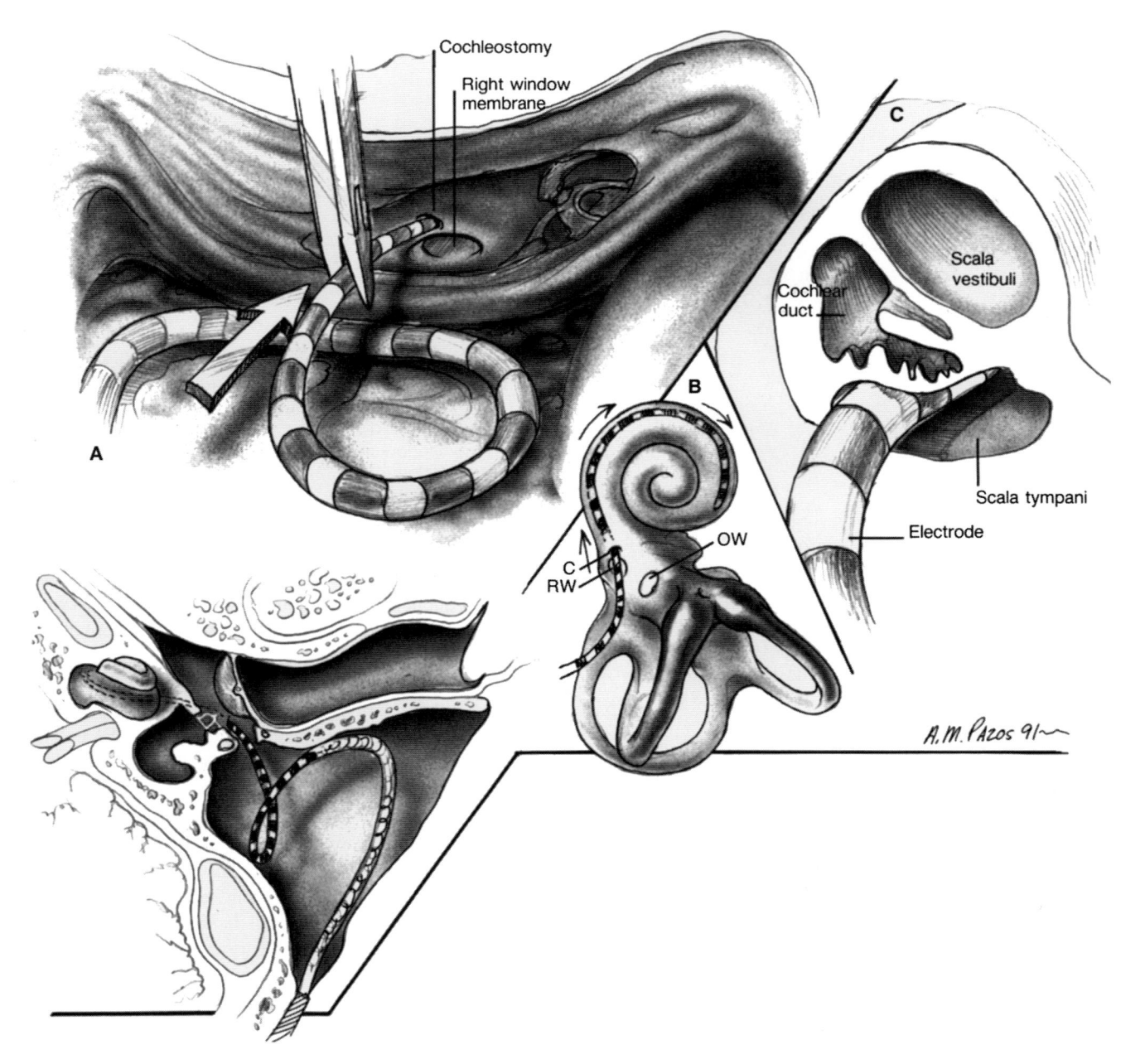

FIG. 5. A: Electrode introduced into basal turn of cochlea through cochleostomy. **B:** Electrode positioned in basal turn of cochlea. **C:** Electrode in scala tympani (cross section of basal turn of cochlea). **D:** Axial view of electrode passing through mastoid and facial recess and into basal turn of cochlea. *C,* cochlea; *OW,* oval window; *RW,* round window.

achieved by the *majority* of single-channel users was the perception of stress pattern and syllable number in speech.

Performance with Multichannel Implants

The research design most commonly applied to evaluate implant speech perception benefit in children is a within-subjects design wherein the subject serves as his or her own control in the pre-and postimplant conditions. The largest studies of this nature have been conducted as part of the FDA clinical trials of the Nucleus multichannel implant in children (24). After 12 months of multichannel implant use, Staller et al. (24) reported mean scores of 39% (n = 84) on a closed-set word identification test, 23% (n = 42) on a test of open-set sentence recognition, and 12% (n = 25) on a test of open-set, monosyllabic word recognition. Examination of individual data revealed that 13% of the subjects demonstrated significantly above chance closed-set word identification before implantation, whereas, postoperatively, 62% of the subjects achieved this level of perfor-

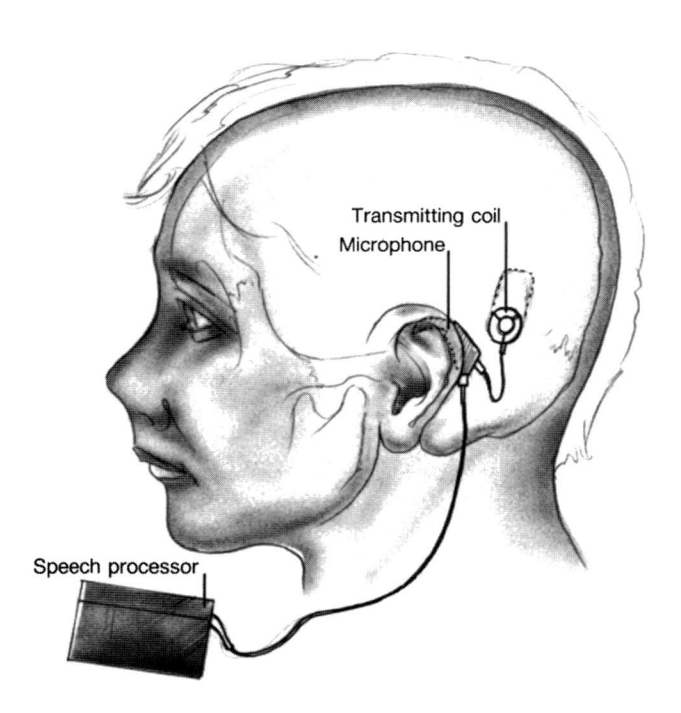

FIG. 6. External system consisting of induction coil, microphone, and speech processor.

mance. Preoperatively, the subjects showed no open-set speech recognition, but 12 months after implantation, 45% of the subjects recognized one or more words in sentences administered in an open set.

Pediatric implant performance also is reported in terms of clinically descriptive categories of benefit. Geers and Moog (25) developed a classification system that describes performance along a hierarchy of speech perception abilities: (a) no pattern perception, (b) consistent pattern perception, (c) inconsistent word identification, (d) consistent word identification, and (e) open-set word recognition. Staller et al. (24) reported that the percentage of children reaching inconsistent word recognition increased from 12% to 80% postoperatively, and roughly half the subjects demonstrated open-set speech recognition. Osberger et al. (26) developed a similar classification scheme, modified to describe performance on the tests in their assessment battery, and reported that roughly one-half the subjects demonstrated open-set speech recognition after they had used their implants for an average of 2 years.

The above results demonstrate that most children receive benefit from cochlear implants. However, the time course during which perceptual skills emerge varies, depending on the population under study or the procedures employed. Recently, Robbins and Kirk (27) reviewed number of studies that investigated the speech perception performance of children with the Nucleus multichannel cochlear implant and reported the following trends.

First, the learning curves of postlingually deafened children who receive a cochlear implant are quite different from those of children with congenital or prelingually acquired deafness (27–29). Postlingually deafened children must map the new signals from the implant onto an existing base of auditory and linguistic knowledge; most of these children show rapid progress in their listening skills within the first 6 months to 1 year of use of the cochlear implant. However, the majority of children who receive a cochlear implant are either congenitally deaf or acquire their hearing loss early, before speech and language skills are established. These children must use the signal provided via a cochlear implant to develop perceptual and expressive representations of spoken language. The ability to understand and to produce speech develops over a relatively long time in children with prelingual hearing loss and may not be accomplished by all children in this group. Therefore, it is important to follow these children for an extended time to determine the eventual communication benefits to be obtained from use of a cochlear implant.

A second trend noted was that closed-set and open-set speech perception abilities emerge in an overlapping fashion, rather than sequentially. On average, children with the Nucleus cochlear implant are able to recognize words from a closed set of responses at levels significantly better than chance only after about 1.5 years of use of the device (26,28,30,31). Mean scores for open-set speech understanding through listening alone show gradual improvements within the first 2 years and increase to approximately 40% by 4 years of use (32). Robbins and Kirk (27) also noted that evidence of substantial auditory-visual enhancement is seen prior to the time that children demonstrate closed- or open-set speech understanding in the auditory-only modality (27). Across all tasks, mean group scores increased over time, even as long as 5 years after implant (29,30), which suggests that learning takes place over an extended time course. Finally, studies of children implanted at very early ages (less than six years) suggest that high levels of speech perception performance may be obtained by many of these children (33).

Variables Affecting Performance

Large individual differences among children with implants have been documented by speech-perception measures. Some children demonstrated relatively high levels of speech recognition; others perceived primarily prosodic speech information from their devices (24,26). Age at onset of deafness, duration of deafness before implantation, and educational setting were the independent variables most often examined to explain such performance differences. Studies by Staller et al. (24,28) reported that two factors, age at onset of deafness and duration of deafness, were significantly related to speech perception performance in children who used the Nucleus multichannel cochlear implant. These authors found that subjects with later onset and shorter duration of deafness performed better on measures of speech perception than did subjects who had early onset of deafness but relatively long duration of deafness at the time of implantation.

The effect of age at onset of deafness on speech perception skills was examined by Osberger et al. (29) in children who received a single- or multichannel cochlear implant. No significant differences in the mean postoperative speech perception scores as a function of age at onset of deafness were found unless the subjects were postlingually deafened (i.e., onset of deafness at or after age 5). Subjects with postlingual deafness achieved significantly higher speech-perception scores on all measures than did the subjects with prelingually deafness (i.e., congenital or acquired deafness). In a study that included only children with multichannel implants (i.e., the Nucleus device) with prelingual deafness who received implants before age 10, the results showed no significant difference between the speech perception scores of a group of subjects with congenital deafness and the mean scores of a second group of subjects with deafness acquired before age 3 (34).

The finding of similar performance between children with congenital and early acquired deafness is probably influenced by the secondary effects of meningitis (e.g., neurologic problems and cochlear ossification) on the performance of the children with acquired deafness. These results indicate that children who are born deaf have the potential to derive the same benefit from multichannel implants as do children who had some exposure to spoken language before the onset of their deafness from meningitis.

The postimplant performance of children with postlingual deafness (i.e., onset of deafness at age 5 or later) differs from that of children with prelingual deafness in several important respects. Children with relatively late onset of deafness typically show rapid and marked improvement in speech-perception abilities after they receive an implant (18,29). As noted earlier, speech perception performance improves very gradually in prelingually implanted children.

A significant relationship between the communication method used by the child and performance on speech perception measures has been shown by several investigations. In these studies, more children who used oral communication achieved higher levels of implant performance than did children who used total communication (i.e., signs plus speaking and listening) (23,26). The relationship between communication mode and implant performance is less clear in other studies. For example, Miyamoto et al. (34) found that children who used oral communication obtained significantly higher scores on only 2 of 13 speech-perception measures. Additional research is needed to clarify this issue.

Comparison of Cochlear Implants, Hearing Aids, and Tactile Aids

Children with profound hearing impairments demonstrate a wide range of auditory capabilities (35). A within-subjects research design is influenced by this variability, thus confounding the evaluation of various sensory aids. Therefore, the establishment of a control group is desirable. Using the results of previous investigators as a guide, Osberger et al. (36) developed a descriptive system to classify the range of hearing levels in children with profound hearing impairments. Hearing aid users were divided into three groups on the basis of their unaided, better-ear pure-tone thresholds at 500, 1,000, 2,000 Hz. Subjects classified as *gold* hearing aid users demonstrated pure-tone thresholds of 90 to 100 dB at two of the three frequencies (with no thresholds greater than 105 dB). *Silver* hearing aid users demonstrated hearing levels of 101 to 110 dB at two of the three frequencies, and *bronze* hearing aid users demonstrated two of three thresholds greater than 110 dB. Using this approach, the gold hearing aid users were viewed as setting the ''gold standard of performance'' for children with profound hearing impairments because children with this amount of residual hearing developed the most intelligible speech. At the other end of the continuum were bronze hearing aid users who appeared to respond to auditory stimuli on the basis of vibrotactile sensation. To date, the majority of children who have received implants probably would be classified as bronze hearing aid users. The unaided pure-tone thresholds of the silver hearing aid users were intermediate to those of the other two groups.

The benefits of multichannel cochlear implantation in prelingually deafened children can be demonstrated only by comprehensive longitudinal studies. Valid performance trends may not become apparent for 1 to 3, or even more years, postoperatively. Studies in our laboratory have documented that deaf children who could not detect sound with conventional hearing aids preoperatively (bronze hearing aid users) have achieved scores with their multichannel implants comparable to those of the gold hearing aid users on most tests (except on a test of open-set speech recognition).

The intermediate group of children, silver hearing aid users (i.e., pure-tone thresholds between 100–105 dB HL), clearly might derive more benefit from multichannel implants than from continued use of hearing aids. Extension of implant candidacy to this group, and even to some gold hearing aid users, is the target of future research. Improved implant technology and earlier implantation promise to widen the candidacy window.

An important issue in sensory aid research with profoundly deaf children has been determination of the benefits derived from noninvasive alternatives to cochlear implants, such as tactile aids. The results of a recent study by Miyamoto et al. (37) demonstrated that children who used multichannel implants derived substantially more speech perception benefit from their devices than did children who used multichannel tactile aids. The performance of two groups of subjects who received either a Nucleus implant or a multichannel vibrotactile aid (Tactaid 7; Audiological Engineering Corporation, Somerville, MA) were compared. There were ten subjects in each group, matched on the basis of age at onset of deafness, age fit with a multichannel device, and nonverbal intelligence. Subjects were tested on a battery of speech perception measures in the predevice interval and at one postdevice interval (i.e., after an average of roughly 1.5 yr of device use). The results revealed that the scores of the implant users improved significantly between the pre- and postdevice intervals on all measures. Moreover, the scores of the Nucleus users were significantly higher than those of the Tactaid users on all measure.

In contrast, the scores of the tactile aid users showed negligible change over time except on a test that evaluated open-set recognition of phrases with both auditory *and* visual cues. The results suggested that children with a multichannel implant learned to recognize words and understand speech without lipreading; children who used a multichannel tactile aid demonstrated evidence of speech recognition only if tactile cues were combined with visual ones.

Speech Production

Although the primary role of a cochlear implant is to make speech sounds accessible auditorily, cochlear implants also serve as aids to speech production. Osberger et al. (38) demonstrated that the phonetic repertoires of profoundly hearing-impaired children increase after the children receive a multichannel cochlear implant. Improvements in the production of consonant and vowel features that are typically difficult for children with profound hearing losses to master (e.g., high vowels, diphthongs, alveolar consonants, and fricatives) have been documented. Improvements in speech production have also been documented by Tobey et al. (39).

Children who are postlingually deafened and children who receive implants at an early age generally demonstrate large improvements in speech, but children with early onset of deafess who are not implanted until adolescence typically show limited improvements in speech production.

The scores for the subjects with implants showed gradual improvement over time. After 2.5 years of use of a cochlear implant, the average speech intelligibility of the subjects began to exceed that of the silver hearing aid users. After 3.5 to 4 years of use of the device, the average intelligibility of the users was 40%, which is approximately 20% higher than that for silver hearing aid users. The majority of the children in this study did not receive implants until they were 5 to 8 years old. Further studies are under way to examine changes in speech intelligibility in children who were implanted at a younger age.

SUMMARY

The aural rehabilitation of deaf and hard-of-hearing individuals is an exceedingly complex process involving a wide range of health-care hearing specialists. The application of time-honored principles has been augmented by the introduction of a broad array of new technologies that continue to advance the field to heights previously deemed unattainable.

ACKNOWLEDGMENT

Supported in part by research grant 2 RO1 DC00064-06 and RO1 DC00423 from the National Institute on Deafness and Other Communication Disorders, National Institutes of Health.

REFERENCES

1. Clark G. The University of Melbourne Nucleusmulti-electrode cochlear implant. *Adv Otol Rhinol Laryngol* 1987;38:V–IX, 1–181.
2. Schindler RA, Kessler DK, Rebscher SJ, Yanda JL, Jackler RK. The UCSF/Storz multichannel cochlear implant: Patient results. *Laryngoscope* 1986;96(6):597–603.
3. Wilson BS, Finley CC, Lawson DT, Wolford RD, Eddington DK, Rubinowitz WM. Better speech recognition with cochlear implants. *Nature* 1991;352:236–238.
4. Schindler RA, Kessler DK, Barker M: Clarion patient performance: An update on the clinical trials. *Ann Otol Rhinol Laryngol* (Suppl. 166), 1995;104:269–272.
5. Matsushima JI, Shepard RK, Seldon HL, Xu SA, Clark GM. Electrical stimulation of the auditory nerve in deaf kittens: effects on cochlear nucleus morphology. *Hear Res* 1991;56:133–142.
6. Donaldson JA, Duckert LG, Lambert PM, Rubel EW, eds. Surgical anatomy of the temporal bone. 4th ed. New York: Raven, 1992.
7. Yune HY, Miyamoto RT, Yune ME. Medical imaging in cochlear implant candidates. *Am J Otol* 1991;12(Suppl):11–17.
8. Jensen S. Malformation of the inner ear in deaf children. *Acta Radiol* 1969;286(Suppl):1–97.
9. Mangabeira-Albernaz PL. the Mondini dysplasia: from early diagnosis to cochlear implant. *Acta Otolaryngol* 1983;95:627–631.
10. Miyamoto RT, Robbins AJM, Myres WA, Pope ML. Cochlear implantation in the Mondini inner ear malformation. *Am J Otol* 1986;7(4):258–261.
11. Jackler RK, Luxford WM, House WF. Sound detection with the cochlear implant in five ears of four children with congenital malformations of the cochlea. *Laryngoscope* 1987;97(Suppl40):15–17.
12. Silverstein H, Smouha E, Morgan N. Multichannel cochlear implantation in a patient with bilateral Mondini deformities. *Am J Otol* 1988;9:451–455.
13. Schuknecht HF. Mondini dysplasia: a clinical and pathological study. *Ann Otol Rhinol Larynol* 1980;89(Suppl 65):3–23.
14. Hinojosa R, Marion M. Histopathology of profound sensorineural deafness. *Ann NY Acad Sci* 1983;405:459–484.
15. Kirk KI, Sehgal M, Miyamoto RT. Speech perception performance of Nucleus multichannel cochlear implant users with partial electrode insertions. *JSHR* (In press).
16. Gantz BJ, McCabe BF, Tyler RS. Use of multichannel cochlear implants in obstructed and obliterated cochleas. *Otolaryngol Head Neck Surg* 1988;98:72–81.
17. Steenerson RL, Gary LB, Wynens MS. Scala vestibuli cochlear implantation for labyrinthine ossification. *Am J Otol* 1990;11:360–363.
18. Fryauf-Bertschy H, Tyler RS, Kelsay DM, Gantz BJ. Performance over time of congenitally deaf and postlingually deafened children using a multichannel cochlear implant. *J Speech Hear Res* 1992;35:913–920.
19. Miyamoto RT, Osberger MJ, Robbins AM, Myres WA, Kessler K, Pope ML. Longitudinal evaluation of communication skills of children with single-or multichannel cochlear implants. *Am J Otol* 1992;13:215–222.
20. Waltzman SB, Cohen NL, Gomolin RH, Shapiro WH, Ozdamar SR, Hoffman RA. Long-term results of early cochlear implantation in congenitally and prelingually deafened children. *Am J Otol* 1994;15 (Suppl. 2):9–13.
21. Miyamoto RT, Kirk KI, Todd SL, Robbins AM, Osberger MJ. Speech perception skills of children with multichannel cochlear implants or hearing aids. *Ann Otol Rhinol Laryngol* 1995;104(Suppl.):334–337.
22. Osberger MJ, Robbins AM, Miyamoto RT, Berry SW, Myres WA, Kessler KS, Pope ML. Speech perception abilities of children with cochlear implants, tactile aids, or hearing aids. *Am Jour Otol* 1991;12(Suppl.):105–115.
23. Berliner KI, Tonokawa LM, Dye LM, House, WF. Open-set speech recognition in children with a single-channel cochlear implant. *Ear Hear* 1989;10:237–24S.

24. Staller SJ, Dowell RC, Beiter AL, Brimacombe JA. Perceptual abilities of children with the Nucleus 22-channel cochlear implant. *Ear Hear* 1991;12 (Suppl.):34S–47S.
25. Geers AE, Moog JS. *Early speech perception test.* St. Louis: Central Institute for the Deaf; 1990.
26. Osberger MJ, Miyamoto RT, Zimmerman-Phillips S, Kemink JL, etal. Independent evaluation of the speech perception abilities of children with the Nucleus 22-Channel cochlear implant system. *Ear Hear* 1991; 12 (Suppl.):66S–805.
27. Robbins AM, Kirk KI. Speech perception assessment and performance in pediatric cochlear implant users. *Sem Hear* 1996;17:353–369.
28. Staller SJ, Beiter AL, Brimacombe JA, Mecklenburg DJ, Arnot P. Pediatric performance with the Nucleus 22-Channel Cochlear Implant System. *Am J Otol* 1991;12 (Suppl.):126–136.
29. Osberger MJ, Todd SL, Berry SW, Robbins AM, Miyamoto RT. Effect of age at onset of deafness on children's speech perception abilities with a cochlear implant. *Ann Otol Rhinol Laryngol* 1991;100:883–888.
30. Gantz BJ, Tyler RS, Woodworth GG, Tye-Murray N, Fryauf-Bertschy H. Results of multichannel cochlear implants in congenital and acquired prelingual deafness in children: five year followup. *Am J Otol* 1994; 15:(Suppl.)1–7.
31. Miyamoto RT, Osberger MJ, Todd SL, Robbins AM, Stroer BS, Zimmerman-Phillips, Cathey BE. Variables affecting implant performance in children. *Laryngoscope* 1994;104:1120–1124.
32. Miyamoto RT, Kirk KI, Robbins AM, Todd S, Riley A. Speech perception and speech production skills of children with multichannel cochlear implants. *Acta Otolaryngol* 1996;116(2):240–243.
33. Waltzman SN, Cohen NL, Gomolin RH, Shapiro WH, Ozdamar SR, Hoffman RA. Long-term results of early cochlear implantation incongenitally and prelingually deafened children. *Am J Otol* 1994; 15(Suppl):9–13.
34. Miyamoto RT, Osberger MJ, Robbins AM, Myres WA, Kessler K. Prelingually deafened children's performance with the Nucleus multichannel cochlear implant. *Am Jour Otol* 1993;14:437–445.
35. Boothroyd A. Auditory perception of speech contrasts by subjects with sensorineural hearing loss. *J Speech Hear Res* 1984;27:134–144.
36. Osberger MJ, Maso M, Sam LK. Speech intelligibility of children with cochlear implants, tactile aids, or hearing aids. *J Speech Hear Res* 1993; 36:186–203.
37. Miyamoto RT, Robbins AM, Osberger MJ, Todd SL, Riley AI, Kirk KI. Comparison of multichannel tactile aids and multichannel cochlear implants in children with profound hearing impairments. *Am J Otol* 1995;16:8–13.
38. Osberger MJ, Osberger, MJ, Robbins, AM, Berry SW, Tood SL, Hisketh LJ, Sedey A. Analysis of the spontaneous speech samples of children with cochlear implants or tactile aids. *Am J Otol* 1991;12 (Suppl):151–164.
39. Tobey EA, Andriette S, Murchison C, Nicosia, J. Sprague S, Staller SJ, et al. Speech production performance in children with multi-channel cochlear implants. *Am J Otol* 1991;12(Suppl):165–173.

PART XIV

Dilemmas, Perplexing Problems, and Controversies

CHAPTER 41

Mixed Hearing Loss in Children

Ken Henry and Kenneth M. Grundfast

Evaluation and management of the child presenting with a mixed (conductive and sensorineural) hearing loss can be challenging. The key to diagnosis and appropriate management of mixed hearing loss (MHL) lies in the ability to determine the air- and bone-conduction thresholds of each ear using pure-tone and/or speech stimuli. The relationship between bone-conduction and air-conduction thresholds allow differential diagnosis between conductive, sensorineural, and mixed hearing losses. A loss of hearing sensitivity by bone conduction, accompanied by an even greater loss of sensitivity by air conduction, is characteristic of MHL. When a child has both conductive hearing loss (CHL) and sensorineural hearing loss (SNHL), interpretation is difficult, and assessing the relative contributions of each component is sometimes impossible.

The ability to diagnose MHL in children can be problematic for many reasons. Some audiologic test methods commonly utilized to differentiate CHL from SNHL may be difficult to administer with the pediatric population. A child's reluctance or inability to cooperate for behavioral testing may mean that strategies other than conventional ones have to be used to determine which components of the child's hearing loss are conductive versus sensorineural. The identification of MHL, however, presents a greater challenge. Reliance on a battery of audiologic tests, including immittance audiometry, auditory brainstem response (ABR), otoacoustic emissions (OAEs), otoscopy, and case history information may still be inadequate to assess the extent of cochlear deficit in a child with MHL. The purpose of this chapter is to focus on the complexities involved in audiologic assessment and the medical and surgical decision making in management of children with MHL.

K. Henry: Professional Hearing Services, The Dizziness and Balance Center, Falls Church, Virginia 22044.
K.M. Grundfast: Department of Otolaryngology and Pediatrics, Georgetown University School of Medicine, Washington, DC 20007.

PROBLEM ASPECTS

Evaluating the child with MHL can be far more complicated than evaluation of a child with CHL or SNHL alone. Further, evaluating the child with MHL is almost always more difficult than evaluation of an adult with MHL. The problems encountered with both the audiologic evaluation and the medical diagnosis of the child with MHL are related to patient, technical and procedural variables. Some of the problems often encountered are summarized here and are further discussed throughout this chapter. A review of some audiologic challenges encountered in the differential diagnosis of MHL are summarized in Table 1.

First, there is the problem of obtaining accurate information from audiologic testing that is sufficient to differentiate the magnitude of the conductive and sensorineural components in a child presenting with MHL. Although determining accurate air- and bone-conduction hearing thresholds in adults is a straightforward matter, determining the air- and bone-conduction thresholds for each ear in a child can be challenging and fraught with difficulty. Even if a child is cooperative and eager to please during audiologic assessment, differentiating an auditory from a vibrotactile stimulus can be extremely difficult for the child. During play audiometry, children may have a tendency to respond to a vibrotactile stimulus even though they have been advised to respond only to sound that is heard in the ear rather than "feeling" the sound. In general, with behavioral testing techniques, the younger the child, the more difficult the task of quantifying separately the magnitude of the conductive and sensorineural components.

Second, there is the problem of early detection of a child who has SNHL. A child with congenital mild bilateral SNHL may be perceived by the parents and pediatrician as a normal-hearing child during the first 2 or 3 years of life. Then, when the child develops otitis media and a CHL is superimposed on the already existing (but previously undetected) SNHL, the child is identified as having a significant hearing problem. In such a case, if initial audiologic tests do not

TABLE 1. *Audiologic challenges in the assessment of children with mixed hearing loss*

Behavioral assessment
  Child unable or unwilling to cooperate for behavioral testing
  Inability to obtain ear-specific information
    Child will not accept placement of headphones, insert earphones and/or bone-conduction oscillator.
    Child can be tested only under sound field.
  Difficulties in masking
    Child might not tolerate headphones or insert receivers to conduct masking of the nontest ear.
    Pure-tone stimulus is difficult to differentiate from masking noise.
    Masking dilemma in bilateral CHL or severe MHL
      Overmasking
      Undermasking
  Technical limitations of bone-conduction testing
    Vibrotactile artifact and airborne radiation of bone-conducted stimulus at high intensities
    Child's inability to differentiate between auditory and tactile stimulus during bone-conduction testing (responds when he or she feels vibration rather than hears stimulus)

Electrophysiologic techniques
  Acoustic immittance
    When findings show abnormal tympanograms and/or absent ARTs, middle ear pathology is suspected. However, quantification of conductive and sensorineural components is not possible based solely on immittance findings.
    Bone-conduction must be done either behaviorally or with ABR if immittance findings are abnormal.
    Sensitivity of ART is excellent for CHL and MHL, but specificity is limited.
      Reflexes and/or tympanograms may be abnormal due to nonpathologic conditions or pathologies not involving the middle ear.
  Otoacoustic emissions
    Otoacoustic emissions will not provide additional diagnostic information with MHL. Emissions (DPOAE or TEOAE) will be absent secondary to either the middle ear transduction deficit or the sensorineural component.
  Auditory brainstem response
    Auditory brainstem response provides limited frequency specific information.
      Click ABR provides information regarding the high-frequency portion (2,000–4,000 Hz) of the cochlea.
      Tone bursts to assess lower frequencies (e.g., 500-Hz tone bursts) are difficult to assess and interpret.
    Elevated wave V thresholds can be secondary to CHL, MHL, or SNHL.
    Wave I of ABR is frequently absent with MHL, rendering interpretation or differential diagnosis of results difficult.
    Peripheral conduction delays in the absolute latency of waves I, III, and V can also be secondary to CHL, SNHL, or MHL.
    Bone-conducted ABR must be performed if air-conducted responses show significant absolute latency delays or if wave I is absent.

ART, acoustic reflex threshold; DPOAE, distortion-product OAE; TEOAE, transient-evoked OAE.

include both air- and bone-conduction testing, the underlying congenital SNHL may go undetected. Even if air and bone thresholds are determined accurately, arriving at an accurate medical diagnosis may have to wait until after the middle ear effusion resolves with medical management or is aspirated from the middle ear. That is, when a child with MHL has an evident middle ear effusion in the affected ear at the time of initial diagnosis of MHL, there really is no way to determine with assurance that the conductive component of the MHL is caused by the middle ear effusion rather than from congenital ossicular abnormality. The problem of delay in detection of possible congenital SNHL is made all the more difficult for children with unilateral SNHL. When a child's SNHL is in only one ear, the hearing loss may go undetected until the child develops otitis media with CHL in the opposite ear or when there is otitis media in the ear with SNHL. In this instance, the parent may then notice that the child seems to be relying on only one ear.

Third, there is the problem in diagnosing an MHL, which may be dynamic in nature. Even if electrophysiologic or behavioral audiologic tests are deemed to be highly accurate, the degree to which the sensorineural and conductive components are contributing to the MHL may change, thus making interpretation of test results and medical diagnosis extremely difficult.

For example, a child with a congenital stable SNHL can have an ephemeral CHL loss that is present, at times, and superimposed on the underlying SNHL, while at other times is not present, so that the MHL changes to a straightforward SNHL when the otitis media resolves. Conversely, the child with persistent middle ear effusion might have a progressive SNHL, in which case the conductive component of the MHL will remain constant, while the magnitude of the sensorineural component will increase with time. Or, a child with a perilymph fistula might have fluctuating SNHL and intermittent otitis media, so that both the sensorineural and conductive components of the MHL will vary over time, making interpretation of test results extremely difficult.

BEHAVIORAL AUDIOLOGIC ASSESSMENT

Procedures used in the assessment of a child will be dictated by the responses he or she is capable of making. The behavioral evaluation should use the most sensitive test to which the child can respond. The sophistication of the child's response will depend on factors such as mental age, chronologic age, neurologic status, hearing level, willingness to perform, prior exposure to auditory testing, the motivational assessment devices used, and the test environment itself (1). Depending on the mental age of the child, behavioral observation audiometry (BOA), visual reinforcement audiometry (VRA), or play audiometry can be considered.

Prior to the age of 6 months, BOA can be utilized. Behavioral observation audiometry is an approach to hearing screening that utilizes a high-intensity (e.g., 90-dBA) narrow-band noise presented by a speaker or hand-held instrument positioned near the infant. The expected response by the infant includes localization, changes in facial expression, cessation of activity, startle, or crying. Because of the high-stimulus intensity used, BOA techniques can miss an infant with a mild-to-moderate bilateral hearing loss or a unilateral impairment (2). The reliability and validity imposed by the stimulus, the type of behavioral response, and observer bias make BOA unacceptable, even for the purpose of general infant screening (2,3). Preferably, electrophysiologic techniques such as ABR testing and OAE testing should be utilized to obtain ear-specific and frequency-specific information on a child 6 months of age or younger.

Once an infant reaches the cognitive age of about 6 months, the use of VRA can be successfully accomplished (4). Visual reinforcement audiometry has emerged as a valid and reliable behavioral procedure for children 6 to 24 months of age (5). It is based a child's natural inclination to direct his or her attention toward a novel sound source. A visual reinforcer is used when the child notices the acoustic stimulus and turns his or her eyes or head. Through operant conditioning, the child anticipates the activation of a light or animation of a toy or animal following the detection of an acoustic stimulus.

Visual reinforcement audiometry should be attempted with earphones and via bone conduction but is frequently conducted via sound field. Unfortunately, headphones, insert earphones, or a bone oscillator often are not tolerated by the young child. In this case, it is possible to obtain frequency-specific information sound field but not ear-specific information. A unilateral hearing loss may be overlooked unless additional diagnostic techniques are used. Also, sound field VRA does not provide a differential diagnosis between CHL, SNHL, and MHL. Without bone-conduction testing, one cannot determine the magnitude of the conductive component or the extent of cochlear reserve. Immittance audiometry and otoscopy will be important in the identification of any external or middle ear abnormality in cases in which bone-conduction testing is not successfully accomplished.

Play audiometry is the test of choice for the majority of children between the ages of 25 and 48 months. The goal in play audiometry is to obtain frequency-specific and ear-specific information by way of air conduction and bone conduction. Play audiometry involves teaching the child to respond to an auditory stimulus as part of a game (e.g., dropping a block into a bucket when the tone is heard). A visual, verbal, or other tangible reinforcement to the auditory stimulus is an integral part of the procedure. Attempts to apply pure-tone techniques to 2- to 3-year old children, even with play techniques, also can often prove frustrating. Often, children simply will not wear earphones of any kind, and if they do, they may not cooperate with a stranger to play a "game." A series of audiometric studies over time may be necessary to establish a good rapport between the child and the audiologist before air- and bone-conduction testing can be successfully accomplished.

BONE-CONDUCTION ASSESSMENT

While the aforementioned procedures can obtain frequency-specific information in children, they do not provide differential information about middle ear status unless bone-conduction or immittance testing is conducted. Many clinics have abandoned bone-conduction testing and use immittance audiometry to rule out middle ear pathology (6). However, bone-conduction testing should be eliminated from the pediatric test battery only when immittance measures clearly and consistently demonstrate normal middle ear function.

Clinical bone-conduction testing is based on two assumptions: First, the threshold for bone-conducted signals is a measure of the integrity of the sensorineural system, and, second, the air-conduction threshold reflects the function of the total hearing system both conductive and sensorineural (7). The difference between the air- and bone-conducted thresholds (air–bone gap) provides the magnitude of the CHL. As previously mentioned, when a child has an MHL, assessing the relative contributions of each component may not be possible. Bone conduction may not be tolerated, leaving interpretation to sound field or air-conduction thresholds along with information from otoscopy, immittance, case history, or other diagnostic techniques. Even if bone-conduction testing is well tolerated and successful, there are a number of technical factors that must be considered. Regardless of the position of the oscillator on the skull, bone-conduction testing results in stimulation of both cochleas. Interaural attenuation (IA) is negligible for a bone-conducted stimulus (except in the higher frequencies), so one cannot be certain which cochlea is responding to the signal. It is necessary to remove the contralateral ear (nontest ear) from the test procedure whenever air–bone gaps are present. This is accomplished by administering an air-conducted masking noise of adequate intensity to elevate the threshold of the nontest ear. Attending to a bone-conducted signal while masking is introduced via air conduction to the contralateral ear is a difficult task for even the most cooperative and attentive child. For pediatric assessment, it is often faster and more reliable to conduct masked bone-conduction testing using speech stimuli instead of relying on the conventional method of pure-tone air- and bone-conduction audiometry. The utilization of spondees is more meaningful and easier to differentiate from the masking stimulus for most children. A comparison of conventional and bone-conducted speech reception thresholds will give a good estimate of the air–bone gap in the primary speech frequencies.

If MHL is suspected prior to audiometry, it may be prudent to pursue testing bone-conduction thresholds *before* air-conduction thresholds. This will give an estimate of SNHL (i.e., cochlear reserve). Earphone or sound field testing can then be pursued to assess any contribution of the outer and middle ear to the hearing loss. This approach should be entertained if case history, radiologic findings, otoscopy, or acoustic immittance findings suggest MHL prior to testing or if participation on the part of the child is limited. The importance of bone-conduction testing in the diagnosis of MHL cannot be overemphasized. Bone-conduction testing is the only technique that can differentiate and quantify the magnitude of conductive and sensorineural pathology in the presence of MHL. Fortunately, bone-conduction assessment can be conducted electrophysiologically as well as behaviorally. The utilization of bone-conduction ABR is discussed later in this chapter.

MASKING

When testing children, the use of masking to prevent participation by the nontest ear is as necessary as it is in audiometry with adults. The same principles of stimulus crossover and IA of the signal apply. When conducting audiologic assessment, unmasked bone-conduction testing evaluates cochlear reserve of the *better* cochlea. Masking is necessary to obtain ear-specific information about sensorineural function. Masking should be utilized when air- and/or bone-conduction thresholds are not similar bilaterally. Its use is dictated by the type of stimulus delivered to the test ear (air conduction vs. bone conduction), the stimulus modality employed (headphones, insert earphones, or bone oscillator), the frequency of the test stimulus, and the anticipated effect of the stimulus on the nontest ear. In MHL, masking should always be used to evaluate the extent of cochlear reserve individually for each ear. This is extremely critical if surgicalintervention is to be considered for MHL.

A common problem encountered in masking is the issue of masking dilemma (8). Masking dilemma is seen clinically in maximum bilateral CHL, in which air–bone gaps of 50 to 60 dB are present. It also may be seen in severe MHL with maximal air–bone gaps and when bone-conduction thresholds show a SNHL of 40 to 50 dB. In the former, overmasking is a concern because of the excellent cochlear reserve bilaterally and the potential for crossover of the masking signal to the test ear, which could artificially elevate the bone-conduction threshold. In the latter case, insufficient masking can be encountered because of the magnitude of the hearing loss. The output of the audiometer may be insufficient to allow minimum effective masking levels. The use of ER-3A insert earphones (a.k.a. tubephones) minimizes the risk of overmasking by increasing interaural attenuation (9). For conventional TDH headphones, IA is approximately 45 to 50 dB. The IA for insert earphones is 80 dB or better in the low frequencies and 60 dB or better in the high frequencies. The risk of overmasking and crossover, particularly in the low frequencies, is therefore minimized.

The use of ER-3A insert earphones provides additional advantages, such as minimizing risk of ear canal collapse (which occurs frequently with children) using TDH earphones with MX-41/AR ear cushions. A collapsed canal results in elevated air-conduction thresholds in the high-frequencies and erroneous high frequency air–bone gaps. The use of insert earphones also is more comfortable and attenuates external noise in the test environment. For these reasons, the use of insert earphones is strongly recommended for pediatric assessment.

There are other technical and procedural variables that substantially influence bone-conduction assessment. Artifactual responses can be obtained during high-intensity bone-conduction presentation levels. Harmonic distortion (ringing) can occur, resulting in acoustic radiation of the sound resulting in false responses. Vibrotactile stimulation (feeling rather than hearing the sound vibrations) also can be encountered during low-frequency (i.e., 250-Hz and 500-Hz) bone-conduction testing, resulting in false air–bone gaps. The placement of the vibrator and the force of the vibrator (headband pressure, which is configured for an adult head) can affect the accuracy of bone-conduction results. These technical difficulties may result in misinterpretation regarding the nature and etiology of the hearing loss.

SPEECH TESTING

Speech testing is extremely important in the differential diagnosis of MHL in infants and children. An infant's response may be more reliable to a speech stimulus because it is more meaningful. With VRA, habituation to the stimulus may be less likely with speech than with a pure-tone or narrow-band stimulus. Conducting speech awareness, picture identification, body part identification, or spondee thresholds with insert earphones as well as with the bone oscillator is faster and more efficient than conducting pure-tone bone-conduction thresholds. The utilization of masking is almost always easier for speech than for pure tones with children. Frequently we find that the best estimate of hearing levels is obtained from speech assessment. Air- and bone-conducted speech assessment may be the only behavioral means to determine the contributions of the middle ear and the cochlea in the child with MHL.

IMMITTANCE AUDIOMETRY

Acoustic immittance studies have been used for over 20 years to evaluate the integrity of the auditory system. Tympanometry and the acoustic stapedial reflex are diagnostically helpful in differentiating between CHL and SNHL as well as in distinguishing some etiologies of CHL. Used in conjunction with pure-tone audiometry, tympanometry, and the acoustic reflex threshold (ART) (i.e., the lowest stimulus intensity levels that activate the stapedial reflex) can usually establish whether the middle ear is involved. It has been demonstrated that ART findings demonstrate greater sensitivity to middle ear pathology than do traditional threshold air- and bone-conduction tests.

The most valuable implication of immittance to MHL is the fact that ARTs are obscured when the probe is coupled to an ear with even a slight middle ear pathology. According to Jerger et al. (10) an air–bone gap of only 10 dB in the probe ear is sufficient to obscure the ART greater than 80% of the time. While ART testing has a very high sensitivity to conductive pathology (11), it has a low specificity, because an absent ART can result from a number of other pathologic as well as nonpathologic conditions (12,13).

When used in conjunction with other immittance measures, such as peak compensated acoustic admittance and tympanometric gradient, the sensitivity and specificity of immittance in the identification of CHL is quite good (14,15). Studies have demonstrated that static compliance, tympanometric gradient, and tympanometric width were better at separating children without middle ear effusion than children with surgically confirmed middle ear effusion (16,17).

When MHL is suspected, tympanometry along with ipsilateral and contralateral ART testing should always be performed. If these findings are normal, a safe assumption may be made that any existing hearing loss is of sensorineural origin and bone conduction is not necessary. When findings do suggest middle ear involvement, immittance does not, unfortunately, quantify the extent of conductive pathology or whether there is an existing sensorineural component. In these instances bone-conduction testing is essential for differential diagnosis.

AUDITORY BRAINSTEM RESPONSE

An important technique in the diagnosis of hearing loss in the pediatric population is the auditory brainstem response (ABR). The procedure is a safe, noninvasive means to assess auditory function in patients who do not or cannot participate in behavioral audiometry. ABR is also commonly used as a cross-check when behavioral findings suggest significant hearing loss. It is important to remember that the ABR should not be used in lieu of audiometric studies in children who are capable of providing reliable behavioral responses. The ultimate goal should be to determine hearing sensitivity with audiometry. When this is not possible, however, medical management can be pursued based on electrophysiologic findings.

Pediatric ABR testing is usually conducted by employing air-conducted clicks, tone bursts, or both clicks and tone burst stimuli for each ear. Frequently, the utilization of air-conducted click ABRs and immittance is all that is necessary to estimate hearing acuity. However, if CHL or MHL is suspected, consideration should be given to both air-conduction click and bone-conduction click ABRs. The ability to conduct bone-conducted as well as air-conducted ABRs may be one of the only ways to differentiate the conductive and sensory components in a child with MHL who cannot cooperate for behavioral assessment. Four considerations should be remembered in administering ABR if middle ear pathology is suspected:

1. The click-evoked ABR has a limited frequency response. The electrophysiologic response arises primarily from the mid- to high-frequency (2,000-Hz to 4,000-Hz) region of the cochlea.
2. Middle ear pathologies typically produce greater low-frequency than high-frequency CHL.
3. Conductive hearing loss essentially attenuates the level of sound reaching the cochlea, which will result in a peripheral conduction delay of the absolute latencies of all air-conducted ABR component waveforms.
4. The extent of absolute latency delay of the ABR waveforms corresponds to the amount of audiometric air–bone gap.

It is well documented that conductive pathology prolongs all ABR waveform component latencies for air-conducted click stimuli (18–21). The most common procedure for predicting the degree of CHL utilizes latency-intensity function of wave V. Much of the early research using electrocochleography and ABR to estimate hearing loss focused on the slope of the wave V latency-intensity function to predict type, degree, and configuration of hearing loss. The threshold of wave V provides an estimate of high-frequency hearing loss, while the absolute latency delay and the amount of horizontal shift in the latency-intensity function help determine the type of hearing loss.

Typically, ABR assessment for audiometric purposes begins at 75 dB using air-conduction unipolarity (e.g., rarefaction) click stimuli. If possible, the absolute, interpeak, and interaural latencies of waves I, III, and V are obtained for neurodiagnostic purposes. If all waveform components are present at 75 dB, click intensity is decreased in 20-dB steps until threshold (lowest discernable level) for wave V is determined. Auditory brainstem response findings in children with suspected MHL must be interpreted with caution, particularly if neurologic interpretation is based solely on the absolute latency of wave V and not on the wave I–V interpeak interval. Failing to take into consideration the contribution of the conductive component may lead to an incorrect interpretation of a central transmission delay (e.g., retrocochlear pathology). Conductive, sensory, and retrocochlear pathologies will produce a delay in wave V latencies at absolute levels. If wave I is clearly identified, there should be no difficulty in differentiating between a peripheral conduction delay (e.g., conductive vs. cochlear) and a central conduction delay (e.g., eighth nerve vs. caudal pontine auditory dysfunction). However, when significant hearing loss secondary to MHL or SNHL is present, wave I may not be readily identified. The inability to obtain a wave I with a significant delay in the absolute latency of wave V at high-intensity levels should make the diagnostician immediately suspect a significant SNHL or MHL. A reliance solely on the absolute latency of wave V could lead to misinterpretation in these instances. Retrocochlear pathology might be suspected when, in fact, the delay of wave V was peripheral in nature.

If CHL or MHL is suspected or if there are absolute latency delays of component waveforms at high stimulus intensities (e.g., 75 dB nHL), both air- and bone-conduction measures should be acquired. Air- and bone-conduction ABR is necessary for an accurate assessment of the conductive versus the sensory component. According to Hall (22), bone-conduction ABR assessment is one of the most underutilized ABR measurement techniques. There has been a reluctance on the part of audiologists and neurodiagnosticians to utilize bone conduction as part of pediatric hearing assessment, even though this procedure may be one of the best tools for the accurate assessment of the degree of cochlear reserve. There are probably a number of number of reasons for this. Technically, the response is more difficult to obtain than a conventional air-conducted ABR. Stimulus artifact or electromagnetic radiation from the bone oscillator can cause artifact, which sometimes obscures wave I, making interpretation difficult. Also, the spectrum of the bone-conducted click is somewhat different from that of air-conducted clicks because of differences in the frequency response of the two transducers. The response obtained by bone conduction will rarely show the familiar five-wave complex seen at high intensities on conventional air-conducted ABR. There also is a reduction in the dynamic range of a bone-conduction ABR. This is similar to conventional bone-conduction audiometry, in which the dynamic range the bone oscillator is significantly smaller than the dynamic range of TDH headphones. The dynamic range for bone-conducted ABRs is generally around 55 to 60 dB, and the output of the bone oscillator will not match the "dial reading" of the evoked potential instrumentation. A bone-conducted ABR stimulus at the limits of the instrumentation (e.g., 100 dB) will be similar to an ABR obtained from air-conducted clicks in the 50-dB range. A summary of the problems encountered in conducting bone-conducted ABR is shown in Table 2.

Auditory brainstem response testing is the best available technique for evaluation of children with suspected MHL when behavioral methods have been unsuccessful. A summary of the ABR protocol for air- and bone-conducted stimulus is shown in Table 3. Even with air- and bone-conducted click ABR testing, it still may not be possible to accurately assess sensorineural integrity if the degree of hearing loss is substantial. The two-part ABR examination should be used in conjunction with other electrophysiologic procedures, such as tone burst ABR, to further evaluate cochlear function, particularly for low-frequency stimuli. Immittance findings and OAE findings should always be included as part of the diagnostic battery when possible. If the child has been sedated for the ABR examination, every opportunity should be taken to obtain as much information as possible.

OTOACOUSTIC EMISSIONS

Otoacoustic emissions are sounds generated within the normal cochlea, either spontaneously or in response to acoustic stimulation (23). Otoacoustic emissions, like the ABR, allow electrophysiologic assessment of the auditory system in unique ways. Both techniques offer site-specific

TABLE 2. *Reasons for limited acceptance of bone-conducted auditory brainstem response in the evaluation of conductive or mixed hearing loss*

Electromagnetic oscillations from the bone vibrator can cause stimulus artifact and obscure wave I.
Reduced dynamic range of transducer
   A bone vibrator has a dynamic range of 55–60 dB
   Evoked potential instrument attenuator is not calibrated for a bone oscillator (correction factors for transducer are necessary).
Masking
   It is assumed that masking will be necessary and problematic. Like conventional audiometry, masking should be employed in the presence of CHL or MHL. There is also concern about overmasking (masking dilemma), which usually can be circumvented.
Response morphology
   Bone-conducted ABRs have a characteristic morphology and latency that is different from high-intensity air-conducted click ABR.
Increased time in test administration
   A threshold search using both air-conduced and bone-conducted ABR can be time consuming.
Procedural differences in bone-conduction protocol
   Stimulation and acquisition parameters have to be modified as a consequence of using a different transducer.

evaluation of the auditory system, utilizing clicks or tone bursts. However, evoked OAEs are considered preneural cochlear responses, while the ABR is considered a test of neural synchrony of the VIIIth nerve and brainstem auditory pathway. Specifically, the test measures the biomechanical activity of outer hair cell function. The measurement of OAEs are dependent on both the inward propagation of energy to the cochlea through the outer and middle ear and the outward propagation of energy from the cochlea through the middle and external ear to the recording microphone in the ear canal. Otoacoustic emissions are physiologically vulnerable to any insults affecting the cochlea, which makes them unique for assessing cochlear function. When the outer hair cells are structurally damaged or nonfunctional, OAEs cannot be elicited by acoustic stimulation (24). Any hearing loss greater than 30 to 40 dB at any given frequency will result in a diminished or absent physiologic response at that frequency. Consequently, OAEs are exquisitely sensitive for the screening of SNHL, particularly in the neonate or pediatric population.

Otoacoustic emissions are actually more sensitive to subtle or mild hearing loss than is the ABR. However, when OAEs are absent, the findings do not provide information about the degree of hearing loss other than that the loss may be greater than 30 to 40 dB. Without other audiologic procedures, such as immittance, OAEs also do not provide information about the type of hearing loss (conductive vs. mixed vs. sensory). Otoacoustic emissions will be unaffected by neural hearing loss, which may also provide extremely useful diagnostic information.

Before stable OAEs can be recorded from the ear canal, it is essential that the middle ear system be normal. Oto-

TABLE 3. *Typical ABR protocol utilized for infants and children*

	Test type	
	Air-conduction ABR	Bone-conduction ABR
Stimulus parameters		
Transducer	Etymotic Research ER-3A insert earphones	Radioear B-70 bone oscillator on mastoid
Stimulus	0.1-msec click	0.1-msec click
Intensity	Begin at 75 nHL (maximum intensity of 100 dB)	Begin at 55–60 dB nHL (maximum intensity of 60 dB)
Polarity	Rarefaction and/or condensation	Alternating
Rate	27.7	9.7
Masking	Not necessary if absolute latencies are normal	Required when wave I is delayed or absent
Recording parameters		
Time base	15 milliseconds	20 milliseconds
Filtering	100 Hz–3,000 Hz	30 Hz–3,000 Hz
Sweeps	1,000–2,000	2,000 or more
Electrode	Channel 1: Cz-A1/A2	Channel 1: Cz-A1/A2
Montage	Channel 2: Cz-A2/A1	Channel 2: Cz-A2/A1

acoustic emissions depend on the inward and outward propagation of energy to and from the cochlea, so any abnormality in the middle ear will affect the transduction of energy. Subtle middle ear dysfunction, such as negative middle ear pressure or a mild low-frequency conductive loss, does not obliterate the OAE (25). However, any substantial middle ear involvement will result in absent OAEs secondary to a transduction deficit and not as a consequence of any sensory hearing loss. In children with significant CHL or MHL, the emissions will be absent and will provide little or no additional diagnostic information than that provided by immittance audiometry. However, if an OAE is observed, there can be only minimal middle ear dysfunction or cochlear dysfunction. Observable OAEs in the presence of hearing loss observed behaviorally or with ABR would suggest the possibility of a neural hearing loss. Otoacoustic emissions in conjunction with ABR testing are proving to be a sensitive method to separate hearing loss of neural origin from hearing loss of cochlear origin. In summary, OAEs should be incorporated into the test battery, especially if one is not certain of the status of either the middle ear or cochlea. Prior to conducting OAEs, it is mandatory to evaluate middle ear status with tympanometry and ART testing.

SYNDROMES THAT INCLUDE MIXED HEARING LOSS

Numerous syndromes include MHL. Although Chapter 22 provides information about how to detect syndromes that include hearing loss of *all* types, several of those syndromes in which MHL is a salient or common feature are described here.

X-linked Mixed Hearing Loss with Stapes Gusher (Nance Deafness/DFN3)

Although this is an inherited syndrome that includes MHL, the X-linked mode of inheritance, often a characteristic shape of the internal auditory canal seen on temporal bone computed tomography (CT) scan, and the finding of a gush of perilymph (or CSF) on fenestrating the footplate or removing the stapes during stapedotomy or stapedectomy surgery. The best way to make a diagnosis of this inherited disorder is *before* operating on an involved ear. Therefore, in evaluation of a male child with MHL, think of this syndrome and take a careful history. If there are two or more males in a family who have MHL and no apparent cause, think of this inherited syndrome and obtain a CT scan of the temporal bones, looking carefully at the shape of the internal auditory canals. If a male with MHL has no siblings and few or no cousins, the family pedigree may not provide helpful information, and you will still need to consider that the patient might have this hereditary hearing syndrome. The gene for X-linked MHL with stapes gusher has been located, and therefore a clinical test for the gene defect might soon be available.

Treacher Collins Syndrome (Mandibulofacial Dysostosis)

Treacher Collins syndrome is a relatively common autosomal dominant craniofacial disorder characterized by constricted midface, cup-shaped ears, down-slanting palpebral fissures, and hearing loss that frequently is mixed. Often, a child with Treacher Collins syndrome will have a small constricted middle ear space and markedly retracted eardrum, so that the conductive component of the MHL may be interpreted as being the result of adhesive otitis media. However, the ossicles often are abnormally formed and the stapes footplate may be fixed within the oval window. Therefore, the otologic surgeon is advised to be cautious in attempting to help a child with Treacher Collins syndrome by operating on an ear with MHL with the intention of improving function of the middle ear ossicular conduction mechanism. Achieving success in terms of lessening or eradicating the conductive component of an MHL in a child with

Treacher Collins syndrome is extremely difficult. Careful analysis of the ossicles and oval window on a preoperative CT scan of the temporal bones can help in selecting for surgery only those patients with the most favorable anatomy. However, in general, good results from ossiculoplasty surgery are difficult to achieve and binaural hearing aids are a reasonable alternative to surgery in many cases.

Stickler Syndrome

The child with Stickler syndrome typically has a flat midface, cleft palate, severe myopia often requiring thick glasses, and progressive SNHL. Children with Stickler syndrome tend to be tall and thin, almost having a marfanoid body habitus. Although the hearing loss that is part of the syndrome is sensorineural, the fact that Stickler syndrome incudes a cleft palate means that a child with the syndrome also is likely to have middle ear effusion with CHL. Therefore, until tympanostomy tubes are inserted to help ventilate the middle ears, a child with Stickler syndrome is likely to have an MHL.

Branchio-oto-renal Syndrome

Children with branchio-oto-renal (BOR) syndrome have branchial cleft, fistulae or cysts; otologic abnormalities, including malformed pinna, preauricular pits, or sinuses; hearing loss; and renal abnormalities, such as an abnormally shaped kidney or an abnormal renal collecting system. In about half of the cases of BOR, the hearing loss is mixed conductive and sensorineural (26).

SUMMARY

This chapter has provided information demonstrating that evaluation and management of the child with MHL can be difficult. The audiologist and otologic surgeon need to communicate effectively in evaluating a child with MHL. The multiple confounding variables make subjective and objective assessment of hearing problematic, and the medical and/or surgical decision making likewise is fraught with difficulties. Some helpful hints follow.

The child presenting with MHL requires special medical attention. The hearing acuity may change dynamically due to the conductive or sensorineural component. Multiple audiologic test techniques may be required to determine accurately the magnitude of the conductive and sensorineural components of MHL for each ear. An accurate diagnosis may require serial studies over time to assess the reliability of findings.

Especially in young children, be careful not to assume that responses to low-frequency sound stimuli are always indicators of the sensorineural (bone-conduction) hearing threshold. At the frequencies of 250 Hz and 500 Hz, the child may be responding to the vibrotactile sensation of the test stimulus on the skin over the mastoid rather than the true auditory sensitivity of the cochlea. Mistakenly interpreting vibrotactile responses as responses to auditory stimulus will give the incorrect impression that a child has an MHL when the actual hearing loss may be purely sensorineural. Do not operate unless you are sure that there is a conductive component and you have a reasonable chance that ossiculoplasty will improve the hearing.

When a child with otitis media is found to have MHL in the ear with middle ear effusion, congenital ossicular abnormality or ossicular erosion as a sequela of the otitis media cannot be ruled out until hearing is tested in the ear after the middle ear effusion has resolved spontaneously, resolved in response to medical management, or been evacuated at the time of myringotomy with insertion of a tympanostomy tube.

Although improving a child's hearing by closing the air–bone gap in an ear with MHL is a desirable goal and may mean that the child could then have acceptable hearing without need for a hearing aid, the otologic surgeon is advised to be cautious in attempting ossiculoplasty surgery in children. MHL may suggest that the temporal bone has developed in an abnormal way. Although there may not be sufficient data to prove the notion scientifically, many experienced otologic surgeons believe that the child with MHL is at higher risk of developing worse sensorineural hearing loss after ossiculoplasty than children who have purely CHL due to an isolated ossicular abnormality. Further, if the child with MHL has an abnormality involving the stapes footplate, many otolgic surgeons believe that there is significant risk for loss of hearing when attempting to remove or fenestrate the stapes footplate.

Although the proper name for one type of hereditary MHL is "X-linked mixed hearing loss with stapes gusher," there is no longer a need to encounter in the operating room a gush of perilymph or CSF in order to recognize and diagnose this disorder. When a male without stigmata of a dysmorphic syndrome is found to have MHL, the stapes gusher syndrome should be suspected. History taking should then be focused on eliciting information about other male family members who might also have MHL, and a CT scan of the temporal bones should be obtained, looking for the bulbous shape of the lateral aspect of the internal auditory canal that is known to be associated with the gusher syndrome. If there is sufficient suspicion that a male with MHL might have the gusher syndrome, recommendation for use of a hearing aid in the affected ear is likely to be preferable to the attempt at stapedotomy or stapedectomy surgery, which might result in the stapes gusher and lead to the postoperative outcome of hearing that is worse than the hearing prior to surgery.

Be careful in recommending ossiculoplasty for patients with Treacher Collins syndrome and MHL. Significant hearing improvement is difficult to achieve, and the risks of hearing loss following surgery are probably greater for patients with MHL and Treacher Collins syndrome than for other patients with MHL. In management of a child with

MHL, when in doubt about the magnitude of each component of the hearing loss, wait, do not operate.

REFERENCES

1. Hodgson WR. Evaluating infants and young children. In: Katz J, ed. *Handbook of clinical audiology* Baltimore: Williams & Wilkins; 1994: 465–75.
2. Diefendorf AO. Screening for hearing loss: behavioral options. In: Bess F, and Hall J, eds. *Screening children for auditory function.* Nashville: Bill Wilkerson Center Press; 1992:243–60.
3. Jacobson JT, Morehouse CR. A comparison of auditory brain stem response and behavioral screening in high risk and normal newborn infants. *Ear Hear* 1984;5:247–53.
4. Liden G, Kankkunen A. Visual reinforcement audiometry. *Acta Otolaryngology* 1969;67:281–92.
5. Wilson WR, Thompson G. Behavioral audiometry. In: Jerger J, ed. *Pediatric audiology.* San Diego: College Hill Press;1984:1–44.
6. Hall JW, Ghorayeb BY. Diagnosis of middle ear pathology and evaluation of conductive hearing loss. In: Jacobson J, Northern J, eds. *Diagnostic audiology.* Austin TX: Pro-Ed; 1991;161–98.
7. Dirks D. Bone-conduction threshold testing. In: Katz J, ed., *Handbook of clinical audiology* Baltimore: Williams & Wilkins; 1994:132–46.
8. Naunton R. A masking dilemma in bilateral conductive deafness. *Arch Otolaryngol Head Neck Surg* 1960;72:753–7.
9. Killion M, Villchur E. Comments on ''Earphones in audiometry.'' *J Acoust Soc Am* 1989;85:1775–8.
10. Jerger JF, Anthony L, Jerger S, Crump B. Studies in impedance audiometry. III Middle ear disorders. *Arch Otolaryngol* 1974;99:165–71.
11. Silman S, Silverman C, Arick D. Acoustic-immittance screening for detection of middle-ear effusion in children. *J Am Acad Audiol* 1992; 3:262–8.
12. Liden G, Renvall U. Impedance audiometry for screening for middle ear disease in school children. In: Harford ER, Bess FH, Bluestone CD. eds. *Impedance screening in middle ear disease in children.* New York: Grune & Stratton; 1978:197–206.
13. Renvall U, Liden G, Jungert S, Nilsson E. Impedance audiometry in the detection of otitis media. *Scand Audiol* 1975;4:119–24.
14. Smith PS, Wiley TL, Pyle MG. Screening for middle-ear effusion in children. *ASHA* 1992;34:154.
15. Smith PS, Wiley TL, Pyle MG. Efficacy of ASHA guidelines for screening middle-ear function. *ASHA* 1993;35:114.
16. Nozza RJ, Bluestone CD, Kardatzke D. Sensitivity, specificity, and predictive value of immittance measures in the identification of middle-ear effusion. In: Bess FH, Hall JW eds. *Screening children for auditory function.* Nashville: Bill Wilkerson Center Press; 1992:315–28.
17. Nozza RJ, Bluestone CD, Kardatzke D, Bachman R. Towards the validation of aural acoustic immittance measures for diagnosis of middle-ear effusion in children. *Ear Hear* 1992;13:442–53.
18. Fria TJ, Sabo DL. The use of brainstem auditory electric responses in children: practical considerations. *Hear Aid J* 1979;32:20–3.
19. Fria TJ, Sabo DL. Auditory brainstem responses in children with otitis media with effusion. *Ann Otol Rhinol Laryngol* 1978;89:200–6.
20. McGee TJ, Clemis JD. Effects of conductive hearing loss on auditory brainstem response. *Ann Otol Rhinol Laryngol* 1982;91:304–9.
21. Hall J. *Handbook of auditory evoked responses.* Boston: Allyn and Bacon; 1991:360–1.
22. Hall JW. Bone-conduction ABR: clinically feasible and clinically valuable. *Hear J* 1992;47:10–37.
23. Kemp DT. Stimulated acoustic emissions from within the human auditory system. *J Acoust Soc Am* 1978;64:1386–91.
24. Norton SJ. Application of transient evoked otoacoustic emissions to pediatric populations. *Ear Hear* 1993;14:64–73.
25. Owens JJ, McCoy MJ, Lonsbury-Martin BL, Martin GK. Influence of otitis media on evoked otoacoustic emissions in children. *Semin Hear* 1992;13:53–65.
26. Gorlin RJ, Cohen MM, Levin LS. *Syndromes of the head and neck.* New York: Oxford University Press; 1990:658.

CHAPTER 42

Fluctuating and Progressive Sensorineural Hearing Loss

Patrick E. Brookhouser

Educationally significant sensorineural hearing loss (SNHL) in childhood is sudden in onset, is fluctuating or progressive (or both); it enhances parental concern and complicates medical management, hearing aid selection, and individualized educational planning for the hearing-impaired child. In spite of intensive multidisciplinary evaluation and intervention (which could entail corticosteroid treatment or exploratory ear surgery in search of a perilymphatic fistula), threshold fluctuation, a gradual decrease in auditory acuity, or both may proceed unabated in a significant percentage of these children. Most published reports estimate the likelihood of progressive loss of acuity in a child's ear with SNHL at 2% to 6% (1–3). Other authors project a substantially higher risk of progression.

Both genetic and nongenetic etiologies have been implicated in fluctuating and progressive SNHL in children (3–4). The availability of effective preventive measures, including vaccines against major nongenetic causes of SNHL such as measles, rubella, mumps and *Haemophilus influenzae* meningitis, should increase the relative prevalence of genetic SNHL among future cohorts of hearing-impaired children. A reasonable prediction of auditory threshold behavior in these patients can often be inferred from the audiologic records of other affected family members. In some types of genetic SNHL, the likelihood of progressive auditory threshold deterioration is nearly 100%; thresholds in other varieties remain stable over extended periods.

FACTORS AFFECTING AUDITORY THRESHOLD DETERMINATION

When considering serial auditory threshold behavior in children with SNHL, one must make allowance for intrinsic and extrinsic factors, apart from an actual change in auditory sensitivity over time, which can contribute to audiometric threshold variation. Exposure to sufficiently intense sound (including inappropriately adjusted hearing aids) or some otoactive drugs or chemicals can produce a temporary threshold shift and should be ruled out by the patient's history. Retesting after a period of rest from hearing aid use may be advisable. Apart from simple occlusion of the external auditory canal with cerumen or foreign body, small canal size, excessive tortuosity, and variable resiliency can lead to pinna or canal collapse under earphones and a factitious conductive loss. Inappropriate size, placement, or both of a circumaural earphone can also contribute to errors. Careful cleaning of the canal, selection of appropriately sized circumaural earphones, and utilization of insert-type earphones, when appropriate, can remedy these problems.

Undetected middle ear dysfunction is a common source of audiometric variance in children and must be excluded by careful otologic examination (e.g., pneumatic otoscopy) and concurrent immitance measures at each audiologic evaluation. As the basis for therapeutic and rehabilitative decisions, accurate determination of the degree and audiometric configuration of a SNHL should be accomplished in an effusion-free ear. In a study population of 437 children who had bilateral SNHL of moderate degree or poorer and who were diagnosed prior to age 5 years, the mean threshold shift observed during middle-ear effusion was 25.0 dB at 250 Hz, 28.5 dB at 500 Hz, 29.5 dB at 1,000 Hz, 24.5 dB at 2000 Hz, and 27.5 dB at 4000 Hz (5) (Table 1) (Fig. 1).

Other potential sources of error may involve the examiner or the patient. Gross attentional and fine auditory attentional deficits in a young child can yield inconsistent conditioned responses, which makes threshold determination challenging. If the testing technique or materials are linguistically or developmentally inappropriate, inconclusive or misleading responses can be elicited. Changes in criteria can occur over

---

P.E. Brookhouser: Boys Town National Research Hospital, Department of Otolaryngology and Human Communication, Creighton University School of Medicine, Omaha, Nebraska 68131.

TABLE 1. *Air conduction threshold shifts at time of effusion*

Category	Frequency (Hz)				
	250	500	1,000	2,000	4,000
Mean threshold shift (dB)	25	28.5	29.5	24.5	27.5
Ears < 20 dB (%)	33	10	21	33	30
Ears 20–30 dB (%)	33	59	46	39	30
Ears > 30 dB (%)	33	31	33	28	40
Ears ≥ 40 dB (%)	15	20	23	23	27

Data from Brookhouser et al. (5).

time in both the patient and examiner. The young patient may learn to "tune in" more attentively to very soft sounds and thus achieve better thresholds not reflective of an actual change in auditory acuity. Age-appropriate normative behavioral audiologic data for infants and preschoolers should be utilized for comparative purposes before reaching conclusions regarding the degree, configuration, and stability of a childhood hearing loss. Different examiners may employ diverse criteria, from a head turn in visual reinforcement audiometry to an auditory stimulus, for judging a young child's positive conditioned response. This type of error is particularly likely with multihandicapped, hearing-impaired children whose repertoire of responses may be limited by a coexisting handicap (e.g., cerebral palsy).

Methodologic differences can also contribute to test–retest variation among different examiners and across multiple tests administered by the same examiner. Evaluating children often entails presentation of not only an auditory stimulus but also an effective reinforcement (e.g., visual stimulus, praise for good performance, etc.) to achieve and maintain a conditioning bond. The best protection against inadvertent errors resulting from methodologic differences is to arrange for the same audiologists to evaluate a particular child's hearing over time. Although this approach does not exclude the possibility of measurement error, it helps ensure that such errors are consistent in monitoring threshold variation. To minimize other potential sources of error, threshold variation at 250 Hz should be accorded less relative importance because background conditions in the test environment can affect low-frequency responses.

At the opposite end of the frequency spectrum, serial thresholds obtained, in the author's practice, on normal hearing contralateral ears of children having unilateral SNHL revealed the greatest test-to-test threshold variation outside the allowable 10 dB envelope (±5 dB) at 8000 Hz. Only 1 of 100 threshold determinations at 500, 1,000, 2,000, and 4,000 Hz in these normal-hearing ears varied by more than 10 dB from the previous threshold; none varied by more than 20 dB. Accordingly, evidence of significant threshold change at the four middle test frequencies should elicit

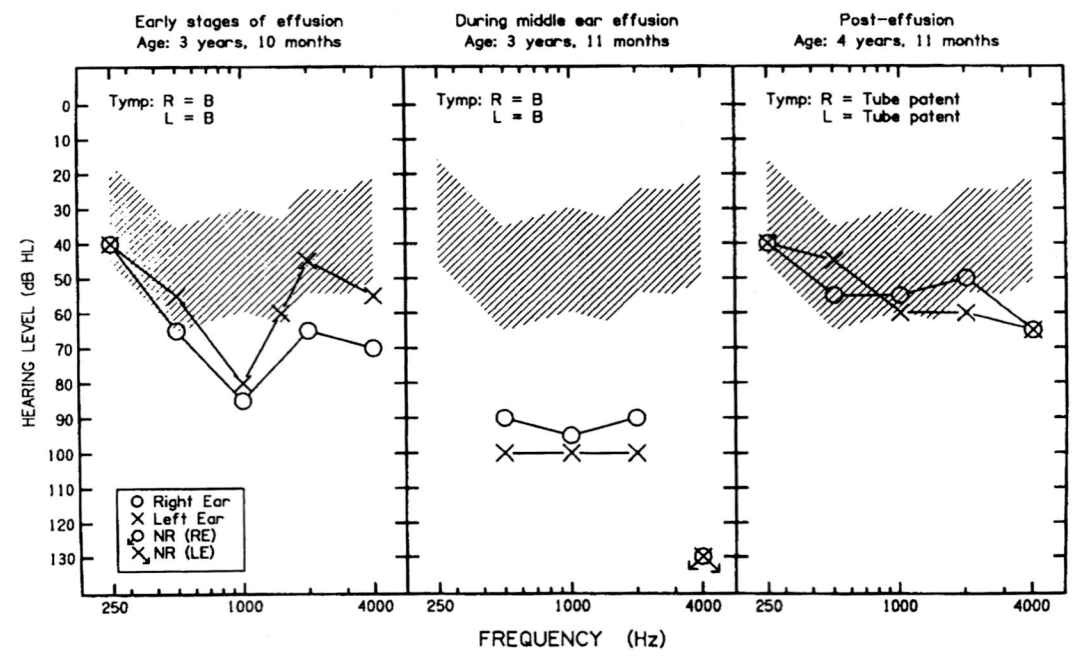

FIG. 1. Effect of middle-ear effusion on a patient with moderate to severe sensorineural hearing loss. Reprinted with permission from Brookhouser et al. (5).

TABLE 2. *Recessive genes causing nonsyndromic hereditary hearing loss*

Locus name	Type of loss	Location	Gene	Reference
DFNB1	Congenital	13q12	Unknown	Guilford et al. (7)
DFNB2	Congenital	11q13.5	Unknown	Guilford et al. (7)
DFNB3	Congenital	17p11.2-q12	Unknown	Friedman et al. (8)
DFNB4	Congenital	7q31	Unknown	Baldwin et al. (9)
DFNB5	Congenital	14q12	Unknown	Fukushima et al. (10)
DFNB6	Congenital	3p14-p21	Unknown	Fukushima et al. (10)
DFNB7	Congenital	9q13-q21	Unknown	Jain et al. (11)
DFNB8	Congenital	21q22	Unknown	Veske et al. (12)
DFNB9	Congenital	2p22-p23	Unknown	Chaib et al. (13)
DFNB10	Congenital	21q22.3	Unknown	Bonné-Tamir et al. (14)
DFNB11	Not available	9q13-q21	Unknown	Scott et al. (15)
DFNB12	Congenital	10q21-22	Unknown	Chaib et al. (16)
DFNB15	Not available	3q21-q25 19p13	Unknown	Chen et al. (17)

greater concern by the clinician than should intertest variation at 250 and 8,000 Hz. Fluctuation or deterioration of thresholds or absent middle-ear dysfunction by 15 dB or more at these frequencies should prompt careful reevaluation of the affected hearing-impaired child.

Behavioral thresholds cannot be compared precisely to threshold information obtained by electrophysiologic methods such as auditory brainstem response (ABR) testing. Although ABR thresholds correlate best with high-frequency behavioral thresholds, evoked potential measurements are not as sensitive as behavioral threshold measures. Behavioral thresholds for click stimuli, which are commonly used in ABR testing, typically occur at 30 to 36 dB peak sound pressure, yet few normal-hearing patients demonstrate ABRs to such low level stimuli in the usual clinical test paradigm.

ETIOLOGIC FACTORS

Both genetic and nongenetic etiologies merit diagnostic consideration in children with fluctuating and progressive SNHL (3,4). As much as 70% to 75% of genetic hearing loss is nonsyndromic, and 80% of these losses are inherited as recessive traits, thus making definitive diagnosis in singleton cases particularly challenging. Nonsyndromic, hereditary, progressive SNHL was broadly categorized by Konigsmark and Gorlin (6) according to age at onset, involved frequencies (low, middle, high) and mode of inheritance (dominant, recessive, X-linked). Recent gene linkage studies have localized a number of genes for syndromic and nonsyndromic hearing loss to specific chromosomal regions. The eventual identification and sequencing of these genes should pave the way for greater diagnostic and prognostic precision in the management of children with this pervasive type of genetic hearing loss. Although estimates of the number of genes involved in nonsyndromic hearing loss have ranged as high as 200, most geneticists predict that no more than 20 genes may account for the majority of these hearing losses (Table 2) (7–17).

Syndromic disorders associated with fluctuating and progressive SNHL include anhidrosis, ataxia, branchial fistulas, optic atrophy, piebald trait, and preauricular pits (3,4). Acoustic neuromata associated with neurofibromatosis, particularly NF2, can present in younger patients (18–21). Inner-ear anomalies such as Mondini's aplasia and enlarged vestibular aqueduct, detectable by temporal bone imaging, have been linked with fluctuating and progressive SNHL in children and are often exacerbated by minimal head trauma (22–24). The differential diagnosis should also include ototoxic drugs and chemicals (22–24); noise trauma (27,28); ear or head trauma (29); mumps and congenital infections such as rubella, cytomegalovirus, toxoplasmosis and syphilis (30–33); bacterial meningitis (34,35); hyperlipidemia, thyroid dysfunction, diabetes, hypercoagulability state (36,37); sickle cell disease, leukemia, autoimmune inner-ear disease (38–42); and perilymphatic fistula (43).

The role of immune-mediated inner-ear disease in fluctuating and progressive SNHL in childhood is not yet sufficiently clear to warrant extensive immunologic evaluation in the majority of patients. In addition, current adult treatment regimens for this disorder, extended high-dose corticosteroids and cytotoxic drugs, would have to overcome serious ethical and health-related concerns regarding complications before being judged safe for administration to a child or adolescent.

Several authors have addressed the possible role of perilymphatic fistulae (PLF) in children with fluctuating and progressive hearing loss (44–46). The unavailability of a sensitive and specific diagnostic technique to confirm the presence of PLF preoperatively has necessitated invasive procedures, either middle-ear exploration or myringotomy with otoendoscopy, to assess the integrity of the perilymphatic compartment. Definitive confirmation of PLF at surgery can also be challenging, and has prompted an ongoing search for perilymph-specific biochemical markers to distinguish perilymph from other clear middle-ear fluids when the child is seen in the clinic or during surgery. Generally accepted indications for exploratory ear surgery in children

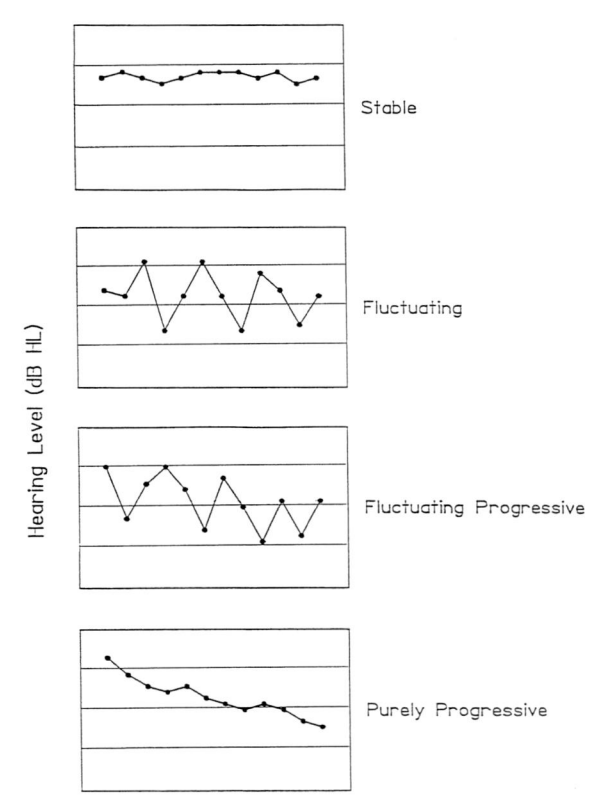

FIG. 2. On the basis of serial audiogram, each abnormal ear was assigned to a category of auditory threshold variation according to specific criteria. Reprinted with permission from Brookhouser et al. (4).

with fluctuating and progressive SNHL have yet to be elucidated and debates in the literature concerning the topic have been contentious (47–52). An often-cited measure of effective surgical treatment is postoperative auditory threshold stability or improvement, (or both) which is invoked to support the advisability of prophylactic graft placement to reinforce the oval and round windows even if a PLF is not visualized. More appropriately, evidence regarding the efficacy of intervention should be weighed against the likelihood of threshold stability or improvement during a comparable follow-up period in the absence of therapeutic intervention, that is, according to the natural history of the disorder.

PATTERNS OF AUDITORY THRESHOLD VARIATION

If audiologic evaluations are obtained infrequently in a child with SNHL, clinicians and parents might presume that any observed loss of auditory acuity has occurred gradually over time, unabated by any relative threshold recovery. Recent studies suggest that progressive deterioration of auditory acuity without intercurrent improvement is an uncommon occurrence in children and adolescents. In one study (4) of 229 children and adolescents (392 ears—132 boys, 97 girls) with etiologically heterogeneous SNHL and normal middle-ear function, who demonstrated fluctuating or deteriorating (or both) auditory thresholds at one or more standard audiologic test frequencies (SATF) (250, 500, 1,000, 2,000, 4,000 and 8,000 Hz) over a mean follow up of 5.75 years, only 22 (6%) of 365 study ears with progressive or fluctuating thresholds demonstrated purely progressive losses of 10 dB or greater. Of the remaining 343 ears, 135 (39%) experienced serial threshold fluctuations of 10 dB or greater without progression. The remaining 208 (61%) demonstrated threshold fluctuation coupled with permanent progression of the hearing loss (Fig. 2) (Tables 3, 4).

Initial audiometric thresholds were obtained before age 6 years for 194 of the 392 ears (49%); only 3 of these 194 ears demonstrated purely progressive losses during follow-up. A fluctuating or progressive pattern was found in 122 of 194 ears (62.5%), and fluctuation without threshold progression occurred in the remaining 70 (36%). Children who were initially evaluated at ages 6 through 14 years were significantly more likely to show fluctuation with progression than without progression. Among youth who were age 14 or older at first audiogram (34 ears), fluctuation without progression was the single most common pattern of variation, occurring in 17 (50%) of the ears.

A companion study (53) involving a subset of the 229 participants (4), documented the natural history of ear-specific auditory threshold behavior during a 6-month follow-up of 95 children (62 boys, 33 girls) with SNHL of diverse etiology who sustained a 20 dB or greater decrement in auditory acuity at one or more of the frequencies (500, 1,000, 2,000 or 4,000 Hz.) Children who had undergone medical or surgical intervention were excluded from this retrospective review. Each 20 dB or greater drop at any of the four target

TABLE 3. Fluctuation without progression, by frequency

Fluctuation	Test frequencies (%)					
	250	500	1,000	2,000	4,000	8,000
≤10 dB	33	37	44	43	47	53
15–20 dB[a]	29	28	25	26	30	22
25–30 dB[a]	16	15	16	12	7	14
35–40 dB[a]	9	6	4	9	7	6
>40 dB[a]	13	14	11	10	9	5

N = 135 ears.
[a] Min–max fluctuation.
Data from Brookhouser et al. (4).

TABLE 4. *Fluctuation with progression only, by frequency*

Fluctuation	Test frequencies (%)					
	250	500	1,000	2,000	4,000	8,000
≤10 dB	175	179	178	188	184	173
15–20 dB[a]	29	22	30	20	28	35
25–30 dB[a]	11	11	8	11	7	14
35–40 dB[a]	7	9	6	8	3	6
>40 dB	8	9	8	3	8	2

N = 230 ears.
[a] Initial–final progression.
Data from Brookhouser et al. (40).

frequencies was designated as an "episode" and 429 separate episodes were identified for 138 ears that met these criteria. Frequency-specific serial thresholds obtained during the 6 months following each episode were classified as stable (±5 dB), improved (10 dB or more), or worse (10 dB or more) (Table 5). These data confirm a significant propensity (approximately 50%) for spontaneous recovery of some auditory acuity during the 6 months following a 20-dB decrement at one of the study frequencies. A 10-dB or greater improvement was observed after 52.4% of the episodes, threshold stability occurred after 31% and additional loss (10 dB or more) was seen in 16.6% of episodes. The percentage of losses followed by either threshold stability or improvement ranged from 80% at 4,000 Hz to 88.5% of episodes at 1,000 Hz. Further hearing loss during follow-up was most likely to occur at 4,000 Hz (20%) and least likely at 1,000 Hz (11.4%). Episodic losses occurred in both ears in 45% of 95 children, but these losses were not necessarily simultaneous or symmetrical.

Of the 95 children in the second study (53), 65 (41 boys, 24 girls) experienced sufficiently severe decrements during 110 episodes to sustain a 20 dB or greater deterioration of the test frequency average (TFA). An improvement of 10 db or more in the TFA was subsequently documented in 51% of these cases, the TFA remained stable in 45%, and a 10 dB or greater decline occurred in only 4% during 6 months of follow-up. Recovery to pre-episodic levels occurred after only 14% of these episodes although at least 20 dB of improvement was achieved 24% of the time. These results provide a natural history benchmark against which the efficacy of therapeutic intervention in cases of fluctuating and progressive childhood SNHL can be compared.

AUDIOGRAM CONFIGURATION

Initial audiogram configuration was examined in these studies (4,53) for possible correlation with subsequent auditory threshold behavior. Three different approaches to audiogram classifications were explored: audiologists' best judgment, determination of low-frequency and high-frequency slope, and use of a computerized Quick Cluster (SPSS Reference Guide, 1990; SPSS, Inc. Chicago, IL) algorithm that assigned initial and final audiograms to one of six categoric patterns. Table 6 compares the audiologists' classification of 2262 ears with all degrees of SNHL in the hospital's clinical database with 358 ears from the first study (4), which demonstrated fluctuating or progressive threshold behavior according to the study's criteria. The audiologists' audiogram classification is also listed for 110 of the 358 ears that sustained a permanent drop of 10 dB or greater in the TFA. For obvious reasons, fragmentary losses (i.e., severe to profound losses in which only low-frequency responses were measurable) demonstrated less potential to fulfill study criteria for threshold fluctuation and progression. The other configuration categories do not differ significantly among the three patient groups, which confirms that this particular classification scheme does not provide clinical guidance regarding which ears with SNHL are at increased risk for threshold instability.

In the second classification method, an audiogram configuration was assigned to one of nine subclasses on the basis of the mathematically determined slope in the low frequencies (250, 500, 1,000 Hz) and the high frequencies (2,000, 4,000, 8,000 Hz) (Fig. 3). Slopes within each frequency region were categorized as flat (slope < 10 dB/octive); rising (upward slope > 10 dB/octive); or sloping (downward slope < 10 dB/octive). Under this classification scheme, 43% of the ears were assigned flat configurations and another 47% had some degree of downward slope. Table 7 reveals that nearly 43% of the ears with flat configuration demonstrated fluctuating thresholds without progressive loss during follow-up as compared with only 22% of ears with

TABLE 5. *Outcome episodes, by frequency*

Outcome (n = 429)	500 Hz (%)	1,000 Hz (%)	2,000 Hz (%)	4,000 Hz (%)
Improved	63 (52.1)	64 (56.1)	49 (49.5)	49 (51.6)
Stable	38 (31.4)	37 (32.5)	31 (31.3)	27 (28.4)
Worse	20 (16.5)	13 (11.4)	19 (19.2)	19 (20.0)
No. of episodes	121	114	99	95

Data from Brookhouser et al. (53).

TABLE 6. *Audiologist classification of audiometric configuration*

Configuration	Ears with SNHL (n = 2,262) (%)	Progression or fluctuation threshold (n = 358) (%)	Progression or fluctuation permanent loss of ≥10 dB (%)[a]
Flat	30.5	31.3	28.4
Gradual slope	21.5	23.2	22.4
Sharp slope	17.7	19.6	20.7
Fragmentary	10.1	2.8	2.6
Saucer-shaped	9.4	8.7	11.2
Rising	8.2	10.9	9.5
Jagged	2.6	3.6	5.2

[a] By test frequency averages.
Data from Brookhouser et al. (4, 53).

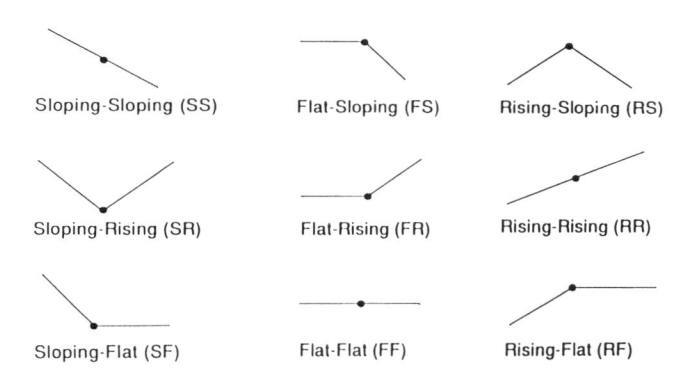

FIG. 3. Configuration assignment on the basis of audiogram's slope in the low-frequency and high-frequency regions. Reprinted with permission from Brookhouser et al. (4).

TABLE 7. *Threshold variation versus initial configuration*

Configuration	Stable	Fluctuation	Fluctuation or progression	Progression	Total
Sloping-sloping	2	3	22	2	29
Sloping-flat	0	34	49	2	85
Sloping-rising	0	0	2	0	2
Flat-sloping	5	15	42	7	69
Flat-flat	17	71	71	9	168
Flat-rising	2	5	12	1	20
Rising-sloping	0	0	3	0	3
Rising-flat	1	7	5	1	14
Rising-rising	0	0	2	0	2
Total	27	135	208	22	392

N = 392 ears.
Data from Brookhouser et al. (4, 53).

TABLE 8. *Initial versus final configuration*

		Final								
		SS	SF	SR	FS	FF	FR	RS	RF	RR
Initial	SS	18	6	0	3	2	0	0	0	0
	SF	7	58	1	2	17	0	0	0	0
	SR	0	1	1	0	0	0	0	0	0
	FS	17	5	1	36	10	0	0	0	0
	FF	0	15	3	9	132	3	1	5	0
	FR	0	0	0	0	9	11	0	0	0
	RS	0	1	0	0	1	0	1	0	0
	RF	0	0	0	0	6	1	0	7	0
	RR	0	0	0	0	1	0	0	0	1

F, flat; R, rising; S, sloping.
Data from Brookhouser et al. (4, 53).

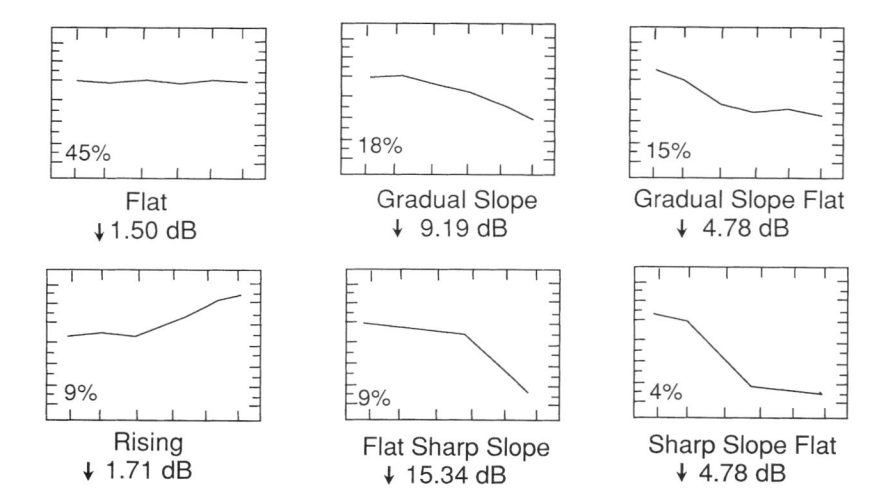

FIG. 4. Audiometric configurations of 389 ears demonstrating fluctuation or progression of 10 dB or greater.

Flat 45% ↓ 1.50 dB
Gradual Slope 18% ↓ 9.19 dB
Gradual Slope Flat 15% ↓ 4.78 dB
Rising 9% ↓ 1.71 dB
Flat Sharp Slope 9% ↓ 15.34 dB
Sharp Slope Flat 4% ↓ 4.78 dB

a flat configuration in the low frequencies and a downward slope in the high frequencies. When the initial and final configurations are compared, 68% of all ears retained the same audiogram configuration. The flat-flat (FF), sloping-flat (SF), and sloping-sloping (SS) categories were most likely to remain unchanged, but nearly 50% of the flat-sloping (FS) configurations changed, most commonly to SS (Table 8).

The results of the Quick Cluster classification method are displayed in Figures 4 and 5. Of the 389 ears (4) that had sufficient information for classification, 78% fell into one of three categories: flat, gradual slope, and gradual SF. The average additional loss in TFA thresholds (see Fig. 4) was greatest for the flat-rising group. Comparison of the initial and final configurations revealed a nearly 75% likelihood of the flat and gradually sloping configurations remaining unchanged, but two thirds of the 60 ears with gradual SF patterns assumed a different final configuration. Additional analyses focused on 107 of the ears that demonstrated a 10 dB or greater deterioration in the TFA. These ears were much less likely to retain their initial audiogram configuration as hearing loss progressed (Figs. 6, 7).

HEARING LOSS ETIOLOGY AND SERIAL THRESHOLD PATTERNS

In spite of a diligent search by a multidisciplinary clinical team for presumptive SNHL etiology in the 229 original study patients, the etiology remained uncertain in fully 40% of the children (Fig. 8). In 14% of cases, a clear hereditary pattern could be identified, but it is likely that a significant number of losses classified as uncertain etiology represent singleton nonsyndromic hereditary losses. Among the subgroup of 95 children in the second study who experienced the most significant additional hearing loss, an even higher percentage (47.3%) were labeled as uncertain etiology (Table 9). It is also likely that some losses attributed to perinatal high-risk factors (HRF) are genetic and that the HRFs were coincidental. Hearing losses were attributed to endolymphatic hydrops only if the patients had a positive response to a diuretic challenge test and PLF was diagnosed when demonstrated at surgery. The unavailability of a definitive laboratory test to confirm congenital cytomegalovirus infection in infants and children older than 4 to 6 weeks of age further clouded diagnostic accuracy among the nongenetic etiologies.

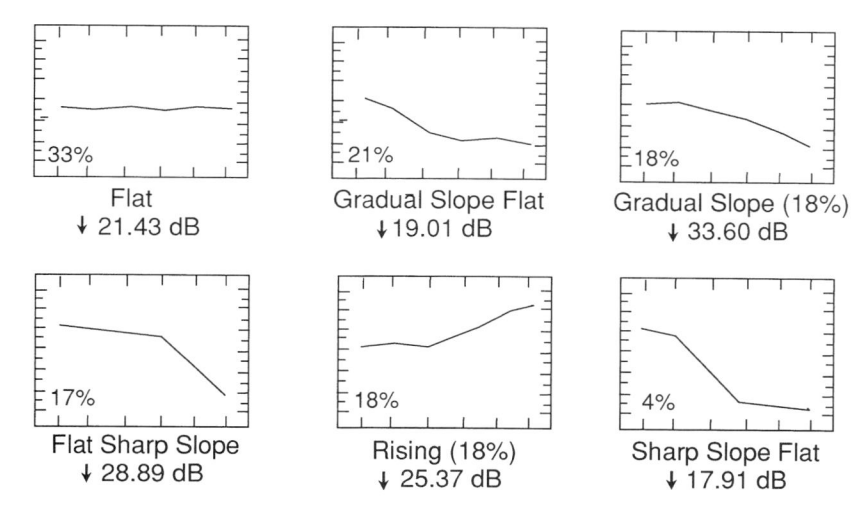

Flat 33% ↓ 21.43 dB
Gradual Slope Flat 21% ↓ 19.01 dB
Gradual Slope (18%) ↓ 33.60 dB
Flat Sharp Slope 17% ↓ 28.89 dB
Rising (18%) 18% ↓ 25.37 dB
Sharp Slope Flat 4% ↓ 17.91 dB

FIG. 5. Audiometric configurations of 107 ears demonstrating 10 dB or greater decrease in the three frequency average (500, 1,000 and 2,000 Hz).

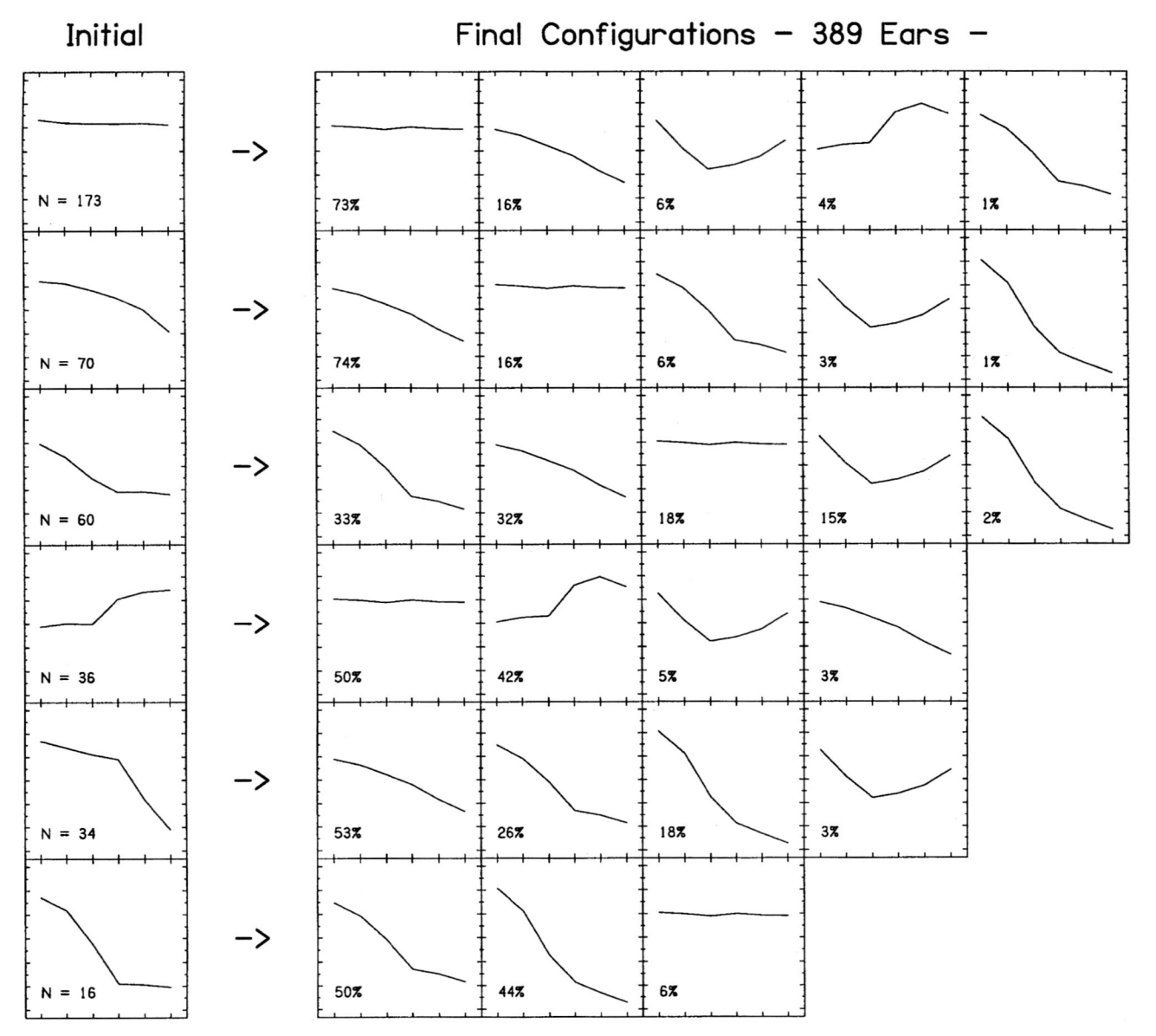

FIG. 6. Comparison of initial and final configuration categories for 389 ears.

TABLE 9. *Threshold patterns, by etiology*

Etiology	Loss of ≤20 dB[a] (n = 95) (%)	Permanent loss of ≥20 dB (n = 65) (%)
Head trauma	5 (5.3)	2 (3.1)
Meningitis	6 (6.63)	3 (4.6)
Hydrops	2 (2.1)	0 (0)
Perinatal HRF	16 (16.8)	11 (16.9)
Hereditary	15 (15.8)	11 (16.9)
Other	6 (6.3)	4 (6.2)
Uncertain	45 (47.3)	34 (52.3)

HRF, high-risk factor.
[a] At 500, 1,000, 2,000, or 4,000 Hz.
Data from Brookhouser et al. (53).

Although the likelihood of threshold instability affecting both of a youngster's ears was quite high, and both ears tended to demonstrate the same general pattern of threshold behavior (i.e., fluctuating vs. progressive), the time course of threshold variation might be asymmetrical (Table 10). The greatest degree of asymmetry was associated with etiologies most likely to occur unilaterally in adults (e.g., endolymphatic hydrops, PLF), and these patients were predominantly in the adolescent age group.

The current state of knowledge of genetic hearing loss precludes definitive diagnosis of nonsyndromic recessive SNHL except in multigenerational families with several affected individuals. Because of the heterogeneity of the losses, prognostic guidance cannot be gleaned from one family and applied to another. Rapid advances in gene localization and eventually gene identification in these families,

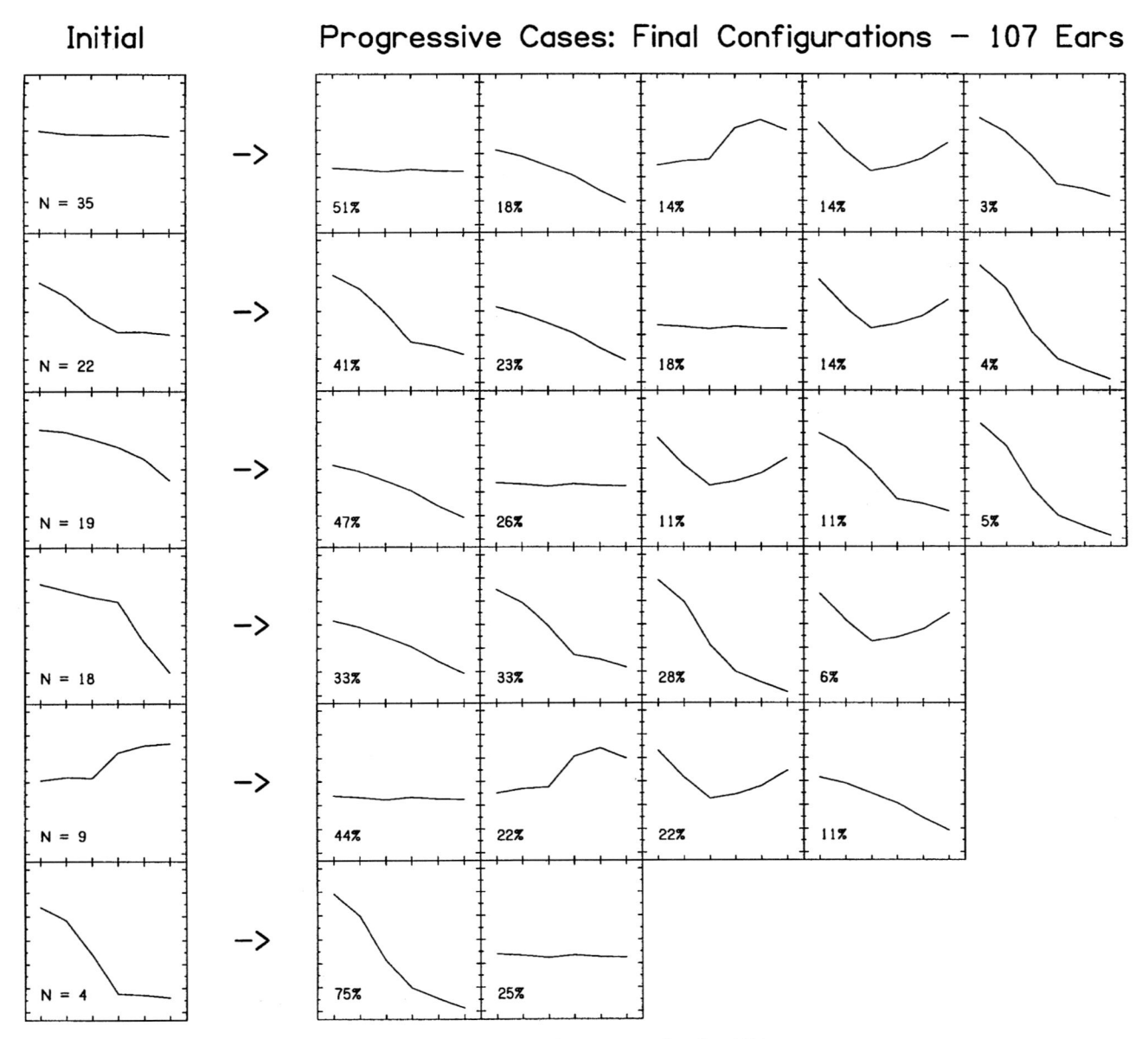

FIG. 7. Comparison of initial and final configuration catetgories for 107 ears.

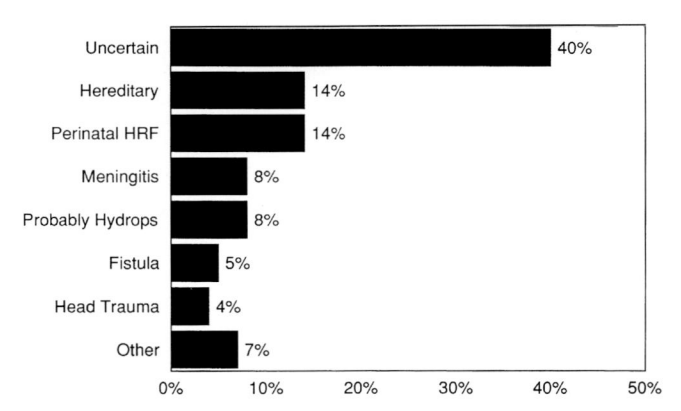

FIG. 8. Presumptive etiology for SNHL in 229 study patients. HRF, High-risk factors. Modified from Brookhouser et al. (4).

TABLE 10. *Symmetry of threshold variation, by etiology*

Etiology	Symmetrical (%)	Asymmetrical (%)	Total
Uncertain	41 (44.6)	51 (55.4)	92
Hereditary	16 (51.6)	15 (48.4)	31
Perinatal HRF	13 (40.6)	19 (59.4)	32
Meningitis	3 (15.8)	16 (84.2)	19
Presumptive hydrops	3 (16.7)	15 (83.3)	18
PLF	2 (18.2)	9 (81.8)	11
Head trauma	1 (10.0)	9 (90.0)	10
Other	9 (56.3)	7 (43.7)	16
Total	88 (38.4)	141 (61.6)	229

HRF, high-risk factor; PLF, perilymph fistula.
Data from Brookhouser et al. (4).

however, promises future availability of diagnostic tools to subclassify childhood genetic SNHL into categories that are prognostically meaningful. Although clinicians must currently speculate regarding the risk of further threshold deterioration in most childhood SNHL, the ultimate goal should be to base decisions regarding rehabilitative intervention, both medical and educational, not only on a child's initial auditory acuity but also on a predictable pattern of threshold behavior to be expected over time, given the child's specific diagnosis.

REFERENCES

1. Parving A. Longitudinal study of hearing-disabled children. A follow-up investigation. *Int J Ped Otorhinolaryngol* 1988;15:233–244.
2. Ruben RJ, Fishmann G. Otological care of the hearing impaired child. In: SE Gerber, GT Mencher, eds. *Early management of hearing loss*. San Francisco: Grune & Stratton; 1981:105–118.
3. Meyerhoff WL, Cass S, Schwaber MK, Sculerati N, Slattery WH. Progressive sensorineural hearing loss in chidlren. *Otolaryngol Head Neck Surg* 1994;110:569–579.
4. Brookhouser PE, Worthington DW, Kelly WJ. FLuctuating and/or progressive sensorineural hearing loss in children. *Laryngoscope* 1994; 104:958–964.
5. Brookhouser PE, Worthington DW, Kelly WJ. Middle ear disease in young children with sensorineural hearing loss. *Laryngoscope* 1993; 103:371–378.
6. Konigsmark BW, Gorlin RJ. *Genetic and Metabolic Deafness*. Philadelphia: WB Saunders; 1976:7–48.
7. Guilford P, Ben Arab S, Blanchard S, et al. A non-syndrome form of neurosensory, recessive deafness maps to the pericentromeric region of chromosome 13 q. *Nat Genet* 1994;6(1):24–28.
8. Friedman TB, Liang Y, Weber JL, et al. A gene for congenital, recessive deafness DFNB3 maps to the pericentromeric region of chromosome 17. *Nat Genet* 1995;(1):86–91.
9. Baldwin CT, Weiss S, Farrer LA, et al. Linkage of congenital recessive deafness (DFNB4) to chromosome 7q31 and evidence for genetic heterogeneity in the Middle Easter Bruze population. *Hum Mol Genet* 1995; 4(9):1637–1642.
10. Fukushima K, Ramesh A, Srisailapathy CR, et al. An autosomal recessive nonsyndromic form of sensorineural hearing loss maps to 3p-DFNB6. *Genome Res* 1995;5(3):305–308.
11. Jain PK, Fukushima K, Deshmukh D, et al. A human recessive neurosensory nonsyndromic hearing impairment locus is a potential homologue of the murine deafness (dn) locus. *Hum Mol Genet* 1995;4: 2391–2394.
12. Veske A, Oehlmann R, Younus F, Mohyuddin A, et al. Autosomal recessive non-syndromic deafness locus (DFNB8) maps on chromosome 21q22 in large consanguineous kindred from Pakistan. *Hum Mol Genet* 1996;5:165–168.
13. Chaib H, Place C, Salem N, et al. A gene responsible for a sensorineural nonsyndromic recessive deafness maps to chromosome 2p22-23. *Hum Mol Genet* 1996a;5:155–158.
14. Bonne-Tamir B, DeStefano AL, Briggs CE, Adair R, et al. Linkage of congenital recessive deafness (gene DFNB10) to chromosome 21q22.3. *Am J Hum Genet* 1996;58(6):1254–9.
15. Scott DA, Carmi R, Elbedour K, Yosefsberg S, Stone EM, Sheffield VC. An autosomal recessive nonsyndromic-hearing-loss locus identified by DNA pooling using two inbred Bedouin kindreds. *Am J Hum Genetic* 1996;59:385–391.
16. Chaib H. Mapping of DFNB12, a gene for nonsyndromal automsomal recessive deafness to chromosome 10q21-22. *Hum Mol Genet* 1997b; 5(7):1061–1064.
17. Chen AH, Ni L, Kikushima K. et al. Linkage of a gene for dominant non-syndromic deafness to chromosome 19. *Hum Mol Genetic* 1995; 4(6):1073–1076.
18. Chen TC, Maceri DR, Giannotta SL, Shih L, McComb JG. Unilateral acoustic neuromas in childhood without evidence of neurofibromatosis: case report and review of the literature. *Am J Otol* 1992;13:318–322.
19. Evans DG, Huson SM, Donnai D, et al. A clinical study of type 2 neurofibromatosis. *Q J Med* 1992;84:603–618.
20. Wigand ME, Haid T, Goertzen W, Wolf S. Preservation of hearing in bilateral acoustic neurinomas by deliberate partial resection. *Acta Otolaryngol (Stockh)* 1992;112:237–241.
21. Miyamoto RT, Roos KL, Campbell RL, Worth RM. Contemporary management of neurofibromatosis. *Ann Otol Rhinol Laryngol* 1991; 100:38–43.
22. Seltzer S, McCabe B. Perilymph fistula: The Iowa experience. *Laryngoscope* 1986;94:37–49.
23. Levenson MJ, Parisier SC, Jacobs M, Edelstein DR. The large vestibular aqueduct syndrome in children. *Arch Otolaryngol Head Neck Surg* 1989;115:54–58.
24. Jackler RK, De la Cruz A. The large vestibular aqueduct syndrome. *Laryngoscope* 1989;99:1238–1242.
25. Fee WE. Aminoglycoside ototoxicity in the human. *Laryngoscope* 1980;90(Suppl.):24:1–19.
26. Quick CA. Chemical and drug effects on the inner ear. In: MM Paparella, DA Shumrick. eds. *Otolaryngology*. Vol. 2. *The Ear*. Philadelphia: WB Saunders; 1980:1804–1827.
27. Brookhouser PE, Worthington DW, Kelly WJ. Noise-induced hearing loss in children. *Laryngoscope* 1992;102:645–655.
28. Eviatar L, Eviatar A. Aminoglycoside ototoxicity in the neonatal period: Possible etiologic factor in delayed postural control. *Otolaryngol Head Neck Surg* 1981;89:818–821.
29. Feldmann H. Sudden hearing loss with delayed onset following head trauma. *Acta Otolaryngol (Stockh)* 1987;103:379–383.
30. Brookhouser PE, Bordley JE. Congenital rubella deafness. *Arch Otolaryngol* 1973;98:252–257.
31. Bordley JE, Alford BR. The pathology of rubella deafness. *Int Audiol* 1970;9:58–67.
32. Stagno S, Pass RF, Dworsky ME, Henderson RE, Moore EG, Walton PD, et al. Congenital cytomegalovirus infection: the relative importance of primary and recurrent maternal infection. *N Engl J Med* 1982;306: 945–949.
33. Hughes GB, Rutherford I. Predictive value of serologic tests for syphilis in otology. *Ann Otol Rhinol Laryngol* 1986;95:250–259.
34. Brookhouser PE, Auslander MC, Meskan ME. The pattern and stability of post-meningitic hearing loss in children. *Laryngoscope* 1988;98: 940–948.
35. Vernon M. Meningitis and deafness: the problem, its physical and audiological, psychological and educational manifestations in deaf children. *Laryngoscope* 1967;77:1856–1874.
36. Spencer JT. Hyperlipoproteinemia in the etiology of inner ear disease. *Laryngoscope* 1973;83:639–678.
37. Strome M, Topf P, Vernick DM. Hyperlipidemia in association with childhood sensorineural hearing loss. *Laryngoscope* 1988;98:165–169.
38. McCabe BF. Autoimmune sensorineural hearing loss. *Ann Otol* 1979; 88:585–589.
39. Bernstein JM, Ogra P, eds. *The immunobiology of autoimmune disease of the inner ear*. New York: Raven; 1987.
40. McCabe BF. Treatment of autoimmune inner-ear disease. In: GE Shambaugh Jr, JJ Shea eds. *Proceedings of the sixth shambaugh international workshop on otomicrosurgery and third shea fluctuant hearing loss-symposium*. Huntsville, AL: Strode; 1981:289–290.
41. Nadol JB, Jr. Medical progress-hearing loss. *New Engl J Med* 1993; 329:1092–1102.
42. Hughes GB, Kinney SE, Barna BP, Calabrese LH. Practical versus theoretical management of autoimmune inner ear disease. *Laryngoscope* 1984;94:758–767.
43. Pappas DG, Simpson LC, Goodwin GH. Perilymphatic fistula inchildren with preexisting sensorineural hearing loss. *Laryngoscope* 1988; 98:507–510.
44. Kubo T, Kohno M, Naramura H, Itoh M. Clinical characteristics and hearing recovery in perilymphatic fistulas of differentetiologies. *Acta Otolaryngol (Stockh)* 1993;113:307–311.
45. Naiberg JB, Flemming E, Patterson M, Hawke M. The perilymphatic fistula: the end of an enigma? *J Otolaryngol* 1990;19:260–263.
46. Pappas DG, Schneiderman TS. Perilymphatic fistula inpediatric patients with a preexisting sensorineural loss. *Am J Otol* 1989;10: 499–501.
47. Supance JS, Bluestone CD. Perilymph fistulas in infants and children. *Otolaryngol Head Neck Surg* 1983;91:663–671.
48. Plath P. Surgery of the round window. *Am J Otology* 1988;9:142–143.
49. Potter CR, Conner GH. Hydrops following perilymph fistula repair. *Laryngoscope* 1983;93:810–812.
50. Bluestone CD, Stool SE, eds. *Pediatric Otolaryngology*. Philadelphia: WB Saunders; 1983.
51. Reilly JS, Kenna MA. Congenital perilymphatic fistula: an overlooked diagnosis? *Am J Otol* 1989;10:496–498.
52. Reilly JS. Congenital perilymphatic fistula: a prospective study in infants and children. *Laryngoscope* 1989;99:393–397.
53. Brookhouser PE, Worthington DW, Kelly WJ. *The natural history of progressive/fluctuating SNHL in children*. Presented at American Society of Pediatric Otolaryngology annual meeting, Palm Beach, FL, May 12, 1994.

CHAPTER 43

The Cleft Palate Ear

John P. Bent III and Richard J.H. Smith

The association between cleft palate and middle ear disease was observed prior to the twentieth century. However, early and active otologic management of the cleft patient did not begin until the 1950s, when the relationship between middle ear disease and cleft palate became "a statistical certainty" (1). By the late 1960s, it became apparent that almost all young cleft palate patients had continuous otitis media with effusion (OME) (2). As the medical community recognized the problems associated with the cleft palate ear, otologists have become integral members of multidisciplinary cleft palate teams.

The significance of ear disease in the cleft palate patient is augmented by the numerous physical and social handicaps that these children already face. The cleft frequently extends into the lip, causing a cosmetic embarrassment. Severe medical disabilities, including mental retardation and congenital cardiac anomalies, also may be present. Even children with an isolated cleft palate are at risk for speech disorders. The fact that children need adequate speech and hearing for learning mandates a minimization of otologic disease. Young children often manifest no symptoms of conductive hearing loss, complicating the physician's task. Studies showing that cleft children tend to have lower IQs and less creativity than noncleft controls emphasize the need for intervention (3).

This chapter contains sections on the epidemiology, pathophysiology, clinical manifestations, management options, and treatment recommendations regarding the cleft palate ear. Hopefully, it will serve as a useful reference to otolaryngologists participating in the care of cleft palate patients.

J.P. Bent III: Surgery Division of Otolaryngology, Medical College of Georgia, Augusta, Georgia 30912-4060.
R.J.H. Smith: Department of Otolaryngology, Division of Pediatric Otolaryngology, Molecular Otolaryngology Research Laboratories, The University of Iowa Hospitals and Clinics, Iowa City, Iowa 52242.

EPIDEMIOLOGY

Environmental and genetic factors both contribute to cleft formation. Palatal clefts occur when the secondary palatal shelves fail to fuse by the 12th week of gestation. Figure 1 demonstrates the different forms of cleft palate. The incisive foramen defines the junction between the primary and secondary palates, and extension of a velar defect anteriorly into the lip creates a combined cleft palate and unilateral or bilateral cleft lip. In approximately 25% of patients the palatal cleft is associated with other syndromic features (4), such as Pierre-Robin sequence or Crouzon's syndrome.

A review of the University of Iowa Cleft Palate Clinic database, tabulated from 1950 to 1991, reveals the data shown in Table 1. This information was generated from a homogeneous population of Northern European ancestry mixed with a small group of Asian immigrants, and it appears similar to other numbers generated in the United States (5).

PATHOPHYSIOLOGY

The auricle and external canal are normally developed in 98% of cleft palate cases (6), and there is no association between cleft palate and inner ear dysplasias. Cleft palate otopathology involves the middle ear, secondary to a constellation of dynamic and static abnormalities that hinder eustachian tube performance.

Dynamic Abnormalities

Figure 2 demonstrates the relevant muscles affecting eustachian tube patency. The tensor veli palatini muscle (TVPM) originates from two heads, one from the inferior skull base at the pterygoid fossa and a larger bundle from the anterior hook of the eustachian tube lateral lamella (7). The muscle heads then converge into a common tendon that passes around the pterygoid hamulus before inserting into the lateral palate. Most authorities believe that the TVPM functions as the primary dilator of the eustachian tube

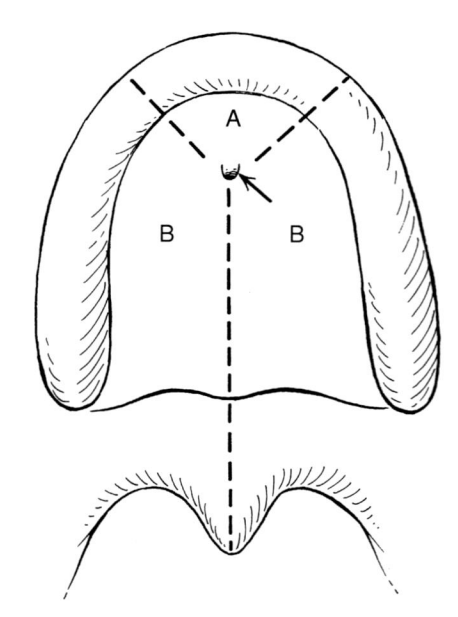

FIG. 1. Potential paths of cleft lip and/or palate. Arrow marks the incisive foramen. A, primary palate; B, secondary palate.

(8–10). The levator veli palatini muscle (LVPM) also contributes to eustachian tube dilation. It arises from the skull base anterior and lateral to the TVPM and passes inferior to the eustachian tube before merging into the palatine aponeurosis. Although it does not insert into the eustachian tube, it functions as a sling, raising the eustachian tube floor as it contracts and accentuating eustachian tube lumen (11).

With a dehiscent palatal aponeurosis, the TVPM and LVPM lose their midline insertions. Consequently, the typical vectors used to open the eustachian tube no longer function. Casselbrant et al. (8) demonstrated the importance of velar musculature by inducing botulinum toxin–mediated TVPM paralysis in six Rhesus monkeys, which caused flat tympanograms in 10 of 12 ears. Additionally, surgically created clefts caused OME in 100% of 20 chinchillas within 24 hours (12). Most evidence indicates that the size of cleft deformity does not affect the extent of middle ear disease (1,6,10,12,13), although at least two studies found the opposite to be true (3,14).

Static Abnormalities

Comparison studies have shown that cleft palate fetuses have altered skull base anatomy with wider nasopharynges

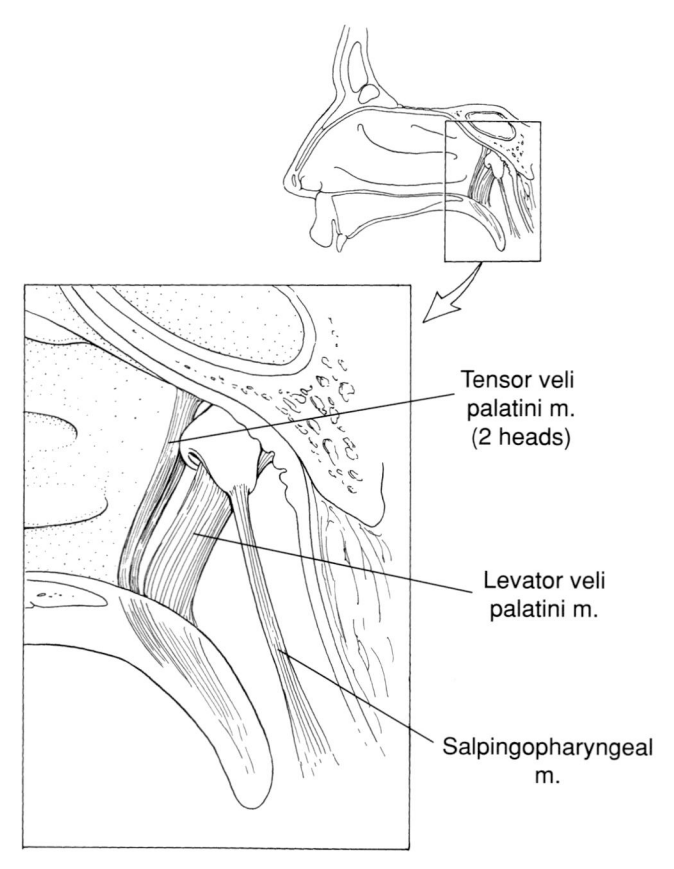

FIG. 2. Velopharyngeal musculature relevant to eustachian tube function.

and narrower, convoluted eustachian tubes (15). Subsequent investigations have confirmed that cleft palate eustachian tubes lack width and have abnormally narrow angles with the TVPM (16). Cadaver dissections have demonstrated the TVPM to be hypoplastic (17), with little or no insertion into the eustachian tube lateral lamella (17,18). A histologic study also demonstrated that cleft palate children have significantly less eustachian tube elastin, predisposing them to noncompliant and collapsed tubal lumens (19). Another abnormality shared by cleft palate patients is the common nasopharyngeal-oropharyngeal cavity, which exposes the eustachian tube to constant oral contamination (1). Graham, Schweiger, and Olin (20) demonstrated that hearing either improved or remained unchanged after the insertion of a

TABLE 1. *Cleft lip and palate incidence, University of Iowa Cleft Palate Clinic database*

	High (yr)	Low (yr)
Range of clefts/newbors in Iowa (1950–1991)		
All clefts	1:604 (1981)	1:1008 (1984)
All palate cleft (with or without lip)	1:748 (1989)	1:1508 (1979)
Relative frequencies		
Cleft lip and palate:cleft palate:cleft lip (1979–1988) = 1.53:1.18:1.00		

palatal obturator, supporting the notion that this common cavity may produce detrimental effects.

CLINICAL MANIFESTATIONS

The anatomic and physiologic derangements of a cleft palate manifest as middle ear disease. Cleft palate clearly predisposes to OME. Normal tympanograms performed during the first days of life indicate that cleft palate neonates have well-aerated middle ears (21). Several months after birth, however, the rate of OME exceeds 90%. The vast majority of these effusions will be mucoid rather than serous (22,23). Table 2 demonstrates prospective data obtained via myringotomy, which defines the prevalence of OME in young cleft palate patients. Other studies that did not use myringotomy, reviewed patients retrospectively, or studied older patients have cited lower rates of effusion (6,20,24), but this information probably underestimates actual OME prevalence. Middle ear disease also is elevated in patients with submucous clefts (25), but not in clefts limited to the lip and primary palate (23). No difference exists between the prevalence of middle ear disease in patients with cleft lip and palate and those with isolated cleft palate (26).

Otorrhea is a frequent complication during the first decade of life. Paradise and Bluestone (27) reported otorrhea after myringotomy and tympanostomy (M&T) in 68% of 130 cleft palate patients under 24 months old. Muntz's review (25) indicates a 6% rate of chronic otorrhea. These figures substantially exceed the otorrhea and chronic suppurative otitis media rates (21–50% and 1.6–.03%, respectively) experienced after M&T by noncleft children (28).

Untreated OME in young children typically translates into a conductive hearing loss (CHL) of 15 to 20 dB (24,25). Although Bennett (29) reported a high incidence of sensorineural hearing loss (SNHL) in 27 of 100 older cleft palate patients, other reviews have indicated only 1% to 2% SNHL in the cleft palate ear (24,30). As children make the transition into teenage years and early adulthood, hearing loss secondary to OME becomes less common, although more serious middle ear pathology may develop. Gould (31) reported that regardless of treatment method, hearing improved with advancing age. This correlates with Moller's finding (30) that OME rates decreased to 19% by 6 years of age and to 6% by 15 years. Crysdale (24) compared 71 children ages 3 to 9 with 47 children ages 10 to 26. The younger group had a much higher rate of middle ear effusion and CHL, whereas tympanosclerosis and perforations predominated in the older group. Clinical studies confirm that hearing improves with age (14,32), while otopathology stabilizes sometime after preschool, between 5 and 10 years (14,26,33,34). In terms of typical long-term outcome, 20% to 50% of adults will have speech thresholds greater than 20 to 30 dB, and approximately half will have otoscopic abnormalities (1,3,13,30,35). Despite the usual stabilization of middle ear disease by the end of the first decade, some children do acquire otologic complications, such as cholesteatoma and tympanic membrane (TM) perforations, usually in the later phase of childhood.

Although cholesteatoma and perforations occur with greater frequency in cleft than noncleft patients, for unknown reasons cleft patients develop significantly fewer otologic complications (TM perforations and cholesteatoma) than noncleft patients with chronic middle ear disease. Active otologic management has certainly helped reduce poor outcomes. Dominguez and Harker (36) reported that organized interdisciplinary care reduced the number of cleft patients developing cholesteatoma from 9.2% to 2.6%. Table 3 illustrates cholesteatoma and perforation rates from several different retrospective or cross-sectional investigations. As expected, advanced age is associated with more complications. The disease incidence in a population that received essentially no otologic care is reflected by Albert et al.'s review (32) of Sri Lankans with cleft palate. Fortunately, a minority of cleft palate patients experience these problems. Although cholesteatoma and TM perforations are more common in the cleft palate ear, they should respond well to conventional management once adequate eustachian tube function develops.

MANAGEMENT OPTIONS

Myringotomy with Tympanostomy

The greatest controversy surrounding management of the cleft palate ear lies in the question, "To tube or not to tube?" All authorities agree that myringotomy by itself, without tympanostomy, yields no benefit (23). However, tympanostomy enables middle ear ventilation, with all of its advantages, until the tube extrudes. Given these advantages, most otolaryngologists have advocated routine, early tympanostomy tube (T-tube) insertion since the widespread nature of OME in cleft palate became fully appreciated (3,23,27).

However, there has not been universal agreement on this issue. Other otolaryngologists have supported a more conservative approach to tympanostomy. In 1976, Crysdale (24) argued that routine and repetitive M&T might result in more adverse middle ear sequelae than untreated OME. He recom-

TABLE 2. *Otitis media with effusion prevalence in the cleft palate ear*

Investigator	Year	Age of patients	Ears examined	% OME
Stool and Randall (2)	1967	9 days–12 mo	50	96
Grant et al. (22)	1988	2–20 mo	116	97
Robinson et al. (40)	1992	2–18 mo	300	92

TABLE 3. Prevalence of cholesteatoma and tympanic membrane perforations in the cleft palate ear

Investigator	Year	Patient age (yrs)	No. of patients	% Cholesteatoma*	% Perforations*
Moller (30)	1975	6	68	1.5	4.4
Moller (30)	1975	15	45	2.2	4.4
Muntz (25)	1993	3	132	0.8	12.9
Dominguez and Harker (36)	1988	≥10	153	2.6	—
Goldman, Martinez, and Ganzel (4)	1993	≥5	110	2.7	—
Caldarelli (48)	1975	≥16	31	19.4	9.7
Skolnick (6)	1958	Children	337	—	27
Albert et al. (32)	1990	≥10	182	2.8	23.1

* Expressed as percentage of diseased ears per patients studied.

mended M&T at 18 months only in those children with significant retraction, hearing loss, otalgia, or poor access to medical care. These concerns were reinforced by several retrospective studies. Gordon, Jean-Louis, and Morton (13) found a higher rate of abnormal audiograms, tympanograms, and otoscopic findings in 48 cleft palate patients who had received M&Ts than in a cohort of 50 cleft palate patients who never had tympanostomy (mean age at follow-up, 12 yr). Robson et al. (37) performed a similar comparison and noted higher audiologic thresholds and more otologic complications in the tympanostomy group. Both studies contained potential treatment bias, in that the more severely diseased ears may have been the ones treated with M&T.

Other studies have supported the more aggressive approach to tympanostomy, as originally espoused by Paradise and Bluestone. Gould (31) retrospectively analyzed 1,699 audiologic records and demonstrated superior hearing in cleft palate patients treated with routine M&T compared with those treated more conservatively. In 1985 Hubbard et al. (38) performed a cross-sectional analysis of two closely matched groups of 24 cleft palate children, ages 5 to 11 years, who had undergone M&T at relatively early and late ages (3.0 and 30.8 mon, respectively). The different ages of initial M&T reflected two conflicting philosophies regarding tympanostomy indications at adjacent medical centers. This study design eliminated the possibility of the more severely affected ears being selected for M&T. They found that hearing acuity and consonant articulation were less impaired in the early M&T group, while otoscopic findings and psychosocial variables were equivalent (38). Unfortunately, the study population may have been too young for serious otologic disease to develop. To date, no prospective study comparing routine and conservative tympanostomy has followed patients into adulthood. Given this contradictory information and the lack of a conclusive study, one must rely on personal experience and good judgment. The most compelling reason to insert T-tubes may be to spare children the frustration and misery associated with continuous OME.

Palatoplasty

A second management controversy concerns the timing of palate closure. In 1974 Paradise and Bluestone (27) noted a statistically significant decrease in myringotomies performed after cleft palate repair in their series of 92 patients. Bluestone et al. (39) then established that the eustachian tube opened at lower positive pressures after palatoplasty. This sentiment that palatoplasty favorably impacts eustachian tube function was echoed by Chaudhuri and Bowen-Jones (14), who noted a decrease from 63% to 10% in long-term hearing loss when they repaired cleft palates before 12 months of age. The particular type of palate repair has not been shown to impact otologic outcome (40), although hamulus fracture has been discouraged, because it may further disable the TVPM (41). Early palate repair also offers several obvious advantages for speech and swallowing. However, palatoplasty alters blood supply and splints the developing maxilla, translating into altered midface growth and occlusal abnormalities. To maximize normal maxillary growth, Frable, Brandon, and Theogard (42) suggested early soft palate closure while delaying hard palate closure until children reach 5.5 years of age. They reported soft palate closure combined with M&T in 36 patients, of whom 81% required no additional myringotomy.

Although these findings suggest that reapproximation of velar musculature lessens middle ear disease, other evidence contradicts this notion. Skolnick (6) reviewed 41 palates closed before age 1 year and 48 closed after age 2 years and noted no significant difference in middle ear pathology (73% vs. 75%, respectively). Adult patients who used obturators in lieu of palate closure have hearing thresholds comparable to patients with surgically closed clefts (26). A report of 68 Malaysians with cleft palate, many of whom had never had cleft closure, found that cleft palate repair did not influence rates of OME (43). In a similar study Albert et al. (32) compared 49 patients with closed cleft palates with 124 who had not undergone repair. In patients older than 10 years, there was no difference in the percent of otoscopically normal ears. This information suggests that improved eustachian tube function may be an inevitable consequence of physical maturation rather than a result of palatoplasty. To clarify this issue, Dhillon (44) prospectively followed 50 patients after performing unilateral M&T simultaneous with palatoplasty. Ninety-seven percent of ears had OME at palatoplasty, and 80% of control ears still had an effusion at

24 months' follow-up. Robinson et al. (40) performed an equivalent prospective study and discovered that 3 years after palatoplasty, 70% of 140 children had OME in the nonintubated ear. Children whose palates were closed prior to 12 months of age had no advantage over those closed 6 months later.

Doyle et al. (45) measured active and passive eustachian tube dynamics before and after palatoplasty and emphasized that although palatoplasty facilitates passive opening of the eustachian tube, it does not appreciably change a patient's ability to *actively* perform tubal dilation. They attributed these findings to improved positioning of the LVPM and believed that palatoplasty does not significantly affect the primary tubal dilator, the TVPM. More recently, Smith, Di-Ruggiero, and Jones (46) studied 81 cleft palate patients, and their data suggested that eustachian tube function does improve after palate repair, but not until an average of 6 years has elapsed. Thus, it appears that palate repair addresses some but not all of the factors influencing eustachian tube dysfunction.

Alternatives to Management

Children with eustachian tube dysfunction that persists into adolescence pose a dilemma. Medical therapy with decongestants, antihistamines, or nasal steroids can be attempted, but no data exist to support their efficacy. If one suspects sinusitis, allergy, or other aggravating medical conditions, appropriate therapy should be undertaken. Adenoidectomy, although commonly used to treat chronic eustachian tube dysfunction, is considered taboo in cleft palate patients because of the potential to worsen velopalatine insufficiency (VPI). Limited lateral adenoidectomy has been used with minimal effect (1). Endoscopically guided lateral adenoidectomy may allow precise removal of obstructing adenoid tissue, but this technique has not gained widespread acceptance.

TREATMENT RECOMMENDATIONS

All cleft palate patients should receive regular otologic examinations, including screening audiometry, as part of their routine follow-up in the cleft palate clinic. Input and intervention are invariably required from the otolaryngologist. Figure 3 depicts our approach to the management of the cleft palate ear.

Palatoplasty

The timing of palate closure should be chosen in consultation with the family and other members of the cleft team without regard to otologic status.

Tympanostomy

We perform tympanostomies for the same indications as in noncleft children, specifically OME that persists beyond 3 months, or three or more episodes of recurrent acute otitis media (AOM) in 6 months. An exception to this criteria occurs if a child has OME when seen for the first time immediately prior to cleft lip repair; in this case, we favor placement of T-tubes without documenting a chronic effusion because of the high likelihood that the effusion will persist

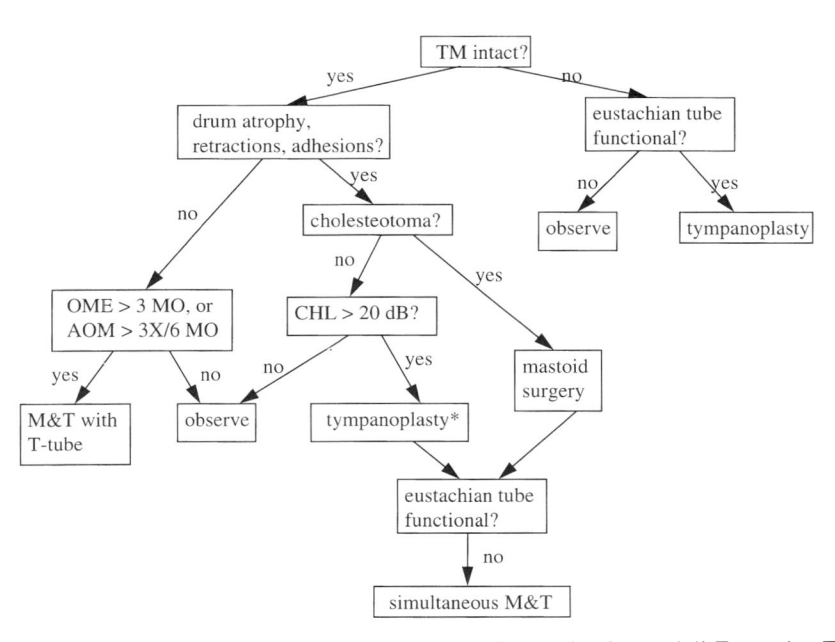

FIG. 3. Otologic management of the cleft palate ear. (See discussion in text.) (* Extensive TM retraction may require mastoid surgery, precluding straightforward tympanoplasty. Hearing aids and observation should be considered as alternatives to surgery.)

during the early years of life. Even though T-tubes are associated with more frequent complications (47), we recommend them because of lower extrusion rates. The finding by Smith, DiRuggiero, and Jones (46), that T-tube use translates into fewer myringotomies supports this practice. Occasionally, narrow external auditory canals make T-tube insert impractical, in which case we use conventional collar button tubes. If the middle ear space is severely atelectatic, transtympanic injection of saline into the anterior mesotympanum with a 30-gauge needle raises the tympanic membrane off the promontory and facilitates atraumatic myringotomy. We generally do not remove functional tubes from the TM but simply allow them to extrude spontaneously.

Tympanic Membrane Perforation

If a perforation occurs, adequate eustachian tube function should be verified before considering tympanoplasty, because the perforation may function physiologically, like a T-tube. This can be accomplished by filling the external ear with saline and asking the patient if the salty taste becomes apparent in the mouth during swallowing. Patients may already have observed this phenomenon with topical ear antibiotic drops. Alternatively, the patient may be able to autoinflate the middle ear and create an audible squeak. Any of these signs suggest a better prognosis for tympanoplasty. However, if the patient is younger than 10 years, the eustachian tube function may fluctuate, threatening successful tympanoplasty.

Chronic Changes in an Intact Tympanic Membrane

A retracted, atrophic, or atelectatic TM commonly develops in the cleft palate adolescent or young adult. When hearing thresholds are below 20 dB, we suggest observation, because the chronic middle ear adhesions are difficult to correct. However, if conductive hearing loss exceeds 20 dB, tympanoplasty could be attempted. This should not be undertaken casually, because one may encounter incus erosion, requiring a partial ossicular replacement prosthesis and resulting in no significant hearing improvement. Also, the patient may have myringostapedopexy, which cannot be reversed because of TM adherence to the stapes superstructure. If a retraction pocket extends into the sinus tympani, a modified or radical mastoidectomy may be necessary. Given unchanging otopathology, hearing aids should be offered as an alternative. A daily Valsalva maneuver may help with middle ear aeration. Ultimately, nonsurgical management may be in the patient's best interest.

If a retraction extends superiorly, so that it can no longer be safely examined, tympanoplasty should be performed, in combination with a simple mastoidectomy if necessary, to avoid the sequelae of cholesteatoma. A cartilage underlay graft to the posterior-superior quadrant helps avoid recurrent retractions into the epitympanum. Certainly, if a cholesteatoma is diagnosed, the appropriate mastoid procedure should be performed.

When performing a mastoid procedure or tympanoplasty on a previously intact drum, the surgeon should consider performing a simultaneous tympanostomy. In preschool children or those who have not evidenced return of eustachian tube function, such a tympanostomy will reduce recurrent middle ear disease.

CASE HISTORY

Case History 1

A plastic surgeon consults you to consider an M&T in a 6-year-old girl who is scheduled to have a pharyngeal flap the following day as treatment of VPI. She is status post-repair of a cleft lip and palate. She has previously had three sets of M&Ts, the most recent set having extruded 9 months previously. Since the tubes extruded, she has had no episodes of AOM. Figure 4 shows her audiogram. Her TMs appeared similar; Fig. 5 demonstrates the right side.

In this setting, there are four indications to intervene:

1. Cholesteatoma
2. Retraction of the pars flacida with possible cholesteatoma
3. Three or more episodes of AOM in 6 months
4. Otitis media with effusion or chronic TM changes associated with CHL $\geq$ 20 dB.

This patient has tympanosclerosis and retraction onto the promontory but no significant hearing impairment. Because none of the criteria apply, a, M&T is not necessary. The tympanosclerosis in the posterior-superior quadrant serves a protective function in that it strengthens the TM, reducing the likelihood of retraction.

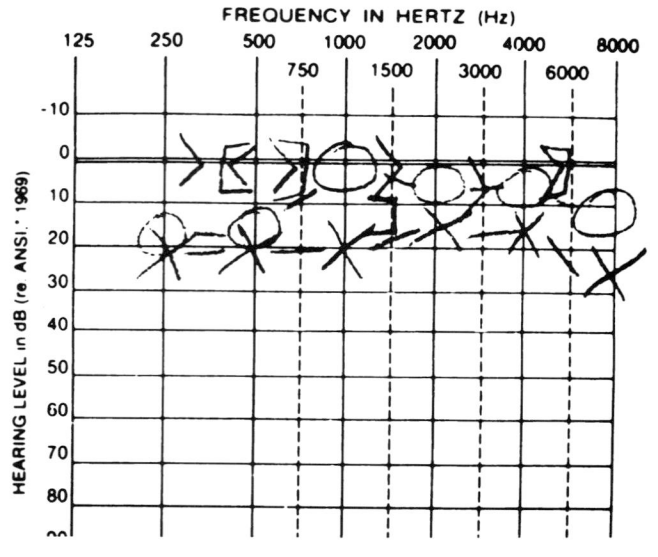

FIG. 4. Audiogram demonstrating bilateral mild CHL.

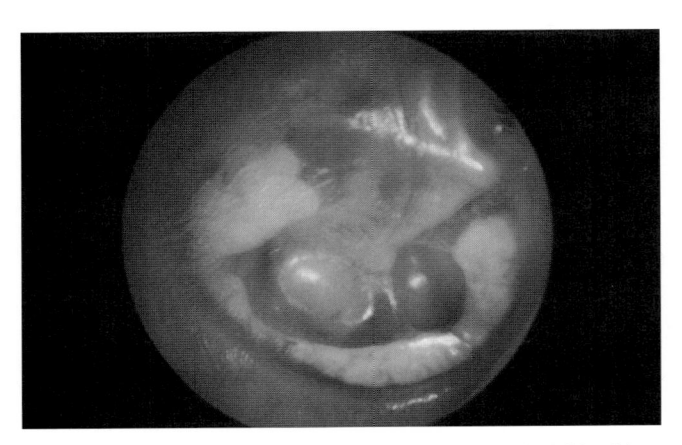

FIG. 5. Extensive tympanosclerosis of the right TM with a retraction onto the promontory.

Case History 2

A 3-year-old boy with a repaired cleft isolated to the soft palate presents with right-sided otorrhea. The otorrhea has persisted for 6 weeks despite treatment with various oral and topical antibiotics. The child has previously had one set of T-tubes when his palate was repaired 1.5 years ago. Examination reveals OME and a slightly retracted, tympanosclerotic left TM without a T-tube. After cleaning the right canal, a deep retraction pocket can be seen behind a granulation pocket in the posterior-superior TM (Fig. 6). Purulence is draining from a right T-tube.

This patient has a cholesteatoma of the right middle ear and mastoid with dysfunctional eustachian tubes. He should have the cholesteatoma removed via a right tympanomastoidectomy, using a facial recess approach, if possible. A T-tube should be placed in the left TM. On the right side, the in dwelling tube should be removed because it may be a source of squamous debris. A new tube must be placed in the salvageable right TM. A cartilage underlay should be used to prevent recurrent retraction, and a second-look procedure will be necessary in approximately 6 months. A modified radical mastoidectomy may be required if the cholesteatoma can not be controlled without removing the posterior canal wall.

SUMMARY

The prevalence of otitis media in patients with congenital cleft palate greatly exceeds that seen in the general pediatric population. This predisposition to otitis media stems from velar and skull base anatomic anomalies with subsequent functional abnormalities of the eustachian tube. The ensuing otopathology adds an additional burden to the already handicapped cleft patients. Intensive and thoughtful management of the cleft palate ear will help reduce the sequelae of middle ear disease and allow these patients to function at their highest level.

CONCLUSIONS

Cleft palate patients, due to static and dynamic factors influencing eustachian tube function, have a higher incidence of middle ear disease. Otolaryngologists must be actively involved on cleft palate teams in order to minimize the consequences of untreated middle ear disease. The prevalence of OME in cleft palate children under 2 years old exceeds 90%. Myringotomy tubes should be inserted for the same indications that apply to noncleft patients. Cleft palate closure may improve eustachian tube function but does not rectify all of the abnormal pathophysiology. Middle ear disease generally stabilizes or improves by the end of the first decade. Tympanic membrane perforations and cholesteatoma usually present after preschool age. Although long-term hearing loss frequently exists, disabling otologic sequelae in the adult patient are uncommon.

REFERENCES

1. Masters FW, Bingham HG, Robinson DW. The prevention and treatment of hearing loss in the cleft palate child. *Plast Reconstr Surg* 1960; 25:503–9.
2. Stool SE, Randall P. Unexpected ear disease in infants with cleft palate. *Cleft Palate J* 1967;4:99–103.
3. Paradise JL. Management of middle ear effusions in infants with cleft palate. *Ann Otol* 1976;85(Supp 2, Pt 2):285–8.
4. Goldman JI, Martinez SA, Ganzel TM. Eustachian tube dysfunction and its sequelae in patients with cleft palate. *South Med J* 1993;86:1236–7.
5. Mattucci KF. Cleft palate patients: otologic management. *NY State J Med* 1979;79:333–9.
6. Skolnik EM. Otologic evaluation in cleft palate patients. *Laryngoscope* 1958;68:1908–49.
7. Ross MA. Functional anatomy of the tensor palatini. *Arch Otol* 1971; 93:1–8.
8. Casselbrant ML, Cantekin EI, Dirkmaat DC, Doyle WJ, Bluestone CD. Experimental paralysis of tensor veli palatini muscle. *Acta Otolaryngol* 1988;106:178–85.
9. Cantekin EI. Effect of surgical alterations on the tensorveli palatini muscle on eustachian tube function. *Ann Otol* 1980;89:47–53.
10. Doyle WJ, Cantekin EI, Bluestone CD. Eustachian tube function in cleft palate children. *Ann Otol Rhinol Laryngol* 1980;89:34–40.
11. Proctor B. Anatomy of the eustachian tube. *Arch Otol* 1973;97:2–8.

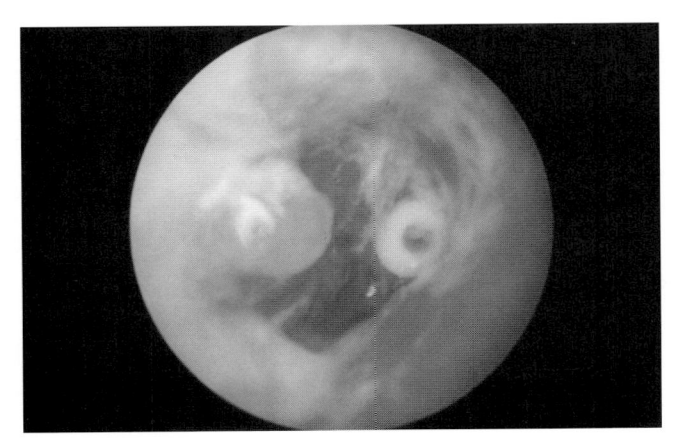

FIG. 6. Granulation polyp and posterior-superior retraction of the right TM, indicating an underlying cholesteatoma.

12. Meyerhoff WL, Shea DA, Foster CA. Otitis media, cleft palate,and middle ear ventilation. *Otolaryngol Head Neck Surg* 1981;89:288–93.
13. Gordon ASD, Jean-Louis F, Morton RP. Late ear sequelae in cleft palate patients. *Int J Pediatr Otorhinolaryngol* 1988;15:149–56.
14. Chaudhuri PK, Bowen-Jones E. An otorhinological study of children with cleft palates. *J Laryngol Otol* 1978;92:29–40.
15. Dickson DR. Anatomy of the normal and cleft palate eustachian tube. *Ann Otol* 1976;85(Supp 25):25–9.
16. Shibahara Y, Sando I. Histopathologic study of eustachian tube in cleft palate patients. *Ann Otol Rhinol Laryngol* 1988;97:403–8.
17. Kriens O. Anatomy of the velopharyngeal area in cleft palate. *Clin Plast Surg* 1975;2:261–83.
18. Matsune S, Sando I, Takahashi H. Insertion of the tensor velipalatini muscle into the eustachian tube cartilage in cleft palate cases. *Ann Otol Rhinol Laryngol* 1991;100:439–46.
19. Matsune S, Sando I, Takahashi H. Elastin at the hinge portion of the eustachian tube cartilage in specimens from normal subjects and those with cleft palate. *Ann Otol Rhinol Laryngol* 1991;100:439–46.
20. Graham MD, Schweiger JW, Olin WH. Hearing loss and ear disease in cleft palate patients with obturators. *Plast Reconstr Surg* 1962;30:348–58.
21. Too-Chung MA. The assessment of middle ear function and hearing by tympanometry in children before and after early cleft palate repair. *Br J Plast Surg* 1983;36:295–9.
22. Grant HR, Quiney RE, Mercer DM, Lodge S. Cleft palate and glue ear. *Arch Dis Child* 1988;63:176–9.
23. Paradise JL, Bluestone CD, Felder H. The universality of otitis media of infants with cleft palate. *Pediatrics* 1969;44:35–42.
24. Crysdale WS. Rational management of middle ear effusions in the cleft palate patient. *J Otolaryngol* 1976;5:463–7.
25. Muntz HR. An overview of middle ear disease in cleft palate children. *Facial Plast Surg* 1993;9:177–80.
26. Anthony PF, Anthony LS. Hearing loss in prosthetically treated adults with cleft palate. *Arch Otol* 1976;102:151–3.
27. Paradise JL, Bluestone CD. Early treatment of the universal otitis media of infants with cleft palate. *Pediatrics* 1974;53:48–54.
28. Kenna MA. Treatment of chronic suppurative otitis media. *Otolaryngol Clin N Am* 1994;27:457–72.
29. Bennett M. The older cleft palate patient. *Laryngoscope* 1972;82:1217–25.
30. Moller P. Long-term otologic features of cleft palate patients. *Arch Otol* 1975;101:605–7.
31. Gould HJ. Hearing loss and cleft palate: the perspective of time. *Cleft Palate J* 1990;27:36–9.
32. Albert DM, Garrett J, Specker B, Ho M. The otologic significance of cleft palate in a Sri Lanka population. *Cleft Palate J* 1990;27:155–161.
33. Young A. The state of the ears in children with a cleft palate deformity. *J Laryngol Otol* 1968;82:707–15.
34. Yules RB. Hearing in cleft palate patients. *Arch Otol* 1970;91:319–23.
35. Yules RB. Current concepts of treatment of ear disease in cleft palate children and adults. *Cleft Palate J* 1975;12:315–21.
36. Dominguez S, Harker LA. Incidence of cholesteatoma with cleft palate. *Ann Otol Rhinol Laryngol* 1988;97:659–60.
37. Robson AK, Blanshard JD, Jones K, Albery EH, Smith IM, Maw AR. A conservative approach to the management of otitis media with effusion in cleft palate children. *J Laryngol Otol* 1992;106:788–92.
38. Hubbard TW, Paradise JL, McWilliams BJ, Elster BA, Taylor FH.Consequences of unremitting middle-ear disease in early life. *N Engl J Med* 1985;312:1529–34.
39. Bluestone CD, Beery QC, Cantekin EI, Paradise JL. Eustachian tube ventilatory function in relation to cleft palate. *Ann Otol* 1975;84:333–8.
40. Robinson PJ, Lodge S, Jones BM, Walker CC, Grant HR. The effect of palate repair on otitis media with effusion. *Plast Reconstr Surg* 1992;89:640–5.
41. Virtanen H, Palva T. Surgical treatment of patulous eustachian tube. *Arch Otol* 1982;108:735–9.
42. Frable MA, Brandon GT, Theogaraj SD. Velar closure and ear tubings as a primary procedure in the repair of cleft palates. *Laryngoscope* 1985;95:1044–6.
43. Lokman S, Loh T, Said H, Omar I. Incidence and management of middle ear effusion in cleft palate patients. *Med J Malaysia* 1992;47:51–5.
44. Dhillon RS. The middle ear in cleft palate children pre and post palate closure. *J R Soc Med* 1988;81:710–13.
45. Doyle WJ, Reilly JS, Jardini L, Rovnak S. Effect of palatoplasty on the function of the eustachian tube in children with cleft palate. *Cleft Palate J* 1986;23:63–8.
46. Smith T, DiRuggiero DC, Jones KR. Recovery of eustachian tube function and hearing outcome in patients with cleft palate. *Otolaryngol Head Neck Surg* 1994;111:423–9.
47. Brockbank MJ, Jonathon DA, Grant HR, Wright A. Goode T-tubes: do the benefits of their use outweigh their complications? *Clin Otolaryngol* 1988;13:351–6.
48. Caldarelli DD. Incidence and type of otologic disease in the older cleft-palate patient. *Cleft Palate J* 1975;12:311–14.

CHAPTER 44

Perilymphatic Fistula

Bradley F. Marple and William L. Meyerhoff

Perilymphatic or labyrinthine fistula (PLF) is an abnormal communication between the perilymphatic space of the inner ear and the middle ear and mastoid. Manifestations of PLF vary in severity and complexity, range from mild to incapacitating, and may or may not include hearing loss, tinnitus, aural fullness, dysequilibrium, vertigo, or any combination of these symptoms. There are obvious difficulties, therefore, in establishing the diagnosis of PLF. Not until the late 1970s was PLF implicated as an etiologic factor in sensorineural hearing loss within the pediatric population (1). It is now estimated that 6% to 11% of unexplained pediatric sensorineural hearing loss is a result of PLF. In data for children suffering progressive sensorineural hearing loss, estimates of PLF increase to 25% (2,3).

Prior to the advent of surgery for otosclerosis, reports of perilymph fistula were infrequent. Publications describing PLF following stapedectomy began to appear in the mid-1960s (4,5). As the signs and symptoms of iatrogenic PLF became more widely recognized, its diagnosis was considered in patients who had not undergone previous stapes surgery. After Fee's 1968 report (6) of three patients with surgically confirmed PLF following head trauma, subsequent reports began to appear linking PLF with abrupt increases in intracranial pressure (7,8). Goodhill (9,10) further clarified the pathogenisis of PLF by describing the impact of implosive and explosive forces on the fluid filled inner ear. Not until 1978, when Grundfast and Bluestone reported surgical confirmation of PLF in five children with sensorineural hearing loss, however, was PLF considered a factor in that population (1). Numerous retrospective studies of pediatric patients have supported this discovery and have not only clarified its association with progressive or fluctuating hearing loss, but have also showed its association with recurrent meningitis, anomalies of the inner and middle ear, and craniofacial and skeletal abnormalities (1,11).

B.F. Marple and W.L. Meyerhoff: Department of Otolaryngology, University of Texas Southwestern Medical Center at Dallas, Dallas, Texas 72535.

ANATOMY

A thorough knowledge of inner-ear anatomy is paramount to understanding the dynamics of this system and the potential sites for perilymph escape. For the most part, the inner ear is almost completely housed within a rigid bony framework. There are, however, at least two sites of communication between the inner ear and the subarachnoid space. One well-recognized communication is the cochlear aqueduct (Fig. 1), which directly links the subarachnoid space with the basal turn of the scala tympani and, when patent, has been implicated as the cause of stapes "gushers" and PLF (12). Anatomic observations reveal that cochlear aqueduct patency is present in about 70% of the population, but varies in degree between subjects. Although some authors suggest that this patency tends to decrease with increasing age as arachnoid tissue that lines the aqueduct becomes more dense, others have found that cochlear aqueduct patency is independent of age (12–14).

Another area identified as a locus for fluid and pressure exchange between the subarachnoid space and the inner ear is the fundus of the internal auditory canal at the lamina cribrosa and cochlear modiolus. This site of communication was suggested by Glasscock (15), who reported three patients with stapes gushers that were controlled only after occlusion of the internal auditory canal. Subarachnoid pressure can also be imparted upon the inner ear through the vestibular aqueduct.

The middle-ear space is also susceptible to wide and sometimes abrupt changes in pressure which, in turn, create pressure, gradients across the partition between the middle and inner ear. The oval and round windows are obvious points of weakness between the middle ear and the perilymphatic space and are therefore vulnerable to development of PLF (9,10). In addition, other areas of potential weakness or dehiscence between the middle and inner ear may exist. The fissula ante fenestram lies anterior to the annulus of the stapes footplate and exists as a transcapsular channel formed by the resorption of precartilage in the fetus and infant (16). Dehiscence at this site creates a direct channel from the vesti-

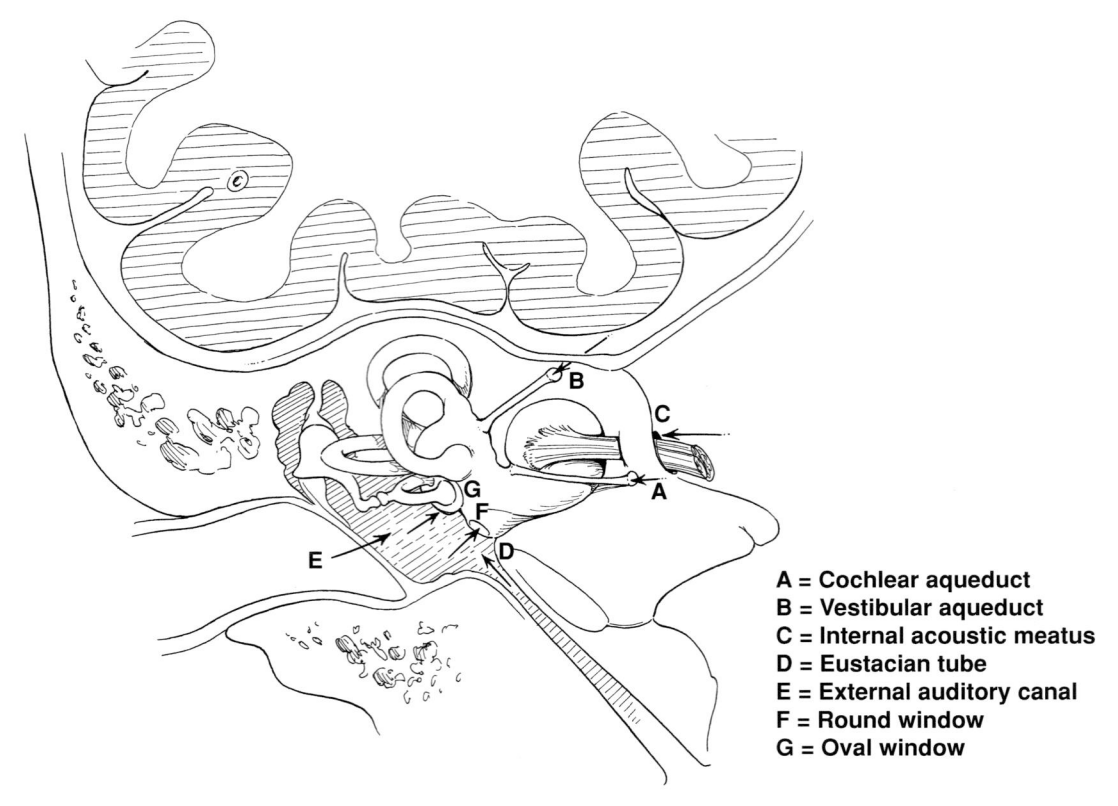

FIG. 1. Schematic diagram depicting sites of potential perilymph egress within the middle ear. Modified from Goodhill V.(ref. 9).

A = Cochlear aqueduct
B = Vestibular aqueduct
C = Internal acoustic meatus
D = Eustacian tube
E = External auditory canal
F = Round window
G = Oval window

bule to the tympanic cavity. Microfissures extending from the ampulla of the posterior semicircular canal to the floor of the round window niche are consistently noted on histologic sections of temporal bones and indicate another possible route for PLF. The histologic appearance of the microscopic channels suggests that they are stress fractures, possibly caused by the forces of mastication upon the temporal bone (17–19). The tympanomeningeal fissure, sometimes referred to as Hyrtl's fissure, is also recognized as a rare site of cerebrospinal fluid (CSF) otorrhea. Its normal course parallels the cochlear aqueduct from the inferior round window niche to the posterior cranial fossa, and it is open only during early embryonic life (20). When patent, this tract bypasses the inner ear and is therefore a site for CSF otorrhea rather than true PLF.

In addition, a strong correlation between nontraumatic CSF otorrhea and other craniofacial or temporal bone anomalies has been recognized since the mid-20th century (21–24). Although such anomalies can be severe, including complete agenesis of the cochlea, the more subtle deformities of the ossicular chain are most frequently seen with PLF. Weber, Perez, and Bluestone (25) described the oval window as the most common site of perilymph leak among 80 pediatric ears with surgically confirmed PLF. Their study showed 86.3% of these ears to have a deformity of the middle or inner ear, but in only 25 of the 80 ears was a malformation detectable on preoperative computed tomography (CT). This study, among others, identified a malformation of the stapes as the most common congenital middle ear anomaly associated with pediatric congenital PLF (Fig. 2).

PATHOPHYSIOLOGY

Any breech in continuity of the bony inner ear provides a point at which perilymph can escape from the inner ear

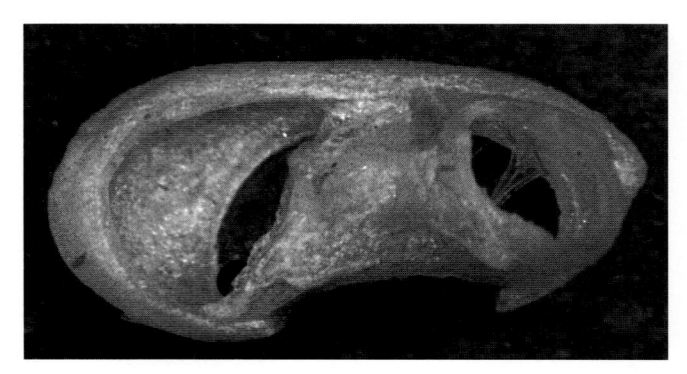

FIG. 2. Photograph of dehiscent stapes footplate retrieved from patient with recurrent otogenic meningitis. Large dehiscence seen in center of stapes footplate. Courtesy of C.G. Wright, Ph.D.

and air can enter. Goodhill (9,17) categorized hydrodynamic forces on the inner ear as *implosive* and *explosive*. Everyday activities such as lifting, straining, coughing, and sneezing are associated with increase in CSF pressure. Pressure increase (3) can then be transmitted to the inner ear via various routes (15), but several inherent anatomic factors decrease the real effects of sudden pressure changes. The length of the cochlear aqueduct and the presence of arachnoid within its lumen dampen the effects of sudden changes in subarachnoid pressure, thus providing a somewhat protective barrier (12). Further, a concurrent increase in pressure imparted on the endolymphatic sac protects the intracochlear membranes by equalizing endolymphatic and perilymphatic pressure (26). Nonetheless, sudden increases in inner-ear fluid pressure are transmitted to the oval window annulus and the round window membrane. These are the pressures termed *explosive* by Goodhill (9,17).

Pressure changes can also be applied to the inner ear in an opposite fashion. Pressure within the middle ear can fluctuate widely through changes in barometric pressure, compression trauma to the ear (27), Valsalva maneuvers, and pinched-nose sneezing (28). Pressure within the middle ear exerts a force on the oval window annulus, round window membrane, fissula ante fenestram, microfissures, Hyrtl's fissure, and so on (9,17). Goodhill termed these forces *implosive*.

Hearing loss and vestibular symptoms are known to result from active loss of perilymph, but the mechanism responsible for these symptoms is not well understood. Change in auditory function is thought by some investigators to occur from decompression of the perilymphatic space. Decrease in the perilymph volume creates a secondary endolymphatic hydrops (ELH) and the constellation of symptoms known to occur with this condition (29). Secondary ELH has been histologically identified in experimental animals with PLF (30), and the concept is indirectly supported by several clinical studies and reports. Walsted, Salemon, and Olson (31), performing audiograms before and after spinal anesthesia on 34 patients, identified one patient who suffered significant but reversible sensorineural hearing loss. Hardy, (32) in 1988, reported similar findings in two patients with sensorineural hearing loss after spinal anesthesia who demonstrated resolution of auditory function after subarachnoid injection of 20 ml of normal saline. In these patients, worsening of auditory function likely occurred because decreased CSF volume and hydrostatic pressure resulted in loss of perilymph through a patent cochlear aqueduct, thus causing secondary endolymphatic hydrops (12,13,33,34).

Despite clinical evidence that decompression of the perilymphatic space can result in auditory changes (26,30), simple loss of perilymph as a cause of sensorineural hearing loss in the experimental setting has yielded conflicting results. Addressing this question, Bohmer (35) demonstrated no changes in auditory thresholds among guinea pigs with simple round window membrane perforations. These findings agree with those of Simmons, Barton, and Beatty (36), but other investigators have demonstrated changes in auditory function in experimentally induced PLF. Robertson (37), in 1974, showed changes in the tuning curves of single spiral ganglion cells emanating from the basilar membrane after removal of perilymph from the tympanic scala of the guinea pig. Flint et al. (38) in 1988 showed a 10 to 15 dB increase in auditory brain stem response (ABR) thresholds in guinea pigs with artificially created PLF.

Evidence of change in auditory function has also been provided by electrocochleography (ECochG) performed before and after creation of PLF. Ackley (30) demonstrated consistent increases in the summating potential-action potential (SP/AP) ratio following creation of PLF in guinea pigs with obstructed cochlear aqueducts. The increases occurred in the absence of changes in other measures of auditory function. Campbell and Savage (39) produced similar results in guinea pigs with artificially induced PLF. In the latter study, ECochG demonstrated increased SP/AP ratio during the active period of fluid leak but gradual return to normal SP/AP ratio following healing of the round window membrane.

Given the inconsistency of reports regarding auditory function in association with experimental PLF, mechanisms other than simple loss of perilymph have been sought to explain the auditory findings observed in that condition. Simmons (40) proposed that sudden fluid loss from the oval window or round window could lead to concurrent rupture in Reissner's membrane. The internal fistula in this case is secondary to rapid changes in the pressure gradient across Reissner's membrane and results in auditory symptoms. Oshiro, Shelton, and Lusted (41) compared the effects of round window membrane perforations in the guinea pig with and without discrete lesions in Reissner's membrane. In animals with only PLF, the action potential showed little or no change, but severe decreases in action potential amplitude and increases in latency were found in animals with perforations of both the round window membrane and Reissner's membrane. The latter condition allows alteration of the normal balance between longitudinal and radial flow of fluids within the cochlea as well as mixture of perilymph and endolymph.

Several reports of PLF describe gas bubbles within the scala tympani. The bubbles were identified during exploratory tympanotomy (42,43) or high-resolution imaging (44,45). Nishioka and Yanaghara (43) studied the effects of air in the cochlea of the guinea pig by measuring AP before and after removal of perilymph from the scala tympani. The AP action threshold increased significantly with the introduction of air into the scala tympani but returned to normal after the air was eliminated. It is not surprising that the presence of compressible gas within the perilymph space may lead to sudden and fluctuating hearing loss, as has been identified in some patients with PLF.

Review of the literature reveals little consensus but tends to support the concept that change in auditory function associated with active PLF is the result of more than a simple communication between the perilymphatic space and the middle ear. Multiple factors are required to create a significant change in auditory function.

DIFFERENTIAL DIAGNOSIS

The signs and symptoms of PLF are relatively nonspecific and overlap greatly with those seen in many other otologic and neurologic diseases. The auditory and vestibular sequelae of PLF may resemble those seen in genetic or syndromal disorders, metabolic disease, Meniere's disease, congenital syphilis, autoimmune inner-ear disease, ototoxicity, labyrinthitis, and retrocochlear lesions such as neoplasms or demyelinating diseases. The pathophysiologic similarities between PLF and Meniere's disease make the two difficult to differentiate, although Ménière's disease is uncommon within the pediatric population (46,47).

Clinical Presentation

Perilymph fistula can be either congenital or acquired. When congenital, it is associated with inner-ear dysgenesis or birth trauma. When acquired, it is usually the result of trauma (e.g., barotrauma, acoustic trauma, blunt or sharp trauma) or bone erosion secondary to infection or neoplasm (including cholesteatoma). Patients with PLF generally complain of auditory symptoms, vestibular symptoms, or both, but there is no constellation of complaints or findings pathognomonic of PLF. The diagnosis, which is difficult enough to establish in adults, is particularly so difficult among children and infants and depends on a high degree of clinical suspicion.

Labyrinthine fistula in children may present in a variety of ways. Meningitis and its association with nontraumatic CSF otorrhea has been recognized since the turn of the century (48). Grundfast and Bluestone, in 1978, drew attention to the relationship between trauma and the development of PLF and sensorineural hearing loss in children (1). Combinations of dysequilibrium, vertigo, and tinnitus also occur as sequelae of PLF in young children. Among children, however, PLF most commonly presents as sensorineural hearing loss, which may be preexistent, sudden in onset, fluctuating, or progressive (11).

Identification of infants and children likely to suffer from PLF presents a significant dilemma. Failure to consider PLF as an underlying cause of progressive sensorineural hearing loss is as great a concern as overzealous exploration of all children with hearing loss. In an effort to resolve both concerns, numerous studies have been performed to help identify factors that are associated with an increased risk of PLF. Antecedent head trauma, including birth trauma, and progressive hearing loss, although challenged by some, are believed by most to be risk factors. High-resolution computed tomography (HRCT) allows noninvasive examination of the temporal bones. Bony anomalies, occasionally detectable on such studies, are associated with a significantly increased likelihood that PLF may be present. This is presumably due to further weaknesses in an inherently delicate system (49). Despite the accuracy of such studies, many anomalies are beyond resolution. Ossicular chain anomalies, which are commonly discovered during exploration of the middle ear or suggested by other craniofacial anomalies, are also more likely in conjunction with PLF. In a 1989 review, Weber, Perez, and Bluestone (25) reported the results of 117 pediatric exploratory tympanotomies for PLF. Of the 80 ears that were shown to have PLF, 65 demonstrated malformations of the middle ear, including malformed stapes (39 ears), deformed round windows (20 ears), deformed incudi (11 ears), and deformed promontories (2 ears). Despite these findings, only 25 ears yielded an abnormality on HRCT. Pappas, and Schneiderman (50), on the basis of results of 36 ears explored for progressive sensorineural hearing loss in children, suggested exploration of only ears that demonstrated hearing loss in association with an anomalous finding on temporal bone HRCT or with a clear history of trauma, exertion, or barometric changes. Considering the impact of hearing loss on the child and family, Myer et al. recommended the slightly more aggressive approach of exploratory tympanotomy for all children with sensorineural hearing loss who have a history of trauma, other sensory handicaps, documented fluctuation of hearing, or radiologic abnormalities of the temporal bones (51).

History and Physical Examination

The sometimes vague presentation of pediatric PLF places a premium on historical data, which should emphasize the presence or absence of recognized risk factors. Concurrent medical problems, infectious diseases, use of ototoxic medications, other sensory deficits, perinatal history, and familial craniofacial anomalies or hearing loss should be investigated and recorded. It is also important to determine whether hearing loss, when present, is progressive and whether there are associated vestibular signs or symptoms. The parents are usually very helpful in this regard. Although historical data are essential to the diagnosis of PLF, physical examination may also provide information important to the diagnosis. A comprehensive examination of the head and neck, focusing on neurotologic function and craniofacial architecture, often yields few abnormalities but is particularly important to eliminate other possible etiologies for the patient's symptoms. Vestibular signs are difficult to recognize in young children and may manifest as clumsiness or frequent falling. Spontaneous nystagmus should be noted if present. Otologic examination for concurrent middle-ear disease should also be performed. Testing with the tuning fork is usually valuable in children older than 6 years of age. Pneumatic otoscopy occasionally reveals nystagmus in pediatric patients with PLF.

Testing

Despite much effort, a single noninvasive test diagnostic for PLF has not been identified. Instead, information gathered during the history and physical examination must be coupled with a battery of tests to arrive at the presumptive diagnosis. Pure-tone audiometry is an important initial diagnostic test. Unfortunately, a characteristic pure-tone audiometric configuration does not exist, thus making the diagnosis from a single audiogram impossible. Serial audiograms may reveal fluctuation or progression of hearing loss and are of help in supporting the diagnosis of PLF if care is taken to ensure consistency when the audiograms are recorded (51).

ECochG has been reported to be an indicator of endolymphatic hydrops (52–54) and was first used for the detection of Ménière's disease. Arenberg et al. (55) introduced the use of ECochG in patients with PLF and demonstrated an increase in the SP/AP ratio in more than half their patients with surgically confirmed PLF. These findings have also been supported by subsequent studies in both human and animal subjects (39,55,56). Meyerhoff and Yellin (57) demonstrated active PLF in 16 of 20 patients undergoing exploratory tympanotomy after obtaining SP/AP ratios in excess of 0.37. Furthermore, the SP/AP ratio returned to normal in 18 of the 20 patients after grafting the oval and round windows. Overall, ECochG provides useful information that aids in the diagnosis of inner-ear fluid imbalance, but its lack of sensitivity precludes its use as a definitive diagnostic test.

Vestibular tests, including conventional electronystagmography (oculomotor screening and positional and caloric testing), platform posturography, the fistula test, and sinusoidal harmonic acceleration, involve cooperation on the part of the patient and are therefore sometimes difficult to perform in the pediatric population. As with audiometric testing, no single vestibular test diagnostic for PLF has emerged. Caloric testing in search of unilateral or bilateral weakness, commonly shows normal results, and the classic fistula test often provides minimal useful information and gives low sensitivity (35%–80%) and specificity (38%–50%) (11,58). Suspance and Bluestone (11) reported some promise in the results of platform posturography and positional testing because these tests were most likely to show abnormal results in patients with PLF (11).

Preoperative laboratory tests should show relatively normal results in the presence of PLF and should be obtained only to eliminate other diagnostic possibilities. Routine screening for congenital syphilis and autoimmune inner-ear disease should be performed by obtaining syphilis serology and erythrocyte sedimentation rate. Additional studies should be obtained when indicated by the history and physical examination and should include complete blood count, renal profile, thyroid function tests, fasting glucose, and additional autoimmune screening, if indicated (59,60). Viral serology may be obtained but is often minimally helpful after the neonatal period.

Imaging is a crucial step in the evaluation of an unexplained progressive sensorineural hearing loss or presumed PLF. Reilly, using multiplanar tomography, found that 20% of the 244 children he was following for sensorineural hearing loss had temporal bone anomalies (49). These results are in agreement with numerous other studies. Currently, multiplanar HRCT using 1.5 mm slices is the imaging procedure of choice because it most accurately assesses the anatomy of the temporal bone. Abnormalities commonly encountered with HRCT include labyrinthine malformation of the pars superior, pars inferior, or both, an enlarged vestibular or cochlear aqueduct, malformations of the oval or round window, and gross ossicular anomalies.

Further search for a definitive test to preoperatively diagnose PLF has led investigators to attempt visualization of the middle ear in search of a fistula prior to exploratory tympanotomy. After the introduction of endoscopic middle-ear visualization by Nomura (61), Poe et al. (62) performed middle-ear endoscopy in 20 patients with suspected PLF. Failing to demonstrate active fistulas in any patients, they placed autologous blood patches in eight patients at both the oval and round windows. No change in hearing loss was noted, but three of four patients with preoperative vertigo had relief of symptoms, and two of three patients showed normalization of preoperative positive fistula tests. The most troublesome difficulty described by Poe et al. (62) was obscured vision of the oval window and round window niche secondary to mucosal adhesions.

The gold standard for the diagnosis of PLF has traditionally been exploratory tympanotomy, but even this procedure is not foolproof. Transudate, irrigation, or injected anesthetic collected within the dependent oval window or round window niche is difficult to differentiate from perilymph. In an attempt to differentiate perilymph from other fluids collected in the dependent oval window and round window niche, Applebaum (63) used the differential clearance of fluorescein from fluid compartments of the body. Bojrab and Bhansali (64), however, later refuted these findings by showing that fluorescein remained present within the soft tissue and transudate of the feline middle ears for no less than 3.5 hours. Intrathecal fluorescein shows more promise for identifying an active leak, although use of this test requires installation of fluorescein within the subarachnoid space and thus places the patient at risk for chemical arachnoiditis (7).

Specific markers have shown promise for identification of perilymph but have been difficult to assay owing to the minute amounts of liquid collected at the site of the leak. β_2 transferrin is specific for human aqueous humor, CSF, and perilymph (65,66). Western blot assay for β_2 transferrin now allows identification with very small amounts of dilute fluid. Unfortunately, the time required to perform the test prevents its use for intraoperative decision making. Preoperative irrigation of the middle ear via a myringotomy has been suggested as a method of obtaining dilute perilymph that could be tested by Western blot assay for the presence of β_2 transferrin, thus providing preoperative evidence of PLF. Inactive or intermittent PLF would be overlooked by this test, and its risk to the patient would approach the risk of exploratory tympanotomy, thus making the efficacy of such a procedure questionable.

GOALS OF MANAGEMENT

Treatment of PLF is best performed with a specific goal in mind. Except in the rare case of recurrent meningitis, PLF poses minimal threat to life or general health. It does, however, significantly affect the psychosocial and educational development of the child and the quality of life of the entire family. In such cases, treatment would ideally be directed toward restoring the patient to his or her premorbid level of audiovestibular function. Although restoration of auditory function to premorbid levels has been reported among a small group of patients, it is generally considered the exception rather than the rule because many of the effects of the disease are irreversible. Realistic expectations for both the family and the surgeon should be stabilization of preexisting hearing levels. Vestibular dysfunction, on the other hand, responds well to repair of PLF (11,58).

Recurrent meningitis, the most life-threatening problem associated with PLF, results from repeated bacterial innoculations of the subarachnoid space. The site of perilymph egress serves as a locus for retrograde inflammation and infection. Auditory function is often quite poor in the affected ear due to concurrent episodes of suppurative labyrinthitis. Surgical treatment is intended to limit bacterial access to the subarachnoid space and prevent subsequent episodes of meninigitis.

Recommended Approach

Once the diagnosis of PLF becomes highly suspected, treatment should be discussed with the family. Surgical exploration of the middle ear offers both the opportunity to confirm the diagnosis and repair the leak, but because surgery for PLF is a quality-of-life issue, the decision must ultimately be made by the family. Such a decision can be made intelligently only after all the potential risks (including cost) and benefits have been carefully explained.

The surgical method of PLF repair has been well described (67,68). Exploratory tympanotomy in children is performed under general anesthesia. Hemostasis is provided by injecting the external auditory canal vascular strip with 1% lidocaine containing 1:50,000 to 1:100,000 partsepinephrine. A tympanomeatal flap is developed and reflected anteriorly and the posterosuperior bony overhang is removed with a curette to enable adequate visualization of the oval window and round window niche. To minimize confusion, which may result from the collection of transudate within the dependent areas of the middle ear, the oval and round windows, fissula ante fenestrum, and the region of Hyrtle's fissure should be inspected prior to instrumentation of the mucosa of the middle ear. These areas are then carefully observed for repeated accumulation of clear fluid, and any anomalies of the ossicular chain or middle ear should be noted. Provocative testing to confirm PLF, advocated by some (69), includes the Valsalva maneuver, Trendelenburg positioning, increase in ventilatory positive pressure, and compression of the internal jugular vein. Others, who routinely graft the oval and round windows, regardless of findings, do not perform provocative testing (18). Preparation for grafting is performed by denuding the mucosa overlying the oval window area and round window niche. This can be done mechanically or with a laser. Autogenous tissue grafts either with or without tissue glue are positioned at the site of the prepared bed, and the ear is closed.

Minor variations in technique have emerged during the development of the operation. Adipose tissue was originally used as graft material, but its use resulted in an unacceptably high rate of recurrent fistula (46,67). Temporalis fascia, preparotid fascia, tragal perichondrium, and areolar tissue are among the materials currently used and are reported to have decreased the incidence of recurrent fistula (46,70,71). To further decrease this incidence, Black et al. (70) have begun using fibrin glue in conjunction with the argon laser to ensure secure adherence of grafts to their recipient site. Weider (47) uses loose areolar tissue because of its superior ability to conform to irregular surfaces; fibrin glue is then added, and the graft is covered with a layer of absorbable gelatin sponge.

Controversy exists regarding the wisdom of placing graft material around the oval and round windows if no active PLF can be demonstrated. Althaus (67) recommended performing provocative maneuvers in an attempt to elicit perilymph leak from the inner ear. If no active leak was found, no grafting was performed. Others support grafting all ears undergoing exploratory tympanotomy in search of PLF (46,71) This stance recognizes the possible intermittent presence of the leak. According to a poll of 167 members of the American Otologic Society and the American Neurotologic Society, 78% advocate placing grafts in all patients undergoing exploratory tympanotomy for PLF, regardless of whether fistula is demonstrated at operation (72). Those who oppose grafting in the absence of an identifiable fistula express concern about potential hearing loss caused by fibrosis around the stapes footplate and the round window niche (2,69,72).

Postoperative care is directed at maintaining the integrity of the graft. Patients are instructed to avoid for a minimum of 6 weeks heavy lifting, straining, and activities that place the head in a dependent position (all of which could lead to increases in intracranial pressure). Antinausea medications are used as necessary.

Alternate Strategies

Among adult patients, alternate management options are available. Nonsurgical options, often advocated for the acute treatment of posttraumatic PLF, include strict bed rest, sedation, elevation of the head of the patient's bed, and the use of stool softeners, coupled with regular audiometric monitoring. These methods are rarely used in the care of pediatric patients with PLF due to the active nature of most children (59).

CONTROVERSIES

Since first recognized as a clinical entity, PLF has been shrouded in some degree of controversy, primarily because of the vagueness of its presenting symptoms, the subjective nature of the intraoperative diagnosis, and the lack of pathologic specimen to confirm the diagnosis (73). Although few challenge the existence of PLF (72), opinions vary with respect to the actual incidence of the disorder and to the preoperative criteria required for surgical exploration. The controversy has served as a catalyst, propelling investigators to improve diagnosis and treatment of PLF. It is now hoped that the increasing availability of β_2 transferrin testing will establish an objective measurement for the presence of PLF.

COMPLICATIONS

In the hands of an experienced otologic surgeon, complications associated with exploratory tympanotomy and repair of PLF are rare. Perforation of the tympanic membrane, injury to the ossicular chain or facial nerve, vertigo, tinnitus, alteration of taste, and sensorineural hearing loss are explained to the patient during the discussion prior to obtaining informed consent. In our experience, postoperative perforation of the tympanic membrane is uncommon, ocurring in less than 1% of patients. Delayed, transient facial palsy has also been observed following repair of PLF but, like perforation of the tympanic membrane, is quite rare. Sensorineural hearing loss following surgery is extremely rare and often represents the progression of the underlying disease process. Conductive hearing loss, on the other hand, has been observed among a minority of patients following the placement of graft material around the oval and round windows (74). The most common postoperative complaint has been temporary dysgeusia and mild xerostomia, both of which resolve over a period of months and are associated with manipulation of the chorda tympani nerve and the tympanic plexus, respectively.

CASE HISTORY

Case History 1: Recurrent Meningitis

A 5-year-old boy presented to the pediatric otolaryngology clinic for evaluation of left-sided hearing loss and otitis media with effusion. His medical history was significant for two previous episodes of bacterial meningitis requiring hospitalization and intravenous antibiotics. Otologic examination revealed left-sided middle-ear effusion, and a behavioral audiogram confirmed a profound left-sided sensorineural hearing loss but normal auditory function in the right ear. Serology, renal profile, and autoimmune tests were normal. Mondini's dysplasia of the cochlea was found on HRCT and the patient was taken to surgery for exploratory tympanotomy. At the time of surgery, a large defect was discovered in the stapes footplate, through which a steady flow of CSF was noted. Stapedectomy was performed, and the enlarged vestibule was tightly packed with temporalis muscle and fascia. A separate fascial graft was placed over the oval window and held in place by a stapes replacement prosthesis. The child subsequently did well and has suffered no further episodes of meningitis.

Case History 2: Posttraumatic Perilymphatic Fistula

A 10-year-old boy presented to the otolaryngology clinic with a history of right-sided sensorineural hearing loss, progessive for 2 years. At the time of presentation, the boy noted accelerated loss of auditory function in the right ear following mild head trauma. His otologic history and family history were otherwise uneventful. Neurotologic examination was within normal limits with the exception of the Weber test lateralizing to the left ear. Audiogram, as compared to previous tests, revealed a stable, moderate high-frequency sensorineural hearing loss in the left ear. The right ear, however, was found to have changed significantly from previous audiograms, showing a 35 dB sensorineural hearing loss coupled with a discrimination of 28%. Laboratory survey and radiologic evaluation were normal. The presumptive diagnosis of PLF was made on the basis of the boy's history. At the time of exploratory tympanotomy, no middle ear anomaly or active fistula could be identified. The oval and round windows, fissula ante fenestram, and Hyrtl's fissure were grafted with preparotid fascia tissue and autologous fibrin glue. Postoperative audiogram demonstrated improvement of pure-tone average to 5 dB and discrimination to 76% in the right ear (Fig. 3). The patient has shown no further deterioration of hearing during the past 2 years.

SUMMARY AND CONCLUSIONS

Progressive sensorineural hearing loss among the pediatric population has a devastating affect on the life and development of a child and his or her family. Historically, the etiology of this problem has been attributed to heredity, antecedent viral disease, or other factors largely beyond control. With the recognition of PLF as a cause of progressive sensorineural hearing loss comes the hope that treatment can be offered to a subgroup of this population. Identification, however, of infants and children likely to suffer from PLF continues to present a significant dilemma. At our institution, we have found that employing the open and active participation of the family and child in diagnostic decision making has significantly aided in the treatment process. Children found to be at risk of PLF on the basis of historical evidence, physical examination, audiovestibular testing, and radiologic findings are offered exploration. On the basis of our experience, we have reached the conclusions listed below.

1. From 6% to 11% of pediatric patients with sensorineural hearing loss and 25% with progressive sensorineral hearing loss may possess occult PLF.
2. Diagnosis of pediatric PLF is difficult and depends on a high degree of suspicion.

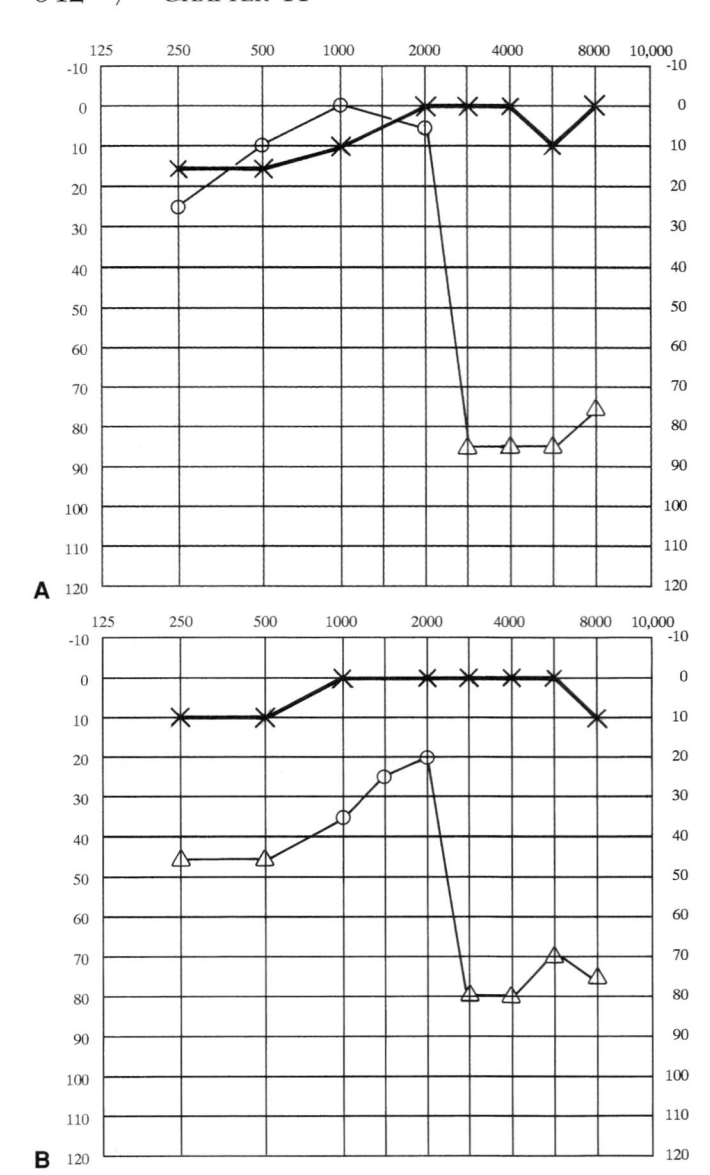

FIG. 3. Audiograms of patient with occult PLF. **A:** Audiogram obtained prior to surgery. **B:** Audiogram obtained following exploratory tympanotomy and oval and round window grafting. Courtesy of W.L. Meyerhoff, MD PhD.

3. Risk factors for pediatric PLF include (60):
   A. History of antecedent trauma
   B. Hearing loss in the presence of craniofacial anomalies
   C. Radiographic evidence of inner ear dysgenesis
   D. Unexplained vestibular or balance abnormalities coupled with hearing loss
   E. Progressive or fluctuating hearing loss
   F. History of previous meningitis or labyrinthitis
4. Patients who suffer hearing loss in a single hearing ear or in the presence of other sensory deficits should be aggressively evaluated for the presence of PLF.
5. Repair of PLF is intended to prevent further loss of hearing, ameliorate vestibular disturbances, and prevent recurrent meningitis.
6. New tests, such as β_2 transferrin assays, should produce objective data on which outcome studies in the future can be based.

REFERENCES

1. Grundfast KM, Bluestone CD. Sudden or fluctuating hearing loss and vertigo in children due to perilymph fistulas. *Ann Otol* 1978;87:761–771.
2. Pappas DG, Simpson LC, Godwin GH. Perilymphatic fistula in children with preexisting sensorineural hearing loss. *Laryngoscope* 1988;98:1507–1510.
3. Reilly JS. Congenital perilymph fistula: a prospective stud yin infants and children. *Laryngoscope* 1989;99:393–397.
4. Harrison WH, Shambaugh GE, Derlacki EL, et al: Perilymph fistula in stapes surgery. *Laryngoscope* 1967;77:836–849.
5. House HP: The fistula problem in otosclerosis surgery. *Laryngoscope* 1967;77:1410–1426.
6. Fee GA. Traumatic perilymph fistula. *Arch Otolaryngol* 1968;88:477–480.
7. Rauch SD. *Intrathecal fluorescein for intraoperative detection of perilymph fistula.* Presented at the International Perilymph Fistula Conference, Portland, OR, September 7, 1990.
8. Simmons FB. Theory of membrane breaks in sudden hearing loss. *Arch Otolaryngol (Stockh)* 1968;88:41–48.
9. Goodhill V. Sudden deafness and round window rupture. *Laryngoscope* 1972;81:1462–1474.
10. Goodhill V. Harris I, Broderman SJ, et al. Sudden deafness and labyrinthine window ruptures: audio and vestibular observations. *Ann Otol Rhinol Laryngol* 1973;82:2–12.
11. Suspance JS, Bluestone CD. Perilymph fistulas in infants and children. *Otolaryngol Head Neck Surg* 1983;91:663–671.
12. Allen GW. Fluid flow in the cochlear aqueduct and cochlear hydrodynamic considerations in PLF, stapes gusher and secondary endolymphatic hydrops. *Am J Otol* 1987;8:319–322.
13. Wtodyka J. Studies on cochlear aqueduct patency. *Ann Otolaryngol* 1978;87:22–28.
14. Palva T, Dammert K: Human cochlear aqueduct. *Acta Otolarygol Suppl (Stockh)* 1969;246,1–58.
15. Glasscock ME. The stapes gusher. *Arch Otolaryngol* 1973;98:82–92.
16. Anson BJ, Donnelson, JA. *Surgical anatomy of the temporal bone and ear.* 3rd ed. Philadelphia: WB Saunders; 1978:55.
17. Goodhill V. Leaking labyrinth lesions, deafness, tinnitus, and dizziness. *Ann Otol* 1981;90:99–105.
18. Kamerer D, Sando I, Hirsh B, et al. Perilymph fistula resulting from microfissures. *Am J Otol* 1987;8:489–494.
19. Sato H, Takahashi H, Sando I: Computer aided 3-D reconstruction and measurement of microfissures. *Am J Otol* 1992;13:141–145.
20. Schuknecht HF, Gulya AJ. *Anatomy of the temporal bone with surgical implications.* Philadelphia: Lea & Febiger; 1986:135.
21. Nenzelius C. On spontaneous cerebrospinal otorrhea due to congenital malformations. *Acta Otolaryngol (Stockh)* 1951;39:314–328.
22. Barr B, Wersall J. Cerebro-spinal otorrhea with meningitis incongenital deafness. *Arch Otolaryngol* 1965;81:26–28.
23. Crook JP. Congenital fistula in the stapedial footplate. *South Med J* 1967;60:1168.
24. Rice WJ, Waggoner LG. Congenital cerebrospinal fluid otorrheavia a defect in the stapes footplate. *Laryngoscope* 1967;77:341–361.
25. Weber PC, Perez BA, Bluestone CD. Congenital perilymphatic fistula and associated middle ear abnormalities. *Laryngoscope* 1993;103:160–164.
26. Allen GW. *Perilymph fistula.* Presented at First International Symposium on Inner Ear Surgery, Snowmass, CO, 1982.
27. Pullen FW. Perilymph fistula induced by barotrauma. *Am J Otol* 1992;13:270–273.
28. Schuknecht HF, Witt RL. Suppressed sneezing as a cause of hearing loss and vertigo. *Am J Otol* 1985;6:468–470.
29. Allen GW. Clinical manifestations of experiments on alterations of labyrinthine fluid pressure: Symposium on inner ear surgery. *Otol Clin North Am* 1983;16:3–26.

30. Ackley RS. *Electrocochleographic and histopathological observation of experimental perilymphatic fistula in guinea pigs* [Dissertation]. UMI Dissertation Information Service, University of Colorado, Boulder, CO, 1985
31. Walsted A, Salemon G, Olsen KS. Low frequency hearing loss after spinal anesthesia: perilymph hypotonia? *Scand Audiol* 1991;20:211–215.
32. Hardy PA. Influence of spinal puncture and injection on Cranial nerves VIII nerve function. *J Laryngol Otol* 1988;102:452.
33. Parisier SL, Barhan SA. Recurrent meningitis secondary to idiopathic oval window leak. *Laryngoscope* 1976;86:1503–1515.
34. Syms CA, Atkins JS, Murphy TP. *Intravenous fluorescein for the detection of perilymph fistulae.* Presented at the International Perilymph Fistula Conference, Portland, OR, September 7, 1990.
35. Bohmer A. On the pathomechanism of cochlear dysfunction inexperimental perilymph fistulas. *Laryngoscope* 1991;101:1307–1312.
36. Simmons FB, Barton RD, Beatty D: Round window injury: auditory behavioral and electrophysiological consequences in the cat. *Trans Am Acad Ophthalmol Otolaryngol* 1962;66:715–722.
37. Robertson D. Cochlear neurons: frequency selectivity altered by perilymph removal. *Science* 1974;186:153–154.
38. Flint P, Duckert L, Dobie R, et al. Chronic perilymph fistula: experimental model in the guinea pig. *Otolaryngol Head Neck Surg* 1988;99:380–387.
39. Campbell KC, Savage MM. Electrocochleographic recordings inacute and healed perilymphatic fistula. *Arch Otolaryngol* 1992;118:301–304.
40. Simmons FB. The double membrane break syndrome in sudden hearing loss. *Laryngoscope* 1979;89:59–64.
41. Oshiro EM, Shelton C, Lusted TS. Role of perilymph fistula in sudden hearing loss: an animal model. *Ann Otolaryngol* 1989;98:491–495.
42. Hazell JWP, Fraser JG, Robinson PJ. Positional audiometry in the diagnosis of perilymph fistula. *Am J Otol* 1992;13:263–269.
43. Nishioka I, Yanaghara N. Role of air bubbles in the perilymphas a cause of sudden deafness. *Am J Otol* 1986;7:430–438.
44. Mafee MF, Valvassori GE, Kumar A, et al. Pneumolabyrinth: a new radiologic sign for fracture of the stapes footplate. *Am J Otol* 1984;5:374–375.
45. Pashey NR. Simultaneous round and oval window fistulae in a child. *Ann Otolaryngol* 1982;91:332–335.
46. Seltzer S, McCabe B. Perilymph fistula: the Iowa experience. *Laryngoscope* 1984;94:37–49.
47. Weider DJ. Treatment and management of perilymph fistula: a New Hampshire experience. *Am J Otol* 1992;13:158–166.
48. Escat E. Ecoulement spontane de liquide cephalorchidien parle conduit auditif extreme: fistule congenitale probable. *Arch Int Laryngol* 1897;10:653–659.
49. Reilly JS, Kenna MA. Congenital perilymph fistula: An overlooked diagnosis. *Am J Otol* 1989;10:496–498.
50. Pappas DG, Schneiderman TS. Perilymphatic fistula in pediatric patients with a preexisting sensorineural hearing loss. *Am J Otol* 1989;10:449–450.
51. Myer CM, Farrer SM, Drake AF, Cotton RT. Perilymphatic fistulas in children: Rationale for therapy. *Ear Hear* 1989;10:112–116.
52. Coats AC. The summating potential and Meniere's disease. *Arch Otolaryngol* 1981;107:199.
53. Gibson WPR, Moffat DA, Rensden RT. Clinical electrocochleography in diagnosis and management of Meniere's disease. *Audiology* 1977;16:389–401.
54. Goin DW, Staller SJ, Asher DL, et al. Summating potential in Meniere's disease. *Laryngoscope* 1982;92:1383.
55. Arenberg IK, Ackley RS, Ferraro J, et al. ECochG results inperilymphatic fistula: clinical and experimental study. *Otolaryngol Head Neck Surg* 1988;99:435–443.
56. Black FO, Lilly DJ, Nashner LM, et al. Quantitative diagnostic test for perilymph fistulas. *Otolaryngol Head Neck Surg* 1987;96:125–134.
57. Meyerhoff WL, Yellin W: SP/AP ratio in perilymph fistula. *Otolaryngol Head Neck Surg* 1990;2:678–682.
58. Ruben RJ, Yankelowitz SM: Spontaneous perilymphatic fistula in children. *Am J Otol* 1989;10:198–207.
59. Strunk CL. Perilymphatic fistula in children. In: Gates GA, ed. *Current therapies in otolaryngology—head and neck surgery.* Chicago: Mosby; 1994:84–85.
60. Shott SR, Pensak ML. Perilymphatic fistula. *Ear Nose Throat J* 1992;71:568–572.
61. Nomura Y. Effective photography in otolaryngology—head and neck surgery: endoscopic photography of the middle ear. *Otolaryngol Head Neck Surg* 1982;90:395–398.
62. Poe DS, Rebeiz EE, Pankeator MM. Evaluation of perilymphatic fistulas by middle ear endoscopy. *Am J Otology* 1992;13(6):529–533.
63. Applebaum EL. Fluorescein kinetics in perilymph and blood: a fluorophotometric study. *Laryngoscope* 1982;92:600–671.
64. Bojrab DI, Bhansali SA: Fluorescein use in the detection of perilymph fistula: a study in cats. *Otolaryngol Head Neck Surg* 1993;108:348–355.
65. Bassiouny M, Hirsch BE, Kelly RH, et al. Beta-2 transferrin application in otology. *Am J Otol* 1992;13:552–555.
66. Weber PC, Kelly RH, Bluestone CD, Bassiouny M. Beta-2 transferrin confirms perilymphatic fistula in children. *Otolaryngol Head Neck Surg* 1994;110:381–386.
67. Althaus SR. Perilymph fistula. *Laryngoscope* 1981;91:538–562.
68. Glasscock ME, McKennan KX, Levine SC. Persistent traumatic perilymph fistula. *Laryngoscope* 1987;97:860–864.
69. Althaus SR. Long-term results of perilymph fistula repair. *Laryngoscope* 1973;23:1502–1507.
70. Black FO, Pesznecker S, Norton T, et al: Surgical management of perilymph fistulas: a new technique. *Arch Otolaryngol* 1991;117:641–648.
71. Shelton C, Simmons FB: Perilymph fistula: the Stanford experience. *Am J Otolaryngol* 1988;97:105.
72. Hughes GB, Sismanis A, House JW. Is there consensus in perilymph fistula? *Otolaryngol Head Neck Surg* 1990;102:111–117.
73. Balkany T. Controversies in pediatric otology: Point/counterpoint—perilymph fistula. *Am J Otol* 1989;10:493.
74. Parell GS, Becker GD, Results of surgical repair of inapparent perilymph fistulas. *Otolaryngol Head Neck Surg* 1986;95:344.

CHAPTER 45

The Atelectatic Ear

Lisa M. Elden and Kenneth M. Grundfast

Common sequelae of otitis media include middle ear atelectasis, localized or total eardrum atrophy, and eardrum retraction. The sequelae, once present, may remain stable or progress and become worse. A problematic aspect of managing children with middle ear atelectasis is the inability to predict outcome once eardrum abnormalities are detected. That is, a retraction pocket can remain stable and never cause significant problems, or the retraction pocket may become progressively deeper, causing hearing loss, and ultimately can become cholesteatoma.

DEFINITIONS AND CLASSIFICATIONS

Many confusing terms have been used to describe observed structural abnormalities of the eardrum. The following are descriptors of significant eardrum pathology from a review of relevant literature.

Atelectasis

Atelectasis is incomplete expansion of the middle ear space, associated with medial displacement of eardrum toward the promontory. The eardrum is atrophic in most cases (1).

Retraction

Local retraction is medial displacement of a portion of the eardrum toward the promontory; it can be fixed or mobile (2). Localized retraction pockets occur most frequently in the posterior-superior portion of the pars tensa (Fig. 1) and in the pars flaccida (Fig. 2) (1,3,4–7).

Diffuse retraction is a term often used interchangeably with the term *atelectasis* (1). The whole eardrum is usually atrophic and retracted toward the promontory (Fig. 3) (8).

In ears that are atelectatic or have retracted eardrums, the middle ear pressure is almost always negative (mean value, -153 mm H_2O), suggesting that an underlying middle ear ventilation disorder is present (5,9). Mobility of the eardrum is observed with use of the pneumatic otoscope, and impedance measures vary with the degree of negative pressure in the middle ear. Tympanogram configurations either have reduced peaks or are flat (type C and type B, respectively).

Atrophy

Local atrophy a portion of the eardrum is thin and transparent or translucent (3,8). A small area of atrophy commonly develops at the site where a ventilation tube or perforation has been. The eardrum mobility is usually normal or hypermobile with pneumatic otoscopy, and impedance measurements are normal. Depending on the size and location of the atrophic area, impedance testing may reveal a biphasic (double-peak) tympanogram.

Diffuse atrophy indicates that an entire eardrum is translucent, thin, and mobile or hypermobile with pneumatic otoscopy. Compliance measurements are hyperdynamic, and the tympanogram configuration is tall, with or without a peak (type Ad) (Fig. 4).

Adhesive Otitis Media

Local adhesive otitis media is a nonmobile portion of an atrophic eardrum that is fixed by adhesions to the promontory and may be fixed to other middle ear structures, including the incus (myringoincudopexy), and in more severe

---

L.M. Elden: Department of Pediatric Otolaryngology, McMaster University Medical Center, Hamilton, Ontario L8N 3Z5 Canada.
K.M. Grundfast: Department of Otolaryngology and Pediatrics, Georgetown University School of Medicine, Washington, DC 20007.

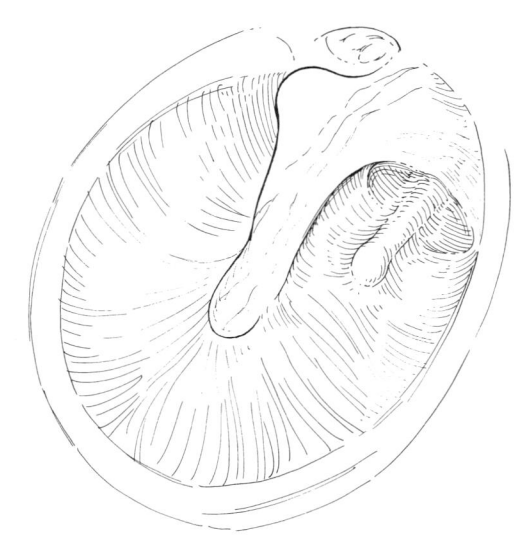

FIG. 1. Left eardrum, demonstrating localized retraction in posterior-superior quadrant pars tensa. The eardrum touches long process of the incus and the lenticular process.

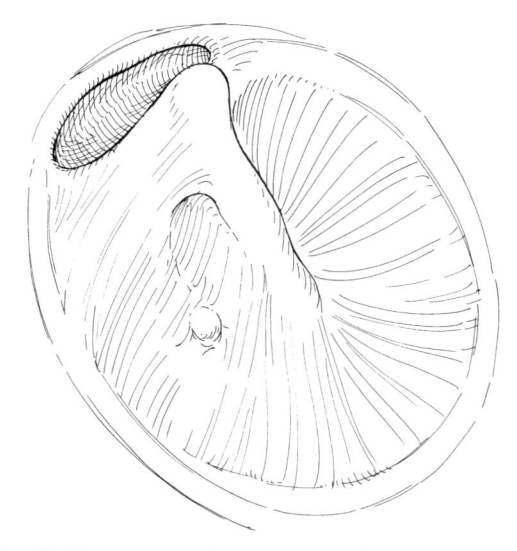

FIG. 2. Right eardrum, demonstrating localized retraction in pars flaccida. The eardrum is adherent to the lenticular process of the incus.

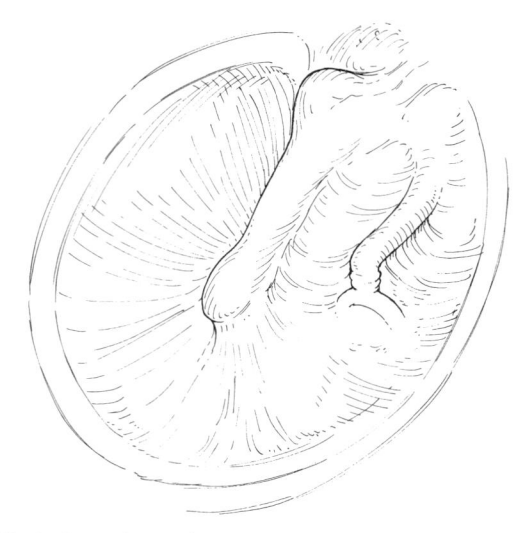

FIG. 3. Left eardrum, demonstrating diffuse retraction involving the whole eardrum with "skeletonized" ossicles. The eardrum is adherent to the incudostapedial joint and stapes suprastructure.

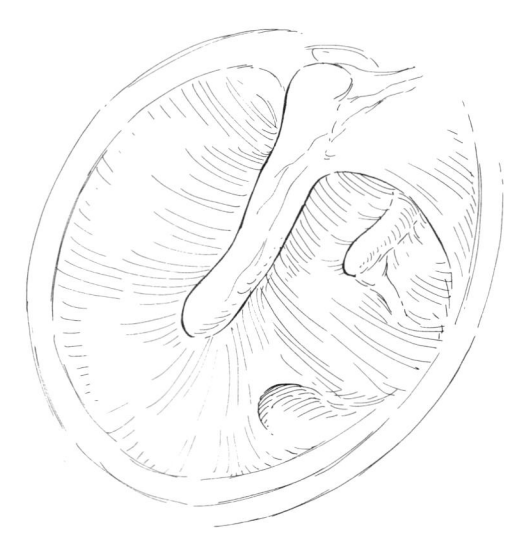

FIG. 4. Left eardrum: diffuse atrophy and retraction. The eardrum is retracted onto the incudostapedial joint and round window niche. Pneumatic otoscopy, impedance measurements, and installation of saline into middle ear may be necessary to differentiate from diffuse adhesive otitis media.

cases, the incudostapedial complex (myringostapedopexy) (1). The adhesions develop as a result of inflammation (3,8). This is an end stage of the continuum that begins with acute otitis media. The tympanogram is usually flat (type B), sometimes causing audiologists or inexperienced clinicians to think there is fluid in the middle ear.

Diffuse adhesive otitis media (The Shrinkwrap Ear) is a condition characterized by a markedly atrophic eardrum with severe adhesive otitis media, in which the whole eardrum is adherent to the middle ear structures, including the ossicles, the promontory, and the round window niche (Fig. 4). The eardrum may be draped so that it appears to be a subtotal eardrum perforation. Hearing in the involved ear is usually normal, or near normal with an air-bone gap of no more than 10 to 15 dB.

Perforation

Perforation is defined as a hole in the eardrum, which can easily be confused with a deep translucent or transparent eardrum retraction. Eversion of the pocket with pneumatic otoscopy and low or normal volume impedance measurements help to differentiate retraction pocket from perforation.

Retraction Pocket/Incipient Cholesteatoma

Over time, and with infection and inflammation; some localized eardrum retraction pockets undergo change and evolve into acquired cholesteatoma. Once the rate of proliferation and other aspects of biologic activity of epithelial cells within the eardrum pocket undergo change, the retraction pocket that previously had merely been a topographic indentation in the eardrum converts to become the slowly enlarging potentially destructive (osteolytic) matrix sac of an acquired cholesteatoma (10) (see the section, Pathophysiology). The conversion from retraction pocket to cholesteatoma occurs before damage to the middle ear structures occurs. Incipient cholesteatoma is more likely to be present when the full extent of the pocket cannot be visualized (especially posteriorly in a pars tensa retraction), the pocket cannot be everted with insufflation using pneumatic otoscopy, and one or more of the following are present:

Flakes or sheets of dry brownish debris within the pocket
Flaky shiny, oily sheet or film covering the epithelium of the pocket
Collection of white or yellowish-white liquid within the pocket, often observed after swimming, water sports, or bathing
Granulation tissue in or near the retraction pocket (11)

Myringosclerosis/Tympanosclerosis

Myringosclerosis and tympanosclerosis are degenerative changes affecting the middle collagenous layer of the eardrum (lamina propria) and less frequently, the middle ear and mastoid mucosa in response to repeated episodes of acute otitis media, respectively. Myringosclerosis and tympanosclerosis are thought to be reparative response to these repeated infections. Histologic studies demonstrate that in myringosclerosis, the normal collagen is replaced by disoriented, thicker collagen fibrils. Hyaline degeneration occurs and deposits of calcium and phosphorus form, creating chalky, thick, white plaques that are most often found in the inferior half of the eardrum (Fig. 5). Tympanosclerosis

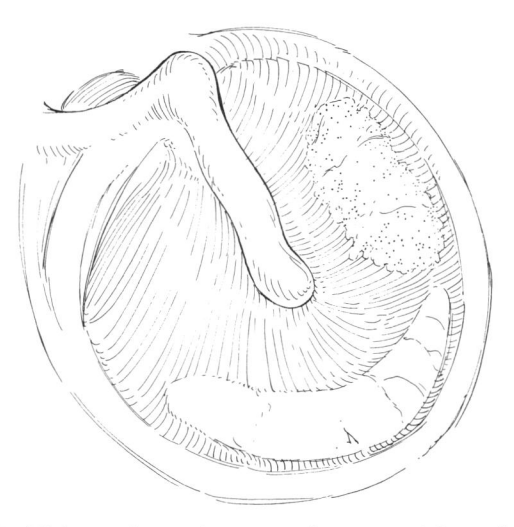

FIG. 5. Right eardrum, demonstrating two patches of myringosclerosis (patchy and discoid types).

occurs when smoother, onion-like deposits are found in the middle ear and mastoid mucosa (12,13). Hearing is rarely affected, except when ossicular fixation occurs, as in some middle ear mucosa lesions.

STAGING

Staging classifications for pars tensa retractions and pars flaccida retractions have been developed based on clinical and otomicroscopic findings (Tables 1, 2) (1,3,4,7). Although these systems are helpful in grading severity of atelectasis, the stages are arbitrary and difficult to remember. Documentation using descriptive terms with diagrams and photographs provides more information and affords comparisons over time of changes that occur (Fig. 6).

EPIDEMIOLOGY

Although much significance is attributed to eardrum atrophy, adhesions, and middle ear atelectasis, the degree to which these findings actually represent pathology requiring treatment remains uncertain. To investigate the significance of eardrum abnormalities, Tos and others have studied pars tensa retractions in otherwise healthy children and found that the prevalence ranges from 2.4% to 9.2%, with higher values

TABLE 1. *Staging classification for the atelectatic ear: pars tensa retractions*

Grade/Stage	Investigation	
	Sade (8)	Charachon, Barthez, and Lejeune (7)
I	Slightly retracted	Mobile retraction
II	Reclined over incus	Fixed and controllable (totally visible)
III	Reclined over promontory	Fixed and uncontrollable (full extent not visible)
IV	Adherent to promontory (adhesive otitis media)	
V	Eardrum adherent and perforated	

TABLE 2. *Staging classifications for the atelectatic eardrum: pars flaccida retraction*

Type I	Slight retraction between Shrapnell's membrane and the neck of the malleus
Type II	Retraction extends to the neck of malleus; no air present
Type III	Retraction extends beyond the bony annulus (implying bone erosion); area of Shrapnell's membrane is enlarged, but air can be seen in attic
Type IV	Pronounced bone resorption and Shrapnell's membrane is adherent to the heads of malleus and incus; bottom of retraction still visible secondary to bone erosion
Type V	Attic cholesteatoma: once the bottom of the retraction is no longer visible

From Tos M, Hvid G, Stangerup S-C, Andreassen UK. Prevalence and progression of sequelae following secretory otitis. In: Bluestone CD, Casselbrant M, Schietz MD, eds. Ann Otol Rhinol Laryngol 1990; 99(Suppl 149):13. (Ref. 3)

reported when otomicroscopy with pneumatoscopy was used compared with pneumatic otoscopy alone (3,4,6). Pars flaccida retractions were seen more frequently (11.5–21%) compared with pars tensa retractions, but most of these pars flaccida retractions were milder and reversible (3,4,6,14). The prevalence of severe pars flaccida retractions with evidence of scutal bone erosion was low in all age groups (0.3–5.8%), as was the prevalence of significant pars tensa abnormalities, such as atrophy with fixation (0.7–2.3%) (3,4). Other structural changes in the eardrum that have been recorded in school-aged children include dry perforation which is seen in 0.3% to 0.8 % of ears examined, and tympanosclerosis, which is seen in 1.2% to 8.6 % of ears examined (6).

Tos followed a cohort of these otherwise healthy children annually from the ages of 5 to 10 years to assess the rate at which these changes develop and found that the prevalence of eardrum changes plateaued from the ages of 6 to 10 years (3,4). Although these incidence and prevalence studies done by Tos and others provide worthwhile information, they did not prospectively follow a cohort that was at risk and for a long enough duration to determine fate or outcome of the observed eardrum abnormalities.

In separate studies, Tos and other investigators have followed at-risk children and adults who had chronic serous otitis media with and without retractions over time. The rate of development of serious structural changes was difficult to assess because the severity of structural changes at initial diagnosis varied greatly from patient to patient, as did the number and type of surgical procedure(s) performed to treat the chronic effusions and eardrum changes (12,15–17) (Table 3). However, it is clear from these studies that a history of previous chronic serous otitis media is the greatest risk factor for the development of atelectatic ears in children (7,17). In addition, the studies demonstrate that retraction pockets tend to be dynamic in nature, and many stabilize or revert to normal with time. Retractions are less likely to normalize and more likely to progress to cholesteatoma if they are severe at the onset of observation, especially if adhesions are present (15,16).

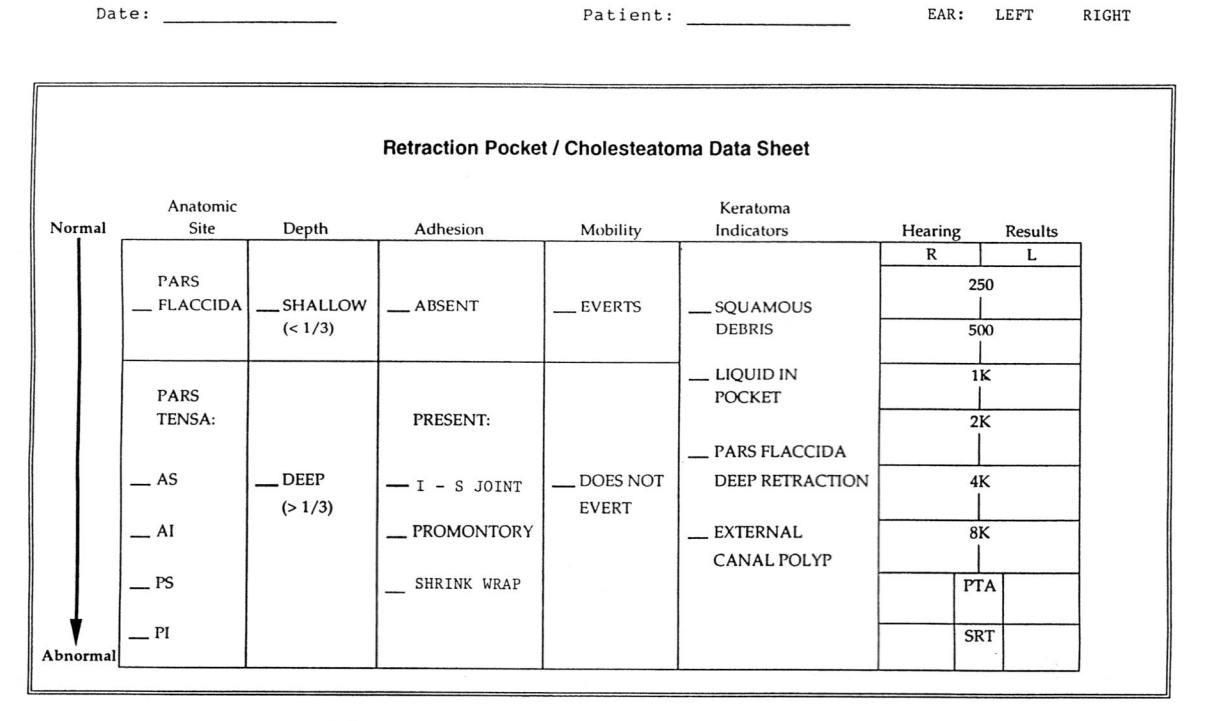

FIG. 6. Retraction pocket/cholesteatoma data sheet.

TABLE 3. Longitudinal studies on progression of retraction pockets/atelectasis (Children ± Adults)

	Moller (12)	Charachon, Barthez, and Lejeune (7)	Tos, Stangerup, and Larsen (15)
No. of eardrums	100	78	362
Population type	Adults/children with retractions	Adults/children with early retraction	Children with retractions
Previous treatments	N/S	Medical	Repeat M&Ts Adenoidectomy
Follow-up time	1–15 yr	1–5 yr	10–15 yr
Outcome (eardrum status)			
Normalized or stabilized	N/S	23%[a]	73% pars flaccida[b] 68% pars tensa[b]
Perforation or worsening retraction (all posterior-superior)	10%	16%	N/C
Retraction with cholesteatoma	5%	0	0.8%

N/S, not stated; N/C, not calculated; M&T, myringotomy and tube.
[a] Reflects percentage that remained normalized (percentage that remained stable not reported).
[b] As calculated from data presented in paper.

PATHOPHYSIOLOGY

Table 4 summarizes stages in the continuum that begins with otitis media and can lead to cholesteatoma in children.

Stage I: Middle Ear Ventilation Disorder, Inflammation, Infection

Normally, the eustachian tube is closed at rest and periodically opens with swallowing and jaw movements, allowing air to enter the middle ear, thereby keeping middle ear pressure equilibrated with ambient atmospheric pressure. Likewise, periodic eustachian tube opening, along with mucociliary action, allows egress of fluid from the middle ear into the nasopharynx (18). Thus, eustachian tube dysfunction results in impaired middle ear ventilation, which may lead to the development of structural changes of the eardrum. Bluestone, Casselbrant, and Cantekin (18) have studied children with retraction pockets by using various tests of the ventilatory function of the eustachian tube (modified inflation-deflation technique, forced-response test, Toynbee maneuver) and concluded that many of these patients have functional obstruction of the eustachian tube, whereby the eustachian tube constricts rather than dilates during swallowing and other such ventilating maneuvers. Alternatively, Magnusun (19), using direct middle ear measurements, suggested that in some situations, tubal dysfunction is caused by persistent tubal patency, which may explain why some children with eustachian tube dysfunction have the habit of recurrent sniffing. The sniffing may provide a means of temporarily closing the eustachian tube, while also creating damaging transient increases in negative middle ear pressure. Regardless of the mechanism causing the eustachian tube dysfunction, both studies concur that the ventilation of the middle ear–mastoid air-cell system becomes impaired such that there is fluctuating or sustained high negative middle ear pressure that leads to stress and eventual weakening of the eardrum, which can lead to retraction pocket formation.

TABLE 4. Factors contributing to the development of structural changes of the eardrum: sequelae of otitis media

Stage I: Middle Ear Ventilation Disorder, Infection, and Inflammation
  Middle ear ventilation disorder: intermittent or chronic negative middle ear pressure
  Eustachian tube dysfunction
    Anatomic/developmental
      Cartilage
      Angle/juxtaposition to nasopharynx and middle ear
    Failure to open on Valsalva maneuver
    Persistently patent tube
  Infection
    Acute otitis media: degradative enzymes from neutrophils
  Inflammation
    Persistent otitis media with effusion: cytokines from mononuclear cells
Stage II: Structural Changes of Eardrum
  Lamina propria changes: loss of collagen and elastin, leading to atrophy
  Changes affect vascular areas the most: posterior-superior pars tensa
Stage III: Invagination
  Mechanically disadvantaged sites: pars flaccida and posterior-superior pars tensa
  Fixed attachment of eardrum (adhesions) to middle ear structures
    Promontory
    Lenticular process of incus
    Incudostapedial joint
    Stapes/stapedius tendon
Stage IV: Proliferation and Desquamation
  Cellular changes: ingrowth of invaginated epithelium
  Mononuclear cell inflammatory changes
  Incipient cholesteatoma
Stage V: Ossicular Erosion (with and without cholesteatoma)
  Inflammatory cell effect: cytokines
    Release of bone-degrading enzymes from fibroblasts and osteoblasts
    Stimulation osteoclasts
  ?Direct pressure effect (granulation tissue)

Experiments on animals support the concept that eustachian tube dysfunction is an underlying cause of eardrum atrophy and retraction. When the eustachian tubes of gerbils and rabbits are ligated or cauterized, eardrum atrophy and retraction and even cholesteatoma are observed (20–22).

Abrahamson, Asarch, and Litton (23) demonstrated that an important factor that causes cholesteatoma (and presumedly its retraction pocket precursor) to form is the presence of inflammation. One of the most reliable ways to create an experimentally induced cholesteatoma is to use direct chemical irritation to cause inflammation. Therefore, both eustachian tube dysfunction and inflammation appear to be important in the development of cholesteatoma.

The mechanism by which chronic and recurrent middle ear inflammation and infection contribute to the development of atelectasis and, in fewer cases, cholesteatoma is suggested by studies on the contents of human middle ear effusions (MEEs) and on the histologic changes seen in retracted eardrums. Supporting collagen and elastin are found to be absent in pars tensa and pars flaccida retractions, respectively, and are replaced by increased inflammation (mostly mononuclear cells) (8,24–27). Neutrophils and cytokines found in the MEEs are likely to play important roles in causing significant eardrum changes. Potent oxidizing enzymes and proteolytic enzymes, including collagenase, elastase, and gelatinase released by neutrophils, most likely degrade fibrous collagen in the pars tensa and elastic fibers in the pars flaccida, respectively. Cytokines (interleukin-1-beta, interleukin-6, interferon-gamma, and tumor necrosis factor-alpha) have also been found in high concentrations in MEE. These immunoregulatory glycoproteins are probably secreted by mononuclear cells and are known to cause pathologic changes such as fibrosis, mucosal hypertrophy, and ossicular erosion (28). The posterior-superior portion of the pars tensa and the pars flaccida are more susceptible to changes caused by inflammation because they are more vascular than the rest of the eardrum. This may help to explain the propensity for retraction pockets (and acquired cholesteatoma) to develop in these areas.

A study of temporal bones in children suggests that instead of degradation of the supporting structures in the lamina propria from enzymes and immunoregulatory proteins in the MEE, retraction pockets may form because these important structural components (collagen and elastin) fail to develop in susceptable patients. The authors observed that mesenchyme in the lamina propria of the pars flaccida and posterior-superior pars tensa remained and did not develop into mature elastin and collagen, respectively, in patients with a history of early middle ear inflammation (29).

Stage II: Structural Abnormalities of the Eardrum

As a result of the microscopic changes in the eardrum caused by chronic inflammation and middle ear ventilation disorders, observable structural changes in the eardrum occur that may or may not be permanent. Microscopically, the eardrum becomes atrophic, changing from a tense trilayer to a thin bilayer with a thicker outer (lateral) squamous epithelium and thin inner (medial) mucosal layer, with intervening inflammation rather than a middle fibrous layer (Fig. 7) (8). Atrophy and retractions are dynamic in nature, as demonstrated by Sade, Avraham, and Brown (1), who prospectively followed children and adults and found that less severe retractions of the pars tensa remained stable or normalized with time, whereas only 10% to 20% progressed to more severe retractions. Therefore, in the majority of cases, these eardrum retractions can be considered innocuous. Perforations occur most often in areas of the eardrum that are atrophic.

Tympanosclerosis (myringosclerosis) is the most common structural abnormality of the eardrum occurring in 4% to 7% of children with a history of secretory otitis media, and in 19% to 33% of the cases, the sclerotic plaques disap-

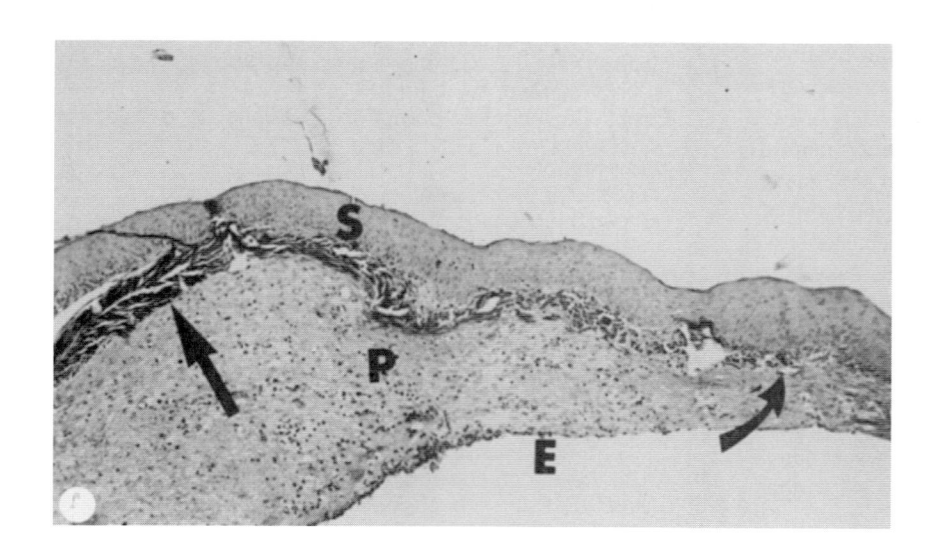

FIG. 7. Histogram. Pars tensa, showing transition of nonatelectatic to atelectatic areas. Note the absence of collagenous backbone in the atelectatic part (*curved arrow*) and the presence of this organized collagenous structure in the nonatelectatic part (*straight arrow*). E, medial side of middle ear presenting flat epithelium; S, thick squamous epithelium; P, edematous lamina propria infiltrated with round cells (8).

pear with time (15,30). These white plaques in the eardrum are even more commonly seen in children who have had ventilation tubes (21–55%), but the mechanism of development is not clear and hearing is rarely affected (1,30).

Stage III: Invagination: Why Are Some Areas of the Eardrum More Likely to Develop Retractions Than Others?

Not only is the posterior-superior portion of the pars tensa more prone to the effects of inflammation and consequent weakening (because it is more vascular than the rest of the eardrum), but this same area and the pars flaccida are structurally more compliant than the rest of the eardrum when exposed to mechanical stress from negative middle ear pressure. Tonndorf and Khanna's (31) and Ars and deCraemer's (32) hologram and viscoelasticity experiments on otherwise normal human cadaver eardrums demonstrate that the site of maximal vibrational amplitude and stress occurs in the posterior-superior aspect of the pars tensa when the eardrum is exposed to either low-frequency sounds or constant negative or positive pressure, respectively. Therefore, ventilation disorders that cause recurrent or chronic negative middle ear pressure are likely to affect the posterior-superior eardrum and, with time, cause weakening that leads to invagination and formation of retraction pockets (31,32).

Stage IV: Proliferation and Desquamation

Why Do Cholesteatomas Form?

As the eardrum invaginates and becomes adherent to the middle ear mucosa, the lateral squamous epithelial layer becomes thicker and grows medially to form papillae. In addition, increased keratin desquamation occurs (26,27). Once the pocket becomes noncleansing (i.e., when the neck of the pocket is more narrow than the pocket itself), keratin debris can fill the pocket (26). Immunohistologic analyses of retraction pockets and cholesteatoma reveal that inflammatory cells adjacent to matrix cells display characteristics of delayed-type hypersensitivity. Specifically, class II–producing cells, mast cells, and IgA-producing cells are seen in the areas with maximal inflammation, suggesting that the components of the mucosal immune system are activated and may be important in initiating the abnormal epithelial migration that causes cholesteatoma (33). Squamous-lined sacs, which may be the direct precursor of cholesteatoma, have been identified microscopically within adherent retraction pockets (2,26,34).

Stage V: Ossicular Erosion

A commonly held belief is that pressure of the eardrum resting on the lenticular process of the incus causes ossicular erosion; however, inflammation more than simple mechanical pressure is likely to be the cause of erosion. A layer of inflamed granulation tissue is almost always observed microscopically between an eroded ossicle and the retracted eardrum (35). In addition, because microscopic ossicular erosion is seen almost as often in patients with and without cholesteatoma, direct-pressure necrosis from an adjacent cholesteatoma is less likely the primary cause. Cytokines, especially, interleukin-1, have been found in increased quantities near eroded bone, both in cases of erosion associated with chronic otitis media and in cases in which the erosion obviously was from cholesteatoma. Further, this lymphokine has been shown to stimulate local bone-cell resorption by recruiting monocytes for osteoclastic bone resorption and by stimulating osteoblasts and fibroblasts to release bone-degrading enzymes (36).

GOALS FOR MANAGEMENT

Because adhesive otitis media and primary acquired cholesteatoma are the adverse end-stage outcomes in the continuum of disorders starting with otitis media, the primary goal in management of all disorders within the continuum should be early detection, to prevent hearing loss and cholesteatoma formation.

CLINICAL MANIFESTATIONS AND DIAGNOSIS

During the child's preschool years, both the primary care physician and ear specialist are likely to see the patient who is having recurrent episodes of otitis media. Once the child enters school, the number of acute symptomatic ear infections declines, and the threshold for visiting the physician is lowered because most parents prefer their child not miss school for a nonurgent problem. An important concept to remember is that structural eardrum changes that can lead to cholesteatoma usually do not cause symptoms in preschool children (3 to 7 years of age). Therefore, detection of those eardrum changes that might be the harbingers of developing cholesteatoma might be detected first by pediatricians and other primary care physicians, who perform the annual physical examination of school-aged children. Advancements in the management of childhood-acquired cholesteatoma probably can be achieved as more pediatricians and primary care physicians understand better the nature of the continuum and focus on subtle changes in topography of the eardrum that could be precursors for cholesteatoma. In addition, primary care physicians need to identify those children who are at higher risk. Children who need to have their eardrums inspected carefully at the time of each primary care office visit are those children who have had tympanostomy tubes (VT-tubes) inserted two or more times, a family history of cholesteatoma, perforated eardrum two or more times, and/or a repaired cleft palate, Turner's syndrome, Treacher Collins syndrome, and other craniofacial deformities, particularly those that adversely affect eustachian tube function.

Notably absent from the aforementioned risks or indicators is hearing loss. For optimum management and, in many instances, prevention of acquired cholesteatomas in children, precursors should be identified and intervention undertaken before ossicular erosion or fixation has occurred.

Symptoms likely to be present if middle ear atelectasis and eardrum abnormalities have progressed to incipient or frank cholesteatoma include subjective hearing loss, malodorous discharge, dizziness, and, otalgia. Therefore, advancement in management and prevention of childhood cholesteatoma should be related to the diagnostic acumen of the primary care physician and his or her ability to differentiate subtle eardrum changes that are likely to be innocuous from those that are potentially ominous. Optimal treatment of a retraction pocket that is in the early stages of developing into acquired cholesteatoma depends on clarity of thinking on the part of the otologic surgeon, who must interpret the significance of observed findings.

Pneumatic otoscopy with a Siegel or Breuning otoscope is most helpful in assessing the important characteristics of the eardrum retraction. These observations include the following:

Retraction pocket
Size
Location (pars flaccida or posterior-superior pars tensa)
Depth
Ability to evert
Adhesion to ossicle (usually lenticular process of incus or stapes suprastructure)
Other
Visible ossicle erosion (scooping of caudal long process or lenticular process of incus)
Granulation or polyp
Perforation
Sclerosis

Observations need to be recorded (diagrammed or photodocumented) so that changes over time will be apparent when interval data are compared. Figure 6 is a checklist that can be photocopied and used in the office to facilitate documentation and comparison of observations at the time of each office visit.

Objective Data

Objective tests such as audiograms and impedance testing cannot be relied on to detect middle ear atelectasis and do not replace a careful physical examination. Routine school screening levels set at 25 dB will miss up to 50% of patients with MEE, because these children have an average hearing loss of 27 dB (37). In addition, testing conditions are less reliable because the audiogram is performed in an environment that is not controlled for backgound noise (5,38).

The use of impedance testing as a screening device to detect silent MEEs and diffusely retracted eardrums is more helpful but only in conjunction with an examination with pneumatic otoscopy. In the diffusely retracted eardrum, tympanograms are most likely to be flat or reveal negative pressure tracings (average value, -153), whereas eardrums with localized retractions may have normal or only slightly negative middle ear pressure (average value, -70 mm H_2O) (5). Therefore, localized retraction pockets can easily be missed if impedance testing alone is used to screen for atelectatic ears.

Imaging

Imaging of the atelectatic eardrum is not routinely necessary. Most necessary information can be obtained simply from a thorough clinical examination. Those cases in which imaging might be helpful in case management include

1. diagnosing suspected underlying cholesteatoma or cholesterol granuloma when one or more of the following are present:

   recurrent/chronic otorrhea
   unexplained conductive hearing loss (greater than 30 dB if chronic serous otitis media is present)
   granulation or polyp in medial external auditory canal (especially posteriorly-superiorly)
   debris in pocket

2. preoperative planning to assess if the mastoid is sclerotic or opacified. Of course, the matter of deciding when to combine mastoidectomy with tympanoplasty in operating on children without cholesteatoma is controversial. Many experienced otologic surgeons do routinely combine mastoidectomy with tympanoplasty when operating on an atelectatic ear, while others believe that opening the mastoid adds little to overall success from tympanoplasty (see sections, Management, and Problems and Pitfalls). For those surgeons who consider the mastoidectomy an important adjunct procedure in surgical management of the atelectatic ear, a preoperative radiologic study would be superfluous. Alternatively, some surgeons prefer to base the decision to add mastoidectomy on the radiographic finding of a mastoid that is sclerotic and poorly pneumatized.

Computed tomography (CT) of the temporal bones, rather than magnetic resonance imaging (MRI) is the preferable imaging study. By comparing preoperative imaging studies and operative findings, Koltai et al. (39) demonstrated that MRI is less helpful than CT in determining the extent of disease and bony destruction, because bone is not imaged well by MRI. In addition, CT was found to be more accurate than MRI in detecting the presence of cholesteatoma in patients with chronic otitis media and granulation tissue (39).

MANAGEMENT

Successful management of the atelectatic ear in a child depends on a series of decisions that enhances the likelihood of achieving the goals of maintaining normal hearing and avoiding development of cholesteatoma. Middle ear atelectasis, alone, is not necessarily an otologic disorder with dire consequences. However, when middle ear atelectasis is followed by localized eardrum atrophy, retraction, and adhesion, ossicular erosion and cholesteatoma can develop. Therefore, the challenge in management of the child with middle ear atelectasis is one of deciding whether any intervention is warranted and choosing among the many seemingly unproven or controversial recommended approaches to management (Table 5). Further, because the eardrum changes that can lead to development of ossicular erosion, cholesteatoma, or both, are likely to develop slowly over time, successful case management depends as much on the otologist's ability to detect subtle changes in condition of the eardrum as on his or her ability to surgically strengthen the eardrum or reconstruct the ossicular chain. In fact, perhaps more than in management of any other otologic disorder, management of an atelectatic ear in a child is a matter of detecting subtle changes and then assigning relative import to the observed changes in a way that allows the otolgic surgeon to assess the risks and benefits of a proposed surgical procedure, compared with the risks and benefits of continuing an expectant approach without any surgical intervention.

TABLE 5. *Interventions available for treatment of the atelectatic eardrum*

Mechanical: aerodynamic, pneumatic
  Middle ear inflation (active)
    Valsalva maneuver
    Politzerization
    Autoinflation (Otovent balloon)
Medical
  Antimicrobial
  Antiinflammatory (steroids)
  Decongestants, antihistamines
  Allergy management (hyposensitization)
Surgical
  Adenoidectomy (improve eustachian tube dysfunction; diminish source of chronic bacterial infection?)
  Middle ear ventilation (passive)
    Ventilation (tympanostomy) tube
  Lysis of adhesions
    Bolus saline injection
  Maintaining the middle ear space; avoiding recurrent adhesions
    Absorbable protein gel (Gelfilm)
    Nonabsorbable synthetic (Silastic)
  Strengthening the eardrum
    Medial fascia graft tympanoplasty
    Medial cartilage graft tympanoplasty
  Replacing the eardrum
    Lateral graft tympanoplasty
    Homograft tympanoplasty
  Creating an enlarged air reservoir
    Mastoidectomy (canal wall up)
  Repairing damaged ossicles
    Ossiculoplasty

Figure 8 is a decision-making algorithm that has been developed to assist in deciding when and how to intervene. In applying this algorithm to case management, it is important to keep in mind the following principles:

1. The goal is to preserve, or keep as normal as possible, structural integrity and function of the ossicular chain. *Corollary:* Delaying or deferring surgical intervention until ossicular erosion, hearing loss, or both, have developed may not ultimately be of maximum benefit to the patient (see section, Otologist's Dilemma).

2. Although compromised middle ear ventilation is a key factor in initial pathogenesis of the atelectatic ear, improving middle ear ventilation alone may not avert further eardrum changes, leading to development of a cholesteatoma if adhesions have already developed between the eardrum and the middle ear structures.

3. Although there is some information available on natural history for the atelectatic ear (see Table 3), deciding what to do in each case is difficult because there are numerous factors that can affect what will happen once an eardrum has developed areas of atrophy, retraction, and adhesion. Factors that can affect the course of an atelectatic ear include mastoid pneumatization, inflammation, infection, immunity, and ability and willingness to use autoinflation techniques.

4. Long-term follow-up is needed, especially after a localized eardrum retraction pocket has developed. The potential for progression from retraction pocket to acquired cholesteatoma must be assessed on the basis of several observations over time.

5. Even in ears that are changing from atelectasis to formation of a retraction pocket, or from a retraction pocket to cholesteatoma, there may be no symptoms whatsoever. That is, the child may experience no ear discomfort or hearing loss.

Deciding what to do when confronted with a child who has signs of a developing atelectatic ear is difficult. If the child is referred by a pediatrician because of abnormal appearance of the eardrum, and the child is asymptomatic, with normal hearing in the involved ear, then there is usually little justification for intervention of any kind. However, the abnormal finding observed by the pediatrician could well be the early signs of a developing deep eardrum retraction with significant possibility for progression to cholesteatoma. How, then, can the otologist decide what should be done? A first step that is helpful in sorting out some of the confusion about management of the child with middle ear atelectasis is to divide ears in children evaluated into four categories based on history, otomicroscopic findings over time, and results of audiologic testing.

1. *Safe stable ear:* looks bad, works well, low risk for developing into cholesteatoma; eardrum does not change with time, and hearing remains normal.
2. *Uncertain:* looks bad, works well, risk for developing into cholesteatoma not clear; changes, such as progressively deepening retraction, are observed over time, but hearing remains normal.
3. *High risk:* looks bad, works well, high risk for develop-

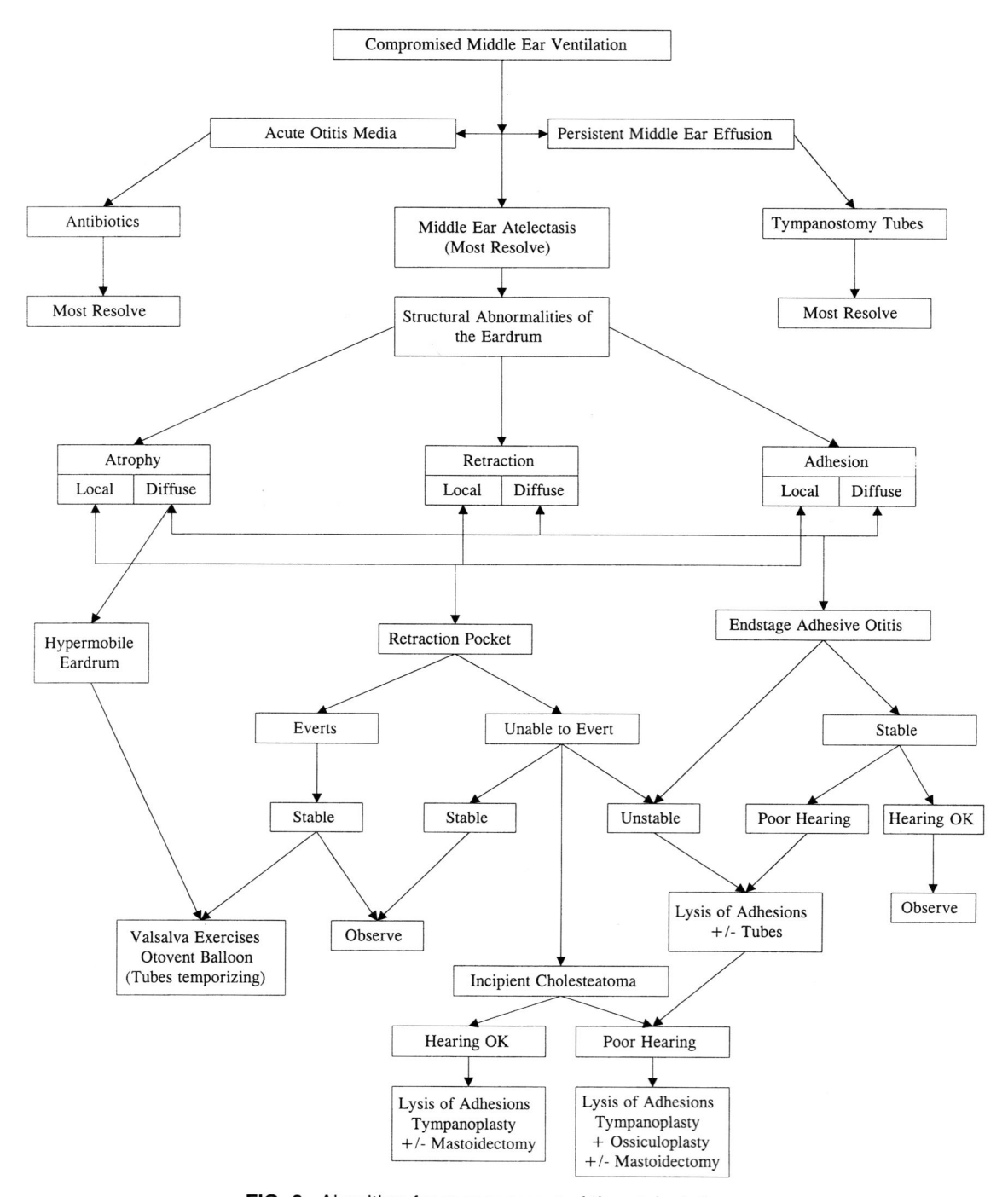

FIG. 8. Algorithm for management of the atelectatic ear.

ing into cholesteatoma; in addition to changes, such as progressively deepening retraction, there are features of an incipient cholesteatoma (see section, Definitions and Classifications), but the hearing is normal or near-normal.

4. *Dysfunctional*: looks bad, works poorly; eardrum changes are occurring or have stabilized, with symptoms that may include otorrhea, bleeding, and discomfort, and an associated conductive hearing loss is usually present.

Treatment

Safe, Stable Ear

Normal Hearing

Expectant therapy is recommended if the retraction appears to be low risk for cholesteatoma and the hearing is normal. This should include interval otomicroscopic examinations with photodocumentation or accurate diagrams and audiologic assessments and tympanograms at 3- to 6-month intervals initially. If the pocket does not progress, the child should continue to be followed, with examinations and audiology assessments (usually for 5 yr) until the pocket has either disappeared or stabilized.

Intermittent or Mild Unilateral Hearing Loss

In many of these cases, there may be an associated conductive hearing loss, because the middle ear space is not fully aerated and/or the mobility of the tympanic membrane is reduced. In situations in which the pocket can be everted in the office with a pneumatic otoscope, mechanical therapy (autoinflation) may be helpful. The Valsalva maneuver can be taught to cooperative children (older than 5–7 yr of age) as a means to keep the middle ear well aerated. Children who are able to use the Valsalva and autoinflate their ears report improvement in hearing, but some children will stop using the autoinflation technique if they experience ear discomfort associated with the sudden middle ear aeration. The Otovent (Invotech International, Inc., Jacksonville, FL) balloon device can be used as an alternative in younger children. This device is a simple, commercially produced "kit" consisting of a piece of plastic, with one end that accepts the rubber band of a balloon and another end that is to be pressed against a nostril. Balloons and simple-to-read instructions are included in the package. The Otovent device is manufactured specifically to be used for autoinflation of a child s middle ear(s) and generally is easy to use, especially in children over the age of 3 years. (The Otovent device costs around $20 and can be ordered from Invotec International, Incorporated, 11221-5 St. Johns Industrial Parkway South, Jacksonville, Florida 32246.) Controlled trials to determine the efficacy of this device demonstrate short-term, significant improvement in otomicroscopic examinations and tympanograms (64% normalized with the device vs. 15% of controls) when the apparatus is used three times per day on a regular basis. Unfortunately, the rate of long-term compliance is poor, and the rate of resolution of the MEE/atelectasis tends to plateau after 1 month of treatment (40,41). For patients who can not autoinflate their ears, politerization has been used with variable success; however, this maneuver is often frightening and rarely well tolerated by young children.

Few authors have addressed the effects of medical treatment, such as decongestants, antihistamines, and steroids, on the atelectatic ear. Most extrapolate efficacy of these treatments from studies on chronic MEEs. Specific studies that addressed these questions include a double-blinded, randomized trial conducted by Cantekin and colleagues (42), which demonstrated that a decongestant–antihistamine combination was no more effective than placebo in clearing chronic MEEs in children. Rosenfeld, Mandel, and Bluestone (43) reported a meta-analysis assessing the efficacy of a short course of systemic steroids for chronic otitis media with effusion and concluded that steroids have advantages, but these benefits could not be proven statistically on a consistent basis. Although eustachian tube dysfunction and inflammation are the most likely common causes for the pathologic findings in children with MEEs and those with atelectasis, the two populations of children are different. Recommendations from studies on children with effusions should be applied with caution to children with atelectatic ears. Children with atelectasis tend to be older and presumably may have irreversible structural changes of the eardrum and more severe eustachian tube problems than children with MEEs alone. In children with atelectatic ears who have chronic nasal symptoms, such as is seen in allergic and nonallergic rhinitis, a trial of medical therapy (usually nasal steroids) with or without consultation by an allergist is recommended to try to optimize eustachian tube function. Likewise, adenoidectomy should be considered if symptoms and signs of hypertrophy or chronic infection are present.

Persistent Hearing Loss (Secondary to Fluid or Nonfixed Retracted Eardrums: The Tube Truce)

To any otologist with significant experience in management of middle ear atelectasis, the attempt to maintain middle ear ventilation and eardrum integrity can seem like a treacherous and frustrating battle. If the young child with middle ear atelectasis grows up to have normal or near-normal eardrums with normal hearing, the battle is won. On the other hand, if the young child with middle ear atelectasis ultimately develops end-stage adhesive otitis media, cholesteatoma, ossicular erosion, or eardrum perforation, the battle is lost. An otologist whose attempts at case management seem to be meeting with little success can get the sense that the atelectatic ear is doing what it wants to do instead of what the otologist wants the ear to do. That is, sometimes, despite all attempts, adequate middle ear ventilation cannot be achieved and sustained, so progressive retraction, adhesions, and even cholesteatoma develop.

In the otologist's war against deleterious effects of atelectasis, insertion of a VT-tube can be viewed only as a truce that staves off MEE and nonfixed retractions, not necessarily as the ultimate weapon that is decisive in winning the war. The truce (VT-tube) is beneficial to the patient only to the extent that function of the eustachian tube improves during the time that the VT-tube remains within the eardrum, because, after tube extrusion, the child has to depend once again on the eustachian tube for middle ear ventilation. If eustachian tube function has not improved sufficiently, atelectasis recurs. In longitudinal studies, there appears to be no long-term preventive benefit with tube use, because there is no change in the rate of retraction formation once the tube extrudes. Although tubes do not contribute to the development of "high-risk" posterior-superior pars tensa retractions, they are more likely to cause localized retractions at the tube site (16). In addition, the rates of tympanosclerosis and perforation with tube use (at the tube site) are elevated (44). In the atelectatic ear, "permanent" tubes such as T-tubes, butterfly tubes, and Paparella type II tubes, with average time to extrusion greater than 2 years are preferable compared with the usual grommet-type tube that extrudes after an average time of 1.0 to 1.5 years (45,46). However, the chance of persistent perforation following tube extrusion is significantly higher compared with long-term tubes: 5% to 12% with permanent tubes versus 0% to 1% with grommet-like tubes (44,45).

In some instances, when a tube cannot be placed because the diffusely atrophic eardrum has become draped over and adherent to the middle ear structures, and there is no obvious air-containing space, or when a pocket cannot be everted with insufflation, saline injected into the middle ear, using a 25-gauge spinal needle, will help to elevate the eardrum. In general, insertion of a VT-tube probably should not be the primary method of treatment when the eardrum has become adherent to middle ear structures such as the ossicles or promontory (adhesive otitis media).

High-Risk Retraction with Normal or Near-Normal Hearing

The major problem in management of the atelectatic ear is not actually doing the otologic surgery required, but deciding when surgery might be indicated and which surgical procedure is most appropriate for the child. Decision making regarding indications for surgery is so difficult because the atelectatic ear in a child may remain stable and be relatively innocuous, become associated with adhesions between the eardrum and middle ear mucosa, ultimately developing into end-stage adhesive otitis media, or become a progressive, deepening retraction pocket with hyperproliferation of eardrum epithelium, ultimately developing into cholesteatoma. Thus, it is not simply the findings observed at one point in time that need to be considered in making the decision to operate, but also changes *over* time that need to be considered in choosing the timing to intervene surgically. The algorithm depicted in Fig. 8 demonstrates the different pathways that can be encountered in the management of the atelectatic ear. The choice of operation depends on the status of the ear and how much eardrum is available for reconstruction (see Table 5).

Adhesions, rather than ossicular erosion or discontinuity, are usually the initial cause of mild-to-moderate conductive hearing loss in an atelectatic ear. When there are adhesions only to the lenticular process of the incus or to the incudostapedial joint, there may be little or no hearing loss. However, when an atrophic eardrum becomes adherent to the stapes suprastructure, oval window niche, and promontory, there may be a more noticeable conductive hearing loss. When the goals of surgery on an atelectatic ear are strengthening the eardrum and lysis of adhesions, there are several alternative surgical approaches.

If the whole eardrum is salvageable, and the problem is maintaining middle ear space to avoid recurrent adhesions, then elevation of the eardrum and placement of a stentlike structure, such as Gelfilm or Silastic, on the promontory has been used with variable success. Gelfilm is recommended in this situation because it is biocompatible and eventually resorbs with time. The greatest chance of developing recurrent adhesions is presumedly just after surgery when the eardrum or middle ear mucosa is more likely to be inflamed. The long-term benefit has not been studied. Use of Silastic has been reported by many authors (47). Although relatively inert, delayed extrusion and infection from Silastic have been seen in patients up to 4 years after placement and, therefore, is not recommended unless a second surgery is planned, at which time the Silastic can be removed.

In the majority of cases, a portion of the eardrum is atrophic (usually the posterior-superior pars tensa), and, therefore, only this area needs to be excised. The eardrum heals in 90% of the cases that are treated by excising the retraction pocket without primary grafting, but the healed area remains weak, and retraction recurs in all but 40% of cases (48). Therefore, medial grafts are important for providing structural support to the eardrum. Many options are available for grafting, but results from various retrospective series suggest that an underlay temporalis fascia and cartilage ensemble provides the most strength and lowest recurrence rate of medial grafts when repairing retraction pocket defects (47,49) (Table 6).

TABLE 6. Results of surgery in the management of the atelectatic ear

Author	Luntz et al. (53)	Paparella and Jung (47)	Charachon, Barthez, and Lejeune (7)
Patient population	48 adults 36 children	58 children and adults	150 children and adults
Follow-up (yr)	4.0–4.5	2.3	>1
Procedure(s)	Tympanoplasty ± tube	Tympanoplasty ± tube	Tympanoplasty (cartilage) ± mastoidectomy ± ossicular reconstruction
Results			
Recurrence	18.8% (children) 22.1% (adults)	15%[a]	16%
Hearing	Not reported	48% better 39% no change 13% worse	Preop PTA 55.4[b] Postop PTA 36.6

[a] Five needed a ventilation tube, and four needed revision tympanoplasty.
[b] PTA, puretone average at 0.5, 1.0, and 20 Hg. These hearing results were calculated from data on children only.

Lateral and homograft tympanoplasties are options if the whole eardrum is atrophic, such as is seen in diffuse adhesive otitis media. Gelfilm placed on the promontory is especially helpful in these cases to prevent adhesion reformation.

With both medial and lateral grafts, some otologists advocate the placement of a VT-tube at the time of surgery (50,51). Although the tube helps to keep the middle ear aerated it does not alter the reformation rate of the retraction (51).

Addition of Mastoidectomy to Create an Enlarged Air Reservoir

In many instances, ipsilateral mastoidectomy appears to be helpful in maintaining or improving aeration of the middle ear (52). Chronic pathologic tissue, including granulations and cholesteatoma in the middle ear and mastoid that obstruct the aditus ad antrum, has been found more frequently in patients with atelectatic ears (52,53). Theoretically, aeration of the middle ear should be improved by removing this obstructing tissue to create a larger reservoir for air, especially in a sclerotic cavity (50,54). The presence of a sclerotic cavity is of unknown significance, but the degree of pneumatization of the mastoid cavity has been shown often to be asymmetric and decreased in the ipsilateral ear in patients with one atelectatic ear (55,56). Whether this is a result or cause of chronic eustachian tube dysfunction and/or chronic otitis media remains unclear and continues to be debated. Evidence that favors inflammation as the cause of mastoid sclerosis includes Ikarashi and Nakano's (57) studies demonstrating that middle ear inflammation in 5-day-old pigs results in severe inhibition of ipsilateral pneumatization of the tympanic bulla. Regardless of the mechanism of development, many believe that poor pneumatization of the mastoid does contribute to eardrum retraction and the development of cholesteatoma. Therefore, it would be logical to assume that adding mastoidectomy would prevent cholesteatoma from developing. However, Avraham, Luntz, and Sade (58) compared postoperative middle ear aeration in patients with retractions of similar severity who had tympanoplasty alone with those who had tympanoplasty and mastoidectomy and found that aeration was actually better in the tympanoplasty-alone group (60.7% vs. 22.2%, respectively; $p = 0.0048$) (58). Although the severity of retraction pockets was similar in each group compared in this retrospective study, the decision to perform mastoidectomy was not random, and the type of mastoidectomy varied considerably from atticotomy to modified radical mastoidectomy. Therefore, the results of this study should be validated before recommending that mastoidectomy is not necessary in the treatment of the atelectatic ear.

Based on evidence taken from the animal study and assuming that improved aeration of the mastoid–middle ear complex will increase the likelihood of successful tympanoplasty, cortical mastoidectomy should be considered if

1. the lateral plain film or CT scan of the mastoid demonstrates a sclerotic, poorly pneumatized mastoid ipsilateral to the retraction pocket and/or a density is present within the epitympanum–mastoid antrum that is suggestive of cholesteatoma or cholesterol granuloma
2. progressive eardrum retraction or chronic perforation persists or recurs following previous tympanoplasty, or
3. intraoperatively if
   a. cholesteatoma is seen extending into the epitympanum, facial recess, or sinus tympani with inability to completely remove the cholesteatoma through a middle ear approach alone
   b. granulation tissue is seen obstructing the aditus ad antrum

Dysfunctional Ear, Repairing Damaged Ossicles

The two most important outcomes to assess with respect to the surgical treatment of the atelectatic ear are (a) recurrence rates and (b) hearing levels, preoperatively and postoperatively. From the literature, optimal hearing is achieved if the ossicles are intact at exploration. Therefore, the primary goal should be ossicular preservation rather than reconstruction, so it is best to intervene before significant ossicular erosion has occurred. However, if ossicles are missing, the outcome is still good if the stapes and malleus are present and available for autograft reconstruction (7).

Ossicular reconstruction usually should be accomplished at the time of tympanoplasty unless there is cholesteatoma in or around the oval window and so on. In general, reconstruction with autograft ossicles (usually incus crutch from stapes to malleus or to drum) is preferable. An exception is when there is a fibrous union of the incudostapedial joint, in which situation a prosthetic incudostapedial joint replacement (Applebaum prosthesis) gives excellent results.

The need for second-look surgery after tympanomastoidectomy for atelectasis is controversial but should remain the prerogative of the surgeon. Second-look surgery is indicated either to improve hearing (if primary ossiculoplasty was not successful) or in cases in which there is a high likelihood of leaving trapped epithelium in the operated ear. In some cases, the surgeon is able to remove a sac as a whole, but if the epithelium tears apart during dissection, there is a good chance that cholesteatoma may later develop. Small rigid telescopes (1.9 mm) and flexible telescopes (1.0 mm) are available that allow for exploration of the middle ear through myringotomy incisions. The rigid scopes are more helpful because the optics, resolution, and field of view are superior to that of the flexible scopes (59).

Alternatively, Rosenberg and colleagues (60) have recommended the use of larger rigid telescopes (2.7 mm and 4.0 mm) to replace an open second-look procedure. This necessitates a 1-cm incision postauricularly and elevation of a tympanomeatal flap. They demonstrated that the risk of missing residual or recurrent disease is low when using this technique.

PROBLEMS AND PITFALLS

This chapter has stressed that successful management of the atelectatic ear is largely a matter of choosing from among the array of alternatives those approaches that are most beneficial to the patient. In making these decisions, it is important to keep in mind the desired outcome: The outcome sought for each patient with middle ear atelectasis severe enough to warrant management by an otologist or otolaryngologist should be hearing as near to normal as possible and avoidance of development of cholesteatoma in the affected ear.

With this in mind, decision making is more the key to achieving the desired outcome than is technical surgical expertise. While there are almost always many different approaches that can lead to successful outcome, there are also pitfalls and decisions that can be made that are likely to lead to unsuccessful outcome. Some of the potential problems and pitfalls are discussed next.

Failure to Communicate Effectively to the Primary Care Physician the Ominous Aspect of the Condition of the Ear

Perhaps the most common problem in managing the atelectatic ear is miscommunication between the otologist or otolaryngologist and the primary care physician, who is likely to be a pediatrician or family doctor. Successful outcome for the patient really depends on close observation, over time, of the affected ear and early detection of subtle but significant changes in the eardrum. At the point in time when hyperproliferation of eardrum epithelium is beginning and epithelial debris is collecting in an eardrum retraction, surgical intervention may be warranted. To detect these subtle but significant changes, the patient may need to be examined with an otomicroscope. If a patient who has developed significant eardrum atelectasis with a progressively deepening eardrum retraction is not examined carefully for months or years by an otologist or an otolaryngologist, ominous changes may go undetected until such time that a frank cholesteatoma with ossicular erosion has developed. In general, primary care physicians do not comprehend the complex concepts and nuances related to development of acquired cholesteatoma. Therefore, in the best interest of the patient, the otologist or otolaryngologist who had detected eardrum changes that could lead to cholesteatoma has the responsibility of describing to the referring primary care physician the observed findings and the ultimate significance of those findings.

Avoiding This Pitfall

Once a posterior superior pars tensa or pars flaccida eardrum retraction has been detected, call or send a letter to the referring physician, explaining that these eardrum abnormalities can be the early signs of a developing cholesteatoma. Stress the importance of close follow-up and decide who is going to see the patient and how often the visits will be scheduled. In general, a period of observation of 1 year, with four repeated ear examinations, preferably with the otomicroscope, 3 months apart, is sufficient for determining if the eardrum retraction is remaining stable and is relatively innocuous, or if changes are occurring that indicate a cholesteatoma or hearing loss may be developing.

Tube Insertion Beyond the Time That Tube Insertion Will Help

The patient with an atelectatic ear is almost always a patient who has a history of having had inadequate eustachian tube function with otitis media and middle ear ventilation problems that required tube insertion. That is, early in the patient's course, inadequate middle ear ventilation and middle ear infection are the main physiologic problems that needed to be solved. However, as the disorder progresses and the ear becomes more atelectatic, adhesions between the eardrum and middle ear structures are likely to develop. Once a deep eardrum retraction with significant adhesions between the eardrum and middle ear structures has developed, there is little likelihood that insertion of a VT-tube in the ear, alone, will be definitive management leading to successful outcome. More specifically, if the eardrum is adherent to structures in addition to the incudostapedial joint, such as the facial recess, the promontory, or the sinus tympani, inserting a tube without lysing the adhesions will not necessarily improve hearing or achieve the desired outcome of avoiding development of cholesteatoma. After all, it is probably the adhesions rather than inadequate middle ear ventilation that is causing the conductive hearing loss, and once the tube becomes extruded, the progression toward development of cholesteatoma has a chance of occurring. Therefore, simply inserting a VT-tube in the atelectatic ear with adhesions should be viewed more as a temporizing intervention than as definitive treatment.

Avoiding This Pitfall

If insertion of a tube is believed to be a reasonable next step in management, attempt to lyse the adhesions and return the eardrum to a more normal position by using a 25-gauge pediatric spinal needle to inject saline into the middle ear. Also, insert a long-term ventilating tube, such as the (Goode) T-tube or (Paparella II) larger-lumen grommet. Explain to the patient that close follow-up will be required for approximately 1 year after the tube has been removed or becomes extruded. The danger zone for progression from atelectasis to acquired cholesteatoma is the 1- or 2-year period after extrusion or removal of a VT-tube that previously had been inserted in a severely atelectatic ear with significant eardrum atrophy.

Fixing the Eardrum and Middle Ear, Ignoring the Mastoid

Otologists have debated for years whether mastoid pneumatization is a significant factor in determining outcome from tympanoplasty surgery. Often, the debate becomes an issue of the chicken and the egg. Is the ear atelectatic because the mastoid is poorly pneumatized, or is the mastoid poorly pneumatized because chronic middle ear infection has interfered with the normal process of mastoid pneumatization? Although there is not a definitive correct answer, pneumatization of the mastoid should be considered in planning surgery for middle ear atelectasis, especially when the middle ear problems have been mostly unilateral. If a CT scan has been obtained to look for evidence of scutum erosion or signs of cholesteatoma, the degree of mastoid pneumatization can be assessed. When there is a deep retraction in the posterior-superior area of the pars tensa or in the pars flaccida, opening the mastoid allows the surgeon to look for eardrum epithelium that may have extended into the fossa incudis or the epitympanum. Furthermore, opening the facial recess may provide another route for air to enter the middle ear from the mastoid, possibly helping to overcome the deleterious effect of poor eustachian tube function.

Avoiding This Pitfall

When planning tympanoplasty surgery for a patient with an atelectatic ear, at least consider that opening the mastoid might be helpful. When in doubt, also obtain an operative permit for mastoidectomy. Do not hesitate to open the mastoid, even if you do not find eardrum epithelium extending into the facial recess. Quite possibly, opening the mastoid air cells will enhance aeration of the middle ear and increase the chances for successful tympanoplasty.

Fixing the Eardrum and the Middle Ear, Not Dealing with Ossicular Erosion

A progressively deepening retraction pocket in the posterior-superior aspect of the pars tensa can be thought of as potentially being an incipient cholesteatoma. The complex matter of deciding when to operate and repair the deep posterior-superior retraction pocket has been discussed previously in this chapter. In cases in which a decision to perform a tympanoplasty has been made to treat the incipient cholesteatoma, the preoperative hearing test will be normal or near-normal because the eardrum is markedly adherent to the incudostapedial joint. After dissecting the eardrum off of the joint, it may become evident that the lenticular process of the incus has become eroded and there may be only a fibrous union between the long process of the incus and the capitulum of the stapes. Because the hearing in the ear was normal preoperatively, the otologic surgeon will often hesitate to transect the fibrous tissue joining the incus to the stapes. However, in doing a cartilage-graft tympanoplasty to repair the eardrum retraction (incipient cholesteatoma), leaving the fibrous connection without creating a better mechanical conducting mechanism risks having postoperative hearing that is worse than the preoperative hearing.

Avoiding This Pitfall

When the lenticular process of the incus is eroded and only a fibrous union is found between the incus and stapes, do not hesitate to use an incudostapedial joint prosthesis, or, alternatively, remove and sculpt the incus to be used as an incus interposition graft. Once the eardrum has been dissected off of a fibrous incudostapedial connection to which it has become adherent, insertion of a cartilage graft alone will achieve the outcome of avoiding cholesteatoma formation, but the chances for achieving normal or near-normal hearing postoperatively are enhanced if a bone-to-bone or bone-to-prosthesis-to-bone connection is created at the time of surgery.

Operating on the Shrink Wrap Eardrum

The shrinkwrap eardrum (in the section, Definitions and Classifications) is a severely atrophic eardrum that is diffusely draped and fixed to the underlying promontory and ossicles. Patients with the shrinkwrap eardrum are often referred to an otologic surgeon because a primary care physician is concerned about the appearance of the eardrum even though the patient is likely to have few of no troublesome symptoms. Indeed, the eardrum looks bad, but, in most cases, the hearing is near normal and no surgery is indicated. After all, unless there is evidence of a progressively deepening eardrum retraction pocket or collection of desquamated epithelium, the likelihood of a cholesteatoma developing in a shrinkwrap eardrum is minimal.

Avoiding This Pitfall

Because the patient with a shrinkwrap eardrum usually has minimal to no hearing impairment, an intact eardrum, and no otorrhea or discomfort; there is little to be gained by operating on the ear. In fact, operating on the shrinkwrap eardrum can be technically difficult, and there is little benefit for the patient in trying to create a middle ear space and a thicker eardrum. You can make the eardrum look better, thereby addressing the concern of the referring physician that the eardrum looks horrible, but in changing the appearance of the eardrum, you run the risk of having postoperative results that include eardrum perforation, otorrhea, and recurrence of adhesions. Therefore, unless the patient referred to you has some specific symptoms that would be alleviated by surgery, do not recommend surgery. Instead, assess the patient's hearing, and if the hearing is close to normal, discuss with the patient the condition that has developed and reassure that although the appearance of the eardrum may be of concern to the primary care physician, there is little that needs to be done. Offer to follow the patient, along with the primary care physician, for a year or so, but do not be quick to operate.

Loss of Follow-up

This chapter has described management of the patient with middle ear atelectasis and eardrum retraction. Most patients with middle ear atelectasis do not require surgery, but they do require close observation over time. After all, the information provided in this chapter has stressed the importance of looking for subtle changes in the appearance of the eardrum that may mean that a stable retraction pocket is changing into an early cholesteatoma. Inadequate eustachian tube function is the underlying problem and major factor leading to the development of the atelectatic ear. Even those patients who have had cartilage-graft tympanoplasty with mastoidectomy may continue to have middle ear atelectasis with recurrence of the retraction. After all, the cartilage graft and opening of the mastoid may be helpful in counteracting the deleterious effects of poor eustachian tube function, but, in many cases, the poor eustachian tube function remains as a formidable factor that needs to be considered in future management. Those otologic surgeons who are experienced in management of the atelectatic ear develop a degree of skepticism about short-term surgical results that appear successful. Unfortunately, many patients who have had surgery on an atelectatic ear are delighted with the initial postoperative results and either are not asked to return for or fail to come in for a scheduled 1- or 2-year follow-up visit. Sometimes, when these patients return years later, not only has atelectasis recurred, but also a cholesteatoma has developed.

Avoiding This Pitfall

Yearly follow-up visits for up to 3 years after surgery are warranted to ensure that atelectasis and eardrum retraction have not recurred. At the time that the consent for surgery is obtained, the risk of recurrence of eardrum retraction and possible future development of cholesteatoma should be discussed with the patient or parent of the patient. The need for regular follow-up appointments should be stressed. In addition, a letter should be sent to the referring physician at the conclusion of the postoperative period after the postoperative hearing test has been obtained. This letter should explain the appearance of the eardrum (which may have a visible white cartilage graft) and the reasons why repeat office examination will be needed at least once a year over the next 3 years. The patient should be referred back to the surgeon promptly if the patient complains of ear discomfort, worsening hearing, or discharge from the ear.

SUMMARY

In this chapter, the complex subject of management of the atelectatic ear has been discussed. The atelectatic ear is not a single, clearly defined disorder that develops as a result of inadequate eustachian tube function and inflammation, which also cause early childhood otitis media. When middle ear atelectasis has developed, eardrum retraction, atrophy, and adhesions of varying severity may also develop, and the ear is at risk for developing significant hearing loss and acquired cholesteatoma. The key to successful management of the atelectatic ear is careful observation over time, with early detection of changes that could signal that a cholesteatoma is beginning to develop. Deciding when to operate on the atelectatic ear and choosing which surgical procedure to perform is extremely difficult. In fact, despite published dogma and strong opinions expressed by experienced otologists, there probably is not one best method for management. Each case must be analyzed carefully, and decisions need to made on the basis of each patient s history, physical findings, and results of audiologic assessment. In making decisions, the otologist will often confront a situation that can best be described as the otologist s dilemma.

THE OTOLOGIST'S DILEMMA

There is no generally accepted correct time to recommend surgery in management of the atelectatic ear. This being the case, the otologist faces a dilemma. If the surgeon recommends a procedure such as cartilage-graft tympanoplasty early in the course when hearing is normal, but telltale changes in the eardrum suggest that a cholesteatoma is beginning to develop, the structural abnormalities in the eardrum are likely to be surgically corrected and the hearing after surgery is likely to remain normal. On the other hand, if the surgeon waits until later in the course, when ossicular erosion and conductive hearing loss have developed, the need for surgery is clearly apparent, and the patient or parent of the patient will be satisfied if the hearing in the involved ear returns to normal or near normal after tympanoplasty with ossicular reconstruction. Stated succinctly, when operation occurs early in the course of progressive eardrum retraction with incipient cholesteatoma, the surgeon is more at risk because the hearing is normal preoperatively. Conversely, waiting until later in the course, when the eardrum retraction has turned into a cholesteatoma sac and there is ossicular erosion, puts the patient at risk for loss of hearing and a need for more extensive surgery. In general, there is a tendency for otologic surgeons to wait until there is a clear indication, such as hearing loss, before recommending surgery. This approach is defensible, at least in the medicolegal sense. However, earlier intervention would be more beneficial if we could find some way to determine which atelectatic ears are most likely to develop hearing loss or cholesteatoma. Once we have that ability, the dilemma will be resolved.

REFERENCES

1. Sade J, Avraham S, Brown M. Dynamics of atelectasis and retraction pockets. In: Tos M, ed. *Cholesteatoma and mastoid surgery*. 2nd ed. Amsterdam: Kugler; 1982:267.
2. Akyildiz N, Akbay C, Ozgirgin ON, Bayramoglu I, Sayin N. The role of retraction pockets in cholesteatoma development: an ultrastructural study. *Ear Nose Throat J* 1993;72;210.
3. Tos M, Hvid G, Stangerup SE, Andreassen UK. Prevalence and progression of sequelae following secretory otitis. *Ann Otol Rhinol Laryngol* 1990;99 [Suppl 149]:13.
4. Tos M. Incidence, etiology and pathogenesis of cholesteatoma in children. *Adv Otorhinolaryngol* 1988;40:110.
5. Axelson A, Lewis C. The comparison of otoscopic findings and impedance measurements. *Scand Audiol* 1976;5:149.
6. Haapaniemi J, Suonpaa J, Virolainen E. Tympanic membrane changes in school-aged children. *Ear Nose Throat J* 1995;74:278.
7. Characon R, Barthez M, Lejeune JM. Spontaneous retraction pockets in chronic otitis media medical and surgical therapy. *Ear Nose Throat J* 1992;71:578.
8. Sade J. Atelectatic tympanic membrane: histological study. *Ann Otol Rhinol Laryngol* 1993;102:712.
9. Holmquist J, Lindeman P. Tympanometric studies in ears with cholesteatoma and retraction pockets. In: Tos M, ed. *Cholesteatoma and mastoid surgery*. 2nd ed. Amsterdam: Kugler; 1982:225.
10. Yoon TH, Schachern PA, Paparella MM, Aeppl DM. Pathology and pathogenesis of tympanic membrane retraction. *Am J Otolaryngol* 1990;11:10.
11. Grundfast KM, Smith RV. Otitis media, structural abnormalities of the eardrum, and cholesteatoma in children. Presented at Ninth Shambaugh/Shea Weekend of Otology. Chicago, Illinois, March 6, 1992.
12. Moller P. Tympanosclerosis of the eardrum in children. *Int J Pediatr Otolaryngol* 1984;7:247.
13. Paparella MM, Shumrick DA, Gluckman JL, Meyerhoff WL, eds. In: *Otolaryngology*. 3rd ed. Philadelphia: WB Saunders; 1991:1270.
14. Mills RP. Management of retraction pockets of the pars tensa. *J Laryngol Otology* 1991;105:525.
15. Tos M, Stangerup SE, Larsen P. Dynamics of eardrum changes following secretory otitis. *Arch Otolaryngol Head Neck Surg* 1987;113:380.
16. Tay HL, Mills RP. Tympanic membrane atelectasis in childhood otitis media with effusion. *J Laryngol Otology* 1995;109:495.
17. Tos M. Upon the relationship between secretory otitis in childhood and chronic otitis and its sequelae in adults. *J Laryngol Otology* 1981;95:1011.
18. Bluestone CD, Casselbrant ML, Cantekin EI. Functional obstruction of the eustachian tube in the pathogenesis of aural cholesteatoma in children. In: Tos M, ed. *Cholesteatoma and mastoid surgery*. 2nd ed. Amsterdam: Kugler; 1982:211.
19. Magnusun B. Eustachian tube pathophysiology. *Am J Otolaryngol* 1983;4:123.
20. Chole RA, Kodama K. Comparative histology of the tympanic membrane and its relationship to cholesteatoma. *Ann Otol Rhinol Laryngol* 1989;98:761.
21. Wolfman DE, Chole RA. Experimental retraction pocket cholesteatoma. *Ann Otol Rhinol Laryngol* 1986;95:639.
22. Steinbach E. Experimental studies on cholesteatoma formation. *Acta Otorhinolaryngol (Belg)* 1980;34:56.
23. Abramson M, Asarch RG, Litton WB. Experimental aural cholesteatoma causing bone resorption. *Ann Otol Rhinol Laryngol* 1975;84:425.
24. Lim DJ, Saunders WH. Acquired cholesteatoma. Light and electron microscopic observation. *Ann Otol Rhinol Laryngol* 1972;81:2.
25. Lim DJ. Tympanic membrane: electron microscopic observation. *Acta Otolaryngolol (Stockh)* 1968;66:181.
26. Paparella MM, Yoon TH, Schachern PA. Pathology and pathogenesis of retraction pockets and cholesteatoma. In: Tos M, Thomsen J, Peitersen E, eds. *Cholesteatoma and mastoid surgery*. 3rd ed. Amsterdam: Kugler; 1989:401.
27. Paparella MM, Schachern PA, Yoon TH, Abdelhammid MM, Sahni R, DaCosta SS. Otopathologic correlates of the continuum of otitis media. *Ann Otol Rhinol Laryngol* 1990;99:17.
28. Yellon RF, Doyle WJ, Whiteside TL, Diven WF, March AR, Fireman A. Cytokines, immunoglobulins and bacterial pathogens in middle ear effusions. *Arch Otolaryngol* 1995;121:865.
29. Ruah CB, Schachern PA, Paparella MM, Zelterman D. Mechanisms of retraction pocket formation in the pediatric tympanic membrane. *Arch Otolaryngol Head Neck Surg* 1992;118:1298.
30. Moller P, Dingsor G, Breck P, et al. Tympanic membrane changes and retraction pockets after secretory otitis media. In: Tos M, Thomsen J, Peitersen E, eds. *Cholesteatoma and mastoid surgery*. 3rd ed. Amsterdam: Kugler; 1989:351.
31. Tonndorf J, Khanna SM. Tympanic membrane vibrations in human cadaver ears studied by time averaged holigraphy. *J Acoust Soc Am* 1972;52(4pt 2):1221.
32. Ars B, deCraemer W. Tympanic membrane lamina propria and middle ear cholesteatoma. In: Tos M, Thomsen J, Peitersen E, eds. *Cholesteatoma and mastoid surgery*. 3rd ed. Amsterdam: Kugler; 1989:429.
33. Mayot D, Bene MC, Faure GC, Wayoff M, Perrin C. Immunohistologic analysis of the cholesteatoma matrix in children. *Int J Pediatr Otorhinolaryngol* 1991;22:115.
34. Wells MD, Michaels L. Role of retraction pockets in cholesteatoma formation. *Clin Otolaryngol* 1983;8:39.
35. Sade J, Berco E. Bone distruction I chronic otitis media. A histopathological study. *J Laryngol Otol* 1974;88:413.
36. Ahn JM, Huang CC, Abrahamson M. Interleukin 1 causing bone destruction in middle ear cholesteatoma. *Otolaryngol Head Neck Surg* 1990;103:528.
37. Fria TJ, Cantekin EI, Probst G. Validation of an automatic otoadmittance middle ear analyzer. *Ann Otol Rhinol Laryngol* 1980;89:200.
38. Bluestone CD, Klein JO. Otitis media and eustachian tube dysfunction. In: Bluestone CD, Stool SE, eds. *Pediatric Otolaryngology* 2nd ed. Philadelphia: WB Saunders, 1990:320.
39. Koltai PJ, Eames FA, Parnes SM, Wood GW, Bie B. Comparison of computed tomography and magnetic resonance imaging in chronic otitis media with cholesteatoma. *Arch Otolaryngol Head Neck Surg* 1989;115:1231.
40. Stangerup SE, Sederberg-Olsen J, Balle V. Autoinflation as a treatment of secretory otitis media. *Arch Otolaryngol Head Neck Surg* 1992;118:149.
41. Blanshard JD, Maw AR, Bawden R. Conservative treatment of otitis media with effusion by autoinflation of the middle ear. *Clin Otolaryngol* 1993;18:188.
42. Cantekin EI, Mandel EM, Bluestone CD, et al. Lack of efficacy of a decongestant-antihistamine combination for otitis media (secretory otitis media) in children. *N Engl J Med* 1983;308:297.
43. Rosenfeld RM, Mandel Em, Bluestone CD. Systemic steroids for otitis media with effusion in children. *Arch Otolaryngol Head Neck Surg* 1991;117:984.
44. Stangerup SE, Tos M. Do grommets affect hearing? In: Tos M, Thomsen J, Peitersen E, eds. *Cholesteatoma and mastoid surgery*. Amsterdam: Kugler; 1989:377.
45. Grundfast KM. Tympanostomy tubes. In: Pillsbury HC, Goldsmith MM, eds. *Operative challenges in otolaryngology—head and neck surgery*. St. Louis: Year Book Medical; 1990:1.
46. Weigel MT, Parker MY, Goldsmith MM, Postma DS, Pillsbury HC. A prospective randomized study of four commonly used tympanostomy tubes. *Laryngoscope* 1989;99:252.
47. Paparella MM, Jung TTK. Experience with tympanoplasty for atelectatic ears. *Laryngoscope* 1981;91:1472.
48. Stewart IA. Surgical treatment of retraction pockets. In: Tos M, Thomsen J, Peitersen E, eds. *Cholesteatoma and mastoid surgery*. 3rd ed. Amsterdam: Kugler; 1989:443.
49. Levinson RM. Cartilage-perichondrial composite graft tympanoplasty in the treatment of posterior, marginal and attic retraction pockets. *Laryngoscope* 1987;97:1069.
50. Harvey SA, Paparella MM, Sperling NM, Alleva M. The flexible (conservative surgical) approach for chronic otitis media in young children. *Laryngoscope* 1992;102:1399.
51. Avraham S, Luntz M, Sade J. The influence of ventilating tubes on the surgical treatment of atelectatic ears. *Eur Arch Otorhinolaryngol* 1991;248:259.
52. Jackler RK, Schindler RA. Myringoplasty with simple mastoidectomy: results in eighty-two consecutive patients. *Otolaryngol Head Neck Surg* 1983;91:14.

53. Luntz M, Avraham S, Sade J. The surgical treatment of atelectatic ears and retraction pockets in children and adults. *Eur Arch Otorhinolaryngol* 1991;248:400.
54. Schachern P, Paparella MM, Sano S, Lamey S, Guo Y. A histopathological study of the relationship between otitis media and mastoiditis. *Laryngoscope* 1991;101:1050.
55. Nakano Y, Sato Y. Prognosis of otitis media with effusion in children and size of the mastoid air cell system. *Acta Otolaryngol (Stockh)* 1990;471:56.
56. Sato Y, Nakano Y, Takahasi S. Suppressed mastoid pneumatization in cholesteatoma. *Acta Otolaryngol (Stockh)* 1990;471:62.
57. Ikarashi H, Nakano Y. The effect of chronic middle ear inflammation on the pneumatization of the tympanic bulla in pigs. *Arch Otolaryngol (Stockh)* 1987;104:130.
58. Avraham S, Luntz M, Sade J. The effect of mastoid surgery on atelectatic ears and retraction pockets. *Eur Arch Otorhinolaryngol* 1991;248:335.
59. Poe DS, Rebeiz EE, Pankeraton MS, Shapshay SM. Transtympanic endoscopy of the middle ear. *Laryngoscope* 1992;102:993.
60. Rosenberg SI, Silverstein H, Hoffer M, Nichols M. Use of endoscopes for chronic surgery in children. *Arch Otolaryngol Head Neck Surg* 1995;121:870.

CHAPTER 46

Intact Canal Wall Versus Canal Wall Down Mastoidectomy

Paul R. Lambert, Edward E. Dodson, and George T. Hashisaki

A consensus exists regarding the principal goals of cholesteatoma surgery in the pediatric age group: (a) disease eradication and (b) preservation or restoration of hearing. Controversy, however, characterizes many other facets of this disease process. For example, are there certain anatomic or physiologic parameters in the child that cause a cholesteatoma to be more aggressive than the same condition in the adult? Is the intact canal wall (ICW) mastoidectomy or canal wall down (CWD) mastoidectomy the preferred surgical approach for pediatric cholesteatomas? Why? Are there differences in pre- and postoperative complications in children and adults?

The controversy that has received the most attention in the literature concerns the optimal surgical treatment of cholesteatomas in children. The obvious conclusion that can be drawn from this body of data is that experienced surgeons strongly disagree and that they are not influenced by reports advocating a different operative approach. A number of factors contribute to this situation. Unquestionably, biases exist because of differences in surgical training and personal experience with cholesteatoma surgery in adults. Secondly, clinical studies presented in the literature are difficult to interpret because of their retrospective nature. For example, comparing one surgeon's experience with both ICW and CWD mastoidectomy is compromised because of inherent biases in patient selection. A prospective, randomized clinical trial would provide insight into surgical management. Such a study would be difficult to conduct, however, because of the variables of mastoid anatomy and extent of disease, and because there are specific settings in which an ICW or CWD approach is definitely indicated. In the final analysis, technical ability and judgment are more important than operative approach.

This chapter does not attempt resolution of the ICW versus CWD controversy. Pertinent literature is reviewed, however, and generalizations summarized. The principal goal is to outline surgical guidelines we have found helpful in treating more than 90 pediatric cholesteatomas during a 12-year period. The discussion is framed within the context of several important considerations unique to the pediatric patient, including disease biology, hearing restoration, and postoperative care.

BIOLOGY OF PEDIATRIC CHOLESTEATOMA

Most studies that have analyzed the incidence of residual and recurrent cholesteatoma have noted an increased rate in children compared with the rate for adults (1–6). The hypothesis that the biology of cholesteatomas in children is different—that is, more aggressive—has been proposed to explain these observations. It is probable that the fundamental disease process is similar in children and adults but that associated factors contribute to the more recalcitrant nature of pediatric cholesteatomas. For example, adults with cholesteatoma frequently have sclerotic temporal bones secondary to childhood infections, but children often have well-pneumatized temporal bones with deep air-cell tracks, which complicates complete disease removal. Also, poor eustachian tube function in children predisposes to otitis media and secondary infection of the cholesteatoma as well as to recurrence of retraction pockets. It is acknowledged, though, that the growth potential of tissues is greater in children than in adults and that various growth factors normally elaborated in childhood may cause a cholesteatoma to progress at an increased rate. Whatever the reason(s) for the behavior of pediatric cholesteatomas, it has been consistently observed

---

P.L. Lambert and G.T. Hashisaki: Division of Otology-Neurotology, Department of Otolaryngology—Head and Neck Surgery, University of Virginia Medical Center, Charlottesville, Virginia 22908.

E.E. Dodson: Department of Otolaryngology, The Ohio State University, Columbus, Ohio 43210.

that the incidence of preoperative intracranial and intratemporal complications is lower than that in adults and this fact may relate to the earlier detection and treatment of this disease in children.

GENERAL CONSIDERATIONS

Residual or Recurrent Cholesteatoma

Cholesteatoma may not be eradicated permanently following an initial surgery, regardless of whether an ICW or CWD technique is used. Both residual and recurrent disease recidivism are possible. Residual disease is defined as persistence of cholesteatoma following an incomplete removal. Occasionally, cholesteatoma is deliberately left on a labyrinthine fistula or the stapes to be removed at a planned, second-stage procedure when conditions (e.g., sterility) are more favorable. In most cases, though, incomplete disease removal is inadvertent, and the minute focus of residual squamous epithelium grows to form a "squamous pearl." As the name suggests, this residual focus of cholesteatoma is spherically shaped, and it usually has a less aggressive growth potential and pattern than did the original cholesteatoma. Recurrent cholesteatoma is a newly developed cholesteatoma secondary to a retraction pocket into the mesotympanum or the epitympanum or antrum. Canal wall defects, created by the original disease process or by the surgeon during removal of the initial cholesteatoma, predispose to retraction pockets. Recurrent cholesteatoma is primarily a concern with ICW mastoid surgery.

Advantages and Limitations

ICW and CWD mastoidectomy each have inherent limitations and advantages that involve ease of disease removal, incidence of recurrent or residual disease, and the extent of postoperative care. For cholesteatomas involving the middle ear, epitympanum, and mastoid, the canal wall partially obscures the disease. Maintaining the canal wall, therefore, necessitates more surgical manipulations (e.g., facial recess approach and alternately working on the canal and epitympanic sides of the canal wall) and usually more operative time, especially for removing disease in the epitympanum and around the stapes. Cholesteatoma that has extended into the sinus tympani and adjacent recesses may be difficult to remove, regardless of whether the canal wall is left intact or removed.

Because disease exposure is more difficult when the canal wall is left intact, the incidence of inadvertently leaving a focus of squamous epithelium is increased. Maintenance of the canal wall also predisposes to the possibility of formation of a retraction pocket. Thus, both residual and recurrent cholesteatoma are more common following ICW than CWD mastoidectomy. As a result, the decision to maintain the canal wall to ensure disease eradication may necessitate more surgical procedures than would a canal wall down technique.

Detection of residual disease postoperatively is easier with a CWD mastoidectomy. When the canal wall has been removed, only disease in the mesotympanum, hidden by the tympanic membrane, may be difficult to see. Although the epitympanum and mastoid cavity are covered by a membrane, the close approximation of this tissue layer to the underlying bone enables early detection of any cholesteatoma pearl in these areas. An exception to this condition are cases in which tissue flaps, bone paté, or both have been used to partially obliterate the mastoid cavity. With an intact canal wall, the mastoid and epitympanum are not accessible to postoperative inspection. Planned second-stage surgery mitigates this postoperative concern in ICW mastoid surgery.

The principal advantages of the ICW technique are more rapid healing postoperatively and, most important, the obviation of many long-term postoperative concerns. Epithelialization of the mastoid cavity in CWD cases may be a slow process (months) and certain areas may require special attention to promote healing. Once healing is complete, the mastoid bowl may require periodic cleaning because of irregular contours and the inability of desquamated epithelium to migrate effectively to the meatus. This condition predisposes to mastoid bowl infection (especially if water exposure has occurred). By contrast, healing of the ICW mastoidectomy is usually rapid, periodic ear cleanings are not necessary, the incidence of external ear infections is not increased, and no limitations of water activities are imposed. As one considers the lifestyle of the pediatric patient, these factors become quite significant. In addition, an ICW approach provides more options for a hearing aid (e.g., canal type), if required, and its use is usually more trouble free (e.g., fewer canal infections).

LITERATURE REVIEW

During the past decade, a number of publications have addressed the controversy of ICW versus CWD mastoidectomy for treatment of pediatric cholesteatoma (1–21). Because of the retrospective nature of these studies, biases in patient selection and surgeon preference (i.e., type of mastoidectomy, staging), and inconsistencies in reporting functional results, a consensus remains elusive, although several generalizations are apparent. First, the recidivism rate, combining the residual and recurrent cholesteatoma rates, was worse for the cumulative ICW cases, 42%, compared with the rate for the cumulative CWD cases, 22%. In some reports, the residual rate includes cholesteatoma intentionally left to be removed at a second stage (7,8). More important, the data demonstrate significant recidivism rates in children as follow-up time lengthens. The average recidivism rate was 30%, ranging from 7% to 57%. Regardless of mastoidectomy technique, the failure rate is significant.

Many authors believe that cholesteatomas in children behave in a more aggressive manner than in adults (5,8–14). This opinion was generally based on the frequent finding in as much as 70% of cases of ossicular erosion at the initial surgery (9,12,14). Also, mastoid air-cell development was frequently normal and is believed to be conducive to insinuation of cholesteatoma projections. On the other hand, several authors note that preoperative complications of cholesteatoma and chronic otitis media were infrequent in their patients. Only Cruz et al. reported a significant number of preoperative intra- and extratemporal complications (11). The lack of complications from cholesteatoma was attributed to a shorter duration of disease in children before presentation and treatment, rather than to a less aggressive nature. Sanna, et al believe that cholesteatomas in children behave as they do in adults, with no differences in aggressiveness of growth (15).

Hearing results were published in such different terms that analysis is inconclusive. Results were reported variously as coming from tests of preoperative speech receeption thresholds (SRT), pure-tone averages (PTA), or air–bone gap; postoperative SRT, PTA, or air–bone gap; and improved, no change, or worsened SRT, PTA, or air–bone gap. Results were stratified differently in each study, with descriptors such as stapes intact, crura absent, ossicular reconstruction, no ossicular reconstruction, canal wall intact, canal wall down, tympanoplasty performed, and tympanoplasty not performed. For studies providing sufficient stratification, the functional status of the ossicular chain seemed to be a better predictor of hearing outcome than did type of mastoidectomy. When ossicular reconstruction was performed, an intact stapes afforded much better hearing results than having only a mobile footplate (6–10). A summary of studies is presented in Table 1.

DATA ANALYSIS

A review of the otologic database at the University of Virginia revealed 71 pediatric patients who underwent surgery by Lambert for cholesteatoma between January 1984 and December 1994. The patient group ranged in age from 10 months to 18 years, with a mean age of 10.4 years (median, 10 years). There were 33 girls and 38 boys. Eight patients had bilateral disease requiring surgery; therefore, the total number of operated ears was 79. The mean follow-up was 36.9 months (range, 1.3 mo–11 yr).

The ICW mastoidectomy with tympanoplasty was used in 43 ears as the initial operative procedure. In three of these patients the ossicular chain was reconstructed primarily, and in the remaining 40 patients a planned second-stage was used to reinspect the middle ear and mastoid and reconstruct the ossicular chain. Six ears required more than two procedures for complete eradication of cholesteatoma, and four of these patients were eventually converted to CWD cases. Three other ears that were converted to CWD cases, required only two surgeries for complete removal of disease. Thus, of the original 43 ICW procedures, 16% eventually required conversion to a CWD. Residual cholesteatoma was found in eight patients (19%) at the time of the planned second stage, but only one patient required a third procedure. In addition, two ears (5%) were successfully managed by purposely leaving a small remnant of cholesteatoma around the footplate at the time of the first procedure, removing it at the planned second-stage surgery. Recurrent cholesteatoma occurred in ten ears (23%). Included in this group were the seven patients subsequently converted to a CWD.

Nineteen patients underwent CWD mastoidectomy with

TABLE 1. *Results of surgery for cholesteatoma, by technique*

Study (date)	n	ICW	CWD	ICW res/rec	CWD res/rec	Recidivism rate (%)	Preferred technique	Follow-up time
Charachon (1987)	141	99	37	38/7	12/2	42	ICW	3.0 yr (min)
Sanna (1987)	124	114	4	37/2	10/1	40	ICW	15 mo (min)
Wetmore (1987)	142	66	8	48 total		32	—	short
Edelstein (1988)	125	39	66	14 total		11	—	3.9 yr (avg)
Cruz (1990)	101	26	75	0/12	0/10	22	CWD	2.0 yr (min)
Schuring (1990)	88	88	0	17/18	—	28	ICW	7.1 yr (avg)
Crellin (1991)	67	5	60	4/0	0/18	33	—	18 mo (min)
Marco-Algarra (1991)	55	40	15	15/2	0/0	31	ICW	7.1 yr (avg)
Mills (1991)	54	3	27	1/0	3/0	7	CWD	50 mo (avg)
Rigner (1991)	19	10	9	7 total		37	CWD	4.0 yr (min)
Schloss (1991)	71	11	48	28 total		39	CWD	—
Schmid (1991)	57	17	40	4/3	3/2	21	—	7.0 yr (avg)
Rosenfeld (1991)	232	46	53	—	—	57	—	2.5 yr (avg)
Stern (1992)	53	19	21	10/0	0/1	21	—	29 mo (avg)
Vartiainen (1992)	50	9	35	2/0	0/6	15	CWD	7.1 yr (avg)
Brackmann (1993)	35	26	9	11 total		31	ICW	4.0 yr (avg)
Mutlu (1995)	73	73	0	27/8	—	48	ICW	4.0 yr (avg)
Total	1,487	691	507			30		
Available ICW res/rec		493		155/52		42		
Available CWD res/rec			314		29/39	22		

CWD, canal wall down; ICW, intact canal wall; rec, recurrent cholesteatoma; res, residual cholesteatoma.

TABLE 2. *Change in hearing level, by technique*

		Intact canal wall		Canal wall down		Middle ear surgery only		
Test	Hearing level (dB)	Intact stapes (n = 11) (%)	Footplate only (n = 15) (%)	Intact stapes (n = 4) (%)	Footplate only (n = 8) (%)	Intact ossicular chain (n = 6) (%)	Intact stapes (n = 2) (%)	Footplate only (n = 2) (%)
Postoperative SRT	≤25	9 (82)	8 (53)	3 (75)	5 (62.5)	6 (100)	2 (100)	0
	26–50	2 (18)	6 (40)	1 (25)	3 (37.5)	0	0	2 (100)
	>50	0	1 (7)	0	0	0	0	0
Postoperative ABG	≤20	7 (64)	8 (53)	2 (50)	2 (25)	5 (83)	2 (100)	0
	21–30	3 (27)	2 (13)	1 (25)	5 (62.5)	1 (17)	0	1 (50)
	>30	1 (9)	5 (33)	1 (25)	1 (12.5)	0	0	1 (50)

ABG, air–borne gap; SRT, speech reception threshold.

tympanoplasty as their first surgery. This decision was made at the time of surgery, primarily on the basis of the size of the mastoid cavity and anatomic relationships of the tegmen mastoideum and sigmoid sinus. In two ears there was extensive erosion of the posterior-superior canal wall, thus precluding the use of the ICW technique. Horizontal semicircular canal fistula and contralateral deafness were not present to serve as indications for CWD mastoidectomy in this patient group. As with the ICW procedure, staging was common, with only two ears reconstructed primarily. There were no cases of recurrent cholesteatoma, and only two patients had unsuspected residual cholesteatoma found at second-stage surgery. Only one patient in the CWD group required a third procedure for complete eradication of disease.

In a third group of 17 ears, no mastoidectomy was required, because cholesteatoma was limited to the mesotympanum. Ears treated with a middle-ear approach only were less often staged (5 cases), and only one patient suffered a recurrent tympanic membrane retraction with cholesteatoma formation. No more than two procedures were necessary for any ear treated with this technique, and no cases of residual cholesteatoma were identified.

Hearing data was available on 48 patients and is shown in Table 2. The data were subdivided according to status of the ossicular chain. Postoperative SRT and air–bone gap were analyzed. In 17 ears (35%), reconstruction of the ossicular chain to an intact stapes was possible, and in 25 ears (52%), only a mobile footplate was present. The ossicular chain remained intact in six ears (13%). Revision ossiculoplasty was required on five ears in the ICW group, one ear in the CWD group, and one ear in the middle-ear surgery group.

When compared to preoperative hearing levels, the postoperative SRT improved 15 dB or more in 38% of ICW ears, remained unchanged in 52%, and worsened in only 10%. In CWD ears, the postoperative SRT improved 15 dB or more in 70% of ears when compared to preoperative hearing levels and remained unchanged in 30%. The middle-ear surgery group showed an improvement in postoperative SRT of 15 dB or more in 50% of ears, and no change in 50%, when compared to preoperative hearing levels. In three patients (6%) a decrease of 10 to 20 dB occurred in the high-frequency bone conduction hearing level. Otherwise, sensorineural hearing levels remained unchanged.

In summary, 43 (69%) pediatric cholesteatoma cases requiring mastoidectomy were managed with the ICW technique. Thirty-six (84%) of the ICW patients are free of disease without a mastoid cavity (mean follow-up, 39 mo), although two of the patients required more than two procedures to achieve this result. Nineteen (31%) cases were initially treated with the CWD technique, and of these, only one patient required more than two procedures for eradication of disease (mean follow-up, 43 mo).

Case History

A 10 year-old-boy was referred for evaluation of chronic otitis media. During the past several years there had been no ear infections although his history was significant for three sets of ventilation tubes and numerous courses of antibiotics. On physical examination, the right tympanic membrane was mildly atelectatic. On the left side, there was severe atelectasis of the tympanic membrane but no drainage or accumulation of debris. An audiogram showed normal hearing in the right ear but an SRT of 15 dB in the left ear with a 20 dB conductive hearing loss in the lower frequencies. Close follow-up was recommended.

Two years later, the child was seen with a 3-month history of intermittent left otorrhea. In the left ear, there was squamous debris coming from the posterior mesotympanum. An audiogram again showed normal hearing in the right ear but increased conductive hearing loss in the left ear (Fig. 1).

Surgery was recommended and an intact canal wall mastoidectomy with tympanoplasty was performed. The surgical findings included extensive cholesteatoma of the middle-ear space extending into the hypotympanum and posteriorly into a deep sinus tympani. The long process of the incus and the superstructure of the stapes were absent. Because of the uncertainty of complete cholesteatoma removal, silastic

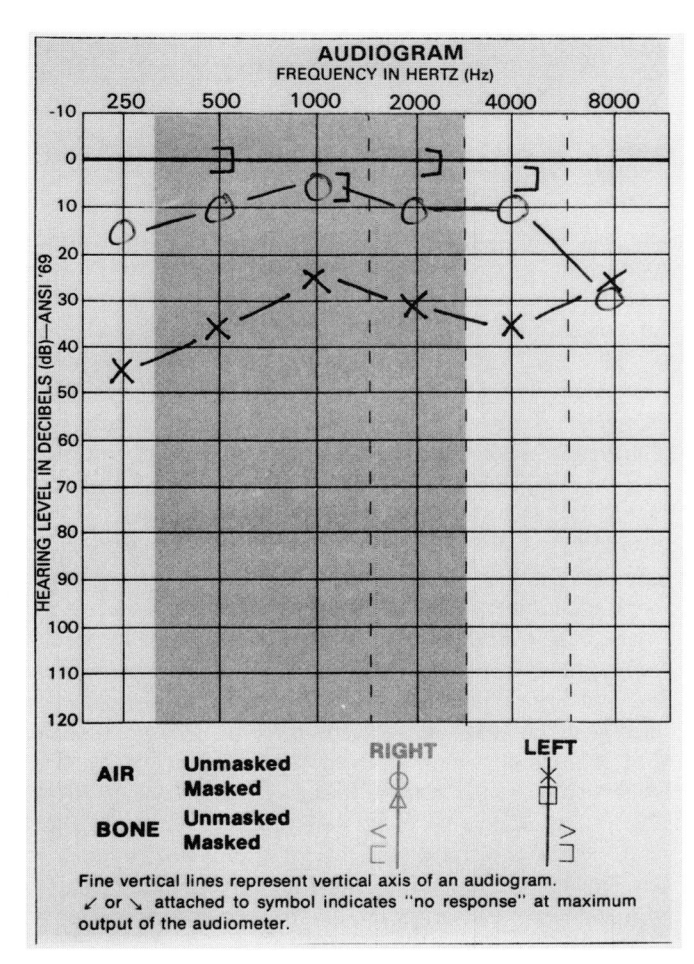

FIG. 1. Audiogram showing normal hearing in the right hear but conductive hearing loss in the left ear.

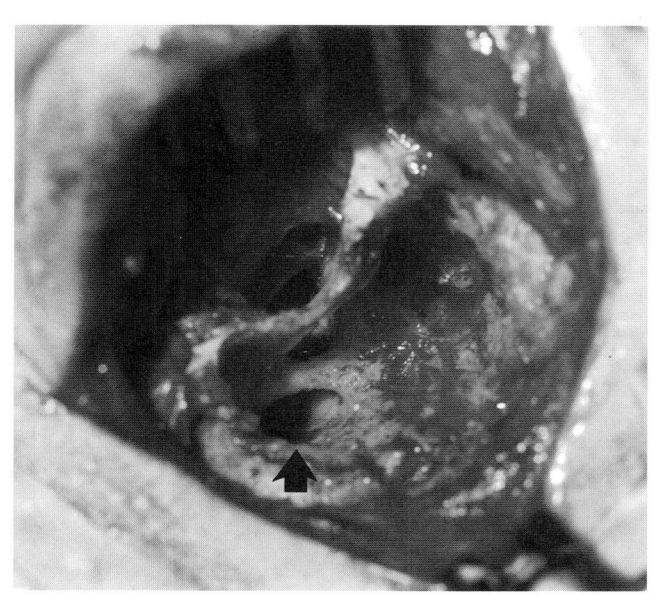

FIG. 2. Intraoperative photograph showing a wide opening into retrofacial aircell tract (*arrow*). This tract communicated with sinus tympani and was filled with cholesteatoma. Note skeletonization of facial nerve.

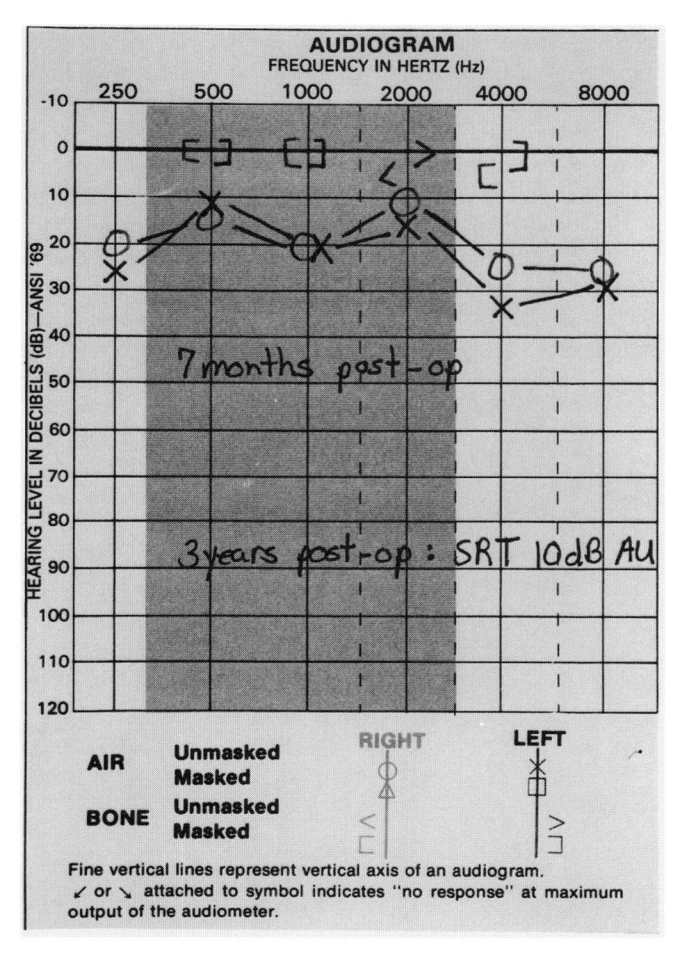

FIG. 3. Follow-up audiogram after ossicular reconstruction, showing improvement in left ear conductive hearing loss.

sheeting was placed in the middle ear and a second stage planned.

At the second-stage procedure 10 months later, residual cholesteatoma in the sinus tympani was encountered. Granulation tissue was noted in the retrofacial air cells of the mastoid and, on opening this area with the drill, the back of the sinus tympani cholesteatoma sac was encountered. With this exposure, all cholesteatoma was confidently removed from the posterior recesses and ossicular reconstruction was accomplished with a total ossicular replacement prosthesis (TORP) (Fig. 2). A 7-month postoperative audiogram showed improvement in the conductive deficit (Fig. 3). The patient has been periodically followed, and an audiogram 5 years after surgery showed an SRT of 15 dB in the left ear.

This case illustrates the difficulty of removing cholesteatoma from the deep posterior recesses of the middle ear. A second-look procedure is always recommended in this circumstance. Although it is uncommon for the disease to extend into the retrofacial air cells of the mastoid, this possibility should be considered when the depths of the sinus tympani cannot be probed.

SURGICAL PHILOSOPHY

Pediatric cholesteatomas are approached with the intent of performing an ICW procedure. A CWD technique, however, may be preferable in certain preoperative settings or if specific intraoperative findings are encountered. Preoperative concerns that would dictate a CWD procedure include operating on the only ear that has hearing, a child who is a poor anesthetic risk, or a child in whom follow-up is problematic. In these circumstances, it is desirable to eradicate disease and preserve or restore function in a single operation. Because the CWD approach has a lower incidence of recurrent and residual disease, it is preferred.

In most cases, the decision to remove the canal wall is made intraoperatively, on the basis of mastoid anatomy or specific disease findings. For example, a low-lying middle cranial fossa dura and an anteriorly positioned sigmoid sinus create a small mastoid and limit access into the anterior epitympanum. Maintaining the canal wall in this circumstance can complicate disease removal. Furthermore, if proper attention is given to creating the mastoid cavity (e.g., saucerization, lowering the facial ridge), the resulting cavity is likely to be trouble free.

The finding of a fistula into the horizontal semicircular canal may also necessitate removal of the canal wall. Depending on the extent of bone erosion over the semicircular canal, it may be prudent to maintain the cholesteatoma matrix over the fistula. In this circumstance, the canal wall must be removed, and the cholesteatoma over the labyrinth becomes part of the epithelial coverage of the mastoid cavity. This decision-making philosophy is summarized in Fig. 4.

Extensive erosion of the scutum by cholesteatoma predisposes to recurrent disease. Options for addressing this problem include removal of the canal wall or reconstruction of the canal wall by cartilage or bone. Our approach is to use autologous cartilage to repair the defect if the mastoid is large but to remove the canal wall if the cavity is small. The intraoperative considerations that dictate canal wall removal do not include extent or size of the cholesteatoma per se.

Mesotympanic Cholesteatoma

In the majority of cases, the most difficult aspect of cholesteatoma surgery is removal of disease from the mesotympanum. Occasionally, a cholesteatoma in a child is limited to the middle ear. Included in this group are the majority of congenital cholesteatomas, which tend to be circumscribed, thus facilitating their complete removal. Extensive involvement of the mesotympanum by a cholesteatoma may, however, occur with acquired cholesteatomas and also with some congenital cholesteatomas. Those that deeply infiltrate the posterior recesses, especially the sinus tympani, or envelop an intact stapes present a special challenge.

The size and depth of extension, both posterior and inferior, are the most variable features of the sinus tympani. In some cases, the sinus is little more than an indentation medial to the bone overlying the fallopian canal, and the cholesteatoma can be easily removed. Conversely, the sinus tympani may be large, extending deep and posterior to the posterior canal wall and mastoid segment of the facial nerve (Fig. 5). In this situation, access to the posterior aspects of the sinus is difficult. As the patient's head is rotated posteriorly to allow the surgeon to see into the recess, the anterior canal wall begins to obstruct the line of sight. In an attempt to circumvent this limitation, Goodhill advocated a change in the position of the surgeon so that the microscope is directed anteriorly to posteriorly (22). Visualization with repositioning of the microscope, however, is still limited by the height of the external auditory canal anteriorly, and this approach can be disruptive to the sterile surgical field. Performing a CWD mastoidectomy also affords only modest benefits, because the overlying facial canal continues to limit access into the sinus tympani. Therefore, our preference is to main-

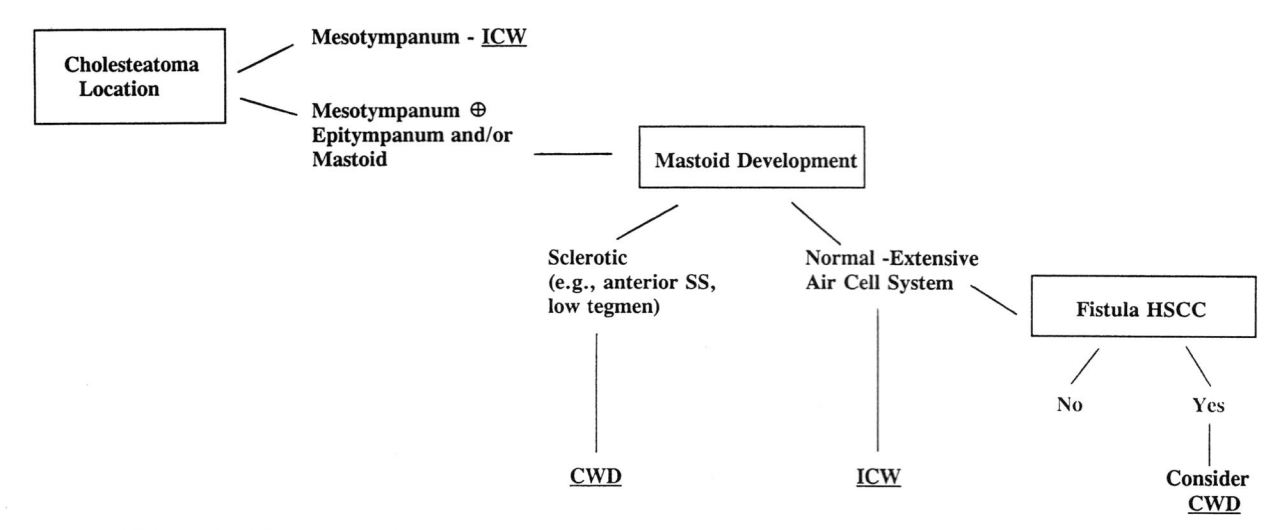

FIG. 4. Decision tree for ICW versus CWD mastoidectomy. *SS*, sigmoid sinus; *HSCC*, horizontal semicircular canal.

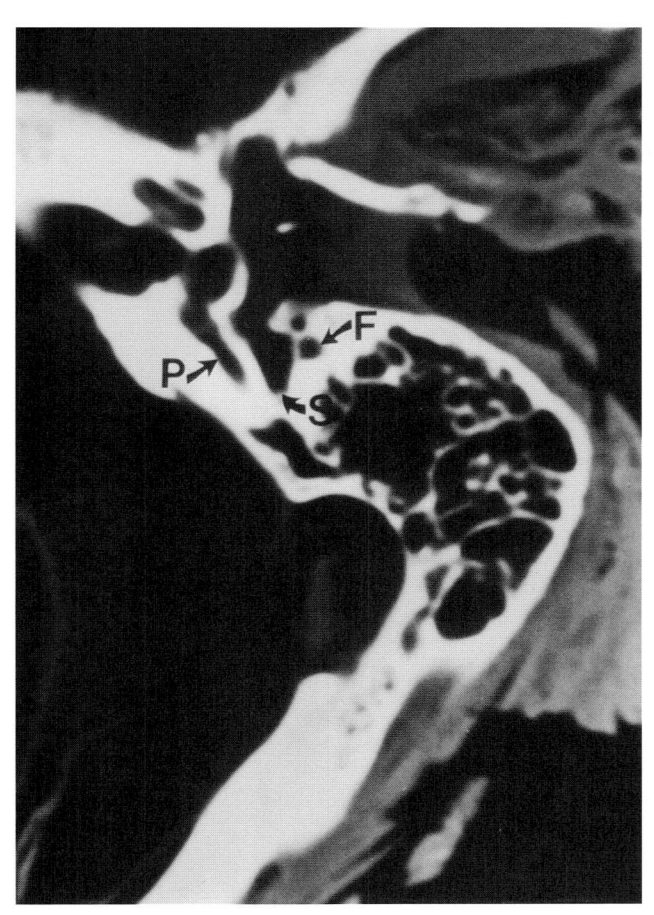

FIG. 5. Large sinus tympani extending deep and posterior to the canal wall and mastoid segment of the facial nerve. F, facial nerve; P, posterior semicircular canal; S, sinus tympani.

tain the canal wall intact, regardless of the extent of middle ear disease. Techniques to improve exposure include drilling away the posterior annulus and skeletonizing the anterior aspect of the mastoid segment of the facial nerve. Even with removal of the lateral lip of the opening into the sinus tympani, however, blind instrumentation is still required to eradicate cholesteatoma if the sinus is extensive. Rigid telescopes are advised for inspecting the posterior recesses after removal of cholesteatoma is considered complete. A second-look procedure 6 to 12 months later is always recommended, and the use of telescopes again facilitates thorough inspection for residual disease. In selected cases, it may be possible to expose the posterior recesses of a well-developed sinus tympani through a retrofacial approach (as discussed in the case report) (23). This approach can be utilized in both ICW and CWD mastoidectomies. Although some have suggested that a well-pneumatized sinus tympani is uncommon in patients with chronic ear disease, embryologic studies predict no correlation. Those studies showed that the adult size and configuration of the sinus tympani is obtained at birth, at a time when chronic ear disease does not exist (24,25). The bone that surrounds these sinuses, lying medial to the facial nerve, is dense and of Reichert's cartilage origin. This bone does not grow or remodel. Therefore, it is likely that variation in size and posterior extension of the sinus tympani is a result of developmental processes, not pathologic processes.

RESTORATION OF HEARING

As noted in the literature review section, neither a CWD nor an ICW approach has much impact on hearing results following middle-ear reconstruction. Our data support that contention. Instead, success depends primarily on middle-ear parameters such as mucosal status, (e.g., presence or absence of adhesions), condition of the tympanic membrane (e.g., thickness, contour), depth of the middle ear cleft, and the presence or absence of the stapes superstructure. To a large extent, these variables depend on eustachian tube function. As noted elsewhere in this book, however, the ability to quantify eustachian tube function in humans or predict eustachian tube function after tympanoplasty remains elusive. Success in hearing restoration is also directly related to the variables of ossicular chain reconstruction: the appropriate selection of an implant (autograft, homograft, or allograft), precision of its placement, and its long-term stability. These parameters mainly depend on the surgeon.

Staging

Although the ability to affect eustachian tube function is limited, we believe that placement of silastic sheeting (0.04 inch thick) in the middle-ear space and delaying the ossicular chain reconstruction for 6 to 12 months optimizes the chance for achieving a good functional result for many patients. The healing process of a middle ear with active infection, granulation tissue, or areas of absent mucosa is variable. Formation of adhesions between the medial wall of the mesotympanum and the tympanic membrane or the ossicular implant can promote tympanic membrane retraction, implant displacement, or both. We recommend staging, therefore, for all ears with abnormal or absent middle ear mucosa or in ears in which residual cholesteatoma is a concern (Fig. 6). If the canal wall has been removed, the silastic sheeting covers the entire mesotympanum, extending superiorly to the horizontal segment of the facial nerve and posteriorly to the facial ridge. In the ICW approach, the silastic extends into the epitympanum and through the facial recess into the mastoid cavity.

CONCLUSION

Eradication of cholesteatoma and restoration of hearing function in the pediatric age group present unique surgical challenges. Given the incidence of recidivism and the degree of ossicular damage found in pediatric cholesteatomas, it is evident that this disease exhibits a more aggressive behavior than its counterpart in the adult. It is, therefore, important for the surgeon to counsel the parents regarding the probable

```
                    Disease Removal
                   /              \
            Uncertain          Complete ────────── ME Mucosal Status
      (e.g., stapes/OW,                             /            \
       posterior recesses ME)                    Good            Poor
              |                                    |        (e.g., granulation tissue,
            Stage                                  |              bare bone)
      (silastic sheeting,                    Single Stage              |
         delay OCR)                              OCR                 Stage
                                                               (silastic sheeting,
                                                                  delay OCR)
```

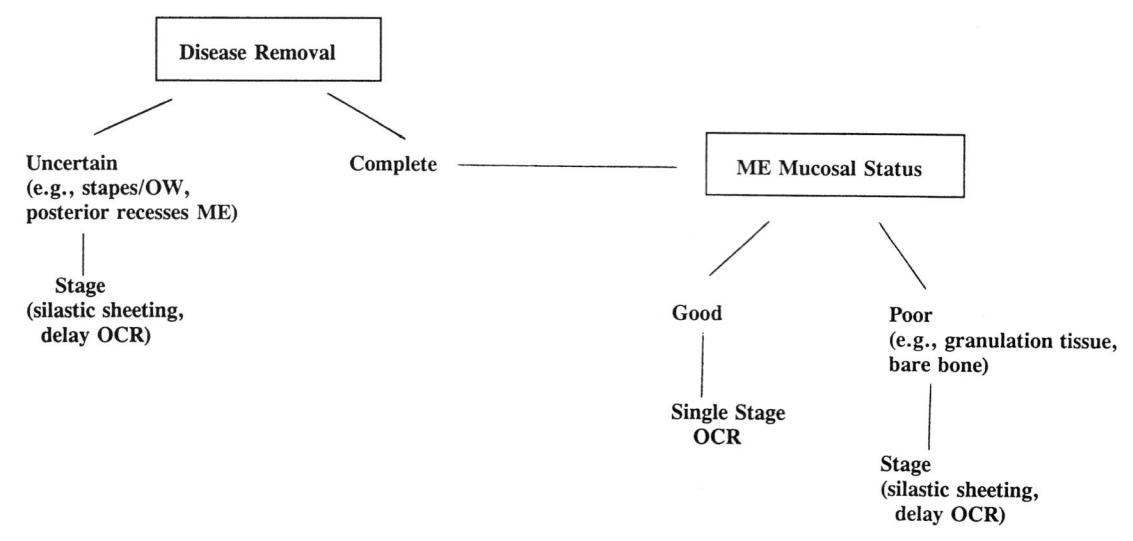

FIG. 6. Decision tree for staging tympanoplasty with an ICW or CWD mastoidectomy. *OW*, oval window; *ME*, middle ear; *OCR*, ossicular chain reconstruction.

need for multiple surgeries, especially if an ICW mastoidectomy is performed. Fortunately, intratemporal and intracranial complications, such as inner ear fistula, facial nerve paralysis, and epidural or intracerebral abscess, are rare in children.

The literature supports the use of either ICW or CWD techniques. The ICW mastoidectomy is our preferred approach, simply because a lifelong concern for water restriction is avoided. Even with this philosophy, however, 30% of our patients were initially treated with a CWD approach because of anatomic factors. In children who have an ICW procedure, more than 80% are free of disease without having to undergo subsequent removal of the canal wall. Although almost 15% of these patients have required more than two surgeries for complete disease eradication, we believe that the extra morbidity and cost, amortized over decades, are acceptable.

Optimal outcomes for pediatric cholesteatomas will result from surgeons with seasoned judgment, sound technical skills, and the ability to utilize multiple operative strategies (ICW vs. CWD; staging vs. single operation; allografts vs. autografts), depending on their patients' anatomic, pathologic, and socioeconomic conditions.

REFERENCES

1. Sheehy JL. Cholesteatoma surgery in children. *Am J Otol* 1985;6:170–172.
2. Glasscock ME, Dickens JRE, Wiet R. Cholesteatoma in children. *Laryngoscope* 1981;91:1743–1753.
3. Sanna M, Zini C, Scandellari R, Jemmi G. Residual and recurrent cholesteatoma in closed tympanoplasty. *Am J Otol* 1984;5:277–282.
4. Kinney SE. Intact canal wall tympanoplasty with mastoidectomy for cholesteatoma: Long-term follow up. *Laryngoscope* 1988;98:1190–1194.
5. Schuring AG, Lippy WH, Rizer FM, Schuring LT. Staging for cholesteatoma in the child, adolescent, and adult. *Ann Otol Rhinol Laryngol* 1990;99:256–260.
6. Brackmann DE. Tympanoplasty with mastoidectomy: canal wall up procedures. *Am J Otol* 1993;14:380–382.
7. Mutlu C, Khashaba A, Saleh E, et al. Surgical treatment of cholesteatoma in children. *Otolaryngol Head Neck Surg* 1995;113(1):56–60.
8. Vartiainen E, Nuutinen J. Long-term results of surgery for childhood cholesteatoma. *Int J Pediatr Otorhinolaryngol* 1992;24:201–208.
9. Charachon R, Gratacap B. The surgical treatment of cholesteatoma in children. *Clin Otolaryngol* 1985;10:177–184.
10. Edelstein DR, Parisier SC, Ahuja GS, et al. Cholesteatoma in the pediatric age group. *Ann Otol Rhinol Laryngol* 1988;97:23–29.
11. Cruz OLM, Takeuti M, Neto SC, Miniti A. Clinical and surgical aspects of cholesteatomas in children. *Ear Nose Throat J* 1990;69:530–536.
12. Marco-Algarra J, Gimenez F, Mallea I, Armengot M, De La Fuente L. Cholesteatoma in children: results in open versus closed techniques. *J Laryngol Otol* 1991;105:820–824.
13. Mills RP, Padgham ND. Management of childhood cholesteatoma. *J Laryngol Otol* 1991;105(5):343–345.
14. Rosenfeld RM, Moura RL, Bluestone CD. Predictors of residual-recurrent cholesteatoma in children. *Arch Otolaryngol Head Neck Surg* 1992;118:384–391.
15. Sanna M, Zini C, Gamoletti R, et al. The surgical management of childhood cholesteatoma. *J Laryngol Otol* 1987;101:1221–1226.
16. Crellin RP, Wilson JA, Cowan DL. Mastoid surgery in childhood. *Clin Otolaryngol* 1991;16:39–42.
17. Rignér P, Renvall U, Tjellström A. Late results after cholesteatoma surgery in early childhood. *Int J Pediatr Otorhinolaryngol* 1991;22:213–218.
18. Schloss MD, Terraza O. Cholesteatoma in children. *J Otolaryngol* 1991;20:43–45.
19. Schmid H, Dort JC, Fisch U. Long-term results of treatment for children's cholesteatoma. *Am J Otol* 1991;12:83–87.
20. Stern SJ, Fazekas-May M. Cholesteatoma in the pediatric population: prognostic indicators for surgical decision making. *Laryngoscope* 1992;102:1349–1352.
21. Wetmore RF, Konkle DF, Potsic WP, Handler SD. Cholesteatoma in the pediatric patient. *Int J Pediatr Otorhinolaryngol* 1987;14:101–112.
22. Goodhill V. Circumferential tympanomastoid access: the sinus tympani area. *Ann Otol Rhinol Laryngol* 1973;82:547–554.
23. Pickett BP, Cail WS, Lambert PR. Sinus tympani. anatomic considerations, computed tomography, and a discussion of the retrofacial approach for removal of disease. *Am J Otol* 1995;16:741–750.
24. Saito R, Igarashi M, Alford BR, Guilford FR. Anatomical measurement of the sinus tympani. *Arch Otolaryngol Head Neck Surg* 1971;94:418–425.
25. Bast TH, Anson BJ, Richany SF. The development of the second branchial arch (Reichert's cartilage), facial canal, and associated structures in man. *Q Bull Northw U Med School* 1956;30:235–250.

PART XV

The Deaf Child

CHAPTER 47

Early Intervention

Janice C. Gatty

One in 1,000 children is born deaf. Ninety percent of deaf children have parents who hear normally and have had little or no personal experience with deafness. The intimacy of the relationship they will have with their child is at risk. Intellectual and language capacities are normally distributed in this population of children. Hearing loss puts the acquisition of knowledge and language at great risk.

There is no medical cure for deafness at this time. Although advances in technology, medicine, and surgery have improved the treatment of hearing impairments, deafness remains primarily a developmental and educational issue. Intervention cannot begin until hearing impairment is identified and diagnosed. The sooner it begins, the greater the potential benefits for the development of the child and the family. Pediatricians and otolaryngologists are in a fine position to direct parents toward sources of evaluation and early intervention. The purpose of this chapter is to discuss (a) the reasons for early intervention, (b) the goals of an early intervention program, (c) the issues surrounding early identification, (d) the philosophies and approaches to early intervention, (e) the components of a program of early intervention, (f) resources for early intervention, and (g) evidence that early intervention is effective.

RATIONALE

Without intervention, hearing impairment can lead to delays in perceptual, cognitive, language, social, and emotional development. Without skills in these areas, children have little access to the educational system and ultimately have few vocational choices. The instinctive reactions of hearing parents are counterproductive. *Intervention* refers to any modifications in the child's environment that serve to reduce the potential limitations deafness imposes on the developmental process. It includes direct services provided to the child and counseling and educational services provided to parents. The goal of intervention is to ensure that development and quality of life is the best that it can be for the child and the family; it is *not* to create the child or family as they would have been if deafness were not a part of their lives.

ISSUES SURROUNDING EARLY IDENTIFICATION

Early intervention requires early identification and diagnosis of hearing loss. Hearing can be measured objectively and reliably soon after birth, and yet some children, even though their parents have voiced concerns about hearing status, are not seen for their first hearing test until they are 2 years of age (1). Reports from parents to primary care physicians should always be followed with a referral for a hearing test. Examples of parent reports are as follows:

1. Delayed auditory responses: "I was vacuuming under her crib during her nap, and she didn't wake up."
2. Capricious behavior: "Although she's a very alert baby, she always seems 'surprised' to see me when I walk in her room."
3. Inattention to voice: "I can't seem to calm him with my voice when he's upset."
4. Delays in receptive language development: "He seems to hear my voice, but he doesn't answer to his name or understand any simple directions."
5. Delays in expressive language development: "He's not talking."

Reports such as these should always be followed with a referral for a hearing test. The observant physician will note that high levels of motor activity, prolonged visual attention to the face, or visual scanning can also be subtle signs of an undiagnosed hearing-impaired child's adaptation to his or her environment.

In summary, to ensure that hearing loss is diagnosed early so that intervention can begin the physician should:

J.C. Gatty: Education and Child Study, Smith College, Northampton, Massachusetts 01060.

1. Listen to parents when they express concerns about their child's hearing or describe behaviors that may be indicative of hearing loss.

2. *Refer* the child for a hearing test at center which specializes in testing children.

PHILOSOPHIES AND APPROACHES TO EARLY INTERVENTION

Models of Intervention

Models of intervention vary across the United States, depending on the social and political milieu of a particular demographic area. There are three fundamental models of early intervention: (a) the medical model, (b) the cultural model, and (c) the educational model (Fig. 1). These models differ primarily in terms of their perspective of and outcome criteria for the hearing-impaired child who lives in a world where most people hear.

The goal of the medical model is to make deaf children hear. A deaf child in this model is viewed as a hearing and speech problem. Rectifying these secondary issues essentially eliminates the deafness as a problem for the child and family. Children are fit with hearing aids, stimulated auditorily, and receive speech and language therapy, usually in a clinical or hospital setting. Parents are taught to teach their children "to listen" and "to hear." Measures of success are based on the child's performance in the area of spoken language. The criterion for success is how closely spoken language approximates that of normally hearing children.

The strength of the medical model is that it narrows the issue of hearing impairment so that it seems manageable for hearing parents. The therapy is usually adult-directed, controlled, and highly structured so that parents view their child as succeeding and achieving in sessions with the therapist. This approach is effective for children who have sufficient residual hearing to acquire spoken language primarily through the sense of hearing.

The limitations of the medical model are that it does not address those areas of development affected by auditory deprivation and language delay, such as cognitive, social, and emotional development, which are equally important in the development of the child. The therapeutic nature of instructional sessions does not make carryover in the home obvious to parents, increasing the likelihood of their dependence on the therapist. In reality, the parents' role extends far beyond that of a therapist or teacher. Their role is to provide the child with an environment at home that is rich in experience and language and supportive in terms of emotional development, with opportunities for social interaction. Parents need information about deafness, choices, and support in decision making in order to feel confident about their ability to parent their child.

The goal of the cultural model is to make the child's world deaf. The deaf child is immersed in a world of deaf people where the sense of hearing has little or no value and communication relies only on the sense of vision. Parents learn to communicate in American Sign Language (ASL), and that becomes the primary language of the home. Use of voice is discouraged. Measures of success are based on the child's ability to communicate effectively in ASL. Success also is measured by how closely performance in the area of cognitive, social, and emotional development approximates that of normally hearing children of the same age.

The strength of the cultural model is that it provides the child with an environment that gives great value to the very aspect of development that makes the child different from most other children. It is more likely that children will feel connected to and part of a culture that is fully accessible to them. In addition, this model does not require deaf children to adapt in ways that are difficult and sometimes impossible in terms of their auditory capacities. The focus of the model is on the developmental strengths of the child rather than on the shortcomings. This approach is very effective for chilren who have deaf parents who are native ASL communicators and who have access to an extended community of deaf people.

The limitation of the cultural model is that most deaf children (90%) have hearing parents, who have little knowledge

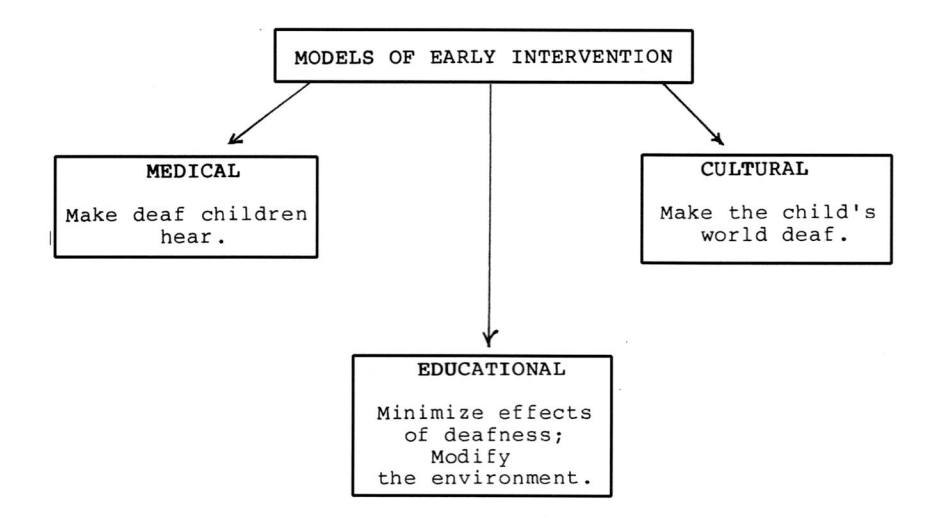

FIG. 1. Models of early intervention.

```
          EDUCATIONAL MODEL of EARLY INTERVENTION
                    │                │
              ┌─────┴─────┐    ┌─────┴─────┐
              │   CHILD   │    │  FAMILY   │
              └─────┬─────┘    └─────┬─────┘
                    ▼                ▼
          ┌───────────────────┐  ┌──────────────────────────┐
          │Evaluate Capabilities│ │Identify values & resources│
          └─────────┬─────────┘  └─────────┬────────────────┘
                    ▼                      ▼
          ┌───────────────────┐  ┌──────────────────────────┐
          │Reduce effects of deafness│ │Choose system of communication│
          └─────────┬─────────┘  └─────────┬────────────────┘
                    ▼                      ▼
          ┌───────────────────┐  ┌──────────────────────────┐
          │  Establish a system│◄─►│ Parent Guidance: Modify │
          │  of communication │  │ behavior with the child  │
          └───────────────────┘  └──────────────────────────┘
```

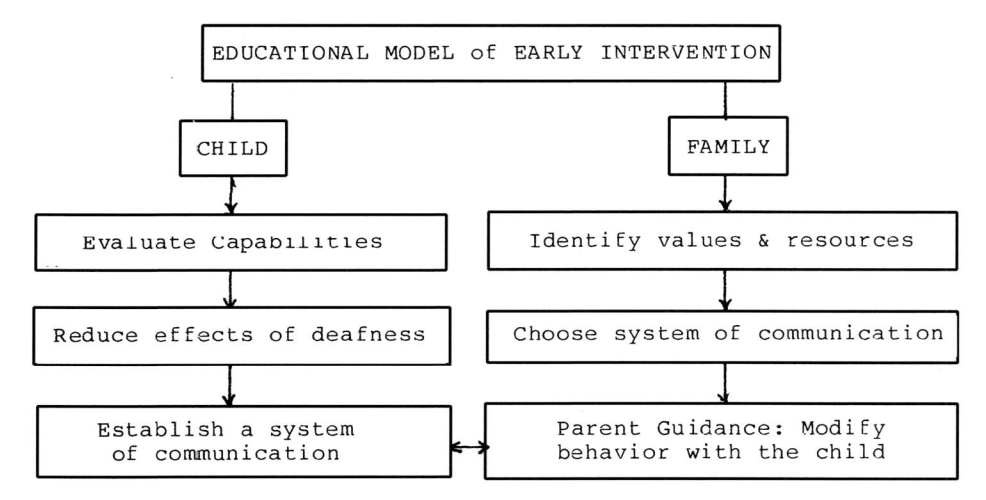

FIG. 2. Educational model of early intervention.

of or access to a deaf community. Like any other language, ASL is learned by interacting with people who use it. Hearing parents are likely to be in the position of having to learn a language that is foreign to them and master it with sufficient fluency to establish and maintain an intimate relationship with their child. Because of their limited experience with Deaf culture, language, and values, parents may feel inadequate in their ability to provide the child with a nurturing environment that will foster acquisition of language and world knowledge. The first language of the child is unfamiliar not only to the parents, but also to the extended family and mainstream culture. It is also a language for which there is no orthography, which increases the likelihood that the child will not have immediate access to the literature of the culture. Without access to information in books and ideas in the minds of others, the child is at risk of acquiring limited world knowledge.

The medical and the cultural models are seldom practiced in a pure form. In their purest form, both models fundamentally deny the perspective that deafness is a disability requiring formidable adaptation by the deaf child to an environment in which most people hear. (Fig. 1).

The goal of the educational model is to promote optimal development in children and to enhance the quality of their life and their family's life. Using sensory aids and establishing an effective system of communication minimize the effects of hearing loss on the child. Educating the parents increases their understanding of deafness and allows them to adapt their home environment to meet the communication, learning, and social, and emotional needs of their hearing-impaired child (Fig. 2). The educational model is the model of choice because it is dynamic and takes into account the capabilities of the individual child as well as the values and resources of a particular family.

Language and Cognition: Philosophical Controversies

Within educational programs of early intervention there is great philosophical and ideologic controversy over the best way for deaf children to learn. Even after hearing-impaired children are fit with appropriate sensory aids, they may not have sufficient access to auditory information to develop spoken language spontaneously. The acquisition of language and cognitive skills is central to methodologic controversies about the best way to educate deaf children. The issue is raised in this chapter because parents often ask their physician for his or her professional opinion on the best way to educate a hearing-impaired child.

The greatest risk faced by hearing-impaired children with hearing parents is that of growing up without language competence and with limited world knowledge. The process of acquiring spoken language is often slow, tedious, incomplete, and out of step with other developmental processes. Without language, deaf children are tied to the here-and-now, unable to understand the ideas and wishes of others, unable to express their own thoughts, and unable to engage in conversational exchange or dialogue. The result is that their world model is incomplete.

There is no simple, straightforward solution to this language dilemma. The issue of language accessibility is affected directly by the degree of the hearing impairment. To the extent that sensory aids, in combination with lipreading, can provide children with access to the spoken language code, these children can interact linguistically and master spoken language. Many children with profound hearing losses, however, may not be able to detect and discriminate linguistic symbols adequately enough to use them and extract rules for their use. Parents of hearing-impaired children may be advised to enrich the acoustic and linguistic environment of their child at home by increasing the amount of time they talk to the child. Without accessibility, however, fluency and enrichment are not effective.

American Sign Language is a complete and rich language, the symbols and rules of which are fully accessible through vision. Unfortunately, 90% of the children who have hearing impairments are born to parents who have no knowledge of or experience with this language. The rate of linguistic mastery is limited not by accessibility of the linguistic code, but by the family's, and later the mainstream culture's, limitation in using the language richly and fluently with the child.

There are a variety of oral approaches to communication. A purely oral approach, by definition, uses only spoken language as a medium for communication (2). In addition to ASL, there are a variety of manual communication systems that are designed to be used in combination with spoken English to support the spoken code. (The next chapter in this book deals with the choosing the appropriate method of communication in greater depth.)

The polarization of linguists, educators, and other professionals on the best way to teach deaf children, has impeded research in education of the deaf for 200 years (3,4) leaving us with few truths or irrefutable facts about how to manage cognitive and linguistic development in young deaf children. In spite of this controversy and dearth of quantitative data, well-established educational programs for the deaf have developed curricula addressing cognitive and language learning needs of hearing-impaired children based on extended observation and interaction with deaf children (5–7). Their successful graduates are living testimony that different linguistic approaches are appropriate for different children and families.

The best way for parents to educate themselves and make decisions about methodologic and communication choices is to visit established educational programs for the deaf who have had a history of experience using a particular approach to teach children. Parents can judge for themselves the effectiveness of a particular approach based on knowledge of their child's capabilities and temperament in light of the values and expectations they have for their family and children. Physicians can identify programs for the deaf in their area and recommend that parents observe there. A comprehensive list of programs across the nation may be found in any annual April issue of the *American Annals of the Deaf.*

THE COMPONENTS OF AN EARLY INTERVENTION PROGRAM

Comprehensive Evaluation

The first step is evaluation. A hearing test, alone, establishes candidacy for a program of early intervention, but it does not give information about the potential impact the loss can have on the child's development. The comprehensive educational evaluation is the vehicle by which specific goals are established for a particular child. The purpose of the comprehensive evaluation is to identify the child's capacities, strengths, and weaknesses in all areas of development. Typically, auditory, intellectual, linguistic, and speech capabilities are measured. Factors such as temperament and learning style, although difficult to measure, are also important factors in establishing expectations for the development of a particular child. Comprehensive evaluations are most helpful when they are conducted by a team of professionals (e.g., audiologists, speech-language pathologists, and teachers of the deaf) who have expertise in and experience with deafness and its effects on development, as well as their specific academic disciplines. There are few test instruments that measure the capabilities and performance of very young deaf children. There is, however, a body of knowledge about the specific effects of deafness on development (8–10). Accurate interpretation of test results, diagnostic teaching, and observation rely heavily on the team members' knowledge of and experience with hearing loss in children (11).

The results of the comprehensive evaluation should provide accurate diagnostic information about the child in a way that makes it accessible to everyone who is responsible for management. This includes the physician, audiologist, speech pathologist, teacher of the deaf, and most importantly, the parent.

Audiological Management

The next step in early intervention is to reduce the primary effects of hearing impairment by fitting the child with a hearing aid. A program of audiologic management is supported by a team that includes the audiologist, the parent, and the teachers and clinicians who work with the child. The goal of audiologic management in the first few years of life is to ensure stability of the hearing loss by (a) monitoring middle ear function, (b) ensuring that the child has most appropriate hearing aid, and (c) advising parents about the efficacy of alternative sensory aids, such as FM systems, vibrotactile aids, or cochlear implants. The audiologist is able to fit a child with a hearing aid adequately, using results from brainstem and behavioral testing. The audiologist can evaluate hearing aid performance after the child has worn the aid for a period of time, has had experience with sound, and has had an opportunity to develop a system of auditory perception. Feedback from the parents and teacher-clinicians is required for information about functional use of hearing so that the audiologist can make adjustments in the hearing aid fitting. Such feedback is also needed should alternatives to conventional hearing aids, such as cochlear implants, be considered.

Part of the job of the audiologist is to monitor the status and function of the middle ear. Children under the age of 5 years are more prone to eustachian tube and, therefore, middle ear dysfunction. A temporary hearing loss, as a result of middle ear problems, is relatively inconsequential in the development of a child who has an intact cochlea. Fluid or chronic negative pressure, which prevents the hearing aid from transmitting sound to the cochlea, may mean a total loss of hearing for the child with a profound sensorineural hearing loss. The process of developing an auditory perceptual system requires consistent transmission of sensory stimuli to the brain. Hearing-impaired children who receive no auditory stimulation or intermittent stimulation do not have the basic building blocks for developing an auditory perceptual system. While there is no medical cure for sensorineural hearing loss, there are many medical interventions that can ensure stability of middle ear function. Using tympanometry to measure middle ear performance, the audiologist plays an important role in helping the parents and physician to ensure medical management of the middle ear.

Audiologic management during the early years of life requires frequent formal testing, informal observations, and consistent communication of information about auditory development among members of the audiologic team. As children mature neurologically, they can give more precise information about their abilities to perceive and use sound. Children who have progressive hearing losses need to be monitored closely for any change in hearing status so that their amplification can be adjusted. Children with chronic otitis media also need to be closely monitored to ensure middle ear function. In general, hearing-impaired children under the age of 5 years should receive complete audiologic assessments every 3 months. Any change in auditory performance as reported by a parent or teacher should be investigated by the audiologist.

To establish realistic performance goals and expectations, parents and professionals need to know if children are reaching their auditory potential once they have been wearing appropriate amplification for a period of time. It may take as long as a year to be able to answer questions about how a child is using his or her hearing compared with children with similar hearing losses. Although there is not a one-to-one correlation between results on an audiogram and a child's ability to use his or her hearing, there is a body of knowledge that exists on auditory performance as it relates generally to auditory capacity in children (12). Professionals in schools for the deaf who value hearing and give priority to audiologic management and auditory stimulation also develop standards for auditory performance based on their knowledge of the child's auditory capabilities. They are in a position to evaluate the child's use of hearing and are able to make judgements about how closely the child is functioning to his or her auditory potential. If there is a discrepancy between auditory performance and capacity, they are in an ideal position to diagnose the reason for the discrepancy. Reasons might include inappropriate hearing aids or earmolds, inconsistent use of hearing aids, chronic middle ear dysfunction, progressive hearing loss, an impoverished environment for auditory stimulation, or auditory processing difficulties.

Before leaving the topic of audiologic management, it is important to remind the physician, once again, that "earlier is better." Hearing children are exposed to the sound patterns of their mother's voice while still in the womb. If the goal of audiologic management for hearing-impaired children is to use their auditory capabilities for perceptual development to acquire knowledge about the world and, ultimately, spoken language, then auditory stimulation should begin as soon as a diagnosis of hearing loss is made. Some practitioners talk about "hearing age" (13), referring to the amount of time the hearing-impaired child has been exposed to sound consistently through hearing aids. While there is no scientific definition of this concept, it can be a useful marker in making predictions about when the child will begin to show observable listening, babbling, or imitative speech behavior.

Parent Guidance

The auditory and language needs of the hearing-impaired child are obvious, but it is the parents of that child who have an even greater need when the child is very young. Parents are responsible for making decisions about the management of the hearing impairment. It is the parents who are providing the child with a home environment that will support its growth and development. Parents who have had their own emotional needs met are more likely to be able to take care of their child.

One of the most critical moments for the parents of a deaf child is the moment the results of the hearing test are delivered. If this takes place in a hospital or diagnostic center, the physician may be included in the diagnostic process. If they listen, physicians can be most helpful to parents at this time. Parents who accompany their child to the hearing test generally anticipate a hearing problem. They may even have observed the baby's poor response to sound in the test booth. The tests results, however, may still be shocking to them.

Reactions to Diagnosis

Emotional responses of hearing parents to a diagnosis of hearing loss in their child are well documented (14–17). Reactions follow the stages of grief, which are now considered part of the process of coping with a perceived loss (18). The stages of mourning include shock, denial, anger, and acceptance. During the intervention process, parents may manifest these feelings in different ways at different times. The state of the parents' emotional well-being directly effects the kind of environment they can provide for their family.

Initially, hearing parents perceive a diagnosis of hearing impairment as a threat to the parent-child relationship and their ability to take care of their child. They may even respond to test results as though they were a threat on life itself. Among the changes we have observed as we have counseled parents after a hearing test are loss of facial color, a change in breathing rate, body tensing, gaze avoidance, blank stares, and incoherent speech. Parents may have difficulty looking at or nurturing their child momentarily. Some parents cry. Most are in shock. At this time, the most helpful response is to listen. It is not yet time for reassurance or problem solving. Initial reactions to loss can make professionals feel uncomfortable. You may feel an urgency or responsibility to make the feelings go away to assuage your own discomfort. It is important to note that these reactions are normal, expected, and protective and serve to alert parents that they may need to prepare for an unchartered journey ahead. To ignore parents' feelings or respond to them by giving them directive or didactic information not only is disrespectful, but also contributes to their sense of powerlessness and delays the process of intervention.

In some cases, emotional reactions to a diagnosis of hearing may be delayed. This is a situation in which physicians are more likely to be involved. A diagnosis of hearing loss may seem quite manageable to parents whose baby is tested after surviving bacterial meningitis, in contrast to the life-threatening experience they have just survived. In these families, the reaction is much less dramatic at the time of diagnosis, but parents may report depression or "feeling low" about the deafness 7 to 12 months after the child has recovered from the illness. At this time, the parents begin to see the child as healthy, strong, and growing, and the long-term secondary effects of the deafness, such as auditory, speech, and language delay, become more salient.

Some parents may actually seem relieved at a diagnosis of hearing impairment in their child. These parents usually have suspected and perhaps voiced their concerns about a delay in the development of their child. The cause for the delay, however, has remained undiagnosed. When a diagnosis of hearing impairment is finally made, it may seem more manageable than an unknown cause. The physician, however, should be prepared for the parents to direct any anger as result of the delay in diagnosis to the primary care physician.

For obvious reasons of identification and affiliation, responses to loss at the time of diagnosis are often not observed in deaf parents. In fact, I can report one case in which the parents, who both had hearing impairments, had to counsel and console the physician about the joys of having hearing-impaired children, after the birth of their third hearing-impaired child. In such cases, there is no perceived loss when a hearing impairment is diagnosed. Once again, the advice to physicians involved in initial diagnoses of hearing impairment is to listen actively to parents' emotional reactions to the diagnosis.

Goals for Parents

After parents cope with initial reactions to a diagnosis of hearing impairment, they will continue to need guidance, emotional support, and education to provide their child with a rich and nurturing environment conducive to optimal growth and development. Goals for parents of hearing-impaired children in an early intervention program are as follows:

1. To know and accept their hearing-impaired children
2. To develop appropriate expectations for their child's performance
3. To re-evaluate these expectations periodically
4. To identify family values and resources
5. To establish an effective system of communication to use in their family
6. To provide an acoustically, cognitively, and linguistically enriched home environment
7. To choose an appropriate preschool program

Activities in which parents can address these goals include (a) a comprehensive developmental assessment of their child; (b) counselling from professionals who work directly with their children, such as: physicians, audiologists, speech pathologists, teachers of the deaf, and early childhood specialists; (c) interaction with deaf adults; and (d) participating in a support group with other parents of hearing-impaired children.

Support Groups

Raising a hearing-impaired child in a culture in which most people hear creates additional stress in the family. Sources of stress vary. Audiology and communication therapy may be helpful for the hearing-impaired child, but adding these services complicates family life. In their parents' efforts to meet the needs of the deaf child, other children in the family may perceive their hearing-impaired sibling as getting more attention. Explaining the choices parents have made for their hearing-impaired child to extended family members adds stress to day-to-day family life. As children grow and acquire skills or parents acquire new diagnostic information, they may be faced with new decisions regarding the management of the child's hearing impairment. These decisions are seldom straightforward in terms of the benefits and liabilities for the child, and parents must examine the decisions in terms of the impact they will have on their particular child and family.

The support group is a very effective vehicle for addressing all of these issues. It provides parents with an opportunity to talk about their feelings of inadequacy, frustration, fear, anger, and powerlessness. It reassures them that they are not alone in their feelings or in their struggle to perform well as a parent. It also gives them a sense of control and purpose to be able to help others through a process they are going through themselves. In short, no single professional can provide for parents what they can provide for each other (14,15,19). An example of the use of a parent group for support follows.

Several years ago, I was working with four families, all of whom were coping with the addition of a second hearing-impaired child. These families had relocated to a rural area so that their first-born hearing-impaired child could attend a school for the deaf as day students. Many of them made the choice to move away from extended family, friends, and jobs so that their hearing-impaired child would have a better opportunity for education.

When the second hearing-impaired child was born, it was easy for professionals and the families to minimize the problem. There was an assumption that because parents had dealt with a diagnosis of hearing impairment earlier in their lives that they would not need to do it again. After all, they were familiar with deafness and now had direct experience with it. In fact, what I observed after the diagnosis of the second child was a general depression in the parents and a lack of support from extended family and associated professionals. We started a support group for these parents and called it, "One More Time with Feeling." Some of the issues raised by the group were as follows: (a) Although they felt early diagnosis benefitted their child (usually soon after birth because of the risk factor of having a deaf sibling), they also felt immediately vaulted into decisions about management of the hearing loss and pressure to be an "enlightened, informed, knowledgeable" parent based on their previous experience with hearing loss; (b) educational and communication decisions for the second child were often confounded by the decisions made for the first child; (c) emotional issues surrounding the hearing loss in the first child that went unresolved often resurfaced; (d) the emotional support of family and friends, which was available when the hearing loss of the first child was diagnosed, was less available either because the diagnosis was not "new" to the family or because the family had moved geographically further away from these sources. As the issues were addressed in the group and parents received support from each other, they were in a stronger position emotionally to make decisions and provide adequately for their families.

One-to-One Work with Hearing-Impaired Infants

The primary impact on the child's development is through the parents interaction. It is through direct interaction with the child, however, that the parent-infant teacher can give the parent feedback on the best way to interact with the child to promote growth.

One-to-one work with a hearing-impaired infant (0 to 3 yr of age) usually includes (a) listening activities to maximize use of the hearing aid and residual hearing, (b) babbling or speech activities to help the child gain control of the speech mechanism, and (c) play activities to enhance cognitive and conceptual development, which provide the foundation for and opportunity to develop language.

The purpose of the one-to-one work is twofold: (a) to give parents models for ways to interact with their children and (b) to use diagnostic teaching strategies to give parents information about the capacities of the child in all areas of development so that realistic goals and expectations for performance can be established. All activities are conducted in a context of play or as part of activities of daily life so that carryover at home is obvious to the parents or other caregivers.

AVAILABLE RESOURCES

Early intervention for the hearing-impaired is not a new concept. In 1867, the Clarke School for the Deaf in Northampton, Massachusetts, admitted hearing-impaired children as young as 4 years of age when most state schools for the deaf did not admit children until 10 years of age. The Sarah Fuller Foundation, established in Boston in 1888, sent teachers of the deaf into the homes of parents with very young hearing-impaired children to help their mothers learn how to communicate with them. Private schools and some state schools for the deaf have been in the business of early intervention for a long time. In the last decade, however, early intervention has been mandated by the federal government.

Legal Aspects of Early Intervention

In 1975, the United States Congress passed the Education of All Handicapped Children's Act (the Act: P.L. 94-142). The Act made education the right of all persons with disabilities aged 5 to 21 years. The lower limit of the Act in many states was soon reduced to 3 years of age to include preschool children. P.L. 99-142 is administered at the state level through local educational systems. In 1986, the Act was amended (P.L. 99-457) to include provision of services to all preschoolers, infants, and toddlers with disabilities. P.L. 99-457 is administered at the state level, usually through public health agencies. Administration of these services is not as uniform nationally as are those services to school-age children (20,21).

Early intervention programs that serve all disabilities can be found in the public sector as a result of implementing P.L. 99-457. Early intervention programs that are specifically for the hearing impaired may be found in the private sector in speech and hearing clinics or in schools for the deaf.

Generic Early Intervention Program

Generic programs of early intervention are available regionally to almost all parents. They are usually staffed with early childhood educators, a speech and language pathologist, an occupational therapist, a physical therapist, and perhaps a nurse. The strength of the generic program is the diverse expertise of the staff, which is valuable for both evaluation and provision of direct service, particularly if the child has delays in other developmental areas that are not associated with hearing loss. Local programs also provide parents with referral information for other services.

The limitations of the generic early intervention programs are that the staff seldom has expertise specifically in the management of hearing impairment. Because there are few appropriate formal test instruments to use with hearing-impaired children, this expertise can be particularly important in the interpretation of assessment results. In addition, generic programs of early intervention do not have on-site audiologic evaluation and management facilities. They probably have support groups for parents of disabled children, but these groups do not address the specific needs of parents of children with hearing impairments.

Speech and Hearing Clinics

Speech and hearing clinics may operate independently or be housed in hospitals or rehabilitation centers. The strengths of the speech and hearing clinics lie specifically in their focus on hearing impairment and communication. Audiologic management is provided on site along with one-to-one work in the area of developing auditory and speech and language skills. Parents of hearing-impaired children may also be included in a support group for hearing-impaired adults or parents of children with speech and language delays. The limitation of the speech and language clinic is that the staff providing the therapy for the child is not necessarily trained or skilled at working with the "whole" child or the child in the context of the family. The work with the child may be necessarily adult-directed and controlled, and carryover at home may not be obvious.

Schools for the Deaf

Schools for the deaf, which have parent-infant programs, can be the most comprehensive resource for children and their parents. Their strength lies in the broad educational focus on the whole child, which addresses the acquisition of language competence and world knowledge but not at the expense of social or emotional development. Teachers of the deaf are teachers of language first, and they are trained specifically to teach children for whom hearing may not be the primary modality for language acquisition. Teachers of the deaf in parent-infant programs use a teacher-parent partnership model. Audiologic management is usually provided on site.

A limitation of programs in schools for the deaf is that many have closed at the expense of public mandate to educate deaf children in schools designed for the hearing (P.L. 94-142). Surviving schools may embrace a single communication or educational philosophy that limits or is not in keeping with parent choice. A summary of delivery of services in early intervention models is in Figure 3.

Other Resources

In general, educational programs for the hearing impaired are concentrated in cities or populated areas, with much poorer accessibility in rural areas, because of the low incidence of hearing impairment in the population. There are, however, some programs of early intervention that are designed specifically for greater geographic accessibility.

SERVICE DELIVERY MODELS	Generic Early Intervention Programs	Speech Hearing Clinics	Schools for the Deaf
COMPONENTS of EFFECTIVE EARLY INTERVENTION PROGRAMS			
Comprehensive Evaluation	*		
-Specifically for the deaf			*
Audiological Component		*	*
Child Component			
- Speech	–	*	*
- Language	*	*	*
- Cognition	*	–	*
-Social-Emotional Status	*	–	*
Family Component	*		*
Support Group for Parents of: Developmentally delayed Children	*		
Hearing-Impaired Children			*

FIG. 3. Summary of services provided by models of early intervention.

The John Tracy Clinic

The John Tracy Clinic Correspondence Course answers parents' questions about the effects of hearing loss on their child's development, provides parents with general information about deafness, and provides them with activities and lessons to do with their deaf infant or toddler. The course is free to parents, and they enroll by writing a letter directly to the director of the correspondence course. Parents receive a personal response to their first letter, along with some general information about how to proceed with the management of their hearing-impaired child. Lessons include activities, instructional videotapes, and feedback forms for the parents to complete about the child's performance. Subsequent information is sent to parents, with a personal letter, in manageable packets after they respond to the previous mailing. The course complements any local program of early intervention and any communication method (22,23).

The John Tracy Clinic was started in 1942 by Mrs. Spencer Tracy following her experiences with her own hearing-impaired son. The course is translated into more than 23 languages and is used by parents all over the world. In addition, families can attend a residential program on the Los Angeles campus during the summer months. The summer program provides diagnostic and direct services to hearing-impaired children and support and information to their parents.

Comprehensive Evaluation and Short-Term Intervention Programs

There are several programs of comprehensive and short-term intervention across the United States that are much like the summer program at the John Tracy Clinic. These are programs designed to make resources at established centers for deafness accessible to families who may not live near such a program. Families usually stay at a center for a short period of time and receive comprehensive evaluation, short-term intervention, and recommendations for programming to be implemented by services closer to home.

Our own Visiting Infant and Parent (VIP) Program at the Clarke School for the Deaf in Northampton, Massachusetts, is a short-term program of evaluation, intervention, and parent education for families with deaf and hard-of-hearing children from birth to 5 years of age. Families from all over the world participate in a VIP program. They are housed on campus for several days while children participate in audiologic, psychological, speech, and language evaluations. Parents observe all evaluations, and a substantial portion of their visit includes discussion of test results and the implications for their child's development. In addition, parents discuss their questions about deafness, observe classes for deaf students, eat meals in the dormitories, and meet with deaf adults. Parents leave with a better understanding of hearing loss, the effects it will have on the development of their child, and a list of recommendations for the next phase of intervention.

Parents and professionals can find a list of educational programs for the deaf in the United States in any annual April issue of the American Annals of the Deaf. Other organizations which disseminate information about the education of hearing-impaired children are

Alexander Graham Bell Association for the Deaf, Inc.
3417 Volta Place, NW
Washington, DC 20007
American Society for Deaf Children
814 Thayer Avenue
Silver Spring, MD 20910

DOES EARLY INTERVENTION WORK?

There is a dearth of empirical data on the efficacy of early intervention programs. Several factors make efficacy studies difficult to design: (a) the heterogeneity of the hearing-impaired population, (b) a lack of appropriate evaluation tools, (c) the ethics of control studies, and (d) methodological controversy.

The population of hearing-impaired children is heterogeneous in terms of etiology, age of onset, degree of impairment, and intellectual and social capabilities, making it difficult, if not impossible, to draw conclusions about the positive effects of early intervention programs that apply to all hearing-impaired children.

There is, however, a body of literature on the negative effects of hearing loss on the development of communication in children (24–27). There are also data on the positive effects of auditory stimulation on the development of auditory and speech perception skills in hearing-impaired children. Performance in these areas is narrowly defined and measurable. The correlation between performance in these areas and cognitive development, social cognition, and even language acquisition, however, is not clear. Unfortunately, we lack good tools to evaluate the effects of environmental influences on those aspects of development that affect quality of life.

Superficially, an ideal way to collect data would be to withhold intervention from a control group of hearing-impaired children. While this may lead to more scientific conclusions, it would also be inhumane and is, in fact, against the law. Without direct evidence, we must rely on indirect evidence to make deductions about efficacy. We know that sensory deprivation negatively affects learning in animals (28–30). In addition to studies on the plasticity of the brain (31,32), these data support the theory that sensory deprivation can also have a permanent effect on a human being's capacity to learn and adapt to the environment.

In the absence of control studies, it would be helpful if we had good reporting of practices in early intervention. Philosophical, political, and methodologic controversies in the education of the hearing impaired have restricted the application of scientific method to efficacy studies, as is supported by the Babbidge Report (3) and later the Report to the President and the Congress of the United States completed by the Commission on Education of the Deaf (4).

In spite of the lack of empirical evidence in support of early intervention programs, medical, clinical, and educational practitioners and parents agree that these programs provide hearing-impaired children with the best opportunity to reach their potential for development (33,36). There are few that would recommend against early intervention on the grounds that it is difficult to find empirical data on efficacy.

FINAL COMMENTS

Deafness is fundamentally an issue of development and education. Intervention is necessary to ensure optimal growth and development in the child and the family. The earlier intervention begins, the more likely it is to improve the quality of life of both the child and the family. Intervention cannot occur without early identification and diagnosis. It is in the area of identification and diagnosis that the physician has the greatest impact.

REFERENCES

1. Gravel J. Auditory assessment of infants. *Semin Hear* 1994; 15:100–13.
2. Gatty J. The oral approach, a professional point of view. In: Schwartz S, ed. *Choices in Deafness* Kensington, MD: Woodbine Press; 1987; 57–64.
3. Babbidge H. *Education of the deaf.* Advisory Committee of the Education of the Deaf, DHEW, Washington, DC; 1965.
4. *Toward equality: education of the deaf.* A report to the President and theCongress of the United States. Washington, DC: The Commission of Education of the Deaf; 1988.
5. Cheney H, Compton C, Harder K. *Developmental language curriculum.* Seattle: University of Washington Press; 1988.
6. McAnally P, Rose S, Quigley S. *Language learning practices with deaf children.* Austin, TX: PRO-ED; 1994.
7. Northcott W. *Curriculum guide: hearing-impaired children (0–3 years) and their parents.* Washington, DC: Alexander Graham Bell Association for the Deaf, Inc; 1977.
8. Boothroyd A. *Hearing impairments in young children.* Washington, DC: A.G. Bell Association; 1982.
9. Liben LS. The development of deaf children: an overview of issues. In: Liben LS, ed. *Deaf children: developmental perspectives.* New York: Academic Press; 1978:3–18.
10. Schlesinger H. The effects of deafness on childhood development: an Eriksonian perspective. In: Leiben LS, ed. *Deaf children: developmental perspectives* New York: Academic Press; 1978:157–167.
11. Gatty J. The V.I.P. program: The Clarke School for the Deaf. In: Roush J, Matkin N, eds. *Infants and toddlers with hearing loss.* Baltimore: York Press; 1994:215–35.
12. Boothroyd A, Erickson F, Medwetsky L. The hearing aid input: a phonemic approach to assessing the spectral distribution of speech. *Ear Hear 1994;* December: 432–42.
13. Pollack D. Reflections of a pioneer. *Volta Rev* 1993;95:197–204.
14. Luterman D. *Counseling parents of hearing-impaired children.* Boston: Little, Brown; 1979.
15. Luterman D. *Counseling the communicatively disordered and their families.* Boston: Little, Brown; 1984.
16. Luterman D. The Thayer Lindsley Family-Centered Nursery, Emerson College. In: Roush J, Matkin N, eds. *Infants and toddlers with hearing loss.* Baltimore: York Press; 1994:301–15.
17. Kampfe C. Parental reaction to a child's hearing impairment. *Am Ann Deaf* 1989; October:255–9.
18. Kubler-Ross E. *On death and dying.* New York: MacMillan; 1969.
19. Foster S. Successful parent meetings. *Young Children* 1994; November: 78–80.
20. Power-deFur L, Harvey J. Legal basis for early intervention services. *Semin Hear* 1994;15:65–75.
21. Mauk G, Behrens T. Historical, political and technological context associated with early identification of hearing loss. *Semin Hear* 1993; 14:1–17.
22. John Tracy Clinic. *Correspondence Course for Parents of Deaf Infants.* Los Angeles, CA: John Tracy Clinic; 1980.
23. John Tracy Clinic. *Correspondence Course for Parents of Preschool Deaf Children.* Los Angeles, CA: John Tracy Clinic; 1983.
24. Davis J, Elfenbein J, Schum D, Bentler R. Effects of mild and moderate hearing impairment on language, educational and psychosocial behavior of children. *J Speech Hear Disord* 1986;51:53–62.
25. Kuhl P, Williams K, Lacerda F, Stevens K, Lindblom B. Linguistic experience alters phonetic perception in infants by 6 months of age. *Science* 1992;255:606–8.
26. Markides A. Age at fitting of hearing aids and speech intelligibility. *Br J Audiol* 1986;20:165–8.
27. Ross M. Implications of delay in detection and management of deafness. *Volta Rev* 1990;92:69–79.
28. Knudsen E, Esterly S, Knudsen P. Monaural occlusion alters sound localization during a sensitive period in the barn owl. *J Neurosci* 1984; 4:1012–20.
29. Knudsen E, Knudsen P, Esterly S. A critical period for the recovery of soundlocalization accuracy following monaural occlusions in the barn owl. *J Neurosci* 1984;4:1012–20.
30. Clopton BM, Winfield JA. Effect of early exposure to patterned sound on unit activity in rat inferior colliculus. *J Neurophysiol* 1976;39: 1081–9.
31. Ruben R, Rapin I. Plasticity of the developing auditory system. *Ann Otol Rhinol Laryngol* 1980;89:303–11.
32. Reisen AH. Effects of stimulus deprivation on the development and atrophy of the visual sensory system. *Am J Orthopsychiatry* 1960;30: 23–6.
33. Downs M. The case for detection and intervention at birth. *Semin Hear* 1994;15:75–84.
34. Laughton J. Models and current practices in early intervention with hearing-impaired infants. *Semin Hearing* 1994;15:148–59.
35. Brackett D, Maxon A, Blackwell P. Intervention issues created by successful universal newborn screening. *Semin Hear* 1993;14:89–104.
36. Tingey C. Early intervention: learning what works. *Exceptional Parent* 1986;16:32–7.

CHAPTER 48

Choosing the Appropriate Method for Communication

Sue Schwartz

More than 90% of children who are deaf are born to hearing parents (1). After hearing the diagnosis of deafness in their young child, parents enter a bewildering new world of terminology and conflicting opinion. They may have minimal knowledge of deafness. They may have never met a deaf person. They may only have seen signing on television as part of a presentation. They may have no clear understanding of what is involved in educating an individual with hearing loss or how they can best go about the process of habilitation for their child. It is critical that parents be empowered by knowledge to make the best-informed decisions possible. How can the physician ease the way? There has to be a clear understanding of the parents' frame of reference, what their educational and medical options are for their children, and how the information they need can effectively be communicated to them in a timely fashion.

Parents must have access to information, but they are often overwhelmed with the diagnosis and thus cannot be given a lot of information at one time. The physician may need to schedule several visits with the parents and gently provide more information at each visit.

As one of the primary individuals to give initial information to parents, the physician must know what options are available and must present this information in a nonbiased way. It must be made clear is that no one educational system or communication methodology works for every child. Throughout the history of deaf education, there have been many studies, each proving its own particular perspective, but no study indicates that a particular methodology works unequivocally. Choices must be available and parents must be made aware of the possibilities. See Appendix A of this text for a list of resources.

S. Schwartz: Montgomery County Public Schools—Special Education, Rockville, Maryland 20904.

HISTORICAL OVERVIEW

Deaf children were not educated until the 17th century when Juan Pablo Bonet hired a tutor to work with his employer's deaf son. Bonet watched the teacher work with the boy by using gestures to represent words. This was the first manual teaching system used with the deaf. During the 18th century, two very strong systems for teaching the deaf were developed simultaneously . The Abbé de l'Épée in France developed a system of sign language adapted from a silent order of monks but did not bother teaching articulation, because he believed it would be a waste of valuable teaching time. The technique was known as the French method and became key in the development of education of the deaf in America. At the same time, Samuel Heinicke of Germany was successful with deaf students by using an oral method that encouraged speaking and discouraged sign language. This technique became known as the German method.

In addition to Heinicke and Abbé de l'Épée, Thomas Braidwood, in England, was teaching the deaf what he believed was the natural acquisition of speech through lipreading and writing. However, Braidwood kept secret his approach to teaching language to the deaf.

At this time, American children who were deaf were sent to England to be educated. Therefore, they were educated solely with Braidwood's techniques. Americans knew of no other approach. In the early part of the 19th century, Thomas Hopkins Gallaudet noticed his neighbor's deaf daughter playing in the yard and became interested in learning how to teach her. Her father did not want to send his daughter to England, but he sent Gallaudet to study the methods of teaching the deaf. Because of Braidwood's secrecy about his teaching methods, he delayed meeting Gallaudet. During his wait, Gallaudet met Abbé Sicard, a follower of the Abbé de l'Épée. Sicard befriended Gallaudet and invited him to France to see how the deaf were taught there. Gallaudet was impressed with what he saw and implored a young deaf man,

Laurent Clerc, to accompany him home to the United States. Clerc established the American Asylum for the Deaf in Hartford, Connecticut in 1817 and used the French method to teach his students. The school exists today as the American School for the Deaf, a strong proponent of the use of sign language.

Within a few years, two schools that used the oral method were started in the United States—one in New York, the Lexington School for the Deaf, and one in Massachusetts, the Clarke School for the Deaf. Both schools are still in existence. The oral movement strengthened and in the late 1800s a group of educators of the deaf held a conference in Milan, Italy. After days of debate, it was decided that the best method for educating the deaf was the oral method and that this method should be the preferred method in all countries in which deaf children were educated. Nevertheless, some educators disagreed with this mandate and thus the strong differences of opinion were formed. For decades the debate about oral and manual communication methods has raged, and the controversy has not yet been resolved (2).

ORAL-AURAL COMMUNICATION

There are two primary modes of oral-aural communication: multisensory and unisensory. In both systems, children use spoken language for face-to-face communication.

In the multisensory approach, children use amplification (hearing aids, frequency modulation [FM] systems, cochlear implants) and speechreading, which involves watching the face and mouth of the speaker. Touch is also used sometimes to allow the child to feel where the sound originates (3). For example, a breath sound such as /f/ or /p/ might be demonstrated by having the child feel the flow of air on the back of the hand. A nasal sound such as /n/ or /m/ might be felt on the side of the speaker's nose.

In a unisensory approach, such as auditory verbal therapy, residual hearing supported by amplification or cochlear implant is the primary vehicle for helping the child learn to listen and speak. Speechreading and tactile clues are not encouraged. The therapist often sits behind or to the side of the child to encourage the child to depend solely on hearing for clues as to what is being said. Children with all degrees of hearing loss have been able to benefit from this system of learning (4).

CUED SPEECH

Considered by many to be an oral approach to communication but too "manual" for some oralists, cued speech represents another option for parents to use with their children. Cued speech is often allied with oral proponents because it is a "phonemically-based hand supplement to speechreading . . . ." It is comprised of eight handshapes representing groups of consonant sounds and four positions about the face to represent groups of vowel sounds. Combinations of the hand configurations and placements show the exact pronunciation of words in connected speech by making them clearly visible and understandable to the Cued Speech recipient. Cued Speech allows [a] child to 'see-hear' precisely every spoken syllable that a hearing person hears'' (5). Cued speech advocates the use of amplification and speech. Some children who have received cochlear implants use cued speech to supplement reception of speech. Cued speech is relatively easy to learn because it is a finite system based on the same language that the hearing parents use. Once the system is learned, there is no limit to the language that can be conveyed to the child that is deaf.

In the history of deafness, Cued Speech is a relative newcomer. It was invented in 1966 by Dr. Orin Cornett at Gallaudet University and subsequently has gained in popularity. It is used in many areas of the United States and in several other countries. Because Cued Speech is based on the sounds of spoken languages, languages other than English can be cued.

SIGN LANGUAGE

There are several options within the global category of sign language. Many deaf adults and many hearing educators believe that American Sign Language is the natural language of the deaf and should be used to teach deaf children. By this philosophy, no amplification or speech would be used. American Sign Language is visual; it does not depend on speech or audition. In fact, most adult deaf individuals who use American Sign Language claim that signing and speaking at the same time is impossible because the sign language does not follow English word order. American Sign Language and English are different; each has its own syntax, grammar, and rules of use. Proponents of this method believe that an early language base in American Sign Language, better prepares a deaf child to learn English as a second language through the vehicles of reading and writing (6).

Other educators feel that teaching sign language first makes the child learn language twice when only once is necessary and that using modified American Sign Language with English word order in addition to amplification, speech, and speechreading is the best approach to teaching the deaf child. This system is known as manually coded English or total communication. Proponents of this approach state The language of deaf children who are exposed to signed and spoken language simultaneously develops in the same time frame as hearing children; The knowledge and use of sign language by deaf children does not inhibit the use of speech; Deaf children who are exposed to oral and manual communication methods perform better linguistically, socially, and academically than those exposed to only oral communication (7).

MAKING A CHOICE

Each method has advantages and disadvantages. Each philosophy has professionals and parents who are firmly committed to it. There are students who are highly successful with each system. What is consistently true in almost every case, is that parental commitment to the choice made is crucial. Without family support, the child is not likely to be as successful as he or she could be, regardless of the system chosen. One of the primary obstacles is getting families to learn a system that is completely different from their own language. Asking parents to learn their own language in a new way, such as the methods of cued speech or manually coded English is difficult, but asking parents to become fluent in an entirely different language, such as American Sign Language, is almost impossible (8).

It is also important to consider the role of amplification when parents choose options for their deaf children. With the exception of American Sign Language, each of the other systems expects children who are deaf or hard of hearing to wear hearing aids, FM systems, or have cochlear implants. Parents, physicians, and other hearing-care professionals must understand that children differ in whether amplification will be useful, and the difference is not based on solely audiometric results. Of two children with identical audiograms measuring exactly the same decibel level, one may benefit from amplification and the other may not. All deaf children should be given the opportunity in the early critical learning years to maximize the residual hearing that they do have.

It is also critical that physicians and parents realize that placing a hearing aid, FM system, or cochlear implant in a child who is deaf will not result in perfect hearing. Much habilitation work is required. Sometimes habilitation comes through the use of an oral method and sometimes it is best to use Cued Speech or manually coded English. The choices are left to parents.

Much is said about the success in both academic and social areas of deaf children who have deaf parents and who communicate in a manual way from the beginning. For these families, there may be no question of how to proceed. Because more than 90% of deaf children are born to hearing parents and more than 90% of deaf parents have hearing children, only a small percentage of deaf parents have deaf children. Thus, there are far larger numbers of families that have no idea of which way to proceed. Nevertheless, a physician should not make the choice for families. Despite a physician's own thoughts and biases, the physician should support the parents in whatever decisions they make. The parents must feel comfortable with their choice and must feel a commitment to their choice. They must be willing to put in the work that is involved to implement their choice. Physicians and other hearing-care professionals must empower the parents and give them the freedom to change systems if they see their child's needs change.

THE PHYSICIAN'S ROLE

Critical to empowering parents to make crucial decisions and possible revisions of those decisions is providing a nurturing environment. The physician's office is the beginning. The physician must spend time with the family when the diagnosis is delivered and during follow-up visits. The physician must have the knowledge of the impact of deafness on a child and family and know the communication options available for the child. The physician is a crucial resource of information for parents. The physician must also know what kind of educational programming is available for parents in the area. The physician should also provide guidelines to evaluate the programs that are available in the area.

Guidelines written by members of the International Organization for Education of the Hearing Impaired (the professional section of the Alexander Graham Bell Association for the Deaf) describe what to look for in evaluating programs for deaf children and can be used to evaluate any of the systems of communication. The guidelines are reprinted here as Table 1.

Once the physician has formed a working partnership to help families through this new and unfamiliar territory, what is left to do? For some families, this is all that is needed. These families will pick up the gauntlet and follow through on suggestions, read about and understand their communication options, and make informed decisions. The physician need only continue to support them as they reach new turns in the road.

Often, however, the road is not as smooth as the physician would like. Sometimes, parents hesitate, retreat, and do not follow through on suggestions. They cancel appointments, fail to show up at educational programs, and seem never to read the reference material suggested. These parents may have other issues, such as denial, to work out. The physician must allow them to process information in their own time. A leading psychologist in the area of grieving says that denial is a necessary process that buys the time needed to build inner strength and outer resources (10). The physician must be the constant support to help these families build the inner strengths and outer resources they need. The physician is the facilitator. Although early and appropriate intervention is the key to successful acceptance of deafness, there is a small window of time during which parents can continue to grieve. The physician should continue to encourage a family in denial to enroll in a program and schedule more frequent appointments to continue to deliver the message of the advantages of an early intervention program. Physicians can also contact local social service agencies that may have staff (or volunteers) who are willing to go with the family to visit the local program options. Gently pushing them in the direction they need may facilitate their movement.

Different members of the family may respond in different ways to the diagnosis. Often, although not always, the mother is more easily and more quickly able to accept the diagnosis and move on. Often the mother enrolls the child in the program and follows through on the visits. Often the mother attends the family support group meetings. Therefore, often the mother has a better understanding of the nature of the difficulty and learns to use the communication

TABLE 1. *Guidelines for evaluating programs for deaf children*

I. A commitment to individualizing educational programming to fit the child's strengths and needs through:
  A. Initial and on-going assessment with parents informed and participating, as appropriate.
  B. Setting of goals and objectives with full parental involvement.
  C. Documentation of progress to be shared with parents at regular intervals.
II. Commitment to aggressive audiological management which includes encouraging and teaching the child in ways which will promote to the utmost his or her use of residual hearing. The educational program, school, or district will have immediate access to audiological services. Such audiological management includes:
  A. Periodic assessment of hearing, to include (as a minimum) pure tone threshold (aided and unaided), speech reception, speech discrimination, and impedance measurements.
  B. Appropriate amplification devices for each child, such as hearing aids, FM systems, vibrotactile aids, cochlear implants, or other devices deemed effective.
  C. Assistance and consultation with teachers and parents regarding practical aspects of the use of amplification.
  D. Establishment and use of system(s) for daily monitoring of hearing aids and other amplification devices to ensure proper functioning.
  E. Easy and fast access to minor repair services for amplification devices.
  F. Availability of batteries, loaner aids, loaner FMs, and other reserve equipment.
III. A commitment to helping children with hearing impairments develop intelligible spoken language to the greatest extent possible through:
  A. A concerted focus on using spoken language to communicate.
  B. Assessment, goal-setting, instruction and documentation of progress (all with parental knowledge) on developing speech and language.
  C. A high, as well as realistic, expectation for each child to communicate as clearly as possible using spoken language.
IV. Parent support offered by the program's leaders and staff by way of:
  A. Providing information and education regarding all aspects and implications of the child's hearing loss including as appropriate, unique roles and responsibilities of parents of children who are hearing impaired.
  B. Providing opportunities for parents to share feelings and experiences with other parents in order to best meet the challenges of parenting a child with a hearing loss.
  C. Informing parents of their rights, and of national and local parent support groups.
V. Well-trained, well-nurtured, available staff
  A. All staff have appropriate training and qualifications.
    1. Teachers or aural habilitationists: state or provincial licensure, also CED (Council on Education of the Deaf) or ACEHI (Association of Canadian Educators of the Hearing Impaired) certification encouraged.
    2. Audiologists/Speech language pathologists: state or provincial licensure, also must be certified by the American Speech-Language Association (ASHA) or the Canadian Association of Speech-Language Pathologists and Audiologists (CASLPA). Supervised experience with children who are hearing impaired prior to being hired is strongly recommended.
    3. Psychologists/social workers: state or provincial licensure.
  B. Staff communicates regularly with each other, with parents, and with the community through periodic meetings, phone calls, or in writing as appropriate.
  C. Staff plans cooperatively in order to provide continuity of education programming.
  D. Professional development (inservice training) of the staff is provided as appropriate.
  E. Staff encourages parent input regarding their child, and parent involvement in all aspects of the program and the child's education.
VI. A range of education settings are available including:
  A. Full time regular class
  B. Full time regular class with supportive services
  C. Part time regular class/part time special class
  D. Full time special class in regular school
  E. Full time special class in special school
  F. Residential/day school placement
  G. Home or hospital services if necessary
VII. Placement in one of these settings is accomplished in full compliance with due process procedures and parent/staff development of the individualized education program or individual family service plan, as stipulated by law.
VIII. The range of supportive services available on site or easily accessible may include:
  A. Audiology
  B. Speech-language pathology
  C. Sensory integration/occupational or physical therapist
  D. Counseling services for students and families
  E. Behavioral management
  F. Social work
  G. Academic tutoring
  H. Oral [cued and signed] interpreters
  I. Note takers
  J. Career counseling/placement service (for high school students)
  K. Respite child care
  L. Coordinated service delivery as needed from other agencies
IX. Curricula in all areas are interfaced and in concert with those provided to students in regular schools and classes.
X. Physical and social environment is accessible and conducive to listening and to speech reading because the facility is:
  A. Located in an area where there is minimal outside noise.
  B. Acoustically treated with carpets on the floor, acoustic tiles, curtains.
  C. Equipped with assistive listening devices as appropriate.
  D. Adequately lighted for easy speechreading.
  E. Arranged so that children in the auditory-oral program are not taught in the same class that is implementing total communication (or cued speech) for other children.
XI. Teachers of regular classes in the mainstream:
  A. Have been given a comprehensive orientation regarding their role in meeting the requirements of students who are hearing impaired.
  B. Agree to wear an FM transmitter when appropriate.
  C. Are regularly consulted, assisted, and supported by specialist staff from the auditory-oral educational program to include, as appropriate, teachers of students who are hearing impaired, aural habilitationists, audiologists, speech language pathologists, and psychologists or social workers.

From the Alexander Graham Bell Association for the Deaf (10) with permission.

---

system more effectively. Sometimes a difference of opinion develops among the family members. One member may want to use sign language but another may want to pursue an oral option. The physician is the support individual; the physician cannot make the decisions for the family, cannot make the members of the family participate, and cannot dictate their involvement. The physician can only provide gentle and continuous support with the hope that the parents realize that the way to success is through active involvement of all family members. The physician, therefore, can be the most pivotal person in the family's life as they pursue lifelong decisions for the deaf member of their family.

REFERENCES

1. Williams C, Kantor R, Pinnell GS. 1992. *The language and literacy worlds of profoundly deaf preschool children: informing developmental theory*. Washington, DC: Educational Resource Information Center; Department of Education. Publication no. ED 349715.
2. Schwartz S. Trends in the education of the hearing impaired: an overview. In: Schwartz, Sue, ed. *Choices in deafness: a parents guide*. Bethesda, MD: Woodbine House; 1987.
3. Gatty J. The oral approach: a professional point of view. In: Schwartz, Sue, ed. *Choices in deafness: a parents guide to communication options*. Bethesda, MD: Woodbine House; 1996.
4. Estabrooks W. *Auditory verbal therapy for parents and professionals*. Washington, DC: Alexander Graham Bell Association; 1994.
5. Williams-Scott B, Kipila E. Cued speech: a professional point of view. *Choices in deafness: a parents guide to communication options*. Bethesda, MD: Woodbine House; 1997
6. Stewart D. Bi-Bi to MCE. *Am Ann Deaf*. 1993;138:331–337.
7. Bodner-Johnson B. Total communication: a professional point of view. Schwartz, Sue, ed. *Choices in deafness: a parents guide to communications options*. Bethesda, MD: Woodbine House.
8. Greenwood-Logsdon, M. *Which sign language system should be used with young deaf children?* Washington, DC: Educational Resources Information Center; 1990; Department of Education. Publication no. ED347 716.
9. Moses, K. Fundamentals of grieving. [audiotape]. Evanston, IL: Resource Networks; 1986.
10. Alexander Graham Bell Association for the Deaf. *Guidelines for evaluating auditory-oral programs for children who are hearing impaired*. Washington, DC: International Organization for Education of the Hearing Impaired; 1993.

CHAPTER 49

Mainstreaming

F. David Manning

Until the 1970s, children with significant hearing losses in the United States were educated in special schools and classes. This approach, begun in the nineteenth century, was a product of the times. It was believed that these children were so different in their learning patterns and needs that it was impossible to educate them in regular schools. Starting in the early 1900s, a series of sociologic, educational, and research events occurred that steadily changed the views of the ways children learn, especially those with special needs. The previous approach of having separate schools and classes often meant that the potential of these children was underestimated. Electronic advances during and after World War II produced improved personal hearing aids and, within recent years, the cochlear implant. These have enabled many children who were previously cut off from sound to hear the human voice and language. These advances, coupled with the civil rights movement of the 1950s and 1960s, brought us to the day when, in the 1970s, Congress threw open the doors of the regular school to all children with special needs (1–4).

During the next 25 years, children with disabilities were moved from special schools into their regular neighborhood schools. The number of students in special schools shrank dramatically, but not all of the students made it into regular classrooms. Instead, many schools continued to teach these students in separate classes down the hall from the regular classroom. The opportunity to work with a regular class was often limited to short, nonacademic activities.

In the 1990s, another movement, known as inclusion has become popular. It calls for all children, disabled or not, to be placed in the regular classroom with no separation by age or ability. All support services are supposed to be delivered in the regular classroom, thus eliminating the need for a student to leave the room for extra assistance (5).

Now that schools are working to include children with hearing loss in regular classes, we realize that there is much more to this than good intentions. Hearing loss is a low-incidence disability, meaning that children with this condition are a very small minority of the school-age population. Although they have some learning needs that are similar to all children, they also have needs that are unique to hearing loss. The typical classroom teacher not only is unfamiliar with these learning needs, but also has no knowledge of what to expect from such a student in terms of communication performance, class participation, or written work. Training for teachers, although called for in legislation and regulations, is often inadequate. Thus, there is no assurance that a school practicing inclusion can provide the child who is deaf or hard-of-hearing with an appropriate education.

The Mainstream Center at the Clarke School for the Deaf/Center for Oral Education was established in 1977 in part to provide training and information to people in regular schools. Its establishment was based on the experience the Clarke School for the Deaf had in mainstreaming its graduates for more than 125 years. The Mainstream Center provides assistance to families in locating appropriate schools for their children, in educating the staff in regular schools about hearing loss and its effects, in planning and monitoring a student's educational program, and in evaluating the results. Over the past 18 years, the Center has worked with more than 500 educational programs, both public and private, throughout the United States, Canada, and Bermuda. In that time, an approach to mainstreaming has evolved that focuses on the needs of the student, the family, and the staff of the regular school.

A GENERALIZATION ABOUT HEARING

Before describing the steps to mainstreaming, it is helpful to keep in mind that hearing extends along a continuum from normal to complete deafness (Fig. 1). As a child's sensitivity to sound drops from normal, the child's method of taking in information gradually changes from one in which audition is the dominant channel, increasingly supported by vision,

---

F. D. Manning: The Mainstream Center, The Clarke School for the Deaf, Center for Oral Education, Northampton, Massachusetts 01060-2199.

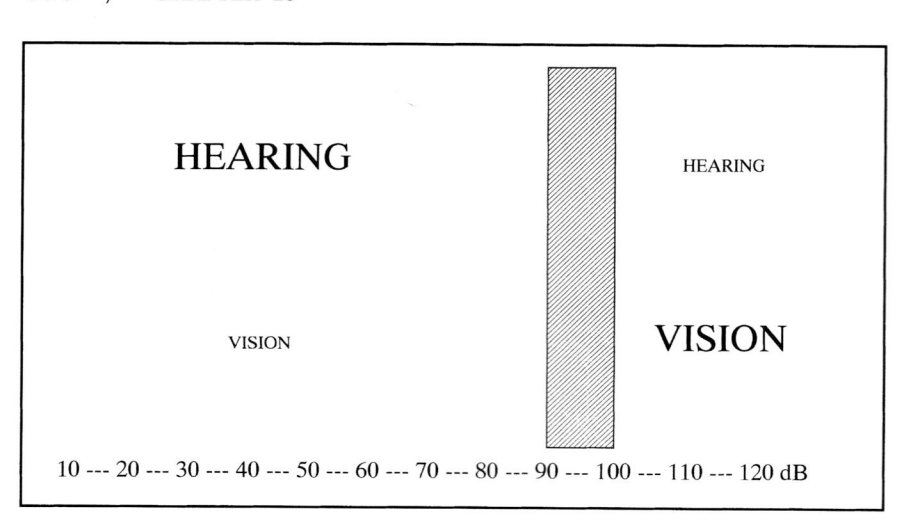

FIG. 1. As the magnitude of a hearing loss increases, a person's dominant receptive sense will change from hearing to vision.

to a completely different system in which vision becomes the dominant mode. It is a misconception to believe that because two children wear hearing aids, they function alike. Children with hearing loss function according to a complex combination of variables, including degree of loss, type of loss, age of onset, ability to perceive and comprehend speech sounds, and psychological factors. Those who function primarily by audition may or may not require support services. As their hearing decreases, the assistance they need may include personal hearing aids, special training to make better use of audition, speech therapy, and remedial language instruction. Those with more serious hearing losses, who depend primarily on vision, will usually require intensive training to make use of their residual hearing, instruction in lipreading, regular speech instruction, special instruction in language by a teacher of the deaf, and perhaps sign language.

EVALUATION

The Student

Before attempting to mainstream a student who is deaf or hard-of-hearing, it is advisable to do a comprehensive educational evaluation to determine the child's intellectual potential, the amount of useful residual hearing she has, her current understanding and use of the English language, and whether she has the necessary communication skill and background of information to be able to participate in and benefit from her placement in a regular classroom. This will provide a basis for deciding whether mainstreaming is a realistic choice to consider at a particular time and will also serve as a baseline for future evaluations.

It is important that the testing be done by professionals who have experience with children of this age and with this type of hearing loss, because they understand the complex interplay between the hearing loss and whatever learning needs are identified. They can then make recommendations for the type of program and any support services that might be needed. In this testing, it is especially important to determine the child's psychological and emotional status, because the mainstreaming experience will be a continuing challenge to her resilience and her psychological and emotional reserves.

This comprehensive testing should be the centerpiece of the mainstreaming effort and should be repeated every 3 years so that the child's parents and educators will have a basis for evaluating progress and planning the next phase of the child's education. Many schools do only partial testing and rely on earned grades as a measure of the student's progress. This is not as reliable because it does not provide a comprehensive view of the child's performance at a single moment in time, and it prevents an evaluation of the interplay among different aspects of the child's performance.

The Family

It is always beneficial to know the family's long range goals for the child, the types of life experiences the child has had, and how readily the family will be able to support the mainstreaming effort. Parents have shown that successful mainstreaming often calls for a large commitment from them in terms of time and energy, because the school system is typically unfamiliar with the needs of such a student. Meetings, evaluations, school visits, and the ongoing need to explain and to educate are just a few of the responsibilities parents have in this effort.

The School

Careful selection of the school is a critical first step toward a successful education. Not every school is appropriate for a student with a hearing loss, and placing such a student in a school without first examining its program is unwise. The intent is to find a match between the abilities and needs of the student (as revealed by the testing described previously) and the key features of the potential school's program, so that the child will have the greatest opportunity to succeed.

In many cases, an appropriate school can be found in the mainstream, but it cannot always be found close to home. Families who find themselves in this position sometimes consider moving to a different area, where the child can enroll in an appropriate mainstream program, but this is a serious step and the needs of other family members also must be considered. If a move is ruled out, it may mean the student either will not mainstream or will undertake it at a more advanced age. The emphasis at this stage is to identify a school where the student will have the best opportunity to participate and grow in an educational program that is appropriate to his abilities and needs.

Basically, there are two types of mainstreaming programs: complete integration with hearing students, which is now referred to as inclusion, or partial integration. In the case of partial integration, the student could be assigned to a class of students with hearing loss for specialized courses in speech and language, while taking the remaining courses in mainstream classrooms. Another variation would be to remain in the special class full time but have contact with hearing students during extracurricular activities. In reality, it is usually difficult to locate a regular program offering inclusion that fits a student with a hearing loss exactly. This is because regular schools were designed for hearing students. Although the student with a hearing loss can often complete such a program, a perfect fit is uncommon.

Part of determining whether a school's program is appropriate for a student is to identify the challenge it will present in terms of classroom communication, the language level of the textbooks, the teachers' classroom expectations, and the amount and type of written work. Will classes involve primarily discussion or lecture? A lecture is usually easier for a child to follow than a discussion. Will the students sit in rows, at a table, or in a large circle? The physical arrangement of the students has implications for lipreading. What is the noise level in most classrooms? High levels of background noise make it difficult for someone using a hearing aid. Is lighting adequate for lipreading purposes? Even in the best of circumstances when most of these factors are controlled, a student with a hearing loss will still miss a great deal of information in the classroom. For this reason, it is best to look for classrooms where information is presented in multiple ways, so that the student will have more than one chance to get the message. It is better to avoid classrooms where the student will be relegated to the role of an observer. Meaningful participation is the goal being sought, not watching from a place on the sidelines.

In addition to the basic school program, consideration must be given to the support services that will probably be needed. These could include one or more of the following: an FM amplification system to pick up the teacher's voice no matter where she is in the classroom, previewing of a new topic, peer note taking, oral or sign language interpreting, and follow-up tutoring. None of these services alone will make an otherwise inappropriate program suitable, but they can make a good program better. Even for students who receive all of these services, there is no guarantee of success. It is a combination of appropriate program, support services, teacher flexibility, student hard work, and family support that produces the best potential for successful results.

PREPARATION

When a specific school has been chosen, the staff of that school should be helped to understand the effect hearing loss will have on the student's ability to participate and should be instructed on the modifications they will need to make to include her. It is often easier to work with a school that has never had a student with a hearing loss than one that has, because inappropriate comparisons will not be made. As mentioned earlier, two students with hearing loss will probably function in very different ways, and comparisons can be misleading or even completely erroneous. The fact that two students wear hearing aids does not mean they are alike in other respects.

In preparing to take the student, the attitude of the staff, not just that of the administrators or admission officer, is critical. A staff that is willing to make a serious effort with the student, is optimistic about the chances for the student's success, and looks at the entire effort as a novel challenge will usually find a way to work successfully with the student. It is not expected that every staff member will be in favor of the attempt to mainstream, but the majority of them should be. If a positive attitude does not predominate among the staff, there is a high likelihood that inflexibility will hamper the program's success.

Once the student has been accepted in the new school, the focus turns to the specific teachers the student will have. On the elementary level, the number of people with whom the student works on a daily basis will be small. On the middle and high school level, it will be much larger. Regardless of level, each teacher needs to know about the student, the support services that will be provided, the type and amount of assistance the student is likely to require in the classroom, and recommendations for teaching modifications. This is usually accomplished through a number of in-service workshops.

At least one study has shown that most teachers are willing to have students with special needs in their classroom if they receive the training they need and have the interest and support of their administrators. In other words, this really needs to be a team effort. One person cannot do it alone. For the effort to succeed, each person needs to know who the other members of the team are and needs to be in touch with them for planning and support. It is interesting to note that this coordinated approach is the one element we most often find missing in schools, even though the staff may tell us they have such a support system in place. Teachers in ordinary schools often work in isolation.

IMPLEMENTATION

Teachers and staff who will be working with the student who is deaf or hard-of-hearing should attend an orientation meeting on or before the first day of school. After that, it is important for teachers to start right in working with the student during the opening days of the school year. They typically report that the first days are spent learning to communicate. As academics get underway, teachers begin to accumulate questions and concerns about how the student is going to manage. A few teachers may feel uncertain about whether the student truly understands the work. There may be questions about setting appropriate expectations. Language difficulties may surface. Teachers learn quickly how the pace of the class is altered simply by having the student in class, yet they do not find it easy to balance the needs of the student who is deaf with those of the others. They quickly develop a list of questions about all aspects of their work with the student.

It is at this time that another visit should be made to the school by a consultant familiar with teaching students with hearing loss. A private talk between consultant and student will usually reveal the student's uncertainties and questions. Observing in the classroom and meeting with each faculty member provides an opportunity for the consultant to uncover other areas where assistance is needed or questions can be answered. There is really no substitute for this type of direct observation and discussion.

MONITORING

From this point on, the consultant's efforts are focused on keeping abreast of the student's progress on a long-term basis. This is done through regular school visits to observe, to answer questions, to participate in planning meetings, to share information about the previous experiences of students with hearing loss, to ensure that everyone involved is informed of the work of the others on the team, and to provide encouragement to all. An attempt is made to identify and root out small difficulties while they are still minor. A series of small adjustments is made to keep the program running smoothly. Each contact with teachers reveals a new set of questions and a deeper appreciation for the ways in which the hearing loss affects almost everything the student does. Helping teachers establish reasonable expectations for the student is perhaps the biggest ongoing task. As they accumulate experience with the student, teachers not only develop a better understanding of the student's potential, but also learn that there are no easy answers to classroom communication difficulties, to the student's persistent language difficulties, or to the lack of ordinary background information that hearing students have.

Most schools treat the mainstreaming of a student who is deaf or hard-of-hearing as an innovation. This is simply because the incidence of hearing loss is so low. Innovations, however, can lead to confusion among staff members, a redefinition of roles and responsibilities, and in some cases to resentment and resistance. In helping a school deal with the situation, a consultant must be sensitive to people's feelings, exercise diplomacy, use negotiating skills, have a vision of what is possible, and be persistent. Teachers need encouragement, guidance, and support to help them continue their work. The student needs an understanding person to encourage her, to help her keep her eye on the goal, and to maintain a reasonable and stable view of her life.

The greatest challenge the student faces in the mainstream is not the academic work. The most demanding task will probably be to develop a sense of belonging—a sense that she is accepted as a full member of the student body within her school. While academic success is the area on which professionals will tend to focus, it is social integration and peer acceptance that will be the top priority for the student. Without that social acceptance, the student is far less likely to work to her academic potential.

A sense of belonging is closely allied to a strong sense of self. For any child, this is an important part of her growth and development within the school community. For a child who is deaf or hard-of-hearing, this is compounded by a continuing need to cope with the hearing loss and all its implications. Her self-esteem is powerfully influenced by her connection to peers. If these connections are inadequate due to a gap in communication and social skills, self-confidence and self-esteem will suffer. Students often tell of feelings of isolation. One student described himself at school as being "invisible. People say hello, but no one really talks to me." Adolescence, a difficult time for any teenager, is especially tough for students with hearing loss. At a time when it is natural to be seeking a place in the world around her, her peers are doing the same and consequently will often appear insensitive and self-absorbed. This is a period when the student is especially vulnerable and in need of a caring adult who can help her to recognize, verbalize, and come to terms with her feelings. The development and nurturing of self-esteem is a critical component to a successful mainstream program and needs to be monitored continually by members of the support team.

With a healthy, growing sense of self-esteem and self-confidence, a student can develop a sense of direction. One of the most important goals throughout the student's educational career is that of developing greater independence. As she grows, she will need to accept more responsibility for her own needs and be better able to advocate on her own behalf. By accepting and coping with her disability, by recognizing and acknowledging her own strengths and weaknesses, and by seeing herself as a member of a community, she will prepare herself for whatever future she sets out to find.

EVALUATION

Bringing the management cycle to full circle (Fig. 2), a periodic evaluation of the student's performance should be done to determine how well the student is coping with the hearing loss and the challenge of mainstreaming. Placing a student with this disability in a regular classroom amounts to placing the student in a system that simply was not designed for him. People in this system, though knowledgeable

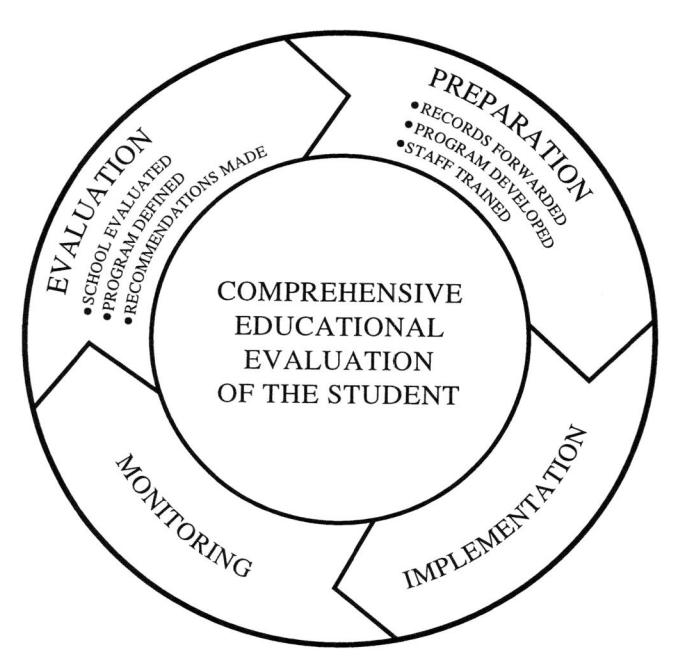

FIG. 2. A careful effort to mainstream a student who is deaf or hard-of-hearing begins with a comprehensive educational evaluation. All other decisions should flow from this, and the educational evaluation should be repeated at least every 3 years.

about normal child development, are unaccustomed to teaching deaf children and do not have familiarity with expectations for them. A thorough evaluation, one that includes psychological, social-emotional, academic, speech, language, oral and written communication, and audition, should be administered every 3 years to document current performance, which in turn will make it possible to document progress and guide the support team and those who are planning the student's future program.

SUGGESTIONS FOR PHYSICIANS

Physicians often view themselves as case managers for a child they identify as having a hearing loss. Once the medical aspects of the hearing loss have been addressed, the matter becomes one of habilitation or rehabilitation. Given the low incidence of the disability, it appears unlikely that the average physician would treat many children with this condition. In addition to being cognizant of the symptoms of hearing loss, physicians have reported that it is useful to become familiar with a local agency that has extensive knowledge of hearing loss and provides a wide array of services to deaf and hard-of-hearing clients. Because of the agency's extensive knowledge, it can assist with issues of testing and rehabilitation.

CASE HISTORIES

The following cases histories illustrate the assistance that a mainstream consulting agency can provide to schools and families.

Jennifer

Jennifer is 8 years old. At the time her mother first contacted our consulting agency, the child was 5 years old and had a severe loss in the right ear, and a profound loss in the left. One month earlier, the child had a moderate loss. The loss resulted from an autoimmune condition.

The parents contacted our agency because they did not think they knew how to manage their daughter's education with her hearing level continually worsening. Also, they had the impression that the school that she was attending also did not know how to manage. The school staff was telling them that the child was doing well, but when the child came home each day, she had difficulty telling them what had happened. The parents were very concerned. After telling their special education director about the consulting services we could provide, we were contacted by the school. Two consultants made a visit to the school to observe the child and talk with the staff.

The consultants found that the child was wearing an FM amplification system that had been purchased by the school without any audiologic direction. They did not know if it was appropriate for her loss, whether it was operating according to the manufacturer's specifications, or if it was working satisfactorily in conjunction with the child's personal hearing aids.

In class, the child was trying to function entirely on her hearing, despite the fact that her hearing level had recently dropped. It was clear that she needed to use lipreading as a support for her hearing, but she was not making the effort, nor was the teacher expecting it. As a result, the child was unsure of what was actually happening and being said in the classroom, her responses were vague, and she was seen copying what other children were writing.

Observing the speech pathologist and the reading specialist, it was noted that each was doing good work with Jennifer, but they never communicated with each other. Opportunities for each of them to reinforce the work of the other were being missed. Additionally, neither of the specialists communicated with the classroom teacher. Everyone was working in isolation, and the parents, who were eager to help at home, were not part of the team at all.

The recommendations of the consultants were that the staff work together more closely so that they could reinforce each other's work. They asked that teachers have the parents work with the child at home. Academically, it was recommended that they move the child into formal reading so that she could use it as a reinforcement for language she was learning in class and could increase her exposure to language she was missing entirely. The principal threw his weight behind these suggestions, and the team came alive.

When the consultants returned 2 months later, there had been a noticeable change in the way the staff was working with Jennifer, and in Jennifer herself. She was no longer giving vague responses and was rapidly learning to read. The principal was deeply involved in her program and took charge of everything.

The agency has continued to follow her over the past 2 years. A consultant makes five visits to the school each year to observe her, talk with her teachers, and make suggestions. Last year, Jennifer went through a comprehensive educational evaluation, which showed that she is above grade level in most subjects. Test results show, however, that she is beginning to have difficulty with some important reading skills as a result of her hearing loss, and so the team is increasing their efforts in these areas to prevent slippage. The staff of the evaluation program concluded that Jennifer is appropriately placed in the mainstream, and they recommended that she continue there. Unfortunately, she is continuing to experience downward changes in her hearing levels.

John

John is 22 years old and is about to graduate from college. He has a congenital, profound loss with a better-ear average of 103 dB. His deafness is of unknown origin. John graduated from a school for the deaf on the eighth grade level and entered a regular ninth grade in a Catholic high school as a fully mainstreamed student.

The mainstream consultant assisted John and his school in this transition to the new school and, through a rather complicated set-up, provided him with the following support services:

- Academic tutoring
- Communication therapy
- Teacher in-service
- Note taking
- FM system
- Periodic school observations
- Periodic telephone contact—student
- Periodic telephone contact—school
- Monthly newsletter on mainstreaming

The consultant required John to be the center of his support program from the very beginning. No service was provided without first talking it over with him and getting his approval. John also assisted in orienting the professionals who worked with him, and the consultant helped him evaluate this support program at the end of each year. John decided which services would be continued the following year. Some of these support services were provided at the expense of his town, others at the expense of his family.

John did his best work in courses in which the emphasis was on factual information. Courses that dealt with abstractions, such as religion and literature, were not beyond his ability but required much more time and work with his tutor. From all reports, John threw himself into the life of the school. He played soccer and joined the ski club. The school commented that he knew a lot of students, but they did not observe development of any real friendships. His group of friends seemed to include former Clarke School students, whom he saw on weekends. Over the course of the next 4 years, his academic tutor died of a heart attack, he had two other tutors, and his guidance counselor changed three times.

The first year in his new school, he decided to run for class treasurer. His history teacher was against the idea and told him and his parents that he would be "a burden to the other officers and would not be able to handle his responsibilities." Most other school staff disagreed and encouraged him to go ahead. The students elected him by a wide margin, and he served with no difficulty.

When he was a sophomore, he signed up to take Spanish. The teacher of the course would not let him enter the classroom because she said it was "a moral issue." The matter finally ended up in the principal's office, and John lost. He waited until the following year, when a different teacher taught the course, and completed it with high marks.

In addition to the aforementioned support services, the consultant's job during these years was to consult regularly with John, his parents, and the school staff; to answer their questions about difficulties in class; and to provide information about the abilities of deaf people. In addition, the consultant helped John and his support team develop a set of realistic goals and maintain their focus through the ups and downs of the daily grind.

When he began looking for colleges during his senior year, he indicated that he wanted to become a lawyer. His guidance counselor advised him against this saying that he was shooting too high. Further, she said it would be better if he just went to a well-known technical college like the other deaf students. John went ahead without her and was accepted at an excellent small college on the East Coast to study pre-law.

He is now a senior in college, having passed all of his courses, having served as the treasurer of his class all 4 years, and having been active in many campus social events. During these years, services provided to facilitate mainstreaming included

- inservice orientation for the teaching staff
- periodic consultation with support staff
- training of oral interpreters
- guidance in peer note taking
- ongoing guidance to John

During John's years in college, he has had the same kind of struggles with doubting staff that he did in high school. Year by year, however, he has made his way through, growing in his sophistication about the best ways to deal with people who do not understand his disability. In his final year of college, our consultant has had only a minor role in John's program because he and the college felt that he could take more responsibility on his own shoulders. At last check, John was doing well and enjoying his senior year. Last summer, John took an LSAT preparation course and found it helpful in preparing him for the real test. He is continuing to look for a suitable program.

These two profiles have illustrated some of the difficulties—even barriers—faced by students with hearing loss. By being in a regular school that was designed for students who can hear, they regularly meet situations in which the sense of hearing plays a critical role. In addition, people who are unfamiliar with the effects of not being able to hear regularly impose preconceived ideas on students' efforts to participate. If we are going to place these students in such a challenging atmosphere, we have a responsibility to make it possible for them to succeed.

SUMMARY

Hearing loss has complex implications. It affects a child's intellectual abilities, self-image, academic strengths and weaknesses, language development, communication abilities, and self-esteem. It influences a child's connection to her family, her community, and her world. Because language is the foundation of all human connections, hearing loss presents one of the most complex disabilities with which a person must cope. It is also one of the most profound challenges that a professional can face.

REFERENCES

1. Birch JW. *Hearing-impaired pupils in the mainstream.* Minneapolis: Leadership Training Institute/Special University of Minnesota; 1975.
2. Nix GW, ed. *Mainstream education for hearing-impaired children and youth.* New York: Grune & Stratton; 1976.
3. Ross M, ed. *Hearing-impaired children in the mainstream.* Parkton, MD: York Press; 1990.
4. Stainback S, Stainback W, Forest M, eds. *Educating all students in the mainstream of regular education.* Baltimore: P.H. Brookes; 1989.
5. Chenoweth, K. *Creating schools for all our students: what 12 schools have to say.* Reston, VA: The Council for Exceptional Children; 1994.

CHAPTER 50

Childhood Deafness

The Complexities of Management

Arthur Boothroyd

Complex problems attract simple solutions. Examples abound in international affairs, economics, government, poverty, crime, and medicine. Whenever the opportunity arises to apply simple solutions, they are ineffective at best and disastrous at worst. In the meantime, any real progress is made by individuals and groups who recognize the complexities of the problems and seek to understand their many dimensions. Progress is usually slow, the solutions are never simple, and the efforts often face criticism and interference from those with simpler views of the world.

So it is with childhood deafness. Absence of the sense of hearing during the early years of development can have multiple, serious, and far-reaching consequences. The severity of the consequences depends on interactions among numerous factors—some internal to the child, some a function of the child's immediate family, some a function of the educational system, and some a function of society at large. Yet, there has never been a shortage of advocates for simple solutions. Hearing aids, tactile aids, cochlear implants, oral education, auditory-verbal therapy, American Sign Language, total communication, signed English, cued speech, residential schools, mainstreaming—each solution has or has had its champions as a blanket solution to the problems of childhood deafness. Examples in which each solution has played a key role in the successful management of specific individuals can be found. But the concept of one best approach to prosthetic, communicative, or educational management for all deaf children is untenable. Management must have many components, each component must be tailored to individual needs, and the components must be coordinated.

With the advent of the cochlear implant as a viable treatment for profound childhood deafness, the medical community has become more involved in management than was previously the case. For this reason, physicians and surgeons have an increasing need for insight into the developmental implications of deafness and the complexities of management. These are the topics of this chapter.

The concept of deafness as a problem, a disorder, a disease, or a handicap is anathema to many members of the deaf community, which exists as an identifiable culture with its own language (in the United States, American Sign Language [ASL]), its own social mores, and even its own brand of humor (1). The more extreme members are opposed to devices such as hearing aids and cochlear implants that seek to reduce deafness, and they are opposed to educational practices that include the teaching of spoken language. To them, deafness is not a liability that needs to be compensated but an asset that is placed at risk by ill-informed physicians, surgeons, parents, and educators. In recent years, some nondeaf authors have provided literary support for the deaf community's point of view (2–4). The arguments are not without merit. The deaf child with deaf parents who are members of the deaf culture will learn sign language as easily and as quickly as a hearing child learns to speak (5). There will be no constraints on the child's ability to communicate, to learn, to work, and to form relationships within the deaf culture. It is unlikely that the child will acquire high levels of competence with written English (6), and this problem may limit the child's opportunities for learning and earning, but it need not stand in the way of a complete, fulfilling life.

Nine of ten deaf children, however, are born to hearing parents who live and work in a hearing speaking culture. Those parents want their child to assimilate into their own culture. They may later realize the benefits of the child's assimilation into the deaf culture, but even then their hope will be a bicultural child with whom they can communicate freely and who has a full range of options for employment and socialization as an adult. The key to membership in the prevailing culture is spoken language and its written deriva-

A. Boothroyd: Department of Speech and Hearing Sciences, Graduate School, City University of New York, New York, New York 10036.

tive hearing is the key to spontaneous acquisition of that language. Herein lies the problem.

HUMAN DEVELOPMENT

Human development is the process by which a dependent newborn is transformed into an independent adult. It occurs through a series of overlapping stages, the transition from one stage to the next determined by the interplay between genetically determined drives and capacities, environmental influences, and skills and knowledge acquired in previous stages (7). Development also takes place in parallel areas—anatomic, motoric, cognitive, linguistic, communicative, social, emotional, and intellectual. Under ideal circumstances, these areas develop in synchrony and to mutual benefit—readiness in one area coincides with needs in another area (8,9). The areas also develop in synchrony and interaction with environmental factors, first in the family, then in school, and later in society at large.

Language plays a pivotal role in the developmental process. Language is, basically, a code by which individuals can externalize and exchange the results of conceptually organized thought. Once acquired, between 2 and 4 years of age, language becomes both the primary avenue for learning and the primary tool for social interaction (10,11). The acquisition of language has no influence on anatomic and motoric development, but in all other areas—cognitive, communicative, social, emotional, and intellectual—it is the key that unlocks the full capacities of the human species (12,14).

Figure 1 encapsulates the developmental process. In response to innate capacities and drives and in interaction with early family environment, the child builds a basic knowledge of the spatial and temporal properties of the world, the materials and objects that occupy that world, their attributes and relationships, the events in which they become involved, and the attributes, relationships, causes, and effects of those events. This aspect of development is called *cognition*. At the same time, the child builds a basic knowledge of the special class of objects called people, and of the attributes, relationships, events, and causes effects that are special to people and their behaviors. This aspect of development is referred to as *social cognition* (15).

In particular, the child learns that *language* is used by people to convey information, request information, and control behavior. The child acquires basic command of that language, as both receiver and sender, by learning its sounds (*phonology*), words (*vocabulary*), and the rules by which words are combined to make sentences (*syntax*). The child also learns the ways in which sounds, words, and sentences are used express meaning (*semantics*), and the ways in which meaningful sentences are used for communication among people (*pragmatics*) (16). Once the basics of language are mastered, language becomes the primary avenue for the acquisition of knowledge and skills and for the development of mature social skills and a healthy self-image. These aspects of development, acquired through interaction within the school, home, and play environments, prepare the way for the competent adult who can earn a living, enter into healthy relationships, and enjoy meaningful leisure activities.

Several things should be noted about Figure 1. First, the arrows are bidirectional to symbolize mutual enhancement. The family environment, for example, not only influences the child's early language and social development but is in turn influenced by it. In a very real sense, the normally developing child helps to create an environment that meets his emerging needs. Perhaps the most beautiful example of this is the infant's smile in response to the mother's face—a

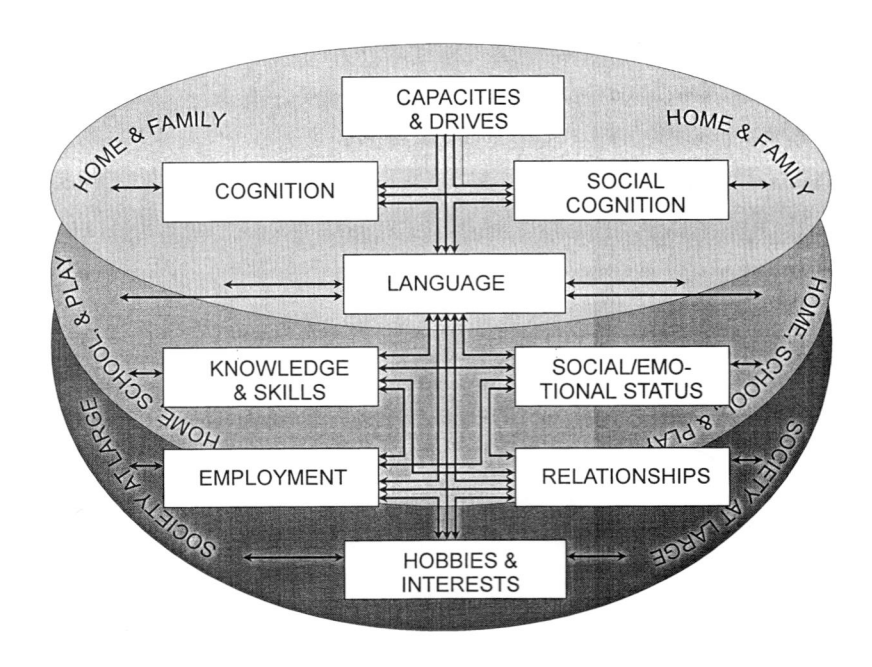

FIG. 1. Schematic representation of the processes involved in human development, emphasizing the key role played by language.

response that helps ensure the continued presence of that face (17). Note, also, the gross division of developmental areas of attainment on the left (intellect, skills, employment) and areas of affiliation on the right (social-emotional status, relationships). In the fully developed individual, these potentially conflicting areas are brought into balance (18). Note finally that, although Figure 1 is intended to stress the central role of language, it remains silent about the form of that language. This basic model applies equally well to the deaf child using sign language as it does to the hearing child learning spoken language (19).

DEVELOPMENTAL CONSEQUENCES OF CHILDHOOD DEAFNESS

For the normally developing child, the capacities in the top box of Figure 1 include normal hearing. Hearing provides access to the sound patterns of spoken language. Through hearing, the child learns the sounds, words, and sentence patterns of his language and learns to control his own speech mechanism to produce the same patterns (20).

For the profoundly deaf child born to hearing parents that vital link is broken. Other drives and capacities are present, and basic cognitive and social development begins; but without auditory access to the speech sounds of self and others, spoken language competence cannot follow—at least, not spontaneously. Thus, without intervention, what begins as a sensory deficit quickly becomes a language deficit (21). A hearing loss of 60 dB is enough to prevent audibility of the speech of others at conversational distance, and a loss of 90 dB is enough to prevent the child from hearing his own speech efforts (22).

Because of the central role of language in development, any language deficit quickly causes deficits in other areas. Learning is slow, difficult, and remains constrained to direct experience. The resulting deficits of knowledge and skill, together with the deficits of language, place severe limitations on opportunities for gainful employment. The asynchrony between developing needs and the language, knowledge, and skills required to meet those needs undermine self-image and interfere with the development of social skills. The resulting social-emotional deficits not only affect the child's ability to develop and sustain relationships, but they also increase the negative implications for employment (5).

As if the internal developmental consequences were not enough, the instinctive reactions of the deaf infant's parents tend to exacerbate the problems caused by the deafness. Because the child does not hear, the parents are less likely to expose the child to meaningful sound. Because the child does not talk, they are less likely to talk to the child. Because the deafness undermines their own self-confidence, the parents' ability to provide the child with the necessary reassurance, discipline, guidance, and support is at risk. And their emotional rejection of the child's deafness can easily come into conflict with the child's need for complete emotional acceptance as he or she is—including the deafness (8).

The instinctive, but counterproductive reactions of the parents are echoed later by society at large—in play, in school, and at work. Sometimes the very professionals who deal with childhood deafness may, in their efforts to solve problems in one area, unwittingly add problems in others areas. Consider, for example, the professional who wishes to emphasize his or her knowledge and competence to reassure parents that the management of their deaf infant is in good hands. The result may be to further undermine the parents' confidence in their own abilities to be effective. Or, consider the concept of mainstreaming, which places the deaf child in the normal educational environment to enhance knowledge, skills, and socialization. If the child lacks the necessary competence with spoken language, the resulting loneliness and isolation is intense and has negative effects on social-emotional development. All these reactions can conspire to exacerbate the problems caused by the child's deafness.

Figure 2 illustrates the unfortunate chain reaction in which the sensory deficit of deafness, by its interference with the development of spoken language, produces deficits of knowledge, skill, and social-emotional status, and eventually limits adult opportunities. The bidirectional arrows that conveyed mutual enhancement in Figure 1 convey mutual interference in Figure 2. Clearly, for the deaf child of hearing parents, intervention is mandatory.

INTERVENTION

If it were possible to restore perfect hearing by hair-cell regeneration, an implantable prosthesis, or a wearable sensory aid, and if it were possible to do so within the first year of life, all the components illustrated in Figure 1 might develop naturally. Most of the negative chain reaction caused by the child's deafness would be prevented; the only intervention required would be that of the surgeon, audiologist, or both. In fact, effective hair-cell regeneration is still only a dream and, even at their most successful, cochlear implants and hearing aids only *improve* sensory capacity—they do not restore it to normal (23,24). Intervention must, therefore, be comprehensive. In effect, each point of negative influence in Figure 2 becomes an opportunity for positive influence through intervention. The exact form of the intervention at each stage must, however, be determined by the needs and characteristics of the child and the child's family. Moreover, intervention should be considered in its totality, not in isolated compartments.

Intervention to Enhance Auditory Capacity

In terms of direct intervention with the child, the first task is to maximize and stabilize auditory capacity. This aspect of intervention is the one that most involves the physician. For that reason, it is explored at some length here, but the emphasis should not be taken as an index of relative importance. Quality sensory management is of little value unless followed by quality management in the other areas.

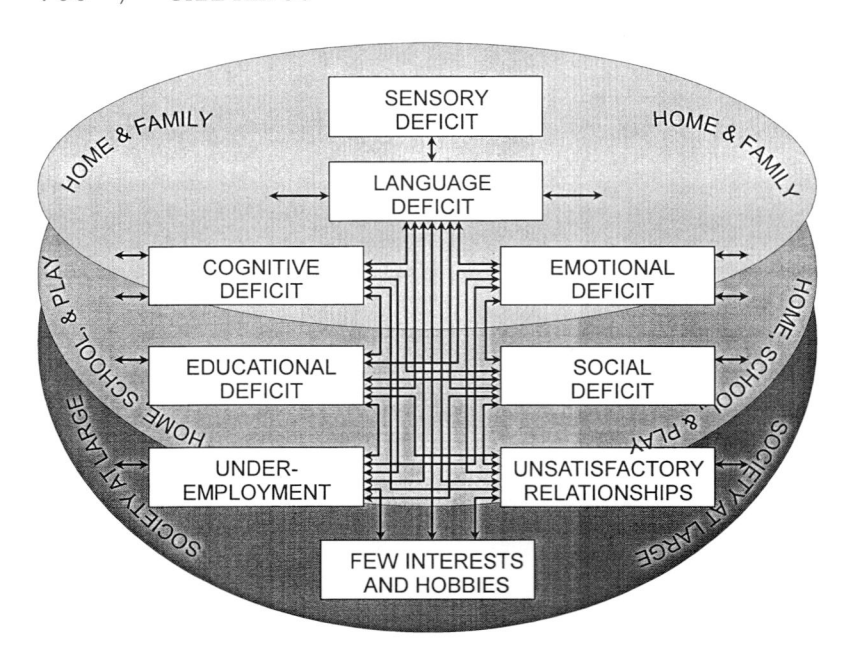

FIG. 2. Schematic representation of the negative consequences of childhood deafness. Note that the effects of deafness on language development are responsible for most negative consequences. Every block represents an opportunity for positive intervention to minimize the effects of deafness.

Components of Sensory Management

The Middle Ear

Middle ear infections should be prevented, if possible, and treated promptly if they occur. Even normally hearing children are known to suffer developmental consequences from the intermittent moderate hearing loss that accompanies recurring otitis media (25). For a deaf child wearing hearing aids, an ear infection can mean the difference between hearing and not hearing.

Hearing Aids

Hearing aids should be fitted promptly and properly. There are four identifiable stages to hearing aid fitting: prescription, selection, confirmation, and validation. *Prescription* involves the specification of desired characteristics on the basis of information about the subject and knowledge of the acoustics of speech and noise; *selection* involves finding or adjusting an instrument to match the prescription as closely as possible; *confirmation* involves measuring acoustic performance on the subject to determine that the goals of prescription have been met; *validation* is the process of determining whether the prescription was appropriate in the first place, that is, that auditory capacity has been brought to the highest possible level (26).

The physician needs to understand that the satisfactory completion of these four steps, even for the cooperative adult, requires considerable skill and knowledge combined with years of experience. Moreover, several prescriptive schemes are in use; the resulting prescriptions are often incompatible with the limitations of hearing aid technology; hearing aid testing in situ is not universally practiced; and clinicians and researchers are still seeking appropriate methods of outcome assessment (27).

Hearing aid fitting is infinitely more difficult in young children than in adults (28). Typically, the only available predictor measure is pure-tone threshold. Measuring threshold in young deaf children is not always easy, even with the development of electrophysiologic indices such as the auditory brain stem response. To make matters worse, the problems of assessment and prescription are often complicated by the presence of other impairments, and the child, unlike the adult, cannot provide the audiologist with verbal feedback about the results of the fitting. In addition, validation for a pediatric hearing aid fitting is a long-term process that occurs over a period of time ranging from months to years.

Proper fitting of hearing aids to young deaf children calls for the highest levels of expertise. If the physician is in the position of referring for a pediatric hearing aid fitting, it is imperative to find a facility with the necessary skills and experience. Ideally, the facility should also be the one in which the child can be seen on a regular basis and in which the other aspects of child and parent management can be handled.

The expected auditory capacity of a deaf child wearing a hearing aid depends, to a great extent, on the degree of hearing loss (22,29,30). Severely deaf children (losses in the 60–90 dB range) can become, essentially, hard of hearing. With hearing aids, they have the opportunity for much spontaneous and incidental learning. Their own speech, though containing errors of vowel and consonant production can have very natural rhythm and melody. These children may be able to hold unstructured conversations over the telephone, and in the absence of other learning disabilities, they may be able to function in schools for hearing children.

Profoundly deaf children (losses in the 90–110 dB range) form a heterogeneous group. With appropriate training, some may meet the description for severely deaf children.

As a group, however, profoundly deaf children are highly dependent on quality instruction for learning, especially of spoken language skills. Their hearing may accelerate that learning and help them attain better results, but it will often be a support to speechreading. Even after good training, their speech may sound unnatural and be difficult for strangers to understand.

When the deafness is near-total (losses in excess of 110 dB) hearing aids provide only minimal help, mainly in terms of environmental sound awareness, perception of temporal patterns, and monitoring of voice level. It is very unlikely that a congenitally deaf or prelingually deafened child, with a hearing loss in excess of 110 dB, wearing hearing aids and being educated in an oral environment, will acquire speech that can be understood by persons other than those with whom the child has regular daily contact.

Thus, although the need for early proper amplification is undeniable, the resulting auditory capacity is very different from child to child. These differences have implications for the severity of the consequences of the hearing impairment and for the type and intensity of intervention needed in other areas of development.

Cochlear Implants

For children whose aided auditory capacity is small, the possibility now exists for the use of cochlear implants. This group includes all children with losses in excess of 110 dB and many children with losses in the range of 90 to 110 dB. The decision to implant must be based on numerous factors in addition to the degree of hearing loss. Not least is the availability of appropriate management once the implant has been provided. As with hearing aids, results differ from child to child. On the basis of results obtained to date, roughly 30% of children who receive implants can be expected to gain auditory capacity similar to that enjoyed by severely deaf children who wear hearing aids (31). Most of the remainder perform like profoundly deaf children who wear hearing aids, and an unfortunate few gain little or no auditory capacity. The exact reasons for intersubject differences are not clear, but the last group probably lacks the necessary stimulable neural tissue (24).

Goals of Sensory Management

The sole purpose of hearing aids and cochlear implants is to increase auditory capacity. Even when this goal has been accomplished successfully, the result is still a child with a serious hearing problem. The subsequent management of the child may have been made easier, and the prognosis for the child's success may have been improved, but the remaining issues of management do not go away once the aid or implant has been fitted. In fact, the need for excellent auditory and spoken language management is, in a sense, increased rather than diminished by successful prosthetic intervention.

Speechreading

When perceiving speech in face-to-face conversation, the deaf child is not limited to the sensory information that can be obtained via hearing aids and cochlear implants. Speechreading (also known as lipreading) provides valuable additional input. When the child receives a lot of information auditorily, speechreading functions as a valuable supplement to hearing. For the child with limited auditory capacity, the situation is reversed; hearing functions as a valuable supplement to speechreading. For the few who have no auditory capacity, speechreading becomes the sole source of sensory evidence about speech (32).

There are many misconceptions about speechreading. Although a fair amount of information about speech can be seen by watching movements of the lips, jaw, and tongue tip, this information is by no means complete. Activities of the breathing mechanism, the larynx, the velum, and the tongue body—all essential to the speech process—are invisible. It is generally estimated that only about one third of the information content of speech is visible to the speechreader. This figure seems at variance with the fact that there are highly proficient speechreaders who seldom make mistakes in face-to-face conversation. These individuals, however, do not see more than the indifferent speechreader. Instead, they are very adept at using the linguistic and situational contexts to fill in the missing information. It is wrong, therefore, to think that speechreading can function as a simple alternative to hearing. The deaf child who has yet to develop spoken language has no idea what is missing from the visual input. Moreover, the absence of information about activities of the breathing mechanism, the larynx, and the velum, make it impossible for the child to learn how to produce intelligible speech via speechreading alone.

In spite of many years of effort, researchers have been unable to identify specific underlying skills or capacities that mark the competent speechreader. Nor have they found a way of converting an indifferent speechreader into a highly proficient speechreader by training. Nevertheless, it is self-apparent that language competence, and an extensive knowledge of the world to which language refers, are prerequisites. In other words, the deaf child acquires competence in speechreading, not by specific training in the art, but as a by-product of language development, cognitive development, general education, and experience with face-to-face communication.

Bimodal Perception

Although the ability to understand speech by speechreading alone appears to be more of a gift than a trainable skill, the ability to *integrate* vision with hearing appears to be a universal trait (33). Normally hearing individuals typically recognize only about 30% of the words in sentences when forced to function by speechreading alone. If, however, they are able to hear just a little of the speech at the same time, their performance typically rises to 70 or 80% correct, without practice (34), and this remains true even when the auditory signal by itself does not permit recognition of any words. One reason for this spontaneous integration is that the most easily observed visual information is exactly that which tends to be lost when one listens in noise or under the constraints of a hearing impairment. In other words, the visual and auditory information tend to be complementary. Another reason is that the visual and auditory information arise from a single source, namely, the speech gestures that represent the sounds, words, and sentences of spoken language. Human beings are particularly adept at integrating information from multiple sources to form a single percept.

Perceptual Training

The foregoing comments may appear to be at variance with the opinions of some educators who believe that the only way to develop effective auditory skills in hearing-impaired children is to withhold visual input.[1] There is, in fact, a school of auditory-verbal therapy in which the therapist covers his or her mouth when talking to the child and encourages parents and classroom teachers to do the same. There is no evidence to show that vision and hearing ever interfere with each other in the development of spoken language in the deaf child. In fact, all the available evidence is of integration (35).[2]

There may, however, be good justification for giving the child opportunities to function by hearing alone during one-on-one training. The goals could be to draw attention to aspects of speech that may be available only through that modality and to give confidence in situations in which visual speech information is simply unavailable from the talker (e.g., the heavily bearded talker, the teacher who talks to the chalkboard, the friend talking over the telephone) (36). When, however, the focus is on the use of spoken language skills for face-to-face communication, learning, or both, the withholding of visual input is counterproductive at best. It is one thing to exercise a weakness in therapy and training but another to deny the use of a strength in everyday life. Physicians and surgeons should be aware of this methodologic issue when counseling parents or referring for management.

Intervention to Optimize the Family and Home Environment

As soon as deafness is identified in a young child, the process of parent guidance must begin. The process is lengthy and requires extreme care and understanding (37).

There are many goals. The parents need support as they deal with issues of guilt and as they work through their grief at the loss of the perfect child; they need to learn about prosthetic and educational options and their strengths and weaknesses; they need to observe different kinds of educational program in action; they need to meet successful deaf adults and to learn that deafness need not compromise quality of life; they need to learn how they can enrich the experiential, auditory, and language environment for their child without giving up the role of parent and taking on that of teacher; they need help in developing strategies to deal with the pressures that will come from well-meaning but ill-informed relatives, friends, and professionals; most of all, they need to develop confidence in their ability to be competent parents of a deaf child.

Numerous research studies have shown that deaf children of deaf parents fare better than do deaf children of hearing parents on a variety of measures including both attainment and social-emotional development (5). The difference is commonly attributed to the early use of sign language. There are, however, a small number of *oral* deaf children of *oral* deaf parents and they, too, tend to fare better than do oral deaf children of hearing parents (38). This finding is explained if one assumes that it is not the form of language that is important but the fact that deaf parents are not troubled by the birth of a deaf child. They are able to get on with the job of parenting, environmental enrichment, and decision making; they know, instinctively, how to establish communication with the child; and they do not have to deal with guilt, insecurity, or the fear that the child will have no future. The goal of parent guidance is, in a sense, to achieve the same result for hearing parents.

Intervention to Enhance Cognitive and Social-Cognitive Development

It was indicated earlier that basic cognitive and social-cognitive development are not at risk when the child is deaf. Nevertheless, the impact of the deafness on language development and on the later stages of cognitive and social-cognitive development can be minimized by providing as solid a cognitive foundation as possible. This goal is addressed by providing the child with a rich physical and social environment. It is also addressed by giving the child the security and self-confidence that encourages and reinforces exploration of, and interaction with that environment. These conditions are established through parent guidance. As the child matures, placement in a stimulating, cognitively oriented preschool or nursery program may help further address the child's cognitive and social-cognitive needs.

Intervention to Promote Language Development

The parents are in the best position to facilitate language development. They do this by talking to the child and reinforcing attempts to talk back. The talk, however, should not

---

[1] Ironically, the first introduction of classroom amplification into schools for the deaf in the 1940s met with opposition because teachers were convinced that the use of hearing would interfere with speechreading.

[2] See, however, the focus issue of *Volta Review* (31), dealing with the auditory-verbal approach.

be indiscriminate but should deal with things the child understands. At the same time, the child should be helped to learn that talking is a good way of giving and getting information and that it is a socially acceptable way of attempting to control the behavior of others. Through parental guidance the appropriate techniques can be demonstrated and practiced. The goal should be to integrate the enriched language environment into the child's activities of daily living and into regular play sessions. It is not the parents' job to be teachers of their child but to make the most of natural opportunities for interaction and communication. As the child matures, there may be good reason to add more formal language work in one-on-one therapy and specialized preschool settings. This becomes especially important if the parents are unable to provide enough input by virtue of work demands or a limited aptitude.

Educators have long disagreed about the appropriate language modality for use with deaf children. Should they learn spoken language only (the oral approach), sign language only (the manual approach), or spoken and signed language together (the total communication approach)? Within these options there are further disagreements about methodologic details. These options, (discussed in more length in the next section), present the hearing parents of deaf children with a confusing set of choices. Each choice offers certain benefits but, at the same time, it carries risks. Good management involves maximizing the benefits while minimizing the risks. Parents need the help of knowledgeable, experienced, objective, caring professionals as they come to terms with these issues and develop the confidence to make long-term choices for themselves and their child.

Educational Intervention

The history of education of the deaf is long and fascinating. It is also filled with disagreement and debate, much of it acrimonious. Most of the disagreement, which continues today, centers around the form of language in which classroom instruction should occur. Oral methods involve the exclusive use of spoken language throughout the period of formal instruction. Sign language methods involve the exclusive use of ASL for instruction but introduce the written form of spoken language as an academic subject. Total communication methods seek a middle road by the simultaneous use of spoken and signed language.

The arguments in favor of an oral approach are that spoken language is the language of the culture; that competence in spoken language is a prerequisite for competence in written language, without which the accumulated knowledge of the world is virtually inaccessible; that spoken and written language competence provide the maximum freedom of vocational and social choice in adult life; that spoken language "immersion" is the only way to ensure functional competence; and that access to sign language in the early years impedes the acquisition of functional competence.

When oral education works well, the benefits cannot be denied. Numerous examples exist of highly successful, orally trained deaf adults. Unfortunately, however, an oral education is no guarantee of competence in spoken and written language. A primary correlate of success is aided (or implanted) auditory capacity. In other words, the less the auditory capacity, the lower the probability of effective spoken and written language. Other correlates include the aptitudes of the child; the absence of secondary impairments; supportive, committed, and informed parents; experienced, competent teachers; and well-managed schools with a coordinated and integrated curriculum. There are, also interactions among these variables. The deafer the child, for example, the more dependent the child becomes on innate aptitude for language and on the qualities of his teachers and the school in which they work. Moreover, the child who does not make adequate progress in an oral environment is exposed to multiple risks. Not the least of these risks is the damage to social and emotional well-being caused by poor communication skills and low attainments. Moreover, if the child fails to acquire adequate competence in spoken and written language, there is no alternative to fall back on.

Not many years ago, there was general adoption of an oral philosophy in American schools for the deaf—regardless of the needs and aptitudes of individual students and in spite of a shortage of adequately trained or supervised teachers. The disappointing results led to general condemnation of the oral philosophy (rather than an indictment of the simplistic approach to a complex problem). The decision to pursue the oral option should not, therefore, be made lightly. Many aspects of the child, the family, and of the available programs must be taken into account.

The arguments in favor of a total communication approach are that the child should be free to use all capabilities both for language learning and for general education; that the acquisition of sign as a primary language enhances rather than impedes the acquisition of speech as a second language; and that the inherent disparity of form between signed and spoken language can be removed by developing a modified sign language whose structures (e.g., sentence patterns and word endings) follow the patterns of spoken language. At its best, the implementation of a total communication philosophy would look like a first-class oral program with the addition of sign language, thus optimizing and accelerating classroom instruction and providing communicative competence to all students, regardless of auditory capacity or spoken language aptitude.

In practice, however, the availability of sign for communication lowers the priority given to auditory management and spoken-language instruction. There is no evidence that the use of artificial sign languages with the syntax of spoken language accelerates the acquisition of spoken or written language competence. As with attempts to mass produce oral education, however, it may not be the philosophy that is at fault as much as its implementation. A characteristic of the normal child is that the child learns in spite of the inadequacies of the educational system. The deaf child, however, fails to learn because of those inadequacies, regardless of stated philosophy.

On the positive side, it should be noted that free use of a fully accessible sign language removes the tensions caused by comprehension problems in the classroom and helps to foster good social-emotional development, at least within the school environment. A deaf child in a mediocre total communication program is likely to fare better, in terms of affiliation and achievement, than does a similar child in a mediocre oral program.

Frustrated by the failure of the wholesale shift from oral to total communication methods to produce significant changes of outcome, many educators now advocate the exclusive use of ASL as the medium for classroom instruction. The arguments are that the child eventually assimilates into the deaf culture; that the child needs the kind of competence in the language of that culture that can only be attained by a first-language learner; that high levels of spoken language competence are unlikely to be attained by the deaf child; that the child will always be relegated to an inferior role within the hearing culture; and that attempts to modify sign language to fit the form of spoken language are not only futile but detract from the inherent power of sign language.

The last argument is not without validity. Languages exist not by edict but as the outcome of evolutionary forces. What works well survives, what does not work well is changed. Structures that work well in spoken language do not necessarily work well in sign language, and vice versa. To put it simply, signed English is neither sign language nor English. The first argument that most deaf children of hearing parents eventually seek assimilation into the deaf culture to the exclusion of the culture of their parents, is open to question. Moreover, the idea that the deaf child of hearing parents can easily acquire sign language as a first language is without merit. Hearing parents who learn sign language to communicate with their deaf infant, regardless of the depth of their commitment, seldom become competent enough to create the kind of language environment that would be available to the deaf child of deaf parents.

For the deaf child with adequate levels of language competence, mainstreaming is often a viable option. As with oral education, however, this is not an option to be taken lightly. The academic demands are likely to be considerable, and there is a serious risk of social isolation. The decision to mainstream should be made only when justified by the child's language competence and social-emotional status. Moreover, it should be accompanied by education and orientation of both the teachers and the students with whom the deaf child interacts. Monitoring and educational support are also called for (see Chapter 49).

In recent years, there has been a trend toward mainstreaming deaf children whose primary language is sign language. Such children are provided with sign language interpreters for classroom instruction. Although the opportunities for learning may be enhanced by this step, the social-emotional risks are self-evident. Once again, this is not an option to be taken lightly.

Intervention to Promote Social-Emotional Development

One of the dangers of childhood deafness and its management is a focus on issues of attainment to the exclusion of issues of affiliation. Parents and professionals can become so involved in promoting the child's language development and educational attainment that the equally pressing needs for a healthy self-image and effective social skills are pushed to the background (39). A major component of effective management at all stages is to promote a balance between the two aspects of development. This is accomplished through parental guidance, careful program choices, and, if necessary one-on-one counseling during the school years. Attention to issues of self-image and social competence within the context of an effective educational program are hallmarks of a first-class school.

Intervention to Promote Vocational Options

Although this chapter is concerned primarily with the young deaf child, physicians should know that the past few decades have seen remarkable improvements in career preparation for young deaf adults. The American Academy of Sciences has a special program to promote careers in science and research for individuals with impairments. Gallaudet University and the National Technical Institute for the Deaf provide opportunities for liberal arts and technical education at the postsecondary level, and the latter has been very effective in developing career training and placement programs for deaf graduates. In addition, universities and colleges around the United States offer tutoring, counseling, note taking, and interpreting services for deaf students. Although it may seem premature to be thinking of college and jobs when a 1-year-old child is found to have a profound sensorineural hearing loss, it will be important in the following months for the child's parents to know that such opportunities exist.

CONCLUSION

The parents of the deaf child must make many choices. These choices are typically made because of the potential gains. But deafness is not simple, and no choice, whether it is prosthetic intervention, therapeutic management, or educational placement, comes without costs. For each choice the parents need to understand the alternatives, their benefits and costs in relation to the characteristics of their own child, and, having made a choice, what they can do to enhance the benefits while minimizing the costs. The physician or surgeon, though not directly involved in decisions beyond those of medical and prosthetic management, can, given an appropriate perspective, play an important role in counseling and referral. That perspective should acknowledge the complexities of the problem and the dangers of offering simple solutions.

ACKNOWLEDGMENT

Preparation of this chapter supported in part by the National Insitute on Deafness and Other Communication Disorders (NIDCD) grant No. DC00178.

REFERENCES

1. Benderley BL. *Dancing without music: deafness in America.* New York: Anchor Press-Doubleday; 1980.
2. Lane H. Cochlear implants are wrong for young deaf children. *Nat Assoc Deaf Broadcaster* 1992;14:1, 5, 9.
3. Lane H. *The mask of benevolence: disabling the deaf community.* New York: Knopf; 1992.
4. Sacks O. *Seeing voices: a journey into the world of the deaf.* Berkeley: University of California Press; 1989.
5. Schlesinger H, Meadow K. *Sound and sign: childhood deafness and mental health.* Berkeley: University of California Press; 1972.
6. Commission on Education of the Deaf. (1988). *Towards equality: report of the Presidential Commission on Education of the Deaf.* Washington, DC: US Government Printing Office; 1988.
7. Craig G. *Human development.* Englewood Cliffs, NJ: Prentice-Hall; 1976.
8. Boothroyd A. *Hearing impairments in young children.* Washington, DC: Alexander Graham Bell Association for the Deaf; 1988.
9. Sroufe A. The coherence of individual development: early care, attachment, and subsequent developmental issues. In: Damon W ed. *Social and personality development: essays on growth of the child.* New York: WW Norton; 1983.
10. Bloom L. *Language development from two to three.* New York: Cambridge University Press; 1991.
11. De Villiers P, De Villiers J. *Language acquisition.* Cambridge: Harvard University Press; 1978.
12. Piaget J. *The language and thought of the child.* New York: World; 1962.
13. Vygotsky L. *Thought and language.* Cambridge: MIT Press; 1962.
14. Wood D. *How children think and learn.* Cambridge: Basil Blackwell; 1989.
15. Butterworth G, Light P. eds. *Social cognition.* Chicago: University of Chicago Press; 1982.
16. Gleason JB. *The development of language.* New York: MacMillan; 1993.
17. Brazelton TB, Tronick E. Preverbal communication between mothers and infants. In: Damon W ed. *Social and personality development: essays on the growth of the child.* New York: WW Norton; 1983.
18. Erikson EH. *Childhood and society.* New York: WW Norton; 1963.
19. Rodda M, Grove C. *Language, cognition, and deafness.* Hillsdale, NJ: Lawrence Erlbaum; 1987.
20. Fry DB. The role and primacy of the auditory channel in speech and language development. In: Ross M, Giolas TG, ed. *Auditory management of hearing-impaired children.* Baltimore: University Park Press; 1978.
21. Paul P, Quigley S. *Language and deafness.* San Diego: Singular Publishing; 1994.
22. Boothroyd A. Profound deafness and cochlear implants. In: Tyler R ed. *Cochlear implants* San Diego: Singular Press; 1993.
23. Studebaker GA, Hochberg I. eds. *Acoustical factors affecting hearing aid performance.* 2nd ed. Boston: Allyn and Bacon; 1993.
24. Tyler RS. ed. *Cochlear implants: audiological considerations.* San Diego: Singular Publishing; 1993.
25. Kavanagh JF. *Otitis media and child development.* Parkton, MD: York; 1986.
26. Skinner MW. *Hearing aid evaluation.* Englewood Cliffs, NJ: Prentice-Hall; 1988.
27. Studebaker GA, Bess FH, Beck LB. *The Vanderbilt hearing aid report II.* Timonium, MD: York; 1991.
28. Feigin JA, Stelmachowicz PG, eds. *Pediatric amplification.* Omaha: Boys Town National Research Hospital; 1991.
29. Boothroyd A. Auditory perception of speech contrasts by subjects with sensorineural hearing loss. *J Speech Hear Res* 1984;27:134–144.
30. Boothroyd A. Speech perception, sensorineural hearing loss, and hearing aids. In: Studebaker G, Hochberg I, eds. *Acoustical factors affecting hearing aid performance.* Boston: Allyn and Bacon; 1993 (277–279).
31. Boothroyd A, Eran O. Auditory speech perception capacity of child implantees expressed as equivalent hearing loss. *Volta Rev* 1995;95 (Suppl.): 151–168.
32. De Filippo CL, Sims DG, eds. *New reflections on speechreading.* Washington, DC: Alexander Graham Bell Association for the Deaf; 1988.
33. Massaro DW. *Speech perception by ear and eye: a paradigm for psychological enquiry.* Hillsdale, NJ: Lawrence Erlbaum; 1987.
34. Boothroyd A, Hnath-Chisolm T, Hanin L, Kishon-Rabin L. Voice fundamental frequency as an auditory supplement to the speechreading of sentences. *Ear Hear* 1988;9:306–312.
35. Boothroyd A. Speech perception and production in hearing-impaired children. In: Bess FH ed. *Amplification for children with auditory deficits.* Memphis: Vanderbilt University; 1995.
36. Wedenberg E. Auditory training of severely hard-of-hearing preschool children. *Arch Otolaryngol* 1954;110:9–82.
37. Luterman D. *Counseling parents of hearing-impaired children.* Boston: Little, Brown; 1979.
38. Corson H. *Comparing deaf children of oral deaf parents, and deaf parents using manual communication, with deaf children of hearing parents on academic, social, and communicative functioning.* [Dissertation] Cincinnati: University of Cincinnati, 1986.
39. Loeb R, Darigiani P. The impact of hearing impairment on self perceptions of children. *Volta Rev* 1986;88:89–100.

Hereditary hearing impairment disorders with eye findings (Alphabetized) Continued

Name and code	Heredity	Eye findings	Type of hearing loss	Other features
Flynn-Aird C, M, RP	AD	Myopia Cataract Retinitis pigmentosa	S	Epilepsy Skin atrophy Baldness Cystic bone changes Ataxia
Friedreich's ataxia O, RO	AR	Optic atrophy Retinal degeneration	S	Spinocerebellar degeneration Limb incoordination
Hunter C, O, RO	X	All features similar to Hurler		
Hurler C, O, RO	AR	Early corneal clouding Subnormal ERG Optic atrophy	S	Gargoyle facies Mental retardation Skeletal abnormalities Hepatosplenomegaly
Kearns-Sayre EOM, P, RP	AR	Ophthalmoplegia Ptosis Retinitis pigmentosa	M	Heart conduction defects
Laurence-Moon—Bardet-Biedl RP	AR	Retinitis pigmentosa	S	Mental retardation Hypogonadism Obesity Short stature
Leopard PC	AD	Hypertelorism	S—Variable	Pulmonary stenosis Hypogonadism ECG change—wide QRS, bundle branch Growth retardation Progressive lentigines
Mandibulofacial dysostosis (Treacher Collins) CE, PC	AD	Downward sloping palpebral fissures Coloboma in outer third of lower lid Ciliary deficiency medial to coloboma	M C—Deformities of ossicles, footplate S—Deformities of labyrinth	85% deformed pinnae EAC atresia Retrognathia Reduced malar bone Sclerotic mastoid Facial nerve anomalies
Marshall C, M	AD	Cataract Myopia	S	Saddle nose
Norrie C, I, RP	X	Cataracts in first decade Atrophic irises Yellow retinal pigment in first few weeks All become blind	S—Second to third decade, mild to severe, one third to two thirds	Mental retardation in two thirds
Osteogenesis imperfecta (van der Hoeve) SC	AD	Blue sclera	C—Otosclerosis with stapes fixation	Fragile bones Loose ligaments
Osteopetrosis (Albers-Schonberg) RO	AR	Retinal degeneration Abnormal ERG	S—Progressive	Defective absorption of immature bone Hepatosplenomegaly Macrocephaly
Oto-palatal-digital II C, Cl, PC	X	Antimongoloid slant of palpebral fissures Corneal clouding Iris coloboma	S—Congenital, severe	Micrognathia Cleft palate Flexed overlapping of fingers with finger and toe syndactyly Hydrocephalus Skeletal abnormalities Cerebellar hypoplasia Mental retardation
Piebaldness I, RP	AR X	Blue irides Fine retinal pigmentation	S	Depigmentation of hair on scalp, face, and trunk
Refsum RP	AR	Retinitis pigmentosa before third decade	S—Less severe than Usher IV Often asymmetrical	Cerebellar ataxia with onset in childhood Ichthyosis Elevated phytanic acid Hypertrophic peripheral neuropathy

(continued)

Hereditary hearing impairment disorders with eye findings (Alphabetized) Continued

Name and code	Heredity	Eye findings	Type of hearing loss	Other features
Richards-Rundel EOM	AR	Horizontal nystagmus to bilateral gazes	S—Begins in infancy	Ataxia Hypogonadism Muscle wasting in early childhood
Spondyloepiphysial dysplasia C, G, M, RO	AD	Myopia Cataracts Glaucoma Retinal degeneration	S—Mild to moderate	Short stature Cleft palate
Stickler RO	AD	Myopic retinal degeneration Retinal detachment Subnormal ERG	S	Cleft palate Micrognathia
Usher I RP	AR	Retinitis pigmentosa Nyctalopia first to second decade ERG nondetectable	S—Congenital, total	No vestibular function
Usher II RP	AR	Retinitis pigmentosa Nyctalopia second to third decade ERG variable	S—Partial	Normal vestibular function
Usher III (Hallgren) RP	AR	Retinitis pigmentosa ERG abnormal	S—Congenital, total	Vestibulocerebellar ataxia Variable psychoses (20%)
Usher IV (infantile phytanic acid storage disease) RP	AR	Retinitis pigmentosa Very abnormal ERG	S—Congenital, total	Hypotonia Mental retardation Elevated phytanic acid (lower than Refsum) No hypertrophic peripheral neuropathy (Refsum)
Unnamed RP	?	Retinitis pigmentosa	S	Enamel dysplasia
Unnamed	AR	Cryptophthalmia (65% bilateral) skin of forehead completely covering one or both eyes	M	Coloboma of nasal alae Syndactyly of toes and fingers Malformed pinnae EAC stenosis or atresia
Unnamed EOM	X	Strabismus External ophthalmoplegia Enophthalmos	S—Congenital, severe	Microcephaly Mental retardation Basal ganglia dysfunction with choreoathetosis
Unnamed C, G, I, O	AR	Aniridia Cataract Glaucoma Optic nerve hypoplasia	S—Moderate to severe	Skeletal deformities Wilm's tumor of kidney
Unnamed M, SC	AD	Myopia Blue sclera	S	Marfanoid
Waardenburg I DC-PC, I, RP, S	AD	Dystopia canthorum Synophrys Heterochromia irides Pigment disturbance of retinal pigmentary epithelium	S—Severe to profound	White forelock, poliosis Vitiligo
Waardenburg II I, RP, S	AD	No dystopia canthorum Other features same as type I	S—Moderate, low to mid frequencies	More common than type I
Waardenburg III I, P, RP, S	AD	Unilateral ptosis Other features same as type I	S	Skeletal abnormalities

AD, autosomal dominant; AR, autosomal recessive; S, sensorineural; C, conductive; M, mixed; EAC, external auditory canal; ERG, electroretinogram.

APPENDIX B

Resources

Sue Schwartz

Abledata
8455 Colesville Road Suite 935
Silver Spring, MD 20910
1-800-227-0216 (V/TTY)
Fax: (301)587-1967
An information and referral project that maintains a database of assistive technology products.

Alexander Graham Bell Association for the Deaf, Inc.
3417 Volta Place NW
Washington, DC 20007
(202)337-5220 (V/TTY)
An organization that advocates for the oral philosophy of education for children who are deaf.

American Society for Deaf Children
1820 Tribute Road, Suite A
Sacramento, CA 95815
1-800-942-ASDC (V/TTY)
An organization of parents and professionals who advocate for the sign language philosophy of education for children who are deaf.

American Speech-Language-Hearing Association
10801 Rockville Pike
Rockville, MD 20852
(301)897-5700 (V/TTY)
A professional and scientific organization for speech-language pathologists and audiologists concerned with communication disorders.

S. Schwartz: Family Services, Montgomery County Public Schools, Special Education Rockville, Maryland 20853.

Auditory-Verbal International, Inc.
2121 Eisenhower Avenue Suite 402
Alexandria, VA 22314
(703)739-1049 (voice only)
(703)739-0874 (TTY)
FAX: (703) 739-0395
An organization that promotes the Auditory-Verbal Therapy approach.

Beginnings for Parents of Hearing Impaired Children
3900 Barrett Drive, Suite 100
Durham, NC 27609
1-800-541-HEAR (V/TTY)
Provides unbiased information about communication approaches and is committed to encouraging parents to make an informed choice in this regard.

Center for Bicultural Studies, Inc.
5506 Kenilworth Avenue Suite 105
Riverdale, MD 20737-3106
(301)277-3945 (voice only)
(301)277-3944 (TTY)
FAX: (301)699-5226
Promotes public education on interaction of deaf and hearing cultures. Promotes an understanding of American Sign Language.

Gallaudet University
800 Florida Avenue NE
Washington, DC 2002-3695
(202)651-5000 (V/TTY)
The world's only 4-year liberal arts university for students who are deaf or hard-of-hearing. Offers more than 50 undergraduate and graduate degree programs in addition to summer courses.

House Ear Institute
2100 W. Third Street 5th Floor
Los Angeles, CA 90057
(213)483-4431 (voice only)
(213)484-2642 (TTY)
FAX: (213)483-8789
Information center for cochlear implants.

John Tracy Clinic
806 W. Adams Boulevard
Los Angeles, CA 90007
(213)748-5481 (voice only)
(213)747-2924 (TTY)
FAX: (213)749-1651
Provides on-site services for preschool-age children with hearing loss. In addition, provides a worldwide correspondence course to parents of children who are deaf.

National Association of the Deaf
814 Thayer Avenue
Silver Spring, MD 20910
(301)587-1788 (voice only)
(301)587-1789 (TTY)
FAX: (301)587-1791
An organization that advocates equal access by people who are deaf or hard of hearing in the areas of employment, education, telecommunication, and rehabilitation.

National Cued Speech Association
1615 B Oberlin Road
P.O. Box 31345
Raleigh, NC 27622
(919)828-1218 (V/TTY)
Provides advocacy and support regarding the use of cued speech.

National Information Center on Deafness
Gallaudet University
800 Florida Avenue NE
Washington, DC 20002-3695
(202)651-5051 (voice only)
(202)651-5052 (TTY)
FAX: (202)651-5054
Serves as a source of information on topics dealing with deafness and hearing loss.

National Institute on Deafness and Other Communication Disorders Information Clearinghouse
9000 Rockville Pike
Bethesda, MD 20892-3456
1-800-241-1044 (voice only)
1-800-241-1055 (TTY)
FAX: (301)907-8830
National resource center for information about hearing, balance, smell, taste, voice, speech, and language.

Self Help for Hard of Hearing People, Inc.
7910 Woodmont Ave. Suite 1200
Bethesda, MD 20814
(301)657-2248 (voice only)
(301)657-2249 (TTY)
FAX: (301) 913-9413
Promotes awareness and information about hearing loss, communication, assistive devices, and alternative communication skills.

Tripod
2901 N. Keystone Street
Burbank, CA 91504-1620
1-800-352-8888 (V/TTY)
FAX: (818)972-2090
Provides a toll-free hotline for parents and other individuals wanting information about rearing and educating deaf and hard-of-hearing children.

Subject Index

A
Abbé de l'épée, 683
ABG (air-bone gap), 306, 307, 609
ABR. *See* Auditory brainstem response
Absolute sensitivity, 32, 32f
Achondroplasia, 357
Acoustic immittance. *See also* Acoustic reflexes; Tympanometry
  with behavioral audiography, 113
  calibration, 123–124
  defined, 113
  in mixed hearing loss evaluation, 610–611
  personnel, 124
  purpose, 103
  screening, 119
  sensitivity, 123
  specificity, 123
  with sweep frequency tympanometry, 119–120
  test battery, 113–114
Acoustic neuromas
  neurofibromatosis type 2. *See* Neurofibromatosis type II
  radiological evaluation, 170
  vertigo and, 436–437, 436f
  vestibular schwannomas, 170, 491f
Acoustic reflex arc, 114, 114f
Acoustic reflexes
  auditory centers in, 121, 121f
  bivariate plotting procedure, 122
  calibration, 123–124
  contralateral, 121, 123
  decay, 123
  defined, 121
  detection of middle ear abnormality, 119
  for hearing-aid fitting, 123
  hearing loss prediction, 122–123
  high-frequency probe tone assessment, 122
  indications, 124
  ipsilateral, 123
  latency, 123
  loudness discomfort and, 123
  measurement, 121
  in mixed hearing loss, 610–611
  personnel, 124
  resistance of child and, 124
  sensitivity, 122, 123
  specificity, 123
  threshold, 121, 121f, 122
  with tympanometry, 113, 114
Acquired hearing loss
  classification, 375, 376t
  diagnosis, 382
  future research, 383
  management, 382–383
  Méniére's disease and, 382
  perinatal, 377–378
  postnatal, 378–380, 379f, 380t

  prenatal, 376–377
  prevention, 382
  surgical treatment, 383
Acquired immunodeficiency syndrome (AIDS). *See also* Human immunodeficiency virus
  acute mastoiditis and, 270
  facial paralysis and, 463
  immunologic defects, 479, 481–482
  sensorineural hearing loss, 484
  temporal bone findings, 483–484
Active function recording, in inflation-deflation test, 21
Acyclovir, for facial paralysis, 466
Adenocarcinoma, temporal bone, 507–508
Adenoidectomy
  complications, 249
  indications, 246
  for otitis media with effusion, 244–245
  postoperative care, 248
  procedure, 248
  technical considerations, 247
Adenomas
  middle ear, 510
  temporal bone, 510
Adhesive otitis media, 255–256, 645–646, 646f
Admittance, 113
ADPAVD (autosomal dominant noncongenital progressive audiovestibular dysfunction), 321–322, 321f–323f
AEPs. *See* Auditory evoked potentials
Age
  for auditory amplification intervention, 586
  for cochlear implantation, 596
  masking level difference and, 34, 35f
  static acoustic admittance and, 120
Agency for Health Care Policy and Research (AHCPR)
  adenoidectomy guidelines, 245
  otitis media guidelines, 252
AIDS. *See* Acquired immunodeficiency syndrome
AIED. *See* Autoimmune inner ear disease
Air-bone gap (ABG), 306, 307, 609
Albers-Schönberg disease (osteopetroses; chalk disease; marble bone disease), 221, 461, 709t
Albinism-deafness, 318
Alexander deformity, 169–170, 203, 399
Alexander Graham Bell Association for the Deaf, Inc., 681
Alignment, ocular, 369
Allele, 67
Allergy, eustachian tube function and, 19, 19t
Alport's syndrome
  candidate gene analysis, 79
  diagnosis, 318

  eye abnormalities, 708t
  hearing loss, 95–96
  types, 358, 358t
  X-linked inheritance, 62, 398
Alstrom syndrome, 708t
American National Standard Institute (ANSI), 113
American Sign Language (ASL), 675–676, 684, 703–704
American Speech-Language-Hearing Association (ASHA), tympanometry guidelines, 116–117, 119, 116f, 117t
Aminoglycoside ototoxicity, 98, 430, 329, 329f
Amoxicillin, for acute otitis media with effusion, 243
Amplification, auditory
  for adults *vs.* children, 584–586
  age of intervention, 586
  assistive listening devices
    follow-up procedures, 592
    hearing aids. *See* Hearing aids
    maximizing signal-to-noise ratio with, 590–592
    personal FM systems, 393, 590–591
  binaural, importance of, 583–584
  candidacy, 585–586
  for deaf children, 685
  diagnostic capabilities for, 584
  direct audio input, 583
  earmolds, 582–583, 583f
  financial management, 585
  hearing aids. *See* Hearing aids
  legal requirements, 585
  pediatric considerations, 590
  selection strategies, 586–587, 587f
  for sensorineural hearing loss, 402
  team members, 584
  telecoils, 583
Amplitude modulation (AM), 33
Anesthesia, for external auditory canal atresia repair, 537–538
Aneuploidy, 51
Angelman's syndrome, 64
Anisocoria, 369
Anosmia, 167
ANSI (American National Standard Institute), 113
Anterior inferior cerebellar artery occlusion, 434–435
Anterior tympanic artery, 89
Antibiotic therapy
  acquired cholesteatoma and, 295
  acute mastoiditis, 272
  acute otitis media with effusion, 243
  chronic otitis media with meningitis, 260
  with myringotomy, for acute mastoiditis, 273
  otitis media with acute perforation, 253
  previous, acute mastoiditis and, 269

Anticipation, 65
Apert's syndrome, 60, 315
Aphysiologic pattern, in computerized dynamic posturography, 180
Apocrine glands, modified, 87
Apoptosis (programmed cell death), 9
Applebaum incudostapedial joint prosthesis, 556, 557f, 657
Aqueduct syndrome, 169
Arachnoid cysts, 495
Arachnoid granulations, temporal bone encephaloceles and, 222
Arches, pharyngeal, 4–5, 6f–7f
Arnold-Chiari malformation (Chiari type II), 211, 212f, 212
ASL (American Sign Language), 675–676, 684, 703–704
Aspergillus fumigatus, otitis media, 483
Assistive listening devices. *See under* Amplification, auditory
Astrocytoma, posterior fossa, 496–497, 497f, 498f
Asymmetric crying facies, 462
Atelectasis
　clinical manifestations, 651–652
　defined, 645
　diagnosis, 651–652
　epidemiology, 647–648, 649t
　eustachian tube dysfunction and, 238–239
　imaging, 652
　management, 656t, 660
　　algorithm for, 653–654, 654f
　　follow-up for, 660
　　general principles for, 652–653
　　goals for, 651
　　with high-risk retraction and normal/near-normal hearing, 656–657
　　interventions for, 653t
　　mastoidectomy for, 657
　　with mild unilateral hearing loss, 655
　　with normal hearing, 654–655
　　ossicle repair for, 657
　　otologist's dilemma and, 660
　　with persistent hearing loss, 655–656
　　problems/pitfalls, 658–660
　pathophysiology, 649–651, 649t, 650f
　staging, 647, 647t, 648t, 648f
Atlantoaxial dislocation/instability, 213–214
Atlanto-occipital fusion abnormalities, 213
Atlas, assimilation/occipitalization abnormalities, 213
Atresia, sensorineural reserve in, 133
Atrophy
　diffuse, 645, 646f
　local, 645
Attic blockade, acute mastoiditis and, 266, 267f
Attic perforation, 254
Audiogram
　atelectasis, 652
　configuration, for fluctuating/progressive SNHL, 621, 623, 622t, 622f, 623f–625f
　U-shaped or "cookie-bite," 334, 335f, 398
Audiologic testing
　for cochlear implantation, 596–597
　in early intervention programs for deafness, 676–677
　syndromic hereditary hearing impairment, 344, 345f
Audiologist, 584
Audiometry
　for acquired cholesteatoma, 302–303
　behavioral. *See* Behavioral observation audiometry

conditioned play, 109–110
cross-check principle, 103
immittance, 29–30. *See also* Acoustic immittance
ossicular malformation, 549
visual reinforcement. *See* Visual reinforcement audiometry
Auditory amplification. *See* Amplification, auditory
Auditory brainstem implants, 493
Auditory brainstem response (ABR)
　automated, for neonatal hearing screening, 157
　bone-conducted, limited acceptance of, 611–612, 612t
　brainstem system integrity and, 129
　case studies, 143–151, 144f–151f
　defined, 30, 127
　detection routines, Fsp and, 130–131, 130f
　for external auditory canal atresia, 533–534
　functions, 128
　hearing level prediction, 133–134, 134f
　interpretation, 129, 129f
　in mixed hearing loss, 611–612, 612t, 613t
　for neonatal hearing screening, 156–157
　protocol, 613t
　role of, 103
　stimuli, 132–133
　thresholds
　　click, 134f
　　pure-tone, 134f
Auditory evoked potentials (AEPs)
　averaging, 132
　for central auditory processing disorder, 392
　characteristics, 127
　early evoked. *See* Auditory brainstem response
　electrocochleography, 127–128, 128f
　electrode placement, 131
　endogenous, 127
　exogenous, 127
　filtering, 131–132, 131f
　in log time scale, 127, 128f
　measurement principles, 130–133, 130f, 131f
　middle latency response, 129–130
　P300 or expectancy wave, 127
　stimuli, 132–133
Auditory Response Cradle, 156
Auditory system
　deprivation, 35–36
　development, 29
　　absolute sensitivity, 32, 32f
　　auditory deprivation and, 35–36
　　binaural processing, 34, 35f
　　frequency processing, 32–33, 33f
　　monaural across-frequency processing, 34
　　perceptual organization of complex sounds, 34–35
　　temporal processing, 33–34
　functional measurement techniques, 29
　　behavioral, 30–32
　　objective, 29–30, 30f
Auditory-training therapy, for central auditory processing disorder, 393
Aural atresia, congenital. *See* External auditory canal atresia
Auricle
　avulsion, 444
　bite wounds, 444–445
　congenital malformations, 9
　construction, for microtia reconstructive surgery, 524–525, 524f
　elevation, for microtia repair, 526, 526f, 527f
　frostbite, 444

hematomas, 443–444
malformations, 517, 520t
　clinical manifestations of, 521
　grade I, 518–519, 519f
　grade II and III, 519–520, 519f
　microtia. *See* Microtia
microvascular replantation, 444
Autoimmune disease, acquired hearing loss and, 379–380
Autoimmune inner ear disease (AIED)
　case reports, 405–406, 408–409, 406f–410f
　diagnosis, 410–412, 412f, 413f
　manifestations, 412–413
　Ménière's disease. *See* Ménière's disease
　non-organ-specific, 414–416
　organ-specific, 409–410
　pathology, 412
　sensorineural hearing loss and, 405, 417
　treatment, 416–417
Automatic gain control, 586
Autosomal dominant inheritance
　description, 59–61, 60f
　syndromes, 342, 397–398. *See also specific syndromes*
Autosomal dominant noncongenital progressive audiovestibular dysfunction (ADPAVD), 321–322, 321f–323f
Autosomal recessive inheritance
　description, 59, 59f
　syndromes, 398. *See also specific syndromes*
　X-linked disorders, 61–62
Averaging, auditory evoked potentials, 132
Avulsion, auricular, 444

B

BAD syndrome, 466
Balance testing, 167
Barr body, 63
Basilar invagination-impression, 212–213, 213f
Basilar membrane, 90
Behavioral observation audiometry (BOA), 110–111
　assessment techniques
　　classification of, 104, 104f
　　for infants/toddlers, 104–109, 105f, 107f, 109f
　　reliability of, 103–104
　for mixed hearing loss, 608–609
　for neonatal hearing screening, 156
　preschool children, 109–110
　school-aged children, 110
　speech measures, 110
Behçet's syndrome, 415
Behind-the-ear hearing aids (BTE), 582, 582f
BEHL (better ear hearing level), 375
Bell's palsy
　magnetic resonance imaging, 186, 189f
　medical therapy, 466
　treatment, 462–463
Benign paroxysmal positional vertigo, Dix-Hallpike test for, 174, 174f
Benign paroxysmal vertigo of childhood (migraine), 424, 435
Benign positional vertigo (BPV), 424–425
Bess-Paradise commentary, on NIH Consensus Conference, 158
Better ear hearing level (BEHL), 375
Bezold abscess, 271
Bimodal perception, 701–702
Binaural summation, 584
Bing-Seibenman syndrome, 202, 399
Bite wounds, auricular, 444–445
Bithermal caloric test, 175, 176–177, 176f

Bivariate plotting procedure, for acoustic reflex, 122
Blepharoptosis, in Goldenhar's syndrome, 349
BOA. *See* Behavioral observation audiometry
Bone-conducting testing, for mixed hearing loss, 609–610
Bone spicules, in Usher syndrome, 371, 372*f*
BOR. *See* Branchio-otorenal syndrome
BPV (benign positional vertigo), 424–425
Brain abscess, after otitis media, 262–263, 262*f*
Brainstem lesions
 gliomas, 497, 499*f*
 vertigo and, 432–433, 433*t*
Brain tumors, of posterior fossa. *See* Posterior fossa tumors
Branchial arches, embryonic development, 4–5, 6*f*–7*f*
Branchio-otorenal syndrome (BOR)
 abnormalities, 359, 360*f*, 397–398
 diagnosis, 318
 frequency, 398
 hearing loss, 96
 mixed hearing loss in, 614
 variable expressivity, 61
Breast feeding, middle-ear infections and, 234
Brudzinski's sign, 259
BTE (behind-the-ear hearing aids), 582, 582*f*

C

Caloric testing, 178
Canal wall down mastoidectomy (CWD)
 advantages/limitations, 664
 for cholesteatoma
  acquired, 295, 302, 304–306, 304*f*
  mesotympanic, 668–669, 669*f*
  results of, 306–307, 307*t*, 308*f*, 308*t*
 data analysis, 665–666, 666*t*
 literature review, 664–665, 665*t*
 postoperative analysis, 309–310
 selection criteria, 564
 for staging tympanoplasty, 669, 670*f*
 surgical philosophy, 668, 668*f*
 vs. intact canal procedure, 663, 669–670
Canal wall up mastoidectomy (CWU). *See* Intact canal wall mastoidectomy
Candidate gene analysis, 79–80
 animal models, 80–81, 81*f*
 molecular approaches, 81–84, 82*f*
CAPD. *See* Central auditory processing disorder
Cardiac response audiometry, 156
Caregiver-child interaction, communication development and, 43
Cartilage
 allografts, for microtia, 522–523, 522*f*
 Meckel's, 5, 92
 for ossicular malformation reconstruction, 558
 for reconstructive surgery, 564
 Reichert's, 5, 6*f*–7*f*, 92
"Cauliflower ear," 443
CCJ. *See* Craniocervical junction
CD4+ lymphocytes, human immunodeficiency virus infection and, 480
CD-ROM databases, for syndromic hereditary hearing impairment diagnosis, 361–362
Central auditory disorders
 audiometric abnormalities, 387
 with identified neuropathology, 387
 idiopathic dysfunction. *See* Central auditory processing disorder
Central auditory processing disorder (CAPD)
 audiologic testing results, 394, 394*f*, 395*f*
 case report, 393–396, 394*f*, 395*f*
 definition
  classification scheme for, 388–389, 389*t*
  controversy/problems, 388
 diagnosis
  problems with, 389–390
  strategies for, 390–392, 391*f*
 etiology, 389
 functional consequences, 392
 overview, 387–388
 sequelae, 393
 terminology, 388
 treatment, 392–395
Central nervous system abnormalities, in Goldenhar's syndrome, 350
Cerebellar dysfunction measurement, 168
Cerebellar hypoplasia, 212
Cerebellar vermal agenesis (Joubert syndrome), 435
Cerebellar vermal atrophy, 435
Cerebellopontine angle tumors (CPA tumors)
 acquired hearing loss and, 381
 arachnoid cysts, 495
 dermoids, 495
 epidermoids, 495, 495*f*
 imaging features, 491, 491*f*
 meningiomas, 494, 494*f*
 neurofibromatosis type II. *See* Neurofibromatosis type II
 vertigo and, 436–437, 436*f*
Cerebral infarction, 434
Cerebrospinal fluid fistula
 radiological evaluation, 171, 172*f*
 risk, 192
 temporal bone fractures and, 451–452
Cerebrospinal fluid leakage, 209, 223, 500
Cerebrovascular disease without structural lesions, vertigo and, 434
Cervico-oculo-acoustic syndrome (Wildervanck triad)
 Duane's retraction syndrome and, 371–372, 372*f*, 373*f*
 eye abnormalities, 708*t*
Chalk disease (osteopetroses; Albers-Schînberg disease; marble bone disease), 221, 461, 709*t*
CHARGE association, 359–360, 360*f*, 400, 461
Chemotherapy, for rhabdomyosarcoma, 506–507
Chest wall deformities, after microtia repair, 529
Chiari malformations
 types, 211–212, 212*f*
 vertigo and, 433–434, 433*f*
Cholesteatomas
 acquired
  diagnosis of, 302–303
  etiology of, 97–98
  historical aspects of, 295
  incidence of, 281
  management of, 295, 306, 306*t*
  mastoid operations for, 304–306, 304*f*
  postoperative analyses, 307–308
  preoperative management, 303–304
  primary, 297–299, 301, 299*f*
  recidivistic/iatrogenic, 300–301, 301*f*, 302*f*
  secondary, 300, 300*f*, 301*f*
  surgical case review, 305–306, 306*f*, 306*t*
  surgical results for, 306–307, 307*t*, 307*f*, 308*f*, 308*t*
  biology, 663–664
  with chronic suppurative otitis media, 239
 classification, 296–297, 296*f*–298*f*, 306, 306*t*
 cleft palate and, 629, 630*t*
 congenital, 7
  age of presentation, 284
  bilateral, 281, 282*f*
  characteristics, 279, 280*f*
  clinical presentation of, 283–284
  definition of, 291
  differential diagnosis, 286, 287*f*
  embryonic cell rest and, 281–283
  epithelial migration and, 281
  facial paralysis and, 284
  giant, 283
  hearing and, 286, 287*f*
  historical aspects, 279–280
  incidence, changes in, 280–281
  location of, 284–285, 284*f*, 285*f*
  management of, 289, 292, 306, 306*t*
  mastoidectomy for, 290–291
  myringotomy and, 289
  ossicular involvement of, 284–285, 284*f*, 285*f*
  otitis media and, 291–292
  posttraumatic implantation and, 281, 292
  radiologic evaluation of, 287, 289, 288*f*
  recurrence, 291
  reexploration, 291
  site of presentation, 285, 286*f*
  squamous metaplasia and, 281, 292
  weakly attached, 281, 281*f*
 etiology, 650, 651
 facial paralysis from, 256
 mesotympanic, 668–669, 669*f*
 middle ear reconstruction, 577
 otic capsule erosion, 169, 170*f*
 from otitis media, 254–255
 recidivistic, 306, 306*t*, 310, 664
 retraction pocket/incipient, 647
 surgical management, 669–670
  advantages, 664
  case report, 666–667, 667*f*
  controversies, 663
  data analysis, 665–666, 666*t*
  goals of, 663
  hearing restoration and, 669, 670*f*
  limitations, 664
  literature review, 664–665, 665*t*
  philosophy for, 668–669, 668*f*, 669*f*
 temporal bone fibrous dysplasia and, 220
Cholesterol granuloma
 from otitis media, 255, 255*f*
 of petrous apex, 499–500, 501*f*
Chondrosarcomas, temporal bone, 509
Chordomas
 cervical, 226, 226*f*
 intracranial, 498–499, 500*f*
Chromatin, 49–51
Chromosome
 analysis, 52
 aneuploidy, 51
 banding patterns, 49–51, 53*f*
 banding techniques, 51–52
 breakpoints, 52
 mutations, 51
 p arm, 50
 q arm, 50
CID (cytomegalic inclusion disease), 376
Clarion multichannel cochlear implant, 595–596
Classroom amplification, maximizing signal-to-noise ratio with, 591
Cleft lip, 627, 628*f*, 628*t*

Cleft palate
  clinical manifestations, 629, 629t
  epidemiology, 627, 628f, 628t
  eustachian tube function and, 19–20
  management, 631, 631f
    alternatives for, 631
    illustrative cases, 632–633, 632f, 633f
    myringotomy with tympanostomy, 629–630
    palatoplasty, 630–631
    tympanostomy, 631–632
  middle ear disease and, 627, 633
  pathophysiology, 627
    dynamic abnormalities, 627–628, 628f
    static abnormalities, 628–629
  tympanic membrane perforation and, 632
Clefts, pharyngeal, 5
Clinical geneticist, SHHL diagnosis and, 347
Closing pressure, of eustachian tube, 21
CMR (comodulation masking release), 34
CMV. *See* Cytomegalovirus infection
Cochlea
  congenital anomalies, 203, 206f, 597
    aplasia, 203
    cochleosaccular dysplasia. *See* Scheibe deformity
    common cavity, 203
    embryogenesis of, 205f
    hypoplasia, 203, 206f
    incomplete partition, 203, 206f
    Mondini's. *See* Mondini's dysplasia
  embryonic development, 4
  function, measurement of, 30
  histology, 90, 90f
  hypoplasia, 93
  incomplete partition, 93, 94f
  ossification, hearing loss and, 97, 97f
Cochlear amplifier, otoacoustic emission and, 134–135
Cochlear aqueduct enlargement, 208
Cochlear band turn dysplasia (Alexander deformity), 169–170, 203, 399
Cochlear duct
  aplasia with high-frequency hearing loss or Alexander deformity, 169–170, 203, 399
  embryonic development, 4, 5f
Cochlear dysplasia, 398–399. *See also specific types of cochlear dysplasia*
Cochlear hearing loss
  acoustic reflexes and, 122
  differential diagnosis, 114
  otoacoustic emissions and, 141–142
Cochlear implants, 99
  for congenital inner ear malformations, 209
  contraindications, 209–210
  for deafness, 701
  evaluation
    audiologic, 596–597
    medical, 597
  multichannel
    benefits of, 603
    performance with, 601–602
    processing strategies, 595–596
    vs. single-channel, 600–601
  for neurofibromatosis type II, 493
  for nonsyndromic hereditary hearing loss, 335
  patient selection, 596–597
  performance variables, 602–603
  recipient categories, 596
  results in children, 598, 600–603
  speech production and, 603
  surgical procedure, 597–598, 598f–601f
  types, 595–596
  vs. hearing aids/tactile aids, 602–603

Cochlear microphonic, 127
Cochlear nerve ganglion, 90, 91f
Cochlear neurons, 90
Cochleosaccular dysplasia. *See* Scheibe deformity
Cochleovestibular neuritis, 170, 171f
Cockayne syndrome, 708t
Codon, 56, 57
Cogan's syndrome, 413, 414–415, 417
Cognition, 698
  development, enhancement for deaf children, 702
  early intervention for deafness and, 675–676
Coloboma, 368f, 370
Common cavity lesions, 192, 194f, 203
Communication
  defined, 39
  expressive, 39
  hearing loss and, 42–46
  nonverbal, 39
  oral-aural, 684
  with primary care physician, in atelectasis management, 658
  receptive, 39
  variables, 43
Comodulation masking release (CMR), 34
Complete penetrance, 60–61
Complex or multifactorial trait, 66
Computed tomography
  acquired cholesteatoma, 303
  acute mastoiditis, 271–272
  inner ear congenital anomalies, 209
  posterior fossa tumors, 489–490
  retraction pocket, *vs.* cholesteatoma, 298–299
  sigmoid sinus thrombosis, 261
  temporal bone, 181–183, 183f–185f
  temporal bone congenital abnormalities, 196
  three-dimensional scanning, temporal bone, 183, 186
Computer, in visual reinforcement audiometry, 108
Computerized dynamic posturography, 179–180, 178f, 179f, 179t
Concha evacuation, for microtia repair, 525
Conditioned head-turn procedure. *See* Visual reinforcement audiometry
Conditioned orienting response (COR), 108–109, 109f
Conditioned play audiometry, 109–110
Conditioned reflexes, 30
Conductive hearing loss
  acoustic reflex and, 122–123
  causes
    chronic otitis media, 548
    congenital, 547–548
    otosclerosis, 548
    trauma, 548
  from congenital stapes fixation. *See* Otosclerosis
  differential diagnosis, 114
  indicators, 160t
  from otitis media, 252
  risk indicators, 158t
  with sensorineural hearing loss. *See* Mixed hearing loss
  unilateral, from otitis media, 252
Congenital malformations. *See also specific congenital malformations*
  causing vertigo, 431–432
Congenital unilateral lower lip palsy (CULLP; asymmetric crying facies), 462
Consanguinity
  autosomal recessive inheritance and, 59, 59f
  genetic hearing loss and, 313

Contig building, 75
Contralateral delayed endolymphatic hydrops, 409
COR (conditioned orienting response), 108–109, 109f
Corneal light reflex, 369
Corticosteroids
  for facial paralysis, 466
  for suppurative labyrinthitis, 257
CPA tumors. *See* Cerebellopontine angle tumors
CpG residue islands, 76
Cranial nerves
  in acute mastoiditis, 271
  in Chiari malformations, 212
  embryonic development, 3
  testing, 167
Craniocervical junction (CCJ)
  abnormalities
    clinical presentation, 215–216, 215t
    congenital/developmental, 211–215, 212f–214f
    evaluation of, 211
    historical aspects of, 211
    radiographic evaluation of, 216
    surgical management of, 216–217, 216f, 216t, 217f–219f
  anatomy, 211
  lymphatic drainage, 214
  surgical decompression, 216, 216t
    anterolateral approach, 217
    postoperative complications, 217
    transoral-transpharyngeal approach, 217, 217f–219f
    transsphenoethmoidal approach, 217
Craniofacial deformity, 517
Craniofacial trauma, 447
Craniometaphysial dysplasia (Pyle's disease), 708t
Craniopharyngioma, 225
Craniosystosis syndromes, 315
Creutzfeldt-Jakob disease, transmission by homografts, 575–577
Crib-O-Gram, 156
Cristae ampullares, 4
Critical periods, 35
Critical period theory, 155
Crouzon's syndrome
  cleft palate and, 627
  gene mutations, 58, 60, 315
  hearing loss, 96
Cryptogenic hearing impairment, 343
Cryptogenitic hearing impairment, 343
Cued speech, 684
CULLP (congenital unilateral lower lip palsy; asymmetric crying facies), 462
Cultural model, for early deafness intervention, 674–675, 674f
Cytomegalic inclusion disease (CID), 376
Cytomegalovirus infection (CMV)
  acquired hearing loss, 376–377
  congenital, sensorineural hearing loss and, 399
  hearing loss and, 96
  prophylaxis, 382
  in temporal bone of AIDS patients, 483–484
Cytotoxan with methotrexate, for autoimmune inner ear disease, 416–417

D

DAI (direct audio input), 583
Deafness
  communication methods
    cued speech, 684

evaluating, guidelines for, 685, 686t
historical overview of, 683–684
oral-aural, 684
physician's role in, 685, 687, 686t
selection of, 684–685
sign language, 684
congenital, incidence, 160
developmental consequences, 699, 700f
early intervention programs, 673–674
audiological management in, 676–677
cognition and, 675–676
comprehensive and short-term, 681
comprehensive evaluation in, 676
efficacy of, 681–682
generic, 679
language skills and, 675–676
legal aspects of, 679
models of, 674–675, 674f, 675f
one-to-one work with infants, 679
parent guidance in, 677–679
rationale for, 673
resources for, 679–681, 680f
education, historical overview of, 683
mainstreaming, 693f
case histories, 693–695
evaluations, 690–691, 692–693
implementation, 691–692
monitoring, 692
physicians and, 693
preparation, 691
management interventions, 704–705
auditory capacity enhancement, 699–702
cognitive/social-cognitive development and, 702
complexities of, 697–698
educational, 703–704
family/home environment and, 702
hair-cell regeneration and, 699
human development and, 698–699, 699f
language development and, 702–703
social-emotional development and, 704
vocational options and, 704
risk factors, 157
Deep tendon reflexes, 167
Degenerative malformations, causing vertigo, 432
Denaturing gradient gel electrophoresis (DGGE), 79
Dermoids
cerebellopontine angle, 495
temporal bone, 511–512, 512f
Desired sensation level approach, for hearing aid fitting, 589
Development
cognitive, enhancement for deaf children, 702
deafness and, 699, 700f
language and, 698–699, 699f
social-cognitive, enhancement for deaf children, 702
social-emotional, of deaf children, 704
Dexamethasone, for bacterial meningitis, 378
DFNA1 gene, 60
DFN3 gene, 62, 327, 331, 80
DGGE (denaturing gradient gel electrophoresis), 79
Dichotic listening, 584
DIDMOAD syndrome (Wolfram syndrome), 361
Diffuse adhesive otitis media (shrinkwrap ear), 646, 646f, 659–660
Digenic inheritance, 314
Digenomic inheritance, 314–315
Direct audio input (DAI), 583

Distortion-product otoacoustic emissions (DPOAEs)
in cochlear hearing loss, 142
DP audiogram, 138, 138f
in infants/children, 140–141, 141f
input/output function or growth rate, 138–139
measurement procedure, 137–139, 137f
in sensorioneural hearing loss, 142–143, 142f
threshold, 138–139
Distraction masking, 33
Diuretics, ototoxicity, 98–99
Dix-Hallpike test, 174, 174f
Dizziness
causes, 424t
evaluation, family history, 163, 165f–166f
with head injury, 449
vs. vertigo, 163–164, 423
DNA
composition, 52–53, 54f
hierarchical structural organization, 49, 50f–51f
replication, 54–55, 55f
sequence alterations, inheritance of, 58
sequence analysis, 68
structure, 52–53, 54f
transcription, 55–56, 56f
DNA-binding proteins, 55
DNA cloning, 83, 82f
cDNA library
construction, 81–83, 82f
screening, tissue-specific, 77
DNA ligase, 54
DNA markers, physical mapping, 76
DNA polymerase, error rate, 57–58
DNA polymerases, 54
DNA probes, 83
Dominant progressive hearing loss (DPHL), 398
"Double ring" sign, 221
Down syndrome, 51, 215, 357
DP audiogram (distortion-product audiogram), 138, 138f, 142–143, 142f
DPOAEs. See Distortion-product otoacoustic emissions
Drift, 168
Drosophila, segmental development, 3
Drugs. See also specific drugs
ototoxic
hearing loss from, 98–99, 380, 380t, 400
usage guidelines for, 431
vertigo and, 429–430, 430–431
Duane's retraction syndrome, 369, 371–372, 372f, 373f
Dyslexia, vertigo and, 435
Dystopia canthorum, 352–353, 353f

E
EAC. See External auditory canal
Ear
abnormalities. See also specific ear abnormalities
in Goldenhar syndrome, 349–350
in Treacher Collins syndrome, 352
in Waardenburg syndrome, 353
development, 93t
dysmorphic vs. dysplastic, 517
embryonic, 3–5, 4f, 5f, 7, 9, 9f
external. See External ear
inner. See Inner ear
middle. See Middle ear
Ear-canal pressure rate, 120

Ear-canal probe, for tympanometry, 115
Ear drainage, cultures, 304
Eardrum. See Tympanic membrane
Ear lobe reconstruction, for microtia repair, 525, 525f, 526f
Earmolds, 582–583, 583f
Ear wax, 87
ECochG (electrocochleography), 127–128, 128f, 637, 639
Education
for acquired hearing loss, 383
for deaf children, historical overview of, 683
of deaf/hearing-impaired children, historical aspects of, 689
interventions, for deaf children, 703–704
Educational model, for early deafness intervention, 675, 675f
Education of All Handicapped Children's Act (P.L. 94–142), 679
Education of the Handicapped Act Amendments (P.L. 99–457), 158
Education specialists, in amplification system management, 585
Edwards syndrome, 708t
Electrocochleography (ECochG), 127–128, 128f, 637, 639
Electromyography, facial nerve, 459
Electronystagmography (ENG), 175–178, 176f
Electro-oculography (EOG), 175, 175f
Embryonic cell rest, congenital cholesteatoma and, 282–283
Encephaloceles, temporal bone or endaural, 222–224
Endolymphatic hydrops. See also Ménière's disease
endolymphatic duct obliteration and, 97, 98f
labyrinthine fistulas and, 174
perilymphatic fistula creation and, 637
secondary, 426–427
Endolymphatic sac surgery, 209
ENG (electronystagmography), 175–176
Enhancer sites, 55
Enlarged vestibular aqueduct (EVA), 191, 192f, 206, 208, 208f
EOAEs (evoked otoacoustic emissions), 157
EOG (electro-oculography), 175, 175f
Eosinophilic granuloma, 509–510
Ependymomas, 497–498, 499f, 500f
Epidermoid cyst implantation, congenital cholesteatoma and, 281
Epidermoids
cerebellopontine angle, 495, 495f
imaging features, 491f
Epistatic effects, 66
Epithelial migration, congenital cholesteatoma and, 281
Epithelium, middle-ear, 88–89
Eponym, 342
Equi test posturography system, 178f
Equivalent ear canal volume, 116–117
Equivalent volume, 115
ER-3A insert earphones, 619
Esotropia, 369
Ethacrynic acid, ototoxicity, 98–99
Ethnicity, tympanic membrane perforation and, 252
Euchromatin, 50–51
Eustachian tube
anatomy, 11–12, 12f, 13f
bony portion, 11
cartilaginous portion, 11–12
clearance function
impairment of, 19
physiology of, 16

Eustachian tube *(contd.)*
  closing pressure, 21
  dysfunction, 17–20, 19t
    middle ear atelectasis and, 238–239
    in otitis media, 23
    in otitis media with effusion, 242
    vestibular symptoms of, 167
  fibrocartilaginous portion, 11, 12
  function
    allergy and, 19, 19t
    assessment of, 114, 305
    cleft palate and, 19–20
    clinical tests of, 20–21, 21f
    indications for testing, 21–22
    otitis media pathogenesis and, 22–24
    tympanometric measure of, 119
  gas pressures, abnormal, 18
  inclination/angulation, 11, 17
  infant, 11, 13f, 15, 15t
  length, 18
  lumen, 12
  mucociliary system, 16
  muscles, 12–14, 14f
  obstruction, 239
    anatomic, 17
    functional, 17
    in otitis media, 23
  occlusion, 305
  opening mechanism failure, 17
  opening pressure, 21
  patency, abnormal, 17–18, 239
  patulous, 239
  pressure regulation
    impairment of, 17
    physiology of, 15–16
  protective function
    loss of, 17–19
    physiology of, 16
  short, 18
  stenosis, 17
  surface tension factors, physiology of, 16–17
  ventilation, middle-ear mucosa and, 305
EVA (enlarged vestibular aqueduct), 191, 192f, 206, 208, 208f
Evoked electromyography, facial nerve, 459
Evoked otoacoustic emissions (EOAEs), 157, 159
Evoked potentials, 30
Ewing's sarcoma, temporal bone, 508–509
Exons, 56
Exon trapping, 76–77
Exotropia, 369
Expressive communication, 39
External auditory canal atresia
  congenital, 95
  evaluation, 533–534
  grading, 534, 534t
  surgical repair
    anesthesia gases and, 537–538
    approach/technique for, 535–537, 536f, 537f
    complications of, 539–540
    goals of, 535
    middle ear pressure and, 537–538, 538f
    patient positioning for, 535
    postoperative care for, 539
    risks of, 535
    skin graft for, 538–539
    timing of, 534
External auditory canal (EAC)
  anatomy, 87, 88f
  development, 93t
  reconstruction, 566–567, 567f–569f
  small, ossicular malformation and, 548

External ear, embryonic development, 9, 9f
Extradural abscess, after otitis media, 261–262, 262f
Extra-dural tumors, 498–500, 500f, 501f
Extraocular motion, measurement, 167, 167f
Eye
  abnormalities
    Goldenhar's syndrome, 349, 370–371, 371f
    recognition of, 365, 367
    Treacher Collins syndrome, 351–352
    Waardenburg syndrome, 352–353, 353f
  anatomy, 365
  embryology, 365, 366f
  external examination, 367
  in hereditary hearing impairment, 707–708
  widely spaced, 367
Eye-care regimen, for facial paralysis, 466

F
Facial abnormalities
  Goldenhar syndrome, 349, 349f
  recognition of, 365, 367
  Treacher Collins syndrome, 351, 350f, 351f
  Waardenburg syndrome, 352, 353f
Facial nerve
  anastomosis, 467–468
  congenital anomalies, 457
  decompression, 466–467
  dysfunction, in osteopetroses, 221
  embryology, 457
  evaluation
    functional tests for, 114, 458–459, 458t, 460
    imaging tests for, 459
  injury
    pathophysiology of, 457–458, 458t
    pediatric diagnostic considerations, 459–460
    with temporal bone fracture, 447, 450–451, 451f
    treatment of, 450–451, 451t
  presentation, 457
  transposition, 468, 469f
Facial nerve paralysis
  from acute otitis media, 256
  from chronic otitis media or cholesteatoma, 256
  congenital, 461–462
  congenital cholesteatoma and, 284
  developmental/inherited, treatment of, 462
  infantile/childhood, 462–466
  management, 466
    case reports of, 468–469, 470f–474f
    eye-care regimen, 466
    medical, 466
    rehabilitative, 467, 467f
    surgical, 466–468, 467f
  secondary, 222
Facial recess, 598, 599f
Facial wounds, facial paralysis and, 465
Facioauriculovertebral dysplasia. *See* Goldenhar's syndrome
Familial conductive hearing loss, 332
Familial periodic cerebellar ataxia and vertigo, 435–436
Family
  consultation, for sensorineural hearing loss, 402
  environment optimization, for deaf child, 702
  evaluation, for mainstreaming, 690
  role, in hearing aid usage, 584–585

Fast spin echo magnetic resonance imaging, 187, 190f
FAV syndrome. *See* Goldenhar's syndrome
Feedback controls, 583
Fetal alcohol syndrome, 354, 354f
Fibroblast growth factor receptor 2 gene (FGRF2), 60, 315
Fibrosarcoma, 509
Fibrous dysplasia, 219–221, 220f
Flask model of eustachian tube-middle ear system, 16, 18, 19
Flynn-Aird syndrome, 709t
FM systems, personal
  for central auditory processing disorder, 393
  maximizing signal-to-noise ratio with, 590–591
FOFIF2 strategy, 595
Forced-choice procedures, 31
Fragile X syndrome, 65, 66
Frameshift mutation, 58
Franceschetti-Zwahlen-Klein syndrome. *See* Treacher Collins syndrome
Fraser syndrome, 521
Frequency
  discrimination, 32, 33
  processing, development, 32–33, 33f
  selectivity, 32–33, 33f
Fresnel lenses, 172–173, 177
Friedreich's ataxia, 709t
Frostbite, auricular, 444
Fsp, auditory brainstem response detection routines and, 130–131, 130f
Functional cloning, 67
Furosemide, ototoxicity, 98–99

G
Gadolinium diethylenetriamine pentaacetic acid (DTPA), MRI enhancement, 186, 189f
GAGs (glycosaminoglycans), in ADPAVD, 322, 323f
Gait analysis, for vestibular function assessment, 168
Gap detection, 33
Gastrointestinal system abnormalities, in Waardenburg syndrome, 353
Gaze test, 175, 177
Gelfilm, for atelectasis, 656
Gene cloning, 67
Gene expression
  replication, 54–55, 55f
  transcription, 55–56, 56f
  translation, 56–57, 57f
Gene mapping/identification, 67–68. *See also* Linkage analysis
  candidate gene analysis for. *See* Candidate gene analysis
  linkage analysis. *See* Linkage analysis
  in linked regions, 76–77
  nonsyndromic hereditary hearing loss, 333, 334t
  of pathogenic mutations, 77, 79, 78f
  physical mapping, 74–76, 75f
  polymerase chain reaction and, 69–70, 70f
  positional cloning and, 74, 74f
  restriction fragment length polymorphism and, 68–69, 69f
  simple sequence repeat polymorphism and, 69–70, 70f
  vs. physical mapping, 74–75, 75f
Genetic counseling, 333–335, 335t, 362
Genetic hearing loss. *See* Hereditary hearing loss
Genetic heterogeneity, 71

Genetic inheritance
　of deafness, 160
　in fluctuating/progressive sensorineural
　　hearing loss, 617, 619
Genetic markers, genetic distance of, 67–68
Genetic mutations, pathogenic, identification
　of, 77, 79, 78f
Genomic imprinting, 63–65, 66f
Gentamicin, ototoxicity, 430
Germ cell tumors, temporal bone, 509
Giant cholesteatoma, 283
Gliomas, brainstem, vertigo and, 433, 433f
Glomus tumors, temporal bone, 511
Glycosaminoglycans (GAGs), in ADPAVD,
　322, 323f
Goldenberg incus prosthesis
　development, 550–551
　placement technique, 552–556, 553f–556f
Goldenhar-Gorlin syndrome. See Goldenhar's
　syndrome
Goldenhar's syndrome
　abnormalities
　　central nervous system, 350
　　ear, 349–350
　　eye, 349, 370–371, 371f, 708t
　　facial, 349, 349f, 370
　　oral, 350
　　renal, 350
　　skeletal, 350, 536
　associated disorders, 342
　bilateral involvement, 521
　diagnosis, 318
　　radiographic studies, 345
　　in subtle cases, 350–351
　incidence, 370
　inheritance, 347, 349
　male-female ratio, 349
　terminology, 347
Gradenigo's syndrome, 259, 271, 273
Gradient echo magnetic resonance imaging,
　187, 190f
Gresinger's sign, 260
Grooves, pharyngeal, 5
Gusher
　diagnosis, 557
　perilymphatic, 329, 331–332, 330f–331f,
　　358, 359f
　poststapedectomy, 545
　stapes, 613, 614, 635

H

Haemophilus influenzae
　mastoiditis, acute, 269–270, 269t
　meningitis, 399
　otitis media
　　acute, 235, 236f, 236, 242
　　with effusion, 238, 238f
Haemophilus influenzae type B vaccine (HIB),
　382
Hair abnormalities, Waardenburg syndrome,
　353
Hair-cell regeneration, 699
Hallgren syndrome (Usher syndrome III), 710t
Hallpike test, 174, 174f, 176, 177, 425
Halogen lighting, for otoscopy, 281
Handicapped Children Act of 1975 (P.L.
　94–142), 585
Hand-Schuller-Christian disease, 509, 510
Haploinsufficiency, 61
Head shadow effect, 583–584
Head trauma
　hearing loss from, 449
　ossicular injuries and, 445–447, 446f
　skull base fractures and, 447

Healthy People 2000, 155
Hearing
　assessments/screenings. See specific
　　assessment/screening methods
　in cholesteatoma
　　congenital, 285–286, 287f
　　postoperative assessment of, 307, 307f,
　　　308f, 308t
　development, 36
　language learning and, 42
　level predictions, auditory brainstem
　　response and, 133–134, 134f
　loss. See Hearing loss; *specific types of
　　hearing losses*
　vision and, 689–690, 690f
Hearing aids
　for acquired hearing loss, 382–383
　candidacy, 585–586
　components, 581, 582f
　confirmation, 700
　for congenital inner ear malformations, 209
　digitally programmable, 587
　fitting, 700–701
　　acoustic reflexes for, 123
　　follow-up procedures for, 592
　　procedures, 587–589, 588f
　　real ear measures for, 588–589, 588f
　　saturation sound pressure level
　　　determination and, 589–590
　flexibility of, 587
　hearing damage from, 592
　maximum output determination, 589–590
　prescription, 700
　selection, 586–587, 587f, 700
　types/styles, 581–582, 582f
　usage, family role in, 584–585
　validation, 700
　vs. cochlear implants/tactile aids, 602–603
　wearing instructions, 591
Hearing loss. See also *specific types of hearing
　loss*
　causes, 95–99. See also *specific causes of
　　hearing loss*
　　from hearing aid, 592
　communication and, 42–46
　defined, 375
　detection, 581
　early identification, 155, 161
　fluctuating, speech/language development
　　and, 45–46
　genetic, incidence of, 58
　incidence, 155, 313
　in infants, 155
　measurement, 375
　prediction, from acoustic reflex, 122–123
　presentation, 375
　speech/language development and, 46–47
　from temporal bone fracture, 448–449
　unilateral, speech/language development and,
　　45
Hearing-screening programs, 155
Helix displacement, after microtia repair, 528
Hematomas
　auricular, 443–444
　postoperative, microtia repair, 527
Hemifacial microsomia. See Goldenhar's
　syndrome
Hemophilia A, 62
Hemotympanum, with temporal bone fracture,
　449
Hereditary Hearing Impairment Resource
　Registry (HHIRR), 362
Hereditary hearing loss
　epidemiology, 314

with eye abnormalities. See Oculoauditory
　syndromes
historical aspects, 313
inheritance patterns, 314–315
nonsyndromic. See Nonsyndromic hereditary
　hearing loss
syndromic. See Syndromic hereditary
　hearing loss
Usher syndromes, 371, 372f
Waardenburg syndromes, 370, 370f
Hereditary Hearing Loss and Its Syndromes,
　361
Herpes simplex, neonatal, 399
Herpes zoster oticus (Ramsey Hunt syndrome),
　427, 428f, 463, 466
Heterochromatin, 50
HHIRR (Hereditary Hearing Impairment
　Resource Registry), 362
HIB (*Haemophilus influenzae* type B vaccine),
　382
High-frequency probe tones, for acoustic reflex
　assessment, 122
High-risk factors of deafness, 157
Hillocks, auricular, 9
Hirduo medicinalis, 444
Hirudin, 444
Histiocytosis X, 509–510
HIV. See Human immunodeficiency virus
HLA allele, MÇniäre's disease and, 413
Home environment, optimization for deaf
　child, 702
Homeobox, 3
Homografts
　antigenicity and, 574–575, 576f
　donor precautions, 576–577
　eardrum-malleus-incus
　　preparation of, 565, 566f
　　transplantation of, 565–566, 566f
　for mastoidectomy, 564–565
　transplantation, 563
　virus transmission and, 575–577
Hox genes, 3
Human development. See Development
Human genome
　mitochondrial or extranuclear, 52
　nuclear, 49–52, 50f, 51f
Human immunodeficiency virus (HIV)
　infection
　　asymptomatic stage of, 481
　　characteristics of, 480
　　classification in children, 481
　　seroconversion, 480–481
　　seropositivity, with otitis media, 482–483
　　transmission
　　　by homografts, 575–577
　　　vertical, 479–480
　　type I, 480
　　type II, 480
Hunter syndrome (mucopolysaccharidosis type
　II), 96, 398
Hurler syndrome (mucopolysaccharidosis type
　I), 96, 398
Huschke, foramen of, 87
Hydrocephalus
　otic, after otitis media, 263
　postoperative, 501
　vertigo and, 437
Hydrops ex vacuo theory, 22, 23
Hydroxyapatite osteointegration, 564
Hyoid arch (Reichert's cartilage), 5, 6f–7f, 92
Hyperbilirubinemia, sensorineural hearing loss
　and, 400
Hypertelorism, 352–353, 353f

Hypertrophic scarring, after microtia repair, 529
Hypertropia, 369
Hyrtl's fissure (tympanomeningeal fissure), 636

I

IAM. *See* Internal auditory meatus
IAM (internal auditory meatus), 182, 208–209
Iatrogenic cholesteatoma, 301–302, 301*f*, 302*f*
IFSP (individualized family service plan), 160–161
IGF-II (insulin-like growth factor), 64
ILO system, for TEOAE measurement, 136
Immittance audiometry, 29–30. *See also* Acoustic immittance
Immune-mediated disease
  AIDS. *See* Acquired immunodeficiency syndrome
  autoimmune
    acquired hearing loss and, 379–380
    inner ear. *See* Autoimmune inner ear disease
  in fluctuating/progressive sensorineural hearing loss, 619
Impedance
  defined, 113
  testing, in atelectasis, 652
Implants
  auditory brainstem, 493
  cochlear. *See* Cochlear implants
  for ossicular reconstruction, 550–551
Imprinting, genomic, 63–65, 66*f*
Inclusion, 689
Incomplete penetrance, 60, 60*f*, 61
Incudostapedial joint
  anatomy, 89
  dislocation, 447
Incudostapedial region, minor discontinuities/fixations, 192, 195*f*
Incus, 89, 446, 563
Independent assortment, 62
Individualized family service plan (IFSP), 160–161
Individuals with Disabilities Education Act (P.L. 102–119), 160, 585
Infant. *See also* Neonatal hearing screening
  ear
    acoustic properties of, 29, 30*f*
    eustachian tube, 11, 13*f*, 15, 15*t*
  hearing
    frequency selectivity, 32–33
    medical aspects of, 160, 160*t*
    middle-ear resonant frequencies, 30, 31*f*
    otoacoustic emissions, 140–141, 140*f*, 141*f*
  hearing impairments
    conductive, indicators of, 160*t*
    delayed-onset sensorineural, indicators of, 160*t*
    incidence of, 155
    one-to-one work with, 679
    sensorineural, herpes simplex infection and, 399
    universal detection of, 158–159, 159*f*
  hearing screening. *See also* Neonatal hearing screening
    behavioral assessment techniques, 30–31, 104–109, 105*f*, 107*f*, 109*f*
    tympanometry for, 120
    visual reinforcement audiometry, 105–108, 105*f*, 107*f*
  language development, 40, 41*f*
  speech development, 40, 41*f*
Infantile phytanic acid storage disease (Usher syndromes IV), 710*t*
Infections. *See also specific infections*
  causing sensorineural hearing disorders, 399–400
  postoperative, microtia repair, 528
Inflation-deflation test, 21
Infrared video system, for electro-oculography, 175, 175*f*
Inheritance. *See also specific inherited syndromes*
  autosomal dominant, 59–61, 60*f*
  autosomal recessive, 59, 59*f*
  DNA sequence alterations, 58
  mitochondrial, 63, 65*f*, 342
  multifactorial, 66–67
  patterns, of genetic disorders, 58–62, 59*f*, 60*f*
Inner ear. *See also specific inner ear structures*
  anatomy, 90–92, 90*f*–92*f*, 635–636, 636*f*
  congenital anomalies
    causes of, 201–202
    classification, 201, 202*t*, 202
    cochleosaccular, 202
    evaluation, 209
    genetic aspects, 201–202
    incidence, 201
    internal auditory meatus, 208–209
    labyrinthine, 203, 206, 207*f*, 208*f*
    management, 209–210
    membranous labyrinth, 202–203
    membranous labyrinth and osseous labyrinths, 203, 204*f*–206*f*
    morphogenetic, 202
    neuroepithelial, 202
    vestibular aqueduct, 206, 208, 208*f*
  embryonic development, 3–4, 4*f*, 5*f*, 93*t*, 201
  hydrodynamic forces, 637
  teratogenesis, 377
Inner hair cell stereocilia, 134
In situ hybridization, 83–84
Insulin-like growth factor (IGF-II), 64
Intact canal wall mastoidectomy (canal wall up procedure)
  advantages/limitations, 663, 669–670
  for cholesteatoma
    acquired, 295, 302, 304–306, 304*f*
    mesotympanic, 668–669, 669*f*
    results of, 306–307, 307*t*, 308*f*, 308*t*
  data analysis, 665–666, 666*t*
  literature review, 664–665, 665*t*
  postoperative analysis, 309–310
  for staging tympanoplasty, 669, 670*f*
  surgical philosophy, 668, 668*f*
  vs. canal wall down procedure, 663, 669–670
Intelligent visual reinforcement audiometry (IVRA), 108
Internal auditory meatus (IAM), 182, 208–209
Interposition grafting, facial nerve, 468
In-the-canal hearing aids (ITC), 582, 582*f*
In-the-ear hearing aids (ITE), 582, 582*f*
Intra-axial tumors, 495–498, 496*f*–499*f*
Intracochlear ossification, cochlear implantation for, 597
Introns, 56
Iris coloboma, 368*f*
ITC (in-the-canal hearing aids), 582, 582*f*
ITE (in-the-ear hearing aids), 582, 582*f*
IVRA (intelligent visual reinforcement audiometry), 108

J

Jackson-Weiss syndrome, 60, 315
Jervell and Lange-Nielsen syndrome, 96, 202, 318, 355, 398
JNA (juvenile nasopharyngeal angiofibroma), 225
The John Tracy Clinic Correspondence Course, 681
Joint Committee on Infant Hearing, 157–159, 158*t*, 161
Joubert syndrome (cerebellar vermal agenesis), 435
Juvenile nasopharyngeal angiofibroma (JNA), 225
Juvenile rheumatoid arthritis, 416

K

Kabuki syndrome, 357, 357*f*
Karyotype, 49–50, 52*f*
Kawasaki disease, 464
Kearns-Sayre syndrome, 342, 358–359, 709*t*
Kernicterus, acquired hearing loss and, 378
Kernig's sign, 259
Kidney abnormalities, in Goldenhar's syndrome, 350
Kinocilium, 91
Klinefelter's syndrome, 51
Klippel-Feil syndrome, 213
K-space, 187

L

Labyrinth
  in acquired cholesteatoma, 302
  anatomy, 182*f*
  malformations
    complete aplasia, 192, 195*f*, 203
    congenital/developmental, 182*f*, 203, 206, 207*f*, 208*f*
    vertigo and, 431
  ossification, 97, 97*f*, 99
Labyrinthine apoplexy (vestibular neuronitis), 427
Labyrinthine fistula, 257, 258*f*
Labyrinthine fistula test, 174
Labyrinthitis
  acute suppurative, vestibular dysfunction and, 429
  acute viral (vestibular neuronitis), 427
  circumscribed, vestibular dysfunction and, 429, 429*f*
  magnetic resonance imaging, 186, 189*f*
  from otitis media, 256–258, 257*f*, 258*f*
  sensorineural hearing loss and, 192, 196, 196*t*
  serous, 257
  vestibular dysfunction and, 428
  suppurative, 257–258, 257*f*, 258*f*
  syphilitic, 377
Labyrinthitis obliterans (ossificans), sensorineural hearing loss and, 196, 197*f*
Lacrimoauriculodentodigital syndrome (LADD), 361
Langerhans' cell histiocytosis, 509–510
Language
  acquisition, otitis media and, 252
  components, 39
  definition of, 39
  development, 39–40
    birth to 1 year, 40
    1 to 2 years, 40, 41*f*
    2 to 3 years, 40, 42, 41*f*

3 to 5 years, 42, 41*f*
  hearing and, 42
  hearing loss and, 46–47
  promotion, for deaf children, 702–703
  in human development, 698–699, 698*f*
  skills, early intervention for deafness and, 675–676
Laser surgery, for ossicular malformation repair, 558
Lateral sinus
  involvement, in cholesteatoma, 297, 298*f*
  thrombosis, after otitis media, 260–261, 261*f*
Late vertex response (LVR), 392
Laurence-Moon-Bardet-Biedl syndrome, 709*t*
Learning disabilities, vertigo and, 435
Leeches, medicinal, 444
Legal issues
  auditory amplification system requirements, 585
  of early intervention, 679
  neonatal hearing screening mandates, 161, 161*t*
Lentiviruses, 480. *See also* Human immunodeficiency virus
Leopard syndrome, 709*t*
Letterer-Siwe disease, 509, 510
Leukemia, temporal bone, 508
Levator veli palatini muscle (LVPM), 14, 628, 628*f*
Linkage, 63, 64*f*
Linkage analysis
  defined, 67, 68
  in disease gene identification, 73–74
  gene identification in linked regions, 76–77
  marker locus and, 70–71
  for nonsyndromic hearing loss, 72–73
  statistical methods, 71–72, 72*f*
  utility/power, 71
  vs. physical mapping, 74–75, 75*f*
Linkage phase, 71
Lipreading, 701
Lobule reconstruction, for microtia repair, 525, 525*f*, 526*f*
LOD score, 71
London Dysmorphology Database, 362
Loudness discomfort, acoustic reflex and, 123
LVPM (levator veli palatini muscle), 14, 628, 628*f*
LVR (late vertex response), 392
Lyme disease, 463
Lyonization, 61, 62, 63

M

McCune-Albright syndrome, 220
McRae's line, 213
Magnetic nerve stimulation, 459
Magnetic resonance angiography
  arterial, 190
  venous, 190–191, 191*f*
Magnetic resonance imaging (MRI), 181
  acute mastoiditis, 272
  fast spin echo, 187, 190*f*
  fat suppressed, 187, 190
  gradient echo, 187, 190*f*
  juvenile nasopharyngeal angiofibroma, 225
  posterior fossa tumors, 490, 490*t*
  sigmoid sinus thrombosis, 261
  temporal bone congenital abnormalities, 196
  temporal bone encephaloceles, 224
Mainstream Center at Clarke School for the Deaf, 689
Mainstreaming
  case histories, 693–695
  evaluation
    family, 690
    school, 690–691
    student, 690
  implementation, 691–692
  monitoring, 692
  physicians and, 693
  preparation, 691
Malleus, 7, 89, 446
Mandibular arch, embryonic development, 5, 6*f*–7*f*
Mandibulofacial dysostosis. *See* Treacher Collins syndrome
Mapping panels, 76
Marble bone disease (osteopetroses; Albers-Schînberg disease; chalk disease), 221, 461, 709*t*
Marshall syndrome, 709*t*
Masking
  dilemma, 619
  for mixed hearing loss evaluation, 610
  in visual reinforcement auditory test protocol, 106
Masking level difference (MLD), 34, 35, 35*f*, 36*f*, 584
Masseter transposition procedure, pedicled, 468
Mastoid
  development, 92, 305
  pneumatization, 181, 182*f*, 268, 659
  surgery. *See also* Mastoidectomy
    postoperative temporal bone encephaloceles, 222–223
Mastoid-air-cell system, 18–19, 265
Mastoid cavity reconstruction, 565–567, 567*f*–569*f*
Mastoidectomy
  for acute mastoiditis, 273
  for atelectasis, 657
  canal wall down. *See* Canal wall down mastoidectomy
  canal wall up. *See* Intact canal wall mastoidectomy
  for congenital cholesteatoma, 290–291
  for facial recess access, 598, 599*f*
  intact canal wall. *See* Intact canal wall mastoidectomy
  postoperative reconstruction. *See* Middle ear reconstruction, postmastoidectomy
Mastoiditis
  acute
    clinical manifestations of, 270–271, 270*f*
    coalescent, 265, 274–275
    complications, 273–274, 274*f*
    defined, 265, 265*t*
    differential diagnosis, 272
    epidemiology, 267–269
    extension, 267, 268*f*, 269*f*
    in immunocompromised host, 270
    incidence, 274
    management, 272–273
    microbiology, 269–270, 269*t*
    from otitis media, 258–259, 258*f*
    pathophysiology, 265–267, 266*f*–269*f*
    with periosteitis, 265, 274
    radiographic evaluation, 271–272
    terminology, 265, 266*t*
  chronic, 266*t*
  coalescent, 266–267, 268*f*, 272–273, 274*f*
    acute mastoiditis and, 266–267, 268*f*
    case study, 273, 274*f*
    management, 272–273
  subacute/silent/masked or latent, 266*t*, 271
Maximal stimulation testing (MST), 458–459
Measles infection, sensorineural hearing loss and, 96, 400

Meckel's cartilage, 5, 92
Medial intercanthal distance measurement, 367, 367*f*
Medical model, for early deafness intervention, 674, 674*f*
Medulloblastomas, posterior fossa, 495–496, 496*f*
MEE. *See* Middle-ear effusion
Meiotic crossovers, 68
Meiotic recombination, 56
Melkersson-Rosenthal syndrome, 464
Membranous labyrinth
  anatomy, 90
  congenital anomalies, 201, 202–203, 204*f*–206*f*
  development, 92
  dysplasia, 202–203
  embryonic development, 4
  physiology, 172, 173*f*
Mendelian genetic principles
  independent assortment, 62
  segregation, 62
  variations on, 63–66, 64*f*–66*f*
Mendelian trait, 66
Ménière's disease
  autosomal dominant inheritance, 322, 324, 323*f*
  bilateral involvement, 425
  etiology, 174, 413–414
  hearing loss, 382, 426, 426*f*
  histology, 425, 425*f*
  vertigo, 425–426
Meningiomas
  imaging features, 491*f*
  skull base, 225–226
  treatment, 494, 494*f*
  vertigo and, 437
Meningitis
  after otitis media, 259–260
  after posterior fossa tumor surgery, 501
  congenital inner ear malformations and, 209
  hearing loss, 97, 97*f*, 378–379, 379*f*
  from mastoidectomy, 260
  prevention, 160
  recurrent, illustrative case, 641
  risk, 192
  temporal bone fractures and, 451–452
  vertigo and, 430
Mental status, in Treacher Collins syndrome, 352
Merin classification, 371
Messenger RNA (mRNA), 56, 57
Metabolic disorders, causing sensorineural hearing loss, 400
Metalinguistic skills, 42
Methionine, 57
Methotrexate, for autoimmune inner ear disease, 416
MHL. *See* Mixed hearing loss
Michel deformity (complete labyrinthine aplasia), 192, 195*f*, 203
Microbiological culture, in otorrhea, 252
Microneurovascular free muscle transfer, 468
Microtia
  anatomy, 517, 518*f*
  atypical, surgical repair of, 526–527, 527*f*, 528*f*
  clinical manifestations, 521
  diagnosis, 521–522
  epidemiology, 517–518
  surgical reconstruction, 522, 532
    alternative approaches, 522–523, 522*f*
    complications/pitfalls, 527–529, 529*f*
    illustrative cases, 529, 530*f*, 531*f*

Microtia (contd.)
   operative technique for, 524–526, 524f–527f
   recommended approach, 523, 523f
Middle ear. *See also specific middle ear structures*
   abnormalities. *See also specific middle ear abnormalities*
      acoustic reflex detection of, 119
   disease. *See also specific middle ear diseases*
      cleft palate and, 627, 629, 629t, 630t, 633
      vestibular symptoms, 167
   effusion. *See* Middle-ear effusion
   embryonic development, 5, 7, 93t
   function
      measurement of, 29–30
      otoacoustic emission and, 139–140
   histology, 88–90, 89f
   infections
      breast feeding and, 234
      prevention, 700
   mucosa, eustachian tubal ventilation and, 305
   nonintact, 18–19
   preparation, for reconstructive surgery, 565
   pressure, 637
      differential, in otitis media with effusion, 242
      external auditory canal atresia repair and, 537–538, 538f
      negative, failure to develop, 22
   reconstruction. *See* Middle ear reconstruction
   resonant frequencies, 30
Middle-ear effusion (MEE)
   atelectasis and, 650
   chronic, tympanometry and, 117
   diagnosis, 114
   eustachian tube function and, 305
   objective testing, 652
   in otitis media. *See* Otitis media with effusion
   otoacoustic emission and, 139–140, 139f
   pathogenesis, hydrops ex vacuo theory of, 22, 23
   persistent, 23, 237
   pure-tone assessment, 116
   resolution failure, 19
   with sensorineural hearing loss, 617, 618f
Middle ear reconstruction, 547
   for cholesteatomas, 577
   postmastectomy
      open radical cavity procedure controversies, 574–577, 576f
   postmastoidectomy
      alternatives, 577
      case histories, 571, 573, 572f–575f
      complications, 569, 571
      controversies, 574–577, 576f
      materials for, 564–565
      outcome, 569, 570t–571t
      postmastoidectomy, 577
      postoperative course/care, 567–569
      procedure for, 565–567, 566f, 567f
      selection criteria for, 564
Middle-ear space, 635–636
Middle ear ventilation disorder, 649–650
Middle fossa craniotomy, 224
Middle latency response (MLR), 129–130, 392
Midwest Ear Foundation, homograft donor precautions, 576–577
Migraine (benign paroxysmal vertigo of childhood), 424, 435
Missense mutation, 58

Mitochondrial inheritance, 63, 65f, 342
Mixed hearing loss (MHL)
   diagnosis, 607
   evaluation, 614
      auditory brainstem response, 611–612, 612t, 613t
      behavioral audiologic, 608–609
      bone-conduction, 609–610
      immittance audiometry for, 610–611
      masking for, 610
      otoacoustic emissions, 612–613
      problem aspects of, 607–608, 608t
      speech testing, 610
   familial, 332
   inheritance, 316
   management, 614–615
   otosclerosis, 332
   speech/language development and, 43–45
   syndromes with, 613–614
   X-linked, with perilymphatic gusher, 329, 331–332, 330f–331f
MLD. *See* Masking level difference
Mobius syndrome, 461
Molecular genetics
   DNA, 52–53, 52f
   gene expression. *See* Gene expression
   human genome, 49–52, 50f–53f
   mutations, 57–58
Monaural across-frequency processing, 34
Mondini's dysplasia
   autosomal dominant, 324–325, 324f, 325f
   cochlear implantation for, 209
   computed tomography, 169, 170f
   endolymphatic sac surgery for, 209
   morphologic abnormalities, 93, 94f, 94t, 399
   in Pendred syndrome, 96, 192, 194f
   radiographic imaging, 191–192, 193f
   vertigo and, 431–432
Moraxella catarrhalis
   in acute otitis media, 235, 236f, 236
   in otitis media with effusion, 235, 236, 236f, 238, 238f
Moro reflex (startle reflex), 156, 169
Motility, ocular, 369
Motion intolerance, vertigo and, 437
mRNA (messenger RNA), 56, 57
MST (maximal stimulation testing), 458–459
Mucociliary defense system, 12, 16
Mucopolysaccharidosis, 96, 398
Multifactorial inheritance, 66–67
Multifactorial trait, 66
MULTIPEAK strategy, 595
Multiple sclerosis, vertigo and, 435
Mumps, 97, 400, 430
Mutations, 57–58
Mycoplasma pneumoniae, in otitis media without effusion, 234
Myotonic dystrophy, facial paralysis, 461
Myringitis, 233, 241
Myringosclerosis. *See* Tympanosclerosis
Myringotomy
   for acute mastoiditis, 272, 273
   for congenital cholesteatoma, 289
   with tympanostomy, 629–630
   with tympanostomy tube insertion, 247

N

Nager syndrome, 521
Nance deafness/DFN3 (X-linked mixed hearing loss with stapes gusher), 613, 614
Nasopharyngeal air pressure, 18
National Collaborative Perinatal Project, 520

National Institute on Deafness and Other Communication Disorders (NIDCD), 362
National Institutes of Health (NIH), 155, 158, 161
NDP (Norrie's disease protein), 52
Neonatal hearing screening
   early intervention, 160–161
   follow-up care, 160–161
   Joint Committee on Infant Hearing and, 157–158, 158t
   legislative mandates, 161, 161t
   location, 155–156
   sensitivity/specificity, 156
   techniques, 156–157
   timing, 155–156
   universal programs, 158–159, 159f, 161–162
Neonatal herpes simplex, sensorineural hearing loss and, 399
Neotragus
   creation, 525–526, 526f
   lateralization, 528
Neurofibromatosis type II
   diagnostic criteria, 491, 491t
   magnetic resonance imaging, 491, 492f
   treatment, 491–494, 492f
   vertigo and, 436–437, 436f
Neurologic deficits, in craniocervical junction abnormalities, 215–216, 215t
Neurologic examination, 163, 167–168
Neuronitis, vestibular, 427
Neuropsychological disorders, 388, 389t
NHHL. *See* Nonsyndromic hereditary hearing loss
NIDCD (National Institute on Deafness and Other Communication Disorders), 362
NIH (National Institutes of Health), 155, 158, 161
Nine-step tympanometric test, 20–21, 21f
Noise-induced hearing loss, 142, 400
Nonsense mutation, 58
Nonsuppurative otitis media. *See* Otitis media with effusion
Nonsyndromic hereditary hearing loss (NHHL)
   candidate gene analysis, 79–80
   chromosomal map, 81, 78f
   classification, 315–316, 315t, 336
   diagnosis, 335–336
      algorithms, 332–333
      considerations for, 317–318, 317f, 318t, 318f
   future research, 336
   gene mapping, 333, 334t
   genetic counseling, 333–335, 335t
   incidence, 341
   inheritance, 316–317, 375
   linkage analysis, 72–73
   rehabilitation, multidisciplinary, 335
   risk, 334–335, 335t
   subtypes, 319–322, 324–329, 319f–329f
Norrie's disease protein (NDP), 52
Norrie's syndrome, 52, 53f, 62, 318, 709t
Northern blot analysis, 77, 83
Northwestern University Children's Perception of Speech (NU-Chips), 110
Nose abnormalities, Treacher Collins syndrome, 352
Notched noise, for auditory brainstem response, 132–133
Notching, on multifrequency tympanogram, 119
NU-Chips (Northwestern University Children's Perception of Speech), 110
Nucleic acid probes, 83

Nucleus multichannel cochlear implant, 595
Nystagmus
  detection, 175–177, 176f
  direction, 172
  elicited, 172
  fixed inhibition of, 177
  optokinetic, 177–178
  pendular, 173
  post-headshake, 173–174
  spontaneous, 172–173, 450
  static positional, 174

O

OAV spectrum. *See* Goldenhar's syndrome
Observer-based Psychoacoustic Procedure (OPP), 31
Ocular movement testing, 369
Oculoauditory syndromes
  diagnosis, 365, 367–370, 367f–369f
  Duane's retraction syndrome, 372, 373f
  eye abnormalities, 707–708
  types, 707t–710t
Oculoauriculovertebral dysplasia. *See* Goldenhar's syndrome
Oculoauriculovertebral syndrome, 461–462
Odontoid process anomalies, 214–215, 214f
Operating microscope, 281
Ophthalmologist consultation, for syndromic hereditary hearing impairment diagnosis, 347
Ophthalmoscopy, 369
OPP (observer-based Psychoacoustic Procedure), 31
Opportunistic organisms, in otitis media of HIV patient, 483
Oral manifestations
  in Goldenhar syndrome, 350
  in Treacher Collins syndrome, 352
  in Waardenburg syndrome, 353
Organ of Corti
  anatomy, 4
  degeneration, in ADPAVD, 322, 323f
  embryonic development, 90, 91f, 92f
Os odontoideum malformation, 214, 214f
Ossicles
  anatomy, 89
  in congenital cholesteatoma, 284–285, 284f, 285f
  damaged, in atelectasis, repair of, 657
  development, 92
  discontinuity, surgical reconstruction for, 552–556, 553f–557f
  dislocation, 557
  embryonic development, 5
  erosion
    in atelectasis, 651
    atelectasis management and, 659
  fixation, surgical reconstruction for, 556–557
  incus, 89, 446, 563
  malformations. *See* Ossicular malformations; *specific malformations*
  malleus, 7, 89, 446
  stapes. *See* Stapes
  traumatic injuries, 445–447, 446f
Ossicular malformations
  chronic otitis media and, 548
  congenital, 95, 547–548
  evaluation, 549–550
  hearing loss, degree of, 550
  medical imaging, 549–550
  surgical reconstruction, 560
    for absence of stapes and/or oval window, 557

alternatives, 558
complications, 558–559
controversial aspects, 558
for discontinuity, 552–556, 553f–557f
for fixation, 556–557
follow-up, 550
goals, 550
illustrative cases, 559–560
implant systems, 550–551
initial assessment, 551
paradigm, 552, 552f
patient selection, 558
staging, 557–558
surgeon selection, 558
technical considerations, 558
Osteitis, post-mastoiditis, 273–274, 274f
Osteogenesis imperfecta
  clinical manifestations, 221–222
  diagnosis, 318
  types, 360–361, 361t, 398
Osteogenesis imperfecta (van der Hoeve syndrome), 709t
Osteopetroses (Albers-Schînberg disease; chalk disease; marble bone disease), 221, 461, 709t
Otalgia, 235
Otic capsule
  development, 92
  dysplasia, 191–192, 192f–196f
  erosion, 169, 170f
Otic hydrocephalus, after otitis media, 263
Otic pits, 4, 92
Otic vesicles (otocysts), 4, 4f
Otitis media. *See also* Otitis media with effusion
  acute, 479
    complications, 251
    diagnosis, 235
    facial paralysis and, 463
    incidence, 234
    microbiology, 235–236, 235f–237f
    otorrhea in, 236–237, 237f
    pathogenesis, 22–23
    risk factors, 234–235
    suppurative. *See* Mastoiditis, acute
  adhesive, 255–256
    diffuse, 646, 646f
    local, 645–646
  chronic, 241
    acquired hearing loss and, 379
    case studies, 143–146, 144f–146f
    etiology, 251
    facial paralysis and, 463
    meningitis and, 259, 260
    ossicular malformation and, 548
    suppurative, 24, 239–240
  classifications, 233, 233t
  complications, 251
    acute mastoiditis, 258–259, 258f
    adhesive otitis media, 255, 255f
    brain abscess, 262–263, 262f
    cholesteatoma, 254–255
    cholesterol granuloma, 255, 255f
    conductive hearing loss, 252
    extradural abscess, 261–262, 262f
    facial paralysis, 256
    labyrinthitis, 256–258, 257f, 258f
    meningitis, 259–260
    otic hydrocephalus, 263
    petrousitis, 259
    sigmoid sinus thrombosis, 260–261, 261f
    tympanic membrane perforation, 252–253
    tympanosclerosis, 253–254, 253f, 254f
  congenital cholesteatoma and, 291–292

defined, 251
fluctuating hearing loss and, 45–46
in HIV-positive child, 482–483
incidence, 233, 234f
pathogenesis
  allergy and, 19, 19t
  eustachian tube function and, 22–24
  hydrops ex vacuo theory of, 22, 23
secretory, 241–242
sequelae, 649–651, 649t, 650f
serous. *See* Otitis media with effusion
with syndromic hereditary hearing impairment, 355
treatment, 233, 241
vertigo and, 163, 427–429, 428f
without effusion, 233–234
Otitis media with effusion (OME)
  acquired hearing loss and, 378
  acute, 237, 241
    antibiotic treatment for, 243–244
    recurrent, 243–245
  chronic, 241, 479, 242–243
    antimicrobial therapy, 244
    corticosteroid therapy, 244
    surgical therapy, 245–246
  cleft palate and, 629, 629t
  diagnosis, 238
  effects on child, 242
  etiology, 251
  hearing loss, 35
  incidence, 237–238
  microbiology, 238, 238f
  otoacoustic emission and, 139–140, 139f
  pathogenesis, 23
  pathophysiology, 242
  risk factors, 242
  surgical therapy, 244–248
    benefits, 246
    complications, 247
    limitations, 246–247
    patient counseling, 246–247
    patient selection, 245–246
    preoperative evaluation, 246
    technical considerations, 247–248
  vestibular dysfunction and, 428
Otoacoustic emissions (OAEs)
  case studies, 143–151, 144f–151f
  cochlear amplifier and, 134–135
  cross-check principle and, 103
  defined, 30
  distortion-product, 137–141, 137f, 141f
  evoked, for neonatal hearing screening, 157
  hearing loss prediction, 133, 141–143, 142f
  in infants/children, 140–141, 140f, 141f
  middle ear function and, 139–140
  in mixed hearing loss, 612–613
  for neonatal hearing screening, 157
  site of lesion testing, 143
  spontaneous, 135, 135f, 140
  transient-evoked, 135–137, 136f, 140, 140f
Otocysts (otic vesicles), 4, 4f
Otolaryngologist, role in syndromic hereditary hearing impairment, 341–342
Otologist
  dilemma, in atelectasis management, 660
  role, in syndromic hereditary hearing impairment, 341–342
Oto-palatal-digital syndrome, eye abnormalities, 709t
Otorhinorrhea, cerebrospinal, temporal bone fractures and, 451–452
Otorrhea
  after tympanostomy tube insertion, 248
  culturing, 252
  purulent, after tympanostomy tubes, 247

Otosclerosis
 classification, 541
 clinical manifestations, 542
 conductive hearing impairment from, 548
 epidemiology, 541
 management, 542–544, 543f, 544f
 pathophysiology, 541–542
 progression, 332
 surgical management, 544–545
Otoscopy, of atelectasis, 652
Otosyphilis, congenital, 97, 98f
Ototoxicity. See Drugs, ototoxic
Outer hair cell, 134
Oval window
 absence, 557
 aplasia, 192, 196f

P

Paget's disease, 318
Palatoplasty, for cleft palate, 630–631
Parachute reflex, 169
Paragangliomas, 65, 511
Parents, of hearing-impaired children
 educational resources for, 676
 goals for, 678
 guidance for, 677–678
 hearing aid wearing instructions and, 591
 reactions to diagnosis, 677–678
 support groups for, 678–679
Parotid surgery, facial paralysis from, 465–466, 466f
Pars flaccida
 anatomy, 87
 retraction, 254, 647–648, 648t
Pars tensa
 anatomy, 87
 eustachian tube function and, 305
 invagination, 651
 retraction, 647t, 647–648
Past pointing, 168
PAX-3 gene, 202
PAX3 gene, 58, 80
Pediatric Speech Intelligibility Test (PSI), 110, 391, 391f
Pedigree
 genomic imprinting, 66f
 mitochondrial inheritance, 65f
 X-linked recessive recombination, 65f
 X-linked recessive trait, 62f
Pendred's syndrome
 clinical manifestations, 96
 diagnosis, 318
 gene, 398
 goiter, 354–355, 355f, 398
 with Mondini cochlea, 192, 194f
Penetrance
 complete, 60–61
 incomplete, 60, 60f, 61
Perception, bimodal, 701–702
Perceptual training, 702
Perilymph, embryonic development, 4
Perilymphatic fistula (PLF)
 acquired hearing loss and, 380–381
 anatomic relationships, 635–636, 636f
 clinical presentation, 638
 congenital inner ear malformations and, 209
 diagnosis, 635, 638–639
 differential diagnosis, 638–639
 etiology, 260, 635
 in fluctuating/progressive sensorineural hearing loss, 619–620
 history, 638
 incidence, 635

management, 641–642
 alternative strategies for, 640
 complications, 641
 controversies, 641
 goals of, 640
 illustrative cases, 641, 642f
 surgical approach for, 640
 pathophysiology, 636–638
 physical examination, 638
 posttraumatic, 641, 642f
 sensorineural hearing loss and, 400
 surgical management, 305
 vertigo and, 432
 vestibular dysfunction and, 429
Perilymphatic space decompression, auditory changes from, 637
Perinatal period, acquired hearing loss in, 377–378
Periosteitis, acute mastoiditis and, 266, 267f
Persistent fetal circulation, acquired hearing loss and, 377–378
Petrous apex lesions, 381, 499–500, 501f
Petrousitis, from otitis media, 259
Pfeiffer's syndrome, 58–59, 60, 315
Pharyngeal apparatus, embryonic development, 4–5, 6f–8f
Phonology, 39, 698
Physician
 mainstreaming and, 693
 otolaryngologist, role in syndromic hereditary hearing loss, 341–342
 otologist. See Otologist
 primary care, atelectasis management and, 658
Picture chart, for visual acuity testing, 368–369, 369f
Pictures of Standard Syndromes and Undiagnosed Malformations (POSSUM), 362
Piebaldness, 709t
Pierre-Robin syndrome, 96, 627
Pinna
 anatomy, 517, 518f
 malpositioned, 521, 521f
Platybasia (basilar invagination-impression), 212–213, 213f
Play audiometry, for mixed hearing loss, 609
PLF. See Perilymphatic fistula
Pneumatization, mastoid, 181, 182f, 268, 659
Pneumocystis carinii otitis media, 483
Polyarteritis nodosa, 413, 414
Polymerase chain reaction assay, of simple sequence repeat polymorphisms, 69–70, 70f
Polymorphisms, 67–68
Positional cloning, 67
Positional testing, 174, 174f, 175–176, 177
POSSUM (Pictures of Standard Syndromes and Undiagnosed Malformations), 362
Posterior fossa arachnoid cysts, vertigo and, 437
Posterior fossa tumors
 cerebellopontine angle. See Cerebellopontine angle
 classification, 489, 490t
 clinical manifestations, 489
 complications, 500–502
 diagnostic evaluation, 489, 490t, 491t
 extra-dural, 498–500, 500f, 501f
 intra-axial, 495–498, 496f–499f
 treatment, general principles of, 490–491
 vertigo and, 432–433, 433t
Post-headshake nystagmus, 173–174

Post-natal bacterial meningitis, sensorineural hearing loss and, 399–400
Posturography, computerized dynamic, 179–180, 178f, 179f, 179t
Pouches, pharyngeal, 5, 8f
POU3F4 gene, 62, 327, 331, 80
Prader-Willi syndrome, 64
Pragmatics, 39, 698
Predisposition, 67
Pre-messenger RNA (pre-mRNA), 56
Prenatal period, acquired hearing loss in, 376–377
Prescription, hearing aids, 700
Pressure regulation, in eustachian tube, 15–16
Probe microphone procedure, for hearing aid fitting, 588–589, 588f
Programmed cell death (apoptosis), 9
Project HEAR, homograft donor precautions, 576–577
Pseudomeningocele, postoperative, 501
Pseudomonas aeruginosa, in chronic suppurative otitis media, 239–240
PSI (Pediatric Speech Intelligibility Test), 110, 391, 391f
Public Law 94-142 (Education of All Handicapped Children's Act), 679
Public Law 99-457, 585, 679
Pupillary examination, 369
Pursuit tests, 177–178
Pyle's disease (craniometaphysial dysplasia), 708t

Q

Quick Cluster algorithm, 621, 623, 621t, 623f–625f

R

Ramsay Hunt syndrome (herpes zoster oticus), 427, 428f, 463, 466
Real ear measure, 29
Real ear saturation response (RESR), 589
Real Ear Unaided Response (REUR), 588–589, 588f
Receptive communication, 39
Receptive language processing disorder, 388, 389t
Recidivism, acquired cholesteatoma, 301–302, 301f, 302f, 303, 307, 307t, 307f, 308f, 308t
Recombination, 63, 64f
Reconstructive ear surgery, historical aspects, 563
Reflexes, developmental progression, 168, 169, 169t
Refsum syndrome, eye abnormalities, 709t
Reichert's cartilage (hyoid arch), 5, 6f–7f, 92
Reissner's membrane, 90, 98f
Relapsing polychondritis, 415
Remote microphone technology, 393
Replication, gene, 54–55, 55f
Replication bubble, 54
Repressor sites, 55
RESR (real ear saturation response), 589
Restriction fragment length polymorphisms (RFLPs), 68–69, 69f
Retina, pigmentary degeneration, 371
Retinal pigment dystrophy, 371
Retinitis pigmentosa (Usher syndrome type I), 371, 432
Retraction
 diffuse, 645, 646f
 local, 645, 646f

Retraction pockets
  extension depth, 298
  fixed, 298
  mobile, 298
  in primary acquired cholesteatoma, 297–299, 301, 299f
  progression, 648, 649t
Retrosigmoid craniotomy, 493
REUR (Real Ear Unaided Response), 588–589, 588f
Reverse transcriptase, 480
RFLPs (restriction fragment length polymorphisms), 68–69, 69f
Rhabdomyosarcoma, temporal bone, 505–507, 506f, 507f
Rheumatoid arthritis, 215, 416
Rhombomeres, 3
Ribosomal RNA (rRNA), 55
Richard-Rundel syndrome, 710t
Righting reflex, 169
Risk, increased, 67
RNA polymerases, 55, 56
RNA probes, 83
RNA transcription, 55–56, 56f
Romano-Ward syndrome, 318
Romberg test, 167–168
Rosenthal's canal, 90
Rotation tests, 178–179
Round window niche, 89, 89f
Rubella infection, 97, 376, 399
Rubeola virus infection, 96, 400

S

SAA (static acoustic admittance), 115, 116, 116f, 120
Saccade test, 177
Saccule, 91
Salpingopharyngeal muscle, 14
Santorini, fissures of, 87
Saturation sound pressure level (SSPL), 589–590
Scala media, 90
Scala tympani, gas bubbles in, 637
Scala vestibuli, 90
SCAN test, 390
Scarpa's ganglion, viral infection, 427
Scheibe deformity (cochleosaccular dysplasia)
  associated syndromes, 399
  clinical manifestations, 202–203
  etiology, 94–95, 95f
  radiological evaluation, 169–170
  vertigo and, 432
Schools
  for the deaf, 680
  evaluation, for mainstreaming, 690–691
  preparation, for mainstreaming, 691
Schwannomas, vestibular, 170, 491f
Sebaceous glands, 87
Secretory otitis media. See Otitis media with effusion
Segmentation abnormalities, 213
Segregation, 62
Segregation analysis, 68
Semantics, 39, 698
Semicircular canal
  aplasia, 206
  cristae, 91
  dysplasia, 203, 206, 207f, 208f
  embryonic development, 4
  functional assessment, 168
  physiology, 172, 173f
Sense strand, 55
Sensitivity, absolute, 32, 32f

Sensitivity prediction with acoustic reflex (SPAR), 122
Sensorineural hearing loss (SNHL)
  abnormal temporal bone morphology and, 93–94
  in AIDS, 484
  autosomal dominant, 319–322, 324, 319f–324f
  autosomal recessive, 325–326, 326f, 327f
  classification, 397
  with conductive hearing loss. See Mixed hearing loss
  congenital
    diagnosis, 317–319, 318t, 318f
    inner ear abnormalities and, 201
    management, 209–210
    mild bilateral, 607–608
    X-linked, 62
  degree, determination of, 401
  delayed-onset infant, indicators for, 160t
  diagnostic algorithm, 368f
  distortion-product otoacoustic emissions, 142–143, 142f
  early identification/intervention, 158–159, 400–401, 401t
  enlarged vestibular aqueduct and, 191, 192f
  epidemiology, 314
  etiology, 401–402
  fluctuating/progressive
    audiogram configuration, 621, 623, 622t, 622f
    auditory threshold determination, 617–619, 618t, 618f
    auditory threshold pattern variations, 620–621, 620f, 620t, 621t
    etiologic factors, 617, 619–620
    etiology, 623–624, 626, 625f, 625t, 626t
    serial threshold patterns, 623–624, 626, 625f, 625t, 626t
  genetic, 397–398
  high-frequency, X-linked, 62
  incidence, 397
  inheritance, 316
  management, 401–402
  medical evaluation, 318t
  metabolic disorders and, 400
  mitochondrial inheritance, 328–329, 329f
  noise-induced, 400
  nongenetic, infections, 399–400
  nonsyndromic, 398
  otoacoustic emissions and, 142
  ototoxic drugs and, 400
  pediatric etiologies, other, 192, 196, 196t, 197f
  perilymph fistula and, 400
  perinatal risk factors, 400
  risk indicators, 158t
  rubella syndrome and, 376
  with temporal bone fracture, 449
  type, determination of, 401
  X-linked, 192, 326–328, 328f
Sensory deprivation, binaural amplification and, 584
Sensory organization test, 179–180, 178f, 179f, 179t
Serous otitis media. See Otitis media with effusion
Shaker 1 mouse deafness model, 81
Sharpened Romberg test, 168
SHHL. See Syndromic hereditary hearing loss
Short tau inversion recovery sequence (STIR), 188
Shprintzen syndrome (velocardiofacial syndrome), 356, 356f

Shrinkwrap ear (diffuse adhesive otitis media), 646, 646f, 659–660
Sickle cell anemia, 66
Sigmoid sinus thrombosis, after otitis media, 260–261, 261f
Signal averaging, auditory evoked potentials, 132
Signal-to-noise ratio (SNR), 130
Sign language
  American, 675–676, 684, 703–704
  historical aspects, 313–314
  parents and, 335
  total communication approach and, 703–704
Simple sequence repeat polymorphisms (SSRPs), 68, 69
Single-stranded-conformational polymorphism (SSCP), 79
Sinusoidal stimulus, for rotational testing, 178
Site of lesion testing, otoacoustic emissions for, 143
Skeletal system abnormalities
  Goldenhar syndrome, 350
  Waardenburg syndrome, 353
Skin
  abnormalities, in Waardenburg syndrome, 353
  of cartilaginous ear canal, 87
  grafting, for external auditory canal atresia repair, 538–539
Skull abnormalities
  craniocervical junction. See Craniocervical junction, abnormalities
  temporal bone
    encephaloceles, 222–224, 223f
    osteodystrophies, 217, 219–222, 220f
    in Treacher Collins syndrome, 351
    tumors, 225–226, 226f
SLE (systemic lupus erythematosus), 415–416
SN10, 129
Snell's Waltzer mouse deafness model, 81
SNHL. See Sensorineural hearing loss
SOAEs (spontaneous otoacoustic emission), 135, 135f
Social cognition, 698
Social-cognitive development, enhancement for deaf children, 702
Somitomeres, 3
Sounds, complex, perceptual organization of, 34–35
Southern blot analysis, 83
SPAR (sensitivity prediction with acoustic reflex), 122
Spectral Peak strategy (SPEAK), 595
Speech
  awareness. See Speech detection threshold
  comprehension, hearing and, 42
  conversational, 42
  cued, 684
  definition of, 39
  development, 39–40
    birth to 1 year, 40, 41f
    1 to 2 years, 40, 41f
    2 to 3 years, 40, 42, 41f
    3 to 5 years, 42, 41f
    hearing loss and, 46–47
  perception
    cochlear implantation effects, 602
    measures of, 110
    production, cochlear implantation and, 603
    testing, for mixed hearing loss, 610
Speech and hearing clinics, 680
Speech audiometry, for central auditory processing disorder, 390–392, 391f
Speech detection threshold, 110

Speech-language specialists, in amplification system management, 585
Speechreading, 701
Speech reception threshold, 110
Spiral ganglion cell count, 209
Spiral limbus, 90
Splice site mutation, 58
Splotch mouse mutation, 58, 80, 202
Spondyloepiphysial dysplasia, eye abnormalities, 710t
Spontaneous nystagmus, 172–173
Spontaneous otoacoustic emission (SOAEs), 135, 135f
Squamous-cell carcinoma, temporal bone, 509
Squamous metaplasia, congenital cholesteatoma and, 281
SSCP (single-stranded-conformational polymorphism), 79
SSPL (saturation sound pressure level), 589–590
SSRPs (simple sequence repeat polymorphisms), 68, 69
Stapedectomy, 361, 541, 544–546
Stapedius muscle
  acoustic reflex and, 121
  anatomy, 89, 89f
  embryonic development, 5
Stapedotomy, for osteogenesis imperfecta, 361
Stapes
  absence, 557
  ankylosis, 192, 541
  congenital fixation. See Otosclerosis
  dehiscence, 636, 636f
  development, 92
  embryonic development, 5
  in external auditory canal atresia repair, 537
  fixation, surgical reconstruction for, 556–557
  subluxation, 446, 446f
  traumatic injury, 446
Staphylococcus aureus
  in acute mastoiditis, 270, 269t
  in acute otitis media, 235, 236f
Staphylococcus epidermidis, in otitis media with effusion, 238, 238f
Startle reflex (Moro reflex), 156, 169
State government mandates, for neonatal hearing screening, 161, 161t
Static acoustic admittance (SAA), 115, 116, 116f, 120
Statoacoustic ganglion, 4
Stereocilia, inner hair cell, 134
Sterocilia, 90–91
Steroids. See also Corticosteroids
  for autoimmune inner ear disease, 416
Sterotactic radiation therapy, for neurofibromatosis type II, 493–494
Stickler syndrome
  clinical manifestations, 355–356, 356f, 398
  eye abnormalities, 710t
  gene mutation, 61
  mixed hearing loss in, 614
Stimuli, auditory evoked potentials, 132–133
Streptococcus pneumoniae
  in acute mastoiditis, 269, 269t
  in acute otitis media, 235–236, 236f, 242
  antibiotic resistance, 236, 237f
Streptococcus pyogenes, in acute mastoiditis, 269, 269t
Stria vascularis
  anatomy, 90
  dysplasia, 94–95, 95f
Stroke incidence, in childhood, 434
Stylomastoid artery, 89

Sudden idiopathic sensorineural hearing loss, 97, 98f
Summating potential, 127
Superficial temporoparietal aponeurotic fascia (STAF), for microtia repair, 526–527, 527f, 528f
Support groups, for parents, 678–679
Surgicel, for sigmoid sinus thrombosis treatment, 261
Susceptibility, 67
Syndromic hereditary hearing loss (SHHL)
  branchio-otorenal syndrome, 359, 360f
  CHARGE association, 359–360, 360f
  chromosomal map, 81, 81f
  diagnosis, 341, 345–347
    audiologic testing, 344, 345f
    blood tests, 345
    clinical geneticist consultation and, 347
    cytogenetics, 345, 345t
    family history, 344
    medical history, 344
    ophthalmologist consultation and, 347
    physical examination, 344
    radiographic studies, 345, 346f
    relativity in, 343
    salient features in, 347
    scoring system for, 347, 348f
  DIDMOAD syndrome, 361
  with difficult detection, 358–359, 358t, 359f
  with facial dysmorphism. See also Goldenhar's syndrome; Treacher Collins syndrome; Waardenburg syndrome
    fetal alcohol syndrome, 354, 354f
  frequently seen, 355–357, 356f, 357f
  genetic counseling, 362
  identification, reasons for, 342–343
  infrequently seen, 354–355, 354f, 355t
  inheritance, 375–376
  lacrimoauriculodentodigital syndrome, 361
  osteogenesis imperfecta, 360–361, 361t
  otologist/otolaryngologist role, 341–342
  resources, 361–362
  sensorineural, 397–398
  terminology, 342
Synostoses, 213
Syntax, 39
Syphilis, congenital
  acquired hearing loss and, 377
  screening, 382
  sensorineural hearing loss and, 399
  treatment, 382
Syphilis, hearing loss, 97, 98f
Systemic lupus erythematosus (SLE), 415–416

T

Tactile aids
  maximizing signal-to-noise ratio with, 591
  vs. hearing aids/cochlear implants, 602–603
Tandem Romberg test, 168
Tandem walking analysis, 168
Tangible reinforcement operant conditioning audiometry (TROCA), 109
Telecoils, 583
Telomeres, 51
Temporal bone
  in AIDS, 483–484
  in Cogan's syndrome, 414
  computed tomography, 181–183, 183f–188f
  congenital abnormalities, 196
  development, 92, 93t
  encephaloceles, 222
  fractures, 445–447, 446f

  acquired hearing loss and, 380, 381t
  cerebrospinal fluid fistula and, 451–452
  complications of, 449t
  facial nerve injury and, 450–451, 451f, 464
  hearing loss from, 448–449
  incidence, 447
  longitudinal, 447, 446f, 447f
  meningitis and, 451–452
  transverse, 447–448, 448f
  vestibular system injury and, 449–450
  magnetic resonance angiography, 190–191, 191f
  magnetic resonance imaging, 186, 189f
    fast spin echo technique, 187, 190f
    fat suppressed technique, 187, 190
    gradient echo, 187, 190f
  middle ear infections and, 251
  morphology, abnormal, 92–95, 94f, 95f
  osteodystrophies, 217, 219–221, 220f
  postnatal changes, 181
  trauma, radiological evaluation of, 171, 171f
  tumors, 505, 506t
    acquired hearing loss and, 381
    benign, 509–512, 512f
    malignant, 505–509, 506f, 507f
Temporalis muscle transposition procedure, pedicled, 468
Temporal modulation transfer function (TMTF), 33–34, 34f
Tension pneumocephalus, in temporal bone encephaloceles, 224
Tensor tympani muscle
  anatomy, 13, 14f, 89–90
  in congenital cholesteatoma, 286, 287f
  embryonic development, 5
Tensor veli palatini muscle (TVPM), 12–14, 14f, 627–628, 628f
Teratogenesis, inner ear, 377
Teratomas, temporal bone, 511–512
TIAs (transient ischemic attacks), 435
Tinnitus, drug-induced, 430
Tissue necrosis, microtia repair, 528
TMTF (temporal modulation transfer function), 33–34, 34f
TOAEs (transient-evoked otoacoustic emissions), 135–137, 136f
Torus, 12
Total ossicular replacement prosthesis (TORP), 667, 667f
Toxoplasmosis, 377, 399
Toynbee test, 18, 19, 20, 22, 119
Transcription, gene, 55–56, 56f
Transcription factors, 55
β_2-Transferrin, 223–224, 639
Transfer RNA (tRNA), 55–56, 57
Transient-evoked otoacoustic emissions (TOAEs)
  in cochlear hearing loss, 142
  in infants/children, 140, 140f
  measurement, 135–137, 136f
  in serous otitis media, 139–140, 139f
  stimulus artifact and, 136
  noise-induced high-frequency hearing loss and, 142
Transient ischemic attacks (TIAs), 435
Translation, gene, 56–57, 57f
Transmastoid craniotomy, 224
Transmastoid-middle fossa craniotomy, 224
Transposition procedures, pedicled temporalis or masseter, 468
Transtympanic tube, patency, tympanometric assessment of, 119
Trauma, hearing loss from, 380, 381t, 548

Traumatic conductive triad, 447
Treacher Collins syndrome (mandibulofacial dysotosis)
    abnormalities, 96
        ears, 352
        eye, 709t
        eyes, 351–352
        facial, 351, 350f, 351f
        nose, 352
        oral, 352
        skeletal, 536
        skull, 351
    bilateral involvement, 521
    clinical manifestations, 398, 521
    diagnosis, 318, 345
    etiology, 341, 351
    inheritance, 351
    mental status, 352
    mixed hearing loss in, 613–614
    parental examination, 342
Trinucleotide repeat expansion, 65–66
TROCA (tangible reinforcement operant conditioning audiometry), 109
Truce tube (T-tube), for atelectasis, 655–656
Tulio phenomenon, 174
Tumarkin, otolithic crisis of
Tumbling "E" chart, 369, 369f
Turner syndrome (Ullrich-Turner syndrome), 356
TW (tympanometric width), 115, 117, 116f, 120
Tympanic membrane
    acoustic reflex and, 121
    anatomy, 87
    assessment. See Tympanometry
    chronic changes, with cleft palate, 632
    in congenital cholesteatoma, 287, 289, 288f
    desquamation, 651
    incompletely healed, 445
    intact, clinical eustachian tube tests and, 20–21, 21f
    invagination, 651
    nonintact, clinical eustachian tube tests and, 21
    perforation, 22, 445
        cleft palate and, 629, 630t, 632
        definition of, 646–647
        marginal, 301
        from otitis media, 252–253
        persistent, 248–249, 253
        secondary cholesteatoma and, 301, 300f, 301f
    rupture, traumatic, 445
    structural abnormalities, 650–651, 650f
    tympanosclerotic plaques, 253
Tympanocentesis, 235, 271
Tympanomastoiditis, acute, 265–266, 266f
Tympanomeningeal fissure (Hyrtl's fissure), 636
Tympanometric width (TW), 115, 117, 116f, 120
Tympanometry
    abnormal, 113–114
    with acoustic reflexes, 113, 114
    assessment
        of eustachian tube function, 119
        of transtympanic tube patency, 119
    calibration, 123–124
    configurations, 115
    definition of, 114
    ear-canal probe, 115
    guidelines, ASHA, 116–117, 119, 116f, 117t
    with higher-frequency probe tones, 120
    indications, 124
    for infants, 120
    interpretation, 115
    multifrequency, 119–120
    nine-step test, 20–21, 21f
    normal, 114–115, 114f
    personnel, 124
    procedure, 115
    referral, 117, 118f
    resistance of child and, 124
    screening, 115–116
    sensitivity, 123
    specificity, 123
    test-retest reliability, 115
Tympanoplasty, postauricular approach, 447
Tympanosclerosis (myringosclerosis)
    assessment, for ossicular reconstruction, 551
    histology, 647, 647f
    incidence, 650–651
    from otitis media, 253–254, 253f, 254f
    treatment, 254
Tympanostomy, 629–632
Tympanostomy tubes
    choice of, 247
    complications, 248–249
    complications from, 247
    insertion
        follow-up visits for, 248
        inappropriate timing of, 658
        with myringotomy, 247
        for otitis media with effusion, 244
        technical considerations for, 247
    tympanic membrane perforation and, 303
Tympanotomy
    for congenital cholesteatoma, 290, 289f–291f
    exploratory, for perilymphatic fistula, 639, 640
    postauricular incision, 290, 289f

U

Ullrich-Turner syndrome (Turner syndrome), 356
Usher syndrome
    animal model, 81
    bony spicules, 372f
    clinical manifestations, 96, 202, 354, 354f, 355t
    diagnosis, 318
    eye abnormalities, 710t
    family members and, 342
    types, 355t, 371, 398
    vertigo and, 432
Utricle, 91

V

Valsalva and Politzer tests, 20
Valsalva maneuver, 119
Vancomycin, ototoxicity, 430
Van der Hoeve syndrome. See Osteogenesis imperfecta
Variable expressivity, 60, 61
Variable number of tandem repeats (VNTRs), 69
Vascular disorders, vertigo and, 434–435
Vasculitis, vertigo and, 434
Velocardiofacial syndrome (Shprintzen syndrome), 356, 356f
Velopharyngeal incompetence, post-adenoidectomy, 249
Velopharyngeal musculature, for eustachian tube function, 627–628, 628f
Vertebral artery occlusion, 435

Vertigo
    benign paroxysmal of childhood (migraine), 424, 435
    benign paroxysmal positional, 424–425
    causes, 424t
    central origin, 432, 433t
        brainstem and posterior fossa lesions, 432–433, 433t
        cerebellopontine angle tumors, 436–437, 436f
        Chiari malformations, 433–434, 433f
        hereditary disorders, 435–436
        multiple sclerosis, 435
        vascular disorders, 434–435
        vs. peripheral origin, 423–424
    defined, 423
    diagnosis, 423
    differential diagnosis, 163, 164f
    genetic origin, 431–432
    peripheral origin, 424t, 429–430
        benign paroxysmal positional, 424–425
        Ménière's disease, 425–426, 425f
        meningitis and, 430
        mumps and, 430
        otitis media, 427–429, 428f
        ototoxicity and, 430–431
        Ramsay Hunt syndrome, 427, 428f
        secondary endolymphatic hydrops, 426–427
        vestibular neuronitis, 427
        vs. central origin, 423–424
    vs. dizziness, 163–164
Vestibular aqueduct
    anatomy, 91
    computed tomography, 182
    congenital anomalies, 206, 208, 208f
    enlargement, 169, 191, 192f
    histology, 206, 208, 208f
    vertigo and, 431
Vestibular neuronitis, 427
Vestibular schwannomas, 170, 491f
Vestibular system
    anomalies, 192, 194f
    dysfunction
        genetic, 431–432
        hematologic examination, 169
        peripheral. See Vertigo, peripheral origin
        physical examination, 169
        posttraumatic, 431
        radiological evaluation, 169–171, 170f–172f
        in temporal bone fractures, 449–450
    embryonic development, 4
    epithelium, 91
    functional assessments, 172–174, 180
        computerized dynamic posturography, 179–180, 178f, 179f, 179t
        electronystagmography, 175–178, 176f
        electro-oculography, 175, 175f
        goals, 171
        initial, 163–164, 167–169, 164f–168f, 169t
        for perilymphatic fistula, 639
        positional, 174, 174f
        rotational, 178–179
    physiology, 172, 173f
Vestibulo-ocular reflex (VOR), 168, 168f, 172
Viomycin, ototoxicity, 430
Viral infections, acquired hearing loss and, 379
Vision, hearing and, 689–690, 690f
Visiting Infant Parent program (VIP), 681
Visual acuity testing, 367–369, 369f
Visual fields confrontation, 369

Visual reinforcement audiometry (VRA)
  conditioned head-turn procedure, 105–106, 105f
  for mixed hearing loss, 609
  test protocol, 31, 106–107
  test suite arrangement/equipment, 107–108, 107f
Visual reinforcement operant conditioning audiometry (VROCA), 109
VNTRs (variable number of tandem repeats), 69
Vocabulary, 698
Vocational options, for deaf children, 704
Vogy-Koyanagi-Harada syndrome, 414
VOR (vestibulo-ocular reflex), 172
VRA. See Visual reinforcement audiometry
VROCA (visual reinforcement operant conditioning audiometry), 109

W

Waardenburg syndrome
  abnormalities, 352
    ear, 353
    eye, 352–353, 353f, 710t
    face, 352, 353f
    hair, 353
    oral, 353
    skeletal system, 353
    skin, 353
  clinical manifestations, 66, 96, 397
  diagnosis, 318, 354
  families, 343
  molecular/genetic analysis, 80–81
  type I, 52, 50f–51f, 53f
    gene mutations, 58
    PAX3 gene mutations, 58
  types, 352, 370, 370f
Wallenberg syndrome, 434
Wegener's granulomatosis, 415
Western blot immunoassay, 83, 411, 412f
White blood count, in acute mastoiditis, 271
Whole nerve action potential, 127
Wildervanck triad. See Cervico-oculo-acoustic syndrome
Wolfram syndrome (DIDMOAD syndrome), 361
Word Intelligibility by Picture Identification test (WIPI test), 110

X

X chromosome, 61, 63
X-linked hearing loss
  congenital sensorineural, 62
  mixed
    gene mutations, 58
    with perilymphatic gusher, 329, 331–332, 330f–331f, 358, 359f
    with stapes gusher, 613, 614
X-linked inheritance, 61–62, 62f
X-linked syndromes, 342, 398. See also specific X-linked syndromes

Y

YAC (yeast artificial chromosome), 74, 75–76
Y chromosome, 61
Yeast artificial chromosome (YAC), 74, 75–76

Z

Zoo blots, of genomic DNA, 77

9780397514663.4